Chapter 14 ▪ ***Cell-Mediated Effector Responses***

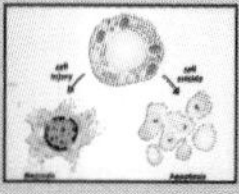

Cell Death ANIMATION

Chapter 15 ▪ ***Leukocyte Migration and Inflammation***

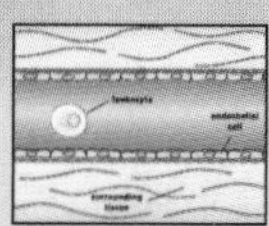

Leukocyte Extravasation ANIMATION

Chapter 16 ▪ ***Hypersensitive Reactions***

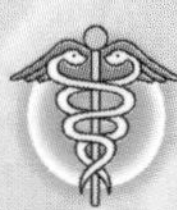

Bee Sting in an Eight-Year-Old Boy CLINICAL CASE STUDY

Chapter 17 ▪ ***Immune Response to Infectious Diseases***

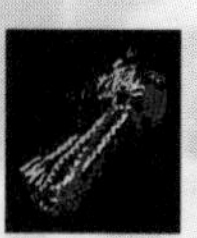

Viral Antigens: Influenza Hemagglutinin and HIV gp120
See Introduction and Flu Virus Hemagglutinin sections. MOLECULAR VISUALIZATION

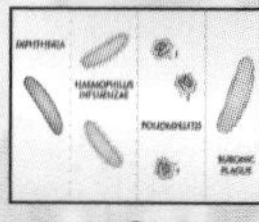

Vaccine Strategies *See pathogenesis sections.* ANIMATION

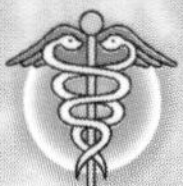

Influenza Outbreak on a Ship CLINICAL CASE STUDY

Chapter 18 ▪ ***Vaccines***

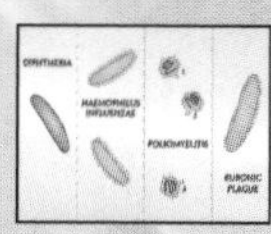

Vaccine Strategies ANIMATION

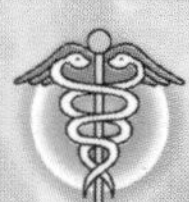

Chicken Pox Vaccine for an Immunosuppressed Fourth-Grade Girl
CLINICAL CASE STUDY

Chapter 19 ▪ ***AIDS and Other Immunodeficiencies***

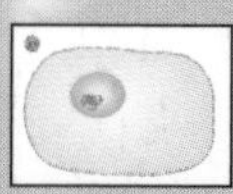

Retrovirus ANIMATION

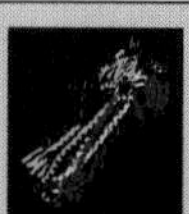

Viral Antigens: Influenza Hemagglutinin and HIV gp120
See Introduction and HIV gp120 sections. MOLECULAR VISUALIZATION

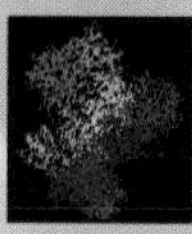

HIV-1 Reverse Transcriptase MOLECULAR VISUALIZATION

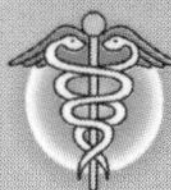

AIDS in a Twenty-Nine-Year-Old Man CLINICAL CASE STUDY

Chapter 20 ▪ ***Autoimmunity***

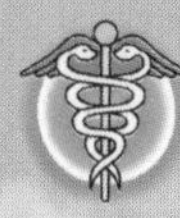

Glomerulonephritis in a Thirty-Five-Year-Old Woman CLINICAL CASE STUDY

KUBY

IMMUNOLOGY

FOURTH EDITION

ICONS USED IN THIS BOOK

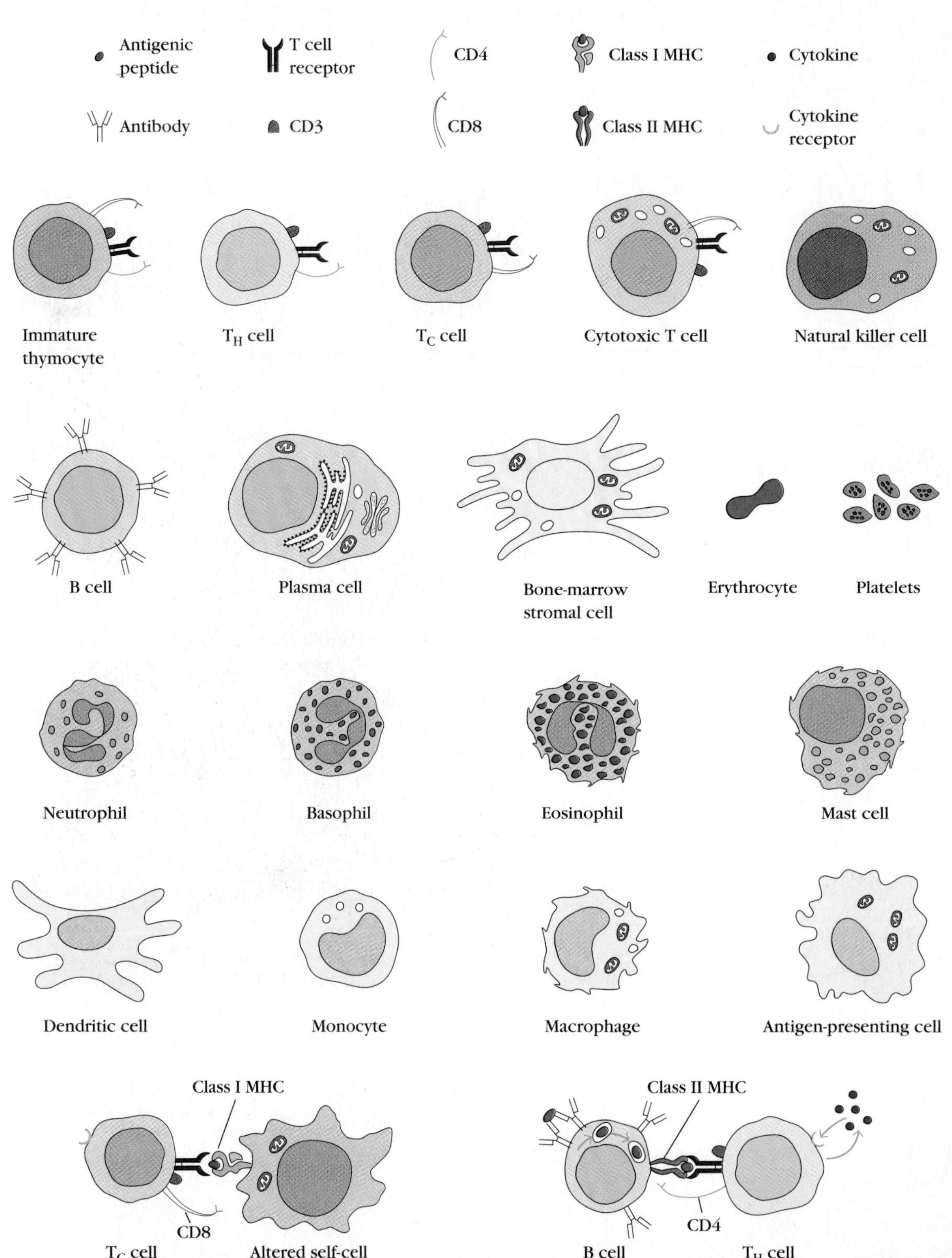

KUBY

IMMUNOLOGY

FOURTH EDITION

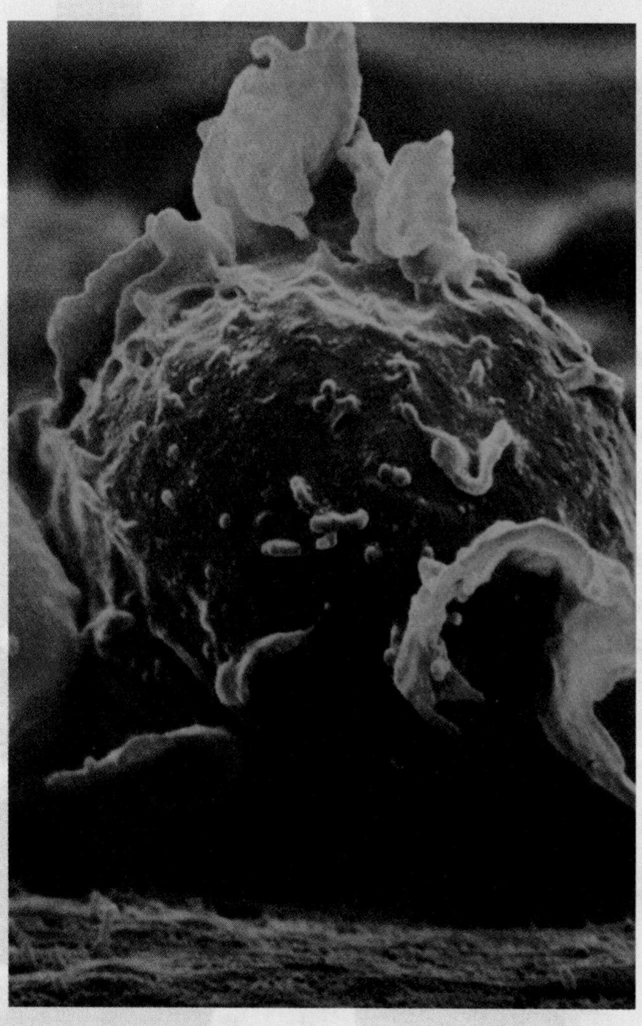

RICHARD A. GOLDSBY
Amherst College

THOMAS J. KINDT
National Institutes of Health

BARBARA A. OSBORNE
University of Massachusetts at Amherst

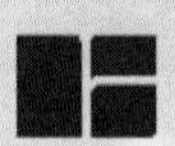

W. H. FREEMAN AND COMPANY

New York

ABOUT THE COVER

Vertebrates are protected by innate and adaptive immunity, two cooperating systems that collaborate to provide an effective defense against a diverse spectrum of pathogens. Invading pathogens are often encountered by macrophages, members of a remarkable family of phagocytic cells. Macrophages can mediate the early and broadly effective processes of innate immunity and play a role in the later highly efficient and exquisitely specific reactions of adaptive immunity. This scanning electron micrograph shows a macrophage in an alveolus of the lung, one of the critical frontiers between the interior of the body and the outside world. (Photograph by D Philips, Science Source/Photo Researchers)

ACQUISITIONS EDITOR: *Nicole Folchetti*
DEVELOPMENT EDITOR: *Janet Tannenbaum*
PROJECT EDITOR: *Georgia Lee Hadler*
LINE EDITOR: *Andrew Kudlacik*
COVER AND TEXT DESIGNER: *Blake Logan*
ILLUSTRATION COORDINATOR: *Bill Page*
ILLUSTRATION: *Fine Line Illustrations*
PHOTO RESEARCHER: *Jennifer MacMillan*
PRODUCTION COORDINATOR: *Paul W. Rohloff*
COMPOSITION: *York Graphic Services, Inc.*
MANUFACTURING: *Von Hoffman Press, Inc.*
MARKETING MANAGER: *John Britch*
SUPPLEMENTS EDITOR: *Bridget O'Lavin*

Library of Congress Cataloging-in-Publication Data
Goldsby, Richard A.
Kuby immunology / by Richard A. Goldsby, Thomas J. Kindt, Barbara A. Osborne.—4th ed.
p. cm.
Includes bibliographical references and index.
ISBN 0-7167-3331-5
1. Immunology I. Kindt, Thomas J. II. Osborne, Barbara A. III. Kuby, Janis. Immunology. IV. Title. V. Title: Immunology.
[DNLM: 1. Immune System—immunology. 2. Immunity. QW 504 G622k 2000]
QR181.K83 2000
616.07'9—dc21
DNLM/DLC 99-32746
for Library of Congress CIP

Printed in the United States of America
Third printing, 2001

This book is dedicated to four gifted teachers:

Janis Kuby, whose approach to teaching inspired and guided the preparation of this edition.

Jeremiah Cameron, whose brilliance and versatility inspired generations of African-American students.

Charles Todd, for his deep insights in immunology and for his ability to infect others with his passion for the field.

James Mitchell, who recognizes potential in students and is a master at instilling his love for scientific inquiry in them.

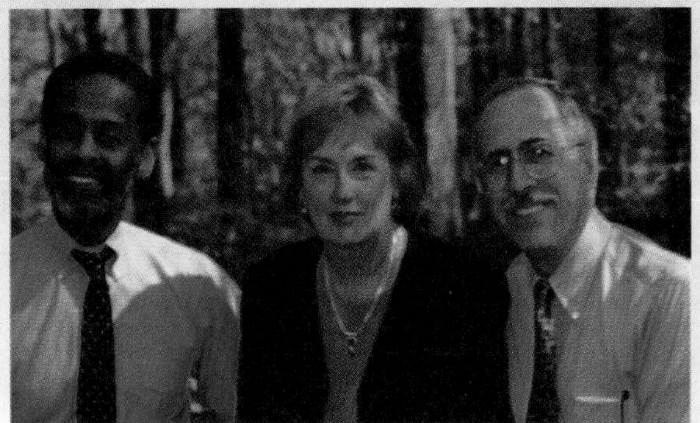

Left to right: Richard A. Goldsby, Barbara A. Osborne, and Thomas J. Kindt.

ABOUT THE AUTHORS

The fourth edition of *Kuby Immunology* is co-authored by Richard A. Goldsby, Thomas J. Kindt, and Barbara A. Osborne. The diverse backgrounds and complementary talents of this new team of authors will carry forward the tradition of fine teaching and scientific excellence the late Dr. Janis Kuby established in the first three editions of her book.

Richard Goldsby, the anchor of the team, is a dedicated teacher and researcher who spends most of his time teaching immunology and other biomedical science courses to undergraduates at Amherst College. Dr. Goldsby's research focus is the somatic mutation of antibody genes in the generation of antibody diversity. Since the 1980s, he has also served as a Course Director in the National Science Foundation-Chautauqua Short Course Program for the education of college teachers, annually presenting a course on current advances in immunology.

Thomas J. Kindt has 30 years of experience in the field of immunology and has made both theoretical and experimental contributions to the field. He currently directs the intramural research program of the National Institute of Allergy and Infectious Diseases, a position that places him in daily contact with the cutting edge of experimental and clinical immunology. As head of the Immunogenetics Research Section, Dr. Kindt studies retroviral infections in animal models to determine how host and viral factors influence the response to infection.

Barbara A. Osborne is an investigator in immunology and a recognized contributor in the fast-moving area of apoptosis, or programmed cell death. Her laboratory is investigating the induction of apoptosis in the mouse thymus. A highly active researcher and frequent participant in national and international meetings, Dr. Osborne also teaches immunology to undergraduate and graduate students at the University of Massachusetts at Amherst.

Drs. Goldsby, Kindt, and Osborne have a friendship that goes back 20 years. In that time they have collaborated on a variety of projects, beginning with a series of workshops on monoclonal antibody technology that the three organized and taught in 1981.

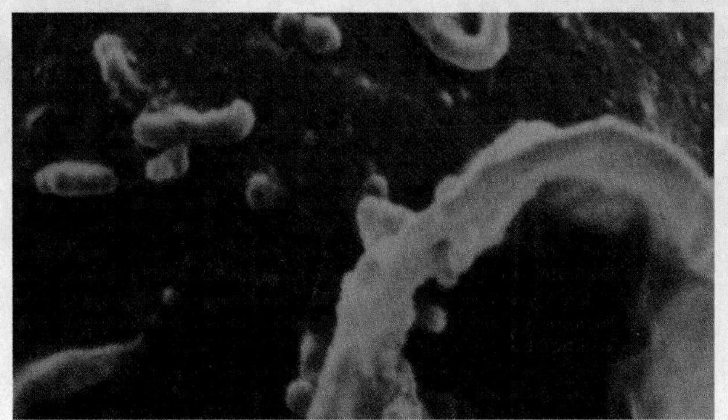

CONTENTS IN BRIEF

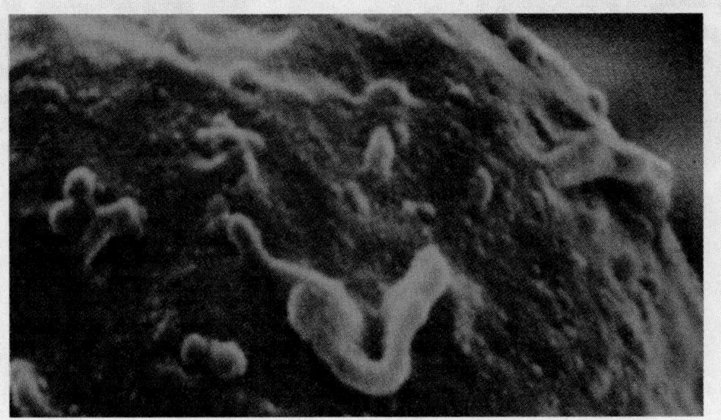

CONTENTS

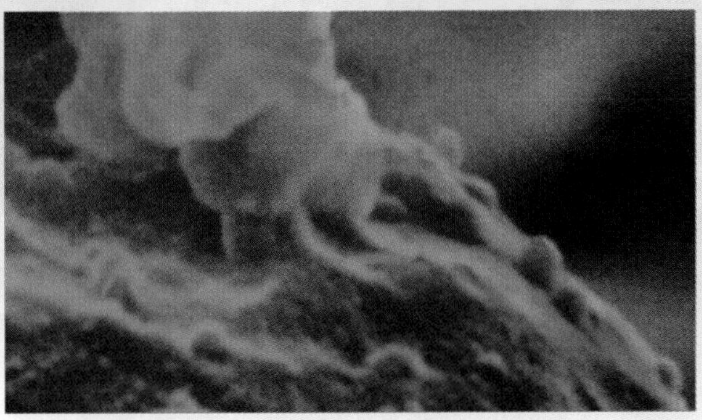

PREFACE

"As a teacher of immunology, I have had the pleasure of watching the field explode from an infusion of new information in the past decade. Each day, newspapers and magazines carry reports of the remarkable advances research in immunology brings to clinical medicine." With these words, Janis Kuby began the preface to the first edition of *Immunology*. In that book, she presented the principles and creative experimental work that underlie the rapid and indeed explosive growth of this exciting field. Over the course of eight years, she created a legacy of three remarkable editions of this book, editions that introduced tens of thousands of students, including our own, to the principles and excitement of immunology. Readability, logical organization, and a strong bias toward experimental examples set Kuby's text apart from the others. In 1997, soon after completing the third edition, Janis Kuby died of cancer. Those who teach and those who learn will miss her clear vision and her explanatory voice. When we undertook preparation of this fourth edition, we resolved to continue the tradition Janis Kuby established for this book, now appropriately renamed *Kuby Immunology* in recognition of her lasting contribution to the teaching of immunology.

Our revision of this classic text maintains the overall organization and tone of previous editions. It presents an up-to-date and comprehensive introduction to the principles and findings of the field. Since the third edition, the continued progress in research has deepened our understanding of important areas of immunology, and the treatment of many topics in the text has been revised to reflect these advances. These topics include cell death, T-cell development, antigen presentation, the mechanism of T- and NK-cell–mediated cytotoxicity, signal transduction, B-cell somatic hypermutation, and cytokine biology. Another pathway of complement activation has been firmly established, and chemokines are taking their place as major players in immunophysiology. As in previous editions, we have continued to exploit opportunities to use an experimental approach to immunology. This edition, like its predecessors, introduces students to many of the landmark experiments that have formed the theoretical framework of immunology.

Although the overall organization of the previous edition has been maintained, we have made some additions and changes that enhance this new edition. The ever-increasing impact of immunology on modern medical practice is reflected in Clinical Focus essays introduced to highlight clinical uses or implications of various topics in immunology. In recognition of the extensive resources available by Internet connection, the list of references for each chapter has been expanded to include selected Web site addresses, annotated to help students choose the sites corresponding to their interests. As detailed in the next few pages, the order and content of several chapters has changed in this edition. Perhaps most noticeable is the shift of the methods chapter from the second to the last of the book, which allows the discussion of experimental systems in that chapter to serve as a resource for students without interrupting the flow of the conceptual presentation. A less noticeable but highly significant change is the reordering of the five chapters that deal with the MHC, antigen presentation, the T-cell receptor, and T- and B-cell maturation and activation (Chapters 7–11). In this edition, the chapter on the B cell has moved from the beginning to the end of the sequence, allowing the molecular concepts to build sequentially and positioning the chapters on T cells and B cells next to each other to accentuate similarities in the activation mechanisms of these cells. As part of this change, the chapter on B-cell maturation and activation now presents unified coverage of B-cell activities by addition of material on the humoral response and its regulation that was previously combined with cell-mediated effector responses in a separate chapter (Chapter 16 in the third edition). The chapter on effector mechanisms in this new edition (Chapter 14) can then focus on cell-mediated mechanisms, including discussion of the Fas–Fas ligand system in T-cell cytotoxicity. Also to unify related topics, we have chosen to merge the coverage of immunodeficiency diseases and of AIDS, which were in separate chapters in the third edition, into a single chapter (Chapter 19). Although not immediately obvious from a glance at the table of contents, the discussion of antigen-antibody interactions in Chapter 6 has shifted its emphasis from precipitation reactions to procedures in wider current use, such as the various methods of ELISA, radioimmunoassay, chemiluminescence assays, fluorescent antibody staining, and flow cytometry. Along with the changes enumerated here and the extensive updating throughout the text, we have also enhanced the illustrations by use of full color and the addition of new diagrams and photographs to reflect new developments. Finally, we have added an annotated table of CD antigens as a useful reference (Appendix).

The recent growth of immunology has been fueled by the increasingly broad application of powerful investigative technologies to questions of immunological interest. These have been joined by Internet-driven improvements in accessing data and communicating new findings and concepts. All this has made it a great challenge to produce a text that is as current as possible in the major areas of immunology but that remains accessible to the beginning student. We hope that this fourth edition of *Kuby Immunology* will invite today's students to acquire a familiarity with the immune system that will make them better doctors, researchers, and teachers.

ORGANIZATION AND CONTENT

The four-part organization introduced by Janis Kuby remains in this edition, with rearrangements of some chapters within the parts. These changes in the order of the chapters are based on the need to develop necessary themes and definitions as a foundation for understanding the immunological functions discussed in subsequent chapters. For example, placing the chapters on MHC, antigen presentation, and the T-cell receptor (Chapters 7, 8, and 9) immediately before those on T- and B-cell development, activation, and differentiation (Chapters 10 and 11) permits use of the latest information concerning molecular interactions in lymphocyte signaling events. This change further strengthens analogies between the responses of T and B cells by placing the descriptions in adjacent chapters. The placement of the methods chapter (Chapter 23) at the end of the text follows our own practice of teaching methods as they are needed to understand experimental advances rather than as a body of isolated information. All chapters contain updated material to give the reader the most current picture of progress in this rapidly evolving area. Changes in this edition are summarized below.

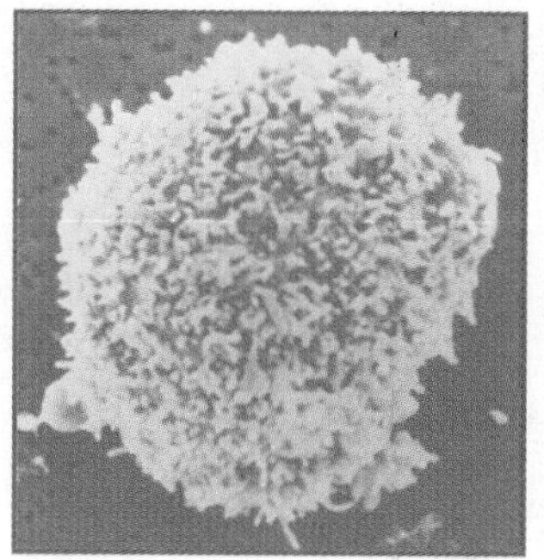

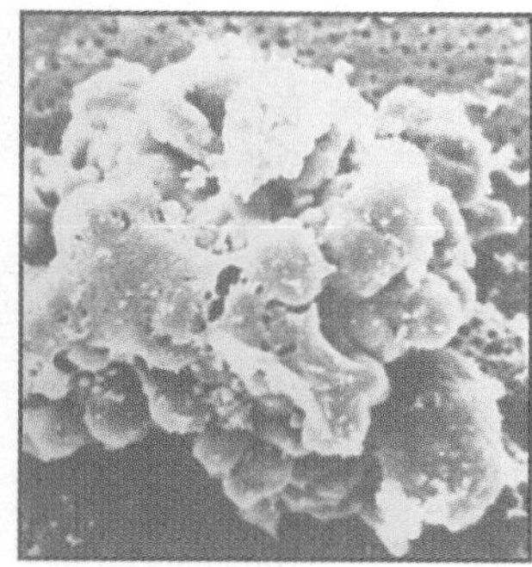

PART I INTRODUCTION

Chapter 1 | *Overview of the Immune System*

This introductory chapter includes some additional consideration of the history of immunology. For example, the discoveries of complement by Bordet and anaphylaxis by Richet focus on facets of immunity that will be developed in later chapters. A new section on immune dysfunction and its consequences signals an increased emphasis on biomedical implications of immunity throughout the text and is intended to tie the introduction to biomedical applications of immunology. In a feature new to this edition, a Clinical Focus essay documents the serious public-health burden caused by allergy and asthma. In recognition of the discovery of innate defense mechanisms in nonmammalian species, a section on comparative immunity has been added, pointing out the existence of alternatives to the mammalian immune system in other species.

Chapter 2 | *Cells and Organs of the Immune System*

The basic description of the cells, organs, and tissues of the immune system has been conserved in this edition. We have continued to include, and have augmented, coverage of the experiments that provide definitive support for key aspects of cellular origins and for the roles of different organs and tissues. Some sections, in particular the one that addresses the rapidly moving area of programmed cell death, have been updated to reflect important new findings. Also, the section on T cells is modified to recognize the existence of NK1-T cells. Hematopoietic stem cell (HSC) transplantation, an important therapy for patients whose hematopoietic systems must be replaced, is discussed, and a Clinical Focus essay describes the applications of this life-saving technology.

PART II GENERATION OF B-CELL AND T-CELL RESPONSES

Chapter 3 | *Antigens*

As in the third edition, this chapter provides an understanding of the nature of antigens and clarifies the differences between antigenicity and immunogenicity. The text of this revision has maintained the combination of explanatory conceptual diagrams and dramatic three-dimensional models based on x-ray crystallographic analysis of antigens and antibodies featured in the third edition. The capacity of some drugs, such as penicillin, to induce allergic reactions in some patients is the subject of a Clinical Focus essay.

Chapter 4 | *Immunoglobulins: Structure and Function*

The basic outline of this chapter is largely maintained. The section on monoclonal antibodies has been shortened by moving the material on the use of recombinant DNA techniques to engineer antibodies to Chapter 5. Such a move allows the introduction of antibody engineering and its possible uses after the students have acquired knowledge of the molecular biology of the rearrangement and expression of antibody genes in Chapter 5. The section on catalytic monoclonal antibodies (abzymes) has been updated. A Clinical Focus essay explores the use of injections of antibody for the treatment of infectious disease and the therapeutic support of patients who have lost the ability to make adequate levels of antibody.

Chapter 5 | *Organization and Expression of Immunoglobulin Genes*

Except for updating the coverage of such topics as the recombinase-activating genes, much of the material in the third edition has been conserved in this revision. An important addition explains the impact that precise knowledge of the number of heavy- and light-chain V-region gene segments has on calculations of the generation of antibody diversity by gene rearrangement. This chapter lays a foundation for understanding applications of recent advances in antibody engineering. Accordingly, the chapter concludes with a description of antibody engineering and, in a Clinical Focus essay, considers its use in designing a new therapy for non-Hodgkin's lymphoma.

Chapter 6 | *Antigen-Antibody Interactions*

This chapter retains material important for understanding the nature and practical application of antigen-antibody interactions. However, we have made changes to provide a balance of coverage that is consistent with modern immunological practice. The presentation of precipitation reactions has been shortened to allow more space for such currently used procedures as radioimmunoassay, ELISA, and the widely used fluorescence-based techniques such as fluorescent-antibody staining and flow cytometry. The use of highly sensitive chemiluminescent assay techniques is introduced and explained in this revision. Also, because so many of the students in an introductory immunology course have strong interests in medicine, the presentation of medically relevant applications of immunoassay has been increased. A Clinical Focus essay on the application of flow cytometry to the characterization of various types of leukemia provides examples of the medical use of this powerful technology.

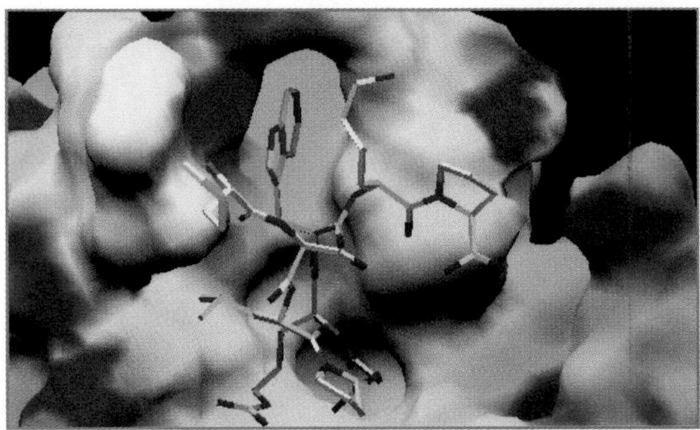

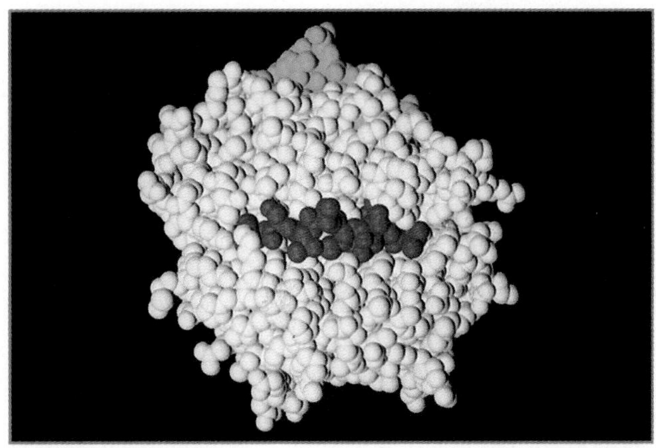

Chapter 7 | *Major Histocompatibility Complex*

We have changed the position of this and the two subsequent chapters in this edition to give the reader information about molecular events in antigen processing and T-cell recognition before discussion of T- and B-cell function. Transplantation, which played a large role in discovery of the MHC, is introduced here. A table listing associations of HLA with certain diseases was moved here from the later chapter on autoimmunity. A Clinical Focus essay highlights the recent discovery of a link between hereditary hemochromatosis and HLA-H. Additions to text and figures place added emphasis on the human MHC.

Chapter 8 | *Antigen Processing and Presentation*

This chapter is updated with new information on pathways for antigen processing. The functions of recently described molecules, such as tapasin and calreticulin, are added and the molecules placed appropriately in revised figures. The role of the MHC molecule DO as an inhibitor of DM function is described, and DO is added to relevant figures. New information clarifying the role of CLIP (the invariant chain fragment) was added along with a three-dimensional structure that compares presentation by class II MHC molecules of CLIP and of several foreign peptides.

Chapter 9 | *T-Cell Receptor*

Recent data on the three-dimensional structure of the TCR-peptide-MHC ternary complex are depicted in full-color models of human and mouse TCR/MHC complexes. The approach taken and the methods used to arrive at these impressive models will give students an appreciation of how modern technologies have led to these advances. These structures conclude the description of the MHC and antigen presentation in Chapters 7 and 8; they set the stage for the description of T-cell activation. Comparisons between the TCR structure and the immunoglobulin structure presented in Chapter 4 are added to show the similarities between these recognition molecules. A general description of affinity constants for biologic systems with an illustrative comparison places the TCR in context as a low-affinity receptor. A Clinical Focus essay describes the use of rearrangements in T-cell–receptor gene segments as markers for lymphoid cell cancers.

Chapter 10 | *T-Cell Maturation, Activation, and Differentiation*

This new edition provides a clear presentation of this central area of immunobiology. The logical organization of the chapter in the third edition contributed significantly to its clarity and has been retained in this revision. However, because many of the areas addressed in this chapter are among the most rapidly evolving in immunology, significant factual and conceptual updating has been necessary. Coverage of many aspects of signal transduction and of TCR-coupled signaling pathways in particular has been extensively revised. The description of T-cell development and selection has been updated to reflect newer findings and changing concepts. The role of apoptosis in maintaining appropriate levels of lymphocyte populations is illustrated in a Clinical Focus essay on the Canale-Smith syndrome, a disease caused by a failure of Fas-mediated cell death.

Chapter 11 | *B-Cell Generation, Activation, and Differentiation*

Although this chapter's overall organization and strong emphasis on basic mechanisms has been preserved, the chapter now includes material on the induction of the antibody response that was formerly part of a later chapter on cell-mediated and humoral effector responses (Chapter 16) in the third edition. Specifically, consideration of primary and secondary responses and the antibody response to hapten-carrier conjugates is now in this earlier chapter. The coverage of signal transduction in B cells has been significantly updated, and a Clinical Focus essay shows the medical consequences of the failure of a critical step in B-cell signal transduction. The section on B-cell differentiation in the third edition covered the germinal-center reaction; in this edition, a major conceptual updating of the coverage reflects the intense research in this area. As experimental underpinnings to this presentation, experiments that directly demonstrated somatic hypermutation within germinal centers have been included.

PART III IMMUNE EFFECTOR MECHANISMS

Chapter 12 | *Cytokines*

The present organization of this chapter provides a framework for the plethora of cytokines and their labyrinthine network of often interconnected functions. Despite the seemingly inexhaustible cornucopia of cytokine effects and interactions, the continual isolation of new cytokines, and the occasional discovery that already well-known ones perform previously unrecognized functions, the passage of each year also seems to bring a deeper understanding of the intracellular pathways responsible for the transduction of cytokine signals. This chapter has been substantially updated to reflect these advances in knowledge. Cytokines are finding wider applications in medicine, and a Clinical Focus essay on the uses of interferon has been added to this chapter to provide examples of successful cytokine therapies.

Chapter 13 | *The Complement System*

A brief description of the experiments leading to the initial discovery of complement has been added to bolster the idea that this is an effector system. Updates include information on the lectin pathway of complement activation and the proteins involved in it. The chapter now reports that there are

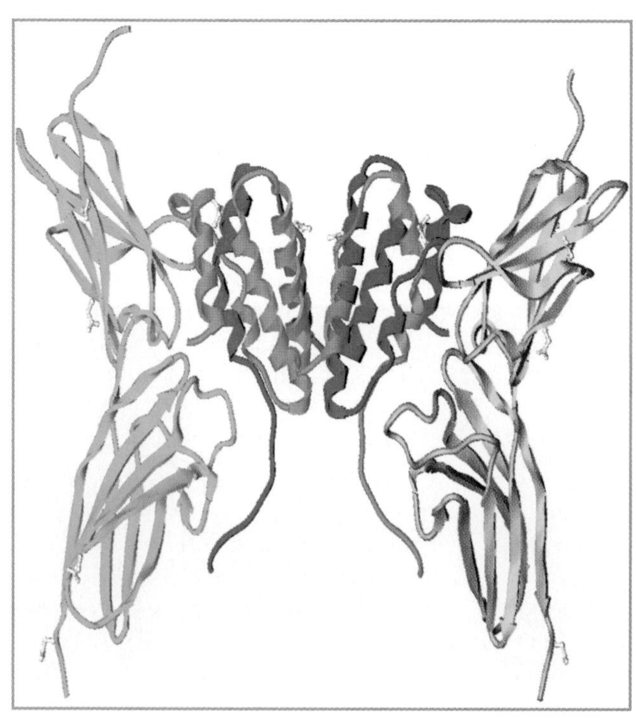

three rather than two complement-activation pathways to consider. Experimental evidence from gene knockout mice with different complement deficiencies is added to define the role of different components more comprehensively and to illustrate redundancy in this system. An effort is made to further define the complement system in terms of its multiple roles; a list of the various functions and an overview figure showing these appear early in the chapter. The critical role of complement in removing immune complexes from serum and the relevance of this process to the development of systemic lupus erythematosus are new topics that indicate the clinical importance of the complement system.

Chapter 14 | *Cell-Mediated Effector Responses*

In the third edition, this chapter included both cell-mediated and humoral effector responses. However, in the interests of integrating the antibody response to immunization with the discussion of B-cell activation and differentiation, we have moved the humoral-response section to Chapter 11 (B-Cell Generation, Activation, and Differentiation). Also, the coverage of cell-mediated cytotoxicity, which presents the roles of perforin and granzymes in killing, has been updated to include the now well-recognized participation of the Fas–Fas ligand system in T-cell–mediated killing. The experiments that demonstrate this point are included in this revision because they clarify thinking about T-cell killing and can be grasped readily by undergraduates.

Chapter 15 | *Leukocyte Migration and Inflammation*

The third edition provided a clear, well-organized, and interesting presentation of inflammation and its central role in organizing and focusing immune responses. Although this organization has been largely maintained, the importance of chemokines and their receptors in regulating leukocyte traffic has become widely appreciated since the writing of the third edition, and our revised chapter reflects this. Also, chemokine receptors have become established as the long-sought "second receptors" for HIV infection. Consequently, there has been an explosion of research and interest in this area. The revision includes some of the important new findings and evolving concepts of this rapidly expanding field. A Clinical Focus essay describes leukocyte adhesion disease, a syndrome in which patients suffer increased rates of infection because of an inability of their leukocytes to undergo adhesion-dependent migration into sites of inflammation.

Chapter 16 | *Hypersensitive Reactions*

The comprehensive overview of a variety of hypersensitive reactions and strong coverage of IgE-mediated reactions has been maintained from the previous edition. Type I, II, III, and IV hypersensitivities are covered in detail. The revision includes a Clinical Focus essay with in-depth coverage of the increase in the incidence of asthma, particularly among inner-city children whose conditions of life place them at risk for this disease.

PART IV THE IMMUNE SYSTEM IN HEALTH AND DISEASE

Chapter 17 | *Immune Response to Infectious Disease*

The chapter contains systematic coverage of immune responses to the four major pathogen groups: viruses, bacteria, protozoa, and roundworms. Although some mechanisms of immune response or pathogen evasion may apply to more than one of these groups, coverage by pathogen category has been maintained in this revision because it conveys a clear picture to the introductory reader. The revision includes a new section on emerging diseases that describes both the emergence of new diseases and the re-emergence of diseases once thought to be under control.

Chapter 18 | *Vaccines*

This chapter includes more information on the practical aspects of vaccine development. Emphasis has been redirected from approaches that have not advanced (such as anti-idiotype vaccines) to currently promising areas of investigation such as DNA vaccines. Passive immunization, which was an early treatment for several major diseases, is revisited in light of new possibilities opened up by genetically engineered antibodies. A Clinical Focus essay describing the new vaccine for the infant diarrhea agent rotavirus has been added. This vaccine is the latest addition to the list of vaccines recommended for all infants, and the story of its development illustrates an imaginative vaccine-development strategy.

Chapter 19 | *AIDS and Other Immunodeficiencies*

This chapter incorporates and updates the material in former Chapter 21 (Immunodeficiency Diseases) and Chapter

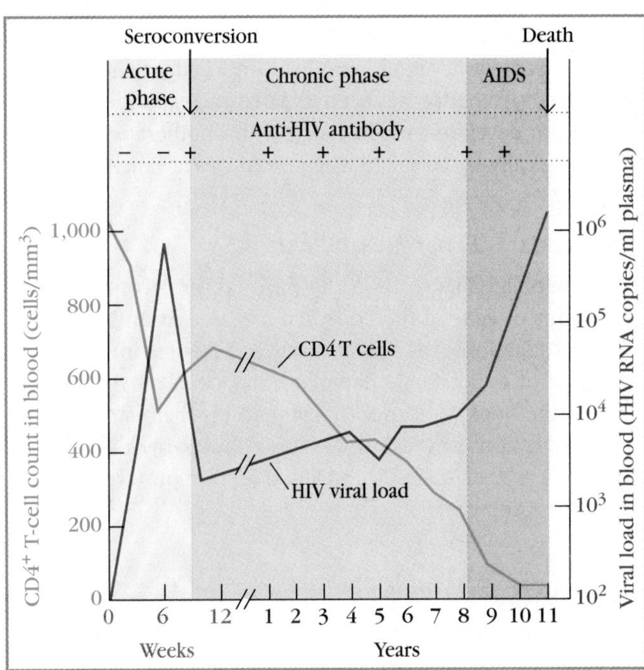

22 (The Immune System in AIDS). This combined chapter begins with a description of the various types of primary immunodeficiencies and their relationship to components of the immune system described in earlier chapters. The description of acquired deficiency highlights AIDS and HIV infection, with recent thinking on the development of HIV/AIDS vaccines and on the drugs that have proven effective in lowering viral load. Statistics on worldwide infection and disease have been updated, and recent progress in understanding the nature of the disease and the virus are recounted. Consideration of hypotheses about the disease that have been disproved has been deleted.

Chapter 20 | *Autoimmunity*

This chapter provides detailed coverage of the most prevalent autoimmune diseases and describes common themes. Some of the factors that contribute to autoimmunity are described and advances in the treatment of autoimmunity are covered. A Clinical Focus essay outlines issues of gender bias in the susceptibility to autoimmune diseases.

Chapter 21 | *Transplantation Immunology*

Additions include the description of new techniques for preventing organ rejection. These techniques are based on immunologic principles developed in earlier chapters for inducing specific tolerance rather than total immunosuppression. Progress in, and barriers to, the use of xenotransplants in humans is considered. The description of specific organ transplantations and the disease conditions for which they offer a viable treatment has been expanded.

Chapter 22 | *Cancer and the Immune System*

The third edition's coverage of this topic remains a good framework for a necessarily abbreviated treatment of a large and still rapidly developing body of knowledge. The section on cancer vaccination has been updated and expanded. Other significant developments in cancer immunotherapy and immunologically based diagnostic procedures are included.

Chapter 23 | *Experimental Systems*

This chapter (Chapter 2 in the third edition) contains descriptions of general methods that are used in immunological investigations. Because its early appearance interrupted the flow of conceptual chapters, it has been moved to the end of the book. A section on protein biochemistry, which includes a nontechnical discussion about x-ray diffraction analysis has been added, as well as a section on targeted expression using Cre/*lox*.

Appendix | *CD Antigens*

A complete annotated table of CD markers is included.

PEDAGOGIC TOOLS

CLINICAL FOCUS ESSAYS

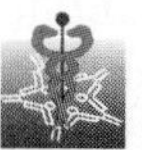

A major difference from the previous edition is the increased coverage of human immunology and the applications of immunology to clinical practice. We believe that examples encountered in everyday life provide incentive to learn the underlying principles and demonstrate the immediate practical value of this knowledge. Although many chapters, especially those in the later section of the book, have clear application to human health and disease, highly relevant examples of clinical importance derive also from material in chapters that describe more basic concepts. Some of these are highlighted in the newly added Clinical Focus essays.

VISUALIZING CONCEPTS

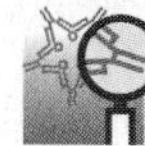

A number of concepts are crucial for students to develop a firm understanding of immunology. These concepts are illustrated in key diagrams called "Visualizing Concepts." These figures summarize important ideas and processes in a way that written text alone cannot convey.

FULL-COLOR ILLUSTRATIONS

The increased use of color and the additional figures will be evident to users of the previous edition. Well-chosen and carefully colored figures enhance the understanding of the text. Recurring elements—such as various immune system cells and important membrane molecules—are depicted consistently by icons, thereby facilitating the recognition of these elements in different contexts. These icons look more realistic than simple, stylized shapes and provide students with an additional intuitive tool to help them construct a more complete picture of the field of immunology. Consistency in the use of icons and of color should aid the student in grasping the larger concepts as the description of the immune system unfolds. A table of these elements now appears as the frontispiece of the book, as an easily accessible guide.

STUDY QUESTIONS

The study questions of earlier editions were popular with both instructors and students. They continue to constitute a useful teaching tool that provides a challenging and thoughtful review for students, and additional questions related to new topics are included in the fourth edition. As before, the answers to the study questions are given at the back of the book.

STUDY AIDS

Key terms appear in boldface type within the text. Definitions of these terms appear in the revised and updated glossary at the end of the book.

Chapter summaries not only present a concise review of the material but also include references to key illustrations and tables that provide an overview of the most important concepts within each chapter.

Updated References at the end of each chapter enable students to sample the primary literature relating to topics of interest.

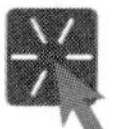

Useful Web Sites are also listed in the References section, a feature new to this edition. Web address updates may be found on the *Kuby Immunology* Web site at www.whfreeman.com/immunology.

SUPPLEMENTS

WEB SITE

The Web site provides students with a chapter-by-chapter online study guide that includes a variety of exercises and resources. Students can apply their knowledge of immunology in a medical context by analyzing **Clinical Case Studies**. **Animations** of key concepts facilitate understanding of complex immunological processes by adding a dimension beyond the printed page. In **Molecular Visualizations** by David Marcy, Kenyon College/California Lutheran University, dynamic guided tours of three-dimensional molecular models make the relationship between molecular structure and function easier to grasp. **Flashcards** allow students to review and then quiz and grade themselves on definitions of key terms from the text. For further exploration, the **News and Notes** section provides related Web links and updates on new developments in the world of immunology.

INSTRUCTOR'S CD-ROM

A CD-ROM available to adopters provides resources for preparing lectures or other presentations. It contains all text images in JPEG and PICT format for use with any presentation software. In addition, the **Presentation Manager Pro** software on the CD-ROM allows instructors to create classroom presentations quickly by incorporating text images, media content from the text Web site, or their own videos, animations, or illustrations. This software can use preloaded content, content saved locally, or content available on the World Wide Web.

ACKNOWLEDGMENTS

We thank the following reviewers for offering their comments and suggestions about the manuscript during preparation of this fourth edition; their expertise and insights have contributed greatly to the book: James Allison, Howard Hughes Medical Institute, University of California, Berkeley; David Allman, College of General Studies, University of Pennsylvania; Cynthia Baldwin, University of Massachusetts, Amherst; Karyl Barron, NIAID, National Institutes of Health; Amer A. Beg, Columbia University; Gilbert Boissoneault, University of Kentucky; A. Malcolm Campbell, Davidson College; Sheldon Cohen, NIAID, National Institutes of Health; Phillip Danielson, University of Denver; Cheryl Davis, Western Kentucky University; Michael Dennis, Montana State University; Betty Diamond, Albert Einstein College of Medicine; Peter Diffley, Notre Dame University; David Drath, California State University, Fullerton; Laurel Eckhardt, Hunter College, City University of New York; Soldano Ferrone, Roswell Park Cancer Institute; Valerie Flechtner, John Carrol University; Juan Gea-Banacloche, NIAID Clinical Center, National Institutes of Health; Richard Hardy, Fox Chase Cancer Center; James Hartman, Florida Atlantic University; Joseph S. Heilig, University of Colorado, Boulder; Pierre Henkart, NCI, National Institutes of Health; Jeffrey L. Henriksen, Bellevue University; Dorothy Hudig, University of Nevada, Reno; Susan H. Jackman, Marshall University School of Medicine; Laura Jenski, Indiana University–Purdue University at Indianapolis; Paul Kincade, Oklahoma Medical Research Foundation; Richard Krause, NIAID, National Institutes of Health; Douglas Lake, University of Arizona; H. Clifford Lane, NIAID, National Institutes of Health; D. H. Lewis, Texas A&M University; Tom Lint, Rush Medical College; Eric Long, NIAID, National Institutes of Health; David H. Margulies, NIAID, National Institutes of Health; Ann Marshak-Rothstein, Boston University School of Medicine; Andrea M. Mastro, Pennsylvania State University; Kathleen McGuire, San Diego State University; Frederick Miller, State University of New York at Stony Brook; Robert Miller, University of New Mexico; Michael Minnick, University of Montana; Larry Pease, Mayo Clinic; Lakshmi Pulakat, Bowling Green State University; Jennifer Punt, Haverford College; Carol Reiss, New York University; Robert C. Rickert, University of California, San Diego; Paul Robbins, NCI, National Institutes of Health; Stephen Rose, NIAID, National Institutes of Health; Tobili Sam-Yellowe, Cleveland State University; Rachel Shefner, Roosevelt University; S. Srikumaran, University of Nebraska; Lisa Steiner, Massachusetts Institute of Technology; Jeff Stott, University of California, Davis; Robert D. Stout, University of Louisville; Douglas Swartzendruber, University of Colorado; James Thompson, LSU Medical Center; Kathryn Vogel, University of New Mexico; Fred Volkert, State University of New York Health Science Center, Brooklyn; Christopher J. Woolverton, Kent State University; Martha Zuniga, University of California, Santa Cruz.

We have been the fortunate beneficiaries of extensive support by the experienced and talented staff at W. H. Freeman and Company. Particular thanks are due Nicole Folchetti, Janet Tannenbaum, Georgia Lee Hadler, Andrew Kudlacik, Blake Logan, Jennifer MacMillan, Bill Page, Paul Rohloff, Bridget O'Lavin, and Michelle Julet.

PART I | INTRODUCTION

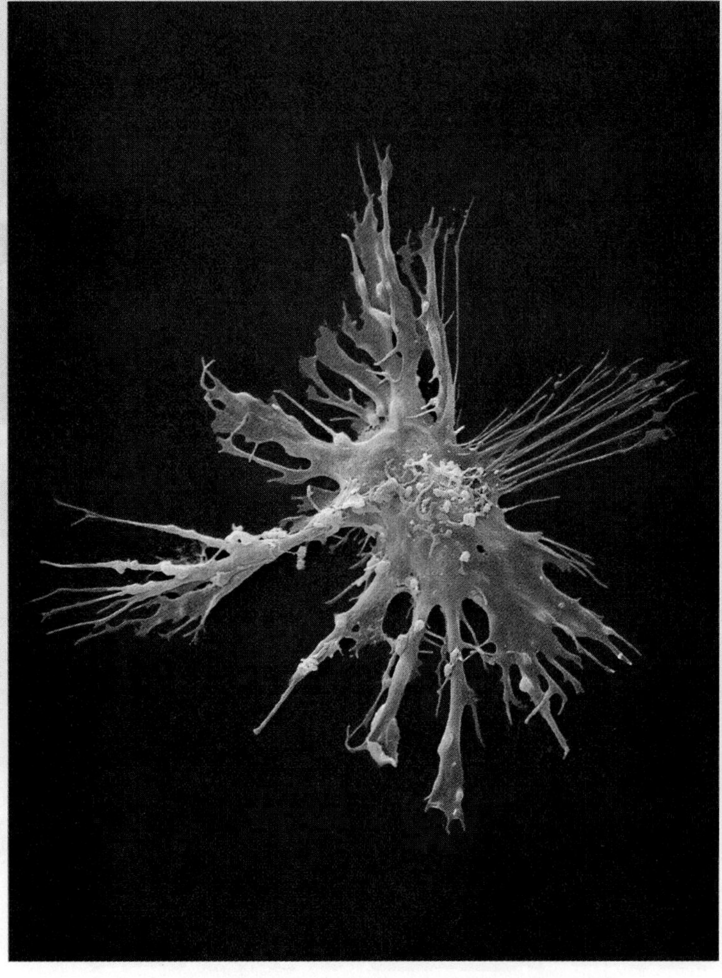

Dendritic cell, an antigen-presenting cell.

From birth, we are exposed to a continuous stream of microorganisms that have the potential to wreak havoc on our bodily processes. Without effective protective mechanisms, each of us would soon succumb to diseases caused by microorganisms or to the harmful effects of foreign substances (e.g., toxins) produced by various plants and bacteria. In the battle with microbial invaders, humans and other vertebrates protect themselves by a complex array of defensive measures collectively termed the immune system. Part I provides a framework for understanding the mechanisms that compose the immune system.

Chapter 1 describes the general properties and development of immunity, the condition of being protected from infection by microorganisms or the effects of foreign molecules. Innate immunity depends on a number of barriers that are effective against a wide variety of pathogens. This nonspecific form of immunity is bolstered and greatly extended by adaptive immunity, which is specific for particular microorganisms or foreign molecules. The key cells in adaptive immunity are B lymphocytes (B cells) and T lymphocytes (T cells). Two major populations of T cells exist: T helper cells and cytotoxic T cells. T helper cells express the membrane glycoprotein called CD4; when activated, these cells secrete numerous low-molecular-weight proteins called cytokines, which exert various effects on other cells of the immune system. T cytotoxic cells express the membrane glycoprotein called CD8; when activated, these cells differentiate into effector cells that can destroy altered self-cells, including cells infected by virus and tumor cells.

An individual contains a large number of immunocompetent clones of B and T lymphocytes. The cells in each clone are capable of recognizing a particular foreign molecule, or antigen. B cells interact with antigen through their membrane-bound immunoglobulin (antibody), and T cells interact with antigen through their T-cell receptors. After the recognition of antigen, lymphocytes proliferate and differentiate, leading them to produce secreted antibodies, which bind to the antigen and help eliminate it (humoral response), and to generate cells that can destroy the invading pathogen (cell-mediated response). When we are first exposed to an invading pathogen, we normally experience some of the early symptoms of an infection because the immune system needs some time to respond and to destroy the pathogen. However, once we have been exposed to a particular pathogen, our immune system "remembers" the encounter and can respond much more quickly to subsequent encounters with it.

Although no evidence for adaptive immunity has been found in invertebrate species, different forms of immunity may be found in diverse invertebrate species, such as insects, and even in plants. These mechanisms, which often utilize elements common to innate immune systems of vertebrates, protect against harmful bacterial or fungal agents.

Although the immune system in its normal function protects from harmful attacks from without, sometimes the system turns against the host, causing symptoms that range from discomfort to debilitating disease or even death. The causes of immune dysfunction include genetic defects and certain infectious agents, as well as the destruction of immune cells or tissues by chemical agents or physical trauma, such as radiation. An important part of the study of immunology is the effort to understand immune dysfunction and the development of means to correct the defects and to alleviate the suffering caused by them.

Chapter 2 covers the basic properties of the cells, tissues, and organs that form the immune system. After reviewing hematopoiesis (the development of blood cells in the bone marrow), it examines the general functions of immune-system cells: lymphocytes, macrophages, granulocytes, mast cells, and dendritic cells. (The details of how these cells participate in immune responses and the ways in which they cooperate with each other are described in later chapters.) Finally, the chapter considers the structures of the primary, secondary, and tertiary lymphoid organs—the sites for the maturation of lymphocytes and their activation by antigen.

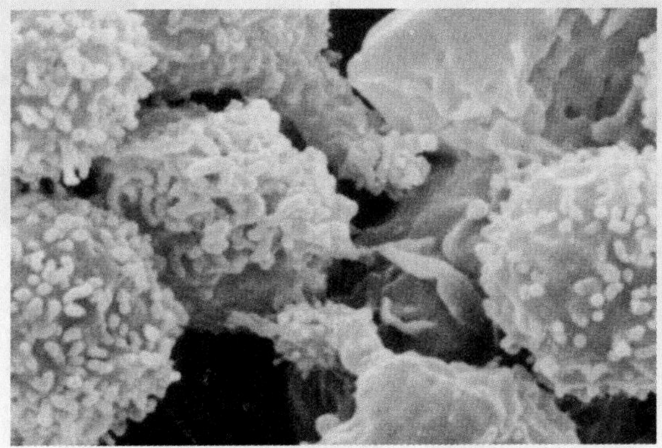

CHAPTER 1 OVERVIEW OF THE IMMUNE SYSTEM

The immune system is a remarkably adaptive defense system that has evolved in vertebrates to protect them from invading pathogenic microorganisms and cancer. It is able to generate an enormous variety of cells and molecules capable of specifically recognizing and eliminating an apparently limitless variety of foreign invaders. These cells and molecules act together in an exquisitely adaptable dynamic network whose complexity rivals that of the nervous system.

Functionally, an immune response can be divided into two related activities—*recognition* and *response.* Immune recognition is remarkable for its specificity. The immune system is able to recognize subtle chemical differences that distinguish one foreign pathogen from another. Furthermore, the system is able to discriminate between foreign molecules and the body's own cells and proteins. Once a foreign organism has been recognized, the immune system enlists the participation of a variety of cells and molecules to mount an appropriate response, called an **effector response,** to eliminate or neutralize the organism. In this way the system is able to convert the initial recognition event into different effector responses, each uniquely suited for eliminating a particular type of pathogen. Later exposure to the same foreign organism induces a **memory response,** characterized by a more rapid and heightened immune reaction that serves to eliminate the pathogen and prevent disease.

This chapter presents a broad overview of the cells and molecules that compose the immune system and the mechanisms by which they protect the body against foreign invaders. Evidence for the presence of very simple immune systems in certain invertebrate organisms then gives an evolutionary perspective on the mammalian immune system, which is the major subject of this book. Finally, in some circumstances, the immune system fails to act as protector because of deficiency in its components; at other times, it becomes an aggressor and turns its awesome powers against its own host. As is always the case with an overview, the details have been simplified to reveal the essential structure and function of the immune system. Substantive discussions, experimental approaches, and in-depth definitions are left to the chapters that follow.

Like some of the later chapters about basic topics in immunology, this one includes a section (called "Clinical Focus") that describes human disease and its relation to immunity. These sections describe the causes, consequences, or treatments of diseases rooted in impaired or hyperactive immune function.

Historical Perspective

The discipline of immunology grew out of the observation that individuals who had recovered from certain infectious diseases were thereafter protected from the disease. The Latin term *immunis,* meaning "exempt," is the source of the English word **immunity,** meaning the state of protection from infectious disease.

Perhaps the earliest written reference to the phenomenon of immunity can be traced back to Thucydides, the great historian of the Peloponnesian War. In describing a plague in Athens, he wrote in 430 BC that only those who had recovered from the plague could nurse the sick because they would not contract the disease a second time. Although early societies recognized the phenomenon of immunity, almost two thousand years passed before the concept was successfully converted into a medically effective practice.

The first recorded crude attempts to induce immunity deliberately were performed by the Chinese and Turks in the fifteenth century. Various reports suggest that the dried crusts derived from smallpox pustules were either inhaled into the nostrils or inserted into small cuts in the skin (a technique called **variolation**). In 1718, Lady Mary Wortley Montagu, the wife of the British ambassador to Constantinople, observed the positive effects of variolation on the native population and had the technique applied to her own children. The technique was significantly improved by the English physician Edward Jenner, in 1798. Intrigued by the fact that milkmaids who had contracted cowpox (a mild disease) were subsequently immune to smallpox (a disfiguring and often fatal disease), Jenner reasoned that introducing fluid from a cowpox pustule into people (i.e., inoculating them) might protect them from smallpox. To test this idea, he inoculated an eight-year-old boy with fluid from a cowpox pustule and later intentionally infected the child with smallpox. As predicted, the child did not develop smallpox. Nevertheless, one cannot help but question the ethical implications of such an experiment!

Jenner's technique of inoculating with cowpox to protect against smallpox spread quickly throughout Europe, but it was nearly a hundred years before it was applied to other diseases. As so often happens in science, serendipity combined with astute observation led to the next major advance in immunology, the induction of immunity to cholera. Louis Pasteur had succeeded in growing the bacterium thought to cause fowl cholera in culture and then had shown that chickens injected with the cultured bacterium developed cholera. After returning from a summer vacation, he injected some chickens with an old culture. The chickens became ill, but, to Pasteur's surprise, they recovered. Pasteur then grew a fresh culture of the bacterium with the intention of injecting it into some fresh chickens. But, as the story goes, his supply of chickens was limited, and therefore he used the previously injected chickens. Again to his surprise, the chickens survived and were completely protected from the disease. Pasteur recognized that aging had weakened the virulence of the pathogen and that such an attenuated strain might be administered to protect against the disease. He called this attenuated strain a **vaccine** (from the Latin *vacca,* meaning "cow"), in honor of Jenner's work with cowpox inoculation.

Pasteur extended these findings to other diseases, demonstrating that is was possible to **attenuate,** or weaken, a pathogen and administer the attenuated strain as a vaccine. In a now classic experiment at Pouilly-le-Fort in 1881, Pasteur first vaccinated one group of sheep with heat-attenuated anthrax bacillus (*Bacillus anthracis*); he then challenged the vaccinated sheep and some unvaccinated sheep with a virulent culture of the bacillus. All the vaccinated sheep lived, whereas all unvaccinated animals died. These experiments marked the beginnings of the discipline of immunology. In 1885, Pasteur administered the first vaccine to a human, a young boy who had been bitten repeatedly by a rabid dog (Figure 1-1). The boy, Joseph Meister, lived and later became a custodian at the Pasteur Institute. In 1940, during the Nazi occupation of Paris, the Nazis asked Meister to give them the keys to Pasteur's crypt. Rather than surrender the keys to the Nazis, Meister took his own life.

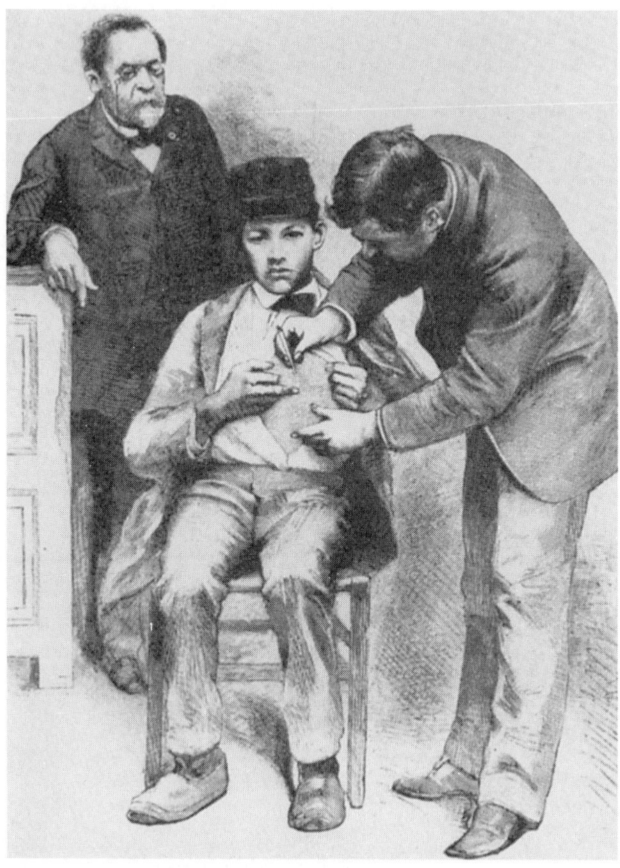

FIGURE 1-1 Wood engraving of Louis Pasteur watching Joseph Meister receive the rabies vaccine. [From *Harper's Weekly* **29:**836; courtesy of the National Library of Medicine.]

Discovery of Humoral and Cellular Immunity

Although Pasteur proved that **vaccination** worked, he did not understand how. The experimental work of Emil von Behring and Shibasaburo Kitasato in 1890 gave the first insights into the mechanism of immunity, earning von Behring the Nobel prize in medicine in 1901 (Table 1-1). Von Behring and Kitasato demonstrated that **serum** (the liquid, noncellular component of coagulated blood) from animals previously immunized to diphtheria could transfer the immune state to unimmunized animals. In search of the protective agent, various researchers during the next decade demonstrated that an active component from immune serum could neutralize toxins, precipitate toxins, and agglutinate (clump) bacteria. In each case, the active agent was named for the activity it exhibited: antitoxin, precipitin, and agglutinin, respectively. Initially, a different serum component was thought to be responsible for each activity, but, during the

TABLE 1-1 NOBEL PRIZES FOR IMMUNOLOGIC RESEARCH

Year	Recipient	Country	Research
1901	Emil von Behring	Germany	Serum antitoxins
1905	Robert Koch	Germany	Cellular immunity to tuberculosis
1908	Elie Metchnikoff Paul Ehrlich	Russia Germany	Role of phagocytosis (Metchnikoff) and antitoxins (Ehrlich) in immunity
1913	Charles Richet	France	Anaphylaxis
1919	Jules Bordet	Belgium	Complement-mediated bacteriolysis
1930	Karl Landsteiner	United States	Discovery of human blood groups
1951	Max Theiler	South Africa	Development of yellow fever vaccine
1957	Daniel Bovet	Switzerland	Antihistamines
1960	F. Macfarlane Burnet Peter Medawar	Australia Great Britain	Discovery of acquired immunological tolerance
1972	Rodney R. Porter Gerald M. Edelman	Great Britain United States	Chemical structure of antibodies
1977	Rosalyn R. Yalow	United States	Development of radioimmunoassay
1980	George Snell Jean Dausset Baruj Benacerraf	United States France United States	Major histocompatibility complex
1984	Cesar Milstein Georges F. Köhler Niels K. Jerne	Great Britain Germany Denmark	Monoclonal antibody Immune regulatory theories
1987	Susumu Tonegawa	Japan	Gene rearrangement in antibody production
1991	E. Donnall Thomas Joseph Murray	United States United States	Transplantation immunology
1996	Peter C. Doherty Rolf M. Zinkernagel	Australia Switzerland	The specificity of the cell-mediated immune response

1930s, mainly through the efforts of Elvin Kabat, a fraction of serum first called gamma-globulin (now **immunoglobulin**) was shown to be responsible for all these activities. The active molecules in the immunoglobulin fraction are called **antibodies.** Because immunity was mediated by antibodies contained in body fluids (known at the time as *humors*), it was called **humoral immunity.**

In 1883, even before the discovery that a serum component could transfer immunity, Elie Metchnikoff demonstrated that cells also contribute to the immune state of an animal. He observed that certain white blood cells, which he termed **phagocytes,** were able to ingest microorganisms and other foreign material. Noting that these phagocytic cells were more active in immunized animals than in nonimmunized animals, Metchnikoff hypothesized that cells, rather than serum components, were the major effector of immunity. The active phagocytic cells identified by Metchnikoff were, likely, blood monocytes and neutrophils (see Chapter 2).

In due course, a controversy developed between those who held to the concept of humoral immunity and those who agreed with Metchnikoff's concept of **cell-mediated immunity.** It was difficult to study the activities of immune cells before the development of modern tissue culture techniques, whereas studies with serum took advantage of established biochemical techniques. Because of these technical problems, information about cellular immunity lagged behind findings that concerned humoral immunity.

In a key experiment in the 1940s, Merrill Chase succeeded in transferring immunity to the tuberculosis organism by transferring white blood cells between guinea pigs. This demonstration helped to rekindle interest in cellular immunity. With the emergence of improved cell culture techniques in the 1950s, the **lymphocyte** was identified as the cell responsible for both cellular and humoral immunity. Soon thereafter, experiments with chickens pioneered by Bruce Glick at Mississippi State University indicated that there were two types of lymphocytes: T lymphocytes derived from the thymus mediated cellular immunity, and B lymphocytes from the bursa of Fabricius were responsible for humoral immunity. The controversy about the roles of humoral and cellular immunity was resolved when the roles were shown to be intertwined, and both systems were shown to be necessary for the immune response.

Early Theories of Immunity

One of the greatest enigmas about the antibody molecule that faced early immunologists was its specificity for foreign material, or **antigen** (the general term for a substance that binds with a specific antibody). Around 1900, Jules Bordet at the Pasteur Institute furthered the concept of immunity by demonstrating specific immune reactivity to nonpathogenic substances. Serum from an animal inoculated with material that did not cause infection would react with this material in a specific manner, and this reactivity could be passed to other animals with serum from the first. The work of Karl Landsteiner and those who followed him showed that injecting an animal with almost any organic chemical could induce production of antibodies that would bind specifically to it. These studies demonstrated that antibodies have a capacity for an almost unlimited range of reactivity, including responses to compounds that had only recently been synthesized in the laboratory and had not previously existed in nature. In addition, it was shown that molecules differing in the smallest detail could be distinguished by their reactivity with different antibodies. Two major theories were proposed to account for this specificity: the selective theory and the instructional theory.

The earliest conception of the *selective theory* dates to Paul Ehrlich in 1900. In an attempt to explain the origin of serum antibody, Ehrlich proposed that cells in the blood expressed a variety of "side-chain" receptors that could react with infectious agents and inactivate them. Borrowing a concept used by Emil Fischer to explain the interaction between an enzyme and its substrate, Ehrlich proposed that binding of the side-chain receptor to an infectious agent was like the fitting of a lock with a key. Ehrlich suggested that interaction between an infectious agent and a cell-bound side-chain receptor would result in release of the side chain and would induce the cell to produce and secrete more side-chain receptors with the same specificity. According to Ehrlich's theory, the side-chain specificity was determined before its exposure to antigen, and the antigen selected the appropriate side-chain receptor.

In the 1930s and 1940s, the selective theory was challenged by various *instructional theories,* in which antigen played a central role in determining the specificity of the antibody molecule. According to the instructional theories, a particular antigen would serve as a template around which antibody would fold. The antibody molecule would thereby assume a configuration complementary to that of the antigen template. This concept was first postulated by Friedrich Breinl and Felix Haurowitz about 1930 and redefined in the 1940s in terms of protein folding by Linus Pauling. The instructional theories were formally disproved in the 1960s, by which time information was emerging about the structure of DNA, RNA, and protein that would offer new insights into the vexing problem of how an individual could make antibodies against almost anything.

In the 1950s, selective theories resurfaced and, through the insights of Niels Jerne, David Talmadge, and F. Macfarlane Burnet, were refined into a theory that came to be known as the **clonal-selection theory.** According to this theory, an individual lymphocyte expresses membrane receptors that are specific for a distinct antigen. This unique receptor specificity is determined before the lymphocyte is exposed to the antigen. Binding of antigen to its specific receptor activates the cell, causing it to proliferate into a **clone** of cells that have the same immunologic specificity as the parent cell. The clonal-selection theory has been further refined and is now accepted as the underlying paradigm of modern immunology. This theory, which has proved to be remarkably accurate, is examined in more depth later in this chapter.

Components of Immunity

Immunity—the state of protection from infectious disease—has both nonspecific and specific components. The nonspecific component, **innate immunity,** is a set of disease-resistance mechanisms that are not specific to a particular pathogen. Phagocytic cells, such as macrophages, play an important role in many aspects of innate immunity. In contrast, the specific component, **adaptive immunity,** displays a high degree of specificity as well as the remarkable property of "memory." Typically, there is an adaptive immune response against an antigen within five or six days after the initial exposure to that antigen. Exposure to the same antigen some time in the future results in a memory response: the immune response to the second challenge occurs more quickly than the first, is stronger, and often is more effective in neutralizing and clearing the pathogen. The major cellular agents of adaptive immunity are lymphocytes and the antibodies and other molecules they produce.

Because adaptive immune responses require some time to marshal, innate immunity provides the first line of defense during the critical period just after the host's exposure to a pathogen. In general, most of the microorganisms encountered by a healthy individual are readily cleared within a few days by nonspecific defense mechanisms before they activate the adaptive immune system. If an invading microorganism eludes innate mechanisms or is not cleared by them, the specific immune response of adaptive immunity is triggered. Adaptive and innate immunity do not operate independently of each other; they function as a highly interactive and cooperative system, producing a total response more effective than either could alone.

Innate (Nonspecific) Immunity

Innate immunity can be seen to comprise four types of defensive barriers: anatomic, physiologic, phagocytic, and inflammatory (Table 1-2).

Anatomic Barriers

Physical and anatomic barriers that tend to prevent the entry of pathogens are an organism's first line of defense against infection. The skin and the surface of mucous membranes are included in this category because they are effective barriers to the entry of most microorganisms. The skin consists of two distinct layers: a thinner outer layer—the **epidermis**—and a thicker layer—the **dermis.** The epidermis contains several layers of tightly packed epithelial cells. The outer epidermal layer consists of dead cells and is filled with a waterproofing protein called keratin. The dermis, which is composed of connective tissue, contains blood vessels, hair follicles, sebaceous glands, and sweat glands. The sebaceous glands are associated with the hair follicles and produce an oily secretion called **sebum.** Sebum consists of lactic and fatty acids, which maintain the pH of the skin between 3 and 5; this pH inhibits the growth of most microorganisms. A few bacteria that metabolize sebum live as commensals on the skin and sometimes cause a severe form of acne. One acne drug, isotretinoin (Accutane), is a vitamin A derivative that prevents the formation of sebum.

Not only does intact skin prevent the penetration of most pathogens, but its low pH also inhibits most bacterial growth. Breaks in the skin, even small ones, resulting from wounds or abrasion are obvious routes of infection. The skin is penetrated also by biting insects (e.g., mosquitoes, mites, ticks, fleas, and sandflies); if these harbor pathogenic organisms, they can introduce the pathogen into the body as they feed. The protozoan that causes malaria, for example, is carried by mosquitoes, who deposit it in humans when they take a blood meal. Similarly, bubonic plague is spread by the bite of fleas, and Lyme disease is spread by the bite of ticks.

The conjunctivae and the alimentary, respiratory, and urogenital tracts are lined by mucous membranes, not by the dry, protective skin that covers the exterior of the body. These membranes consist of an outer epithelial layer and an underlying layer of connective tissue. Although most pathogens enter the body by binding to and penetrating mucous membranes, a number of nonspecific defense mechanisms tend to prevent this entry. For example, saliva, tears, and mucous secretions act to wash away potential invaders and also contain antibacterial or antiviral substances. The viscous fluid called mucus, which is secreted by epithelial cells of mucous membranes, entraps foreign microorganisms. In the lower respiratory tract and the gastrointestinal tract, the mucous membrane is covered by **cilia,** hairlike protrusions of the epithelial-cell membranes. The synchronous movement of cilia propels mucus-entrapped microorganisms from these tracts. In addition, nonpathogenic organisms tend to colonize the

TABLE 1-2 SUMMARY OF NONSPECIFIC HOST DEFENSES

Type	Mechanism
Anatomic barriers	
Skin	Mechanical barrier retards entry of microbes. Acidic environment (pH 3–5) retards growth of microbes.
Mucous membranes	Normal flora compete with microbes for attachment sites and nutrients. Mucus entraps foreign microorganisms. Cilia propel microorganisms out of body.
Physiologic barriers	
Temperature	Normal body temperature inhibits growth of some pathogens. Fever response inhibits growth of some pathogens.
Low pH	Acidity of stomach contents kills most ingested microorganisms.
Chemical mediators	Lysozyme cleaves bacterial cell wall. Interferon induces antiviral state in uninfected cells. Complement lyses microorganisms or facilitates phagocytosis.
Phagocytic/endocytic barriers	Various cells internalize (endocytose) and break down foreign macromolecules. Specialized cells (blood monocytes, neutrophils, tissue macrophages) internalize (phagocytose), kill, and digest whole microorganisms.
Inflammatory barriers	Tissue damage and infection induce leakage of vascular fluid, containing serum proteins with antibacterial activity, and influx of phagocytic cells into the affected area.

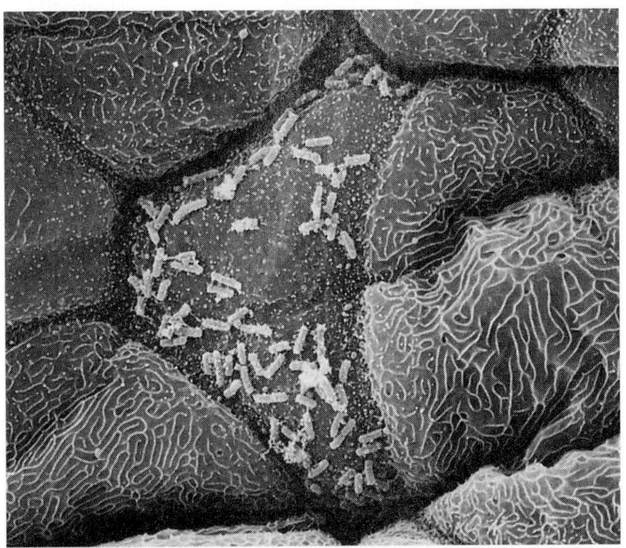

FIGURE 1-2 Electron micrograph of rod-shaped *Escherichia coli* bacteria adhering to surface of epithelial cells of the urinary tract. [From N Sharon and H Lis, 1993, *Sci. Am.* **268**(1):85.]

epithelial cells of mucosal surfaces. These *normal flora* generally outcompete pathogens for attachment sites on the epithelial cell surface and for necessary nutrients.

Some organisms have evolved ways of escaping these defense mechanisms and thus are likely to invade the body through mucous membranes. For example, influenza virus (the agent that causes flu) has a surface molecule that enables it to attach firmly to cells in mucous membranes, preventing the virus from being swept out by the ciliated epithelial cells. Similarly, the organism that causes gonorrhea has surface projections that allow it to bind to epithelial cells in the mucous membrane of the urogenital tract. Adherence of bacteria to mucous membranes is due to interactions between hairlike protrusions on a bacterium, called **fimbriae** or **pili,** and certain glycoproteins or glycolipids that are expressed only by epithelial cells of the mucous membrane of particular tissues (Figure 1-2). For this reason, some tissues are susceptible to bacterial invasion, whereas others are not.

Physiologic Barriers

The physiologic barriers that contribute to innate immunity include temperature, pH, and various soluble factors. Many species are not susceptible to certain diseases simply because their normal body temperature inhibits growth of the pathogens. Chickens, for example, have innate immunity to anthrax because their high body temperature inhibits the growth of the bacteria. Gastric acidity is an innate physiologic barrier to infection because very few ingested microorganisms can survive the low pH of the stomach contents. One reason newborns are susceptible to some diseases that do not afflict adults is that their stomach contents are less acid than those of adults.

A variety of soluble factors contribute to nonspecific immunity, among them the soluble proteins lysozyme, interferon, and complement. **Lysozyme,** a hydrolytic enzyme found in mucous secretions and in tears, is able to cleave the peptidoglycan layer of the bacterial cell wall. **Interferon** comprises a group of proteins produced by virus-infected cells. Among the many functions of the interferons is the ability to bind to nearby cells and induce a generalized antiviral state. **Complement** is a group of serum proteins that circulate in an inactive state. A variety of specific and nonspecific immunologic mechanisms can convert the inactive forms of complement proteins into an active state that enables them to damage the membranes of pathogenic organisms, either destroying the pathogens or facilitating their clearance.

Phagocytic Barriers

Another important innate defense mechanism is the ingestion of extracellular particulate material by **phagocytosis.** Phagocytosis is one type of **endocytosis,** which is the general term for the uptake by a cell of material from its environment. Phagocytosis is the ingestion of particulate material, which may include whole pathogenic microorganisms (Figure 1-3). In phagocytosis, a cell's plasma membrane expands around the particulate material to form large vesicles

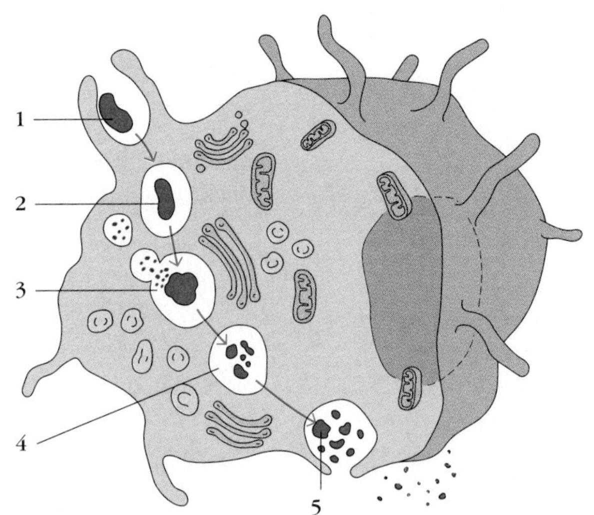

FIGURE 1-3 Phagocytosis of bacteria. Schematic diagram of the steps in phagocytosis: (1) attachment of a bacterium (red) to long membrane evaginations, called pseudopodia; (2) ingestion of bacterium, forms a phagosome, which moves toward a lysosome; (3) fusion of the phagosome and lysosome, releases lysosomal enzymes into the phagosome; (4) digestion of ingested material; and (5) release of digestion products from the cell.

called **phagosomes.** Most phagocytosis is conducted by specialized cells, such as blood monocytes, neutrophils, and tissue macrophages (see Chapter 2). Most cell types are capable of other forms of endocytosis, such as *receptor-mediated endocytosis* wherein extracellular molecules are internalized after binding by specific cellular receptors, and *pinocytosis,* by which cells take up fluid from the surrounding medium and any molecules contained in it.

Inflammatory Barriers

Tissue damage caused by a wound or by an invading pathogenic microorganism induces a complex sequence of events collectively known as the **inflammatory response.** Many of the classic features of the inflammatory response were described as early as 1600 BC, in Egyptian papyrus writings. In the first century AD, the Roman physician Celsus described the "four cardinal signs of inflammation" as *rubor* (redness), *tumor* (swelling), *calor* (heat), and *dolor* (pain). In the second century AD, another physician, Galen, added a fifth sign: *functio laesa* (loss of function). The cardinal signs of inflammation reflect the three major events of an inflammatory response (Figure 1-4):

1. Vasodilation—an increase in the diameter of blood vessels—of nearby capillaries occurs as the vessels that carry blood away from the affected area constrict, resulting in engorgement of the capillary network. The engorged capillaries are responsible for tissue redness (*erythema*) and an increase in tissue temperature.
2. An increase in capillary permeability facilitates an influx of fluid and cells from the engorged capillaries into the tissue. The fluid that accumulates **(exudate)** has a much higher protein content than fluid normally released from the vasculature. Accumulation of exudate contributes to tissue swelling **(edema).**
3. Influx of phagocytes from the capillaries into the tissues is facilitated by the increased capillary permeability. The emigration of phagocytes is a complex series of events, including adherence of the cells to the endothelial wall of the blood vessels **(margination),** followed by their emigration between the capillary-endothelial cells into the tissue **(diapedesis** or **extravasation),** and, finally, their migration through the tissue to the site of the inflammatory response **(chemotaxis).** As phagocytic cells accumulate at the site and begin to phagocytose

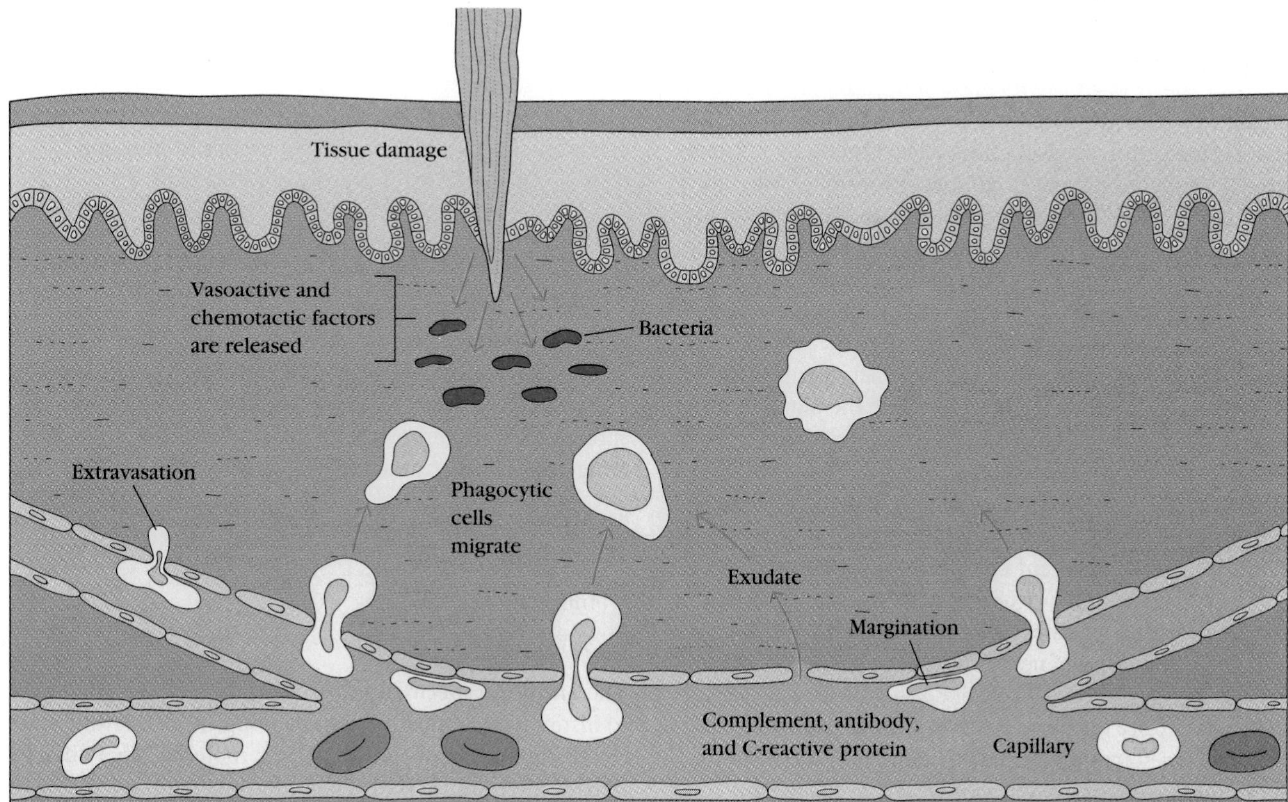

FIGURE 1-4 Major events in the inflammatory response. A bacterial infection causes tissue damage with release of various vasoactive and chemotactic factors. These factors induce increased blood flow to the area, increased capillary permeability, and an influx of white blood cells, including phagocytes and lymphocytes, from the blood into the tissues. The serum proteins contained in the exudate have antibacterial properties, and the phagocytes begin to engulf the bacteria, as illustrated in Figure 1-3.

bacteria, they release lytic enzymes, which can damage nearby healthy cells. The accumulation of dead cells, digested material, and fluid forms a substance called pus.

The events in the inflammatory response are initiated by a complex series of events involving a variety of chemical mediators, whose interactions are still only partly understood. Some of these mediators are derived from invading microorganisms, some are released from damaged cells in response to tissue injury, some are generated by several plasma enzyme systems, and some are products of various white blood cells participating in the inflammatory response.

Among the chemical mediators released in response to tissue damage are various serum proteins called **acute-phase proteins.** The concentrations of these proteins increase dramatically in tissue-damaging infections. C-reactive protein is a major acute-phase protein produced by the liver in response to tissue damage. Its name derives from the fact that it binds to the C-polysaccharide cell-wall component found on a variety of bacteria and fungi. This binding activates the complement system, resulting in increased clearance of the pathogen either by complement-mediated lysis or by complement-mediated increase in phagocytosis.

One of the principal mediators of the inflammatory response is **histamine,** a chemical released by a variety of cells in response to tissue injury. Histamine binds to receptors on nearby capillaries and venules, causing vasodilation and increased permeability. Another important group of inflammatory mediators, small peptides called **kinins,** are normally present in blood plasma in an inactive form. Tissue injury activates these peptides, which then cause vasodilation and increased permeability of capillaries. A particular kinin, called bradykinin, also stimulates pain receptors in the skin. This effect probably serves a protective role, because pain normally causes an individual to protect the injured area.

Vasodilation and the increase in capillary permeability in an injured tissue also enable enzymes of the blood-clotting system to enter the tissue. These enzymes activate an enzyme cascade that results in the deposition of insoluble strands of **fibrin,** which is the main component of a blood clot. The fibrin strands wall off the injured area from the rest of the body and serve to prevent the spread of infection.

Once the inflammatory response has subsided and most of the debris has been cleared away by phagocytic cells, tissue repair and regeneration of new tissue begin. Capillaries grow into the fibrin of a blood clot. New connective tissue cells, called fibroblasts, replace the fibrin as the clot dissolves. As fibroblasts and capillaries accumulate, scar tissue forms. The inflammatory response is described in more detail in Chapter 15.

Collaboration Between Innate and Adaptive Immunity

Innate and adaptive immunity do not operate in total independence of each other. They cooperate in important ways to produce more effective immunity. For example, the encounter between macrophages and microbes can generate "danger" or "warning" signals that stimulate and direct adaptive immune responses. Such encounters can increase the ability of macrophages to display antigen for recognition by antigen-specific T cells. This facilitates the participation of the adaptive immune system in the elimination of the pathogen. As well as displaying antigen in a manner that allows it to be recognized by T cells, macrophages stimulated by encounters with microbes also secrete immunoregulatory hormone-like molecules, called cytokines. The particular cytokines produced direct adaptive immune responses that combat particular intracellular pathogens. These and other signals generated by innate immunity play important roles in triggering lymphocyte responses.

Just as important, the adaptive immune system produces signals and components that stimulate and increase the effectiveness of innate responses. When they encounter appropriately presented antigen, some T cells synthesize and secrete cytokines that increase the ability of macrophages to kill the microbes they have ingested. The production of antibodies against an invading pathogen also has important effects on the recruitment of the complement system to the defense of the host. By binding to the pathogen, antibodies mark it as a target for attack by complement, and the complex of antibody and pathogen is also a potent activator of this attack. Thus, these two systems, nonspecific and specific immunity, form an interactive and mutually supportive network that erects an effective and formidable barrier to infection.

Adaptive (Specific) Immunity

Adaptive, or specific, immunity is capable of recognizing and selectively eliminating specific foreign microorganisms and molecules (i.e., foreign antigens). Unlike innate immune responses, adaptive immune responses are reactions to specific antigenic challenges and display four characteristic attributes:

- Antigenic specificity
- Diversity
- Immunologic memory
- Self/nonself recognition

The **antigenic specificity** of the immune system permits it to distinguish subtle differences among antigens. Antibodies can distinguish between two protein molecules that differ in only a single amino acid. The immune system is capable of generating tremendous *diversity* in its recognition molecules, allowing it to recognize billions of uniquely different structures on foreign antigens. Once the immune system has recognized and responded to an antigen, it exhibits *immunologic memory*; that is, a second encounter with the same antigen induces a heightened state of immune reactivity. Because of this attribute, the immune system can confer lifelong immunity to many infectious agents after an initial encounter. Finally, the immune system normally responds only to foreign antigens, indicating that it is capable of *self/nonself recognition.* The ability of the immune system to distinguish self from nonself and respond only to nonself-molecules is essential, for, as described below, the outcome of an inappropriate response to self-molecules can be fatal.

As noted already, adaptive immunity is not independent of innate immunity. The phagocytic cells crucial to nonspecific immune responses are intimately involved in activating the specific immune response. Conversely, various soluble factors produced by a specific immune response have been shown to augment the activity of these phagocytic cells. As an inflammatory response develops, for example, soluble mediators are produced that attract cells of the immune system. The immune response will, in turn, serve to regulate the intensity of the inflammatory response. Through the carefully regulated interplay of adaptive and innate immunity, the two systems work together to eliminate a foreign invader.

Cells of the Immune System

An effective immune response involves two major groups of cells: *lymphocytes* and *antigen-presenting cells.* Lymphocytes are one of many types of white blood cells produced in the bone marrow by the process of hematopoiesis (see Chapter 2). Lymphocytes leave the bone marrow, circulate in the blood and lymphatic systems, and reside in various lymphoid organs. Because they produce and display antigen-binding cell-surface receptors, lymphocytes mediate the defining immunologic attributes of specificity, diversity, memory, and self/nonself recognition. The two major populations of lymphocytes—**B lymphocytes (B cells)** and **T lymphocytes (T cells)**—are described briefly here and in greater detail in later chapters.

B Lymphocytes

B lymphocytes mature within the bone marrow; when they leave it, each expresses a unique antigen-binding receptor on its membrane (Figure 1-5a). The B-cell receptor is a membrane-bound **antibody molecule.** Antibodies are glycoproteins. An antibody molecule consists of two identical heavy polypeptide chains and two identical light polypeptide chains. One of each are held together in a pair by disulfide bonds, which also hold the two pairs together. The amino-terminal ends of the pairs of heavy and light chains form a Y-shaped cleft within which antigen binds. When a naive B cell, which has not previously encountered antigen, first encounters the antigen that matches its membrane-bound antibody, the binding of the antigen to the antibody causes the cell to divide rapidly; its progeny differentiate into **memory B cells** and **effector B cells** called **plasma cells.**

Memory B cells have a longer life span than naive cells; they continue to express the same membrane-bound antibody as their parent naive B cell. Plasma cells do not express membrane-bound antibody; instead they produce the antibody in a form that can be secreted. Although plasma cells live for only a few days, they secrete enormous amounts of antibody during this time. It has been estimated that a single plasma cell can secrete more than 2000 molecules of antibody per second. Secreted antibodies are the major effector molecules of humoral immunity.

T Lymphocytes

T lymphocytes also arise in the bone marrow. Unlike B cells, which mature within the bone marrow, T cells migrate to the thymus gland to mature. During its maturation within the thymus, the T cell comes to express a unique antigen-binding molecule, called the **T-cell receptor,** on its membrane. Unlike membrane-bound antibodies on B cells, which can recognize antigen alone, T-cell receptors can recognize

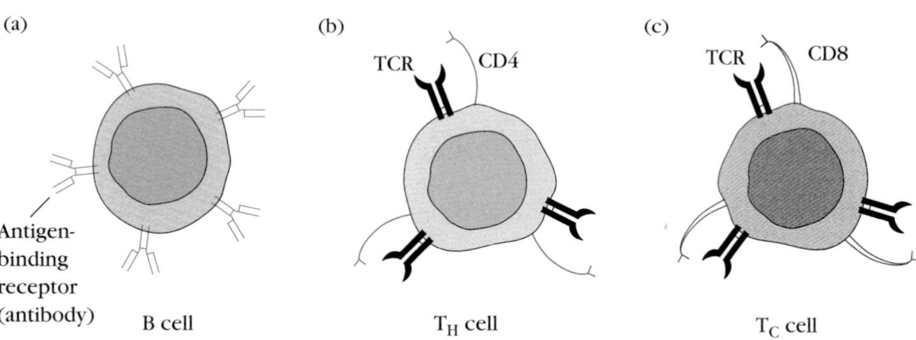

FIGURE 1-5 Distinctive membrane molecules on lymphocytes. (a) B cells have about 10^5 molecules of membrane-bound antibody per cell. All the antibody molecules on a given B cell have the same antigenic specificity and can interact directly with antigen. (b) T cells bearing CD4 ($CD4^+$ cells) recognize only antigen bound to class II MHC molecules. (c) T cells bearing CD8 ($CD8^+$ cells) recognize only antigen associated with class I MHC molecules. In general, $CD4^+$ T cells act as helper cells and $CD8^+$ cells act as cytotoxic cells. Both types of T cells express about 10^5 identical molecules of the antigen-binding T-cell receptor (TCR) per cell, all with the same antigenic specificity.

only antigen that is bound to cell-membrane proteins called **major histocompatibility complex (MHC) molecules.** MHC molecules that function in this recognition event, which is termed "antigen presentation," are polymorphic (genetically diverse) glycoproteins found on cell membranes (see Chapter 7). There are two major types of MHC molecules: Class I MHC molecules, which are expressed by nearly all nucleated cells, consist of a heavy chain linked to a small invariant protein called β_2-microglobulin. Class II MHC molecules, which consist of an α and a β glycoprotein chain, are expressed only by antigen-presenting cells. When a naive T cell encounters antigen combined with an MHC molecule on a cell, the T cell proliferates and differentiates into memory T cells and various effector T cells.

There are two well-defined subpopulations of T cells: **T helper (T_H) and T cytotoxic (T_C) cells.** Although a third type of T cell, called a T suppressor (T_S) cell, has been postulated, recent evidence suggests that it may not be distinct from the T_H and T_C subpopulations. T helper and T cytotoxic cells can be distinguished from one another by the presence of either **CD4** or **CD8** membrane glycoproteins on their surfaces (Figure 1-5b,c). T cells displaying CD4 generally function as T_H cells, whereas those displaying CD8 generally function as T_C cells (see Chapter 2).

After a T_H cell recognizes and interacts with an antigen–MHC class II molecule complex, the cell is activated—it becomes an effector cell that secretes various growth factors known collectively as **cytokines.** The secreted cytokines play an important role in activating B cells, T_C cells, macrophages, and various other cells that participate in the immune response. Differences in the pattern of cytokines produced by activated T_H cells result in different types of immune response.

Under the influence of T_H-derived cytokines, a T_C cell that recognizes an antigen–MHC class I molecule complex proliferates and differentiates into an effector cell called a **cytotoxic T lymphocyte (CTL).** In contrast to the T_H cell, the CTL generally does not secrete many cytokines and instead exhibits cytotoxic activity. The CTL has a vital function in monitoring the cells of the body and eliminating any, such as virus-infected cells, tumor cells, and cells of a foreign tissue graft, that display antigen. Cells that display foreign antigen complexed with a class I MHC molecule are called *altered self-cells.*

Antigen-Presenting Cells

Activation of both the humoral and cell-mediated branches of the immune system requires cytokines produced by T_H cells. It is essential that activation of T_H cells themselves be carefully regulated, because an inappropriate T_H-cell response to self-components can have fatal autoimmune consequences. To ensure carefully regulated activation of T_H cells, they can recognize only antigen that is displayed together with class MHC II molecules on the surface of antigen-presenting cells (APCs). These specialized cells, which include macrophages, B lymphocytes, and dendritic cells, are distinguished by two properties: (1) they express class II MHC molecules on their membranes, and (2) they are able to deliver a co-stimulatory signal that is necessary for T_H-cell activation.

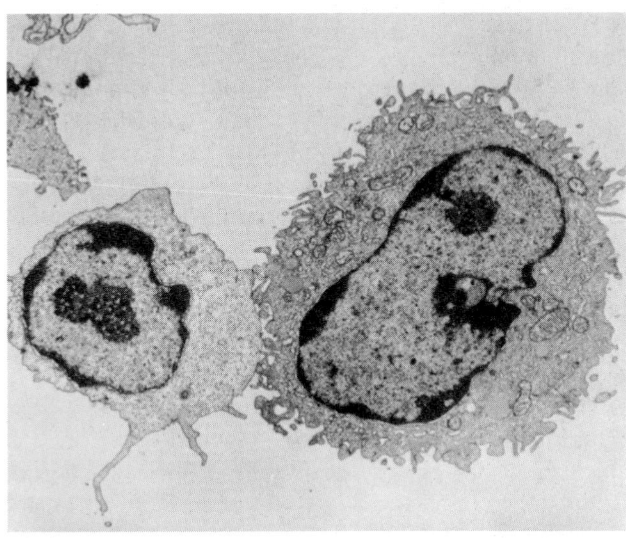

FIGURE 1-6 Electron micrograph of an antigen-presenting macrophage (*right*) associating with a T lymphocyte. [From AS Rosenthal et al, 1982, in *Phagocytosis—Past and Future,* Academic Press, p. 239.]

Antigen-presenting cells first internalize antigen, either by phagocytosis or by endocytosis, and then display a part of that antigen, bound to a class II MHC molecule, on their membrane. The T_H cell recognizes and interacts with the antigen–class II MHC molecule complex on the membrane of the antigen-presenting cell (Figure 1-6). An additional co-stimulatory signal is then produced by the antigen-presenting cell, leading to activation of the T_H cell.

Functions of Humoral and Cell-Mediated Immune Responses

As mentioned above, immune responses can be divided into humoral and cell-mediated responses. Humoral immunity refers to immunity that can be conferred upon a nonimmune individual by administration of serum antibodies from an immune individual. In contrast, cell-mediated immunity can be transferred only by administration of T cells from an immune individual.

The humoral branch of the immune system is at work in the interaction of B cells with antigen and their subsequent proliferation and differentiation into antibody-secreting plasma cells (Figure 1-7). Antibody functions as the effector of the humoral response by binding to antigen and neutralizing it or facilitating its elimination. When an antigen is coated with antibody, it can be eliminated in several ways. For example, antibody can cross-link several antigens, forming clusters that are more readily ingested by phagocytic cells

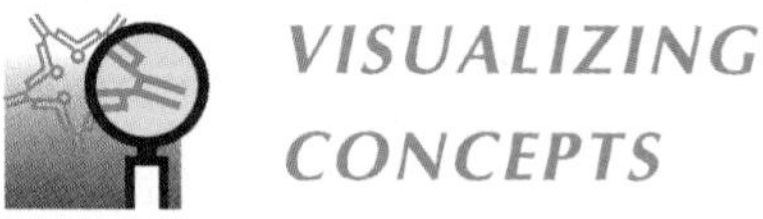

Antigens

Foreign proteins
Viruses
Bacteria
Parasites
Fungi

Vertebrate body

HUMORAL RESPONSE
B cell
+
Antigen
+ T_H-cell cytokines
Ab-secreting plasma cells
Antigen elimination

CELL-MEDIATED RESPONSE
T cell
T_H cell
T_C cell
+ Ag–class II MHC molecule
+ Ag–class I MHC molecule
Activated T_H cell
Cytokine secretion
CTL
Killing of altered self-cells
Altered self-cell

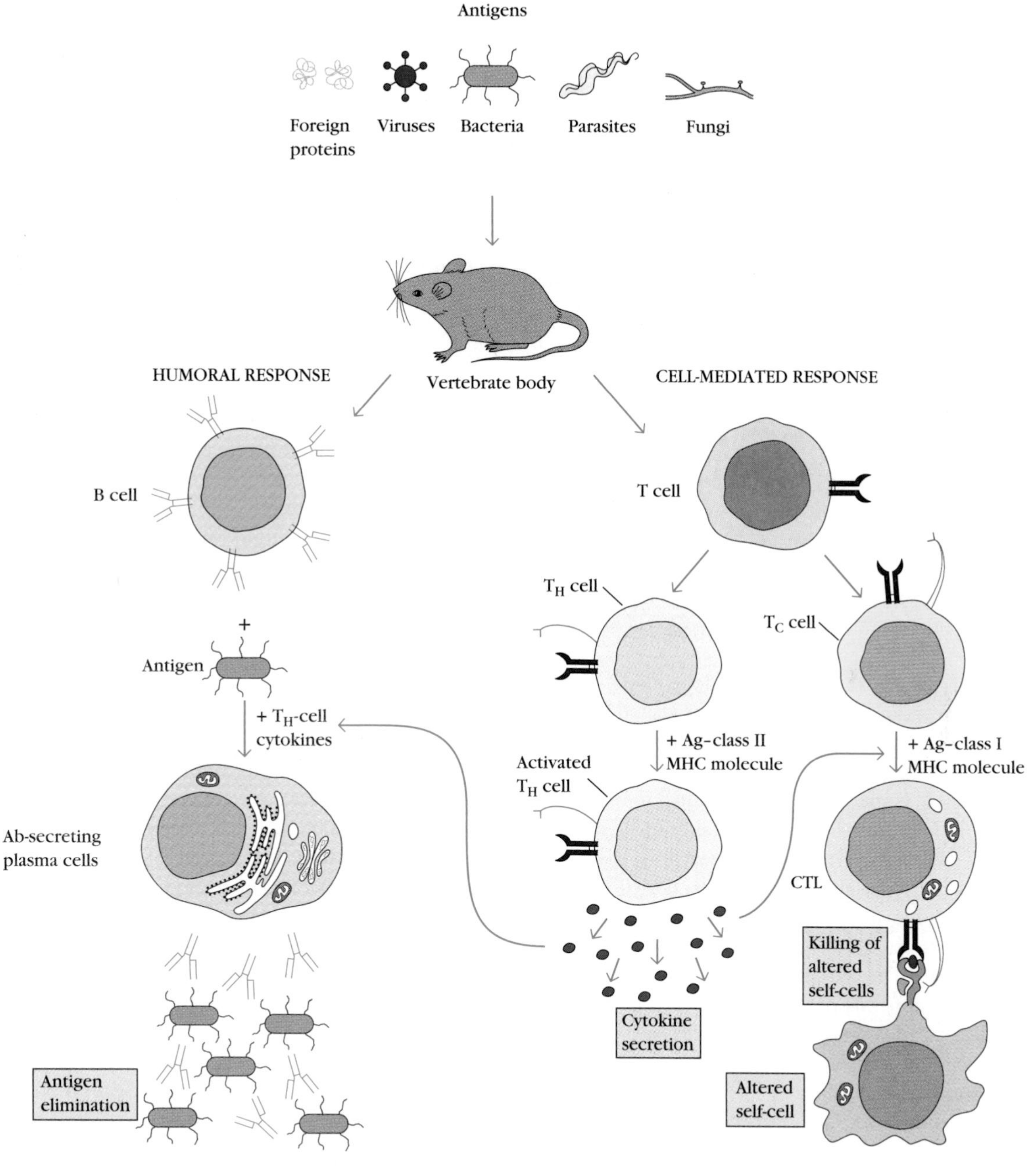

FIGURE 1-7 Overview of the humoral and cell-mediated branches of the immune system. In the humoral response, B cells interact with antigen (Ag) and then differentiate into antibody-secreting plasma cells. The secreted antibody (Ab) binds to the antigen and facilitates its clearance from the body. In the cell-mediated response, various subpopulations of T cells recognize antigen presented on self-cells. T_H cells respond to antigen by producing cytokines. T_C cells respond to antigen by developing into cytotoxic T lymphocytes (CTLs), which mediate killing of altered self-cells (e.g., virus-infected cells).

than a single one. Binding of antibody to antigen on a microorganism also can activate the complement system, resulting in lysis of the foreign organism. Antibody can also neutralize toxins or viral particles by coating them; this prevents them from binding to host cells.

Effector T cells generated in response to antigen are responsible for cell-mediated immunity (see Figure 1-7). Both activated T_H cells and CTLs serve as effector cells in cell-mediated immune reactions. Cytokines secreted by T_H cells can activate various phagocytic cells, enabling them to phagocytose and kill microorganisms more effectively. This type of cell-mediated immune response is especially important also in ridding the host of bacteria and protozoa contained by infected host cells. Cytotoxic T lymphocytes (CTLs) participate in cell-mediated immune reactions by killing altered self-cells; they play an important role in the killing of virus-infected cells and tumor cells.

Recognition of Antigen by B and T Lymphocytes

Antigens, which are generally very large and complex, are not recognized in their entirety by lymphocytes. Instead, both B and T lymphocytes recognize discrete sites on the antigen called **antigenic determinants,** or **epitopes.** Epitopes are the immunologically active regions on a complex antigen, the regions that actually bind to B-cell or T-cell receptors.

Although B cells can recognize an epitope alone, T cells can recognize an epitope only when it is associated with an MHC molecule on the surface of a self-cell (either an antigen-presenting cell or an altered self-cell). Each branch of the immune system is therefore uniquely suited to recognize antigen in a different milieu. The humoral branch (B cells) recognizes an enormous variety of epitopes: those displayed on the surfaces of bacteria or viral particles, as well as those displayed on soluble proteins, glycoproteins, polysaccharides, or lipopolysaccharides that have been released from invading pathogens. The cell-mediated branch (T cells) recognizes protein epitopes displayed together with MHC molecules on self-cells, including altered self-cells such as virus-infected self-cells and cancerous cells.

Thus, four related but distinct cell-membrane molecules are responsible for antigen recognition by the immune system:

- Membrane-bound antibodies on B cells
- T-cell receptors
- Class I MHC molecules
- Class II MHC molecules

Each of these molecules plays a unique role in antigen recognition, ensuring that the immune system can recognize and respond to the different types of antigen that it encounters.

Generation of Lymphocyte Specificity and Diversity

The antigenic specificity of each B cell is determined by the membrane-bound antigen-binding receptor (i.e., antibody) expressed by the cell. The antibody on a B cell can recognize epitopes on macromolecules with incredible precision. For example, protein antigens that differ by only a single amino acid often can be distinguished from each other. As a B cell matures in the bone marrow, its specificity is created by random rearrangements of a series of gene segments that encode the antibody molecule (see Chapter 5). As a result of this process, each mature B cell possesses a single functional gene encoding the antibody heavy chain and a single functional gene encoding the antibody light chain; the cell therefore synthesizes and displays antibody with one specificity on its membrane. All 10^5 antibody molecules on a given B lymphocyte have identical specificity, giving each B lymphocyte, and the clone of daughter cells to which it gives rise, a distinct specificity for a single epitope on an antigen. The mature B lymphocyte is therefore said to be **antigenically committed.**

The fine specificity of the antibody molecule is coupled to an enormous diversity. The random gene rearrangements during B-cell maturation in the bone marrow generate an enormous number of different antigenic specificities. The resulting B-cell population, which consists of individual B cells each expressing a unique antibody, is estimated to exhibit collectively more than 10^8 different antigenic specificities. This enormous diversity in the mature B-cell population is later reduced by a selection process in the bone marrow that eliminates any B cells whose membrane-bound antibody recognizes self-components. This process helps to ensure that self-reactive antibodies (auto-antibodies) are not produced.

The attributes of specificity and diversity also characterize the antigen-binding T-cell receptor (TCR) on T cells. As in B-cell maturation, the process of T-cell maturation includes random rearrangements of a series of gene segments that encode the cell's antigen-binding receptor (see Chapter 9). Each T lymphocyte cell expresses about 10^5 receptors, and all 10^5 receptors on a cell and its clonal progeny have identical specificity for antigen. The random rearrangement of the TCR genes is capable of generating on the order of 10^9 unique antigenic specificities. This enormous potential diversity is later diminished through a selection process in the thymus that eliminates any T cell with self-reactive receptors and ensures that only T cells with receptors capable of recognizing antigen associated with MHC molecules will be able to mature (see Chapter 10).

Role of the Major Histocompatibility Complex

The major histocompatibility complex (MHC) is a large genetic complex with multiple loci. The MHC loci encode two major classes of membrane-bound glycoproteins: **class I** and

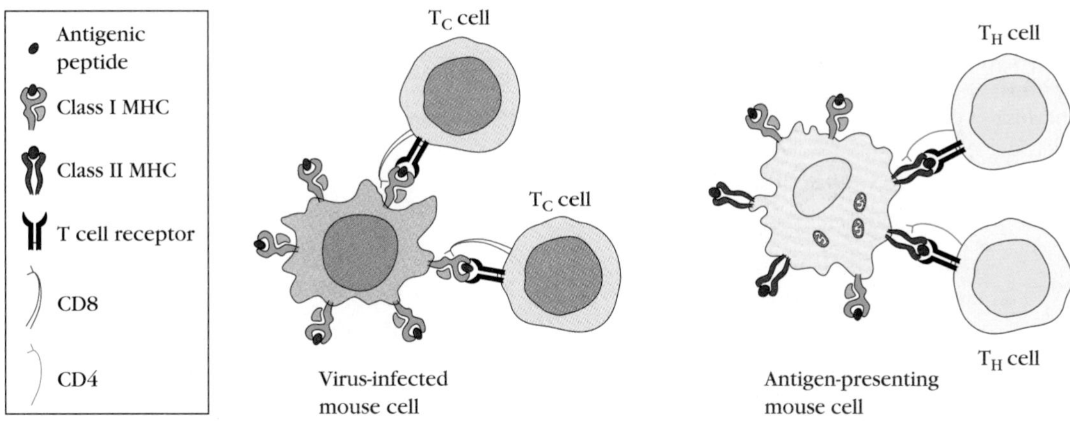

FIGURE 1-8 The role of MHC molecules in antigen recognition by T cells. Class I MHC molecules are expressed on nearly all nucleated cells. Class II MHC are expressed only on antigen-presenting cells. $CD4^+$ T cells recognize only antigenic peptides displayed with a class II MHC molecule; they generally function as T helper (T_H) cells. $CD8^+$ T cells only recognize antigenic peptides displayed with a class I MHC molecule; they generally function as T cytotoxic (T_C) cells.

class II MHC molecules. As noted above, T_H cells generally recognize antigen combined with class II molecules, whereas T_C cells generally recognize antigen combined with class I molecules (Figure 1-8).

Class I MHC molecules associate on the cell membrane with a small protein called β_2-microglobulin. There are three class I genetic loci in humans (*A, B,* and *C*) and two in mice (*K* and *D*). Class II MHC molecules are heterodimeric glycoproteins, consisting of an alpha and a beta chain. There are three class II genetic loci in humans (*DR, DP,* and *DQ*) and two in mice (*IA* and *IE*). Each class II locus encompasses an alpha gene and a beta gene, which respectively encode the alpha and beta chains of the class II MHC molecule. Both class I and class II MHC genes are highly polymorphic; that is, within a species each gene exists in many different forms, called **alleles.** Because an individual inherits one allele from each parent for each locus, multiple class I MHC molecules are expressed on each nucleated cell in the body; in addition, multiple class II molecules are expressed on antigen-presenting cells.

MHC molecules also function as antigen-recognition molecules, but they do not possess the fine specificity for antigen characteristic of antibodies and T-cell receptors. Rather, each MHC molecule can bind to a spectrum of **antigenic peptides** derived from the intracellular degradation of antigen molecules. In both class I and class II MHC molecules the distal regions (farthest from the membrane) of different alleles display wide variation in their amino acid sequences. These distal regions form a cleft within which the antigenic peptide sits and is presented to T lymphocytes (see Figure 1-8). Different allelic forms of the genes encoding class I and class II molecules confer different structures on the antigen-binding cleft with different specificity. Thus the ability to present an antigen to T lymphocytes is influenced by the particular set of alleles that an individual inherits.

Processing and Presentation of Antigens

In order for a foreign protein antigen to be recognized by a T cell, it must be degraded into small antigenic peptides that form complexes with class I or class II MHC molecules. This conversion of proteins into MHC-associated peptide fragments is called antigen processing and presentation. Whether a particular antigen will be processed and presented together with class I MHC or class II MHC molecules appears to be determined by the route that the antigen takes to enter a cell (Figure 1-9).

Exogenous antigen is produced outside of the host cell and enters the cell by endocytosis or phagocytosis. Antigen-presenting cells (macrophages, dendritic cells, and B cells) degrade ingested exogenous antigen into peptide fragments within the endocytic processing pathway. Experiments suggest that class II MHC molecules are expressed within the endocytic processing pathway and that peptides produced by degradation of antigen in this pathway bind to the cleft within the class II MHC molecules. The MHC molecules bearing the peptide then are exported to the cell surface. Since expression of class II MHC molecules is limited to antigen-presenting cells, presentation of exogenous peptide–class II MHC complexes is limited to these cells. T cells displaying CD4 recognize antigen combined with class II MHC molecules and thus are said to be class II MHC restricted. These cells generally function as T helper cells.

Endogenous antigen is produced within the host cell itself. Two common examples are viral proteins synthesized within virus-infected host cells and unique proteins synthesized by cancerous cells. Endogenous antigens are thought

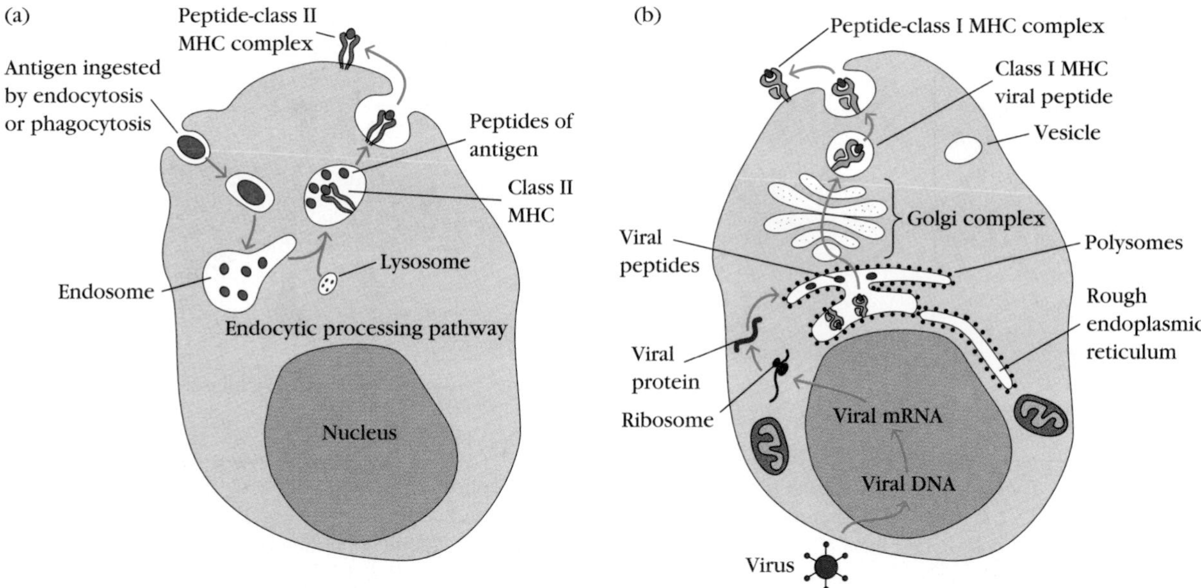

FIGURE 1-9 Processing and presentation of exogenous and endogenous antigens. (a) Exogenous antigen is ingested by endocytosis or phagocytosis and then enters the endocytic processing pathway. Here, within an acidic environment, the antigen is degraded into small peptides, which then are presented with class II MHC molecules on the membrane of the antigen-presenting cell. (b) Endogenous antigen, which is produced within the cell itself (e.g., in a virus-infected cell), is degraded within the cytoplasm into peptides, which move into the endoplasmic reticulum, where they bind to class I MHC molecules. The peptide–class I MHC complexes then move through the Golgi complex to the cell surface.

to be degraded into peptide fragments that bind to class I MHC molecules within the endoplasmic reticulum. The peptide–class I MHC complex is then transported to the cell membrane. Since all nucleated cells express class I MHC molecules, all cells producing endogenous antigen use this route to process the antigen. T cells displaying CD8 recognize antigen associated with class I MHC molecules and thus are said to be class I MHC restricted. These T cytotoxic cells attack and kill cells displaying the antigen–MHC class I complexes for which their receptors are specific.

Clonal Selection of Lymphocytes

A mature immunocompetent animal contains a large number of antigen-reactive clones of T and B lymphocytes; the antigenic specificity of each of these clones is determined by the specificity of the antigen-binding receptor on the membrane of the clone's lymphocytes. As noted above, the specificity of each T and B lymphocyte is determined before its contact with antigen by random gene rearrangements during maturation in the bone marrow or thymus.

The role of antigen becomes critical when it interacts with and activates mature, antigenically committed T and B lymphocytes, bringing about expansion of the population of cells with a given antigenic specificity. In this process of **clonal selection,** an antigen binds to a particular T or B cell and stimulates it to divide repeatedly into a clone of cells with the same antigenic specificity as the original parent cell (Figure 1-10).

Clonal selection provides a framework for understanding the specificity and self/nonself recognition characteristic of adaptive immunity. Specificity is shown because only lymphocytes whose receptors are specific for a given epitope on an antigen will be clonally expanded and thus mobilized for an immune response. Self/nonself discrimination is accomplished by the elimination, during development, of lymphocytes bearing self-reactive receptors or by the functional suppression of these cells in adults.

Immunologic memory also is a consequence of clonal selection. During clonal selection, the number of lymphocytes specific for a given antigen is greatly amplified. Moreover, many of these lymphocytes, referred to as memory cells, appear to have a longer life span than the naive lymphocytes from which they arise. The initial encounter of a naive immunocompetent lymphocyte with an antigen induces a **primary response**; a later contact of the host with antigen will induce a more rapid and heightened **secondary response.** The amplified population of memory cells accounts for the rapidity and intensity that distinguishes a secondary response from the primary response.

In the humoral branch of the immune system, antigen induces the clonal proliferation of B lymphocytes into antibody-secreting plasma cells and memory B cells. As seen in Figure 1-11a, the primary response has a lag of approximately 5–7 days before antibody levels start to rise. This lag is the time required for activation of naive B cells by antigen and T_H cells and for the subsequent proliferation and

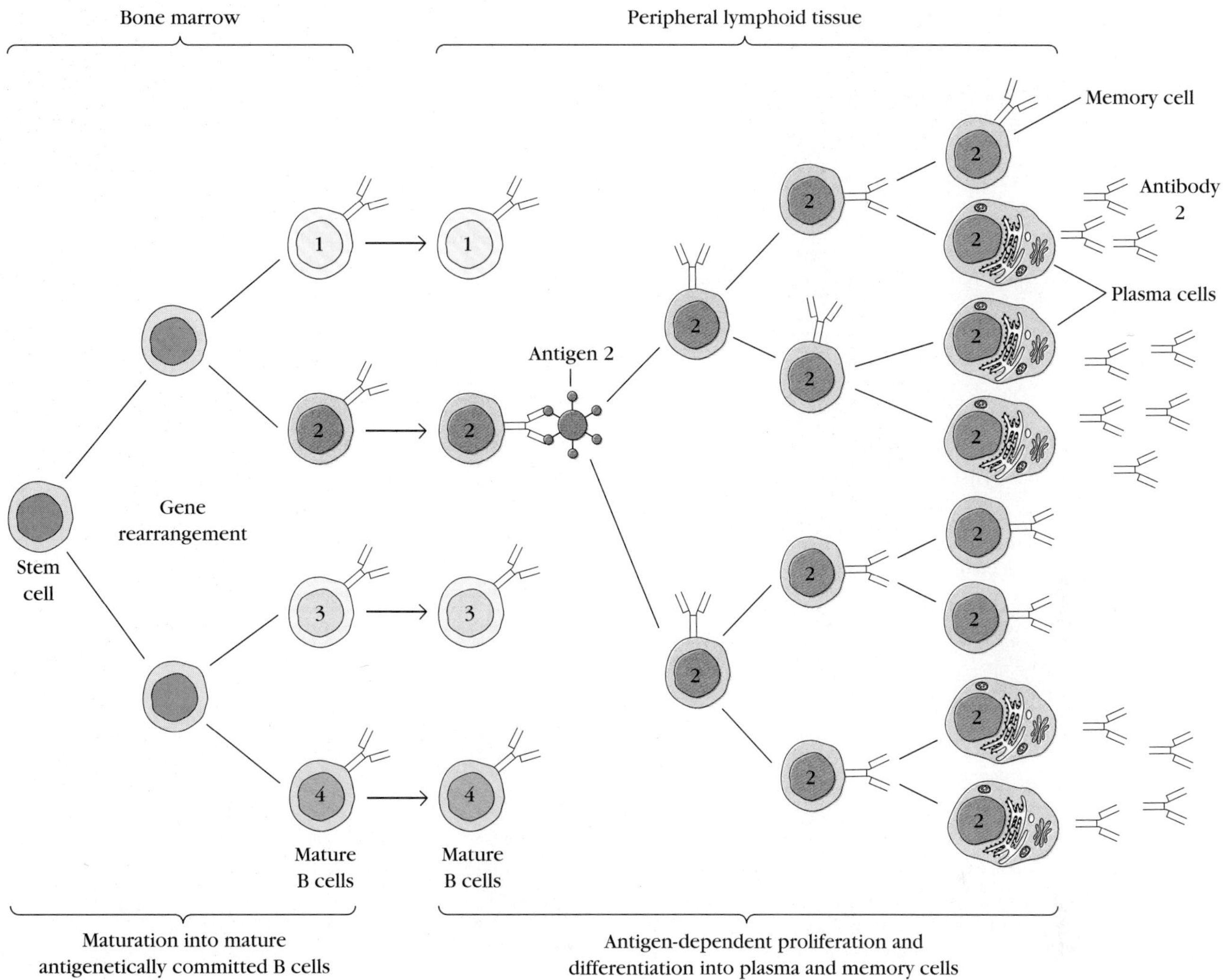

FIGURE 1-10 Maturation and clonal selection of B lymphocytes. Maturation, which occurs in the absence of antigen, produces antigenically committed B cells, each of which expresses antibody with a single antigenic specificity (indicated by 1, 2, 3, and 4). Clonal selection occurs when an antigen binds to a B cell whose membrane-bound antibody molecules are specific for epitopes on that antigen. Clonal expansion of an antigen-activated B cell (number 2 in this example) leads to a clone of memory B cells and effector B cells, called plasma cells; all cells in the expanded clone are specific for the original antigen. The plasma cells secrete antibody reactive with the activating antigen. Similar processes take place in the T-lymphocyte population, resulting in clones of memory T cells and effector T cells; the latter include activated T_H cells, which secrete cytokines, and cytotoxic T lymphocytes (CTLs).

differentiation of the activated B cells into plasma cells. Antibody levels peak in the primary response at about day 14 and then begin to drop off as the plasma cells begin to die. In the secondary response, the lag is much shorter (only 1–2 days), antibody levels are much higher, and they are sustained for much longer. The secondary response reflects the activity of the clonally expanded population of memory B cells. These memory cells respond to the antigen more rapidly than naive B cells; in addition, because there are many more memory cells than there were naive B cells for the primary response, more plasma cells are generated in the secondary response, and antibody levels are consequently 100-fold to 1000-fold higher.

In the cell-mediated branch, the recognition of an antigen-MHC complex by a specific mature T lymphocyte induces clonal proliferation into various T cells with effector functions (T_H cells and CTLs) and into memory T cells. The cell-mediated response to a skin graft is depicted in Figure 1-11b. When skin from strain C mice is grafted onto strain A mice, a primary response develops and all the grafts are rejected in about 10–14 days. If strain C skin is grafted a second time onto the same mice, it is rejected much more vigorously and

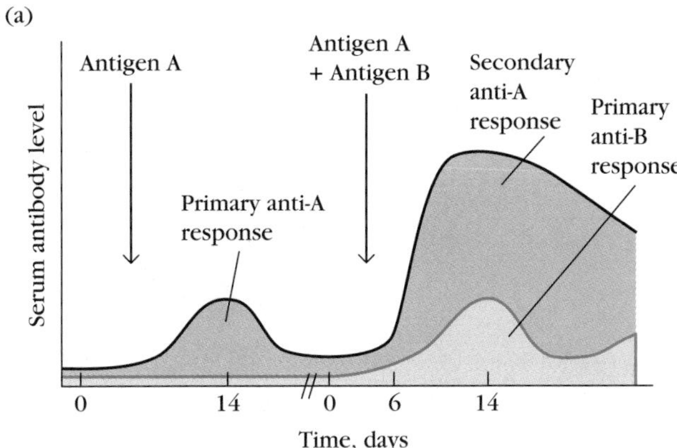

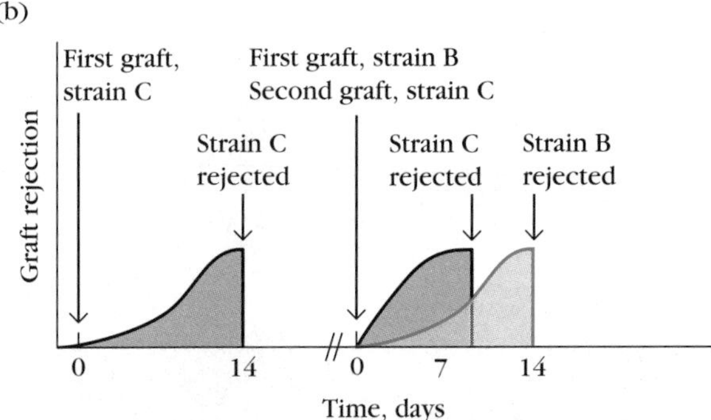

FIGURE 1-11 Differences in the primary and secondary response to injected antigen (humoral response) and to a skin graft (cell-mediated response) reflect the phenomenon of immunologic memory. (a) When an animal is injected with an antigen, it produces a primary serum antibody response of low magnitude and short duration, peaking at about 10–17 days. A second immunization with the same antigen results in a secondary response that is greater in magnitude, peaks in less time (2–7 days), and lasts longer (months to years) than the primary response. Compare the secondary response to antigen A with the primary response to antigen B administered to the same mice. (b) When skin grafts from strain C mice are transplanted to strain A mice, the grafts are rejected in about 10–14 days. If strain C grafts are grafted onto mice previously exposed to strain C skin, the grafts are rejected much more vigorously and rapidly than the first grafts were; compare the rejection of the second strain C graft to the rejection of the first strain B graft.

rapidly than the first grafts. If the animals previously engrafted with strain C skin are next given skin from an unrelated strain, strain B, the response to strain B is a typical of the primary response and is rejected in 10–14 days. That is, graft rejection is a specific immune response. The same mice that showed a secondary response to graft C will show a primary response to graft B. The increased speed of rejection of graft C reflects the presence of a clonally expanded population of memory T_H and T_C cells specific for the antigens of the foreign graft. This expanded memory population generates more effector cells, resulting in faster graft rejection.

Cellular Interactions Required for Generation of Immune Responses

Both the humoral and the cell-mediated branches of the immune system require interaction among several different types of cells to induce a specific immunologic response. These cells include various antigen-presenting cells, T_H cells, and either B cells, for induction of humoral immunity, or T_C cells, for induction of cell-mediated immunity.

Activation and Proliferation of T Helper Cells

The generation of both humoral and cell-mediated immune responses depends on the activation of T_H cells. This process begins when antigen-binding receptors on T_H cells link to antigenic peptide–class II MHC complexes on antigen-presenting cells (Figure 1-12). This interaction generates a signal that, together with a necessary co-stimulatory signal, leads to activation and proliferation of the T_H cells (Figure 1-13a).

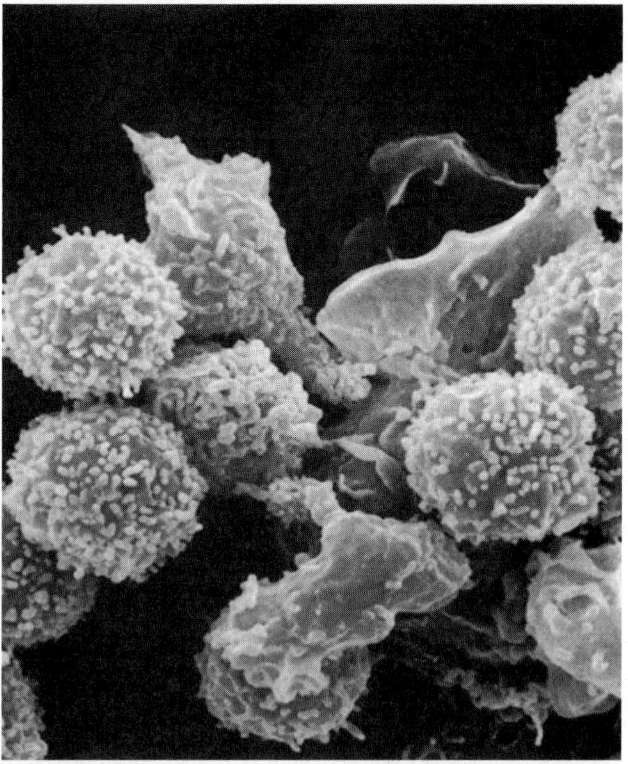

FIGURE 1-12 This scanning electron micrograph reveals numerous T lymphocytes interacting with a single macrophage. The macrophage presents processed antigen combined with class II MHC molecules to the T cells. [From WE Paul (ed.), 1991, *Immunology: Recognition and Response,* W. H. Freeman and Company, New York; courtesy of MH Nielsen and O Werdelin.]

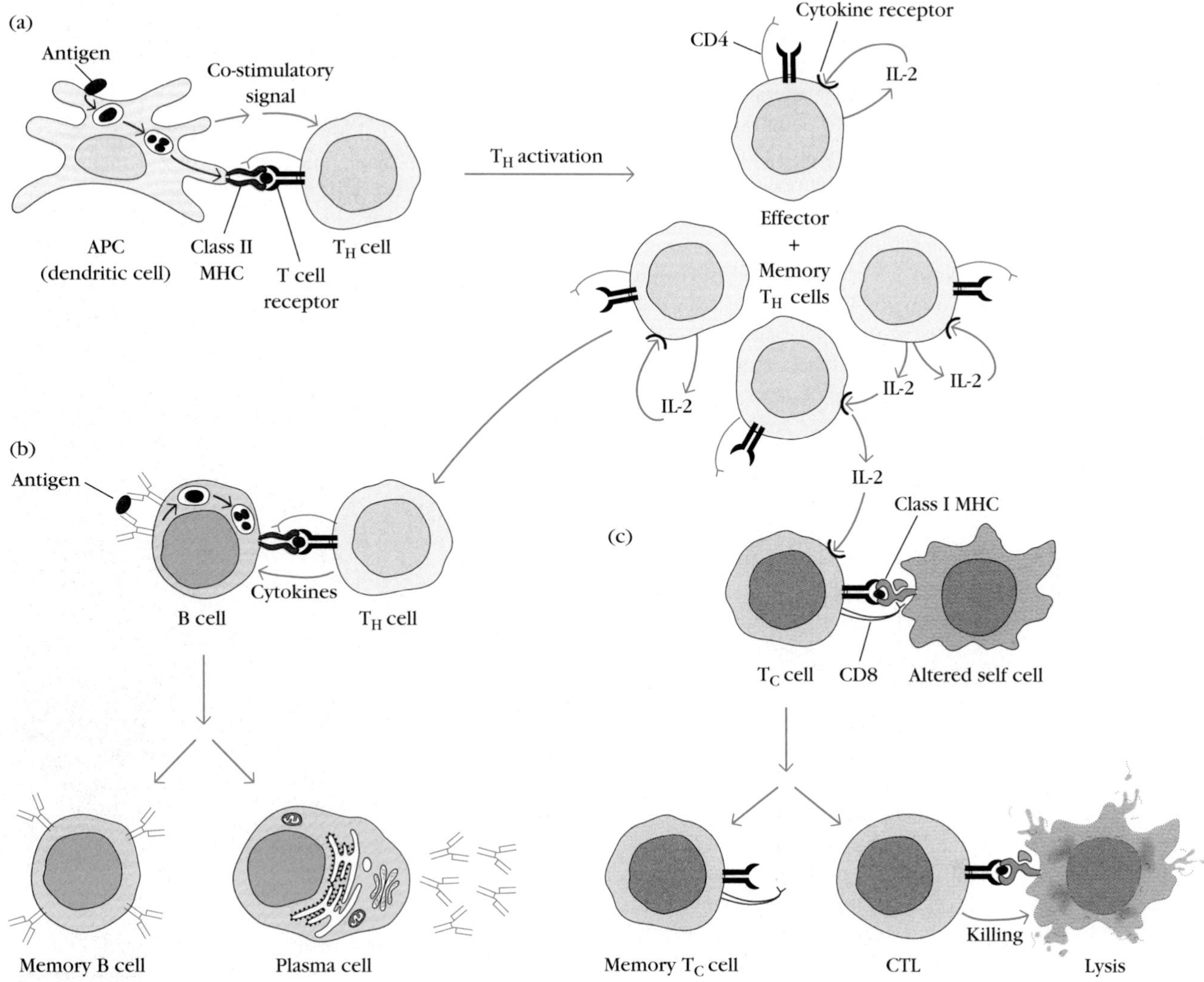

FIGURE 1-13 Cellular interactions involved in induction of immune responses. Activation (APC = antigen-presenting cell) and proliferation of T_H cells (a) is required for generation of a humoral response (b) and a cell-mediated response to altered self-cells (c).

The clonally expanded population of antigen-specific T_H cells can now play a role in the activation of the B and T lymphocytes that generate the humoral and cell-mediated responses, respectively.

Generation of the Humoral Immune Response

Mature antigen-committed B lymphocytes are seeded out from the bone marrow to circulate in the blood or lymph or to reside in various lymphoid organs. Interaction of a mature B cell with antigen triggers its activation, proliferation, and differentiation. This process begins when antigen cross-links membrane-bound antibody molecules on a B cell. Some of the bound antigen is internalized by receptor-mediated endocytosis. After processing the antigen, the B cell presents the resulting antigenic peptides, combined with class II MHC molecules, on its membrane. A T_H cell specific for the presented antigen-MHC complex then binds to the complex; as a result of this interaction, the T_H cell secretes cytokines that stimulate various stages of B-cell division and differentiation. The activated B cell undergoes a series of cell divisions over about 5 days, differentiating into a population of both antibody-secreting plasma cells and memory cells (Figure 1-13b).

Generation of the Cell-Mediated Response

The cell-mediated response is generated by various subpopulations of T lymphocytes. As in the humoral response, a clonally expanded population of antigen-specific activated T_H cells is required. Cytokines secreted by these T_H cells help to activate various T effector cells responsible for cell-mediated responses. For example, after a T_C cell binds to processed antigen combined with class I MHC molecules on the membrane of an altered self-cell, the cytokine interleukin 2 (IL-2), secreted by T_H cells, stimulates proliferation and differentiation of the T_C cell. This process generates cytotoxic T lymphocytes (CTLs), which mediate membrane damage to the altered self-cell, causing cell lysis; it also generates populations of memory T_H and T_C cells (Figure 1-13c).

The cytokines secreted by activated T_H cells also regulate the proliferation and differentiation of a number of nonspecific effector cells that play various roles in cell-mediated immune responses. These nonspecific effector cells do not possess the immunologic attributes of specificity and memory; instead, their activity is regulated by cytokines secreted by antigen-specific T_H cells. Among the nonspecific effector cells in the cell-mediated immune response are natural killer (NK) cells and activated macrophages. These are described in Chapter 2, and their role in cell-mediated immunity is covered in Chapter 14.

Comparative Immunity

The field of immunology is concerned mostly with how innate and adaptive mechanisms collaborate to protect vertebrates from infection. Although many cellular and molecular actors have important roles, antibodies and lymphocytes are the principal players. Despite their prominence in vertebrate immune systems, though, it would be a mistake to conclude that these extraordinary molecules and versatile cells are essential for immunity. In fact, a determined search for antibodies, T cells, and B cells in organisms of many nonvertebrate phyla has failed to find them. The interior spaces of organisms as diverse as fruit flies, cockroaches, and plants do not contain unchecked microbial populations, though, which implies that some sort of immunity exists in most, possibly all, multicellular organisms. Thus the development of some system of immunological defense seems to be an evolutionary imperative of multicellular life. A rich variety of defense mechanisms has arisen, with great variation in the use and importance of particular mechanisms. Although these various mechanisms of immunity differ, in many cases the signal transduction pathways used to invoke immunity are strikingly similar. Some of the key elements of these signaling pathways in vertebrates, insects, and even plants have been found to contain evolutionarily conserved molecules. Considering that plants and vertebrates diverged into separate evolutionary branches at least a billion years ago, this degree of conservation is remarkable.

Insects and plants provide particularly clear and dramatic examples of innate immunity that is not based on lymphocytes. The invasion of the interior body cavity of the fruit fly, *Drosophila melanogaster*, by bacteria or molds triggers the synthesis of small peptides that have strong antibacterial or antifungal activity. The effectiveness of these antimicrobial peptides is demonstrated by the fate of mutants that are unable to produce them. For example, a fungal infection overwhelms a mutant fruit fly that is unable to trigger the synthesis of drosomycin, an antifungal peptide (Figure 1-14).

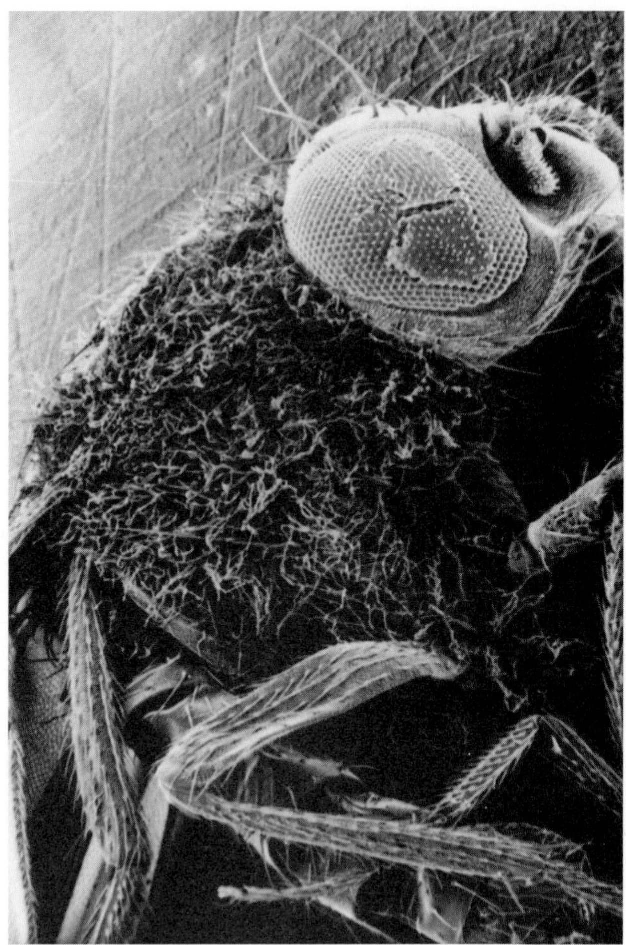

FIGURE 1-14 Severe fungal infection in a fruit fly (*Drosophila melanogaster*) with a disabling mutation in a signal transduction pathway required for the synthesis of the antifungal peptide drosomycin. [From Lemaitre et al, *Cell* **86:**973, 1996; courtesy of JA Hoffman, University of Strasbourg.]

Plants respond to infection by producing a wide variety of antimicrobial proteins and peptides, as well as small nonpeptide organic molecules that have antibiotic activity. Among these agents are enzymes that digest microbial cell walls, peptides and a protein that damage microbial membranes, and the small organic molecules phytoalexins. The importance of the phytoalexins is shown by the fact that mutations that alter their biosynthetic pathways result in loss of resistance to many plant pathogens. In some cases, the response of plants to pathogens goes beyond this chemical assault to include an architectural response, in which the plant walls off cells in the infected area by strengthening the walls of surrounding cells. Table 1-3 compares the capabilities of immune systems in a wide range of multicellular organisms, both animals and plants.

TABLE 1-3 IMMUNITY IN MULTICELLULAR ORGANISMS

Taxonomic group	Innate immunity (nonspecific)	Adaptive immunity (specific)	Invasion-induced protective enzymes and enzyme cascades	Phagocytosis	Antimicrobial peptides	Pattern-recognition receptors	Graft rejection	T and B cells	Antibodies
Higher plants	+	–	+	–	+	+	–	–	–
Invertebrate animals									
Porifera (sponges)	+	–	?	+	?	?	+	–	–
Annelids (earthworms)	+	–	?	+	?	?	+	–	–
Arthropods (insects, crustaceans)	+	–	+	+	+	+	?	–	–
Vertebrate animals									
Elasmobranchs (cartilaginous fish; e.g., sharks, rays)	+	+	+	+	equivalent agents	+	+	+	+
Teleost fish and bony fish (e.g., salmon, tuna)	+	+	+	+	probable	+	+	+	+
Amphibians	+	+	+	+	+	+	+	+	+
Reptiles	+	+	+	+	?	+	+	+	+
Birds	+	+	+	+	?	+	+	+	+
Mammals	+	+	+	+	+	+	+	+	+

KEY: + = definitive demonstration; – = failure to demonstrate thus far; ? = presence or absence remains to be established.

SOURCES: L Du Pasquier, 1993, "Evolution of the immune system," in *Fundamental Immunology,* 3rd ed., WE Paul, ed., Raven, New York. B Fritig, T Heitz, and M Legrand, 1998, "Antimicrobial proteins in induced plant defense," *Curr. Opin. Immunol.* **10:**16. K Soderhall and L Cerenius, 1998, "Role of the prophenoloxidase-activating system in invertebrate immunity," *Curr. Opin. Immunol.* **10:**23.

Immune Dysfunction and Its Consequences

The above overview of innate and specific immunity depicts a multicomponent interactive system that protects the host from infectious diseases and from cancer. This overview would not be complete without mentioning that the immune system can function improperly. Sometimes the immune system fails to protect the host adequately or misdirects its activities to cause discomfort, debilitating disease, or even death. There are several common manifestations of immune dysfunction:

- Allergy and asthma
- Graft rejection and graft-versus-host disease
- Autoimmune disease
- Immunodeficiency

Allergy and asthma are results of inappropriate immune responses, often to common antigens such as plant pollen, food, or animal dander. The possibility that certain substances increased sensitivity rather than protection was recognized in about 1902 by Charles Richet, who attempted to immunize dogs against the toxins of the aquatic organism *Physalia.* He and his colleague Paul Portier observed that dogs exposed to sublethal doses of the toxin reacted almost instantly, and fatally, to subsequent challenge with minute amounts of the toxin. Richet concluded that a successful immunization or vaccination results in *phylaxis,* or protection, and that the opposite result is **anaphylaxis,** in which an initial exposure to antigen can lead to a violent fatal reaction to a subsequent one. Richet received the Nobel Prize in 1913 for his discovery of the anaphylactic response.

Fortunately, most allergic reactions in humans are not rapidly fatal. A specific allergic or anaphylactic response usually involves one immunoglobulin type, called IgE. Binding

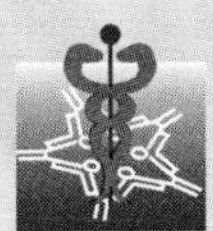

CLINICAL FOCUS
ALLERGY AND ASTHMA AS SERIOUS PUBLIC HEALTH PROBLEMS

Although the immune system serves to protect the host from infectious diseases and from cancer, inappropriate responses of this system can lead to disease. Common among the results of immune dysfunction are allergies and asthma. Together, allergy and asthma make up a serious public health problem. Details of the mechanisms that underly allergic and asthmatic responses to environmental antigens (or allergens) will be considered in Chapter 16. Simply stated, allergic reactions are responses to antigenic stimuli that result in immunity based mainly on the IgE class of immunoglobulin. Exposure to the antigen (or allergen) triggers an IgE-mediated release of chemicals that cause symptoms that range from sneezing and dermatitis to inflammation of the lungs in an asthmatic attack.

The discomfort from common allergies such as plant pollen allergy (often called ragweed allergy) consists of a week or two of sneezing and runny nose, which may seem trivial compared with health problems such as cancer, cardiac arrest, or life-threatening infections. A more serious allergic reaction is asthma, a chronic disease of the lungs in which inflammation, mediated by environmental antigens or infections, causes severe difficulty in breathing. The real importance of asthma and allergy is manifest in the number of visits to the doctor's office, visits to the emergency room, and days spent in the hospital because of these problems. Data on the frequency of care sought for the most common medical complaints in the United States show that asthma and allergy figure prominently.

The single most common reason for a visit to a hospital emergency room is an asthma attack, accounting for one third of all visits. In addition to those treated in the ER, there were about 160,000 hospitalizations for asthma in the past year, with an average stay of 3 to 4 days. Approximately 14.6 million persons in the United States suffer from asthma, and there are about 5000 deaths per year. In the past twenty years, the prevalence of asthma in the Western World has doubled. Although all ages and races are affected, deaths from asthma are 3.5 times more common among African-American children. The reasons for the increases in number of asthma cases and for the higher death rate in African-American children remain unknown, although some clues may have been uncovered by recent studies of genetic factors in allergic disease (see Clinical Focus in Chapter 16).

It is estimated that about one third of all persons in the United States suffer from allergy of some type, and many require treatment. As the data in the table indicate, asthma and allergy together resulted in more than 28 million visits to the doctor in 1995. The data compared in the table include visits by persons of all ages and, as might be expected, common conditions such as respiratory infections, joint and back problems, and heart diseases top the list of reasons for a visit to the doctor. Some perspective on the importance of allergy as a public health problem is given by the fact that the annual number of doctor visits for hypertension, routine medical examinations, or normal pregnancy, are each fewer than the number of visits for the three cited allergic conditions.

In addition to the suffering and anxiety caused by these inappropriate immune responses or allergies to environmental antigens, there is the staggering cost in terms of lost work time and for caregivers. The data on frequency of visits to the doctor or hospital confirm the size of the problem and well justify the extensive efforts by basic and clinical immunologists and allergists to relieve the suffering caused by these disorders.

Annual Ambulatory Care Visits for the Most Common Medical Complaints, 1995

Diagnoses	Office visits (thousands)
Respiratory, sinus, ear, and throat infections	101,800
Joint and back problems	56,600
Heart disease	33,500
Allergies and asthma	28,200
Asthma	12,000
Allergic rhinitis	8,500
Contact dermatitis and other eczema	7,700
Essential hypertension	25,400
General medical examination	22,800
Normal pregnancy	22,800
Health supervision of infant or child	21,300
Cancer	17,200
Diabetes mellitus	15,500
Cataract	8,100

SOURCE: Ambulatory care visits to physician offices, hospital outpatient departments, and emergency departments: United States, 1995. Centers for Disease Control and Prevention, National Center for Health Statistics, 1997, DHHS Publication No. (PHS)97-1790, June 1997.

of IgE to its specific antigen (allergen) releases substances that cause irritation and inflammation. When an allergic individual is exposed to an allergen, symptoms may include sneezing, wheezing, and difficulty in breathing (asthma); dermatitis or skin eruptions (hives); and, in more extreme cases, strangulation due to blockage of airways by inflammation. A significant fraction of our health resources is expended to care for those suffering from allergy and asthma. The frequency of allergy and asthma in the United States place these complaints among the most common reasons for a visit to the doctor's office or to the hospital emergency room (see Clinical Focus).

When the immune system encounters foreign cells or tissue, it responds strongly to rid the host of the invaders. However, in some cases, the transplantation of cells or an organ from another individual, although viewed by the immune system as a foreign invasion, may be the only possible treatment for disease. For example, it is estimated that more than 60,000 persons in the United States alone could benefit from a kidney transplant. Because the immune system will attack and reject any transplanted organ that it does not recognize as self, it is a serious barrier to this potentially life-saving treatment. An additional danger in transplantation is that any transplanted cells with immune function may view the new host as nonself and react against it. This reaction, which is termed graft-versus-host disease, can be fatal. The rejection reaction and graft-versus-host disease can be suppressed by drugs, but this type of treatment suppresses all immune function, so that the host is no longer protected by its immune system and becomes susceptible to infectious diseases. Transplantation studies have played a major role in the development of immunology. A Nobel prize was awarded to Karl Landsteiner, in 1930, for the discovery of human blood groups, a finding that allowed blood transfusions to be carried out safely. In 1980, G. Snell, J. Dausset, and B. Benacerraf were recognized for discovery of the major histocompatibility complex, and, in 1991, E. D. Thomas and J. Murray were awarded a Nobel Prize for advances in transplantation immunity. To enable a foreign organ to be accepted without suppressing immunity to all antigens remains a challenge for immunologists today.

In certain individuals, the immune system malfunctions by losing its sense of self and nonself, which permits an immune attack upon the host. This condition, **autoimmunity,** can cause a number of chronic debilitating diseases. The symptoms of autoimmunity differ depending on which tissues and organs are under attack. For example, multiple sclerosis is due to an autoimmune attack on the brain and central nervous system, Crohn's disease is an attack on the tissues in the gut, and rheumatoid arthritis is an attack on joints of the arms and legs. The genetic and environmental factors that trigger and sustain autoimmune disease are very active areas of immunologic research, as is the search for improved treatments.

If any of the many components of innate or specific immunity is defective because of genetic abnormality or if any loses function because of damage by chemical, physical, or biological agents, the host suffers from **immunodeficiency.** The severity of the immunodeficiency disease depends on the number of affected components. A common type of immunodeficiency in North America is a selective immunodeficiency in which only one type of immunoglobulin, IgA, is lacking; the symptoms may be minor or even go unnoticed. In contrast, a rarer immunodeficiency called severe combined immunodeficiency (SCID), which affects both B and T cells, if untreated, results in death from infection at an early age. Since the 1980s, the most common form of immunodeficiency has been acquired immune deficiency syndrome, or AIDS, which results from infection with the retrovirus human immunodeficiency virus, or HIV. In AIDS, helper cells are infected and destroyed by HIV, causing a collapse of the immune system. It is estimated that 33 million persons worldwide suffer from this disease, which is usually fatal within 8 to 10 years after infection. Although certain treatments can prolong the life of AIDS patients, there is no known cure for this disease.

This chapter has been a brief introduction to the immune system, and it has given a thumbnail sketch of how this complex system functions to protect the host from disease. The following chapters will concern the structure and function of the individual cells, organs, and molecules that make up this system. They will describe our current understanding of how the components of immunity interact and the experiments that allowed discovery of these mechanisms. Specific areas of applied immunology, such as immunity to infectious diseases, cancer, and current vaccination practices are the subject matter of later chapters. Finally, to complete the description of the immune system in all of its activities, a chapter addresses each of the major types of immune dysfunction.

Summary

1. Immunity is the state of protection against foreign organisms or substances (antigens). Vertebrates have two types of immunity, innate and adaptive. The components and mechanisms of innate (nonspecific) immunity are not specific to any one pathogen. Adaptive immunity displays a high degree of specificity. Typically, innate immune responses begin much more quickly than adaptive ones and therefore constitute the first line of defense after the host has been invaded by a pathogen.
2. Innate and adaptive immunity do not operate independently of each other. They act in cooperative and interdependent ways that make them both more effective. The

activation of innate immune responses produces signals that stimulate and direct subsequent adaptive immune responses. In addition, the adaptive immune system generates signals and components that stimulate and increase the effectiveness of innate immune responses.

3. Innate immune responses include anatomic, physiologic, endocytic and phagocytic, and inflammatory barriers that help prevent the entrance and establishment of infectious agents (see Figures 1-3, 1-4). In cooperation with these nonspecific mechanisms, the body mounts an adaptive (specific) immune response.
4. Adaptive immune responses exhibit four immunologic attributes: specificity, diversity, memory, and self/nonself recognition. Functionally, an immune response consists of two interrelated events: recognition of antigen and response to that antigen (i.e., generation of effector cells and molecules). Antigen-presenting cells, B lymphocytes, and T lymphocytes are the primary cells of the immune responses.
5. The cell membranes of both B and T lymphocytes have antigen-binding receptors. The receptors on B cells are antibody molecules, which can recognize and interact directly with antigen. T-cell receptors, in contrast, recognize only antigen that is combined with either class I or class II major histocompatibility complex (MHC) molecules on the surface of a cell. As B and T lymphocytes mature, each cell comes to express receptors that recognize a single antigenic determinant (epitope).
6. The two major subpopulations of T lymphocytes are T helper (T_H) cells and T cytotoxic (T_C) cells. In general, T_H cells express CD4, a membrane glycoprotein, and recognize antigen combined with class II MHC cells, whereas T_C cells express CD8 and recognize antigen combined with class I MHC cells (see Figure 1-8).
7. Exogenous (extracellular) antigens are internalized and degraded by antigen-presenting cells (macrophages, B cells, and dendritic cells); the resulting antigenic peptides complexed with class II MHC molecules then are displayed on the cell surface. Endogenous (intracellular) antigens (e.g., viral and tumor proteins produced in altered self-cells) are degraded in the cytoplasm and then displayed with class I MHC molecules on the cell surface. (See Figure 1-9.)
8. Interaction of a mature, immunocompetent lymphocyte with the antigen it recognizes stimulates the cell to proliferate and differentiate into effector cells and memory cells (see Figure 1-10). Such initial exposure to a particular antigen induces a primary response; the expanded population of memory cells permits a more rapid and intense secondary response to subsequent exposure to the same antigen (see Figure 1-11).
9. The immune system produces both humoral and cell-mediated responses. The humoral response is best suited for elimination of exogenous antigens; the cell-mediated response, for elimination of endogenous antigens. The effector cells of the humoral response are plasma cells, which secrete soluble antibody. The effector cells of the cell-mediated response are activated T_H cells, which secrete various cytokines, and cytotoxic T lymphocytes (CTLs), which can destroy altered self-cells. T_H-cell activation is required for both types of response. (See Figures 1-7 and 1-13.)
10. The signature elements of adaptive immunity, lymphocytes and antibodies, are found only in vertebrates. However, some type of innate immunity appears to be a characteristic of multicellular organisms, and immunity has been demonstrated in organisms as different as insects, earthworms, and higher plants. The mechanisms used by different phyla are highly diverse and include phagocytosis, the generation of antimicrobial peptides, and the induction of protective enzyme cascades.
11. Dysfunction of the immune system can cause debilitating or fatal disease. The most common dysfunctions result in allergy or asthma. If the immune system fails to function because some component is lost or inactivated, the resulting immunodeficiency leaves the host susceptible to infection. In autoimmunity, the immune system attacks host cells or tissues, which leads to serious diseases such as multiple sclerosis and rheumatoid arthritis.

REFERENCES

Ada, GL, and G Nossal. 1987. The clonal selection theory. *Sci. Am.* **257**(2):62.

Burnet, FM. 1959. *The Clonal Selection Theory of Acquired Immunity.* Cambridge University Press, Cambridge.

Cohen, SG, and M Samter. 1992. *Excerpts from Classics in Allergy.* Symposia Foundation, Carlsbad, California.

Desour, L. 1922. *Pasteur and His Work* (translated by AF and BH Wedd). T. Fisher Unwin Ltd., London.

Engelhard, VH. 1994. How cells process antigens. *Sci. Am.* **271**(2):54.

Fearon, DT, and RM Locksley. 1996. The instructive role of innate immunity in the acquired immune response. *Science* **272:**50.

Fritig, B, T Heitz, and M Legrand. 1998. Antimicrobial proteins in induced plant defense. *Curr. Opin. Immunol.* **10:**12.

Grey, HM, A Sette, and S Buus. 1989. How T cells see antigen. *Sci. Am.* **261**(5):56.

Kindt, TJ, and JD Capra. 1984. *The Antibody Enigma.* Plenum Press, New York.

Krause, RM. 1981. *The Restless Tide: The Persistent Challenge of the Microbial World.* Foundation for Infectious Disease, Washington, D.C.

Landsteiner, K. 1947. *The Specificity of Serologic Reactions.* Harvard University Press, Cambridge, Massachusetts.

Lemaitre, B, E Nicolas, JM Reichart, and JA Hoffman. 1996. The dorsoventral regulatory gene cassette *spatzle/Toll/cactus* controls the potent antifungal response in *Drosophila* adults. *Cell* **86:**973.

Life, Death, and the Immune System. 1994. Readings from *Scientific American Magazine.* W. H. Freeman and Company, New York.

Medawar, PB. 1958. *The Immunology of Transplantation. The Harvey Lectures 1956–1957.* Academic Press, New York.

Medzhitov, R, and CA Janeway. 1998. An ancient system of host defense. *Curr. Opin. Immunol.* **10:**12.

Metchnikoff, E. 1905. *Immunity in the Infectious Diseases.* MacMillan, New York.

Roitt, IM, and PJ Delves, eds. 1998. *An Encyclopedia of Immunology,* 2nd ed., vols. 1–4. Academic Press, London.

Sher, A., and R Ahmed. 1995. Immunity to infection. *Curr. Opin. Immunol.* **7:**471.

Useful Web Sites

http://www.umdnj.edu/~acole/main1.html
The Antimicrobial Peptide Web site provides good coverage of the varieties of antimicrobial peptides that play a role in innate immunity.

http://www.sciencexchange.com
The Web site of the American Association of Immunologists contains a good deal of information of interest to immunologists.

http://www.path.ox.ac.uk/sg
The Macrophage Home Page provides an extensive view of the activities and workings of these phagocytic cells, which play such important roles in innate immunity.

http://www.ncbi.nlm.nih.gov/PubMed/
PubMed, the National Library of Medicine database of more than 9 million publications, is the world's most comprehensive bibliographic database for biological and biomedical literature. It is also a highly user-friendly site.

STUDY QUESTIONS

1. Indicate to which branch(es) of the immune system the following statements apply, using **H** for the humoral branch and **CM** for the cell-mediated branch. Some statements may apply to both branches.

a. _____ Involves class I MHC molecules
b. _____ Responds to viral infection
c. _____ Involves T helper cells
d. _____ Involves processed antigen
e. _____ Most likely responds following an organ transplant
f. _____ Involves T cytotoxic cells
g. _____ Involves B cells
h. _____ Involves $CD8^+$ T cells
i. _____ Responds to extracellular bacterial infection
j. _____ Involves secreted antibody
k. _____ Kills virus-infected self-cells

2. Specific immunity exhibits four characteristic attributes, which are mediated by lymphocytes. List these four attributes and briefly explain how they arise.

3. Name three features of a secondary immune response that distinguish it from a primary immune response.

4. Compare and contrast the four types of antigen-binding molecules used by the immune system—antibodies, T-cell receptors, class I MHC molecules, and class II MHC molecules—in terms of the following characteristics:

a. Specificity for antigen
b. Cellular expression
c. Types of antigen recognized

5. Fill in the blanks in the following statements with the most appropriate terms:

a. ________, ________, and ________ all function as antigen-presenting cells.

b. Antigen-presenting cells deliver a _______ signal to _______ cells.

c. Only antigen-presenting cells express class _______ MHC molecules, whereas nearly all cells express class _______ MHC molecules.

d. _________ antigens are internalized by antigen-presenting cells, degraded in the _________, and displayed with class _________ MHC molecules on the cell surface.

e. _________ antigens are produced in altered self-cells, degraded in the ___________, and displayed with class ___________ MHC molecules on the cell surface.

6. Briefly describe the three major events in the inflammatory response.

7. The $CD8^+$ T cell is said to be class I restricted. What does this mean?

8. Match each term related to innate immunity (a–p) with the most appropriate description listed below (1–19). Each description may be used once, more than once, or not at all.

Terms

a. ______ Fimbriae or pili
b. ______ Exudate
c. ______ Sebum
d. ______ Margination
e. ______ Dermis
f. ______ Lysosome
g. ______ Histamine
h. ______ Macrophage
i. ______ Lysozyme
j. ______ Bradykinin
k. ______ Interferon
l. ______ Edema
m. ______ Complement
n. ______ Extravasation
o. ______ C-reactive protein
p. ______ Phagosome

Go to www.whfreeman.com/immunology Self-Test
Review and quiz of key terms

Descriptions

(1) Thin outer layer of skin

(2) Layer of skin containing blood vessels and sebaceous glands

(3) One of several acute-phase proteins

(4) Hydrolytic enzyme found in mucous secretions

(5) Migration of a phagocyte through the endothelial wall into the tissues

(6) Acidic antibacterial secretion found on the skin

(7) Has antiviral activity

(8) Induces vasodilation

(9) Accumulation of fluid in intercellular space, resulting in swelling

(10) Large vesicle containing ingested particulate material

(11) Accumulation of dead cells, digested material, and fluid

(12) Adherence of phagocytic cells to the endothelial wall

(13) Structures involved in microbial adherence to mucous membranes

(14) Stimulates pain receptors in the skin

(15) Phagocytic cell found in the tissues

(16) Phagocytic cell found in the blood

(17) Group of serum proteins involved in cell lysis and clearance of antigen

(18) Cytoplasmic vesicle containing degradative enzymes

(19) Protein-rich fluid that leaks from the capillaries into the tissues

9. Innate and adaptive immunity act in cooperative and interdependent ways to protect the host. Discuss the collaboration of these two forms of immunity.

10. How might an arthropod, such as a cockroach or beetle, protect itself from infection? In what ways might the innate immune responses of an arthropod be similar to those of a plant and how might they differ?

11. Give examples of mild and severe consequences of immune dysfunction. What is the most common cause of immunodeficiency throughout the world today?

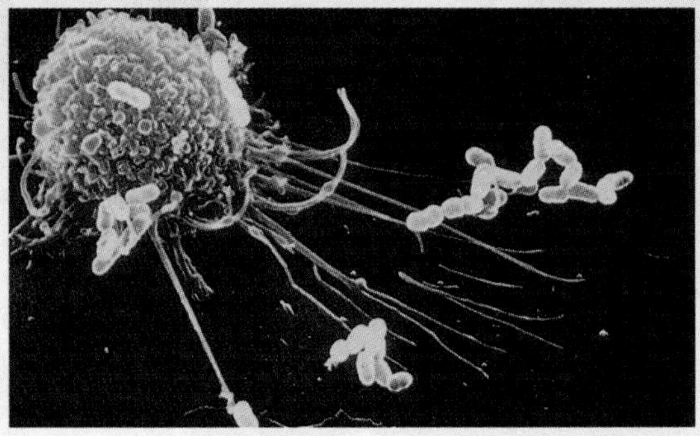

CHAPTER 2
CELLS AND ORGANS OF THE IMMUNE SYSTEM

Hematopoiesis

Cells of the Immune System

Organs of the Immune System

The immune system consists of many different organs and tissues that are found throughout the body. These organs can be classified functionally into two main groups. The *primary lymphoid organs* provide appropriate microenvironments for the development and maturation of lymphocytes. The *secondary lymphoid organs* trap antigen from defined tissues or vascular spaces and are sites where mature lymphocytes can interact effectively with that antigen. The blood vessels and lymphatic systems connect these organs, uniting them into a functional whole.

Carried within the blood and lymph and populating the lymphoid organs are various white blood cells, or **leukocytes,** that participate in the immune response. Of these cells, only the lymphocytes possess the attributes of diversity, specificity, memory, and self/nonself recognition, the hallmarks of an adaptive immune response. All the other cells play accessory roles in adaptive immunity, serving to activate lymphocytes, to increase the effectiveness of antigen clearance by phagocytosis, or to secrete various immune-effector molecules. Some leukocytes, especially T lymphocytes, secrete various protein molecules called cytokines. These molecules act as immunoregulatory hormones and play important roles in the regulation of immune responses. This chapter describes the formation of blood cells; then, the properties of the various immune-system cells; finally, the functions of the lymphoid organs.

Hematopoiesis

All blood cells arise from a type of cell called the **hematopoietic stem cell (HSC). Stem cells** are cells that can differentiate into other cell types; they are self-renewing—they maintain their population level by cell division. In humans, **hematopoiesis,** the formation and development of red and white blood cells, begins in the embryonic yolk sac during the first weeks of development. Here, yolk-sac stem cells differentiate into primitive erythroid cells that contain embryonic hemoglobin. In the third month of gestation, hematopoietic stem cells migrate from the yolk sac to the fetal liver and then to the spleen; these two organs have major roles in hematopoiesis from the third to the seventh months of gestation. After that, the differentiation of HSCs in the bone marrow becomes the major factor in hematopoiesis, and by birth there is little or no hematopoiesis in the liver and spleen.

It is remarkable that every functionally specialized, mature blood cell is derived from the same type of stem cell. In contrast to a *unipotent* cell, which differentiates into a single cell type, a hematopoietic stem cell is *pluripotent,* able to differentiate in various ways and thereby generate erythrocytes, granulocytes, monocytes, mast cells, lymphocytes, and megakaryocytes. These stem cells are few, normally fewer than one HSC per 5×10^4 cells in the bone marrow.

The study of hematopoietic stem cells is difficult both because of their scarcity and because they are hard to grow in vitro. As a result, little is known about how their proliferation and differentiation are regulated. By virtue of their capacity for self-renewal, hematopoietic stem cells are maintained at stable levels throughout adult life; however, when there is an increased demand for hematopoiesis, HSCs display an enormous proliferative capacity. This can be demonstrated in mice whose hematopoietic systems have been completely destroyed by a lethal dose (950 rads; one rad represents the absorption by an irradiated target of an amount of radiation corresponding to 100 ergs/gram of target) of x-rays. Such irradiated mice will die within 10 days unless they are infused with normal bone-marrow cells from a syngeneic (genetically identical) mouse. Although a normal mouse has 3×10^8 bone-marrow cells, infusion of only

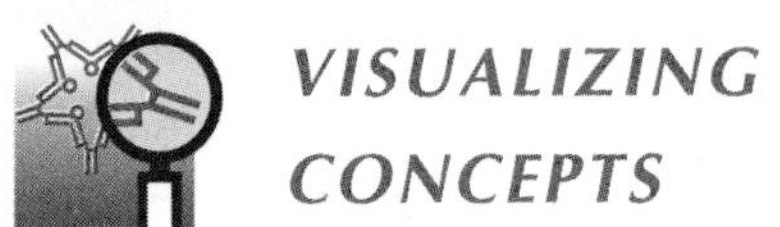

VISUALIZING CONCEPTS

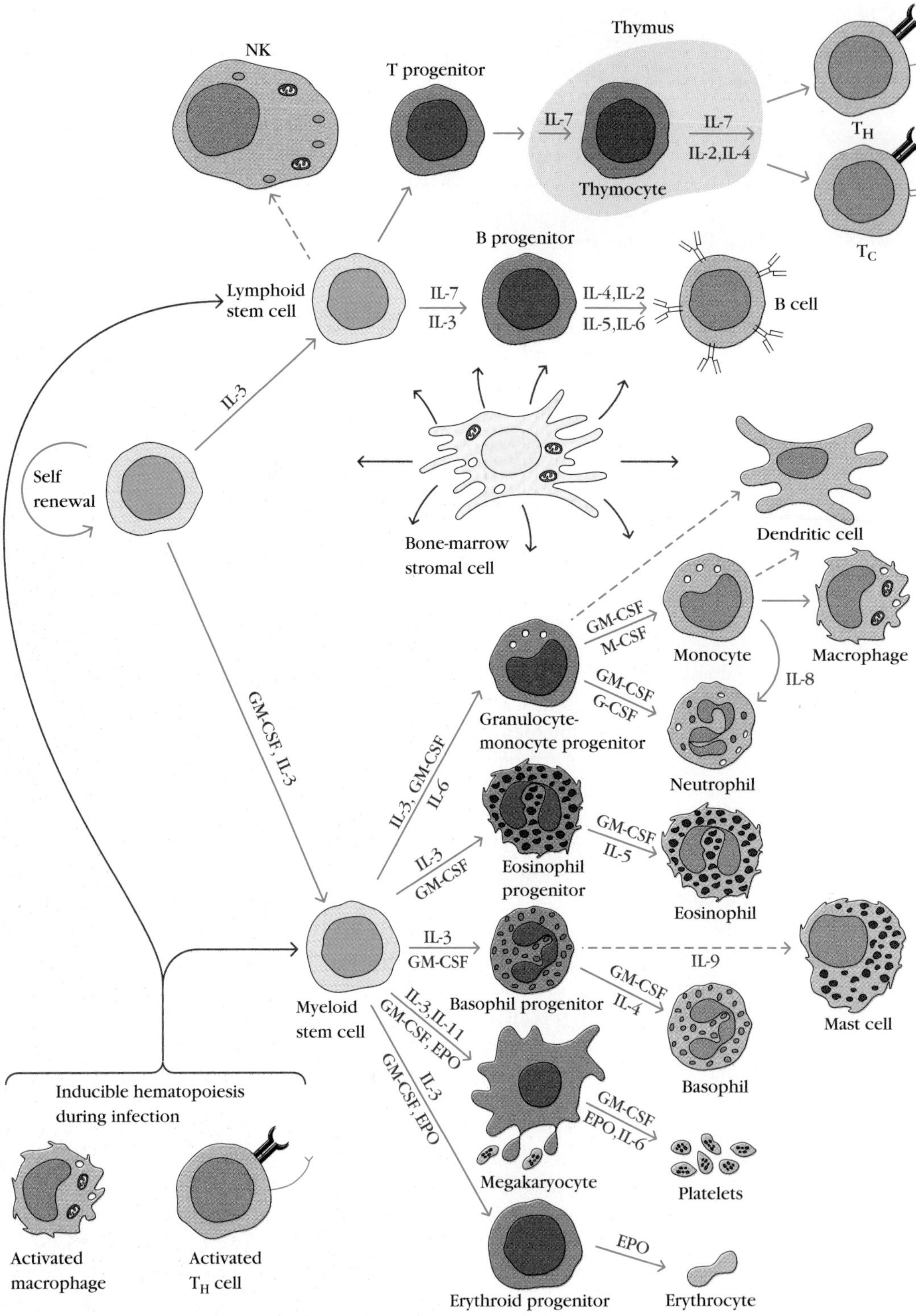

FIGURE 2-1 Regulation of hematopoiesis by cytokines that stimulate the proliferation and/or differentiation of various hematopoietic cells. In the absence of infection, bone-marrow stromal cells are the major source of hematopoietic cytokines (red arrows). In the presence of infection, cytokines (red arrows) produced by activated macrophages and T_H cells induce additional hematopoietic activity, resulting in rapid expansion of the population of white blood cells that fight infection. IL = interleukin: CSF = colony-stimulating factor; EPO = erythropoietin, NK = natural killer cell. Stem cells are shown in blue; progenitor and immature cells in purple; stromal cell in yellow; and mature differentiated cells in tan. Dashed lines indicate likely, but still hypothetical pathways.

10^4–10^5 bone-marrow cells (i.e., 0.01% – 0.1% of the normal amount) from a donor is sufficient to completely restore the hematopoietic system, which demonstrates the enormous proliferative and differentiative capacity of the stem cells.

Early in hematopoiesis, a pluripotent stem cell differentiates along one of two pathways, giving rise to either a common **lymphoid progenitor cell** or a **myeloid stem cell** (Figure 2-1). The types and amounts of growth factors in the microenvironment of a particular stem cell or progenitor cell control its differentiation. During the development of the lymphoid and myeloid lineages, stem cells differentiate into **progenitor cells,** which have lost the capacity for self-renewal and are committed to a particular cell lineage. Common lymphoid progenitor cells give rise to B, T, and NK (natural killer) cells. Myeloid stem cells generate progenitors of red blood cells (erythrocytes), many of the various white blood cells (neutrophils, eosinophils, basophils, monocytes, mast cells), and platelets. Progenitor commitment depends on the acquisition of responsiveness to particular growth factors and **cytokines.** When the appropriate factors and cytokines are present, progenitor cells proliferate and differentiate into the corresponding cell type, either mature erythrocyte, a particular type of leukocyte, or a platelet-generating cell. Red and white blood cells pass into bone-marrow channels, from which they enter the circulation.

In adult bone marrow, hematopoietic cells grow and mature on a meshwork of **stromal cells,** which are nonhematopoietic cells that support the growth and differentiation of hematopoietic cells. Stromal cells include fat cells, endothelial cells, fibroblasts, and macrophages. Stromal cells influence the differentiation of hematopoietic stem cells by providing a **hematopoietic-inducing microenvironment (HIM)** consisting of a cellular matrix and either membrane-bound or diffusible growth factors.

Hematopoietic Growth Factors

Cell-culture systems that can support the growth and differentiation of lymphoid and myeloid stem cells have made it possible to identify many hematopoietic growth factors. In these in-vitro systems, bone-marrow stromal cells are cultured to form a layer of cells that adhere to a petri dish; freshly isolated bone-marrow hematopoietic cells placed on this layer will grow, divide, and produce large visible colonies (Figure 2-2). If the cells have been cultured in semisolid agar, their progeny will be immobilized and can be analyzed for cell types. Colonies that contain stem cells can be replated to produce mixed colonies that contain different cell types; progenitor cells, which cannot be replated, produce lineage-restricted colonies.

Various growth factors are required for the survival, proliferation, differentiation, and maturation of hematopoietic cells in culture. These growth factors, the hematopoietic cytokines, are identified by how they are able to stimulate the formation of hematopoietic cell colonies in bone-marrow cultures. Among the cytokines detected in this way was a family of acidic glycoproteins, the **colony-stimulating factors (CSFs),** named for their ability to induce the formation of distinct hematopoietic cell lines.

Four colony-stimulating factors have been identified: **multilineage CSF (multi-CSF),** also known as **interleukin 3 (IL-3); macrophage CSF (M-CSF); granulocyte CSF (G-CSF);** and **granulocyte-macrophage CSF (GM-CSF).** Another important hematopoietic cytokine detected by this method is a glycoprotein called **erythropoietin (EPO);** produced by the kidney, this cytokine induces the terminal development of erythrocytes and regulates the production of red blood cells. The commitment of a progenitor cell to a particular differentiation pathway is associated with the expression

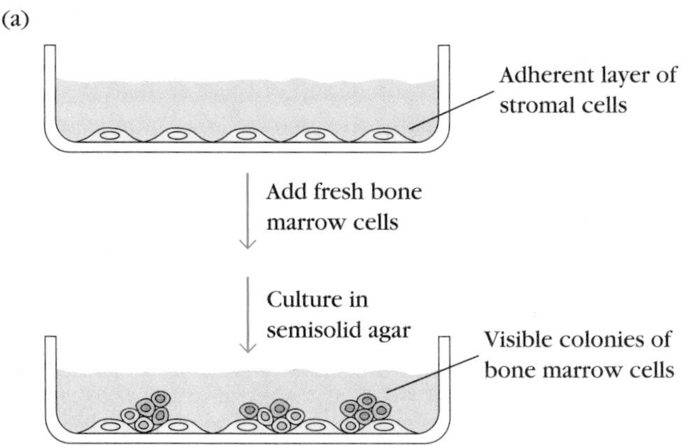

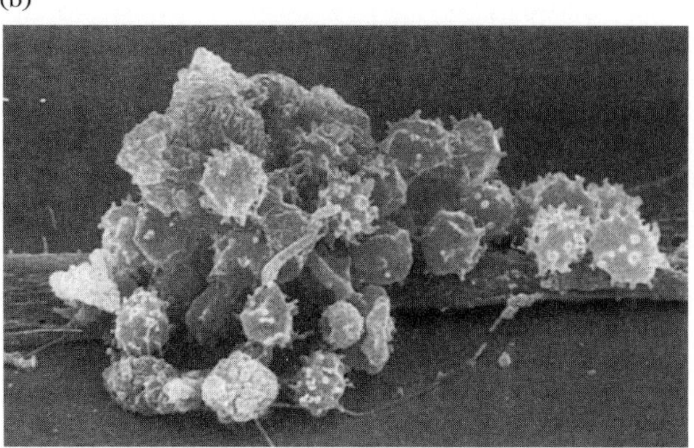

FIGURE 2-2 (a) Experimental scheme for culturing hematopoietic cells. Adherent bone-marrow stromal cells form a matrix on which the hematopoietic cells proliferate. Single cells can be transferred to semisolid agar for colony growth, and the colonies analyzed for differentiated cell types. (b) Scanning electron micrograph of cells in long-term culture of human bone marrow. [Photograph from MJ Cline and DW Golde, 1979, *Nature* **277:**180.]

on the cell of membrane receptors that are specific for particular cytokines. The receptor specific for a cytokine is necessary for the cell to respond to the presence of that cytokine and is therefore required for it to play a role in the cell's differentiation. Many of the cytokines important for hematopoiesis are indicated in Figure 2-1. A variety of cell types, including bone-marrow stromal cells, activated T-helper T_H2 cells, and activated macrophages, produce one or more of these cytokines.

Genes That Regulate Hematopoiesis

The development of pluripotent hematopoietic stem cells into different cell types requires the expression of different sets of lineage-determining and lineage-specific genes at appropriate times and in the correct order. The proteins specified by these genes are critical components of regulatory networks that direct the differentiation of the stem cell and its descendants. Much of what we know about the dependence of hematopoiesis on a particular gene comes from studies of mice in which a gene has been inactivated or "knocked out" by targeted disruption, which blocks the production of the protein that it encodes (see Targeted Disruption of Genes, in Chapter 23). If mice fail to produce red cells or particular white blood cells when a gene is knocked out, we conclude that the protein specified by the gene is necessary for development of those cells.

Although much remains to be done, targeted disruption and other approaches have identified a number of transcription factors (Table 2-1). Some of these transcription factors affect many different hematopoietic lineages, and others affect only a single lineage, such as the developmental pathway that leads to lymphocytes. One transcription factor that affects multiple lineages is GATA-2, a member of a family of transcription factors that recognize the tetranucleotide sequence GATA, a nucleotide motif in target genes. A functional ***GATA-2* gene,** which specifies this transcription factor, is essential for the development of the lymphoid, erythroid, and myeloid lineages. As might be expected, animals in which this gene is disrupted die during embryonic development. In contrast to GATA-2, another transcription factor, **Ikaros,** is required only for the development of cells of the lymphoid lineage. Although Ikaros knockout mice do not produce significant numbers of B, T, and NK cells, their production of erythrocytes, granulocytes, and other cells of the myeloid lineage is unimpaired. Ikaros knockout mice survive embryonic development, but they are severely compromised immunologically and die of infections at an early age.

TABLE 2-1 SOME TRANSCRIPTION FACTORS ESSENTIAL FOR HEMATOPOIETIC LINEAGES

Factor	Dependent lineage
GATA-1	Erythroid
GATA-2	Erythroid, myeloid, lymphoid
PU.1	Erythroid (maturational stages), myeloid (later stages), lymphoid
BM11	Myeloid, lymphoid
Ikaros	Lymphoid
Oct-2	B lymphoid (differentiation of B cells into plasma cells)

Regulation of Hematopoiesis

Hematopoiesis is a continuous process that generally maintains a steady state in which the production of mature blood cells equals their loss (principally from aging). The average erythrocyte has a life span of 120 days before it is phagocytosed and digested by macrophages in the spleen. The various white blood cells have life spans ranging from days, for neutrophils, to as long as 20–30 years for some T lymphocytes. To maintain steady-state levels, the average human being must produce an estimated 3.7×10^{11} white blood cells per day.

Hematopoiesis is regulated by complex mechanisms that affect all of the individual cell types. These regulatory mechanisms ensure steady-state levels of the various blood cells, yet they have enough built-in flexibility so that production of blood cells can rapidly increase tenfold to twentyfold in response to hemorrhage or infection. Steady-state regulation of hematopoiesis is accomplished in various ways, which include:

- Control of the levels and types of cytokines produced by bone-marrow stromal cells
- The production of cytokines with hematopoietic activity by other cell types, such as activated T cells and macrophages
- The regulation of the expression of receptors for hematopoietically active cytokines in stem cells and progenitor cells
- The removal of some cells by the controlled induction of cell death

A failure in one or a combination of these regulatory mechanisms can have serious consequences. For example, abnormalities in the expression of hematopoietic cytokines or their receptors could lead to unregulated cellular proliferation and may contribute to the development of some leukemias. Evidence that such abnormal autostimulation can lead to cancerous proliferation comes from studies of the human adult T-cell leukemia associated with the HTLV-1 retrovirus, which infects human T cells, immortalizes them, and in some cases transforms them into leukemic cells. T cells infected with HTLV-1 begin to increase their expression of forms of the IL-2 receptor that are responsive to low concentrations of IL-2. Secretion of IL-2 by these same cells may be a factor that allows unregulated cellular proliferation, resulting in leukemia.

Ultimately, the number of cells in any hematopoietic lineage is set by a balance between the number of cells removed by cell death and the number that arise from division and differentiation. Any one or a combination of regulatory factors can affect rates of cell reproduction and differentiation. These factors can also determine whether a hematopoietic cell is induced to die.

Programmed Cell Death

Programmed cell death, an induced and ordered process in which the cell actively participates in bringing about its own demise, is a critical factor in the homeostatic regulation of many types of cell populations, including those of the hematopoietic system.

Cells undergoing programmed cell death often exhibit distinctive morphologic changes, collectively referred to as **apoptosis** (Figures 2-3, 2-4). These changes include a pronounced decrease in cell volume, modification of the cytoskeleton to result in membrane blebbing, a condensation of the chromatin, and degradation of the DNA into smaller fragments. Following these morphologic changes, an apoptotic cell sheds tiny membrane-bounded apoptotic bodies containing intact organelles. Macrophages quickly phagocytose apoptotic bodies and cells in the advanced stages of apoptosis. This ensures that their intracellular contents, including proteolytic and other lytic enzymes, cationic proteins, and oxidizing molecules are not released into the surrounding tissue. In this way, apoptosis does not induce a local inflammatory response. Apoptosis differs markedly from **necrosis,** the changes associated with cell death arising from injury. In necrosis the injured cell swells and bursts, releasing its contents and possibly triggering a damaging inflammatory response.

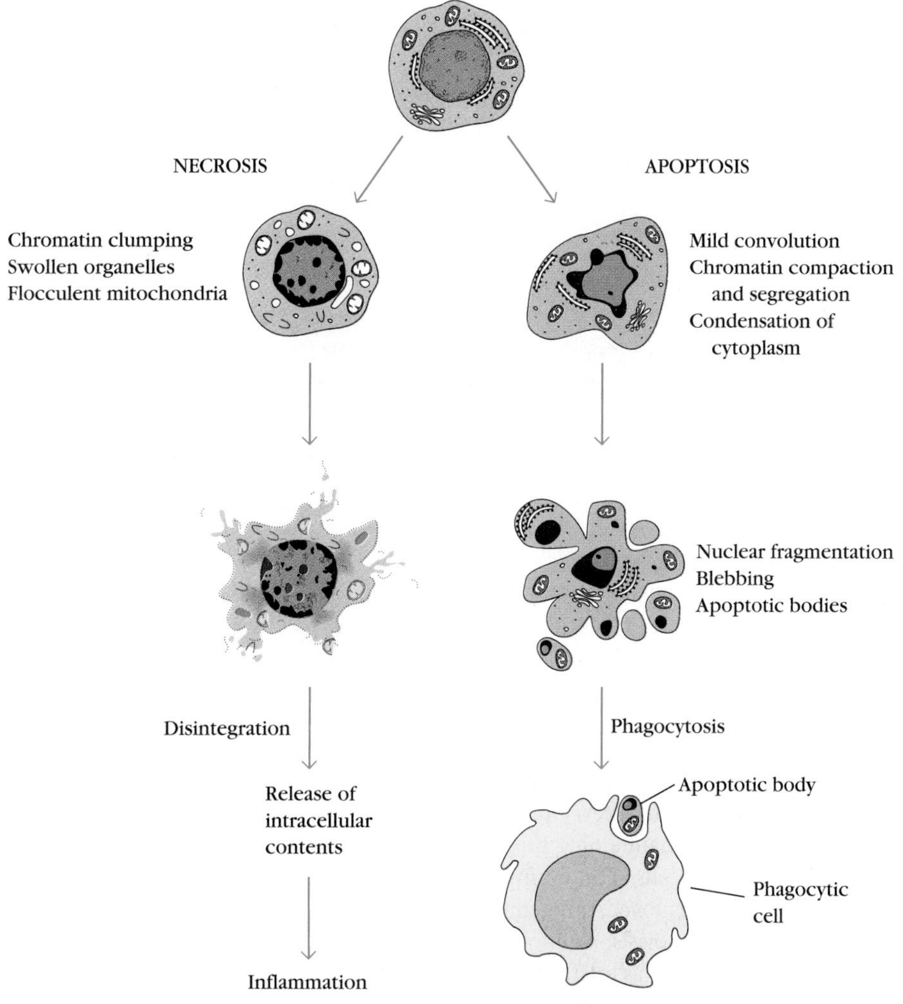

FIGURE 2-3 Comparison of morphologic changes that occur in apoptosis and necrosis. Apoptosis, which results in the programmed cell death of hematopoietic cells, does not induce a local inflammatory response. In contrast, necrosis, the process that leads to death of injured cells, results in release of the cells' contents, which may induce a local inflammatory response.

Go to www.whfreeman.com/immunology **Animation**
Cell Death

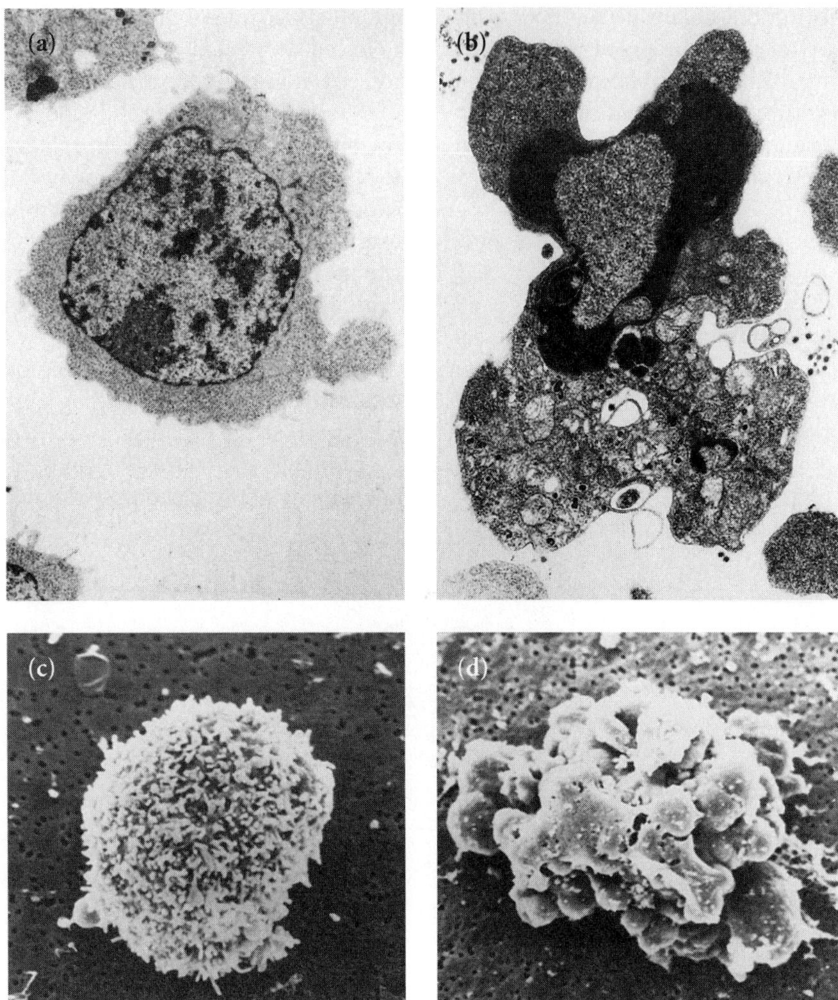

FIGURE 2-4 Apoptosis. Light micrographs of (a) normal thymocytes (developing T cells in the thymus) and (b) apoptotic thymocytes. Scanning electron micrographs of (c) normal and (d) apoptotic thymocytes. [Photographs from BA Osborne and S Smith, 1997, *Journal of NIH Research* **9**:35; courtesy BA Osborne, University of Massachusetts at Amherst.]

Each of the leukocytes produced by hematopoiesis has a characteristic life span and then dies by programmed cell death. In the adult human, for example, there are about 5×10^{10} neutrophils in the circulation. These cells have a life span of only a few days and then die by programmed cell death. This death, along with constant neutrophil production, maintains a stable number of these cells. If programmed cell death fails to occur, a leukemic state may develop. Programmed cell death also plays a role in maintaining proper numbers of hematopoietic progenitor cells. For example, when colony-stimulating factors are removed, progenitor cells undergo apoptosis. Beyond hematopoiesis, apoptosis is important in such immunological processes as tolerance and the killing of target cells by cytotoxic T cells or natural killer cells. Details of the mechanisms underlying apoptosis are emerging; Chapter 14 describes them in detail.

The expression of several genes accompanies apoptosis in leukocytes and other cell types (Table 2-2). Some of the proteins specified by these genes induce apoptosis, others are critical during apoptosis, and still others inhibit apoptosis. For example, the radiation-induced death of thymocytes by apop-

TABLE 2-2 GENES THAT REGULATE APOPTOSIS

Gene	Function	Role in apoptosis
bcl-2	Prevents apoptosis	Inhibits
bax	Opposes *bcl-2*	Promotes
bcl-X$_L$ *(bcl-Long)*	Prevents apoptosis	Inhibits
bcl-X$_S$ *(bcl-Short)*	Opposes *bcl-X*$_L$	Promotes
caspase (several different ones)	Protease	Promotes
fas	Induces apoptosis	Initiates

tosis requires the protein p53; many cell deaths are induced by signals from Fas, a molecule present on the surface of many cells; and proteases known as caspases take part in a cascade of reactions that lead to apoptosis. On the other hand, members of the bcl-2 (B-cell lymphoma 2) family of genes, *bcl-2* and *bcl-*X_L encode protein products that inhibit apoptosis. Interestingly, the first member of this gene family, *bcl-2,* was found in studies that were concerned not with cell death but with the uncontrolled proliferation of B cells in a type of cancer known as B-lymphoma. In this case, the *bcl-2* gene was at the breakpoint of a chromosomal translocation in a human B-cell lymphoma. The translocation moved the *bcl-2* gene into the immunoglobulin heavy-chain locus, resulting in transcriptional activation of the *bcl-2* gene and overproduction of the encoded Bcl-2 protein by the lymphoma cells. The resulting high levels of Bcl-2 are thought to help transform lymphoid cells into cancerous lymphoma cells by inhibiting the signals that would normally induce apoptotic cell death.

Bcl-2 levels have been found to play an important role in regulating the normal life span of various hematopoietic cell lineages, including lymphocytes. A normal adult has about 5 L of blood with about 2000 lymphocytes/mm^3, for a total of about 10^{10} lymphocytes. During acute infection, the lymphocyte count increases 4- to 15-fold, giving a total lymphocyte count of $40–150 \times 10^9$. Because the immune system cannot sustain such a massive increase in cell numbers for an extended period, the system needs a means to eliminate unneeded activated lymphocytes once the antigenic threat has passed. Activated lymphocytes have been found to express lower levels of Bcl-2 and therefore are more susceptible to the induction of apoptotic death than are naive lymphocytes or memory cells. However, if the lymphocytes continue to be activated by antigen, then the signals received during activation block the apoptotic signal. As antigen levels subside, so does activation of the block and the lymphocytes begin to die by apoptosis (Figure 2-5).

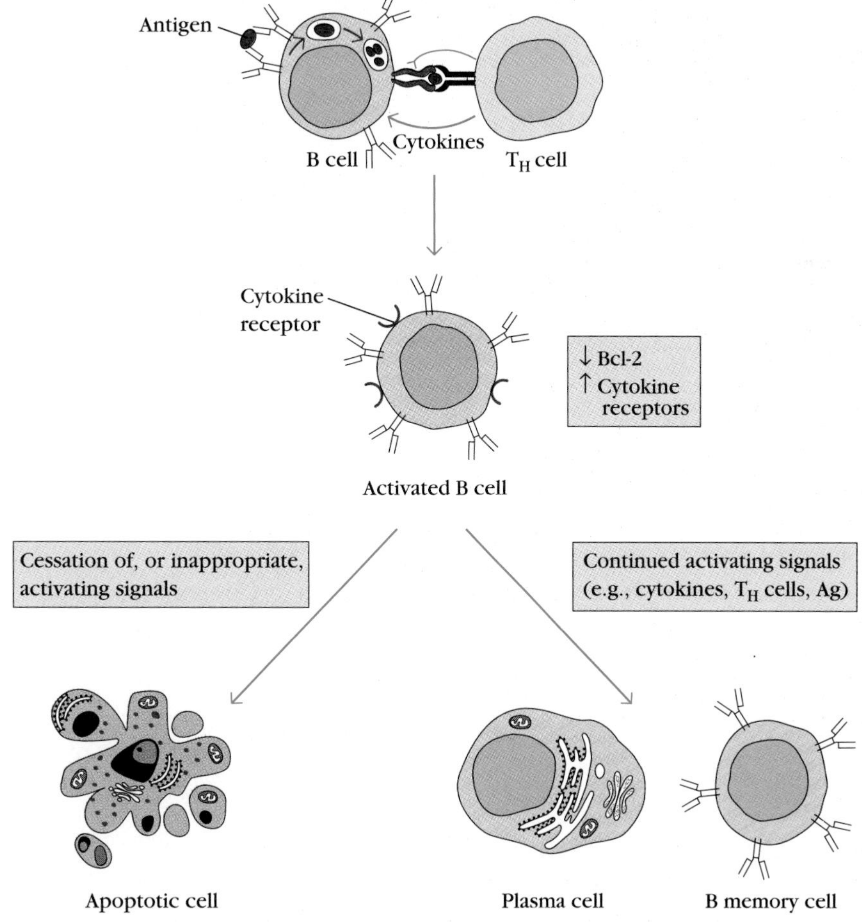

FIGURE 2-5 Regulation of activated B-cell numbers by apoptosis. Activation of B cells induces increased expression of cytokine receptors and decreased expression of Bcl-2. Because Bcl-2 prevents apoptosis, its reduced level in activated B cells is an important factor in increasing their susceptibility to programmed cell death over the susceptibility of naive or memory B cells. A reduction in activating signals quickly leads to destruction of excess activated B cells by apoptosis. Similar processes occur in T cells.

Enrichment of Hematopoietic Stem Cells

I. L. Weissman and colleagues developed a novel way of enriching the concentration of mouse pluripotent stem cells, which normally constitute less than 0.05% of all bone marrow cells in mice. Their approach relied on the use of antibodies specific for molecules known as **differentiation antigens,** which are expressed only by particular cell types. They exposed bone-marrow samples to the antibodies, which had been labeled with a fluorescent compound and were specific for the differentiation antigens expressed on the surface of mature red and white blood cells (Figure 2-6). The labeled cells were then removed by flow cytometry with a fluorescence-activated cell sorter (see Chapter 6). After each sorting, the remaining cells were assayed to determine the number needed for restoration of hematopoiesis in a lethally x-irradiated mouse. As the pluripotent stem cells were becoming relatively more numerous in the remaining population, fewer and fewer cells were needed to restore hematopoiesis in this system. Because stem cells do not express differentiation antigens known to be on developing and mature hematopoietic cells, by removing those hematopoietic cells that express known differentiation antigens, these investigators were able to obtain a 50- to 200-fold enrichment of pluripotent stem cells. To further enrich the pluripo-

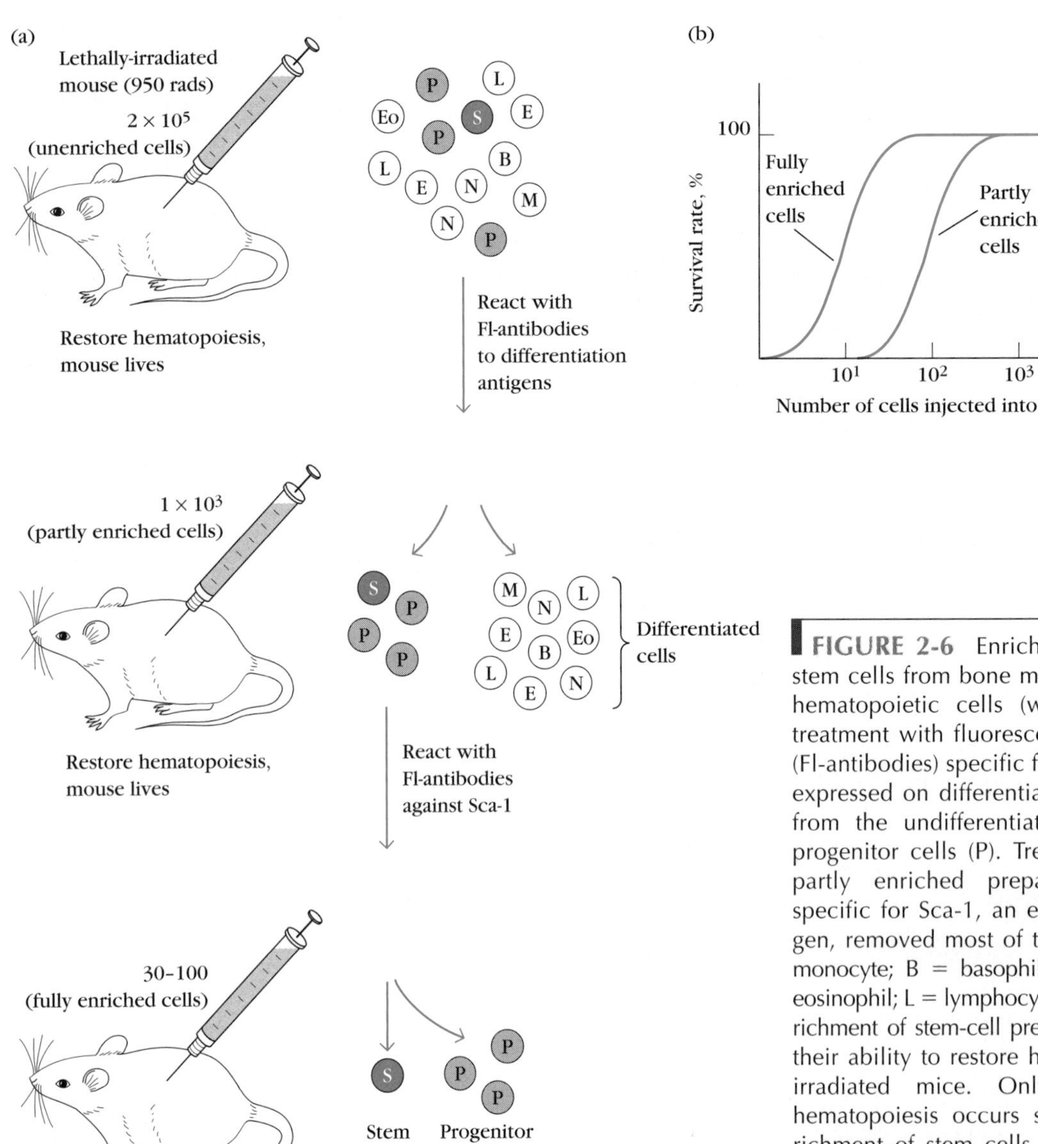

FIGURE 2-6 Enrichment of the pluripotent stem cells from bone marrow. (a) Differentiated hematopoietic cells (white) are removed by treatment with fluorescently labeled antibodies (Fl-antibodies) specific for membrane molecules expressed on differentiated lineages but absent from the undifferentiated stem cells (S) and progenitor cells (P). Treatment of the resulting partly enriched preparation with antibody specific for Sca-1, an early differentiation antigen, removed most of the progenitor cells. M = monocyte; B = basophil; N = neutrophil; Eo = eosinophil; L = lymphocyte; E = erythrocyte. (b) Enrichment of stem-cell preparations is measured by their ability to restore hematopoiesis in lethally irradiated mice. Only animals in which hematopoiesis occurs survive. Progressive enrichment of stem cells is indicated by the decrease in the number of injected cells needed to restore hematopoiesis. A total enrichment of about 1000-fold is possible by this procedure.

tent stem cell, the remaining cells were incubated with various antibodies raised against cells likely to be in the early stages of hematopoiesis. One of these antibodies recognized a differentiation antigen called stem-cell antigen 1 (Sca-1). Treatment with this antibody aided capture of undifferentiated stem cells and yielded a preparation so enriched in pluripotent stem cells that an aliquot containing only 30–100 cells could restore hematopoiesis in a lethally x-irradiated mouse, whereas more than 10^4 nonenriched bone marrow cells were needed for restoration.

It has been found that CD34, a marker found on about 1% of hematopoietic cells, while not actually unique to stem cells, is found on a small population of cells that contains stem cells. Using this marker that is associated with stem cell populations, it has become possible to routinely enrich preparations of human stem cells. The administration of human-cell populations suitably enriched for $CD34^+$ cells can reconstitute a patient's entire hematopoietic system (see Clinical Focus).

One of the obstacles to identifying and characterizing the human pluripotent stem cell is the lack of an in-vivo assay system comparable to the irradiated mouse. One experimental system that is being used to study the human pluripotent stem cell is the **SCID (severe combined immunodeficiency) mouse.** SCID mice do not have B and T lymphocytes and are unable to mount adaptive immune responses such as those that act in the normal rejection of foreign tissues and organs. Consequently, these animals do not reject transplanted human tissues such as thymus and bone marrow (see Chapter 23). SCID mice implanted with fragments of human thymus and bone marrow support the differentiation of pluripotent human hematopoietic stem cells into mature hematopoietic cells. Different subpopulations of $CD34^+$ human bone-marrow cells are injected into these SCID-human mice, and the development of various lineages of human cells in the bone-marrow fragment is subsequently assessed. In the absence of human growth factors, only low numbers of granulocyte-macrophage progenitors develop. However, when human IL-3, GM-CSF, erythropoietin, and mast-cell growth factor are administered along with $CD34^+$ cells, progenitor and mature cells of the myeloid, lymphoid, and erythroid lineages develop. This system has enabled the study of subpopulations of $CD34^+$ cells and the effect of human growth factors on the differentiation of various hematopoietic lineages.

Cells of the Immune System

Lymphocytes are the central cells of the immune system, responsible for acquired immunity and the immunologic attributes of diversity, specificity, memory, and self/nonself recognition. The other types of white blood cells play important but often ancillary roles, engulfing and destroying microorganisms, presenting antigens, and secreting cytokines.

Lymphoid Cells

Lymphocytes constitute 20%–40% of the body's white blood cells and 99% of the cells in the lymph (Table 2-3). There are approximately 10^{11} (range depending on body size and age: $\sim 10^{10}-10^{12}$) lymphocytes in the human body. These lymphocytes continually circulate in the blood and lymph and are capable of migrating into the tissue spaces and lymphoid organs, thereby integrating the immune system to a high degree.

The lymphocytes can be broadly subdivided into three populations—B cells, T cells, and null cells—on the basis of function and cell-membrane components. The null population of lymphocytes does not express surface markers typical of B or T cells. It consists mostly of large, granular lymphocytes which are the **natural killer cells (NK cells).** Resting B and T lymphocytes are small, motile, nonphagocytic cells, which cannot be distinguished morphologically. B and T lymphocytes that have not interacted with antigen—referred to as **naive,** or unprimed—are resting cells in the G_0 phase of the cell cycle. Known as small lymphocytes, these cells are only about 6μm in diameter; their cytoplasm forms a barely discernible rim around the nucleus. Small lymphocytes have densely packed chromatin, few mitochondria, and a poorly developed endoplasmic reticulum and Golgi apparatus. The naive lymphocyte is generally thought to have a short life span. Interaction of small lymphocytes with antigen, in the presence of certain cytokines discussed later, induces these cells to enter the cell cycle by progressing from G_0 into G_1 and subsequently into S, G_2, and M (Figure 2-7a). As they progress through the cell cycle, lymphocytes enlarge into 15-μm-diameter blast cells, called **lymphoblasts;** these cells have a higher cytoplasm:nucleus ratio and more organellar complexity than small lymphocytes (Figure 2-7b).

TABLE 2-3 NORMAL ADULT BLOOD-CELL COUNTS

Cell type	Cells/mm^3	%
Red blood cells	5.0×10^6	
Platelets	2.5×10^5	
Leukocytes	7.3×10^3	
Neutrophil		50–70
Lymphocyte		20–40
Monocyte		1–6
Eosinophil		1–3
Basophil		<1

Go to www.whfreeman.com/immunology Animation
Cells and Organs of the Immune System

(a)

Effector cell G_0
(i.e., plasma cell)
Memory cell G_0
Small, naive
B lymphocyte
G_0
Antigen activation
Early G_1
(gene activation)
Cell division
M
G_2
Lymphoblast S
(DNA synthesis)
Late G_1
(gene activation)

(b)

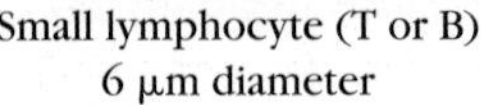

Small lymphocyte (T or B)
6 μm diameter

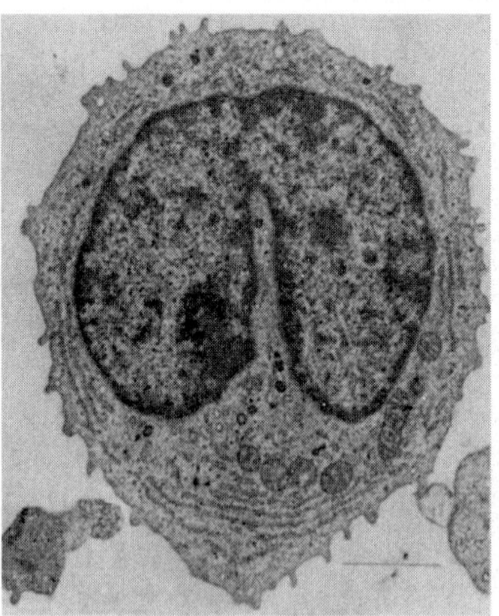

Blast cell (T or B)
15 μm diameter

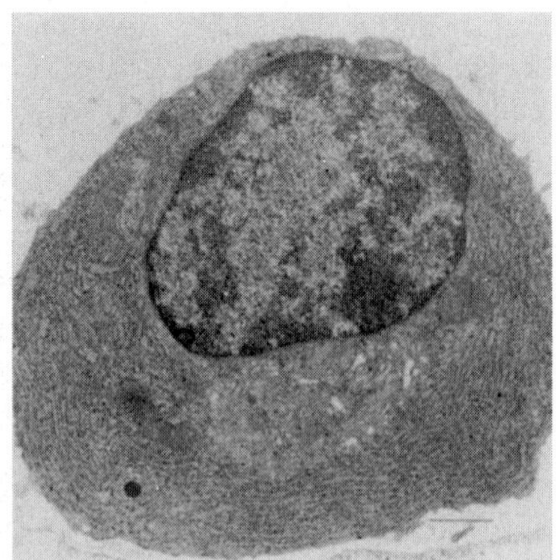

Plasma cell (B)
15 μm diameter

FIGURE 2-7 Fate of antigen-activated small lymphocytes. (a) A small resting (unprimed or naive) lymphocyte resides in the G_0 phase of the cell cycle. At this stage, B and T lymphocytes cannot be distinguished morphologically. After antigen activation, a B or T cell enters the cell cycle and enlarges into a lymphoblast, which undergoes several rounds of cell division and, eventually, generates effector cells and memory cells. Shown here are cells of the B-cell lineage. (b) Electron micrographs of a small lymphocyte (*left*) showing condensed chromatin indicative of a resting cell, an enlarged lymphoblast (*center*) showing decondensed chromatin, and a plasma cell (*right*) showing abundant endoplasmic reticulum arranged in concentric circle and a prominent nucleus that has been pushed to a characteristically eccentric position. The three cells are shown at different magnifications. [Part (b) courtesy of Dr. JR Goodman, Dept. of Pediatrics, University of California at San Francisco.]

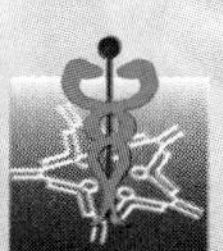

CLINICAL FOCUS

CLINICAL USES OF HEMATOPOIETIC STEM CELLS

The transplantation of hematopoietic stem cells (HSCs) is an important therapy for patients whose hematopoietic systems must be replaced. It has three major applications:

1. Providing a functional immune system to individuals with a genetically determined immunodeficiency, such as severe combined immunodeficiency (SCID).
2. Replacing a defective hematopoietic system with a functional one to cure some patients who have a life-threatening nonmalignant genetic disorder in hematopoiesis, such as sickle-cell anemia or thalassemia.
3. Restoring the hematopoietic system of cancer patients after treatment with doses of chemotherapeutic agents and radiation so high they destroy the system. These high-dose regimens can be much more effective at killing tumor cells than are therapies that use more conventional doses of cytotoxic agents. Stem-cell transplantation makes it possible to recover from such drastic treatment, so this technique is most frequently used in the treatment of cancer. Also, certain cancers, such as some cases of acute myeloid leukemia, can be cured only by destroying the patient's own hematopoietic system, which is the source of the leukemia cells.

Restoration of the hematopoietic system by transplanting stem cells is facilitated by several important technical considerations. First, HSCs have extraordinary powers of regeneration. Experiments in mice indicate that only a few—perhaps, on occasion, a single HSC—can completely restore the erythroid population and the immune system. In humans it is necessary to administer no more than 10% of a donor's bone marrow to provide enough HSCs to completely restore the hematopoietic system. Once injected into a vein, HSCs enter the circulation and find their own way to the bone marrow, where they begin the process of engraftment. There is no need for a surgeon to directly inject the cells into bones. In addition, HSCs can be preserved by freezing. This means that hematopoietic cells can be "banked." After collection, the cells are treated with a cryopreservative, frozen, and then stored for later use. When needed, the frozen preparation is thawed and infused into the patient, where it reconstitutes the hematopoietic system. This cell-freezing technology even makes it possible for individuals to store hematopoietic cells for transplantation to themselves at a later time. Currently, this procedure is used to allow cancer patients to donate cells before undergoing chemotherapy and radiation treatments and then to reconstitute their hematopoietic system from their own stem cells. Hematopoietic stem cells are found in cell populations that display distinctive surface antigens. One of these antigens is CD34, which is present on only a small percentage (~1%) of the cells in adult bone marrow. An antibody specific for CD34 is used to select cells displaying this antigen, producing a population enriched in $CD34^+$ stem cells. Various versions of this selection procedure have been used to enrich populations of stem cells from a variety of sources.

Transplantation of stem cell populations may be **autologous** (the recipient is also the donor), **syngeneic** (the donor is the identical twin of the recipient) or **allogeneic** (the donor and recipient are not genetically identical). In any transplantation procedure, genetic differences between donor and recipient can lead to immune-based rejection reactions. Aside from host rejection of transplanted tissue (host versus graft), lymphocytes in the graft can attack the recipient's tissues, thereby causing **graft-versus-host disease (GVHD).** In order to suppress rejection reactions, powerful immunosuppressive drugs must be used. Unfortunately, these drugs have serious side effects, and immunosuppression increases the patient's risk of infection and further growth of tumors. Consequently, HSC transplantation has fewest complications when there is genetic identity between donor and recipient.

Until recently, bone-marrow transplantation has been the usual way of restoring the hematopoietic system. However, the essential element of bone-marrow transplantation is stem-cell transplantation, and significant numbers of stem cells can be obtained from other tissues, such as peripheral blood and umbilical-cord blood ("cord blood"). These alternative sources of HSCs are attractive because the donor does not have to undergo anesthesia and an invasive procedure that extracts bone marrow. Many in the transplantation community believe that peripheral blood will replace marrow as the major source of hematopoietic stem cells for many applications. To obtain HSC-enriched preparations from peripheral blood, agents are used to induce increased numbers of circulating HSCs, and then the HSC-containing fraction is separated from the plasma and red blood cells in a process called leukopheresis. If necessary, further purification can be done to remove T cells and to enrich the $CD34^+$ population.

(continued)

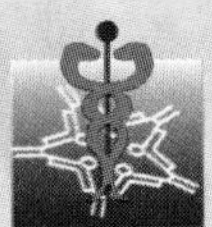

CLINICAL FOCUS (continued)

Umbilical cord blood, which already contains a significant number of stem cells, has also become a source of cells for HSC transplantation. Although HSCs from cord blood fail to engraft somewhat more often than do cells from peripheral blood, grafts of cord blood cells produce GVHD less frequently than do marrow grafts, probably because cord blood has fewer mature T cells.

Beyond its current applications in cancer treatment, many researchers feel that autologous stem-cell transplantation will be useful for gene therapy, the introduction of a normal gene to correct the disorder caused by a defective gene. Rapid advances in genetic engineering may soon make gene therapy a realistic treatment for genetic disorders of blood cells, and hematopoietic stem cells are attractive vehicles for such an approach. The therapy would entail removing a sample of hematopoietic stem cells from a patient, inserting a functional gene to compensate for the defective one, and then reinjecting the engineered stem cells into the donor. The advantage of using stem cells in gene therapy is that they are self-renewing. Consequently, at least in theory, patients would have to receive only a single injection of engineered stem cells. In contrast, gene therapy with engineered mature lymphocytes or other blood cells would require periodic injections because these cells are not capable of self renewal.

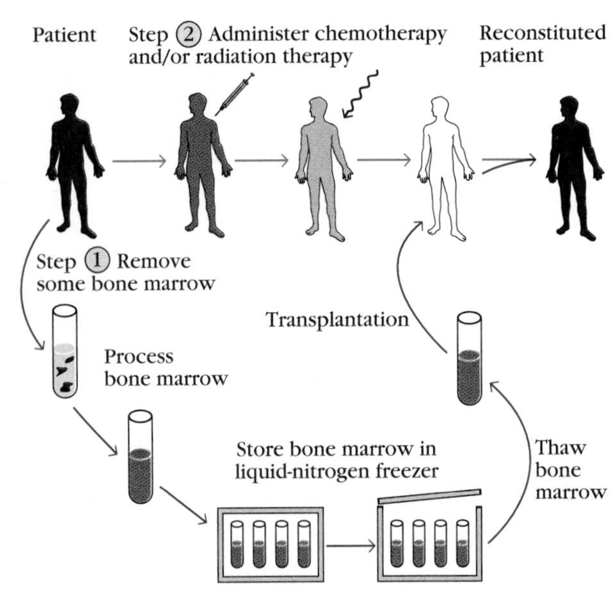

Bone marrow can be used to reconstitute the hematopoietic system of cancer patients whose stem cells and other hematopoietic cells have been killed by radiation and/or chemotherapy. In this procedure, some bone marrow is removed from the patient before treatment, stored, and reinfused at a later time.

Lymphoblasts proliferate and eventually differentiate into **effector cells** or into **memory cells.** Effector cells function in various ways to eliminate the antigen. These cells have short life spans, generally ranging from a few days to a few weeks. **Plasma cells**—the antibody-secreting effector cells of the B-cell lineage—have a characteristic cytoplasm that contains abundant endoplasmic reticulum (to support their high rate of protein synthesis) arranged in concentric layers and also many Golgi vesicles (see Figure 2-7). The effector cells of the T-cell lineage include the cytokine-secreting T helper cell (T_H cell) and the cytotoxic T lymphocyte (T_C or, sometimes, CTL). Some of the progeny of B and T lymphoblasts differentiate into memory cells. The persistence of this population of cells is responsible for life-long immunity to many pathogens. Memory cells look like small lymphocytes but can be distinguished from naive cells by the presence or absence of certain cell-membrane molecules.

Different lineages or maturational stages of lymphocytes can be distinguished by their expression of membrane molecules recognized by particular monoclonal antibodies (antibodies that are specific for a single epitope of an antigen; see Chapter 4 for a description of monoclonal antibodies). All of the monoclonal antibodies that react with a particular membrane molecule are grouped together as a **cluster of differentiation (CD).** Each new monoclonal antibody that recognizes a leukocyte membrane molecule is analyzed

TABLE 2-4 COMMON CD ANTIGENS USED TO DISTINGUISH FUNCTIONAL LYMPHOCYTE SUBPOPULATIONS

CD designation*	Function	B cell	T cell		NK cell
			T_H	T_C	
CD2	Adhesion molecule; signal transduction	−	+	+	+
CD3	Signal-transduction element of T-cell receptor	−	+	+	−
CD4	Adhesion molecule that binds to class II MHC molecules; signal transduction	−	+ (usually)	− (usually)	−
CD5	Unknown	+	+ (subset)	+	−
CD8	Adhesion molecule that binds to class I MHC molecules; signal transduction	−	− (usually)	+ (usually)	+ (variable)
CD16 (FcγRIII)	Low-affinity receptor for Fc region of IgG	−	−	−	+
CD21 (CR2)	Receptor for complement (C3d) and Epstein-Barr virus	+	−	−	−
CD28	Receptor for co-stimulatory B7 molecule on antigen-presenting cells	−	+	+	−
CD32 (FcγRII)	Receptor for Fc region of IgG	+	−	−	−
CD35 (CR1)	Receptor for complement (C3b)	+	−	−	−
CD40	Signal transduction	+	−	−	−
CD45	Signal transduction	+	+	+	+
CD56	Adhesion molecule	−	−	−	+

*Synonyms are shown in parentheses.

for whether it falls within a recognized CD designation; if it does not, it is given a new CD designation reflecting a new membrane molecule. Although the CD nomenclature was originally developed for the membrane molecules of human leukocytes, the homologous membrane molecules of other species, such as mice, are commonly referred to by the same CD designations. Table 2-4 lists some common CD molecules (often referred to as CD markers) found on human lymphocytes. However, this is only a partial listing of the more than 150 CD markers that have been described. A complete list and description of known CD markers is in the appendix at the end of this book.

The general characteristics and functions of B and T lymphocytes were described in Chapter 1 and are reviewed briefly in the next sections. These central cells of the immune system will be examined in more detail in later chapters.

B Lymphocytes

The B lymphocyte derived its letter designation from its site of maturation, in the *b*ursa of Fabricius in birds; the name turned out to be apt, for *b*one marrow is its major site of maturation in a number of mammalian species, including humans and mice. Mature B cells are definitively distinguished from other lymphocytes by their synthesis and display of membrane-bound immunoglobulin (antibody) molecules, which serve as receptors for antigen. Each of the approximately 1.5×10^5 molecules of antibody on the membrane of a single B cell has an identical binding site for antigen. Among the other molecules expressed on the membrane of mature B cells are the following:

- **B220** (a form of CD45, CD45R) is frequently used as a marker for B cells and their precursors. However, unlike antibody, it is not found uniquely on B-lineage cells.
- **Class II MHC molecules** permit the B cell to function as an antigen-presenting cell (APC).
- **CR1** (CD35) and **CR2** (CD21) are receptors for certain complement products.
- **FcγRII** (CD32) is a receptor for IgG, a type of antibody.
- **B7-1** (CD80) and **B7-2** (CD86) are molecules that interact with CD28 and CTLA-4, important regulatory molecules on the surface of different types of T cells, including T_H cells.
- **CD40** is a molecule that interacts with CD40 ligand on the surface of helper T cells. In most cases this interaction is critical for the survival of antigen-stimulated B cells and for their development into antibody-secreting plasma cells or memory B cells.

Interaction between antigen and the membrane-bound antibody on a mature naive B cell, as well as interactions with T-cells and macrophages, selectively induces the activation and differentiation of B-cell clones of corresponding specificity. In this process, the B cell divides repeatedly and differentiates over a 4- to 5-day period, generating a population of plasma cells and memory cells. Plasma cells, which lack membrane-bound antibody, synthesize and secrete one of the five classes of antibody. All clonal progeny from a given B cell secrete antibody molecules with the same antigen-binding specificity. Plasma cells are terminally differentiated cells, and many die in 1 or 2 weeks.

T Lymphocytes

T lymphocytes derive their name from their site of maturation in the *t*hymus. Like B lymphocytes, these cells have membrane receptors for antigen. Although the antigen-binding T-cell receptor is structurally distinct from immunoglobulin, it does share some common structural features with the immunoglobulin molecule, most notably in the structure of its antigen-binding site. Unlike the membrane-bound antibody on B cells, though, the T-cell receptor (TCR) does not recognize free antigen. Instead the TCR recognizes only antigen that is bound to particular classes of self-molecules. Most T cells recognize antigen only when it is bound to a self-molecule encoded by genes within the major histocompatibility complex (MHC). Thus, as explained in Chapter 1, a fundamental difference between the humoral and cell-mediated branches of the immune system is that the B cell is capable of binding soluble antigen, whereas the T cell is restricted to binding antigen displayed on self-cells. To be recognized by most T cells, this antigen must be displayed together with MHC molecules on the surface of antigen-presenting cells or on virus-infected cells, cancer cells, and grafts. The T-cell system has developed to eliminate these altered self-cells, which pose a threat to the normal functioning of the body.

Like B cells, T cells express distinctive membrane molecules. All T-cell subpopulations express the T-cell receptor, a complex of polypeptides that includes CD3; and most can be distinguished by the presence of one or the other of two membrane molecules, CD4 and CD8. In addition, most mature T cells express the following membrane molecules:

- **CD28,** a receptor for the co-stimulatory B7 family of molecules present on B cells and other antigen-presenting cells
- **CD45,** a signal-transduction molecule

T cells that express the membrane glycoprotein molecule CD4 are restricted to recognizing antigen bound to class II MHC molecules, whereas T cells expressing CD8, a dimeric membrane glycoprotein, are restricted to recognition of antigen bound to class I MHC molecules. Thus the expression of CD4 versus CD8 corresponds to the MHC restriction of the T cell. In general, expression of CD4 and of CD8 also defines two major functional subpopulations of T lymphocytes. $CD4^+$ T cells generally function as T helper (T_H) cells and are class-II restricted; $CD8^+$ T cells generally function as T cytotoxic (T_C) cells and are class-I restricted. Thus the ratio of T_H to T_C cells in a sample can be approximated by assaying the number of $CD4^+$ and $CD8^+$ T cells. This ratio is approximately 2:1 in normal human peripheral blood, but it may be significantly altered by immunodeficiency diseases, autoimmune diseases, and other disorders.

The classification of $CD4^+$, class II–restricted cells as T_H cells and $CD8^+$, class I–restricted cells as T_C cells is not absolute. Some $CD4^+$ cells can act as killer cells. Also, some T_C cells have been shown to secrete a variety of cytokines and exert an effect on other cells comparable to that exerted by T_H cells. The distinction between T_H and T_C cells, then, is not always clear; there can be ambiguous functional activities. However, because these ambiguities are the exception and not the rule, the generalization of T helper (T_H) cells as being $CD4^+$ and class-II restricted and of T cytotoxic cells (T_C) as being $CD8^+$ and class-I restricted is assumed throughout this text, unless otherwise specified.

T_H cells are activated by recognition of an antigen–class II MHC complex on an antigen-presenting cell. After activation, the T_H cell begins to divide and gives rise to a clone of effector cells, each specific for the same antigen–class II MHC complex. These T_H cells secrete various cytokines, which play a central role in the activation of B cells, T cells, and other cells that participate in the immune response. Changes in the pattern of cytokines produced by T_H cells can change the type of immune response that develops among other leukocytes. The **T_H1 response** produces a cytokine profile that supports inflammation and activates mainly certain T cells and macrophages, whereas the **T_H2 response** activates mainly B cells and immune responses that depend upon antibodies.

T_C cells are activated when they interact with an antigen–class I MHC complex on the surface of an altered self-cell (e.g., a virus-infected cell or a tumor cell) in the presence of appropriate cytokines. This activation, which results in proliferation, causes the T_C cell to differentiate into an effector cell called a **cytotoxic T lymphocyte (CTL).** In contrast to T_H cells, most CTLs secrete few cytokines. Instead, CTLs acquire the ability to recognize and eliminate altered self-cells.

Another subpopulation of T lymphocytes—called **T suppressor (T_S) cells**—has been postulated. It is clear that some T cells help to suppress the humoral and the cell-mediated branches of the immune system, but the actual isolation and cloning of normal T_S cells is a matter of controversy and dispute among immunologists. For this reason, it is uncertain whether T_S cells do indeed constitute a separate functional subpopulation of T cells. Some immunologists believe that the suppression mediated by T cells observed in some systems is simply the consequence of activities of T_H or T_C subpopulations whose end results are suppressive.

Null Cells

A small group of lymphocytes, called **null cells,** in the peripheral blood do not express the membrane molecules and receptors that distinguish T- and B-cell lineages. These cells also fail to synthesize immunoglobulin and incorporate it into their plasma membrane. Because these cells do not produce antigen-binding receptors, they lack precise immunologic specificity and memory. Most members of the null cell population are large, granular lymphocytes called natural killer (NK) cells: these cells constitute 5%–10% of the lymphocytes in human peripheral blood.

The natural killer cell was first described in 1976, when it was shown that certain null cells display cytotoxic activity against a wide range of tumor cells in the absence of any previous immunization with the tumor. NK cells were subsequently shown to play an important role in host defense both against tumor cells and against cells infected with some, though not all, viruses. NK cells can recognize potential target cells in two different ways. In some cases, an NK cell employs NK cell receptors to distinguish abnormalities, notably a reduction in the display of class I MHC molecules and the unusual profile of surface antigens displayed by some tumor cells and cells infected by some viruses. Another way in which NK cells recognize potential target cells depends upon the fact that some tumor cells and cells infected by certain viruses display antigens against which the immune system has made an antibody response, so that antitumor or antiviral antibodies are bound to their surfaces. Because NK cells express CD16, a membrane receptor for the carboxyl-terminal end of the IgG molecule, called the Fc region, they can attach to these antibodies and subsequently destroy the targeted cells. This is an example of a process known as **antibody-dependent cell-mediated cytotoxicity (ADCC).** The exact mechanism of NK-cell cytotoxicity, the focus of much current experimental study, is described further in Chapter 14.

Several observations suggest that NK cells play an important role in host defense against tumors. For example, in humans the **Chediak-Higashi syndrome**—an autosomal recessive disorder—is associated with impairment in neutrophils, macrophages, and NK cells and an increased incidence of lymphomas. Likewise, mice with an autosomal mutation called *beige* lack NK cells; these mutants are more susceptible than normal mice to tumor growth following injection with live tumor cells.

There has been growing recognition of a cell type, the **NK1-T cell,** that has some of the characteristics of both T cells and NK cells. Like T cells, NK1-T cells have T cell receptors (TCRs). Unlike most T cells, the TCRs of NK1-T cells interact with MHC-like molecules called CD1 rather than with class I or class II MHC molecules. Like NK cells, they have variable levels of CD16 and other receptors typical of NK cells, and they can kill cells. A population of triggered NK1-T cells can rapidly secrete large amounts of the cytokines needed to support antibody production by B cells as well as inflammation and the development and expansion of cytotoxic T cells. Some immunologists view this cell type as a kind of rapid response system that has evolved to provide early help while conventional T_H-cell responses are still developing.

Mononuclear Cells

The mononuclear phagocytic system consists of **monocytes** circulating in the blood and **macrophages** in the tissues (Figure 2-8). During hematopoiesis in the bone marrow, granulocyte-monocyte progenitor cells differentiate into promonocytes, which leave the bone marrow and enter the blood, where they further differentiate into mature monocytes. Monocytes circulate in the bloodstream for about 8 h, during which time they enlarge; they then migrate into the tissues and differentiate into specific tissue macrophages.

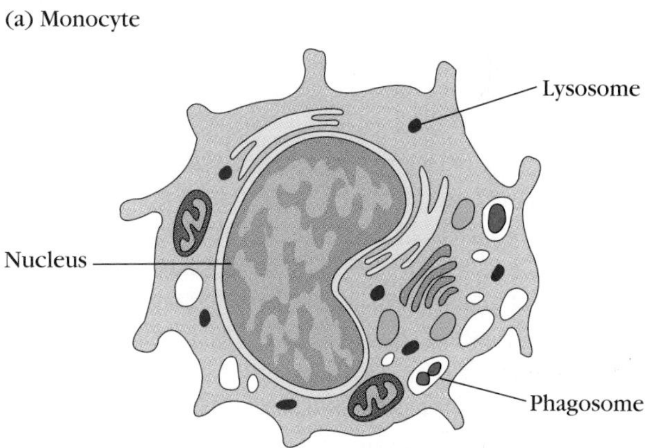

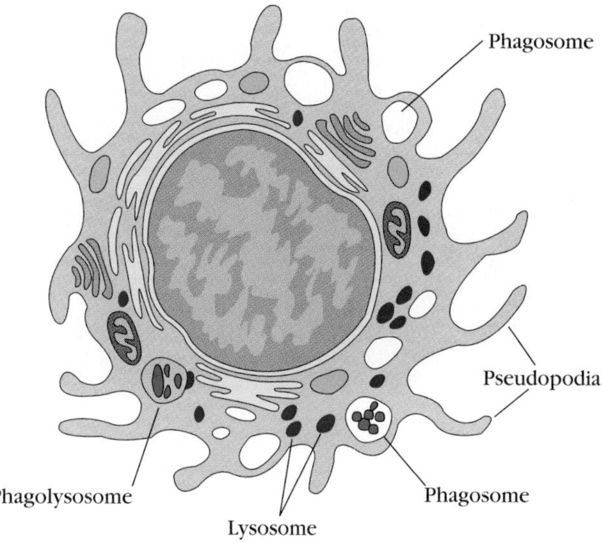

FIGURE 2-8 Typical morphology of a monocyte and a macrophage. Macrophages are five- to tenfold larger than monocytes and contain more organelles, especially lysosomes.

Differentiation of a monocyte into a tissue macrophage involves a number of changes: The cell enlarges five- to tenfold; its intracellular organelles increase in both number and complexity; and it acquires increased phagocytic ability, produces higher levels of hydrolytic enzymes, and begins to secrete a variety of soluble factors. Macrophages are dispersed throughout the body. Some take up residence in particular tissues, becoming fixed macrophages, whereas others remain motile and are called free, or wandering, macrophages. Free macrophages travel by amoeboid movement throughout the tissues. Macrophage-like cells serve different functions in different tissues and are named according to their tissue location:

- **Alveolar macrophages** in the lung
- **Histiocytes** in connective tissues
- **Kupffer cells** in the liver
- **Mesangial cells** in the kidney
- **Microglial cells** in the brain
- **Osteoclasts** in bone

Although normally in a resting state, macrophages are activated by a variety of stimuli in the course of an immune response. Phagocytosis of particulate antigens serves as an initial activating stimulus. However, macrophage activity can be further enhanced by cytokines secreted by activated T_H cells, by mediators of the inflammatory response, and by components of bacterial cell walls. One of the most potent activators of macrophages is interferon gamma (IFN-γ) secreted by activated T_H cells.

Activated macrophages are more effective than resting ones in eliminating potential pathogens, because they exhibit greater phagocytic activity, an increased ability to kill ingested microbes, increased secretion of inflammatory mediators, and an increased ability to activate T cells. In addition, activated macrophages, but not resting ones, secrete various cytotoxic proteins that help them eliminate a broad range of pathogens, including virus-infected cells, tumor cells, and intracellular bacteria. Activated macrophages also express higher levels of class II MHC molecules, allowing them to function more effectively as antigen-presenting cells. Thus, macrophages and T_H cells during the immune response facilitate each other's activation.

Phagocytosis

Macrophages are capable of ingesting and digesting exogenous antigens, such as whole microorganisms and insoluble particles, and endogenous matter, such as injured or dead host cells, cellular debris, and activated clotting factors. In the first step in phagocytosis, macrophages are attracted by and move toward a variety of substances generated in an immune response; this process is called **chemotaxis.** The next step in phagocytosis is adherence of the antigen to the macrophage cell membrane. (Complex antigens, such as whole bacterial cells or viral particles, tend to adhere well and are readily phagocytosed; isolated proteins and encapsulated bacteria tend to adhere poorly and are less readily phagocytosed.) Adherence induces membrane protrusions, called **pseudopodia,** to extend around the attached material (Figure 2-9a). Fusion of the pseudopodia encloses the ma-

(a)

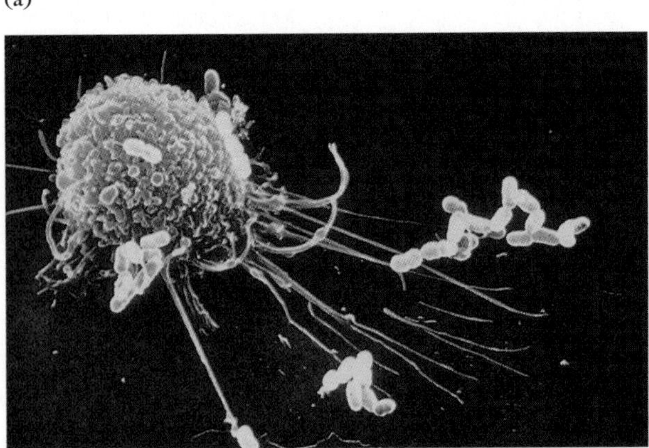

(b)

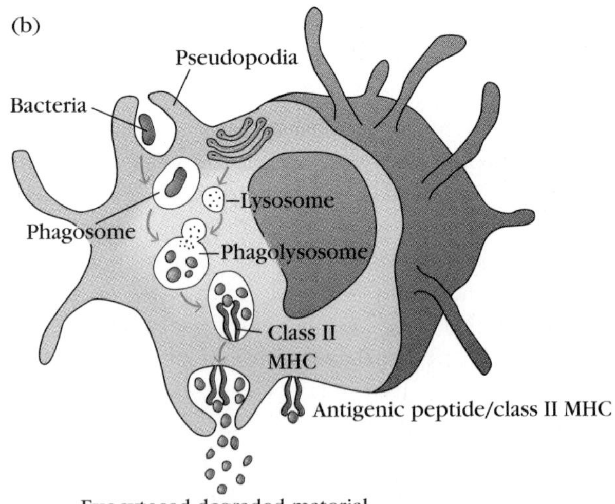

FIGURE 2-9 Macrophages can ingest and degrade particulate antigens, including bacteria. (a) Scanning electron micrograph of a macrophage. Note the long pseudopodia extending toward and making contact with bacterial cells, an early step in phagocytosis. (b) Phagocytosis and processing of exogenous antigen by macrophages. Most of the products resulting from digestion of ingested material are exocytosed, but some peptide products may interact with class II MHC molecules, forming complexes that move to the cell surface, where they are presented to T_H cells. [Photograph by L Nilsson; courtesy of Boehringer Ingelheim International GmbH.]

terial within a membrane-bounded structure called a **phagosome,** which then enters the endocytic processing pathway (Figure 2-9b). In this pathway, a phagosome moves toward the cell interior, where it fuses with a **lysosome** to form a **phagolysosome.** Lysosomes contain lysozyme and a variety of other hydrolytic enzymes, which digest the ingested material. The digested contents of the phagolysosome are then eliminated in a process called **exocytosis** (see Figure 2-9b).

The macrophage membrane has receptors for certain classes of antibody and certain complement components, both of which also can bind to antigen. If an antigen (e.g., a bacterium) is coated with the appropriate antibody or complement component, the antigen binds more readily to the macrophage membrane; as a result, phagocytosis is enhanced. In one study, for example, the rate of phagocytosis of an antigen was 4000-fold higher in the presence of specific antibody to the antigen than in its absence. Thus, antibody and complement function as **opsonins,** molecules that bind to both antigen and macrophages and enhance phagocytosis. The process by which particulate antigens are rendered more susceptible to phagocytosis is called **opsonization.**

Antimicrobial and Cytotoxic Activities

A number of antimicrobial and cytotoxic substances produced by activated macrophages can destroy phagocytosed microorganisms (Table 2-5). Many of the mediators of cytotoxicity listed in Table 2-5 are reactive forms of oxygen.

Oxygen-Dependent Killing Mechanisms Activated phagocytes produce a number of **reactive oxygen intermediates (ROIs)** and **reactive nitrogen intermediates** that have potent antimicrobial activity. During phagocytosis, a metabolic process known as the **respiratory burst** occurs in activated macrophages. This process results in the activation of a membrane-bound oxidase that catalyzes the reduction of oxygen to superoxide anion, a reactive oxygen intermediate that is extremely toxic to ingested microorganisms. The superoxide anion also generates other powerful oxidizing agents, including hydroxyl radicals and hydrogen peroxide. As the lysosome fuses with the phagosome, the activity of myeloperoxidase produces hypochlorite from hydrogen peroxide and chloride ions. Hypochlorite, the active agent of household bleach, is toxic to ingested microbes.

When macrophages are activated with bacterial cell-wall components such as lipopolysaccharide (LPS) or, in the case of mycobacteria, muramyl dipeptide (MDP), together with a T-cell–derived cytokine (IFN-γ), they begin to express high levels of **nitric oxide synthetase (NOS),** an enzyme that oxidizes L-arginine to yield L-citrulline and **nitric oxide (NO),** a gas:

$$\text{L-arginine} + O_2 + \text{NADPH} \longrightarrow \text{NO} + \text{L-citrulline} + \text{NADP}$$

Nitric oxide has potent antimicrobial activity; it also can combine with the superoxide anion to yield even more potent antimicrobial substances. Recent evidence suggests that much of the antimicrobial activity of macrophages against bacterial, fungal, helminthic, and protozoal pathogens is due to nitric oxide and substances derived from it.

Oxygen-Independent Killing Mechanisms Activated macrophages also synthesize **lysozyme** and various hydrolytic enzymes whose degradative activities do not require oxygen. In addition, activated macrophages produce a group of antimicrobial and cytotoxic peptides, commonly known as **defensins.** These molecules are cysteine-rich cationic peptides containing 29–35 amino-acid residues. Each peptide, which contains six invariant cysteines, forms a circular molecule that is stabilized by intramolecular disulfide bonds. These circularized defensin peptides have been shown to form ion-permeable channels in bacterial cell membranes. Defensins can kill a variety of bacteria, including *Staphylococcus aureus, Streptococcus pneumoniae, Escherichia coli, Pseudomonas aeruginosa,* and *Haemophilus influenzae.* Activated macrophages also secrete **tumor necrosis factor α (TNF-α)**, a cytokine that has a variety of effects and is cytotoxic for some tumor cells.

Resistant Pathogens Most phagocytosed microorganisms are killed by the lysosomal contents that are released into phagosomes. Some microorganisms, however, can survive and multiply within macrophages. These **intracellular pathogens** include *Listeria monocytogenes, Salmonella typhimurium, Neisseria gonorrhoeae, Mycobacterium avium, Mycobacterium tuberculosis, Mycobacterium leprae, Brucella abortus,* and *Candida albicans.*

TABLE 2-5 MEDIATORS OF ANTIMICROBIAL AND CYTOTOXIC ACTIVITY OF MACROPHAGES AND NEUTROPHILS

Oxygen-dependent killing	Oxygen-independent killing
Reactive oxygen intermediates	Defensins
$O_2^{\cdot-}$ (superoxide anion)	Tumor necrosis factor α (macrophage only)
$OH^{\cdot}$ (hydroxyl radicals)	Lysozyme
H_2O_2 (hydrogen peroxide)	Hydrolytic enzymes
ClO^- (hypochlorite anion)	
Reactive nitrogen intermediates	
NO (nitric oxide)	
NO_2 (nitrogen dioxide)	
HNO_2 (nitrous acid)	
Others	
NH_2Cl (monochloramine)	

Some intracellular pathogens prevent the fusion of lysosomes with phagosomes and proliferate within phagosomes; others have cell walls that are resistant to the contents of lysosomes; and still others survive by escaping from phagosomes and proliferating within the cytoplasm of infected macrophages. These intracellular pathogens, which have developed a clever defense against the nonspecific phagocytic defense system, are shielded from a specific immunologic response. A unique cell-mediated immunologic defense mechanism, called **delayed-type hypersensitivity (DTH),** combats such pathogens; this mechanism is described in Chapters 15 and 16.

Antigen Processing and Presentation

Although most of the antigen ingested by macrophages is degraded and eliminated, experiments with radiolabeled antigens have demonstrated the presence of antigen peptides on the macrophage membrane. As depicted in Figure 2-9b, phagocytosed antigen is digested within the endocytic processing pathway into peptides that associate with class II MHC molecules; these peptide–class II MHC complexes then move to the macrophage membrane. Activation of macrophages induces increased expression of both class II MHC molecules and the co-stimulatory B7 family of membrane molecules, thereby rendering the macrophages more effective in activating T_H cells. This processing and presentation of antigen, examined in detail in Chapter 8, are critical to T_H-cell activation, a central event in the development of both humoral and cell-mediated immune responses.

Secretion of Factors

A number of important proteins central to development of immune responses are secreted by activated macrophages (Table 2-6). These include a collection of cytokines, such as **interleukin 1 (IL-1),** TNF-α, and **interleukin 6 (IL-6),** that promote inflammatory responses. Typically, each of these agents has a variety of effects. For example, IL-1 activates lymphocytes; and IL-1, IL-6, and TNF-α promote fever by affecting the thermoregulatory center in the hypothalamus.

Activated macrophages secrete a variety of factors involved in the development of an inflammatory response. The **complement proteins** are a group of proteins that assist in eliminating foreign pathogens and in promoting the ensuing inflammatory reaction. The major site of synthesis of complement proteins is the liver, these proteins are also produced in macrophages outside this organ. The hydrolytic enzymes contained within the lysosomes of macrophages also can be secreted when the cells are activated. The buildup of these enzymes within the tissues contributes to the inflammatory response and can, in some cases, contribute to extensive tissue damage. Activated macrophages also secrete soluble factors, such as TNF-α, that can kill a variety of cells. The secretion of these cytotoxic factors has been shown to contribute to tumor destruction by macrophages. Finally, as mentioned earlier, activated macrophages secrete a number of cytokines that stimulate inducible hematopoiesis.

TABLE 2-6 SOME FACTORS SECRETED BY ACTIVATED MACROPHAGES

Factor	Function
Interleukin 1 (IL-1)	Promotes inflammatory responses and fever
Interleukin 6 (IL-6) TNF-α	Promote innate immunity and elimination of pathogens
Complement proteins	Promote inflammatory response and elimination of pathogens
Hydrolytic enzymes	Promote inflammatory response
Interferon alpha (IFN-α)	Activates cellular genes, resulting in the production of proteins that confer an antiviral state on the cell
Tumor necrosis factor (TNF-α)	Kills tumor cells
GM-CSF G-CSF M-CSF	Promote inducible hematopoiesis

Granulocytic Cells

The **granulocytes** are classified as neutrophils, eosinophils, or basophils on the basis of cellular morphology and cytoplasmic staining characteristics (Figure 2-10). The **neutrophil** has a multilobed nucleus and a granulated cytoplasm that stains with both acid and basic dyes; it is often called a polymorphonuclear leukocyte (PMN) for its multilobed nucleus. The **eosinophil** has a bilobed nucleus and a granulated cytoplasm that stains with the acid dye eosin red (hence its name). The **basophil** has a lobed nucleus and heavily granulated cytoplasm that stains with the basic dye methylene blue. Both neutrophils and eosinophils are phagocytic, whereas basophils are not. Neutrophils, which constitute 50%–70% of the circulating white blood cells, are much more numerous than eosinophils (1%–3%) or basophils (<1%).

Neutrophils

Neutrophils are produced by hematopoiesis in the bone marrow. They are released into the peripheral blood and circulate for 7–10 h before migrating into the tissues, where they have a life span of only a few days. In response to many types of infections, the bone marrow releases more than the usual number of neutrophils and these cells generally are the first

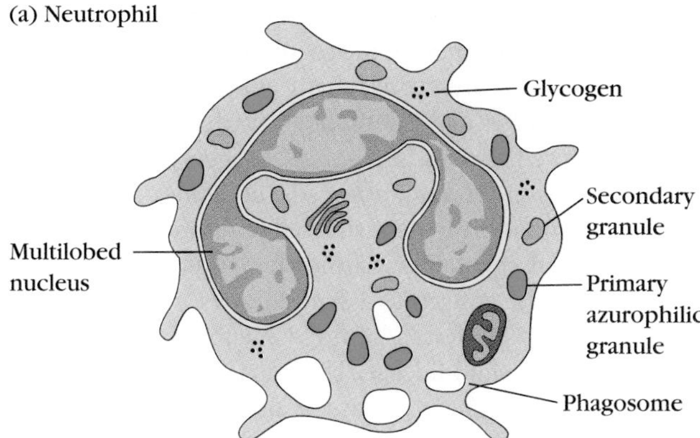

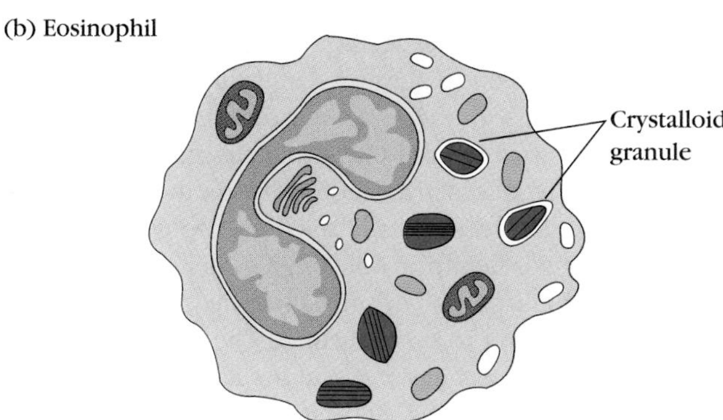

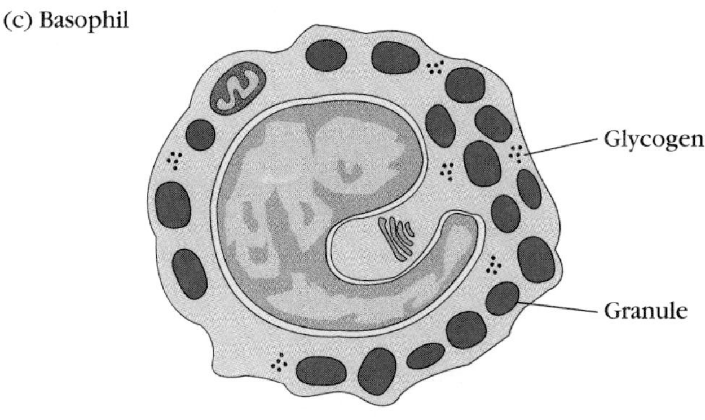

FIGURE 2-10 Drawings showing typical morphology of granulocytes. Note differences in the shape of the nucleus and in the number and shape of cytoplasmic granules.

to arrive at a site of inflammation. The resulting transient increase in the number of circulating neutrophils, called **leukocytosis,** is used medically as an indication of infection.

Movement of circulating neutrophils into tissues, called **extravasation,** takes several steps: the cell first adheres to the vascular endothelium, then penetrates the gap between adjacent endothelial cells lining the vessel wall, and finally penetrates the vascular basement membrane, moving out into the tissue spaces. (This process is described in detail in Chapter 15.) A number of substances generated in an inflammatory reaction serve as **chemotactic factors** that promote accumulation of neutrophils at an inflammatory site. Among these chemotactic factors are some of the complement components, components of the blood-clotting system, and several cytokines secreted by activated T_H cells and macrophages.

Like macrophages, neutrophils are active phagocytic cells. Phagocytosis by neutrophils is similar to that described for macrophages, except that the lytic enzymes and bactericidal substances in neutrophils are contained within primary and secondary granules (see Figure 2-10a). The larger, denser primary granules are a type of lysosome containing peroxidase, lysozyme, and various hydrolytic enzymes. The smaller secondary granules contain collagenase, lactoferrin, and lysozyme. Both primary and secondary granules fuse with phagosomes, whose contents are then digested and eliminated much as they are in macrophages.

Neutrophils also employ both oxygen-dependent and oxygen-independent pathways to generate antimicrobial substances. Neutrophils are in fact much more likely than macrophages to kill ingested microorganisms. Neutrophils exhibit a larger respiratory burst than macrophages and consequently are able to generate more reactive oxygen intermediates and reactive nitrogen intermediates (see Table 2-5). In addition, neutrophils express higher levels of defensins than macrophages do.

Eosinophils

Eosinophils, like neutrophils, are motile phagocytic cells that can migrate from the blood into the tissue spaces. Their phagocytic role is significantly less important than that of neutrophils, and it is thought that they play a role in the defense against parasitic organisms (see Chapter 16). The secreted contents of eosinophilic granules may damage the parasite membrane.

Basophils

Basophils are nonphagocytic granulocytes that function by releasing pharmacologically active substances from their cytoplasmic granules. These substances play a major role in certain allergic responses.

Mast Cells

Mast-cell precursors, which are formed in the bone marrow by hematopoiesis, are released into the blood as undifferentiated cells; they do not differentiate until they leave the blood and enter the tissues. Mast cells can be found in a wide variety of tissues, including the skin, connective tissues of various organs, and mucosal epithelial tissue of the respiratory, genitourinary, and digestive tracts. Like circulating basophils, these cells have large numbers of cytoplasmic granules that contain histamine and other pharmacologically active substances. Mast cells, together with blood basophils, play an important role in the development of allergies.

Dendritic Cells

The **dendritic cell** acquired its name because it is covered with a maze of long membrane extensions that resemble the dendrites of nerve cells. Dendritic cells can be difficult to isolate because the conventional procedures for cell isolation tend to damage their long extensions. The development of isolation techniques that employ enzymes and gentler dispersion has facilitated isolation of these cells for study in vitro.

Most dendritic cells process and present antigen to T_H cells. These cells can be classified by their location:

- **Langerhans cells** found in the epidermis (skin) and mucous membranes
- **Interstitial dendritic cells,** which populate most organs (e.g., heart, lungs, liver, kidney, gastrointestinal tract)
- **Interdigitating dendritic cells** present in T-cell areas of secondary lymphoid tissue and the thymic medulla
- **Circulating dendritic cells** include those in the blood, which constitute 0.1% of the blood leukocytes, and those in the lymph (known as **veiled cells**)

The dendritic cells in different locations have different forms and functions. Despite their differences, all of these dendritic cells constitutively express high levels of both class II MHC molecules and members of the co-stimulatory B7 family. For this reason, they are more potent antigen-presenting cells than macrophages and B cells, both of which need to be activated before they can function as antigen-presenting cells (APCs). After capturing antigen in the tissues by phagocytosis or by endocytosis, dendritic cells migrate into the blood or lymph and circulate to various lymphoid organs, where they present the antigen to T lymphocytes.

Dendritic cells descend from hematopoietic stem cells through the myeloid lineage. The exact developmental path or paths taken by these cells is still under investigation. The major issue is whether dendritic cells belong to the monocyte/macrophage lineage or develop from an entirely separate lineage. Two possible developmental pathways are shown in Figure 2-11. In one pathway, a dendritic cell develops from a myeloid precursor in the bone marrow, then appears in the blood as an immature cell that completes its differentiation in the tissues. An alternative model proposes that a late monocytic-stage cell differentiates in the tissues to generate either a macrophage or dendritic cell. Some evidence suggests that mature macrophages and dendritic cells may interconvert, although this has yet to be confirmed. The morphologic and functional differences observed among Langerhans cells and interstitial, interdigitating, and circulating dendritic cells is

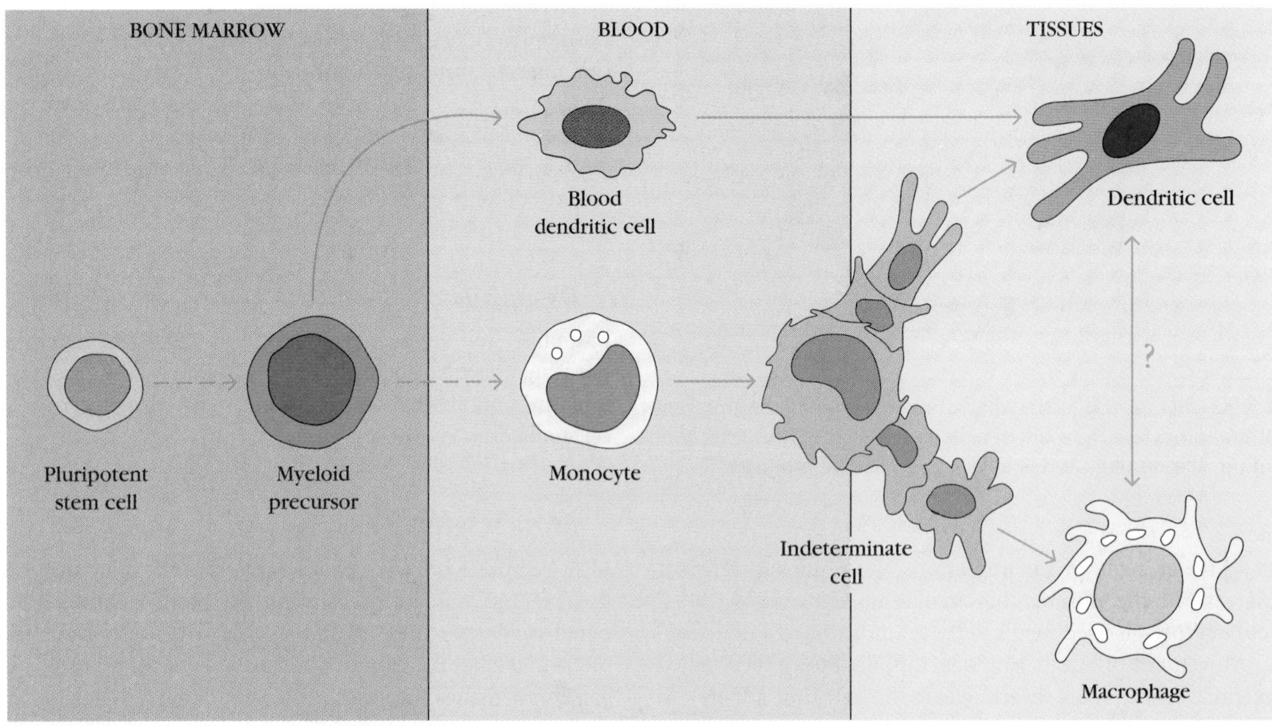

FIGURE 2-11 Two proposed pathways for development of dendritic cells (exclusive of follicular dendritic cells). The dendritic-cell lineage may branch from the monocyte/macrophage lineage at the myeloid precursor stage in the bone marrow. Alternatively, dendritic cells and macrophages may arise from a common late intermediate stage (indeterminate cell). The interconversion of mature dendritic cells and macrophages is suggested by some evidence but is still not confirmed. [Adapted from JH Peters et al, 1996, *Immunol. Today* **17**:273.]

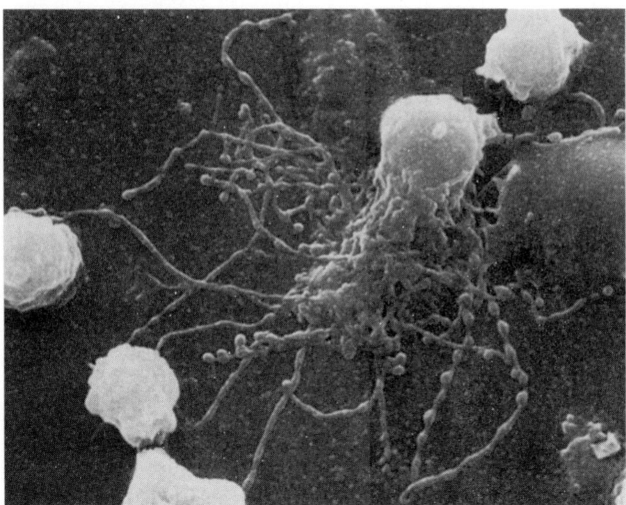

FIGURE 2-12 Scanning electron micrograph of follicular dendritic cells showing long, beaded dendrites. The beads are coated with antigen-antibody complexes. The dendrites emanate from the cell body. [From AK Szakal et al, 1985, *J. Immunol.* **134:**1353; American Association of Immunologists, reprinted with permission.]

thought to reflect different maturational states of the cells and the different microenvironments in which they reside.

Another type of dendritic cell, the **follicular dendritic cell,** appears to have a different origin and function from the antigen-presenting dendritic cells described above. Follicular dendritic cells do not express class II MHC molecules and therefore do not function as antigen-presenting cells for T_H-cell activation. These dendritic cells were named for their exclusive location in organized structures of the lymph node, called lymph follicles, which are rich in B cells. Although they do not express class II molecules, follicular dendritic cells express high levels of membrane receptors for antibody and complement. Binding of circulating antibody-antigen complexes by these receptors is thought to facilitate B-cell activation in lymph nodes. These complexes have been shown to be retained on the dendritic-cell membrane for very long periods of time, ranging from weeks to months or possibly even longer (Figure 2-12). The presence of antigen-antibody complexes on the membrane of follicular dendritic cells is thought to play a role in the development of memory B cells within the follicle.

Organs of the Immune System

A number of morphologically and functionally diverse organs and tissues have various functions in the development of immune responses. These can be distinguished by function as the **primary** and **secondary lymphoid organs** (Figure 2-13). The thymus and bone marrow are the primary (or central) lymphoid organs, where maturation of lymphocytes takes place. The lymph nodes, spleen, and various mucosal-associated lymphoid tissues (MALT) such as gut-associated lymphoid tissue (GALT) are the secondary (or peripheral) lymphoid organs, which trap antigen and provide sites for

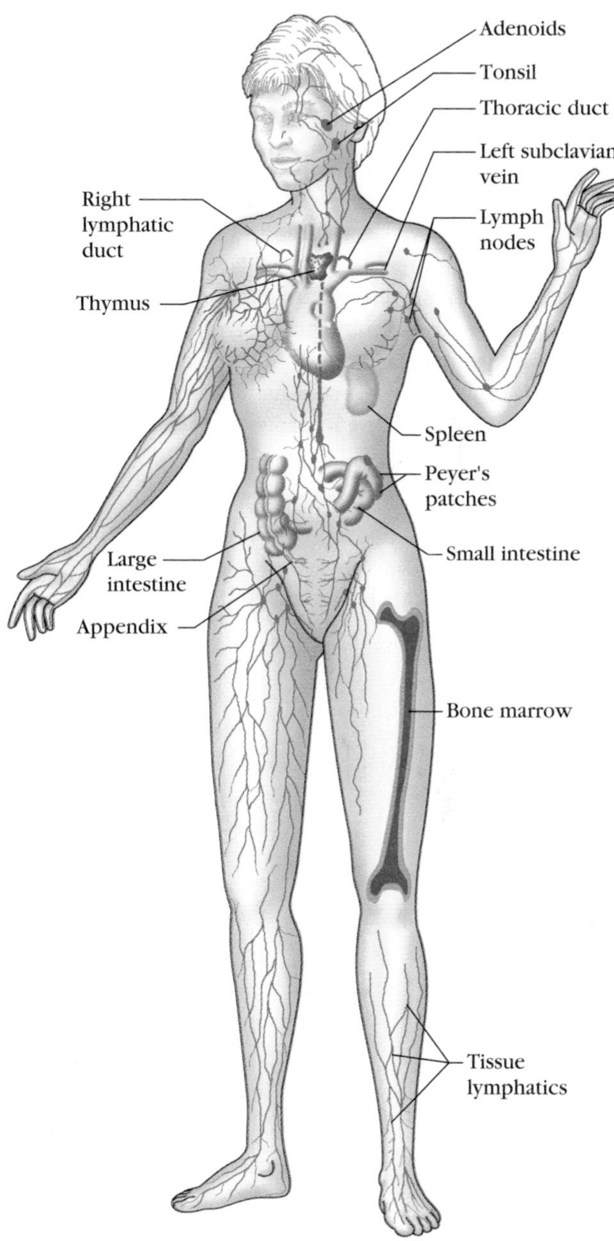

FIGURE 2-13 The human lymphoid system. The primary organs (bone marrow and thymus) are shown in red; secondary organs and tissues, in blue. These structurally and functionally diverse lymphoid organs and tissues are interconnected by the blood vessels (not shown) and lymphatic vessels (purple) through which lymphocytes circulate. Only one bone is shown, but all major bones contain marrow and thus are part of the lymphoid system. [Adapted from Lodish et al, 1995, *Molecular Cell Biology,* 3rd ed., Scientific American Books.]

Go to www.whfreeman.com/immunology Animation
Cells and Organs of the Immune System

mature lymphocytes to interact with that antigen. In addition, **tertiary lymphoid tissues,** which normally contain fewer lymphoid cells than secondary lymphoid organs, can import lymphoid cells during an inflammatory response. Most prominent of these are cutaneous-associated lymphoid tissues. Once mature lymphocytes have been generated in the primary lymphoid organs, they circulate in the blood and **lymphatic system,** a network of vessels that collect fluid that has escaped into the tissues from capillaries of the circulatory system and ultimately return it to the blood.

Primary Lymphoid Organs

Immature lymphocytes generated in hematopoiesis mature and become committed to a particular antigenic specificity within the primary lymphoid organs. Only after a lymphocyte has matured within a primary lymphoid organ is the cell **immunocompetent** (capable of mounting an immune response). In mammals, T cells mature in the **thymus** and B cells mature in the **bone marrow.**

Thymus

The thymus is a flat, bilobed organ situated above the heart. Each lobe is surrounded by a capsule and is divided into lobules, which are separated from each other by strands of connective tissue called trabeculae. Each lobule is organized into two compartments: the outer compartment, or *cortex,* is densely packed with immature T cells, called thymocytes, whereas the inner compartment, or *medulla,* is sparsely populated with thymocytes.

The sequence of T-cell maturation within the thymus is not completely understood. After progenitor T cells formed in hematopoiesis enter the thymus, they are thought to multiply rapidly within the cortex; this rapid proliferation of thymocytes is coupled with an enormous rate of cell death. A small subset of more mature thymocytes are then thought to migrate from the cortex to the medulla, where they continue to mature and finally leave the thymus through postcapillary venules. There appear to be exceptions to this sequence; some studies show that a small subpopulation of cortical thymocytes can mature and leave the thymus without ever entering the medulla.

Both the cortex and medulla of the thymus are crisscrossed by a three-dimensional stromal-cell network composed of epithelial cells, interdigitating dendritic cells, and macrophages, which make up the framework of the organ and contribute to the growth and maturation of thymocytes. Many of these stromal cells interact physically with the developing thymocytes (Figure 2-14). Some thymic epithelial cells in the outer cortex, called **nurse cells,** have long mem-

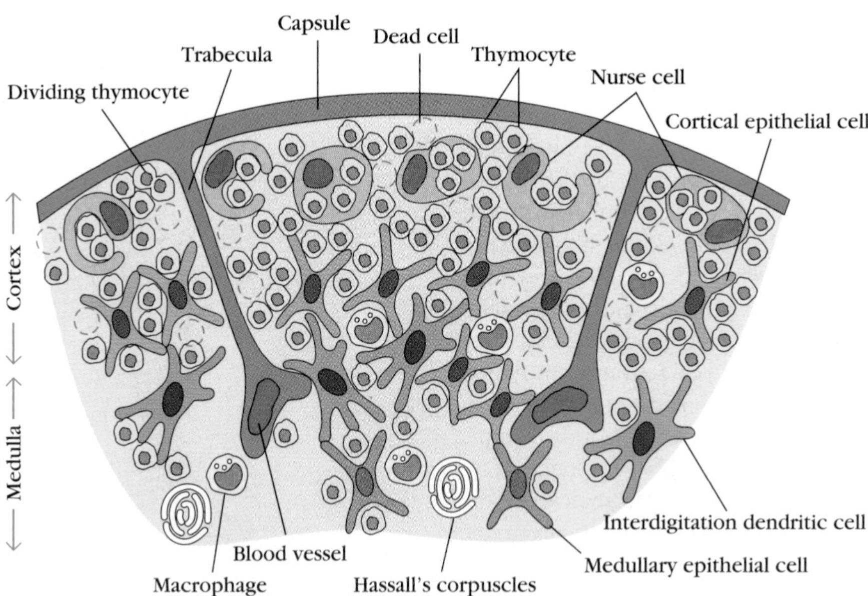

FIGURE 2-14 Diagrammatic cross-section of a portion of the thymus, showing several lobules separated by connective tissue strands (trabeculae). The densely populated outer cortex is thought to contain many immature thymocytes (blue), which undergo rapid proliferation coupled with an enormous rate of cell death. Also present in the outer cortex are thymic nurse cells (gray), which are specialized epithelial cells with long membrane extensions that surround as many as 50 thymocytes. The medulla is sparsely populated and is thought to contain thymocytes that are more mature. During their stay within the thymus, thymocytes interact with various stromal cells, including cortical epithelial cells (light red), medullary epithelial cells (tan), interdigitating dendritic cells (purple), and macrophages (yellow). These cells produce thymic hormones and express high levels of class I and class II MHC molecules. Hassalls corpuscles, found in the medulla, contain concentric layers of degenerating epithelial cells. [Adapted from W van Ewijk, 1991, *Annu. Rev. Immunol.* **9:**591.]

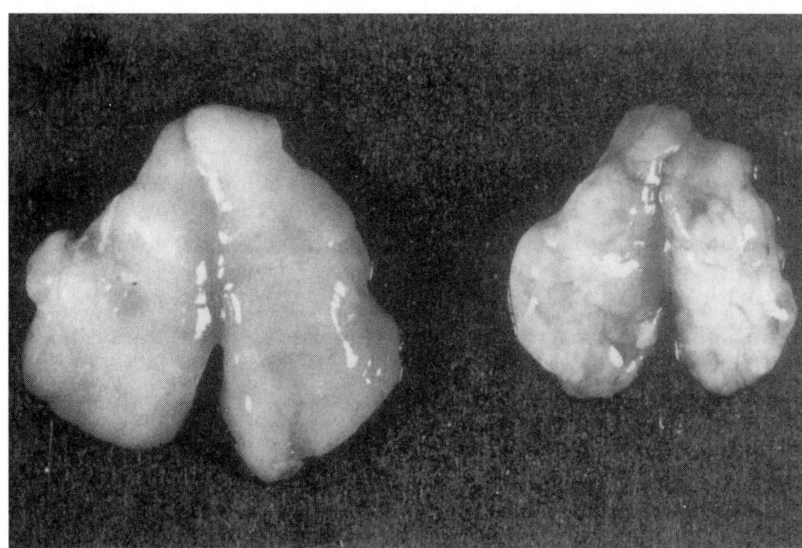

FIGURE 2-15 Effects of corticosteroids on the rat thymus gland. A normal thymus *(left)* compared with the thymus of a rat 48 h after injection of a corticosteroid (5 mg/kg body weight). [From MM Compton and JA Cidlowski, 1992, *Trends Endocrinol. Metabol.* **3:**17.]

brane extensions that surround as many as 50 thymocytes, forming large multicellular complexes. Other cortical epithelial cells have long interconnecting cytoplasmic extensions that form a network and have been shown to interact with numerous thymocytes as they traverse the cortex. Interdigitating dendritic cells, which are located at the junction of the cortex and medulla, also have long extensions that interact with developing thymocytes.

Maturation and Selection of T Cells As thymocytes mature in the thymus, the antigenic diversity of their T-cell receptors is generated by a series of random gene rearrangements (see Chapter 9). After developing thymocytes begin to express antigen-binding receptors, they are subjected to a two-step selection process. Thymic stromal cells, which express high levels of class I and class II MHC molecules, play a role in this process. Any developing thymocytes that are unable to recognize self-MHC molecules or that do have a high affinity for self-antigen plus self-MHC (or self-MHC alone) are eliminated by programmed cell death. Thus, only those cells whose receptors recognize a self-MHC molecule plus foreign antigen are allowed to mature. A detailed description of thymic selection is presented in Chapter 10.

An estimated 95%–99% of all thymocyte progeny undergo programmed cell death within the thymus without ever maturing. This high death rate probably results primarily from the elimination of thymocytes that cannot recognize foreign antigenic peptides displayed by self-MHC molecules and of thymocytes that recognize self-peptides displayed by self-MHC molecules. It is not known whether some sort of external signal (e.g., the presence or absence of a factor) initiates the programmed cell death of those thymocytes. Some have suggested (see Chapter 10) that the death of most nonselected thymocytes may be induced by endogenous glucocorticoids (also known as corticosteroids). It has been known for some time that cortical thymocytes, especially in rodents, are extremely sensitive to glucocorticoids, whereas mature T cells are not. For instance, when mouse thymocytes are incubated with high physiologic levels of glucocorticoids, the cells begin to die within 1–2 h by apoptosis. Injection of glucocorticoids into rats and other experimental animals leads to marked atrophy of the thymus (Figure 2-15).

The Thymus and Immune Function The importance of the thymus in immune function can be studied in mice by examining the effects of neonatal thymectomy, a procedure in which the thymus is surgically removed from newborn mice. These thymectomized mice show a dramatic decrease in circulating lymphocytes of the T-cell lineage and an absence of cell-mediated immunity. Other evidence of the importance of the thymus comes from studies of a congenital birth defect in humans (**DiGeorge's syndrome**) and in certain mice (**nude mice**) in which the thymus fails to develop. In both cases, there is an absence of circulating T cells and of cell-mediated immunity and an increase in infectious disease.

Aging is accompanied by a decline in thymic function. This decline may play some role in the decline in immune function during aging in humans and mice. The thymus reaches its maximal size at puberty and then atrophies, with a significant decrease in both cortical and medullary cells and an increase in the total fat content of the organ. Whereas the average weight of the thymus is 70 g in infants, its age-dependent involution leaves an organ with an average weight of only 3 g in the elderly.

A number of experiments have been designed to look at the effect of age on the immune function of the thymus. In one experiment, the thymus from a 1-day-old or 33-month-old mouse was grafted into thymectomized adults. (For most laboratory mice, 33 months is very old.) Mice receiving the newborn thymus graft showed a significantly larger improvement in immune function than mice receiving the 33-month-old thymus.

Bone Marrow

In birds, a lymphoid organ called the bursa of Fabricius, a gut-associated lymphoid tissue, is the primary site of B-cell maturation. In mammals such as primates and rodents, there is no bursa and no single counterpart to it as a primary lymphoid organ. Instead, in these animals, regions of the bone marrow and possibly of other lymphoid tissues serve as the "bursal equivalent," where B-cell maturation occurs. However, there are mammals, cattle and sheep for example, in which early fetal spleen and a large ($>10^{11}$ B cells) specialized Peyer's patch (a prominent focus of lymphoid tissue embedded in the wall of the intestine), called the ileal Peyer's patch, acts as a primary lymphoid tissue for the maturation, proliferation, and diversification of B cells. The rabbit, too, uses gut-associated tissues such as the appendix as primary lymphoid tissue for important steps in the proliferation, and diversification of B cells.

In those animals whose immature B cells proliferate and differentiate within the bone marrow, stromal cells within the bone marrow interact directly with the B cells and secrete various cytokines that are required for development. Like thymic selection during T-cell maturation, a selection process within the bone marrow eliminates B cells with self-reactive antibody receptors. This process is explained in detail in Chapter 11.

Lymphatic System

As blood circulates under pressure, its fluid component **(plasma)** seeps through the thin wall of the capillaries into the surrounding tissue. Much of this fluid, called **interstitial fluid,** returns to the blood through the capillary membranes. The remainder of the interstitial fluid, now called **lymph,** flows from the spaces in connective tissue into a network of tiny open lymphatic capillaries and then into a series of progressively larger collecting vessels called **lymphatic vessels** (Figure 2-16).

The largest lymphatic vessel, the **thoracic duct,** empties into the left subclavian vein near the heart (see Figure 2-13). In this way, the lymphatic system captures fluid lost from the blood and returns it to the blood, thus ensuring steady-state levels of fluid within the circulatory system. The heart does not pump the lymph through the lymphatic system; instead the flow of lymph is achieved as the lymph vessels are squeezed by movements of the body's muscles. A series of one-way valves along the lymphatic vessels ensures that lymph flows only in one direction.

When a foreign antigen gains entrance to the tissues, it is picked up by the lymphatic system (which drains all the tissues of the body) and is carried to various organized lymphoid tissues such as lymph nodes, which trap the foreign antigen. As lymph passes from the tissues to lymphatic vessels, it becomes progressively enriched in lymphocytes. Thus, the lymphatic system also serves as a means of transporting lymphocytes and antigen from the connective tissues to organized lymphoid tissues where the lymphocytes may interact with the trapped antigen and undergo activation.

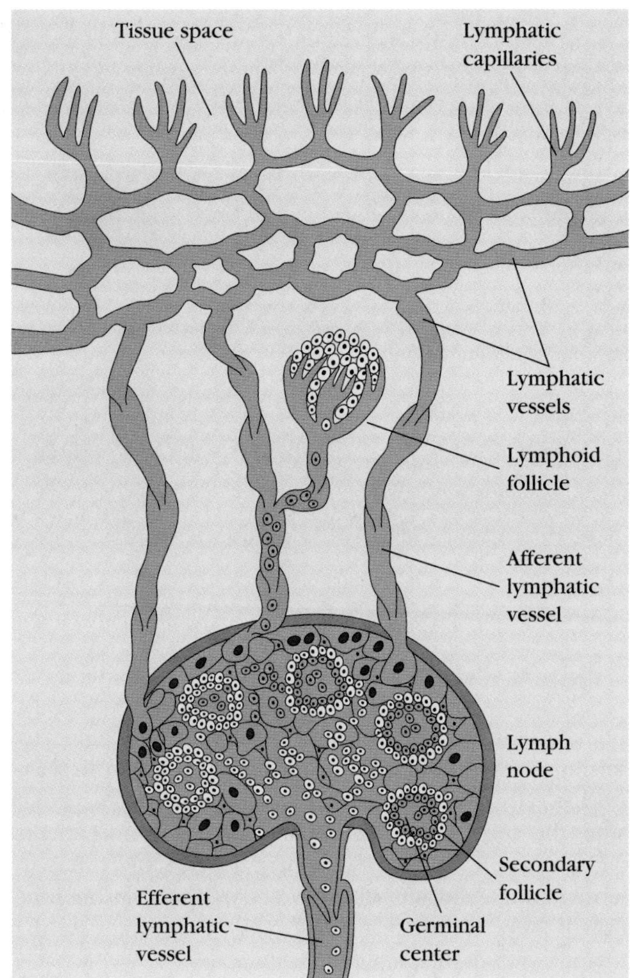

FIGURE 2-16 Lymphatic vessels. Small lymphatic capillaries opening into the tissue spaces pick up interstitial tissue fluid and carry it into progressively larger lymphatic vessels, which carry the fluid, now called lymph, into regional lymph nodes. As lymph leaves the nodes, it is carried through larger efferent lymphatic vessels, which eventually drain into the circulatory system at the thoracic duct or right lymph duct (see Figure 2-13).

Secondary Lymphoid Organs

Various types of organized lymphoid tissues are located along the vessels of the lymphatic system. Some lymphoid tissue in the lung and lamina propria of the intestinal wall consists of diffuse collections of lymphocytes and macrophages. Other lymphoid tissue is organized into structures called lymphoid follicles, which consist of aggregates of lymphoid and nonlymphoid cells surrounded by a network of draining lymphatic capillaries. Until it is activated by antigen, a lymphoid follicle—called a **primary follicle**—comprises a network of follicular dendritic cells and small resting B cells. After an antigenic challenge, a primary follicle becomes a larger **secondary follicle**—a ring of concentrically packed B lymphocytes surrounding a center (the **germinal center**) in which one finds a focus of proliferating B lymphocytes and an area that contains nondividing B cells, and some helper T cells interspersed with macrophages and follicular dendritic cells (Figure 2-17).

Most antigen-activated B cells divide and differentiate into antibody-producing plasma cells in lymphoid follicles, but only a few B cells in the antigen-activated population find their way into germinal centers. Those that do enter a germinal center undergo one or more rounds of cell division, during which the genes that encode their antibodies mutate at an unusually high rate. Following the period of division and mutation, there is a rigorous selection process in which more than 90% of these B cells die by apoptosis. In general, those B cells producing antibodies that bind antigen more strongly have a much better chance of surviving than do their weaker companions. The small number of B cells that survive the germinal center's rigorous selection differentiate into plasma cells or memory cells and emerge. The process of B-cell proliferation, mutation, and selection in germinal centers is described more fully in Chapter 11.

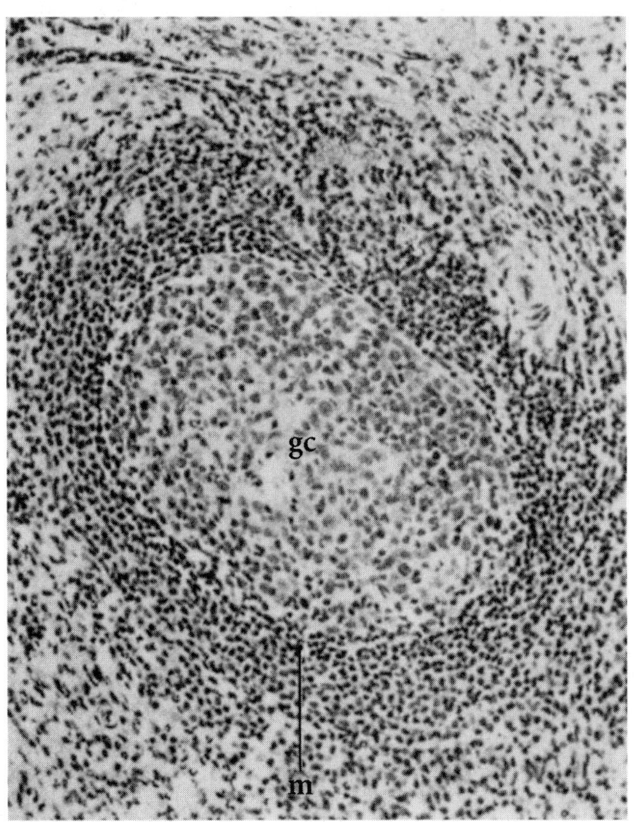

FIGURE 2-17 A secondary lymphoid follicle consisting of a large germinal center (gc) surrounded by a dense mantle (m) of small lymphocytes. [From W Bloom and DW Fawcett, 1975, *Textbook of Histology,* 10th ed., W. B. Saunders Co.]

Lymph nodes and the **spleen** are the most highly organized of the secondary lymphoid organs; they comprise not only lymphoid follicles, but additional distinct regions of T-cell and B-cell activity, and they are surrounded by a fibrous capsule. Less-organized lymphoid tissue, collectively called mucosal-associated lymphoid tissue (MALT), is found in various body sites. MALT includes Peyer's patches (in the small intestine), the tonsils, and the appendix, as well as numerous lymphoid follicles within the lamina propria of the intestines and in the mucous membranes lining the upper airways, bronchi, and genital tract.

Lymph Nodes

Lymph nodes are encapsulated bean-shaped structures containing a reticular network packed with lymphocytes, macrophages, and dendritic cells. Clustered at junctions of the lymphatic vessels, lymph nodes are the first organized lymphoid structure to encounter antigens that enter the tissue spaces. As lymph percolates through a node, any particulate antigen that is brought in with the lymph will be trapped by the cellular network of phagocytic cells and dendritic cells (follicular and interdigitating). The overall architecture of a lymph node supports an ideal microenvironment for lymphocytes to effectively encounter and respond to trapped antigens.

Morphologically, a lymph node can be divided into three roughly concentric regions: the cortex, the paracortex, and the medulla, each of which supports a distinct microenvironment (Figure 2-18). The outermost layer, the **cortex,** contains lymphocytes (mostly B cells), macrophages, and follicular dendritic cells arranged in primary follicles. After antigenic challenge, the primary follicles enlarge into secondary follicles, each containing a germinal center. In children with B-cell deficiencies, the cortex lacks primary follicles and germinal centers. Beneath the cortex is the **paracortex,** which is populated largely by T lymphocytes and also contains interdigitating dendritic cells thought to have migrated from tissues to the node. These interdigitating dendritic cells express high levels of class II MHC molecules, which are necessary for presenting antigen to T_H

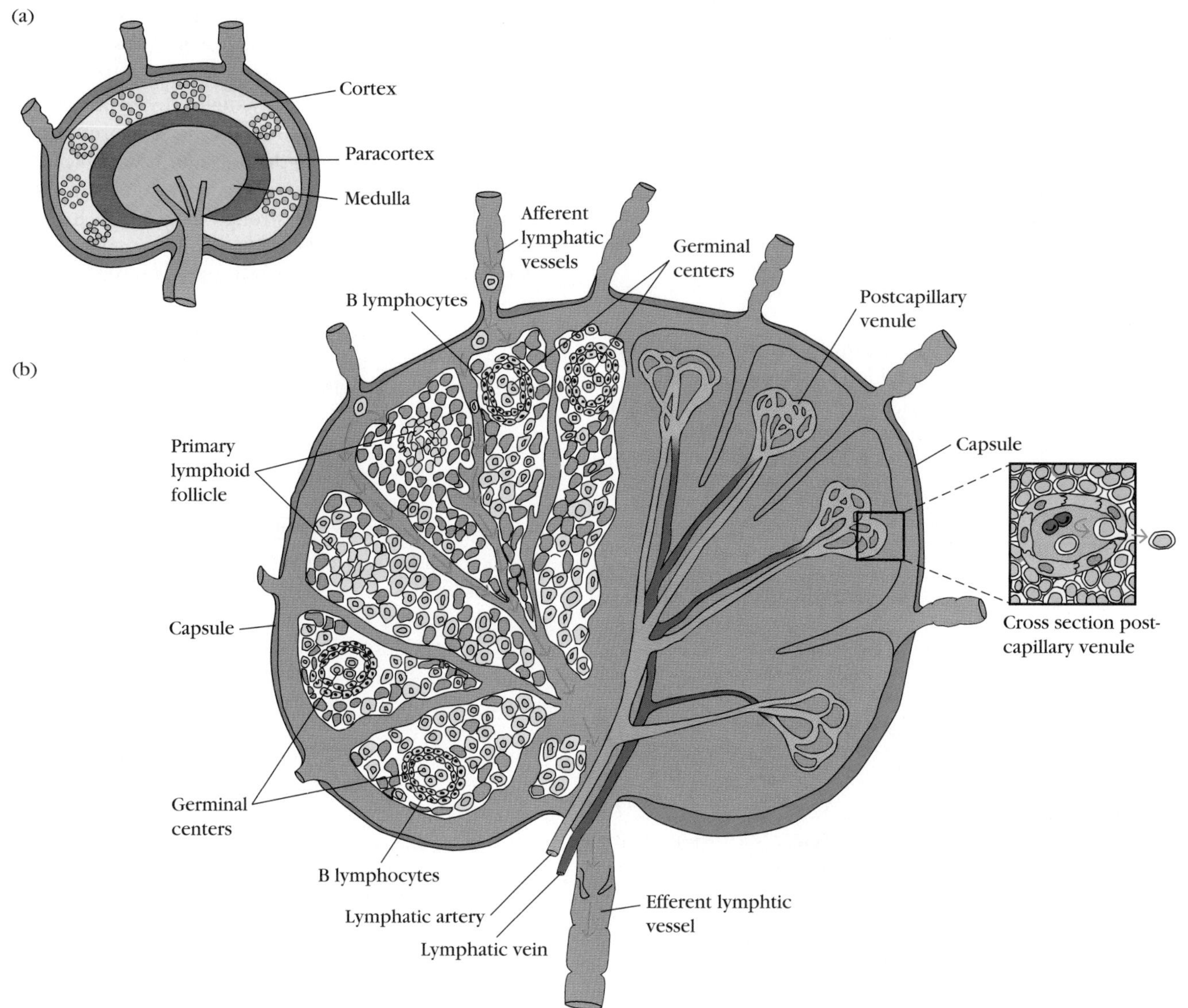

FIGURE 2-18 Structure of a lymph node. (a) The three layers of a lymph node support distinct microenvironments. (b) The left side depicts the arrangement of reticulum and lymphocytes within the various regions of a lymph node. Macrophages and dendritic cells, which trap antigen, are present in the cortex and paracortex. T_H cells are concentrated in the paracortex; B cells are located primarily in the cortex, within follicles and germinal centers. The medulla is populated largely by antibody-producing plasma cells. Lymphocytes circulating in the lymph are carried into the node by afferent lymphatic vessels; they either enter the reticular matrix of the node or pass through it and leave by the efferent lymphatic vessel. The right side of (b) depicts the lymphatic artery and vein and the postcapillary venules. Lymphocytes in the circulation can pass into the node from the postcapillary venules by a process called extravasation (*inset*).

cells. Lymph nodes taken from neonatally thymectomized mice have unusually few cells in the paracortical region; the paracortex is therefore sometimes referred to as a **thymus-dependent area** in contrast to the cortex, which is a **thymus-independent area.** The innermost layer of a lymph node, the **medulla,** is more sparsely populated with lymphoid-lineage cells; of those present, many are plasma cells actively secreting antibody molecules.

As antigen is carried into a regional node by the lymph, it is trapped, processed, and presented together with class II MHC molecules by interdigitating dendritic cells in the paracortex, resulting in the activation of T_H cells. The initial activation of B cells is also thought to take place within the T-cell–rich paracortex. Once activated, T_H and B cells form small foci consisting largely of proliferating B cells at the edges of the paracortex. Some B cells within the foci differentiate into plasma cells secreting IgM and IgG. These foci reach maximum size within 4–6 days of antigen challenge. Within 4–7 days of antigen challenge, a few B cells and T_H cells migrate to the primary follicles of the cortex. It is not known what causes these cells to migrate to the primary follicles. Within a primary follicle, cellular interactions between follicular dendritic cells, B cells, and T_H cells take place, leading to development of a secondary follicle with a central germinal center. Some of the plasma cells generated in the germinal center move to the medullary areas of the lymph node, and many migrate to bone marrow.

Afferent lymphatic vessels pierce the capsule of a lymph node at numerous sites and empty lymph into the subcapsular sinus (see Figure 2-18b). Lymph coming from the tissues percolates slowly inward through the cortex, paracortex, and medulla, allowing phagocytic cells and dendritic cells to trap any bacteria or particulate material (e.g., antigen-antibody complexes) carried by the lymph. After infection or the introduction of other antigens into the body, the lymph leaving a node through its single efferent lymphatic vessel is enriched with antibodies newly secreted by medullary plasma cells and also has a fiftyfold higher concentration of lymphocytes than the afferent lymph.

The increase in lymphocytes in lymph leaving a node is due in part to lymphocyte proliferation within the node in response to antigen. Most of the increase, however, represents blood-borne lymphocytes that migrate into the node by passing between specialized endothelial cells that line the **postcapillary venules** of the node. Estimates are that 25% of the lymphocytes leaving a lymph node have migrated across this endothelial layer and entered the node from the blood. Because antigenic stimulation within a node can increase this migration tenfold, the concentration of lymphocytes in a node that is actively responding can increase greatly; the node swells visibly. Factors released in lymph nodes during antigen stimulation are thought to facilitate this increased migration.

Spleen

The spleen is a large, ovoid secondary lymphoid organ situated high in the left abdominal cavity. While lymph nodes are specialized for trapping antigen from local tissues, the spleen specializes in filtering blood and trapping blood-borne antigens; thus, it can respond to systemic infections. Unlike the lymph nodes, the spleen is not supplied by lymphatic vessels. Instead, blood-borne antigens and lymphocytes are carried into the spleen through the splenic artery. Experiments with radioactively labeled lymphocytes show that more recirculating lymphocytes pass daily through the spleen than through all the lymph nodes combined.

The spleen is surrounded by a capsule that extends a number of projections (trabeculae) into the interior to form a compartmentalized structure. The compartments are of two types, the red pulp and white pulp, which are separated by a diffuse marginal zone (Figure 2-19). The splenic **red pulp** consists of a network of sinusoids populated by macrophages and numerous red blood cells (erythrocytes); it is the site where old and defective red blood cells are destroyed and removed. Many of the macrophages within the red pulp contain engulfed red blood cells or iron pigments from degraded hemoglobin. The splenic **white pulp** surrounds the branches of the splenic artery, forming a **periarteriolar lymphoid sheath (PALS)** populated mainly by T lymphocytes. The **marginal zone,** located peripheral to the PALS, is rich in B cells organized into primary lymphoid follicles.

Blood-borne antigens and lymphocytes enter the spleen through the splenic artery, which empties into the marginal zone. In the marginal zone, antigen is trapped by interdigitating dendritic cells, which carry it to the PALS. Lymphocytes in the blood also enter sinuses in the marginal zone and migrate to the PALS.

The initial activation of B and T cells takes place in the T cell–rich PALS. Here interdigitating dendritic cells capture antigen and present it combined with class II MHC molecules to T_H cells. Once activated, these T_H cells can then activate B cells. The activated B cells, together with some T_H cells, then migrate to primary follicles in the marginal zone. Upon antigenic challenge, these primary follicles develop into characteristic secondary follicles containing germinal centers (like those in the lymph nodes), where rapidly dividing B cells (centroblasts) and plasma cells are surrounded by dense clusters of concentrically arranged lymphocytes.

The effects of splenectomy on the immune response depends on the age at which the spleen is removed. In children, splenectomy often leads to an increased incidence of bacterial sepsis caused primarily by *Streptococcus pneumoniae, Neisseria meningitidis,* and *Haemophilus influenzae.* Splenectomy in adults has less adverse effects, although it leads to some increase in blood-borne bacterial infections **(bacteremia).**

Mucosal-Associated Lymphoid Tissue

The mucous membranes lining the digestive, respiratory, and urogenital systems have a combined surface area of about 400 m^2 (about the floor area of a room 65 ft × 65 ft) and are the major sites of entry for most pathogens. These vulnerable membrane surfaces are defended by a group of organized lymphoid tissues known collectively as **mucosal-associated lymphoid tissue (MALT).** Structurally, these tissues range from loose, barely organized clusters of lymphoid

(a)

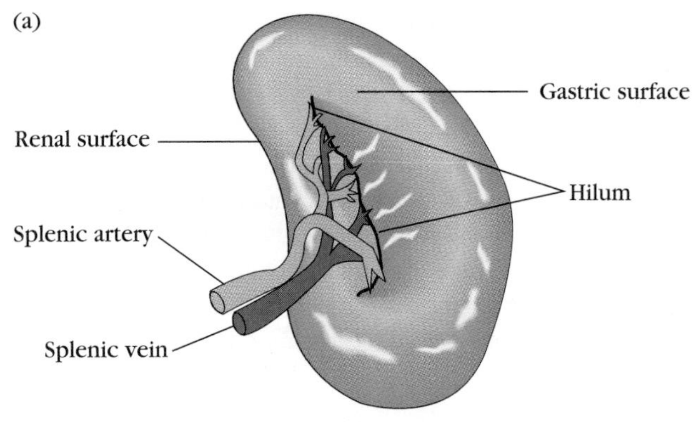

(b)

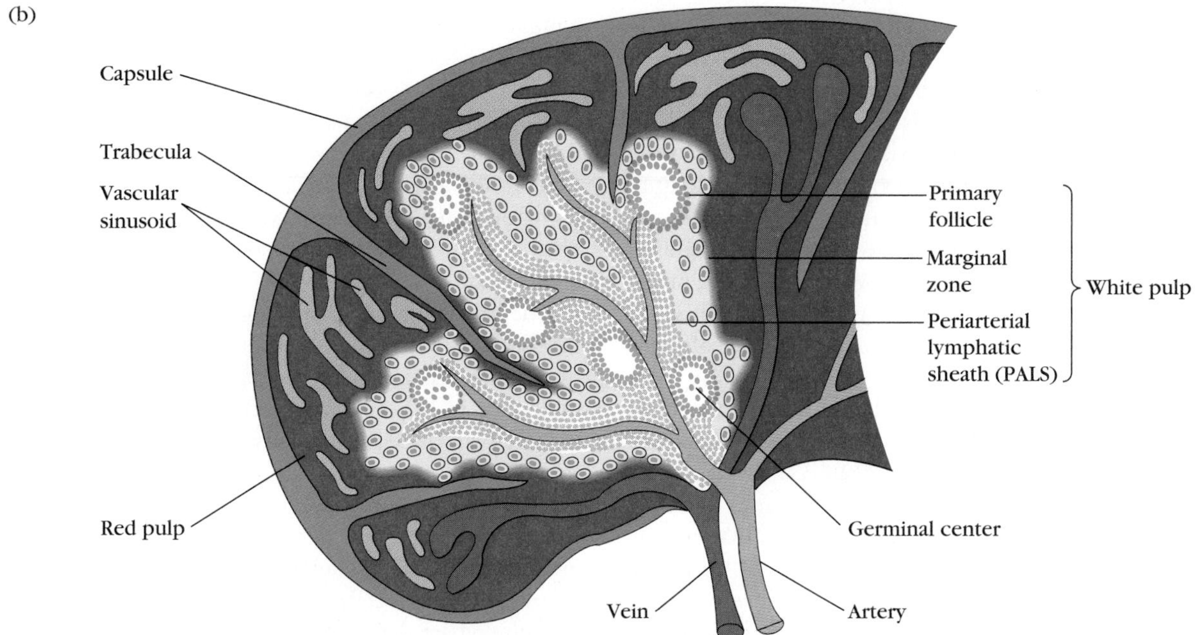

FIGURE 2-19 Structure of the spleen. (a) The spleen, which is about 5 inches long in adults, is the largest secondary lymphoid organ. It is specialized for trapping blood-borne antigens. (b) Diagrammatic cross section of the spleen. The splenic artery pierces the capsule and divides into progressively smaller arterioles, ending in vascular sinusoids that drain back into the splenic vein. The erythrocyte-filled red pulp surrounds the sinusoids. The white pulp forms a sleeve, the periarteriolar lymphoid sheath (PALS) around the arterioles; this sheath contains numerous T cells. Closely associated with the PALS is the marginal zone, an area rich in B cells that contains lymphoid follicles that can develop into secondary follicles containing germinal centers.

cells in the lamina propria of intestinal villi to well-organized structures such as the familiar tonsils and **appendix,** as well as **Peyer's patches,** which are found within the submucosal layer of the intestinal lining. The functional importance of MALT in the body's defense is attested to by its large population of antibody-producing plasma cells, whose number far exceeds that of plasma cells in the spleen, lymph nodes, and bone marrow combined.

The **tonsils** are found in three locations: lingual at the base of the tongue; palatine at the sides of the back of the mouth; and nasopharyngeal (adenoids) in the roof of the nasopharynx (Figure 2-20). All three tonsil groups are nodular structures consisting of a meshwork of reticular cells and fibers interspersed with lymphocytes, macrophages, granulocytes, and mast cells. The B cells are organized into follicles and germinal centers; the latter are surrounded by regions showing T-cell activity. The tonsils defend against antigens entering through the nasal and oral epithelial routes.

The best studied of the mucous membranes is the one that lines the gastrointestinal tract. Lymphoid cells are found in various regions within this tissue. The outer mucosal epithelial layer contains so-called **intraepithelial lymphocytes (IELs).** The majority of these lymphocytes are T cells that express unusual receptors ($\gamma\delta$ T-cell receptors, or $\gamma\delta$ TCRs), which exhibit limited diversity for

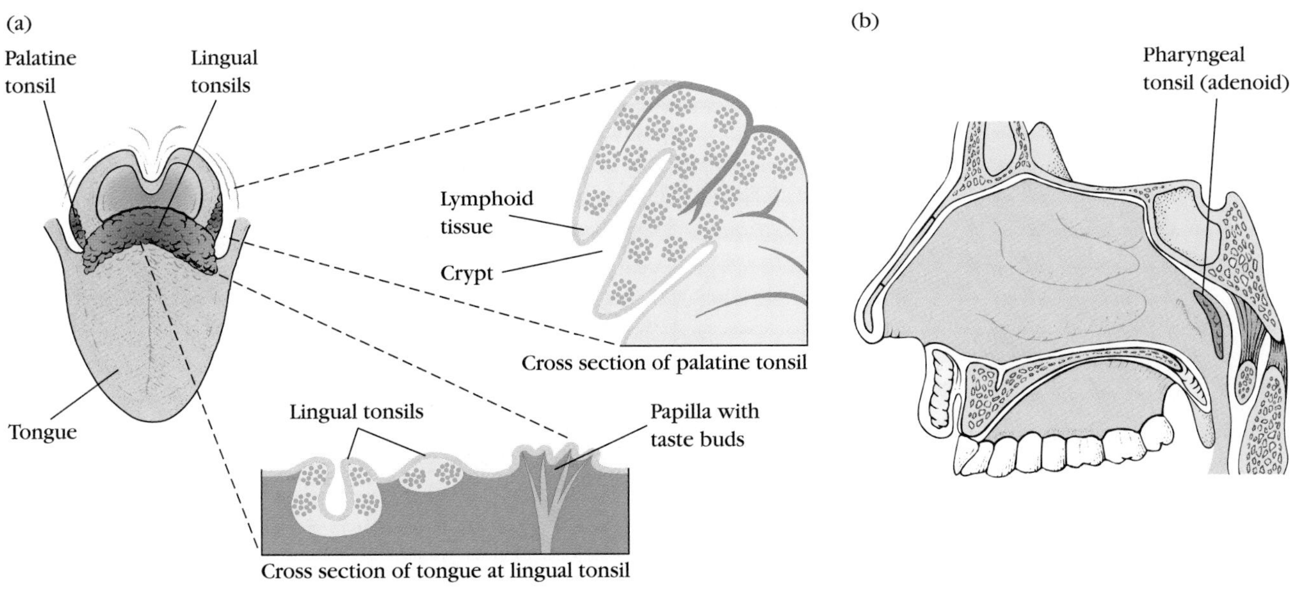

FIGURE 2-20 Three types of tonsils. (a) The position and internal features of the palatine and lingual tonsils; (b) a view of the position of the nasopharyngeal tonsils (adenoids).

antigen. Although this population of T cells is well situated to encounter antigens that enter through the intestinal mucous epithelium, their actual function remains largely unknown (Figure 2-21). The lamina propria, which lies under the epithelial layer, contains large numbers of B cells, plasma cells, activated T_H cells, and macrophages in loose clusters. Histologic sections have revealed more than 15,000 lymphoid follicles within the intestinal lamina propria of a healthy child. The submucosal layer beneath the lamina propria contains Peyer's patches, nodules of 30–40 lymphoid follicles. Like lymphoid follicles in other sites, those that compose Peyer's patches can develop into secondary follicles with germinal centers.

The epithelial cells of mucous membranes play an important role in promoting the immune response by delivering small samples of foreign antigen from the lumina of the respiratory, digestive, and urogenital tracts to the underlying mucosal-associated lymphoid tissue. This antigen transport is carried out by specialized cells, called **M cells.** The structure of the M cell is striking: these are flattened epithelial cells lacking the microvilli that characterize the rest of the mucous epithelium. In addition, M cells have a deep invagination, or pocket, in the basolateral plasma membrane; this pocket is filled with a cluster of B cells, T cells, and macrophages (Figure 2-22a). Luminal antigens are endocytosed into vesicles that are transported from the luminal membrane to the underlying pocket membrane. The vesicles then fuse with the pocket membrane, delivering the potentially response-activating antigens to the clusters of lymphocytes contained within the pocket.

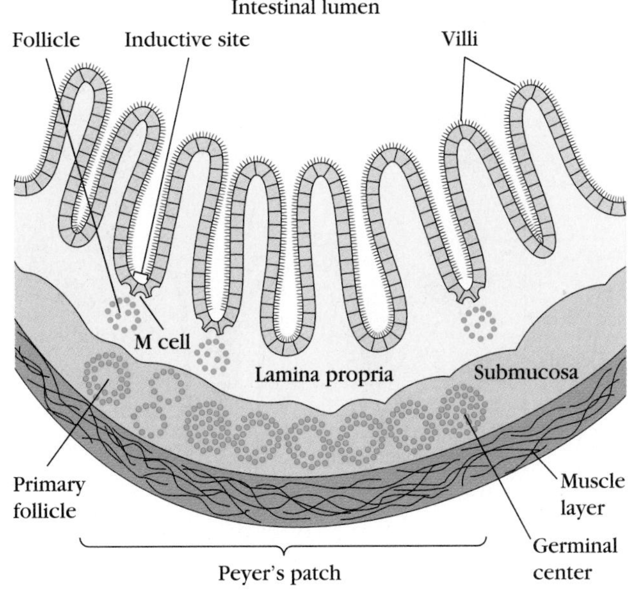

FIGURE 2-21 Cross-sectional diagram of the mucous membrane lining the intestine showing a nodule of lymphoid follicles that constitutes a Peyer's patch in the submucosa. The intestinal lamina propria contains loose clusters of lymphoid cells and diffuse follicles.

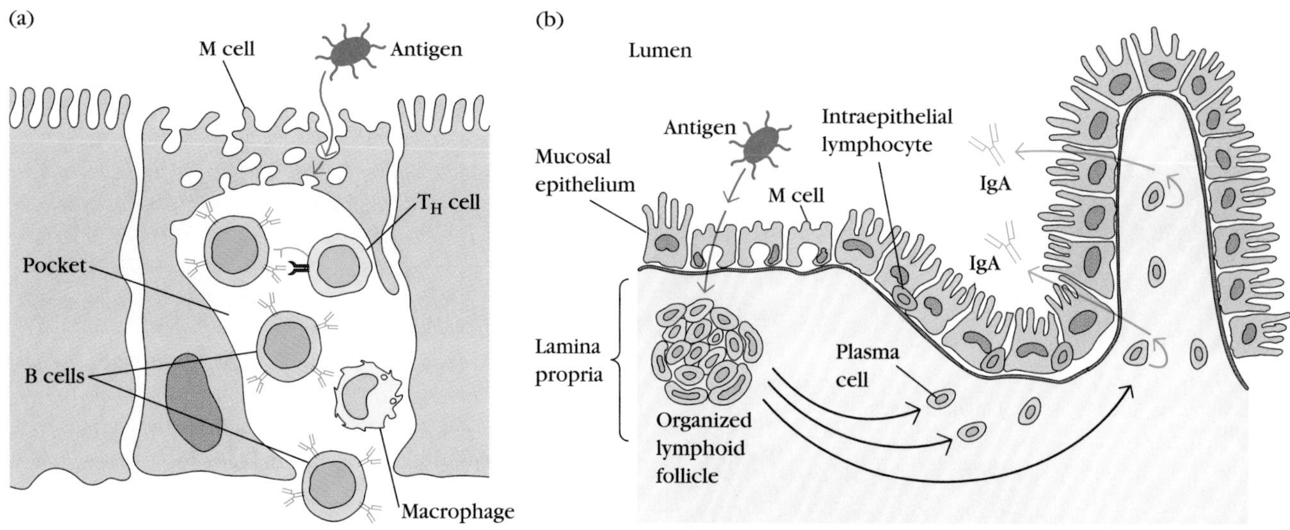

FIGURE 2-22 Structure of M cells and production of IgA at inductive sites. (a) M cells, located in mucous membranes, endocytose antigen from the lumen of the digestive, respiratory, and urogenital tracts. The antigen is transported across the cell and released into the large basolateral pocket. (b) Antigen transported across the epithelial layer by M cells at an inductive site activates B cells in the underlying lymphoid follicles. The activated B cells differentiate into IgA-producing plasma cells, which migrate along the submucosa. The outer mucosal epithelial layer contains intraepithelial lymphocytes, of which many are $CD8^+$ T cells that express $\gamma\delta$ TCRs with limited receptor diversity for antigen.

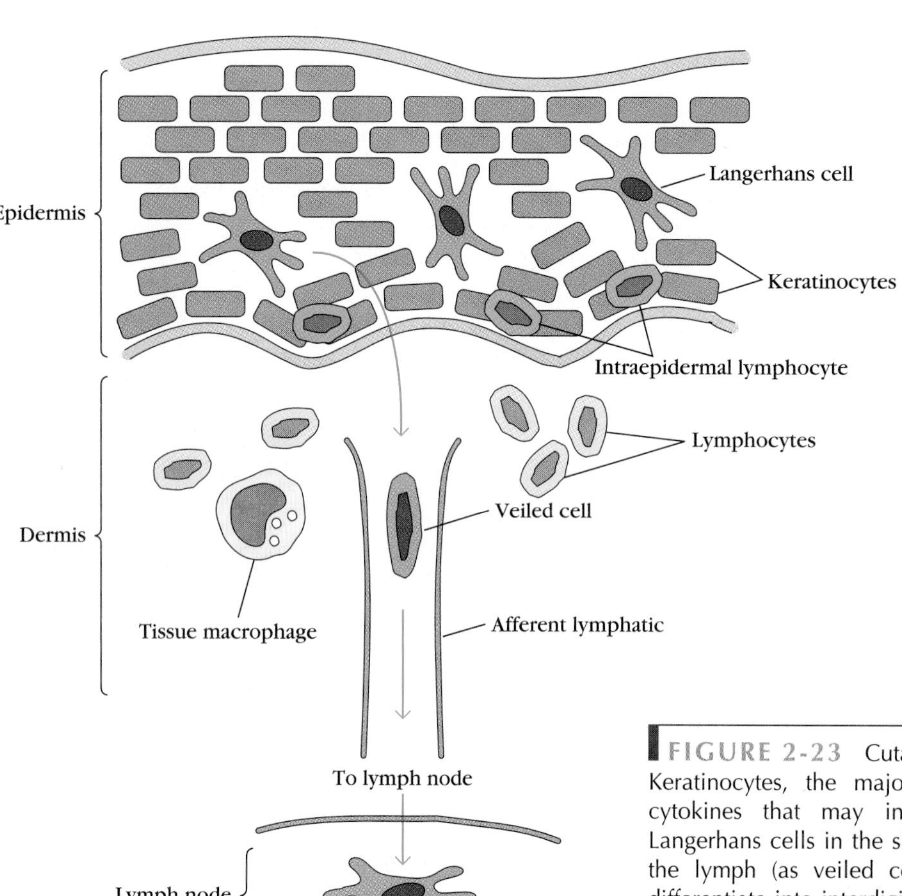

FIGURE 2-23 Cutaneous-associated lymphoid tissue. Keratinocytes, the major cells of the epidermis, secrete cytokines that may induce an inflammatory response. Langerhans cells in the skin internalize antigen and move in the lymph (as veiled cells) to lymph nodes, where they differentiate into interdigitating dendritic cells; these function as potent antigen-presenting cells. Intraepidermal lymphocytes are predominantly T cells that express the $\gamma\delta$ T-cell receptor.

M cells are located in so-called **inductive sites**—small regions of a mucous membrane that lie over organized lymphoid follicles (Figure 2-22b). Antigens transported across the mucous membrane by M cells can activate B cells within these lymphoid follicles. The activated B cells differentiate into plasma cells, which leave the follicles and secrete the IgA class of antibodies. These antibodies then are transported across the epithelial cells and released as **secretory IgA** into the lumen, where they can interact with antigens.

As described in Chapter 1, mucous membranes are an effective barrier to the entrance of most pathogens, which thereby contributes to nonspecific immunity. One reason for this is that the mucosal epithelial cells are cemented to one another by tight junctions that make it difficult for pathogens to penetrate. Interestingly, some enteric pathogens, including both bacteria and viruses, have exploited the M cell as an entry route through the mucous-membrane barrier. In some cases, the pathogen is internalized by the M cell and transported into the pocket. In other cases, the pathogen binds to the M cell and disrupts the cell, thus allowing entry of the pathogen. Among the pathogens that use M cells in these ways are several invasive *Salmonella* species, *Vibrio cholerae,* and the polio virus.

Cutaneous-Associated Lymphoid Tissue

The skin is an important anatomic barrier to the external environment, and its large surface area makes this tissue important in nonspecific (innate) defenses. The epidermal (outer) layer of the skin is composed largely of specialized epithelial cells called keratinocytes. These cells secrete a number of cytokines that may function to induce a local inflammatory reaction. In addition, keratinocytes can be induced to express class II MHC molecules and may function as antigen-presenting cells. Scattered among the epithelial-cell matrix of the epidermis are Langerhans cells, a type of dendritic cell, which internalize antigen by phagocytosis or endocytosis. The Langerhans cells then migrate from the epidermis to regional lymph nodes, where they differentiate into interdigitating dendritic cells (Figure 2-23). These cells express high levels of class II MHC molecules and function as potent activators of naive T_H cells.

The epidermis also contains so-called *intraepidermal lymphocytes.* These are similar to the intraepithelial lymphocytes of MALT in that most of them are $CD8^+$ T cells, many of which express $\gamma\delta$ T-cell receptors, which have limited diversity for antigen. It is thought that these intraepidermal T cells may be uniquely suited to combat antigens that enter through the skin. The underlying dermal layer of the skin contains scattered $CD4^+$ and $CD8^+$ T cells and macrophages. Most of these dermal T cells were either previously activated cells or are memory cells.

Summary

1. The cells that participate in the immune response are white blood cells, or leukocytes. The lymphocyte is the only cell to possess the immunologic attributes of specificity, diversity, memory, and self/nonself recognition.
2. All of the white blood cells develop from a common pluripotent stem cell in hematopoiesis. Various hematopoietic growth factors (cytokines) induce proliferation and differentiation of the different blood cells (see Figure 2-1). The differentiation of stem cells into different cell types requires the expression of different lineage-determining genes. A number of transcription factors (see Table 2-1) play important roles in this regard. Hematopoiesis is closely regulated to assure steady-state levels of each of the different types of blood cell. Cell division and differentiation of each of the lineages is balanced by programmed cell death by apoptosis (see Figures 2-3, 2-4 and 2-5).
3. Lymphoid cells can be subdivided into B lymphocytes, T lymphocytes, and null cells (e.g., NK cells); null cells are much less abundant than B and T cells, and most lack a receptor that is specific for a particular antigen. However, NK1-T cells have both T-cell receptors and many of the markers characteristic of NK cells. Although morphologically indistinguishable, the three types of lymphoid cells can be distinguished on the basis of function and the presence of various membrane molecules (see Table 2-4).
4. Naive B and T lymphocytes, which have not encountered antigen, are small resting cells in the G_0 phase of the cell cycle. After interacting with antigen, these cells enlarge into lymphoblasts, which proliferate and eventually differentiate into effector cells and memory cells (see Figure 2-7).
5. Macrophages and neutrophils are the accessory cells of the immune system that phagocytose and degrade antigens (see Figure 2-9). Phagocytosis is facilitated by opsonins such as antibody and complement, which increase the attachment of antigen to the membrane of the phagocyte. Activated macrophages also secrete various factors that regulate the development of the immune and inflammatory responses (see Table 2-6). Basophils and mast cells are nonphagocytic cells that release a variety of pharmacologically active substances; these cells are critical in hypersensitivity responses.
6. Dendritic cells capture antigen. With the exception of follicular dendritic cells, these cells express high levels of class II MHC molecules. Along with macrophages and B cells, these dendritic cells play an important role in T_H-cell activation by processing and presenting antigen bound to class II MHC molecules and by providing the required co-stimulatory signal. Follicular dendritic cells, unlike the others, facilitate B-cell activation but play no role in T-cell activation.
7. The primary lymphoid organs provide sites where lymphocytes mature and become antigenically committed. T

lymphocytes mature within the thymus (see Figure 2-14), and B lymphocytes mature within the bursa of Fabricius in birds and in the bone marrow of several, but not all, mammalian species. In both cases, a selection process eliminates immature lymphocytes that react with self antigens; in addition, thymocytes that do not recognize self-MHC molecules are eliminated.

8. The secondary lymphoid organs function to capture antigen and to provide sites where lymphocytes interact with that antigen and undergo clonal proliferation and differentiation into effector cells. The lymphatic system drains the tissue spaces and interconnects many organized lymphoid tissues (see Figure 2-16). Lymph nodes are specialized to trap antigen from regional tissue spaces (see Figure 2-18), whereas the spleen traps blood-borne antigens (see Figure 2-19). Lymphoid tissue that is less organized is found in mucous membranes; these tissues include loose clusters of lymphoid follicles in the intestinal lamina propria and Peyer's patches (see Figure 2-21), found on the wall of the intestine. Cutaneous-associated lymphoid tissue constitutes the most important tertiary lymphoid tissue (see Figure 2-23).

REFERENCES

Appelbaum, FR. 1996. Hematopoietic stem cell transplantation: In *Scientific American Medicine.* D Dale, and D Federman, eds. Scientific American Publishers, New York.

Bendelac, A, MN Rivera, S-H Park, and JH Roark. 1997. Mouse CD1-specific NK1 T cells: Development, specificity and function. *Annu. Rev. Immunol.* **15:**535.

Brenner, MK. 1996. Gene transfer to hematopoietic cells. *N. Engl. J. Med.* **335:**337.

Caux, CY, J Liu, and J Banchereau. 1995. Recent advances in the study of dendritic cells and follicular dendritic cells. *Immunol. Today* **16:**2.

Clevers, HC, and R Grosschedl. 1996. Transcriptional control of lymphoid development: lessons from gene targeting. *Immunol. Today* **17:**336.

Cory, S. 1995. Regulation of lymphocyte survival by the BCL-2 gene family. *Annu. Rev. Immunol.* **12:**513.

Golde, DW. 1991. The stem cell. *Sci. Am.* **255** (Dec.):86.

Gordon, S, et al. 1995. Molecular immunobiology of macrophages: recent progress. *Curr. Opin. Immunol.* **7:**24.

Henderson, H, and K Calame. 1998. Transcriptional regulation during B cell development. *Annu. Rev. Immunol.* **16:**163.

Jones, B, L Pascopella, and S Falkow. 1995. Entry of microbes into the host: using M cells to break the mucosal barrier. *Curr. Opin. Immunol.* **7:**474.

Knight, SC, and S Patterson. 1998. Bone-marrow–derived dendritic cells, infection with human immunodeficiency virus, and immunopathology. *Annu. Rev. Immunol.* **15:**593.

Lapidot, T, et al. 1992. Cytokine stimulation of multilineage hematopoiesis from immature human cells engrafted in SCID mice. *Science* **255:**1137.

Lehrer, RI, AK Lichtenstein, and T Ganz. 1993. Defensins: antimicrobial and cytotoxic peptides of mammalian cells. *Annu. Rev. Immunol.* **11:**105.

MacLennan, ICM. 1994. Germinal centers. *Annu. Rev. Immunol.* **12:**117.

Melchers, F, and A Rolink. 1999. B-lymphocyte development and biology. In *Fundamental Immunology,* 4th ed., WE Paul, ed., p. 183. Lippincott-Raven, Philadelphia.

Nathan, C. 1995. Natural resistance and nitric oxide. *Cell* **82:**873.

Russell, DG. 1995. Of microbes and macrophages: entry, survival, and persistence. *Curr. Opin. Immunol.* **7:**479.

Osborne, BA. 1996. Apoptosis and the maintenance of homeostasis in the immune system. *Curr. Opin. Immunol.* **8:**245.

Picker, LJ, and MH Siegelman. 1999. Lymphoid tissues and organs. In *Fundamental Immunology,* 4th ed., WE Paul, ed., p. 145. Lippincott-Raven, Philadelphia.

Schmidt, HH, and U Walter. 1994. NO at work. *Cell* **78:**919.

Spangrude, GJ. 1994. Biological and clinical aspects of hematopoietic stem cells. *Annu. Rev. Med.* **45:**93.

Steinman, RM. 1991. The dendritic cell system and its role in immunogenicity. *Annu. Rev. Immunol.* **9:**271.

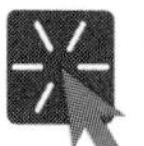

Useful Web Sites

http://www.ncbi.nlm.nih.gov/prow

The PROW Guides are authoritative short, structured reviews on proteins and protein families that bring together the most relevant information on each molecule into a single document of standardized format.

http://hms.medweb.harvard.edu/qry/core/setframe.cfm?crs=HSHeme

This brilliantly illustrated atlas of normal and abnormal blood cells informatively displayed as stained cell smears has been assembled to help train medical students at the Harvard Medical School to recognize and remember cell morphology that is associated with many different pathologies including leukemias, anemias and even malarial infections.

STUDY QUESTIONS

1. Explain why each of the following statements is false.

a. All T_H cells express CD4 and recognize only antigen associated with class II MHC molecules.

b. The pluripotent stem cell is one of the most abundant cell types in the bone marrow.

c. Activation of macrophages increases their expression of class I MHC molecules, making the cells present antigen more effectively.

d. Lymphoid follicles are present only in the spleen and lymph nodes.

e. Infection has no influence on the rate of hematopoiesis.

f. Follicular dendritic cells can process and present antigen to T lymphocytes.

Go to www.whfreeman.com/immunology Self-Test
Review and quiz of key terms

g. All lymphoid cells have antigen-binding receptors on their membrane.

h. All vertebrates generate B lymphocytes in bone marrow.

2. For each of the following situations, indicate which type(s) of lymphocytes would be expected to proliferate rapidly in lymph nodes and where in the nodes they would do so.

a. Normal mouse immunized with a soluble protein antigen

b. Normal mouse with a viral infection

c. Neonatally thymectomized mouse immunized with a protein antigen

d. Neonatally thymectomized mouse immunized with the thymus-independent antigen bacterial lipopolysaccharide (LPS), which does not require the aid of T_H cells to activate B cells

3. Do monocyte progenitor cells secrete M-CSF? Do they express receptors for M-CSF? What would be the likely consequences if a cell and its descendents expressed both M-CSF and the receptor for M-CSF?

4. List the primary lymphoid organs and summarize their functions in the immune response.

5. List the secondary lymphoid organs and summarize their functions in the immune response.

6. What are the two primary characteristics that distinguish hematopoietic stem cells and progenitor cells?

7. What do nude mice and humans with DiGeorge's syndrome have in common?

8. What cell types compose the stroma of the thymus? List two important functions of the thymic stromal cells.

9. At what age does the thymus reach its maximal size?

a. During the first year of life

b. Teenage years (puberty)

c. Between 40 and 50 years of age

d. After 70 years of age

10. Preparations enriched in pluripotent stem cells would be useful for research and in clinical practice. In Weissman's method for enriching pluripotent stem cells, why is it necessary to use lethally irradiated mice?

11. What effect does thymectomy have on a neonatal mouse? On an adult mouse? Explain why these effects differ.

12. What effect would removal of the bursa of Fabricius (bursectomy) have on chickens?

13. Some microorganisms (e.g., *Neisseria gonorrhoeae, Mycobacterium tuberculosis,* and *Candida albicans*) are classified as intracellular pathogens. Define this term and explain why the immune response to these pathogens differs from that to other pathogens such as *Staphylococcus aureus* and *Streptococcus pneumoniae.*

14. Indicate whether each of the following statements about the spleen is true or false. If you think a statement is false, explain why.

a. It filters antigens out of the blood.

b. The marginal zone is rich in T cells, and the periarteriolar lymphoid sheath (PALS) is rich in B cells.

c. It contains germinal centers.

d. It functions to remove old and defective red blood cells.

e. Lymphatic vessels draining the tissue spaces enter the spleen.

15. For each type of cell indicated (a–m), select the most appropriate description (1–16) listed below. Each description may be used once, more than once, or not at all.

Cell Types

a. _____ Myeloid stem cells

b. _____ Monocytes

c. _____ Eosinophils

d. _____ Veiled cells

e. _____ Natural killer (NK) cells

f. _____ Kupffer cells

g. _____ Langerhans cells

h. _____ Mast cells

i. _____ Neutrophils

j. _____ M cells

k. _____ Bone-marrow stromal cells

l. _____ Intraepithelial lymphocytes

m. _____ NK1-T cell

Descriptions

(1) Circulating dendritic cells

(2) Specialized epithelial cells found in MALT

(3) Phagocytic cells important in the body's defense against parasitic organisms

(4) Macrophages found in the liver

(5) Give rise to red blood cells

(6) Dendritic cells found exclusively in lymph nodes

(7) Generally first cells to arrive at site of inflammation

(8) Secrete colony-stimulating factors (CSFs)

(9) Give rise to thymocytes

(10) Circulating blood cells that differentiate into macrophages in the tissues

(11) A type of null cell involved in antibody-dependent cell-mediated toxicity

(12) Dendritic cells found in the epidermis and mucous membranes

(13) $CD8^+$ cells that may be important in combating intestinal pathogens

(14) Nonphagocytic granulocytic cells that release various pharmacologically active substances

(15) White blood cells that migrate into the tissues and play an important role in the development of allergies

(16) These cells sometimes recognize their targets with the aid of an antigen-specific cell-surface receptor and sometimes by mechanisms that resemble those of natural killer cells.

PART II | GENERATION OF B-CELL AND T-CELL RESPONSES

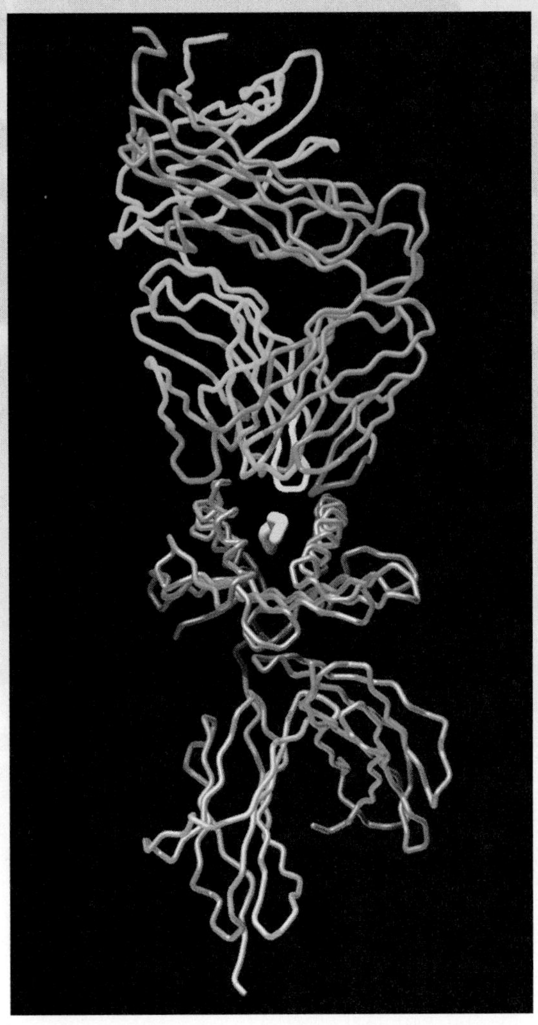

Crystal structure of T-cell receptor (blue) bound to an MHC molecule (red) and peptide antigen (yellow). Hypervariable regions of the T-cell receptor are shown in red, blue, and yellow.

In Part II we take a closer look at how lymphocyte progenitor cells develop into mature B and T cells, how these mature cells recognize foreign substances, and the consequences of recognition. Although there are many similarities between B and T cells, they are fundamentally different in how they recognize antigen.

Chapter 3 focuses on the properties that contribute to immunogenicity, that is, the ability to induce an immune response. Lymphocytes do not recognize, or interact with, an entire antigen molecule, but only with discrete, smaller sites (epitopes) on the antigen. B and T cells recognize quite distinct epitopes because of their different ways of doing so. Not only the nature of the antigen itself but certain other factors influence whether a particular antigen will induce an immune response.

Chapter 4 describes the structure of immunoglobulins, or antibodies, the recognition and effector molecules of humoral immunity. Naive B cells express membrane-bound antibody and an associated signal-transducing membrane-protein complex, which together form the antigen-binding B-cell receptor. Secreted antibody is produced by plasma cells, which are generated from naive B cells that have interacted with antigen. The sequence of the antigen-binding region of the antibody molecule is highly variable, which enables recognition of a great diversity of antigen molecules. The remainder of the antibody molecule, the constant region, has one of a small number of different sequences, which mediate different effector functions. Finally, the production and uses of monoclonal antibody, which is a single molecular species and recognizes a single antigenic determinant (epitope), are described.

We learn in Chapter 5 how the rearrangement and modification of a relatively small number of germ-line genes permits the generation of an incredibly large number of genes that encode antibodies specific for different epitopes. As described in Chapter 11, during maturation of a progenitor B cell in the bone marrow, rearrangement of the germ-line DNA generates a single functional immunoglobulin gene. The resulting mature B cell expresses antibody specific for one or more closely related epitopes. Mature B cells leave the bone marrow and circulate within the bloodstream and lymphatic system. Binding of antigen by the membrane immunoglobulin on a circulating mature B cell and its interaction with an activated T_H cell may take place within the specialized environment of secondary lymphoid organs. These events generate intracellular signals that cause changes in gene expression, leading to activation, proliferation, and differentiation of a naive B cell into memory B cells and antibody-secreting plasma cells. In the initial response to an antigen, the class of antibodies produced may change and the affinity of the antibodies for antigen increase.

The characteristics of antigen-antibody interactions are covered in Chapter 6. The binding of an antibody with an antigen is due to a large number of noncovalent interactions and is highly specific. Although these interactions produce no chemical changes in either the antigen or antibody, they can lead to precipitation of soluble antigens and agglutination (visible clumping) of particulate antigens. The exquisite specificity of antigen-antibody interactions has allowed development of both qualitative and highly sensitive quantitative assays for detecting either antigen or antibody.

The next four chapters in Part II explore the analogous processes in T cells. Unlike B cells, T cells do not recognize soluble antigen; instead, they recognize small peptides, derived from protein antigens, that are displayed on the surface of other body cells in combination with membrane molecules encoded by the major histocompatibility complex (MHC) described in Chapter 7. Thus, antigen recognition by T cells is self-MHC restricted. Chapter 8 describes the two pathways by which endogenous and exogenous antigens are processed and presented with MHC molecules so that they can be recognized by T cells.

Chapter 9 examines the heterodimeric T-cell receptor, which recognizes antigen. Unlike antibodies, T-cell receptors exist only as membrane-bound molecules. But like the antibody molecule, the TCR molecule contains a variable region, which interacts with antigen, and a constant region. Also like membrane-bound antibody, the T-cell receptor cooperates with a signal-transducing membrane-protein complex as well as with other accessory molecules that strengthen the association with antigen and assist in signal transduction. A further similarity between B and T cells is exhibited in the organization of the germ-line DNA that encodes their antigen-binding molecules and in the rearrangement of this DNA to generate functional genes.

Chapter 10 describes T-cell maturation, activation, and differentiation. Activation of T cells requires formation of a ternary complex between the T-cell receptor, an antigenic peptide, and an MHC molecule on an antigen-presenting cell or altered self-cell. This interaction generates a TCR-mediated signal and co-stimulatory signal that induce changes in gene expression, leading to activation, proliferation, and differentiation of T cells into effector and memory T cells. The vast majority of mature T cells express the $\alpha\beta$ T-cell receptor; these cells recirculate extensively and are primarily responsible for cell-mediated immune responses. About 5%–10% of the peripheral T cells express the alternative $\gamma\delta$ T-cell receptor; these cells are located primarily in the skin and intestinal epithelium, do not recirculate, and may form a primitive surveillance system for guarding the body's surfaces against invasion by microorganisms.

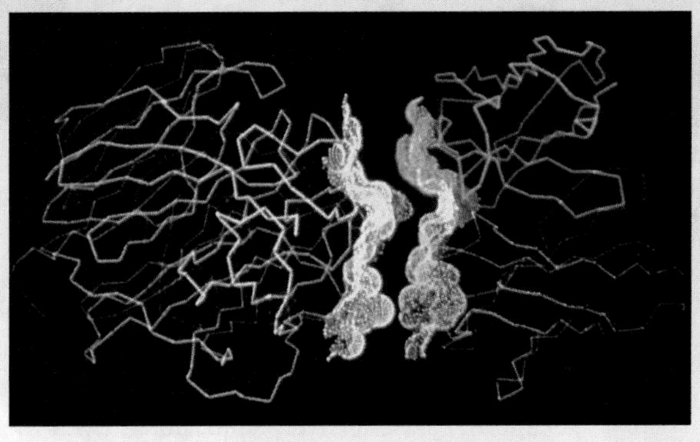

CHAPTER 3
ANTIGENS

Substances capable of inducing a specific immune response are called antigens. The molecular properties of antigens and the way in which these properties ultimately contribute to immune activation are central to our understanding of the immune system. This chapter describes some of the molecular features of antigens recognized by B or T cells. The chapter also explores the contribution made to immunogenicity by the biological system of the host; ultimately the biological system determines whether a molecule that combines with a B or T cell's antigen-binding receptor can then induce an immune response. Fundamental differences in the way T and B lymphocytes recognize antigen determine which molecular features of an antigen are recognized by each branch of the immune system. These differences also are examined in this chapter.

Immunogenicity Versus Antigenicity

Immunogenicity and antigenicity are related, but distinct, immunologic properties that sometimes are confused. **Immunogenicity** is the ability to induce a humoral and/or cell-mediated immune response:

$$\text{B cells} + \text{antigen} \longrightarrow \underset{\substack{\downarrow \\ \text{(plasma cells)}}}{\text{effector B cells}} + \text{memory B cells}$$

$$\text{T cells} + \text{antigen} \longrightarrow \underset{\substack{\downarrow \\ \text{(e.g., CTLs, } T_H\text{s)}}}{\text{effector T cells}} + \text{memory T cells}$$

Although a substance that induces a specific immune response is usually called an **antigen,** it is more appropriately called an **immunogen.**

Antigenicity is the ability to combine specifically with the final products of the above responses (i.e., antibodies and/or cell-surface receptors). Although all molecules that have the property of immunogenicity also have the property of antigenicity, the reverse is not true. Some small molecules, called **haptens,** are antigenic but incapable, by themselves, of inducing a specific immune response. In other words, they lack immunogenicity.

Factors That Influence Immunogenicity

To protect against infectious disease, the immune system must be able to recognize bacteria, bacterial products, fungi, parasites, and viruses as immunogens. In fact, the immune system actually recognizes particular macromolecules of an infectious agent, generally either proteins or polysaccharides. Proteins are the most potent immunogens, with polysaccharides ranking second. In contrast, lipids and nucleic acids of an infectious agent generally do not serve as immunogens unless they are complexed with proteins or polysaccharides. Immunologists tend to use proteins or polysaccharides as immunogens in most experimental studies of humoral immunity (Table 3-1). For cell-mediated immunity, only proteins and some lipids and glycolipids serve as immunogens. These molecules are not recognized directly. Proteins must first be processed into small peptides and then presented

TABLE 3-1 MOLECULAR WEIGHT OF SOME COMMON EXPERIMENTAL ANTIGENS USED IN IMMUNOLOGY

Antigen	Approximate molecular mass (Da)
Bovine gamma globulin (BGG)	150,000
Bovine serum albumin (BSA)	69,000
Flagellin (monomer)	40,000
Hen egg-white lysozyme (HEL)	15,000
Keyhole limpet hemocyanin (KLH)	>2,000,000
Ovalbumin (OVA)	44,000
Sperm whale myoglobin (SWM)	17,000
Tetanus toxoid (TT)	150,000

together with MHC molecules on the membrane of a cell before they can be recognized as immunogens. Recent work shows that those lipids and glycolipids that can elicit cell-mediated immunity must also be combined with MHC-like membrane molecules, called CD1 (see Chapter 8).

Immunogenicity is not an intrinsic property of an antigen but rather depends on a number of properties of the particular biological system that the antigen encounters. The next two sections describe the properties that most immunogens share and the contribution that the biological system makes to the expression of immunogenicity.

Contribution of the Immunogen to Immunogenicity

Immunogenicity is determined, in part, by four properties of the immunogen: its foreignness, molecular size, chemical composition and complexity, and ability to be processed and presented with an MHC molecule on the surface of an antigen-presenting cell or altered self-cell.

Foreignness

In order to elicit an immune response, a molecule must be recognized as nonself by the biological system. Much of the ability to recognize self-molecules is thought to arise during lymphocyte development by exposure of immature lymphocytes to self-components. Any molecule that has not been exposed to immature lymphocytes during this critical period may be later recognized as nonself, or foreign, by the immune system. When an antigen is introduced into an organism, the degree of its immunogenicity depends on the degree of its foreignness. Generally, the greater the phylogenetic distance between two species, the greater the structural (and therefore the antigenic) disparity between them.

For example, the common experimental antigen bovine serum albumin (BSA) is not immunogenic when injected into a cow but is strongly immunogenic when injected into a rabbit. Moreover, BSA would be expected to exhibit greater immunogenicity in a chicken than in a goat, which is more closely related to bovines. There are some exceptions to this rule. Some macromolecules (e.g., collagen and cytochrome *c*) were highly conserved throughout evolution and therefore display very little immunogenicity across diverse species lines. Conversely, some self-components (e.g., corneal tissue and sperm) are effectively sequestered from the immune system, so that if these tissues are injected even into the animal from which they originated, they will function as immunogens.

Molecular Size

There is a correlation between the size of a macromolecule and its immunogenicity. The best immunogens tend to have a molecular mass approaching 100,000 daltons (Da). Generally, substances with a molecular mass less than 5000–10,000 Da are poor immunogens; however, a few substances with a molecular mass less than 1000 Da have proven to be immunogenic.

Chemical Composition and Heterogeneity

Size and foreignness are not, by themselves, sufficient to make a molecule immunogenic; other properties are needed as well. For example, synthetic homopolymers (polymers composed of a single amino acid or sugar) tend to lack immunogenicity regardless of their size. Studies with copolymers composed of different amino acids has shed light on the contribution of chemical complexity to immunogenicity. Copolymers of sufficient size, if they contain two or more different amino acids, are immunogenic. The addition of aromatic amino acids, such as tyrosine or phenylalanine, profoundly enhances the immunogenicity of these synthetic polymers. For example, a synthetic copolymer of glutamic acid and lysine requires a minimum molecular weight of 30,000–40,000 for immunogenicity. The addition of tyrosine to the copolymer reduces the required minimum molecular weight to 10,000–20,000, and the addition of both tyrosine and phenylalanine reduces the minimum molecular weight to 4000. All four levels of protein organization—primary, secondary, tertiary, and quaternary—contribute to the structural complexity of a protein and hence affect its immunogenicity (Figure 3-1).

Susceptibility to Antigen Processing and Presentation

The development of both humoral and cell-mediated immune responses requires interaction of T cells with antigen that has been processed and presented together with MHC molecules. To T_H cells, the antigen must be presented with class II MHC molecules on an antigen-presenting cell; to T_C

– Lys – Ala – His – Gly – Lys – Lys – Val – Leu

Amino acid sequence
of polypeptide chain

PRIMARY STRUCTURE

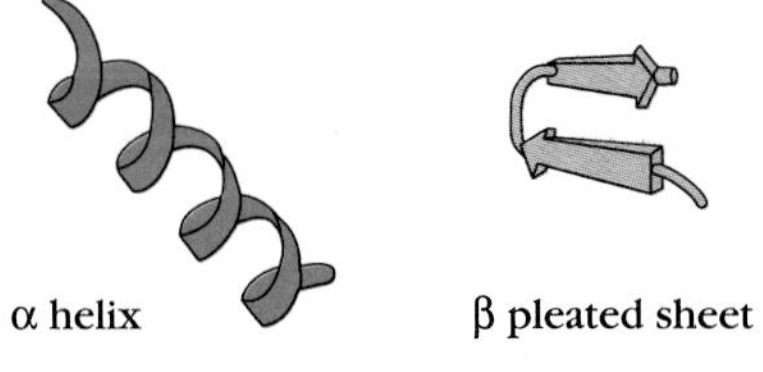

SECONDARY STRUCTURE

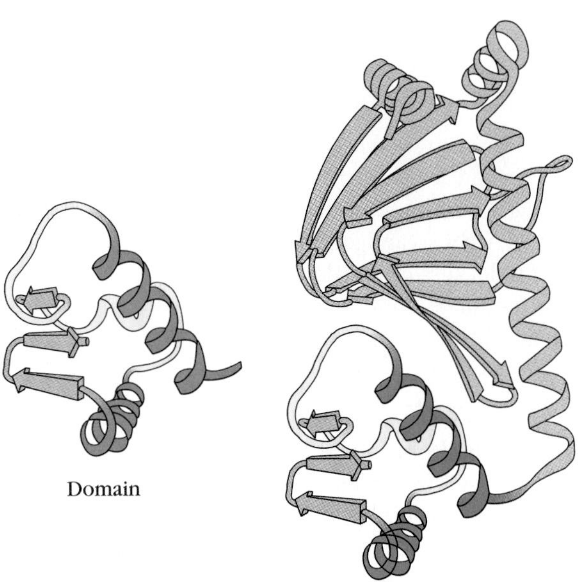

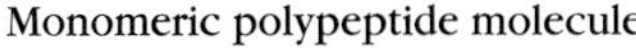

Monomeric polypeptide molecule

TERTIARY STRUCTURE

Dimeric protein molecule

QUATERNARY STRUCTURE

FIGURE 3-1 The four levels of protein organizational structure. The linear arrangement of amino acids constitutes the primary structure. Folding of parts of a polypeptide chain into regular structures (e.g., α helices and β pleated sheets) generates the secondary structure. Tertiary structure refers to the folding of regions between secondary features to give the overall shape of the molecule or parts of it (domains) with specific functional properties. Quaternary structure results from the association of two or more polypeptide chains into a single polymeric protein molecule.

cells, the antigen must be presented with class I MHC molecules on an altered self-cell. Macromolecules that cannot be degraded and presented with MHC molecules are poor immunogens. This can be illustrated with polymers of D-amino acids, which are stereoisomers of the naturally occurring L-amino acids. Because the degradative enzymes within antigen-presenting cells can degrade only proteins containing L-amino acids, polymers of D-amino acids cannot be processed and thus are poor immunogens.

Large, insoluble macromolecules generally are more immunogenic than small, soluble ones because the larger molecules are more readily phagocytosed and processed. Intermolecular chemical cross-linking, induction of aggregation by heating, and attachment to insoluble matrices have been routinely used to increase the insolubility of macromolecules, thereby facilitating their phagocytosis and increasing their immunogenicity.

Contribution of the Biological System to Immunogenicity

Even if a macromolecule has the properties that contribute to immunogenicity, its ability to induce an immune response will depend on certain properties of the biological system that the antigen encounters. These properties include the genotype of the recipient, the dose and route of antigen administration, and the administration of substances, called adjuvants, that increase immune responses.

Genotype of the Recipient Animal

The genetic constitution (**genotype**) of an immunized animal influences the type of immune response the animal manifests, as well as the degree of the response. For example, Hugh McDevitt showed that two different inbred strains of mice responded very differently to a synthetic polypeptide immunogen. After exposure to the immunogen, one strain produced high levels of serum antibody, whereas the other strain produced low levels. When the two strains were crossed, the F_1 generation showed an intermediate response to the immunogen. By backcross analysis, the gene controlling immune responsiveness was mapped to a subregion of the major histocompatibility complex (MHC). Numerous experiments with simple defined immunogens have demonstrated genetic control of immune responsiveness, largely confined to genes within the MHC . These data indicate that MHC gene products, which function to present processed antigen to T cells, play a central role in determining the degree of immune responsiveness.

The response of an animal to an antigen is also influenced by the genes that encode B-cell and T-cell receptors and by genes that encode various proteins of immune regulatory mechanisms. Genetic variability in all of these genes affects the immunogenicity of a given macromolecule in different animals. These genetic contributions to immunogenicity will be described more fully in later chapters.

Immunogen Dosage and Route of Administration

Each experimental immunogen exhibits a particular dose-response curve, which is determined by measuring the immune response to various doses and by different administration routes. Some combination of optimal dosage and route of administration will induce a peak immune response in a given animal.

An insufficient dose will not stimulate an immune response either because it fails to activate enough lymphocytes or because it induces a nonresponsive state. Conversely, an excessively high dose also can fail to induce a response because it causes lymphocytes to enter a nonresponsive state. The immune response of mice to the purified pneumococcal capsular polysaccharide illustrates the importance of dose. A 0.5-mg dose of antigen fails to induce an immune response in mice, whereas a thousand-fold lower dose of the same antigen (5×10^{-4} mg) induces a humoral antibody response. This phenomenon of "immunologic unresponsiveness," or **tolerance,** is discussed in Chapters 10 and 21. A single dose of most experimental immunogens will not induce a strong response; rather, repeated administration over a period of weeks is required to stimulate a strong immune response. Such repeated administrations, or **boosters,** increase the clonal proliferation of antigen-specific T cells or B cells.

Experimental immunogens are generally administered parenterally (*para,* around; *enteric,* gut)—that is, by routes other than the digestive tract. The following administration routes are common:

- Intravenous (iv): into a vein
- Intradermal (id): into the skin
- Subcutaneous (sc): beneath the skin
- Intramuscular (im): into a muscle
- Intraperitoneal (ip): into the peritoneal cavity

The administration route strongly influences which immune organs and cell populations will be involved in the response. Antigen administered intravenously is carried first to the spleen, whereas antigen administered subcutaneously moves first to local lymph nodes. Differences in the lymphoid cells that populate these organs may be reflected in the subsequent immune response.

Adjuvants

Adjuvants (from Latin *adjuvare,* to help) are substances that, when mixed with an antigen and injected with it, enhance the immunogenicity of that antigen. Adjuvants are often used to boost the immune response when an antigen has low immunogenicity or when only small amounts of an antigen are available. For example, the antibody response of mice to immunization with BSA can be increased fivefold or more if the BSA is administered with an adjuvant. Precisely how adjuvants augment the immune response is not entirely known, but they appear to exert one or more of the following effects (Table 3-2):

- Prolong antigen persistence
- Enhance co-stimulatory signals
- Induce granuloma formation
- Stimulate lymphocyte proliferation nonspecifically

Aluminum potassium sulfate (alum) prolongs the persistence of antigen. When an antigen is mixed with alum, the salt precipitates the antigen. Injection of this alum precipitate results in a slower release of antigen from the injection site, so that the effective time of exposure to the antigen increases from a few days without adjuvant to several weeks with the adjuvant. The alum precipitate also increases the size of the antigen, thus increasing the likelihood of phagocytosis.

Freund's water-in-oil adjuvants also prolong the persistence of antigen. **Freund's incomplete adjuvant** contains antigen in aqueous solution, mineral oil, and an emulsifying agent such as mannide monooleate, which disperses the oil into small droplets surrounding the antigen; the antigen is then released very slowly from the site of injection. **Freund's complete adjuvant,** which contains heat-killed *Mycobacteria* in the water-in-oil emulsion, also has this ef-

TABLE 3-2 POSTULATED MODE OF ACTION OF SOME COMMONLY USED ADJUVANTS

	Postulated mode of action			
Adjuvant	Prolongs antigen persistence	Enhances costimulatory signal	Induces granuloma formation	Stimulates lymphocytes nonspecifically
Freund's incomplete adjuvant	+	+	+	−
Freund's complete adjuvant	+	++	++	−
Aluminum potassium sulfate (alum)	+	?	+	−
Mycobacterium tuberculosis	−	?	+	−
Bordetella pertussis	−	?	−	+
Bacterial lipopolysaccharide (LPS)	−	+	−	+
Synthetic polynucleotides (poly IC/poly AU)	−	?	−	+

fect. Muramyl dipeptide, a component of the mycobacterial cell wall, activates macrophages, making Freund's complete adjuvant more potent than the incomplete form. Activated macrophages are more phagocytic than unactivated macrophages, express higher levels of class II MHC molecules and the membrane molecule B7, and secrete increased levels of cytokines such as interleukin 1 (IL-1). Both B7 and the increased cytokine levels enable **co-stimulation** and other signals that favor a maximal activation of T_H cells. Co-stimulation is the enhancement of immune response that results when the cell-surface proteins CD80 and CD86 on a macrophage engage with CD28 on a responding T cell. Thus, antigen presentation and the requisite co-stimulatory signal usually are increased in the presence of adjuvant.

Alum and both Freund's adjuvants also stimulate a local, chronic inflammatory response that attracts both phagocytes and lymphocytes. This infiltration of cells at the site of the adjuvant injection often results in formation of a dense, macrophage-rich mass of cells called a **granuloma.** Because the macrophages in a granuloma are activated, this mechanism also enhances the activation of T_H cells.

Other adjuvants (e.g., synthetic polyribonucleotides and bacterial lipopolysaccharides) stimulate the nonspecific proliferation of lymphocytes and thus increase the likelihood of antigen-induced clonal selection of lymphocytes.

Epitopes

As mentioned in Chapter 1, immune cells do not interact with, or recognize, an entire immunogen molecule; instead, lymphocytes recognize discrete sites on the macromolecule called **epitopes,** or **antigenic determinants.** Epitopes are the immunologically active regions of an immunogen that bind to antigen-specific membrane receptors on lymphocytes or to secreted antibodies. Studies with small antigens have revealed that B and T cells recognize different epitopes on the same antigenic molecule. For example, when mice are immunized with glucagon, a small human hormone of 29 amino acids, antibody is elicited to epitopes in the amino-terminal portion, whereas the T cells respond only to epitopes in the carboxyl-terminal portion.

Lymphocytes and a complex antigen may interact on several levels of antigen structure. An epitope on a protein antigen may involve elements of the primary, secondary, tertiary, and even quaternary structure of the protein (see Figure 3-1). In polysaccharides, extensive side-chain branching by glycosidic bonds affects the conformation of epitopes.

The recognition of antigens by T cells and B cells is fundamentally different (Table 3-3). B cells recognize soluble antigen when it binds to their membrane-bound antibody. Because B cells bind antigen that is free in solution, the epitopes they recognize tend to be highly accessible sites on the exposed surface of the immunogen. As noted previously, most T cells recognize only peptides combined with MHC molecules on the surface of antigen-presenting cells and altered self-cells. Because most T cells recognize antigen only when it is combined with an MHC molecule, T-cell epitopes, as a rule, cannot be considered apart from their associated MHC molecules.

Properties of B-Cell Epitopes

Several generalizations have emerged from studies in which the conformation of the epitope recognized by B cells has been established.

The ability to function as a B-cell epitope is determined by the nature of the antigen-binding site on the antibody molecules displayed by B cells. Antibody binds to an epitope by weak noncovalent interactions, which operate only over short distances. For a strong bond, the antibody's binding site and the epitope must have complementary shapes that place the interacting

TABLE 3-3 COMPARISON OF ANTIGEN RECOGNITION BY T CELLS AND B CELLS

Characteristic	B cells	T cells
Interaction with antigen	Involves binary complex of membrane Ig and Ag	Involves ternary complex of T-cell receptor, Ag, and MHC molecule
Binding of soluble antigen	Yes	No
Involvement of MHC molecules	None required	Required to display processed antigen
Chemical nature of antigens	Protein, polysaccharide, lipid	Mostly proteins, but some lipids and glycolipids presented on MHC-like molecules
Epitope properties	Accessible, hydrophilic, mobile peptides containing sequential or nonsequential amino acids	Internal linear peptides produced by processing of antigen and bound to MHC molecules

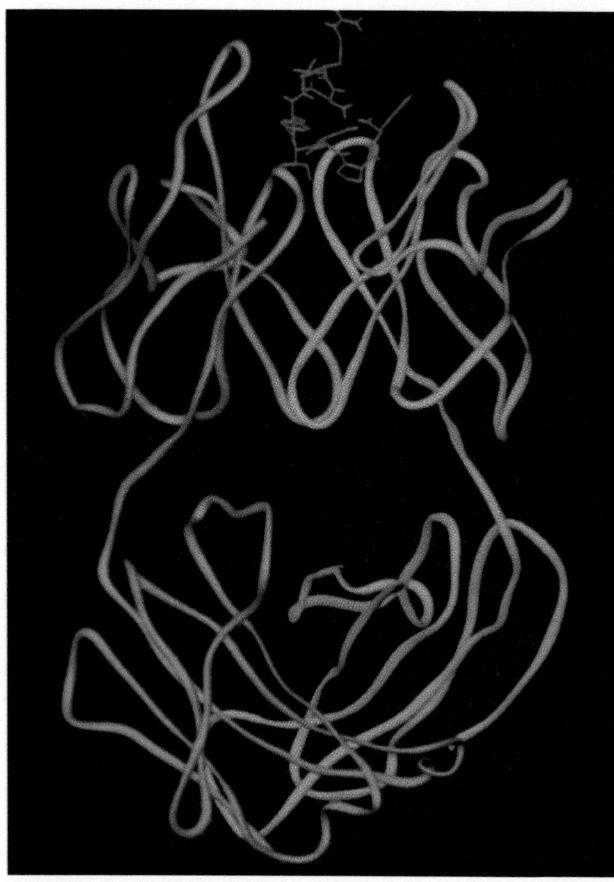

FIGURE 3-2 Three-dimensional structure of an octapeptide hormone (angiotensin II) complexed with a monoclonal antibody Fab fragment, the antigen-binding unit of the antibody molecule. The angiotensin II peptide is shown in red, the heavy chain in blue, and the light chain in purple. [From KC Garcia et al, 1992, *Science* **257**:502.]

groups near each other. This requirement poses some restriction on the properties of the epitope. The size of the epitope recognized by a B cell can be no larger than the size of the antibody's binding site. For any given antigen–antibody reaction, the shape of the epitope that can be recognized by the antibody is determined by the shape assumed by the sequences of amino acids in the binding site and the chemical environment that they produce. A detailed picture of B-cell epitope structure has emerged from x-ray crystallographic analyses of complexes between monoclonal antibodies and various antigens.

Smaller ligands such as carbohydrates, small oligonucleotides, peptides, and haptens often bind within a deep pocket of an antibody. For example, angiotensin II, a small octapeptide hormone, binds within a deep and narrow groove (725 $Å^2$) of a monoclonal antibody specific for the hormone (Figure 3-2). Within this groove, the bound peptide hormone folds into a compact structure with two turns, which brings its amino (N-terminal) and carboxyl (C-terminal) termini close together. All eight amino acid residues of the octapeptide are in van der Waals contact with 14 residues of the antibody's groove.

A quite different picture of epitope structure emerges from x-ray crystallographic analyses of monoclonal antibodies bound to globular protein antigens such as hen egg-white lysozyme (HEL) and neuraminidase (an envelope glycoprotein of influenza virus). These antibodies make contact with the antigen across a large flat face (Figure 3-3). The interacting face between antibody and epitope is a flat or undulating surface in which protrusions on the epitope or antibody are matched by corresponding depressions on the antibody or epitope. These studies have revealed that 15–22 amino acids on the surface of the antigen make contact with a similar number of residues in the antibody's binding site; the surface area of this large complementary interface is between 650 Å^2 and 900 Å^2. For these globular protein antigens, then, the shape of the epitope is entirely determined by the tertiary conformation of the native protein.

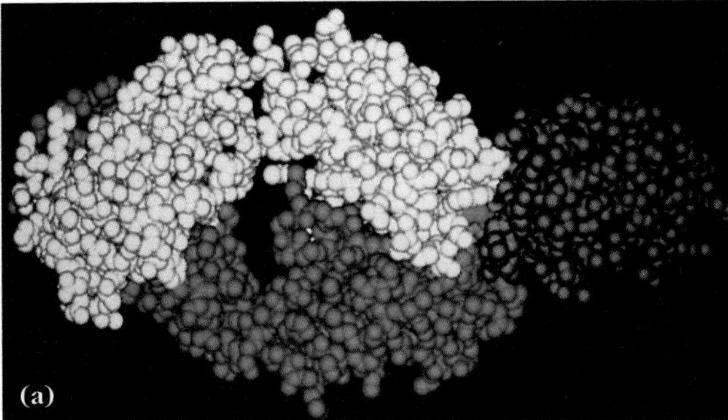

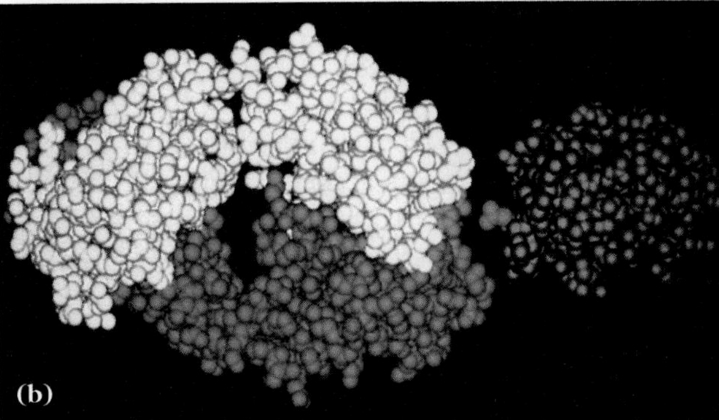

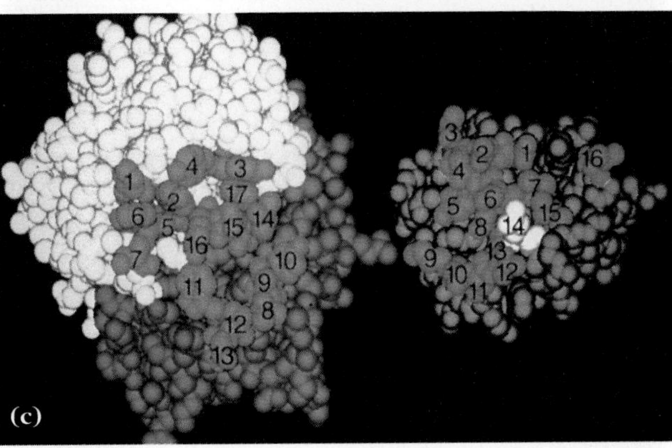

FIGURE 3-3 (a) Model of interaction between hen egg-white lysozyme (HEL) and Fab fragment of anti-HEL antibody based on x-ray diffraction analysis. HEL is shown in green, the Fab heavy chain in blue, and the Fab light chain in yellow. A glutamine residue of lysozyme (red) fits into a pocket in the Fab fragment. (b) Representation of HEL and the Fab fragment when pulled apart showing complementary surface features. (c) View of the interacting surfaces of the Fab fragment and HEL obtained by rotating each of the molecules. The contacting residues are numbered and shown in red with the protruding glutamine (#14) in HEL now shown in white. [From AG Amit et al, 1986, *Science* **233**:747.]

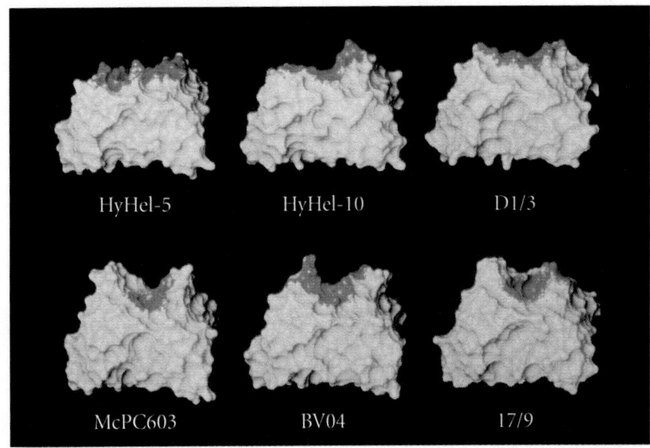

FIGURE 3-4 Models of the variable domains of six Fab fragments with their antigen-binding regions shown in purple. The top three antibodies are specific for lysozyme, a large globular protein. The lower three antibodies are specific for smaller molecules or very small segments of macromolecules: McPC603 for phosphocholine; BV04 for a small segment of a single-stranded DNA molecule; and 17/9 for a peptide from hemagglutinin, an envelope protein of influenza virus. In general, the binding sites for small molecules are deep pockets, whereas binding sites for large proteins are flatter, more undulating surfaces. [From IA Wilson and RL Stanfield, 1993, *Curr. Opin. Struc. Biol.* **3**:113.]

Thus, globular protein antigens and small peptide antigens interact with antibody in different ways (Figure 3-4). Typically, larger areas of protein antigens are engaged by the antibody binding site. In contrast, a small peptide such as angiotensin II can fold into a compact structure that occupies less space and fits into a pocket or cleft of the antibody binding site. This pattern is not unique to small peptides; it extends to the binding of low-molecular-weight antigens of various chemical types. However, these differences between the binding of small and large antigenic determinants do not reflect fundamental differences in the regions of the antibody molecule that make up the binding site. Despite differences in the binding patterns of small haptens and large antigens, all antibody binding sites are assembled from the same regions of the antibody molecule. Chapter 4 will show that all binding sites are made up of the same regions of the antibody molecule—namely, parts of the variable regions of its polypeptide chains.

The B-cell epitopes on native proteins generally are composed of hydrophilic amino acids on the protein surface that are topographically accessible to membrane-bound or free antibody. A B-cell epitope must be accessible in order to be able to bind to an antibody. Amino acid sequences that are hidden within the interior of a protein cannot function as B-cell epitopes unless the protein is first denatured.

Michael Sela demonstrated the importance of this topographical accessibility in experiments with synthetic branched copolymers in which the accessible amino acids attached to the backbone polypeptide chain were varied. One

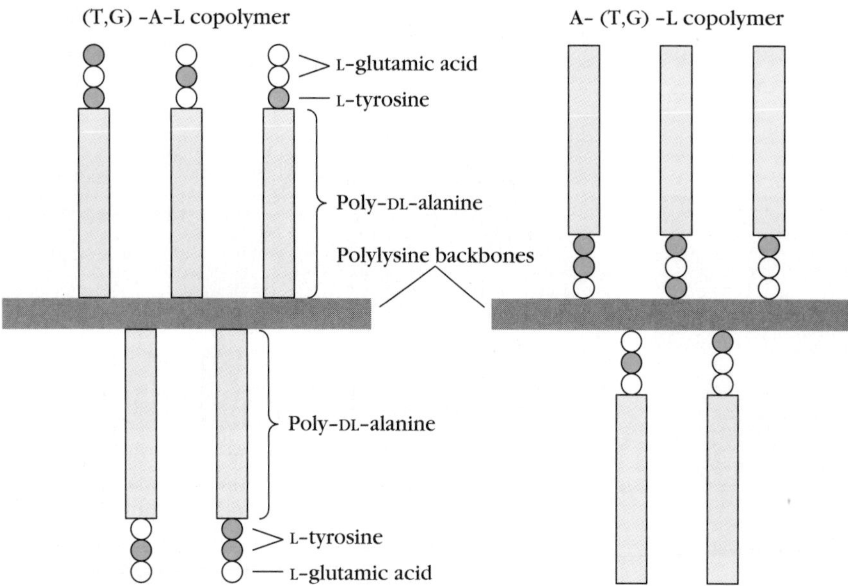

FIGURE 3-5 Antibodies elicited by immunization with the (T,G)-A-L copolymer (*left*) react largely with the exposed tyrosine and glutamic acid residues. Anti-(T,G)-A-L antibodies do not react with the A-(T,G)-L copolymer (*right*) in which the tyrosine and glutamic acid residues are buried. [Adapted from M Sela, 1969, *Science* **166**:1365.]

copolymer, designated (T,G)-A-L, consisted of a poly-L-lysine backbone with poly D,L-alanine side chains whose N-termini were capped with variable amounts of L-glutamic acid and/or L-tyrosine (Figure 3-5). Antibody to (T,G)-A-L reacted largely with the accessible tyrosine and glutamic acid residues at the ends of the side chains. Furthermore, the related synthetic copolymer A-(T,G)-L, in which poly D,L-alanine residues were in the accessible terminal positions and the glutamic acid and tyrosine residues were less accessible, did not react with the antibody to (T,G)-A-L.

The entire surface of globular proteins is thought to be potentially antigenic. In general, regions that protrude on the surface of the protein are recognized as epitopes. Because the residues are accessible, they are often hydrophilic. In the crystallized antigen-antibody complexes analyzed to date, the interface between antibody and antigen shows numerous complementary protrusions and depressions (Figure 3-6). Between 15 and 22 amino acids on the antigen contact the antibody by 75–120 hydrogen bonds as well as by ionic and hydrophobic interactions.

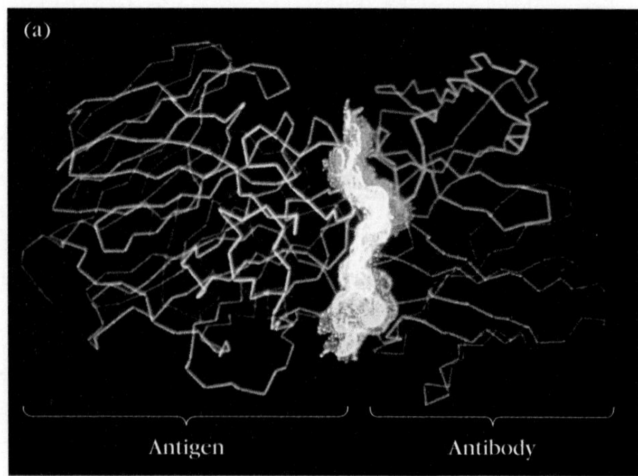

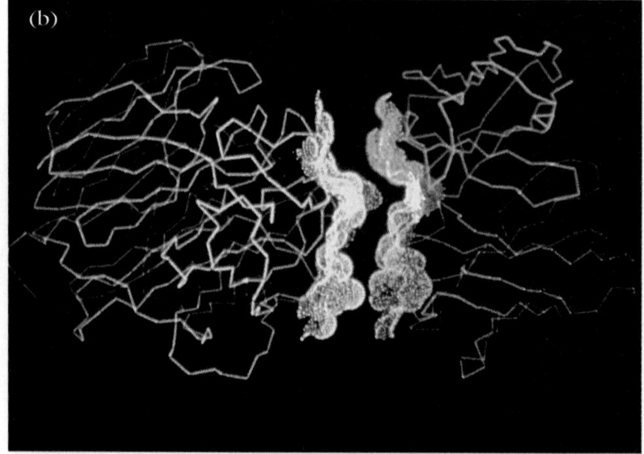

FIGURE 3-6 Computer simulation of an interaction between antibody and influenza virus antigen, a globular protein. (a) The antigen (yellow) is shown interacting with the antibody molecule; the variable region of the heavy chain is red, and the variable region of the light chain is blue. (b) The complementarity of the two molecules is revealed by separating the antigen from the antibody by 8 Å. [Based on x-ray crystallography data collected by PM Colman and WR Tulip. From GJVH Nossal, 1993, *Sci. Am.* **269**(3):22.]

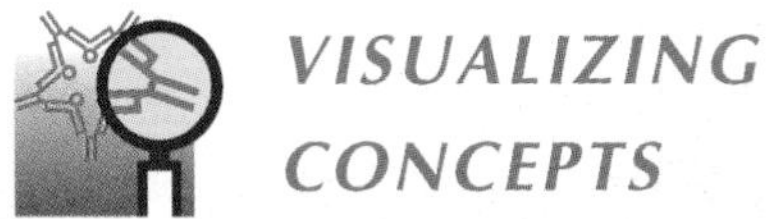

(a)

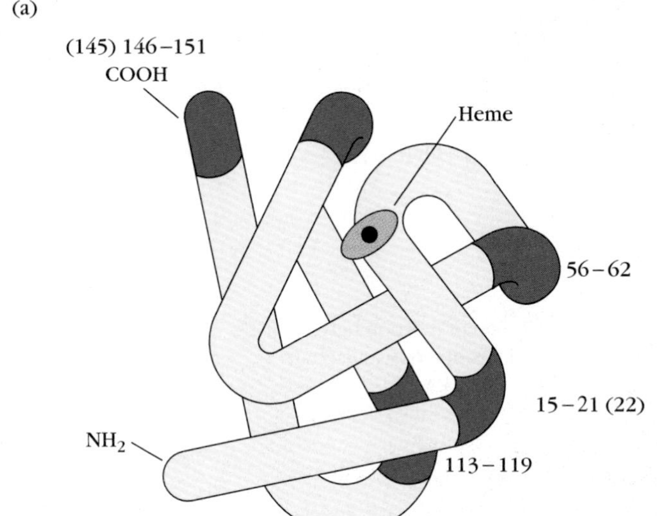

(b)

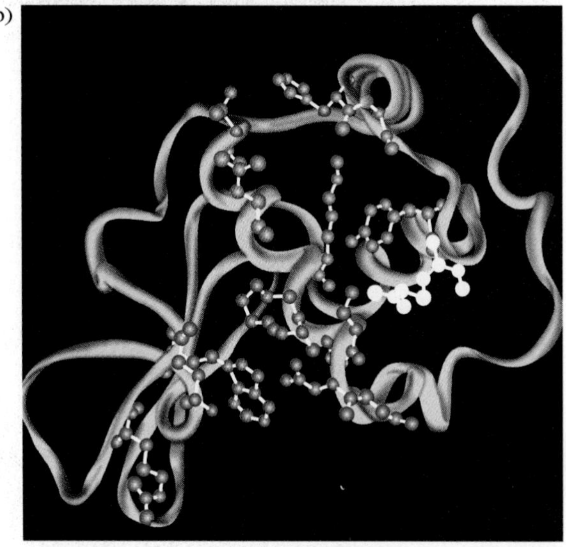

FIGURE 3-7 Protein antigens usually contain both sequential and nonsequential B-cell epitopes. (a) Diagram of sperm whale myoglobin showing locations of five sequential B-cell epitopes (blue). (b) Ribbon diagram of hen egg-white lysozyme showing residues that compose one nonsequential (conformational) epitope. Residues that contact antibody light chains, heavy chains, or both are shown in red, blue, and white, respectively. These residues are widely spaced in the amino acid sequence but are brought into proximity by folding of the protein. [Part (a) adapted from MZ Atassi and AL Kazim, 1978, *Adv. Exp. Med. Biol.* **98:**9; part (b) from WG Laver et al, 1990, *Cell* **61**:554.]

B-cell epitopes can contain sequential or nonsequential amino acids. Epitopes may be composed of sequential contiguous residues along the polypeptide chain or nonsequential residues from segments of the chain brought together by the folded conformation of an antigen. Most antibodies elicited by globular proteins bind to the protein only when it is in its native conformation. Because denaturation of such antigens usually changes the structure of their epitopes, antibodies to the native protein do not bind to the denatured protein.

Sperm whale myoglobin, which has an abundance of α-helical regions, contains five distinct **sequential epitopes,** each containing six to eight contiguous amino acids. Each of these epitopes is on the surface of the molecule at bends between the α-helical regions (Figure 3-7a). Sperm whale myoglobin also contains several **nonsequential epitopes,** or **conformational determinants.** The residues that constitute these epitopes are far apart in the primary amino acid sequence but close together in the tertiary structure of the molecule. Such epitopes depend on the native protein conformation for their topographical structure. One well-characterized nonsequential epitope in hen egg-white lysozyme is shown in Figure 3-7b. Although the amino acid residues that compose this epitope of HEL are far apart in the primary amino acid sequence, they are brought together by the tertiary folding of the protein.

Sequential and nonsequential epitopes generally behave differently when a protein is denatured, fragmented, or reduced. For example, appropriate fragmentation of sperm whale myoglobin can yield five fragments, each retaining one sequential epitope, as demonstrated by the observation that antibody can bind to each fragment. On the other hand, fragmentation of a protein or reduction of its disulfide bonds often destroys nonsequential epitopes. For example, HEL has four intrachain disulfide bonds, which determine the final protein conformation (Figure 3-8a). Many antibodies to HEL recognize eight different epitopes, most of which are conformational determinants dependent on the overall structure of the protein. If the intrachain disulfide bonds of HEL are reduced with mercaptoethanol, the nonsequential epitopes are lost; for this reason, antibody to native HEL does not bind to reduced HEL.

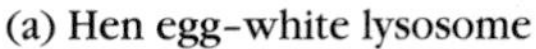

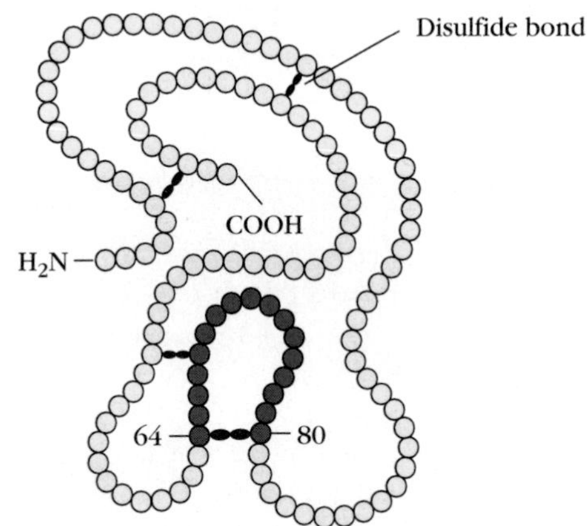

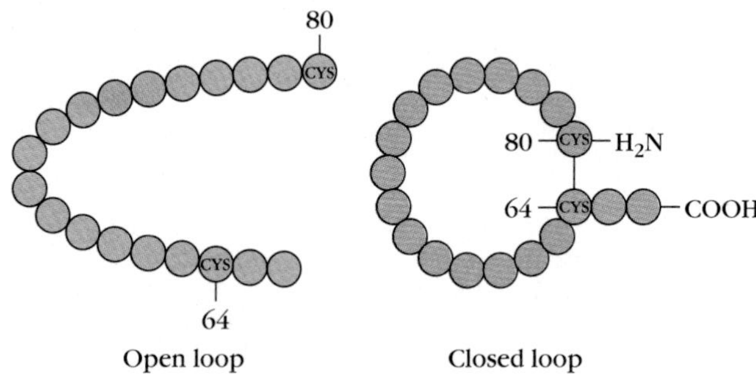

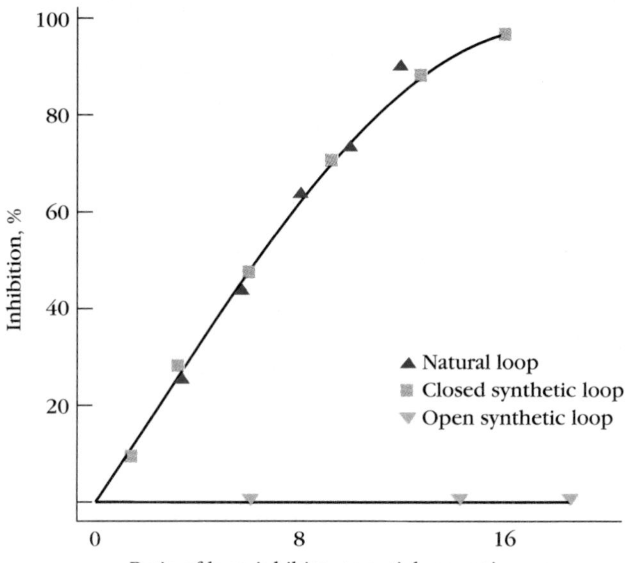

FIGURE 3-8 Experimental demonstration that binding of antibody to conformational determinants in hen egg-white lysozyme (HEL) depends on maintenance of the tertiary structure of the epitopes by intrachain disulfide bonds. (a) Diagram of HEL primary structure, in which circles represent amino acid residues. The loop (blue circles) formed by the disulfide bond between the cysteine residues at positions 64 and 80 constitutes one of the conformational determinants in HEL. (b) Synthetic open-loop and closed-loop peptides corresponding to the HEL loop epitope. (c) Inhibition of binding between HEL loop epitope and anti-loop antiserum. Anti-loop antiserum was first incubated with the natural loop sequence, the synthetic closed-loop peptide, or the synthetic open-loop peptide; the ability of the antiserum to bind the natural loop sequence then was measured. The absence of any inhibition by the open-loop peptide indicates that it does not bind to the anti-loop antiserum. [Adapted from D Benjamin et al, 1984, *Annu. Rev. Immunol.* **2**:67.]

The inhibition experiment shown in Figure 3-8 nicely demonstrates this point. An antibody to a conformational determinant, in this example a peptide loop present in native HEL, was able to bind the epitope only if the disulfide bond that maintains the structure of the loop was intact. Information about the structural requirements of the antibody combining site was obtained by examining the ability of structural relatives of the natural antigen to bind to that antibody. If a structural relative has the critical epitopes present in the natural antigen, it will bind to the antibody combining site, thereby blocking its occupation by the natural antigen. In this inhibition assay, the ability of the closed loop to inhibit binding showed that the closed loop was sufficiently similar to HEL to be recognized by antibody to native HEL. Even though the open loop had the same sequence of amino acids as the closed loop, it lacked the epitopes recognized by the antibody and therefore was unable to block binding of HEL.

B-cell epitopes tend to be located in flexible regions of an immunogen and display site mobility. John A. Tainer and his colleagues analyzed the epitopes on a number of protein antigens (myohemerytherin, insulin, cytochrome *c*, myoglobin, and hemoglobin) by comparing the positions of the known B-cell epitopes with the mobility of the same residues. Their analysis revealed that the major antigenic determinants in these proteins generally were located in the most mobile regions. These investigators proposed that site mobility of epitopes maximizes complementarity with the antibody's binding site, permitting an antibody to react with an epitope that it might not otherwise react with if it were rigid. However, because of the loss of entropy due to binding to a flexible site, the binding of antibody to a flexible epitope is generally of lower affinity than the binding of antibody to a rigid epitope.

Complex proteins contain multiple overlapping B-cell epitopes, some of which are immunodominant. For many years, it was dogma in immunology that each globular protein had a small number of epitopes, each confined to a highly accessible region and determined by the overall conformation of the protein. However, it has been shown more recently that most of the surface of a globular protein is potentially antigenic. This has been demonstrated by comparing the antigen-binding profiles of different monoclonal antibodies to various globular proteins. For example, when 64 different monoclonal antibodies to BSA were compared for their ability to bind to a panel of 10 different mammalian albumins, 25 different overlapping antigen-binding profiles emerged, suggesting that these 64 different antibodies recognized a minimum of 25 different epitopes on BSA. Similar findings have emerged for other globular proteins, such as myoglobin and HEL.

The surface of a protein, then, must present a large number of potential antigenic sites. The subset of antigenic sites on a given protein that is recognized by the immune system of an animal is much smaller than the potential antigenic repertoire, and it varies from species to species and even among individual members of a given species. Within an animal, certain epitopes of an antigen are recognized as immunogenic, but others are not. Furthermore, some epitopes, called **immunodominant,** induce a more pronounced immune response than other epitopes in a particular animal. It is thought that intrinsic topographical properties of the epitope as well as the animal's regulatory mechanisms influence the immunodominance of epitopes.

Properties of T-Cell Epitopes

Studies by P. G. H. Gell and Baruj Benacerraf in 1959 suggested that there was a qualitative difference between the T-cell and the B-cell response to protein antigens. Gell and Benacerraf compared the humoral (B-cell) and cell-mediated (T-cell) responses to a series of native and denatured protein antigens (Table 3-4). They found that when primary immunization was with a native protein, only native protein, not denatured protein, could elicit a secondary antibody (humoral) response. In contrast, both native and denatured protein could elicit a secondary cell-mediated response. The finding that a secondary response mediated by T cells was induced by denatured protein, even when the primary immunization had been with native protein, initially puzzled immunologists. In the 1980s, however, it became clear that T cells do not recognize soluble native antigen but rather recognize antigen that has been processed into **antigenic peptides,** which are presented in combination with MHC molecules. For this reason, destruction of the conformation of a protein by denaturation does not affect its T-cell epitopes.

Because the T-cell receptor does not bind free peptides, experimental systems for studying T-cell epitopes must include antigen-presenting cells or target cells that can display the peptides bound to an MHC molecule. In some systems, synthetic peptides are first allowed to interact with MHC molecules on antigen-presenting cells, and then T-cell proliferation is measured. Only activated T cells will undergo cell division, and activation requires the TCRs of responding cells to recognize peptide-MHC complexes on antigen-presenting cells. Consequently, only those peptides that contain epitopes recognized by the TCRs of responding T cell populations can induce proliferation in these populations.

Antigenic peptides recognized by T cells form trimolecular complexes with a T-cell receptor and an MHC molecule. Before a T cell can be activated, a trimolecular complex must form between its antigen-binding receptor, an MHC molecule, and an antigenic peptide. Antigens recognized by T cells must, therefore, have two distinct interaction sites: one, the epitope, interacts with the T-cell receptor, and the other, called the **agretope,** interacts with an MHC molecule (Figure 3-9). The structures of TCR-peptide-MHC trimolecular complexes have been determined by x-ray crystallography and are described in Chapter 9.

X-ray crystallography of class I or class II MHC molecules crystallized with known T-cell antigenic peptides has shown that the peptide binds to a cleft in the MHC molecule (see Figure 7-8). This bond is due primarily to certain

TABLE 3-4 ANTIGEN RECOGNITION BY T AND B LYMPHOCYTES REVEALS QUALITATIVE DIFFERENCES

		Secondary immune response	
Primary immunization	Secondary immunization	Antibody production	Cell-mediated T_{DTH} response*
Native protein	Native protein	+	+
Native protein	Denatured protein	−	+

*T_{DTH} is a subset of $CD4^+$ T_H cells that mediate a cell-mediated response called delayed-type hypersensitivity (see Chapter 14).

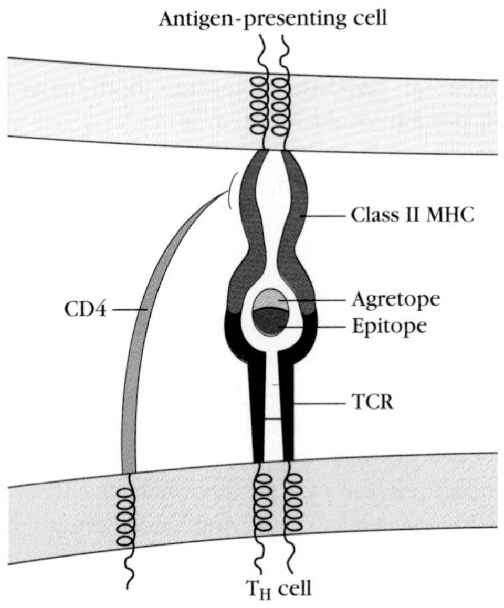

FIGURE 3-9 Schematic diagram of the ternary complex formed between a T-cell receptor (TCR) on a T_H cell, an antigen, and a class II MHC molecule. Antigens that are recognized by T cells have two distinct interaction sites: an agretope, which interacts with an MHC molecule, and an epitope, which interacts with the T-cell receptor. As described in later chapters, CD4 on T_H cells also interacts with MHC molecules. T_C cells form similar ternary complexes with class I MHC molecules on target cells.

key residues of the peptide, which protrude into complementary pockets in the cleft of the MHC molecule (Figures 7-10 and 7-13). Unlike B-cell epitopes, which can be viewed strictly in terms of their ability to interact with antibody, T-cell epitopes must be viewed in terms of their ability to interact with both a T-cell receptor and an MHC molecule.

The antigen-binding cleft on an MHC molecule interacts with various oligomeric peptides that function as T-cell epitopes. The antigen-binding cleft on an MHC molecule determines the nature and size of the peptide(s) that the MHC molecule can bind and consequently the maximal size of the T-cell epitope. Studies of the binding of peptides to class I MHC molecules have revealed that peptides of nine amino acid residues (nonamers) bind most strongly; peptides of 8–11 residues also bind but generally with lower affinity than nonamers. With class II MHC molecules, peptides of 12–25 amino acid residues are preferentially bound.

The binding of an MHC molecule to an antigenic peptide does not appear to have the kind of fine specificity of the interaction between an antibody and its epitope. Instead, a given MHC molecule can selectively bind a variety of different peptides. For example, the class II MHC molecule designated IA^d can bind peptides from ovalbumin (residues 323–339), hemagglutinin (residues 130–142), and lambda repressor (residues 12–26). This broad but selective interaction suggests that the agretopes on these various peptides may share certain structural features, enabling them to bind to the same MHC molecule. Studies revealing structural features, or motifs, common to different peptides that bind to a single MHC molecule are described in Chapter 7.

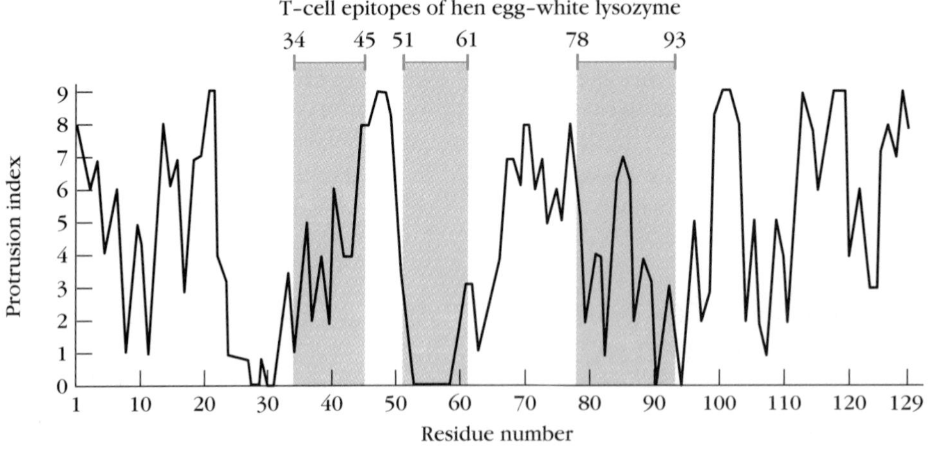

FIGURE 3-10 Experimental evidence that T_H cells tend to recognize internal peptides of antigens. This plot shows the relative protrusion of amino acid residues in the tertiary conformation of hen egg-white lysozyme. The known T-cell epitopes in HEL are indicated by the blue bars at the top. Notice that, in general, the amino acid residues that correspond to the T-cell epitopes exhibit less overall protrusion. In contrast, note that the B-cell epitope consisting of residues 64–80, which form a conformational determinant in native HEL that is recognized by antibody (see Figure 3-8), exhibit greater overall protrusion. [From J Rothbard et al, 1987, *Mod. Trends Hum. Leuk.*, vol. 7.]

Antigen processing is required to generate peptides that interact specifically with MHC molecules. As mentioned in Chapter 1, endogenous antigens and exogenous antigens appear to be processed by different intracellular pathways (see Figure 1-9). Endogenous antigens are processed into peptides within the cytoplasm, while exogenous antigens are processed within the endocytic pathway. Processing yields antigenic peptides that combine with class I or class II MHC molecules; the resulting peptide-MHC complexes are then presented on the cell surface, where they can be recognized by T cells. The details of antigen processing and presentation are described in Chapter 8.

Epitopes recognized by T cells are often internal. T cells tend to recognize internal peptides that are exposed by processing within antigen-presenting cells or altered self-cells. J. Rothbard analyzed the tertiary conformation of hen egg-white lysozyme and sperm whale myoglobin to determine which amino acids protruded from the natural molecule. He then mapped the major T-cell epitopes for both proteins and found that, in each case, the T-cell epitopes tended to be on the "inside" of the protein molecule (Figure 3-10).

Immunodominant T-cell epitopes are determined in part by the set of MHC molecules expressed by an individual. Various experiments have suggested that the MHC plays a significant role in determining which T-cell epitopes in a given antigen will be immunodominant in a given individual. For example, S. Buus and coworkers found a correlation between the ability of a peptide to bind to a particular MHC molecule and the T-cell response to that peptide. These researchers analyzed 14 synthetic peptides, representing overlapping sequences of the entire length of an immunogenic protein. Of these 14 peptides, the three that activated T_H cells also bound to a class II MHC molecule expressed by the same strain of mice (Figure 3-11).

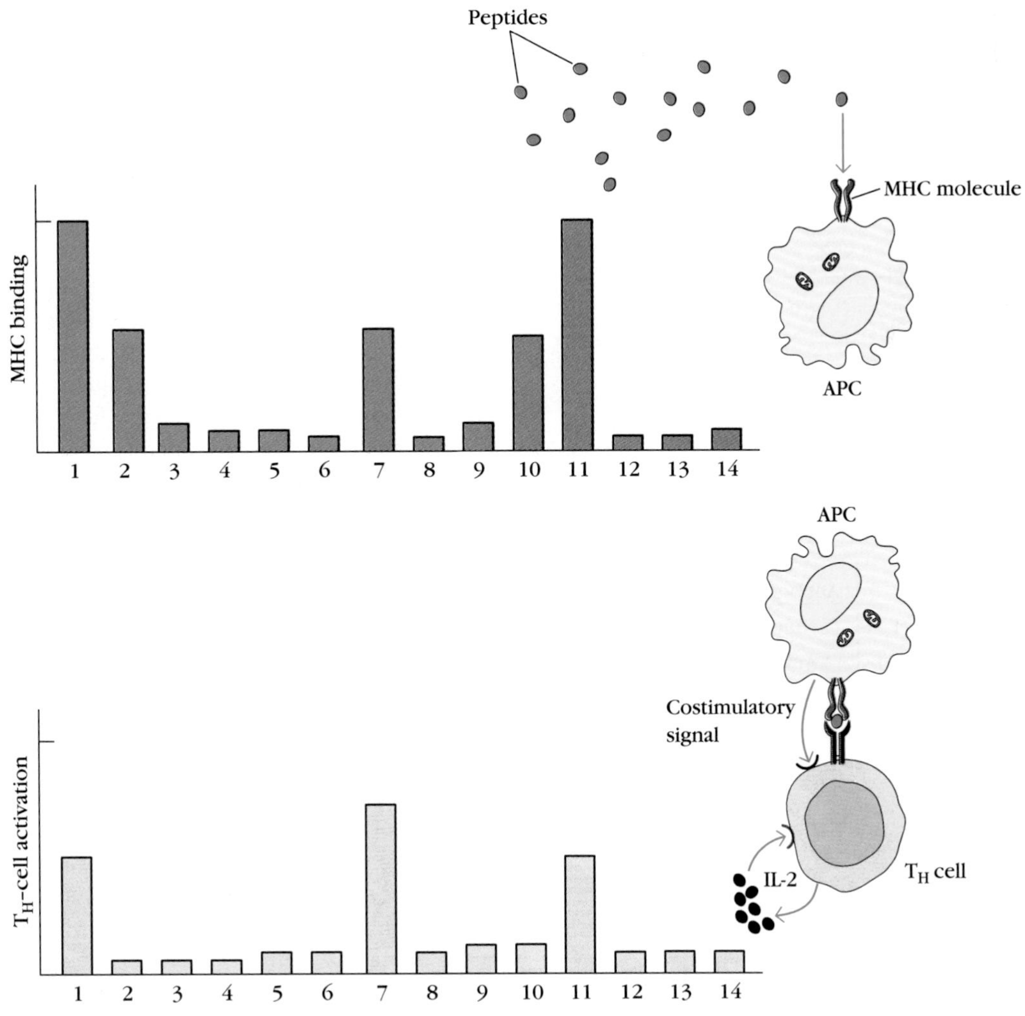

FIGURE 3-11 Correlation of MHC-binding ability and T-cell–activating ability of 14 synthetic peptides representing overlapping sequences of an immunogenic protein. Of the five peptides that bound to MHC molecules on mouse antigen-presenting cells (*top*), three also stimulated T-cell activation (*bottom*). These data suggest that binding to an MHC molecule is necessary, but not sufficient, for a peptide to induce an immune response. [Adapted from HM Grey et al, 1989, *Sci. Am.* **261**(5):59.]

Haptens and the Study of Antigenicity

The pioneering work of Karl Landsteiner in the 1920s and 1930s created a simple, chemically defined system for studying the binding of an individual antibody to a unique epitope on a complex protein antigen. Landsteiner employed various **haptens,** small organic molecules that are antigenic but not immunogenic. Chemical coupling of a hapten to a large protein, called a **carrier,** yields an immunogenic **hapten-carrier conjugate.** Animals immunized with such a conjugate produce antibodies specific for (1) the hapten determinant, (2) unaltered epitopes on the carrier protein, and (3) new epitopes formed by combined parts of both the hapten and carrier (Figure 3-12). By itself, a hapten cannot function as an immunogenic epitope. But when multiple molecules of a single hapten are coupled to a carrier protein (or nonimmunogenic homopolymer), the hapten becomes accessible to the immune system and often functions as the immunodominant determinant.

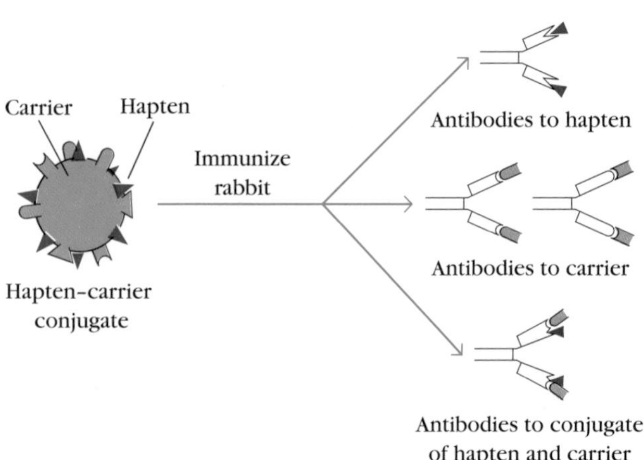

Injection with:	Antibodies formed:
Hapten (DNP)	None
Protein carrier (BSA)	Anti-BSA
Hapten-carrier conjugate (DNP-BSA)	Anti-DNP (major) Anti-BSA (minor) Anti-DNP/BSA (minor)

FIGURE 3-12 A hapten-carrier conjugate contains multiple copies of the hapten—a small nonimmunogenic organic compound such as dinitrophenol (DNP)—chemically linked to a large protein carrier such as bovine serum albumin (BSA). Immunization with DNP alone elicits no anti-DNP antibodies, but immunization with DNP-BSA elicits three types of antibodies. Of these, anti-DNP antibody is predominant, indicating that in this case the hapten is the immunodominant epitope in a hapten-carrier conjugate, as it often is in such conjugates.

The beauty of the hapten-carrier system is that it provides immunologists with a chemically defined determinant that can be subtly modified by chemical means to determine the effect of various chemical structures on immune specificity. In his studies, Landsteiner immunized rabbits with a hapten-carrier conjugate and then tested the reactivity of the rabbit's immune sera with that hapten and with closely related haptens coupled to a different carrier protein. Thus he could measure, specifically, the reaction of the antihapten antibodies in the immune serum and not that of antibodies to the original carrier epitopes. Landsteiner tested whether an antihapten antibody could bind to other haptens having a slightly different chemical structure. If a reaction occurred, it was called a **cross-reaction.** By observing which hapten modifications prevented or permitted cross-reactions, Landsteiner was able to gain insight into the specificity of antigen-antibody interactions.

Using various derivatives of aminobenzene as haptens, Landsteiner found that the overall configuration of a hapten plays a major role in determining whether it can react with a given antibody. For example, antiserum from rabbits immunized with aminobenzene or one of its carboxyl derivatives (*o*-aminobenzoic acid, *m*-aminobenzoic acid, or *p*-aminobenzoic acid) coupled to a carrier protein reacted only with the original immunizing hapten and did not cross-react with any of the other haptens (Table 3-5, *top*). In contrast, if the overall configuration of the hapten was kept the same and the hapten was modified in the para position with various nonionic derivatives, then the antisera showed various degrees of cross-reactivity (Table 3-5, *bottom*). Landsteiner's work not only demonstrated the specificity of the immune system, but also demonstrated the enormous diversity of epitopes that the immune system is capable of recognizing.

Many biologically important substances, including drugs, peptide hormones, and steroid hormones, can function as haptens. Conjugates of these haptens with large protein carriers can be used to produce hapten-specific antibodies. These antibodies are useful for measuring the presence of various substances in the body. For instance, the original home pregnancy test kit employed antihapten antibodies to determine whether a woman's urine contained human chorionic gonadotropin (HCG), which is a sign of pregnancy. However, as shown in the Clinical Focus, the formation of drug-protein conjugates in the body can produce drug allergies that may be life-threatening.

TABLE 3-5 REACTIVITY OF ANTISERA WITH VARIOUS HAPTENS

	Reactivity with			
Antiserum against	Aminobenzene (aniline)	*o*-Aminobenzoic acid	*m*-Aminobenzoic acid	*p*-Aminobenzoic acid
Aminobenzene	+++	0	0	0
o-Aminobenzoic acid	0	+++	0	0
m-Aminobenzoic acid	0	0	++++	0
p-Aminobenzoic acid	0	0	0	+++/++++

	Reactivity with			
Antiserum against	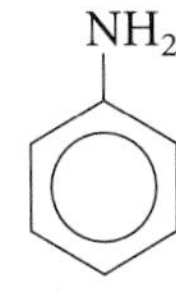 Aminobenzene (aniline)	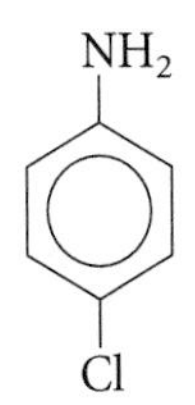 *p*-Chloroamino benzene	*p*-Toluidine	*p*-Nitroamino benzene
Aminobenzene	+/++	+	+±	+
p-Chloroaminobenzene	+++	++	++	+/++
p-Toluidine	++/+	++	++	+
p-Nitroaminobenzene	+	++	+/++	+

KEY: 0 = no reactivity; +++ and ++++ = strong reactivity; ++ and + = lesser degrees of reactivity

SOURCE: Based on K Landsteiner, 1962, *The Specificity of Serologic Reactions,* Dover Press. Modified by J Klein, 1982, *Immunology: The Science of Self-Nonself Discrimination,* John Wiley.

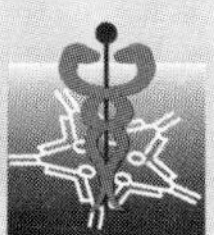

CLINICAL FOCUS
DRUG ALLERGIES—WHEN MEDICINES BECOME IMMUNOGENS

During and after World War II, penicillin came increasingly to be used in the successful treatment of a wide variety of bacterial infections. Although the penicillin family of antibiotics has become a mainstay in the arsenal of antibacterial agents, these powerful drugs are not without their drawbacks. One of these is, of course, the role of penicillins and other antibiotics in the evolution of antibiotic-resistant bacterial strains. The other is their capacity to induce allergic reactions in some patients. Medical science became aware of this when an increasing number of serious allergic reactions, some of which resulted in death, were traced to penicillin exposure. Indeed, penicillin and its relatives are responsible for most of the recorded allergic reactions to drugs and 97% of the deaths caused each year by drug allergies.

Penicillin and other drug allergies can be induced by small doses of the drug; they are not consequences of the pharmacological or physiological effects of the drugs. Typically, an allergic response occurs about a week or so after the patient's first exposure to the agent. The symptoms produced are typically mild, often including hives, some fever, possibly swelling of lymph nodes, and, in some patients, an arthritis-like discomfort. However, subsequent treatments with the drug usually cause much more rapid and, often, more severe reactions. Symptoms can appear within minutes after drug injection and may include swelling of the throat and eyelids. The greatest danger is that these symptoms can progress to anaphylaxis, a grave physiological collapse that often involves the respiratory, circulatory, and digestive systems. Hives are not unusual and there may be gastrointestinal symptoms such as vomiting, abdominal pain, and diarrhea. It is the respiratory and circulatory problems, however, that make anaphylaxis life threatening. There is shortness of breath, wheezing, and, in some cases, mechanical obstruction of airflow by swelling of the larynx and epiglottis. A profound drop in blood pressure causes shock and is frequently accompanied by weakened heart contractions. Treatment of anaphylaxis thus requires immediate medical intervention.

Injection of the drug epinephrine (adrenaline) is the treatment of choice for anaphylaxis. It has two critical effects that intervene to stop and reverse the body's slide into deeper and deeper anaphylaxis. One of these is to raise blood pressure and ease constriction of the air passages, and the other is to inhibit the release from mast cells and basophils of the agents that induce anaphylaxis. Other drugs may also be used to treat the low blood pressure and strengthen heart contractions. For relief of respiratory distress, oxygen and other drugs that open and expand airways are sometimes given. After a case of drug-induced anaphylaxis, the use of the agent responsible is discontinued and the affected individual is advised to carry or wear a notice of his allergy to the offending drug.

Like penicillin, most drugs are low-molecular-weight compounds that are not capable of inducing immune responses unless they are conjugated with a larger molecule. Intensive investigation of allergy to penicillin has provided critical insight into the basis of allergic reactions to this and other drugs. As shown in the accompanying figure, penicillin can react with proteins to form a penicilloyl-protein derivative. The penicilloyl-protein behaves as a hapten-carrier conjugate, with the penicillin-derived penicilloyl group acting as a haptenic epitope. This epitope is readily recognized by the immune system, and antibodies are produced against it. Some individuals respond to penicillin by producing significant amounts of a type of antibody known

Summary

1. Immunogenicity is the ability of an antigen to induce an immune response by either the humoral or the cell-mediated branch of the immune system. Antigenicity is the ability of an antigen simply to interact specifically with free antibody and/or with antigen-binding receptors on lymphocytes. B cells and T cells recognize small sites called antigenic determinants, or epitopes, on a complex immunogen.
2. The foreignness, molecular size, chemical composition and complexity, and susceptibility to antigen processing and presentation influence the immunogenicity of a substance. In addition, several properties of the biological system that an antigen encounters affect its immunogenicity; these include the genotype of the recipient animal, in particular, its set of MHC genes; the immunogen dosage; the route of administration; and the presence or absence of adjuvants.
3. The size of B-cell epitopes ranges widely. Some are quite small (e.g., small peptides or small organic molecules), whereas protein B-cell epitopes are much larger. Protein B-cell epitopes tend to be amino acid sequences that are accessible, hydrophilic, and mobile. In general, a small peptide epitope interacts with a deep, narrow groove in the antibody molecule; a protein epitope interacts with a larger, flatter complementary surface on the antibody

as immunoglobulin E (IgE). Once generated, these IgE antibodies are dispersed throughout the body and are bound by IgE receptors on the surfaces of mast cells and basophils, where they can remain for a long time. If a person with penicillin-specific IgE antibody bound to mast cells is subsequently treated with penicillin, there may be an allergic reaction. In fact, between 1 and 5 percent of people treated with penicillin do develop some degree of allergy to it.

Penicillin is not the only drug against which patients can develop allergies. Others include streptomycin, aspirin, sulfa-containing antibiotics ("sulfa-drugs"), some anesthetics (e.g., succinyl choline), and some opiates. All of these small molecules first react with proteins to form drug-protein derivatives. When this happens, there is a possibility that the immune system will produce an anti-hapten response to the drug, just as with penicillin. This is the basis of a general principle of drug allergy. If a low-molecular-weight drug, or its metabolic products, are capable of forming covalent conjugates with proteins, there is some likelihood that drug allergies will arise. On the other hand, drugs (and their metabolites) that are incapable of forming drug-protein conjugates rarely elicit allergic reactions.

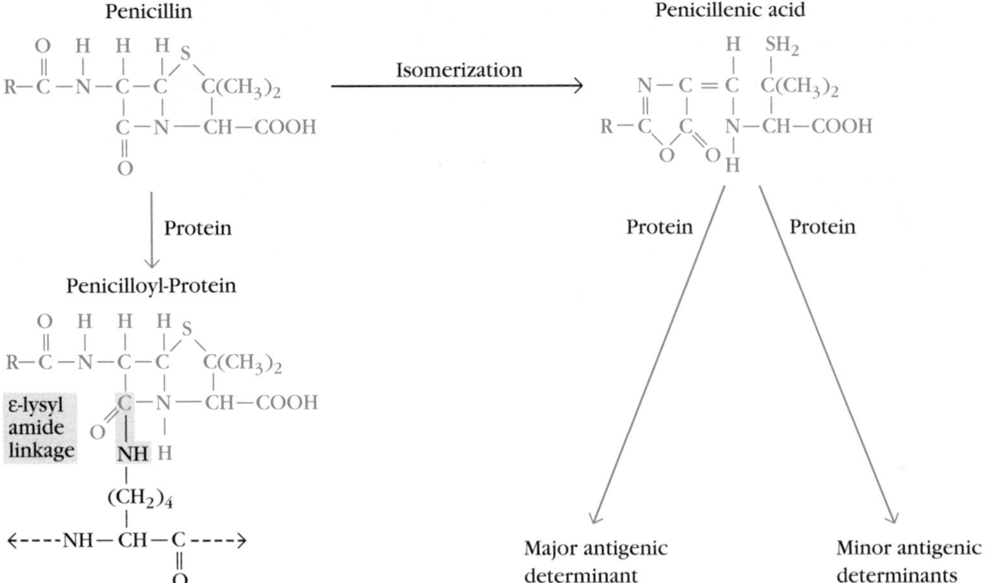

The free amino groups of lysine residues in some proteins can react with penicillin (or with its spontaneously forming isomeric compounds, such as penicillenic acid) to produce protein derivatives, which are the major immunogenic species that elicit immune responses to this antibiotic. However, as indicated, other hapten-carrier conjugates of somewhat different structure are also formed and, because of their structural similarity, can also induce immune responses to penicillin. [Adapted from NF Adkinson, 1995, in *Manual of Clinical Laboratory Immunology,* N Rose et al, eds., American Society for Microbiology, Washington, D.C.]

molecule (see Figures 3-3 to 3-6). Sequential B-cell epitopes consist of amino acid residues contiguous along the polypeptide chain. In contrast, nonsequential B-cell epitopes, also called conformational determinants, are formed from noncontiguous segments of the polypeptide chain that are brought into proximity by the folding of a protein (see Figure 3-7).

4. T-cell epitopes—those epitopes recognized by T-cell receptors—generally consist of internal amino acid sequences. T-cell epitopes are rendered accessible to the immune system by antigen processing, which fragments the protein into small peptides that combine with class I MHC or class II MHC molecules. The resulting peptide-MHC complexes are then displayed on the surface of altered self-cells or antigen-presenting cells. Activation of T cells requires formation of a ternary complex between the T-cell receptor, MHC molecule, and antigenic peptide (see Figure 3-9).
5. MHC molecules have an antigen-binding cleft that selectively binds a variety of antigenic peptides. The T-cell epitopes that are immunodominant within an antigen are determined in part by the particular MHC molecules expressed by an individual.
6. Haptens are small molecules that can bind to antibodies but cannot by themselves induce an immune response. The conjugate formed by coupling a hapten to a large

carrier protein is immunogenic and elicits production of antihapten antibodies when injected into an animal (see Figure 3-12). In the body, the formation of hapten-carrier conjugates is the basis of drug allergies such as penicillin allergy. The study of haptens has allowed immunologists to learn about the structural basis of antibody specificity. Antihapten antibodies can be used in assays for nonimmunogenic biological substances, including drugs, peptide hormones, and steroid hormones.

REFERENCES

Arevalo, JH, MJ Taussig, and IA Wilson. 1993. Molecular basis of crossreactivity and the limits of antibody-antigen complementarity. *Nature* **365:**859.

Berzofsky, JA, et al. 1987. Protein antigenic structures recognized by T cells: potential applications to vaccine design. *Immunol. Rev.* **98:**9.

Berzofsky, JA, and JJ Berkower. 1999. Immunogenicity and antigen structure. In *Fundamental Immunology,* 4th ed., WE Paul, ed. Lippincott-Raven, Philadelphia.

Berzofsky, J, S Brett, H Streicher, and H Takahashi. 1988. Antigen processing for presentation to T lymphocytes: function, mechanisms and implications for the T cell repertoire. *Immunol. Rev.* **106:**5.

Buus, S, A Sette, and HM Grey. 1987. The interaction between protein-derived immunogenic peptides and IA. *Immunol. Rev.* **98:**115.

Dale, D, and D Federman, eds. 1997. Drug allergy. In *Scientific American Medicine.* Chapter VIII, Hypersensitivity and allergy, p. 27.

Demotz, S, HM Grey, E Appella, and A Sette. 1989. Characterization of a naturally processed MHC class II-restricted T cell determinant of hen egg lysozyme. *Nature* **342:**682.

Greenspan, NS. 1992. Epitopes, paratopes, and other topes: Do immunologists know what they are talking about? *Bull. Inst. Pasteur* **90:**267.

Grey, HM, A Sette, and S Buus. 1989. How T cells see antigen. *Sci. Am.* **261**(5):56.

Landsteiner, K. 1945. *The Specificity of Serological Reactions.* Harvard University Press, Cambridge, Massachusetts.

Laver, WG, GM Air, RG Webster, and SJ Smith-Gill. 1990. Epitopes on protein antigens: misconceptions and realities. *Cell* **61:**553.

Rothbard, JB, and ML Gefter. 1991. Interactions between immunogenic peptides and MHC proteins. *Annu. Rev. Immunol.* **9:**527.

Silver, ML, HC Guo, JL Strominger, and DC Wiley. 1992. Atomic structure of a human MHC molecule presenting an influenza virus peptide. *Nature* **360:**367.

Stanfield, RL, and IA Wilson. 1995. Protein-peptide interactions. *Curr. Opin. Struc. Biol.* **5:**103.

Tainer, JA, et al. 1985. The atomic mobility component of protein antigenicity. *Annu. Rev. Immunol.* **3:**501.

Useful Web Sites

http://www.umass.edu/microbio/rasmol/

RASMOL is free software for visualizing molecular structures that can be run on Windows-based or Macintosh PCs. With it one can view three-dimensional structures of many types of molecules, including proteins and nucleic acids.

http://www.expasy.ch/

This is the excellent and comprehensive Swiss Institute of Bioinformatics (SIB) Web site that contains extensive information of protein structure. From it one can obtain protein sequences and three-dimensional structures of proteins.

STUDY QUESTIONS

1. Indicate whether each of the following statements is true or false. If you think a statement is false, explain why.

a. Most antigens induce a response from more than one clone.

b. A large protein antigen generally can combine with many different antibody molecules.

c. A hapten can stimulate antibody formation but cannot combine with antibody molecules.

d. MHC genes play a major role in determining the degree of immune responsiveness to an antigen.

e. T-cell epitopes tend to be accessible amino acid residues that can combine with the T-cell receptor.

f. Many B-cell epitopes are nonsequential amino acids brought together by the tertiary conformation of a protein antigen.

g. Both T_H and T_C cells recognize antigen that has been processed and presented with an MHC molecule.

h. Each MHC molecule binds a unique peptide.

i. All antigens also are immunogens.

2. An antigenic peptide derived from hemagglutinin induces potent proliferation of T_H cells in mice that express the class II MHC molecule designated IA^k. Would this peptide also induce potent T_H-cell proliferation in mice expressing IA^d? Explain your answer.

3. Two vaccines are described below. Would you expect either or both of them to activate T_C cells? Explain your answer.

a. A UV-inactivated ("killed") viral preparation that has retained its antigenic properties but cannot replicate

b. An attenuated viral preparation that has low virulence but can still replicate within host cells

4. For each pair of antigens listed below, indicate which is likely to be more immunogenic. Explain your answer.

a. Native bovine serum albumin (BSA)
Heat-denatured BSA

b. Hen egg-white lysozyme (HEL)
Hen collagen

c. A protein with a molecular weight of 30,000
A protein with a molecular weight of 150,000

Go to www.whfreeman.com/immunology Self-Test
Review and quiz of key terms

d. A synthetic copolymer of two nonaromatic amino acids
A similar copolymer that also includes tyrosine residues

5. Indicate which of the following statements regarding haptens and carriers are true.

a. Haptens are large protein molecules such as BSA.

b. When a hapten-carrier complex containing multiple hapten molecules is injected into an animal, most of the induced antibodies are specific for the hapten.

c. Carriers are needed only if one wants to elicit a cell-mediated response.

d. It is necessary to immunize with a hapten-carrier complex in order to obtain antibodies directed against the hapten.

e. Carriers include small molecules such as dinitrophenol and penicillenic acid (derived from penicillin).

6. For each of the following statements, indicate whether it is true only of B-cell epitopes (B), only of T-cell epitopes (T), or both types of epitopes (BT) within a large antigen.

a. They *always* consist of a linear sequence of amino acid residues.

b. They generally are located in the interior of a protein antigen.

c. They generally are located on the surface of a protein antigen.

d. They lose their immunogenicity when a protein antigen is denatured by heat.

e. Immunodominant epitopes are determined in part by the MHC molecules expressed by an individual.

f. They are present only in protein antigens.

g. Multiple different epitopes may occur in the same antigen.

h. Their immunogenicity may depend on the three-dimensional structure of the antigen.

i. The immune response to them may be enhanced by co-administration of Freund's complete adjuvant.

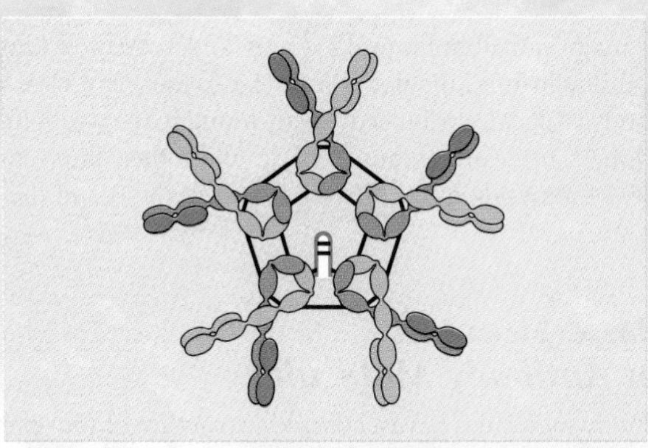

CHAPTER 4

IMMUNOGLOBULINS: STRUCTURE AND FUNCTION

Immunoglobulins function as antibodies, the antigen-binding proteins that are present on the B-cell membrane and also are secreted by plasma cells. Membrane-bound antibody confers antigenic specificity on B cells; antigen-specific proliferation of B-cell clones is elicted by the interaction of membrane antibody with antigen. Secreted antibodies circulate in the blood; they serve as the effectors of humoral immunity by searching out and neutralizing antigens or marking them for elimination. All immunoglobulins share certain structural features, bind to antigen, and participate in a limited number of effector functions. Most of this chapter focuses on how the primary, secondary, and tertiary structures of immunoglobulins contribute to both their specificity and their effector functions.

The serum antibodies produced in response to a particular antigen are heterogeneous. Because most antigens are complex and contain many different antigenic determinants, the immune system usually responds by producing antibodies to several of them. This response requires the recruitment of several clones of B cells. Their outputs are monoclonal antibodies, each of which specifically binds a single antigenic determinant. Together, these monoclonal antibodies make up the polyclonal and heterogeneous serum antibody response to an immunizing antigen. Although the polyclonal antibody produced in vivo is beneficial to the organism, it has numerous disadvantages for immunologic research and clinical applications that demand precise control of antibody quantity, properties, and specificity. The last section of this chapter describes a technology for the production and use of monoclonal antibodies in research. Monoclonal antibodies also have many diagnostic and therapeutic applications.

Basic Structure of Immunoglobulins

It has been known since the turn of the century that antibodies—the effector molecules of humoral immunity—reside in the serum. The first evidence that antibodies were contained in particular serum protein fractions came from a classic experiment by A. Tiselius and E. A. Kabat, in 1939. They immunized rabbits with the protein ovalbumin (the albumin of egg whites) and then divided the immunized rabbits' serum into two aliquots. Electrophoresis of one serum aliquot revealed four peaks corresponding to albumin and the alpha (α), beta (β), and gamma (γ) globulins. The other serum aliquot was reacted with ovalbumin, and the precipitate that formed was removed; the remaining serum proteins, which did not react with the antigen, were then electrophoresed. A comparison of the electrophoretic profiles of these two serum aliquots revealed that there was a significant drop in the γ-globulin peak in the aliquot that had been reacted with antigen (Figure 4-1). Thus, the **γ-globulin fraction** was identified as containing serum antibodies, which were called **immunoglobulins,** to distinguish them from any other proteins that might be contained in the γ-globulin fraction. Advances in electrophoresis technology now make it possible to resolve serum proteins into

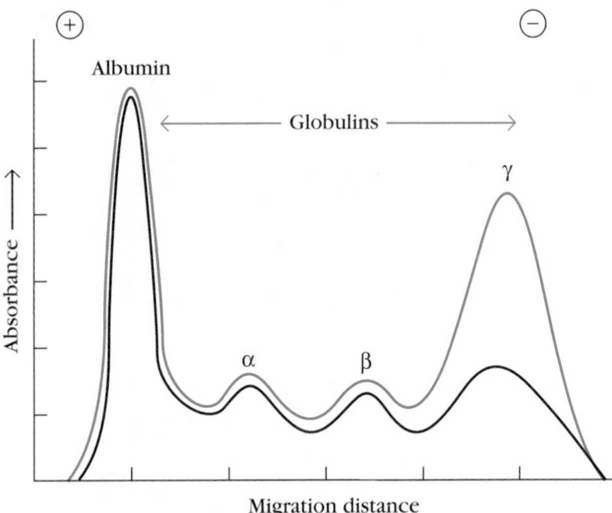

FIGURE 4-1 Experimental demonstration that antibodies are present in the γ-globulin fraction of serum proteins. After rabbits were immunized with ovalbumin (OVA), their antisera were pooled and electrophoresed, which separated the serum proteins according to their electric charge and mass. The blue line shows the electrophoretic pattern of untreated antiserum. The black line shows the pattern of antiserum that was incubated with OVA to remove anti-OVA antibody and then electrophoresed. [Adapted from A Tiselius and EA Kabat, 1939, *J. Exp. Med.* **69:**119.]

three major nonalbumin peaks—α, β, and γ. We now know that although immunoglobulin G (IgG), the main class of antibody molecules, is indeed mostly found in the γ-globulin fraction, significant amounts of it and other important classes of antibody molecules are found in the β and the α fractions of serum.

Basic Structure of Antibody Molecules

Antibody molecules have a common structure of four peptide chains (Figure 4-2). This structure consists of two identical **light (L) chains,** polypeptides of about 25,000 molecular weight, and two identical **heavy (H) chains,** larger polypeptides of molecular weight 50,000 or more. Each light chain is bound to a heavy chain by a disulfide bond, a strong covalent linkage between the two polypeptides, and by a combination of such noncovalent interactions as salt linkages, hydrogen bonds, and hydrophobic bonds. Similar noncovalent interactions and disulfide bridges link the two identical heavy and light (H-L) chain combinations to each other to form the basic four-chain immunoglobulin structure, the dimer $(H–L)_2$. As we shall see, the exact number and precise positions of these interchain disulfide bonds differs among immunoglobulin classes and subclasses.

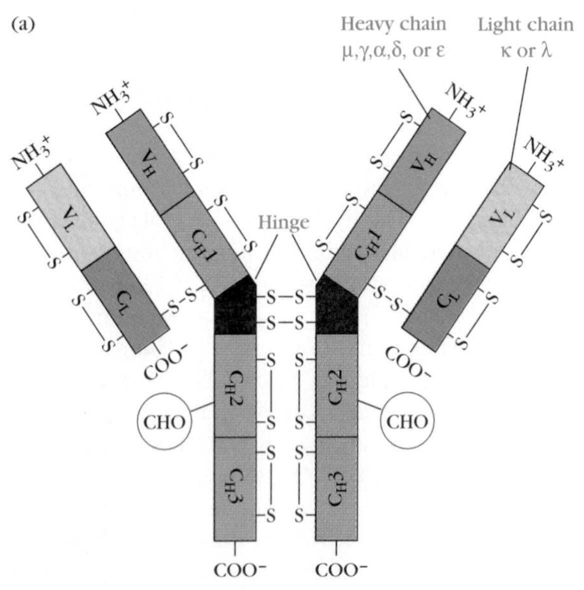

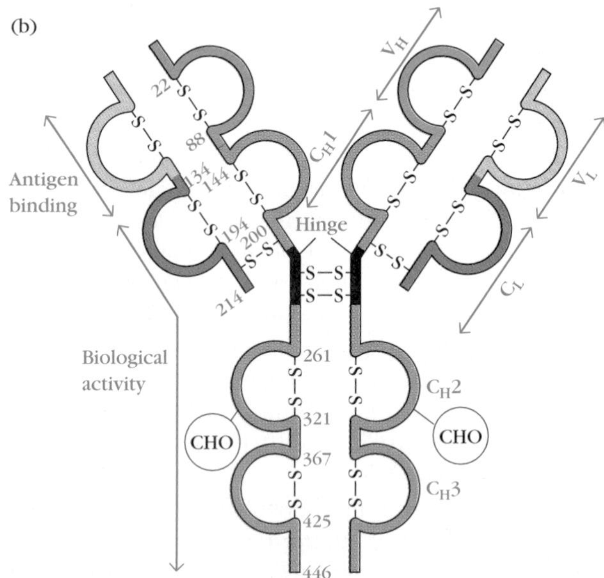

FIGURE 4-2 Schematic diagram of structure of immunoglobulins derived from amino acid sequencing studies. (a) Each heavy and light chain in an immunoglobulin molecule contains an amino-terminal variable (V) region (aqua and tan, respectively) that consists of 100–110 amino acids and differs from one antibody to the next. The remainder of each chain in the molecule—the constant (C) regions (red and purple)—exhibits limited variation that defines the two light-chain subtypes and the five heavy-chain subclasses. Some heavy chains (γ, δ, and α) also contain a proline-rich hinge region (black). (b) Heavy and light chains are folded into domains, each containing about 110 amino acid residues and an intrachain disulfide bond that forms a loop of 60 amino acids. The amino-terminal domains, corresponding to the V regions, bind to antigen; effector functions are mediated by the other domains. The μ and ε heavy chains, which lack a hinge region, contain an additional domain in the middle of the molecule.

Go to www.whfreeman.com/immunology Animation
Immunoglobulins

The first 110 or so amino acids of the amino-terminal region of a light or heavy chain varies greatly among antibodies of different specificity. These segments of highly variable sequence are called **V regions:** V_L in light chains and V_H in heavy. All of the differences in specificity displayed by different antibodies can be traced to differences in the amino acid sequences of V regions. In fact, most of the differences among antibodies fall within areas called complementarity-determining regions (CDRs), and it is these CDRs, on both light and heavy chains, that constitute the antigen-binding site of the immunoglobulin molecule. By contrast, within the same immunoglobulin class, far fewer differences are seen when one compares sequences throughout the rest of the molecule. The regions of relatively constant sequence beyond the variable regions have been dubbed C regions, C_L on the light chain and C_H on the heavy chain. Immunoglobulins are glycoproteins; with few exceptions, the sites of attachment for carbohydrates are restricted to the constant region. We do not completely understand the role played by glycosylation of immunoglobulins, but some effects of carbohydrate attachment have emerged: it affects the rate at which immunoglobulins are cleared from the serum by the liver, and it probably increases the solubility of immunoglobulins.

Deducing Antibody Structure

Our knowledge of basic antibody structure comes from a variety of experimental observations. In the 1950s and 1960s, experiments by Rodney Porter and by Gerald Edelman elucidated the basic structure of the immunoglobulin molecule. (These experiments were considered so significant that the two investigators shared a Nobel prize in 1972.) Edelman's and Porter's experimental approaches were quite different. Porter cleaved the immunoglobulin molecule with enzymes to obtain fragments, whereas Edelman dissociated the molecule by reducing the interchain disulfide bonds. The results attained by these two approaches complemented each other.

Porter and Edelman first separated the γ-globulin fraction of serum into high-molecular-weight and low-molecular-weight fractions. They both studied the low-molecular-weight fraction, which contained a 150,000-MW γ globulin designated as immunoglobulin G (IgG). Porter subjected IgG to brief digestion with the enzyme papain and separated the fragments. Although papain has general, nonspecific proteolytic activity and will eventually digest the entire IgG molecule, brief treatment cleaves only the most susceptible bonds. Papain digestion of IgG produced two identical fragments (each with a MW of 45,000), called **Fab fragments** ("fragment, antigen binding") because they had antigen-binding activity, and one fragment (MW of 50,000) called the **Fc fragment** ("fragment, crystallizable") because it was found to crystallize during cold storage (Figure 4-3). A similar experimental approach, but with the enzyme pepsin, was taken by Alfred Nisonoff. Brief pepsin digestion generated a single 100,000-MW fragment composed of two Fab-like fragments and designated F(ab)$_2$. Unlike the Fab fragments, the **F(ab′)$_2$ fragment** was able to precipitate antigens. However, the Fc fragment was not recovered from pepsin digestion, because it had been digested into multiple fragments (see Figure 4-3).

The multichain structure of IgG was first suggested by experiments of Edelman and his colleagues and later confirmed by Porter. Porter subjected IgG to mercaptoethanol reduction and alkylation, a chemical treatment that irreversibly cleaves disulfide bonds. The sample was then chromatographed on a column that separates molecules by size. This experiment revealed that the 150,000-MW IgG molecule was composed of two 50,000-MW polypeptide chains, designated as heavy (H) chains, and two 25,000-MW chains, designated as light (L) chains (see Figure 4-3).

The remaining puzzle was to determine how the enzyme digestion products—Fab, F(ab)$_2$, and Fc—were related to the heavy-chain and light-chain reduction products. Porter answered this question by using antisera from goats that had been immunized with either the Fab fragments or the Fc fragments of rabbit IgG. He found that antibody to the Fab fragment could react with both the H and the L chains,

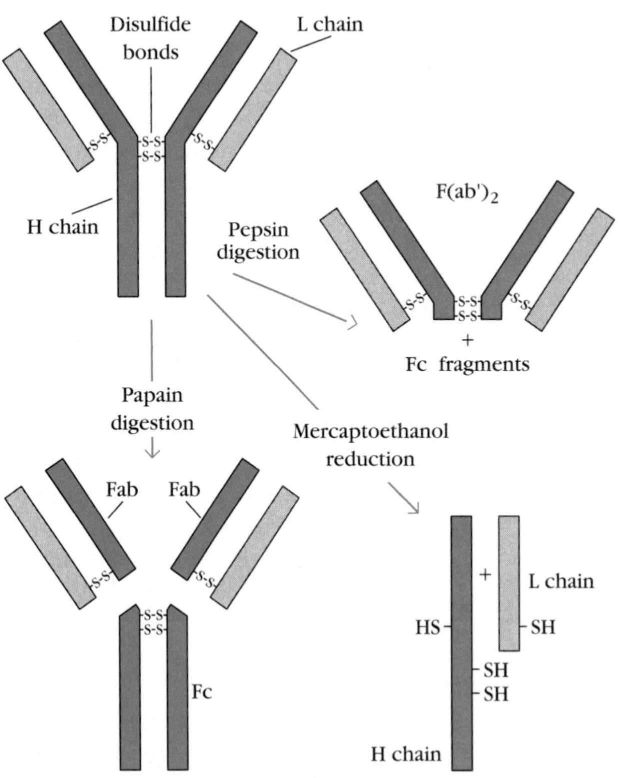

FIGURE 4-3 Prototype structure of IgG, proposed by Rodney Porter in 1962, showing chain structure and interchain disulfide bonds. The fragments produced by various treatments are also indicated. Light (L) chains are in gray and heavy (H) chains in blue.

whereas antibody to the Fc fragment reacted only with the H chain. These observations led to the conclusion that Fab consists of portions of a heavy and a light chain and that Fc contains only heavy-chain components. From these results, Porter and Edelman proposed a structure for IgG (see Figure 4-3). According to this model, the IgG molecule consists of two identical H chains and two identical L chains, which are linked by disulfide bridges. The enzyme papain cleaves just above the interchain disulfide bonds linking the heavy chains, whereas the enzyme pepsin cleaves just below these bonds, so that the two proteolytic enzymes generate different digestion products. Mercaptoethanol reduction and alkylation allow separation of the individual heavy and light chains.

Immunoglobulin Sequencing Studies

Initial attempts to determine the amino acid sequence of the immunoglobulin heavy and light chains were unsuccessful because insufficient amounts of homogeneous protein were available. Although the basic structure and chemical properties of different antibodies are similar, their antigen-binding specificities, and therefore their exact amino acid sequences, are very different. The population of antibodies in the serum γ-globulin fraction consists of a heterogeneous spectrum of antibodies that reflect all the different antigens that have induced an immune response in an animal. Even if immunization is done with a hapten-carrier conjugate, the antibodies formed just to the hapten alone are heterogeneous: they recognize different epitopes of the hapten and have different binding affinities. This heterogeneity of serum immunoglobulin rendered it unsuitable for sequencing studies.

Role of Multiple Myeloma

Sequencing analysis finally became feasible with the discovery of **multiple myeloma,** a cancer of antibody-producing plasma cells. The plasma cells in a normal individual are end-stage cells that secrete specific antibody for a few days and then die. In contrast, the plasma cells in an individual with multiple myeloma have escaped normal controls on their life span and proliferation and are not end-stage cells; rather, they divide over and over in an unregulated way without requiring any activation by antigen to induce clonal proliferation. Although such a cancerous plasma cell, called a **myeloma cell,** has been transformed, its protein-synthesizing machinery and secretory functions are not altered; thus, the cell continues to secrete specific antibody. This antibody is indistinguishable from normal antibody molecules but is called **myeloma protein** to denote its source.

In a patient afflicted with multiple myeloma, myeloma protein can account for 95% of the serum immunoglobulins. In most patients, the myeloma cells also secrete excessive amounts of light chains. These excess light chains were first discovered in the urine of myeloma patients and were named **Bence-Jones proteins,** for their discoverer.

Multiple myeloma also occurs in other animals. In mice it can arise spontaneously, as it does in humans, or it can be induced by injecting mineral oil into the peritoneal cavity. The clones of malignant plasma cells that develop are called **plasmacytomas,** and many of these are designated MOPCs, denoting the mineral-oil induction of plasmacytoma cells. A large number of mouse MOPC lines secreting different immunoglobulin classes are presently carried by the American Type-Culture Collection, a repository of cell lines commonly used in research.

Light-Chain Sequencing

When the amino acid sequences of several Bence-Jones proteins (light chains) from different individuals were compared, a striking pattern emerged. The amino-terminal half of the chain, consisting of 100–110 amino acids, was found to vary among different Bence-Jones proteins. This region was called the **variable (V) region.** The carboxyl-terminal half of the molecule, called the **constant (C) region,** had two basic amino acid sequences. This led to the recognition that there were two light chain types, **kappa (κ)** and **lambda (λ).** In humans, 60% of the light chains are kappa and 40% are lambda, whereas in mice, 95% of the light chains are kappa and only 5% are lambda. A single antibody molecule contains only one light chain type, either κ light chains or λ light chains but never both.

The amino acid sequences of λ light chains show minor differences, on the basis of which λ light chains are classified into subtypes. In mice, there are three subtypes (λ1, λ2, and λ3); in humans, there are four subtypes. Different single amino acids at two or three positions are responsible for the subtype differences.

Heavy-Chain Sequencing

For heavy-chain sequencing studies, myeloma proteins were reduced with mercaptoethanol and alkylated, and the heavy chains were separated by gel filtration in a denaturing solvent. When the amino acid sequences of several myeloma protein heavy chains were compared, a pattern similar to that of the light chains emerged. The amino-terminal part of the chain, consisting of 100–110 amino acids, showed great sequence variation among myeloma heavy chains and was therefore called the variable (V) region. The remaining part of the protein revealed five basic sequence patterns, corresponding to five different heavy-chain constant (C) regions (μ, δ, γ, ε, and α). Each of these five different heavy chains is called an **isotype.** The length of the constant regions is approximately 330 amino acids for δ, γ, and α and

TABLE 4-1 CHAIN COMPOSITION OF THE FIVE IMMUNOGLOBULIN CLASSES IN HUMANS

Class	Heavy chain	Subclasses	Light chain	Molecular formula
IgG	γ	γ1, γ2, γ3, γ4	κ or λ	$\gamma_2\kappa_2$ $\gamma_2\lambda_2$
IgM	μ	None	κ or λ	$(\mu_2\kappa_2)_n$ $(\mu_2\lambda_2)_n$ $n = 1$ or 5
IgA	α	α1, α2	κ or λ	$(\alpha_2\kappa_2)_n$ $(\alpha_2\lambda_2)_n$ $n = 1, 2, 3,$ or 4
IgE	ϵ	None	κ or λ	$\epsilon_2\kappa_2$ $\epsilon_2\lambda_2$
IgD	δ	None	κ or Λ	$\delta_2\kappa_2$ $\delta_2\lambda_2$

440 amino acids for μ and ϵ. The heavy chains of a given antibody molecule determine the class of that antibody: IgM(μ), IgG(γ), IgA(α), IgD(δ), or IgE(ϵ). Each class can have either κ or λ light chains. A single antibody molecule has two identical heavy chains and two identical light chains, H_2L_2, or a multiple $(H_2L_2)_n$ of this basic four-chain structure (Table 4-1).

Minor differences in the amino acid sequences of the α and the γ heavy chains led to further classification of the heavy chains into subclasses. In humans, there are two subclasses of α heavy chains (α1 and α2) and four subclasses of γ heavy chains (γ_1, γ_2, γ_3, and γ_4): in mice, there are four subclasses (γ1, γ2a, γ2b, and γ3).

Immunoglobulin Fine Structure

The structure of the immunoglobulin molecule is determined by the primary, secondary, tertiary, and quaternary organization of the protein. The primary structure, the amino acid sequence, accounts for the variable and constant regions of the heavy and light chains. The secondary structure is formed by folding of the extended polypeptide chain back and forth upon itself into an antiparallel β pleated sheet (Figure 4-4). The chains are then folded into a tertiary structure of compact globular domains, which are connected to neighboring domains by continuations of the polypeptide chain that lie outside the β pleated sheets. Finally, the globular domains of adjacent heavy and light polypeptide chains interact in the quaternary structure (Figure 4-5), forming functional domains that enable the molecule to specifically bind antigen and, at the same time, perform a number of biological effector functions (see Figure 4-2b).

Immunoglobulin Domains

Careful analysis of the amino acid sequences of immunoglobulin heavy and light chains showed that both chains contain several homologous units of about 110 amino acid residues. Within each unit, termed a domain, an intrachain disulfide bond forms a loop of about 60 amino acids. Light chains contain one variable domain (V_L), and one constant domain (C_L); heavy chains contain one variable domain (V_H), and either three or four constant domains (C_H1, C_H2, C_H3, and C_H4), depending on the antibody class (see Figure 4-2b).

X-ray crystallographic analysis revealed that immunoglobulin domains are folded into a characteristic compact structure called the **immunoglobulin fold.** This structure consists of a "sandwich" of two β pleated sheets, each

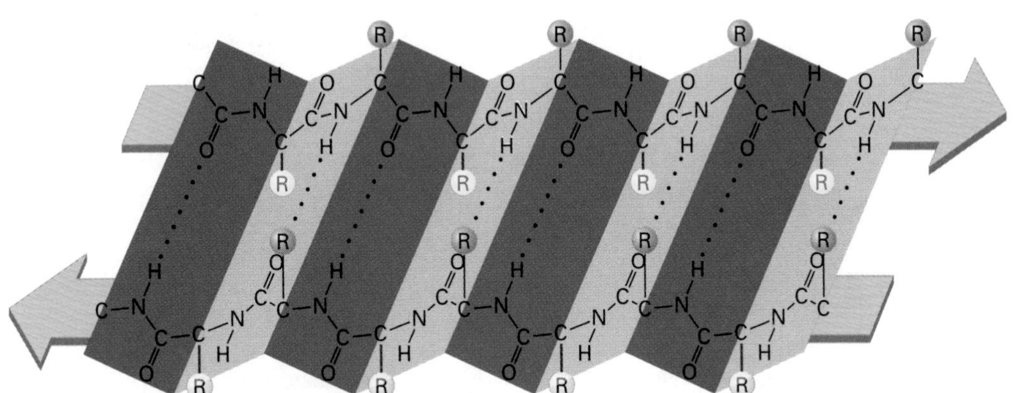

FIGURE 4-4 Structural formula of a β pleated sheet containing two antiparallel β strands. The structure is held together by hydrogen bonds between peptide bonds of neighboring stretches of polypeptide chains. The amino acid side groups (R) are arranged perpendicular to the plane of the sheet. [Adapted from H Lodish et al, 1995, *Molecular Cell Biology*, 4th ed., Scientific American Books, New York.]

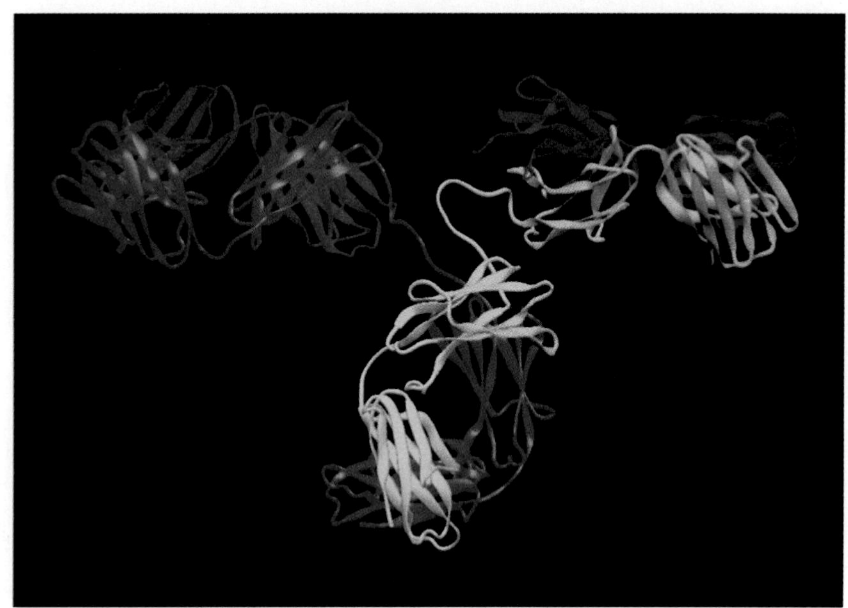

FIGURE 4-5 Ribbon representation of an intact monoclonal antibody depicting the heavy chains (yellow and blue) and light chains (red). The domains of the molecule composed of β pleated sheets are readily visible as is the extended conformation of the hinge region. [The laboratory of A McPherson provided this image, which is based on x-ray crystallography data determined by LJ Harris, 1992, *Nature* **360:**369.]

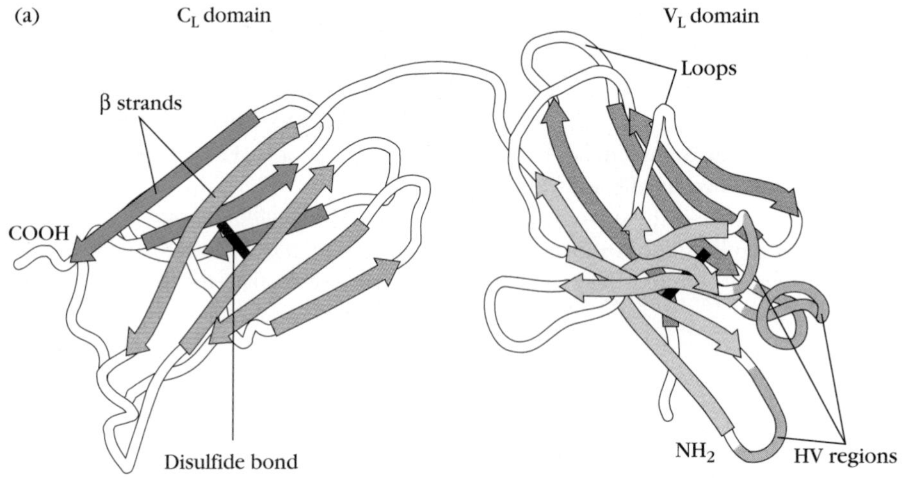

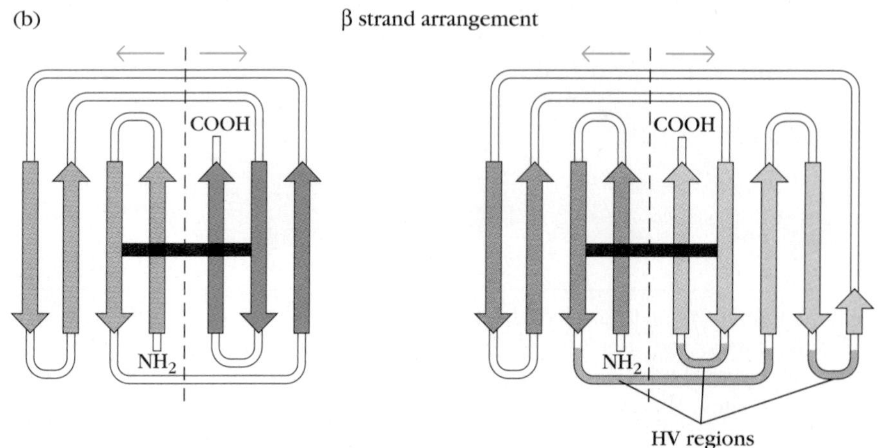

Go to www.whfreeman.com/immunology Molecular Visualization
An Introduction to Immunoglobulin Structure

containing antiparallel β strands of amino acids, which are connected by loops of various lengths (Figure 4-6). The β strands within a sheet are stabilized by hydrogen bonds that connect the –NH groups in one strand with carbonyl groups of an adjacent strand (see Figure 4-4). The β strands are characterized by alternating hydrophobic and hydrophilic amino acids whose side chains are arranged perpendicular to the plane of the sheet; the hydrophobic amino acids are oriented toward the interior of the sandwich, and the hydrophilic amino acids face outward.

The two β sheets within an immunoglobulin fold are stabilized by the hydrophobic interactions between them and by the conserved disulfide bond. An analogy has been made to two pieces of bread, the butter between them, and a toothpick holding the slices together. The bread slices represent the two β pleated sheets; the butter represents the hydrophobic interactions between them; and the toothpick represents the intrachain disulfide bond. Although variable and constant domains have a similar structure, there are subtle differences between them. The V domain is slightly longer than the C domain and contains an extra pair of β strands within the β-sheet structure, as well as the extra loop sequence connecting this pair of β strands (see Figure 4-6).

The basic structure of the immunoglobulin fold contributes to the quaternary structure of immunoglobulins by facilitating noncovalent interactions between domains across the faces of the β sheets (Figure 4-7). Interactions form links between identical domains (e.g., C_H2/C_H2, C_H3/C_H3, and C_H4/C_H4) and between nonidentical domains (e.g., V_H/V_L and C_H1/C_L). The structure of the immunoglobulin fold also allows for variable lengths and sequences of amino acids that form the loops connecting the β strands. As the next section explains, some of the loop sequences of the V_H and V_L domains contain variable amino acids and constitute the antigen-binding site of the molecule.

Variable-Region Domains

Detailed comparisons of the amino acid sequences of V_L and V_H domains revealed that the sequence variability is concentrated in several **hypervariable (HV) regions** (Figure 4-8). Three such hypervariable regions are present in each mouse and human heavy and light chain, constituting 15%–20% of the variable domain. The remainder of the V_L and V_H domains exhibit far less variation; these stretches are called the **framework regions (FRs).** The hypervariable regions form the antigen-binding site of the antibody molecule. Because the antigen-binding site is complementary to the structure of the epitope, the hypervariable regions are also called **complementarity-determining regions (CDRs).**

High-resolution x-ray crystallography has been used to determine the three-dimensional structure of the framework regions and hypervariable regions (or CDRs). The more conserved sequence of the framework regions forms the basic β pleated sheet structure of the V_H and V_L domains. The three heavy-chain and three light-chain CDR regions are located on the loops that connect the β strands of the V_H and V_L domains (see Figure 4-6, right). The wide range of specificities exhibited by antibodies is due to variations in the length and amino acid sequence of the six hypervariable loops in each Fab fragment. The framework region thus acts as a scaffold that supports these six loops. The three-dimensional structure of the framework regions of virtually all antibodies analyzed to date can be superimposed on one another; in contrast, the hypervariable loops (i.e., the CDRs) have different orientations in different antibodies. The three-dimensional structure of the immunoglobulin variable region thus provides a rigid framework, which is necessary for overall antibody function; at the same time, an enormous spectrum of antigen-binding specificities is achieved by the diversity of the six CDRs.

CDRs and Antigen Binding

The earliest evidence demonstrating the role of the hypervariable regions in binding antigen was obtained by L. Wofsy, H. Metzger, and S. J. Singer using an experimental technique called *affinity labeling.* This technique used a chemically reactive hapten as a labeling reagent that would bind specifically to an antibody and form a covalent bond with neighboring residues within the antibody's binding site. Identification of the amino acids covalently bound to the affinity label revealed that amino acids within light- and heavy-chain CDRs constitute the antigen-binding site.

The three-dimensional structure of the antigen-binding site and the role of the CDRs in the binding of antigen have also been investigated by high-resolution x-ray crystallography. To date, crystallographic analysis has been completed for many Fab fragments of monoclonal antibodies complexed either to large globular protein antigens or to a number of

FIGURE 4-6 *(facing page)* (a) Diagram of an immunoglobulin light chain depicting the immunoglobulin-fold structure of its variable and constant domains. The two β pleated sheets in each domain are held together by hydrophobic interactions and the conserved disulfide bond. The β strands that compose each sheet are shown in different colors. The amino acid sequences in three loops of each variable domain show considerable variation; these hypervariable (HV) regions (blue) make up the antigen-binding site. Hypervariable regions are usually called CDRs (complementarity-determining regions). Heavy-chain domains have the same characteristic structure. (b) The β pleated sheets are opened out to reveal the relationship of the individual β strands and joining loops. Note that the variable domain contains two more β strands than the constant domain. [Part (a) adapted from M Schiffer et al, 1973, *Biochemistry* **12:**4620; part (b) adapted from Williams and Barclay, 1988, *Annu. Rev. Immunol.* **6:**381.]

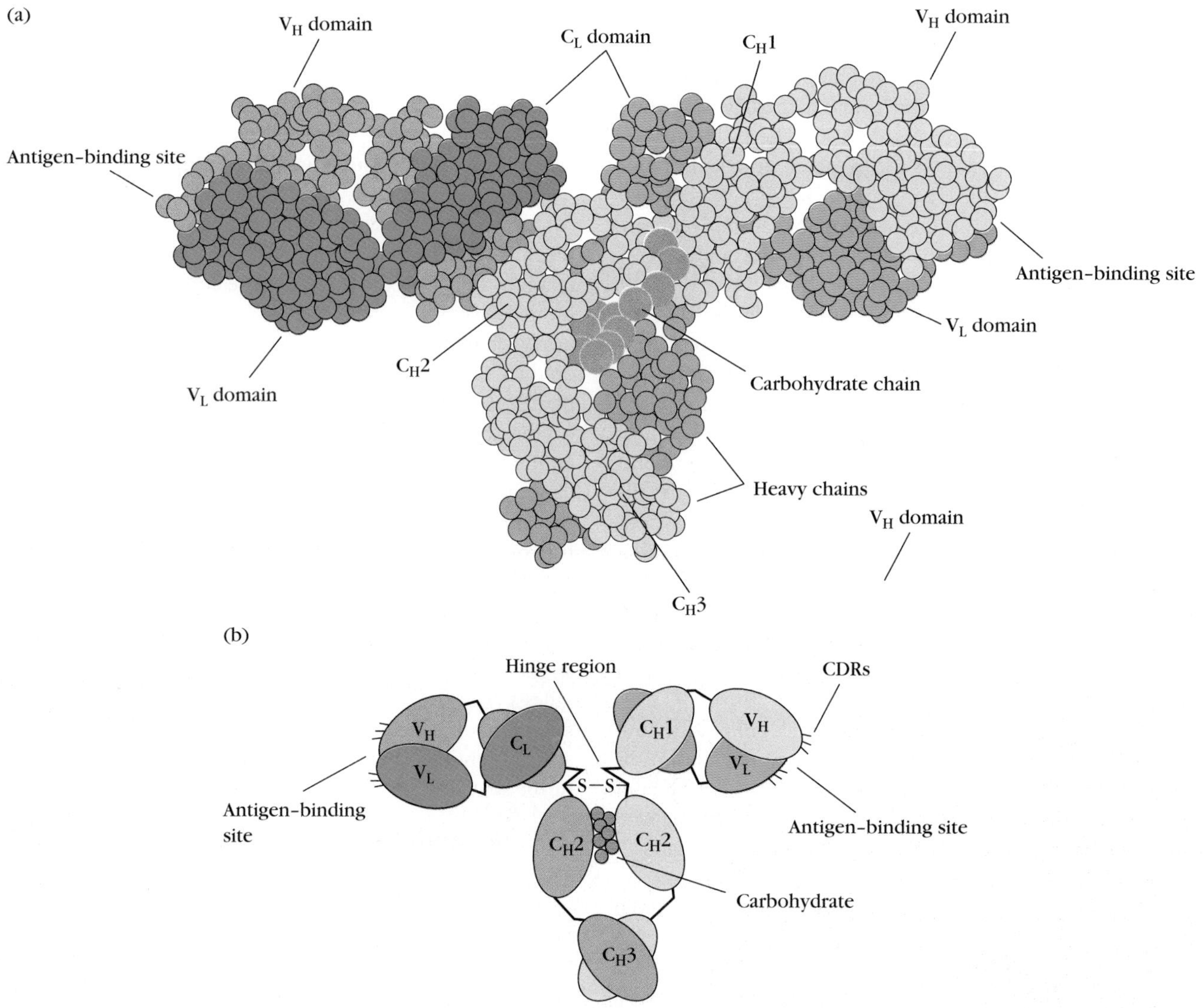

FIGURE 4-7 Interactions between domains in the separate chains of an immunoglobulin molecule are critical to its quaternary structure. (a) Model of IgG molecule, based on x-ray crystallographic analysis, showing associations between domains. Each solid ball represents an amino acid residue; the larger tan balls are carbohydrate. The two light chains are shown in shades of red; the two heavy chains, in shades of blue. (b) A schematic diagram showing the interacting heavy- and light-chain domains. Note that the C_H2/C_H2 domains protrude because of the presence of carbohydrate (tan) in the interior. The protrusion makes this domain more accessible, enabling it to interact with molecules such as certain complement components. [Part (a) from EW Silverton et al, 1977, *Proc. Nat. Acad. Sci. USA* **74:**5140.]

smaller antigens including carbohydrates, nucleic acids, peptides, and small haptens. In addition, complete structures have been obtained for several intact monoclonal antibodies.

The results of these crystallographic studies have provided valuable insights into the structure of the V_H and V_L domains and the interactions between antigen and antibody. As in lysozyme binding with anti-lysozyme antibody (Chapter 3), a large globular protein antigen contacts the antibody molecule across a rather flat, undulating face. In the area of contact, protrusions or depressions on the antigen are likely to match complementary depressions or protrusions on the antibody. The surface area of this large complementary face ranges from about 650 Å^2 to more than 900 Å^2; within this area, some 15–22 amino acids in the antibody contact the same number of residues in the protein antigen. In antibodies that bind smaller antigens, such as small haptens, the antigen-binding site is generally smaller and is more like a deep pocket in which the ligand is buried. This is nicely illustrated by the interaction of the small octapeptide hormone angiotensin II with the binding site of an anti-angiotensin antibody (Figure 4-9).

Go to www.whfreeman.com/immunology **Molecular Visualization**
Antibody Recognition of Antigen

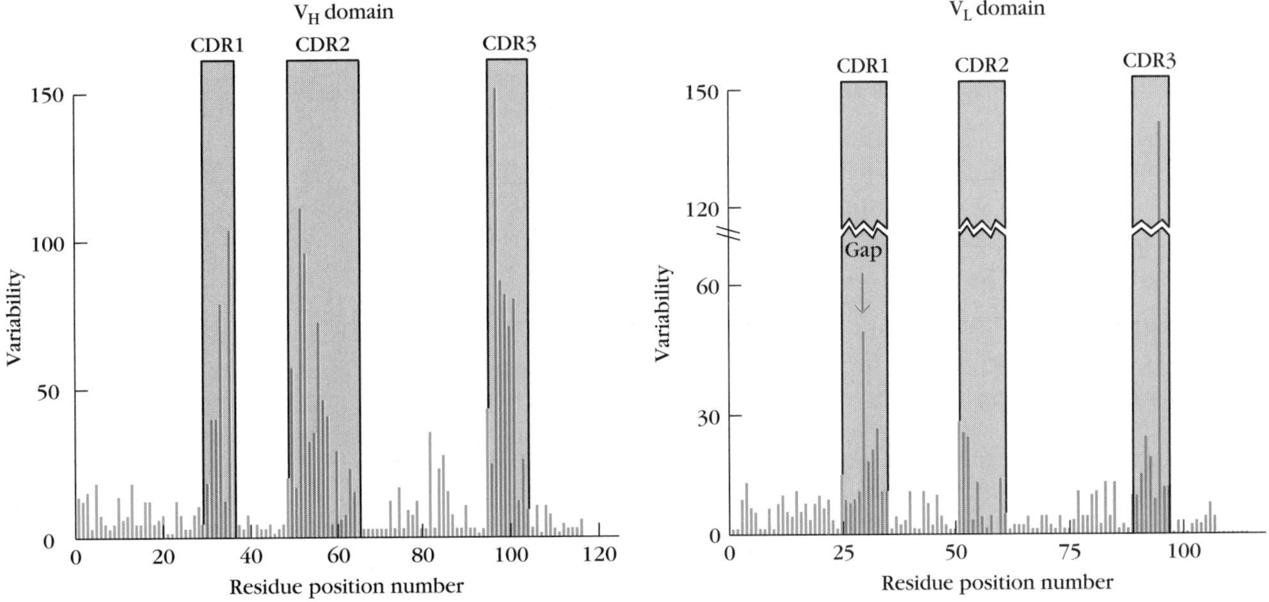

FIGURE 4-8 Variability of amino acid residues in the V_L and V_H domains of human antibodies with different specificities. Three hypervariable (HV) regions, also called complementarity-determining regions (CDRs), are present in both heavy- and light- chain V domains. As shown in Figure 4-6 (*right*), the three HV regions in the light-chain V domain are brought into proximity in the folded structure. The same is true of the heavy-chain V domain. [Based on EA Kabat et al, 1977, *Sequence of Immunoglobulin Chains,* U.S. Dept. of Health, Education, and Welfare.]

X-ray diffraction analysis of antibody Fab–antigen complexes has shown that several CDRs make contact with the antigen, and a number of complexes have been observed in which all six CDRs contact the antigen. In general, more residues in the heavy-chain CDRs appear to contact antigen than in the light-chain CDRs. Thus the V_H domain often contributes more to antigen binding than the V_L domain. The dominant role of the heavy chain in antigen binding was demonstrated in a study in which a single heavy chain specific for a glycoprotein antigen of the human

(a)

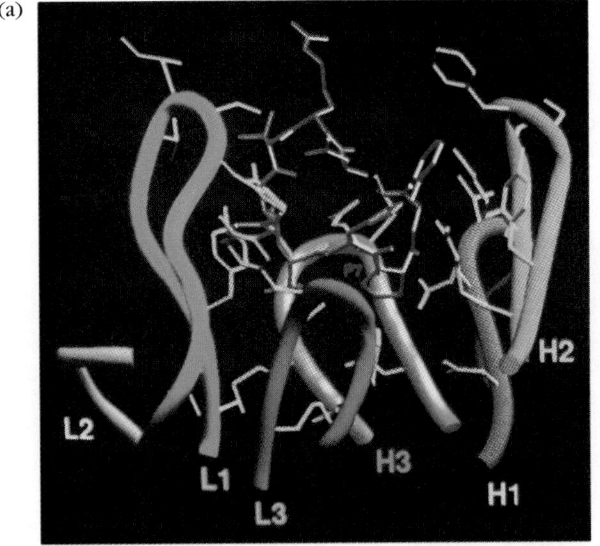

(b)

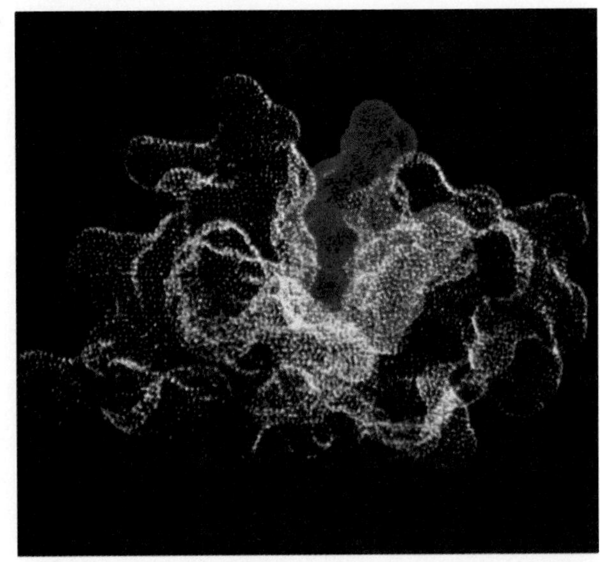

FIGURE 4-9 (a) Side view of the three-dimensional structure of the combining site of an angiotensin II–Fab complex. The peptide is in red. The three heavy-chain CDRs (H1, H2, H3) and three light-chain CDRs (L1, L2, L3) are each shown in a different color. All six CDRs contain side chains, shown in yellow, that are within van der Waals contact of the angiotensin peptide. (b) Side view of the van der Waals surface of contact between angiotensin II and Fab fragment. [From KC Garcia et al, 1992, *Science* **257**:502; courtesy of Mario Amzel, Johns Hopkins University.]

immunodeficiency virus (HIV) was combined with various light chains of different antigenic specificity. All of the hybrid antibodies bound to the HIV glycoprotein antigen, indicating that the heavy chain alone was sufficient to confer specificity. However, one should not conclude that the light chain is largely irrelevant; in some antibody-antigen reactions, the light chain makes the more important contribution.

Conformational Changes Induced by Antigen Binding

As more x-ray crystallographic analyses of Fab fragments were completed, it became clear that in some cases binding of antigen induces conformational changes in the antibody, antigen, or both. Formation of the complex between neuraminidase and anti-neuraminidase is accompanied by a change in the orientation of side chains of both the epitope and the antigen-binding site. This conformational change results in a closer fit between the epitope and the antibody's binding site.

In another example, comparison of an anti-hemagglutinin Fab fragment before and after binding to a hemagglutinin peptide antigen has revealed a visible conformational change in the heavy-chain CDR3 loop (Figure 4-10a) and in the accessible surface of the binding site (Figure 4-10b). Another striking example of conformational change has been seen in the complex between an Fab fragment derived from a monoclonal antibody against the HIV protease and the peptide epitope of the protease. As shown in Figure 4-11, there are significant changes in the Fab upon binding. In fact, upon antigen binding, the CDR1 region of the light chain moves as much as 1 Å and the heavy chain CDR3 moves 2.7 Å. Thus, in addition to variability in the length and amino acid composition of the CDR loops, the ability of these loops to significantly change conformation upon antigen binding enables antibodies to assume a shape more effectively complementary to that of their epitopes.

As already indicated, conformational changes following antigen binding need not be limited to the antibody. Although it is not shown in Figure 4-11, the conformation of

(a)

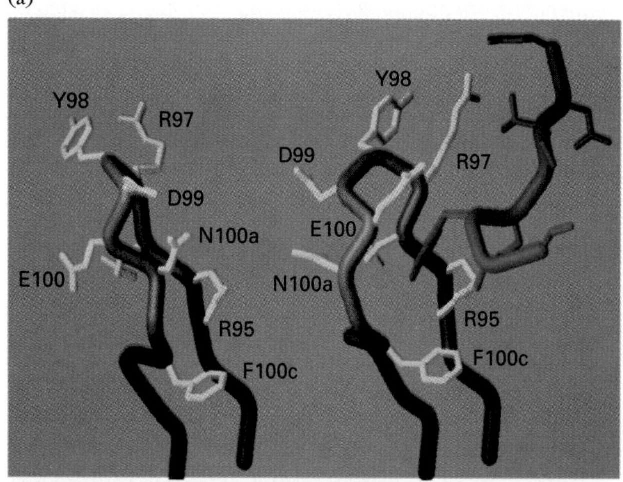

(b)

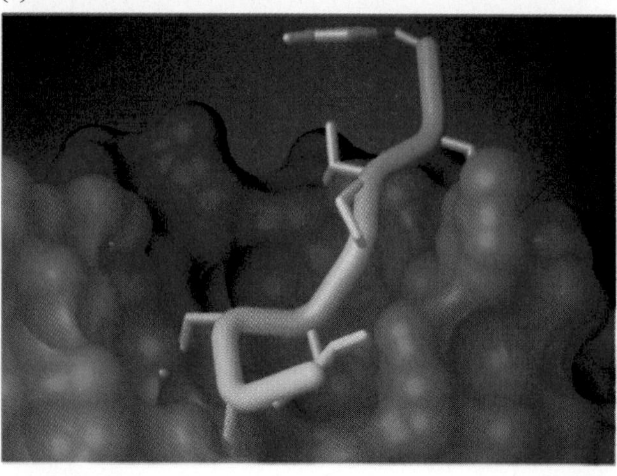

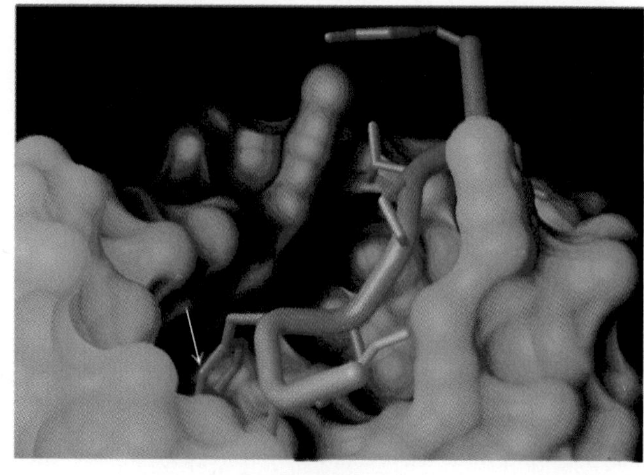

FIGURE 4-10 (a) Model of the heavy-chain CDR3 loops in an unbound (*left*) and bound (*right*) anti-hemagglutinin Fab fragment. Note the major rearrangement in the heavy-chain CDR3 loop (green) that accompanies binding of hemagglutinin peptide (red). The side chains in the CDR3 loop are shown in yellow. (b) Model of the solvent-accessible surface of an unbound (*left*) and bound (*right*) anti-hemagglutinin Fab fragment showing that peptide binding is accommodated by an alteration in the shape of the antibody's binding pocket. In the left panel, the free hemagglutinin peptide (light blue) is positioned over an open, basin-shaped pocket in the unbound Fab fragment. In the right panel, the bound Fab fragment has a prominent channel that interacts with the extended peptide and a pocket that interacts with the tyrosine residue (arrow). [From JM Rini et al, 1992, *Science* **255**:959.]

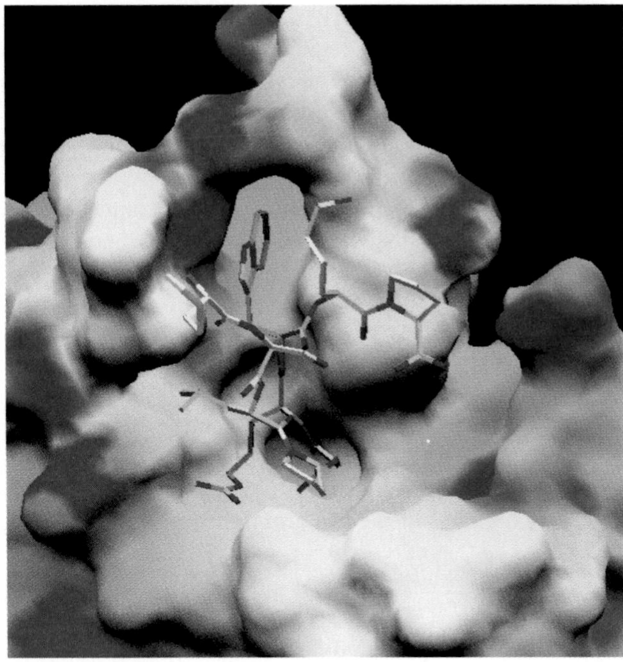

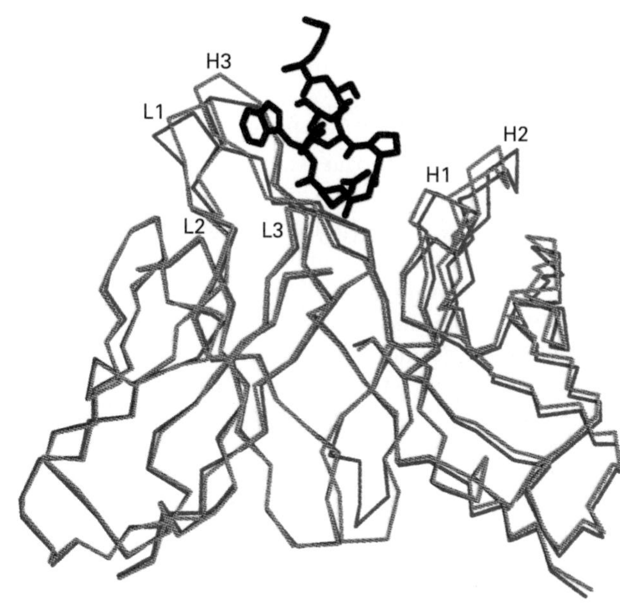

FIGURE 4-11 Structure of a complex between a peptide derived from HIV protease and an Fab fragment from an anti-protease antibody (*left*) and comparison of the Fab structure before and after peptide binding (*right*). In the right panel, the red line shows the structure of the Fab fragment before it binds the peptide and the blue line shows its structure when bound. There are significant conformational changes in the CDRs of the Fab on binding the antigen. These are especially pronounced in the light chain CDR1 (L1) and the heavy chain CDR3 (H3). [From J Lescar et al, 1997, *J. Mol. Biol.* **267:**1207; courtesy of G Bentley, Institute Pasteur.]

the protease peptide bound to the Fab shows no structural similarity to the corresponding epitope in the native HIV protease. It has been suggested that the inhibition of protease activity by this anti-HIV protease antibody is a result of its distortion of the enzyme's native conformation.

Constant-Region Domains

The immunoglobulin constant-region domains take part in various biological functions that are determined by the amino acid sequence of each domain.

C_H1 and C_L Domains

The C_H1 and C_L domains serve to extend the Fab arms of the antibody molecule, thereby facilitating interaction with antigen and increasing the maximum rotation of the Fab arms. In addition, these constant-region domains help to hold the V_H and V_L domains together by virtue of the interchain disulfide bond between them (see Figure 4-2).

The C_H1 and C_L domains also may contribute to antibody diversity by allowing more random associations between V_H and V_L domains than would occur if this association were driven by the V_H/V_L interaction alone. Reassociation experiments have provided some support for this concept. For instance, when V_H and V_L domains from two antibodies having different known specificities (*a* and *b*) were prepared separately and then mixed, each domain reassociated almost exclusively with its original partner to form homogeneous V_La/V_Ha or V_Lb/V_Hb complexes. In another experiment, Fab fragments from antibody *a* and antibody *b* were mildly reduced and denatured to obtain V_HC_H1 and V_LC_L fragments from each antibody. Mixing these longer fragments yielded not only homogeneous complexes containing heavy and light chains from antibody *a* (V_LaC_La/V_HaC_H1a) or heavy and light chains from antibody *b* but also hybrid complexes with one chain from antibody *a* and one from antibody *b* (e.g., V_LaC_La/V_HbC_H1b).

These considerations have important implications for building a diverse repertoire of antibodies. As Chapter 5 will show, random rearrangements of the immunoglobulin genes generate unique V_H and V_L sequences for the heavy and light chains expressed by each B lymphocyte; association of the V_H and V_L sequences then generates a unique antigen-binding site. The presence of C_H1 and C_L domains appears to increase the number of stable V_H and V_L interactions that are possible, thus contributing to the overall diversity of antibody molecules that can be expressed by an animal.

Hinge Region

The γ, δ, and α heavy chains contain an extended peptide sequence between the C_H1 and C_H2 domains that has no homology with the other domains (see Figure 4-7). This region, called the **hinge region,** is rich in proline residues and is flexible, giving IgG, IgD, and IgA segmental flexibility. As a result, the two Fab arms can assume various angles to each other when antigen is bound. This flexibility of the hinge region can be visualized in electron micrographs of antigen-antibody complexes. For example, when a molecule containing two dinitrophenol (DNP) groups reacts with anti-DNP antibody and the complex is captured on a grid, negatively stained, and observed by electron microscopy, large complexes (e.g., dimers, trimers, tetramers) are seen. The angle between the arms of the Y-shaped antibody molecules differs in the different complexes, reflecting the flexibility of the hinge region (Figure 4-12).

X-ray crystallographic analysis of an entire monoclonal antibody specific for canine lymphoma-cell membrane antigen has revealed that the hinge region serves as a sort of tether that allows the Fab components and the Fc to move relative to each other. In this way, the Fab arms can move and twist to align the CDRs with epitopes displayed on cell surfaces, and the Fc can move to maximize various effector functions such as those of the complement system, or bind to cell-surface receptors specific for the Fc region.

Two prominent amino acids in the hinge region are proline and cysteine. The large number of proline residues in the hinge region gives it an extended polypeptide conformation, making it particularly vulnerable to cleavage by proteolytic enzymes; it is this region that is cleaved with papain or pepsin (see Figure 4-3). The cysteine residues form interchain disulfide bonds that hold the two heavy chains together. The number of interchain disulfide bonds in the hinge region varies considerably among different classes of antibodies and between species. Although μ and ε chains lack a hinge region, they have an additional domain of 110 amino acids (C_H2/C_H2) that has hingelike features.

Other Constant-Region Domains

As noted already, the heavy chains in IgA, IgD, and IgG contain three constant-region domains and a hinge region, whereas the heavy chains in IgE and IgM contain four constant-region domains and no hinge region. The corresponding domains of the two groups are as follows:

IgA, IgD, IgG	IgE, IgM
C_H1/C_H1	C_H1/C_H1
Hinge region	C_H2/C_H2
C_H2/C_H2	C_H3/C_H3
C_H3/C_H3	C_H4/C_H4

Although the C_H2/C_H2 domains in IgE and IgM occupy the same position in the polypeptide chains as the hinge region in the other classes of immunoglobulin, the function of this extra domain has not yet been determined.

X-ray crystallographic analyses have revealed that the two C_H2 domains of IgA, IgD, and IgG (and the C_H3 do-

(a)

DNP ligand O_2N–⟨benzene⟩–N∿∿∿N–⟨benzene⟩–NO_2 (NO_2, NO_2)

25Å

Anti-DNP

DNP ligand

Hinge region

Ag-Ab Trimer

(b)

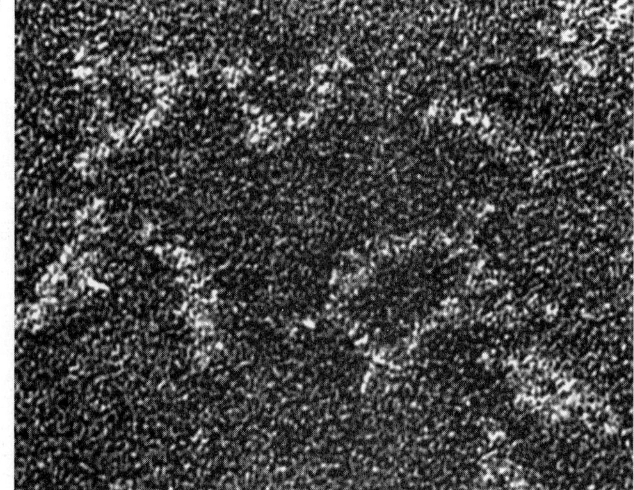

FIGURE 4-12 Experimental demonstration of the flexibility of the hinge region in antibody molecules. (a) A divalent dinitrophenol (DNP) hapten reacts with anti-DNP antibodies to form trimers, tetramers, and other larger antigen-antibody complexes. A trimer is shown schematically. (b) In an electron micrograph of a negatively stained preparation of these complexes, two triangular trimeric structures are clearly visible. The antibody protein stands out as a light structure against the electron-dense background. Because of the flexibility of the hinge region, the angle between the arms of the antibody molecules varies. [Photograph from RC Valentine and NM Green, 1967, *J. Mol. Biol.* **27:**615.]

mains of IgE and IgM) are separated by oligosaccharide side chains; as a result, these two globular domains are much more accessible than the others to the aqueous environment (see Figure 4-7b). This accessibility is one of the elements that contributes to the biological activity of these domains in the activation of complement components by IgG and IgM.

The carboxyl-terminal domain is designated C_H3/ C_H3 in IgA, IgD, and IgG and C_H4/C_H4 in IgE and IgM. Immunoglobulins in the five classes and their subclasses can be expressed either as **secreted immunoglobulin (sIg)** or as **membrane-bound immunoglobulin (mIg).**

The carboxyl-terminal domain in secreted immunoglobulin differs in both structure and function from the corresponding domain in membrane-bound immunoglobulin. Secreted immunoglobulin has a hydrophilic amino acid sequence of various lengths at the carboxyl-terminal end. The functions of this domain in the various classes of secreted antibody will be described later. In membrane-bound immunoglobulin, the carboxyl-terminal domain contains three regions:

- An extracellular hydrophilic "spacer" sequence composed of 26 amino acid residues
- A hydrophobic transmembrane sequence
- A short cytoplasmic tail

Although the length of the transmembrane sequence is constant among all immunoglobulin isotypes, the lengths of the extracellular spacer sequence and the cytoplasmic tail are different.

B cells express different classes of mIg at different developmental stages. The immature B cell, called a pre-B cell, expresses only mIgM; mIgD appears later in maturation and is coexpressed with IgM on the surface of mature B cells before they have been triggered by antigen. A memory B cell can express mIgM, mIgG, mIgA, or mIgE. Even when different classes are expressed sequentially on a single cell, the antigenic specificity of all the membrane antibody molecules is identical, so that each antibody molecule binds to the same epitope. The genetic mechanism that allows a single B cell to express multiple immunoglobulin isotypes all with the same antigenic specificity is described in Chapter 5.

Immunoglobulin Classes and Biological Activities

The various immunoglobulin classes, or isotypes, have been mentioned briefly already. Each class is distinguished by unique amino acid sequences in the heavy-chain constant region that confer class-specific structural and functional properties. In this section, the structure and effector functions of each class are described in more detail. The molecular properties and biological activities of the immunoglobulin classes are summarized in Table 4-2. The structures of the five major classes are diagrammed in Figure 4-13.

Immunoglobulin-Mediated Effector Functions

When considering the role of antibody in defending against disease, it is important to remember that antibodies generally do not kill or remove pathogens solely by binding to them. In order to be effective against pathogens, antibodies not only must recognize antigen, but also must invoke responses—effector functions—that will remove the antigen and kill the pathogen. While variable regions of antibody are the sole agents of binding to antigen, the heavy-chain constant region (C_H) is responsible for a variety of collaborative interactions with other proteins, cells, and tissues that result in the effector functions of the humoral response.

Because these effector functions result from interactions between heavy-chain constant regions and other serum proteins or cell-membrane receptors, not all classes of immunoglobulin have the same functional properties. An overview of four major effector functions mediated by domains of the constant region is presented here. The fifth function, the activation of mast cells, eosinophils, and basophils, which is unique to IgE, will be described later.

Opsonization

Opsonization, the promotion of phagocytosis of antigens by macrophages and neutrophils is an important factor in antibacterial defenses. Protein molecules called **Fc receptors (FcR),** which can bind the constant region of most subclasses of IgG molecules, are present on the surfaces of macrophages and neutrophils. While the interaction between a single FcR and the Fc region of an individual IgG molecule is quite weak, the simultaneous binding of the Fc of several antibody molecules complexed with the same target, such as a bacterial cell, produces an interaction of significant strength. The immediate result is the binding of the pathogen to the phagocyte membrane by these FcR-antibody tethers. This crosslinking of the FcR by binding to an array of antibody Fc regions initiates a signal-transduction pathway that results in the phagocytosis of the antigen-antibody complex. Inside the phagocyte, the pathogen becomes the target of various processes that include enzymatic digestion, oxidative damage, and the membrane-damaging effects of antibacterial peptides. All of these combine to make death a likely fate of organisms phagocytosed because they were recognized.

TABLE 4-2 PROPERTIES AND BIOLOGICAL ACTIVITIES* OF CLASSES AND SUBCLASSES OF HUMAN SERUM IMMUNOGLOBULINS

Property/Activity	IgG1	IgG2	IgG3	IgG4	IgA1	IgA2	IgM‡	IgE	IgD
Molecular weight†	150,000	150,000	150,000	150,000	150,000–600,000	150,000–600,000	900,000	190,000	150,000
Heavy-chain component	$\gamma 1$	$\gamma 2$	$\gamma 3$	$\gamma 4$	$\alpha 1$	$\alpha 2$	μ	ϵ	δ
Normal serum level (mg/ml)	9	3	1	0.5	3.0	0.5	1.5	0.0003	0.03
In vivo serum half life (days)	23	23	8	23	6	6	5	2.5	3
Activates classical complement pathway	+	+/−	++	−	−	−	+++	−	−
Crosses placenta	+	+/−	+	+	−	−	−	−	−
Present on membrane of mature B cells	−	−	−	−	−	−	+	−	+
Binds to Fc receptors of phagocytes	++	+/−	++	+	−	−	?	−	−
Mucosal transport	−	−	−	−	++	++	+	−	−
Induces mast-cell degranulation	−	−	−	−	−	−	−	+	−

*Activity levels indicated as follows: ++ = high; + = moderate; +/− = minimal; − = none; ? = questionable.

†IgG, IgE, and IgD always exist as monomers; IgA can exist as a monomer, dimer, trimer, or tetramer. Membrane-bound IgM is a monomer, but secreted IgM in serum is a pentamer.

‡IgM is the first isotype produced by the neonate and during a primary immune response.

Activation of Complement

IgM and, in humans, most IgG subclasses can activate a collection of serum glycoproteins called the **complement system.** Complement includes a collection of proteins that can perforate cell membranes. An important byproduct of complement activation pathway is the protein fragment called C3b, which binds nonspecifically to cell- and antigen-antibody complexes near the site of activation. Many cell types—for example, red blood cells and macrophages—have receptors for C3b and so bind cells or complexes to which C3b has adhered. Binding of adherent C3b by macrophages leads to phagocytosis of the cells or molecular complexes attached to C3b. Binding of antigen-antibody complexes by the C3b receptors of a red blood cell allows the erythrocyte to deliver the complexes to liver or spleen, where resident macrophages remove them without destroying the red cell. The collaboration between antibody and the complement system is important for the inactivation and removal of antigens and the killing of pathogens. The process of complement activation is described in detail in Chapter 13.

Antibody-Dependent Cell-Mediated Cytotoxicity (ADCC)

The linking of antibody bound to target cells (virus infected cells of the host) with the Fc receptors of NK cells can kill the cell. In this process, called ADCC, the NK cell causes death by apoptosis of the target cell.

Transcytosis

The delivery of antibody to the mucosal surfaces of the respiratory, gastrointestinal, and urogenital tracts, as well as its export to breast milk, requires the movement of immunoglobulin across epithelial layers. The capacity to be transported depends upon properties of the constant region. In humans and mice, although IgM can be transported to mucosal surfaces, IgA is the major antibody species that undergoes such **transcytosis.** Some mammalian species, for example humans and mice, also transfer significant amounts of most subclasses of IgG from mother to fetus.

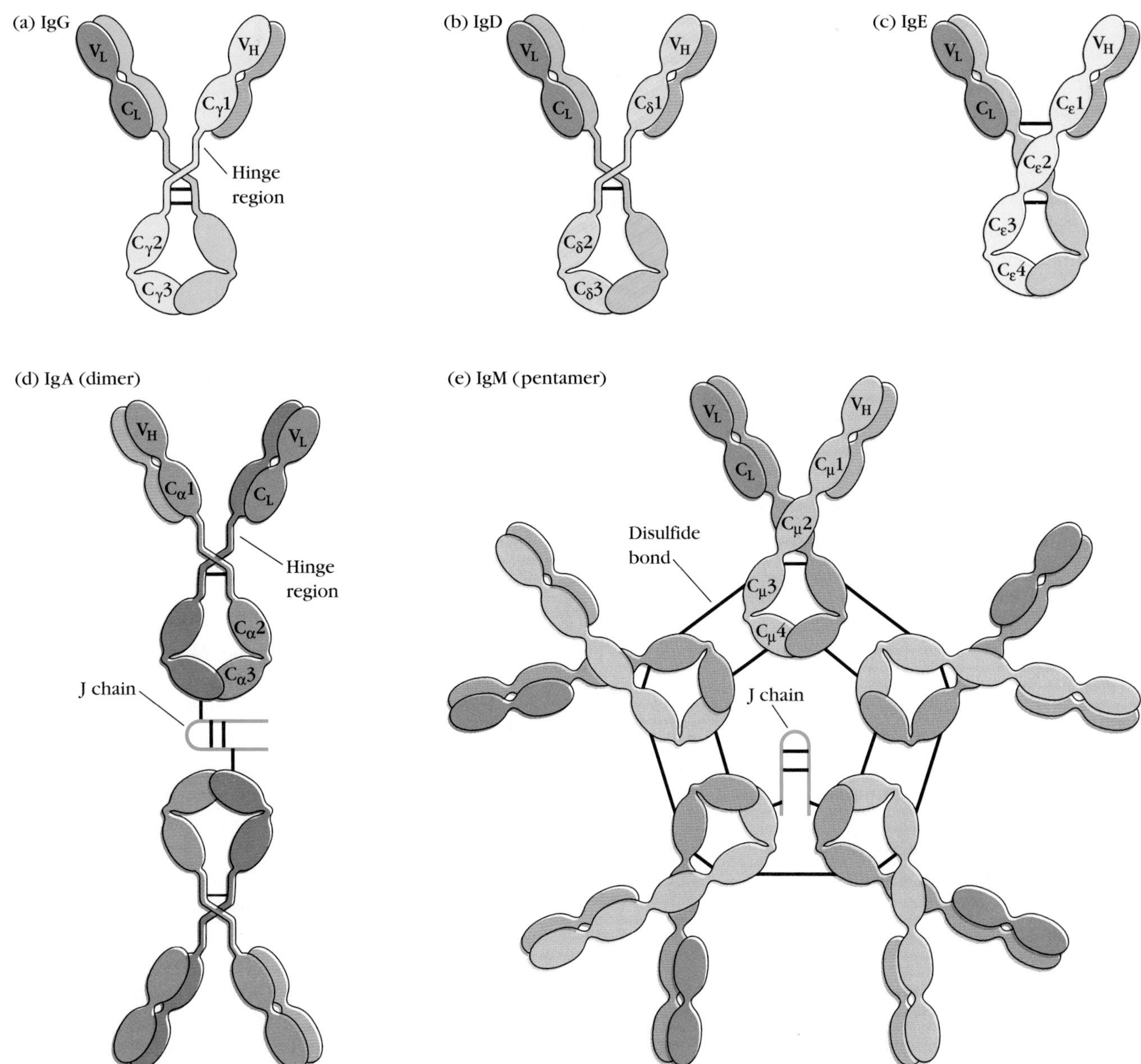

FIGURE 4-13 General structures of the five major classes of secreted antibody. Light chains are shown in shades of pink, disulfide bonds are indicated by thick black lines. Note that the IgG, IgA, and IgD heavy chains (blue, orange, and green, respectively) contain four domains and a hinge region, whereas the IgM and IgE heavy chains (purple and yellow, respectively) contain five domains but no hinge region. The polymeric forms of IgM and IgA contain a polypeptide, called the J chain, that is linked by two disulfide bonds to the Fc region in two different monomers. Serum IgM is always a pentamer; most serum IgA exists as a monomer, although some dimers, trimers, and even tetramers sometimes are present. Not shown in these figures are intrachain disulfide bonds and disulfide bonds linking light and heavy chains (see Figure 4-2).

Since maternal and fetal circulatory systems are separate, antibody must be transported across the placental tissue that separates mother and fetus. In humans, this transfer takes place during the third trimester of gestation. The important consequence is that the developing fetus receives a sample of the mother's repertoire of antibody as protective endowment against pathogens. As with the other effector functions described here, the capacity to undergo transplacental transport depends upon properties of the constant region of the antibody molecule.

This transfer of IgG from mother to fetus is a form of **passive immunization,** which is the acquisition of immunity by receipt of preformed antibodies rather than by active production of antibodies after exposure to antigen. The ability to transfer immunity in this manner is the basis of passive antibody therapy, an important medical tool (see Clinical Focus).

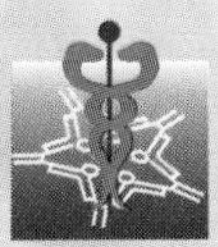

CLINICAL FOCUS
PASSIVE ANTIBODY THERAPY

In 1890, Emil Behring and Shibasaburo Kitasato reported an extraordinary experiment. They immunized rabbits with tetanus and collected serum from these immune animals. Then they injected 0.2 ml of the immune serum into the abdominal cavity of six mice. After 24 hours, they infected the treated animals and untreated controls with live, virulent tetanus bacteria. Although all of the control mice died within 48 hours of infection, the treated mice not only survived but showed no effects of infection. This landmark experiment demonstrated two important points. First, it showed that following immunization, substances appeared in serum that could protect an animal against pathogens. Second, this work demonstrated that immunity could be passively acquired. Immunity could be transferred from one animal to another by taking serum from an immune animal and injecting it into a nonimmune one. These and subsequent experiments did not go unnoticed. Both men eventually received titles (Behring became von Behring and Kitasato became Baron Kitasato). A few years later, in 1901, von Behring was awarded the first Nobel Prize in Medicine.

These early observations and others paved the way for the introduction of passive immunization into clinical practice and, during the 1930s and 1940s, passive immunotherapy, the endowment of resistance to pathogens by transfer of the agent of immunity from an immunized donor to an unimmunized recipient, was used to prevent or modify the course of measles and hepatitis A. During subsequent years, clinical experience and advances in the technology of preparation of immunoglobulin for passive immunization have made this approach a standard medical practice. Passive immunization based on the transfer of antibodies is widely used in the treatment of immunodeficiency diseases and as a protection against the anticipated exposure to infectious agents against which one does not have immunity.

Immunoglobulin for passive immunization is prepared from the pooled plasma of thousands of donors. In effect, recipients of these antibody preparations are receiving a sample of the antibodies produced by many people to a broad diversity of different pathogens. In fact a gram of intravenous immune globulin (IVIG) contains about 10^{18} molecules of antibody (mostly IgG) and may incorporate more than 10^7 different antibody specificities. During the course of therapy, patients receive significant amounts of IVIG, usually 200–400 mg per kilogram of body weight. This means that an immunodeficient patient weighing 70 kilograms would receive 14 to 28 grams of IVIG every 3 to 4 weeks. A product derived from the blood of such a large number of donors carries a risk of harboring pathogenic agents, particularly viruses. The risk is minimized by the processes used to produce intravenous immune globulin. The manufacture of IVIG involves treatment with solvents, such as ethanol, and the use of detergents that are highly effective in inactivating viruses such as HIV and hepatitis. In addition to removing or inactivating infectious agents, the production process must also eliminate aggregated immunoglobulin, because antibody aggregates can trigger massive activation of the complement pathway, leading to severe, even fatal, anaphylaxis.

Passively administered antibody exerts its protective action in a number of ways. One of the most important can be the recruitment of the complement pathway to the destruction or removal of the pathogen. In bacterial infections, antibody binding to bacterial surfaces promotes their opsonization, the phagocytosis and killing by macrophages and neutrophils. Toxins and viruses can be bound by antibody and neutralized. In addition to neutralizing these agents, antibodies mark them for removal from the body by phagocytes and by organs such as liver and kidneys. By the initiation of antibody-dependent cell-mediated cytoxicity (ADCC), antibodies can also mediate the killing of target cells by such cytotoxic cell populations as natural killer cells.

Immunoglobulin G (IgG)

IgG, the most abundant class in serum, constitutes about 80% of the total serum immunoglobulin. The IgG molecule consists of two γ heavy chains and two κ or two λ light chains (see Figure 4-13a). There are four human IgG subclasses, distinguished by differences in γ-chain sequence and numbered according to their decreasing average serum concentrations: IgG1, IgG2, IgG3, and IgG4 (see Table 4-2).

The amino acid sequences that distinguish the four IgG subclasses are encoded by different germ-line C_H genes, whose DNA sequences are 90%–95% homologous. The structural characteristics that distinguish these subclasses from one another are the size of the hinge region and the number and position of the interchain disulfide bonds between the heavy chains (Figure 4-14). The subtle amino acid differences between subclasses of IgG affect the biological activity of the molecule:

- IgG1, IgG3, and IgG4 readily cross the placenta and play an important role in protecting the developing fetus.
- IgG3 is the most effective complement activator, followed by IgG1; IgG2 is less efficient, and IgG4 is not able to activate complement at all.
- IgG1 and IgG3 bind with a high affinity to Fc receptors on phagocytic cells and thus mediate opsonization. IgG4 has an intermediate affinity, and IgG2 has an extremely low affinity.

Immunoglobulin M (IgM)

IgM accounts for 5%–10% of the total serum immunoglobulin, with an average serum concentration of 1.5 mg/ml. Monomeric IgM, with a molecular weight of 180,000, is expressed as membrane-bound antibody on B cells. IgM is secreted by plasma cells as a pentamer in which five monomer units are held together by disulfide bonds that link their carboxyl-terminal heavy chain domains ($C_\mu4/C_\mu4$) and link their $C_\mu3/C_\mu3$ domains (see Figure 4-13e). The five monomer subunits are arranged with their Fc regions in the center of the pentamer and the ten antigen-binding sites on the periphery of the molecule. Each pentamer contains an additional Fc-linked polypeptide called the **J (joining) chain,** which is disulfide-bonded to the carboxyl-terminal cysteine residue of two of the ten μ chains. The J chain appears to be required for polymerization of the monomers to form pentameric IgM; it is added just before secretion of the pentamer.

IgM is the first immunoglobulin class produced in a primary response to an antigen, and it is also the first immunoglobulin to be synthesized by the neonate. Because of its pentameric structure with 10 antigen-binding sites, serum IgM has a higher valency than the other isotypes. An IgM molecule can bind 10 small hapten molecules; however, because of steric hindrance, only 5, or fewer, molecules of larger antigens can be bound simultaneously. Because of its high valency, pentameric IgM is more efficient than other isotypes in binding such multidimensional antigens as viral particles and red blood cells (RBCs). For example, when RBCs are incubated with specific antibody, they clump together into large aggregates in a process called agglutination. It takes 100 to 1000 times more molecules of IgG than of IgM to achieve the same level of agglutination. A similar phenomenon occurs with viral particles: less IgM than IgG is required to neutralize viral infectivity. IgM is also more efficient than IgG at activating complement. Complement activation requires two Fc regions in close proximity, and the pentameric structure of a single molecule of IgM fulfills this requirement.

Because of its large size, IgM does not diffuse well and therefore is found in very low concentrations in the intercellular tissue fluids. The presence of the J chain allows IgM to bind to receptors on secretory cells, which transport it across epithelial linings to the external secretions that bathe mucosal surfaces. Although IgA is the major isotype found in these secretions, IgM plays an important accessory role as a secretory immunoglobulin.

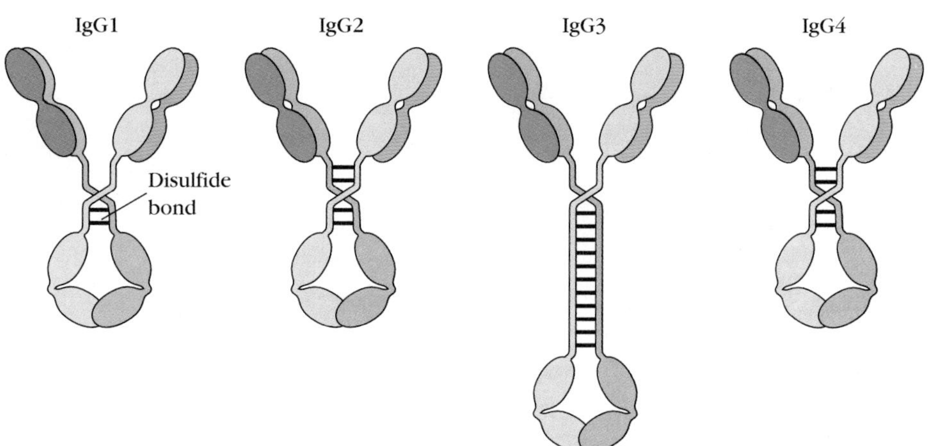

FIGURE 4-14 General structure of the four subclasses of human IgG, which differ in the number and arrangement of the interchain disulfide bonds (thick black lines) linking the heavy chains. A notable feature of human IgG3 is its 11 interchain disulfide bonds.

Immunoglobulin A (IgA)

Although IgA constitutes only 10%–15% of the total immunoglobulin in serum, it is the predominant immunoglobulin class in external secretions such as breast milk, saliva, tears, and mucus of the bronchial, genitourinary, and digestive tracts. In serum, IgA exists primarily as a monomer, but polymeric forms such as dimers, trimers, and even tetramers, all of which contain a J-chain polypeptide, are sometimes seen (see Figure 4-13d). The IgA of external secretions, called **secretory IgA,** consists of a dimer or tetramer, a J-chain polypeptide, and a polypeptide chain called **secretory component** (Figure 4-15a). As is explained below, secretory component is derived from the receptor that is responsible for transporting polymeric IgA across cell membranes. The J-chain polypeptide in IgA is identical to that found in pentameric IgM and serves a similar function in facilitating the polymerization of both serum IgA and secretory IgA. The secretory component is a 70,000-MW polypeptide produced by epithelial cells of mucous membranes. It consists of five immunoglobulin-like domains that bind to the Fc region domains of the IgA dimer. This interaction is stabilized by a disulfide bond between the fifth domain of the secretory component and one of the chains of the dimeric IgA.

The daily production of secretory IgA is greater than that of any other immunoglobulin class. IgA-secreting plasma cells are concentrated along mucous membrane surfaces. Along the jejunum of the small intestine, for example, there are more than 2.5×10^{10} IgA-secreting plasma cells—a number that surpasses the total plasma cell population of the bone marrow, lymph, and spleen combined! Every day, a human secretes from 5 g to 15 g of secretory IgA into mucous secretions.

(a) Structure of secretory IgA

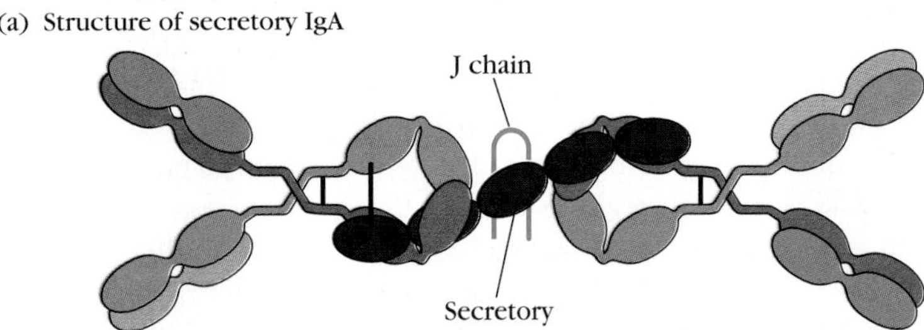

(b) Formation of secretory IgA

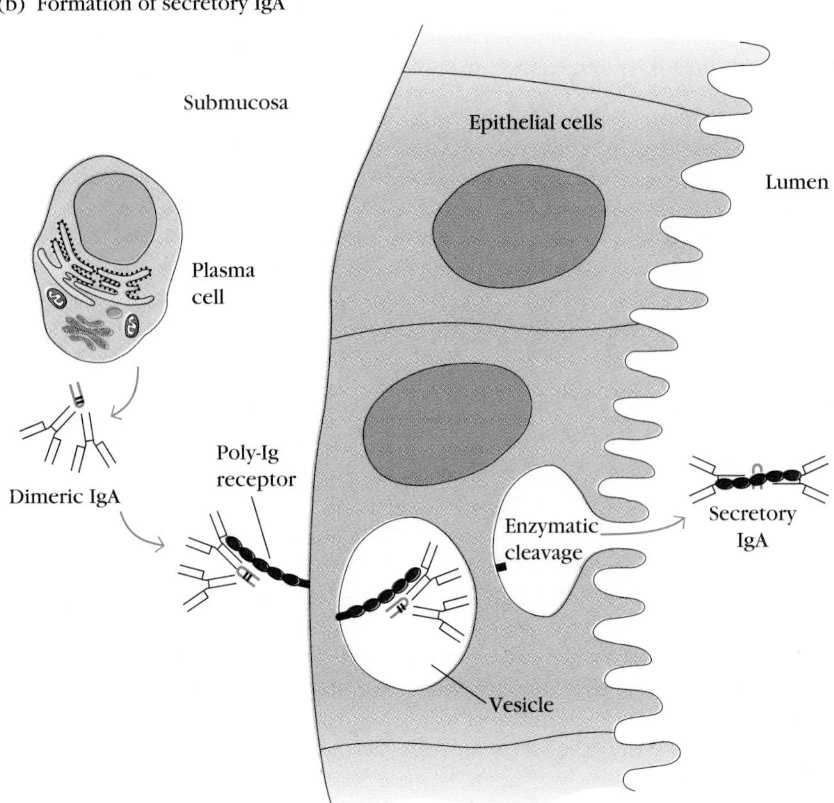

FIGURE 4-15 Structure and formation of secretory IgA. (a) Secretory IgA consists of at least two IgA molecules, which are covalently linked by a J chain and with the secretory component. The secretory component contains five Ig-like domains and is linked to dimeric IgA by a disulfide bond between its fifth domain and one of the IgA heavy chains. (b) Secretory IgA is formed during transport through mucous membrane epithelial cells. Dimeric IgA binds to a poly-Ig receptor on the basolateral membrane of an epithelial cell and is internalized by receptor-mediated endocytosis. After transport of the receptor-IgA complex to the luminal surface, the poly-Ig receptor is enzymatically cleaved, releasing the secretory component bound to the dimeric IgA.

The plasma cells that produce IgA preferentially migrate (home) to subepithelial tissue, where the secreted IgA binds tightly to a receptor for polymeric immunoglobulin molecules (Figure 4-15b). This **poly-Ig receptor** is expressed on the basolateral surface of most mucosal epithelia (e.g., the lining of the digestive, respiratory, and genital tracts) and on glandular epithelia in the mammary, salivary, and lacrimal glands. After polymeric IgA binds to the poly-Ig receptor, the receptor-IgA complex is transported across the epithelial barrier to the lumen. Transport of the receptor-IgA complex involves receptor-mediated endocytosis into coated pits and directed transport of the vesicle across the epithelial cell to the luminal membrane, where the vesicle fuses with the plasma membrane. The poly-Ig receptor is then cleaved enzymatically from the membrane and becomes the secretory component, which is bound to and released together with polymeric IgA into the mucous secretions. The secretory component masks sites susceptible to protease cleavage in the hinge region of secretory IgA, allowing the polymeric molecule to exist longer in the protease-rich mucosal environment than would be possible otherwise. Pentameric IgM is also transported into mucous secretions by this mechanism, although it accounts for a much lower percentage of antibody in the mucous secretions than does IgA. The poly-Ig receptor interacts with the J chain of both polymeric IgA and IgM antibodies.

Secretory IgA serves an important effector function at mucous membrane surfaces, which are the main entry sites for most pathogenic organisms. Because it is polymeric, secretory IgA can crosslink large antigens with multiple epitopes. Binding of secretory IgA to bacterial and viral surface antigens prevents attachment of the pathogens to the mucosal cells. Once attachment is blocked, viral infection and bacterial colonization are inhibited. Complexes of secretory IgA and antigen are easily entrapped in mucus and then eliminated by the ciliated epithelial cells of the respiratory tract or by peristalsis of the gut. Secretory IgA has been shown to provide an important line of defense against bacteria such as *Salmonella, Vibrio cholerae,* and *Neisseria gonorrhoeae* and viruses such as polio, influenza, and reovirus.

Breast milk contains secretory IgA and many other molecules that help protect the newborn against infection during the first month of life (Table 4-3). Because the immune system of infants is not fully functional, breast-feeding plays an important role in maintaining the health of newborns.

Immunoglobulin E (IgE)

The potent biological activity of IgE allowed it to be identified in serum despite its extremely low average serum concentration (0.3 μg/ml2 IgE antibodies mediate the immediate hypersensitivity reactions that are responsible for the symptoms of hay fever, asthma, hives, and anaphylactic shock. The presence of a serum component responsible for allergic reactions was first demonstrated in 1921 by K. Prausnitz and H. Kustner, who injected serum from an allergic person intradermally into a nonallergic individual. When the appropriate antigen was later injected at the same site, a wheal and flare reaction (analogous to hives) developed there. This reaction, called the **P-K reaction,** was the basis for the first biological assay for IgE activity.

Actual identification of IgE was accomplished by K. and T. Ishizaka in 1966. They obtained serum from an allergic individual and immunized rabbits with it to prepare anti-isotype antiserum. The rabbit antiserum was then allowed to react with each class of human antibody known at that

TABLE 4-3 IMMUNE BENEFITS OF BREAST MILK

Antibodies of secretory IgA class	Bind to microbes in baby's digestive tract and thereby prevent their attachment to the walls of the gut and their subsequent passage into the body's tissues.
B_{12} binding protein	Reduces amount of vitamin B_{12}, which bacteria need in order to grow.
Bifidus factor	Promotes growth of *Lactobacillus bifidus*, a harmless bacterium, in baby's gut. Growth of such nonpathogenic bacteria helps to crowd out dangerous varieties.
Fatty acids	Disrupt membranes surrounding certain viruses and destroy them.
Fibronectin	Increases antimicrobial activity of macrophages; helps to repair tissues that have been damaged by immune reactions in baby's gut.
Hormones and growth factors	Stimulate baby's digestive tract to mature more quickly. Once the initially "leaky" membranes lining the gut mature, infants become less vulnerable to microorganisms.
Interferon ⅡFN-γ2	Enhances antimicrobial activity of immune cells.
Lactoferrin	Binds to iron, a mineral many bacteria need to survive. By reducing the available amount of iron, lactoferrin thwarts growth of pathogenic bacteria.
Lysozyme	Kills bacteria by disrupting their cell walls.
Mucins	Adhere to bacteria and viruses, thus keeping such microorganisms from attaching to mucosal surfaces.
Oligosaccharides	Bind to microorganisms and bar them from attaching to mucosal surfaces.

SOURCE: Adapted from J Newman, 1995, How breast milk protects newborns, *Sci. Am.* 273(**6**): 76.

time (i.e., IgG, IgA, IgM, and IgD). In this way, each of the known anti-isotype antibodies was precipitated and removed from the rabbit anti-serum. What remained was an anti-isotype antibody specific for an unidentified class of antibody. This anti-isotype antibody turned out to completely block the P-K reaction. The new antibody was called IgE (in reference to the E antigen of ragweed pollen, which is a potent inducer of this class of antibody).

IgE binds to Fc receptors on the membranes of blood basophils and tissue mast cells. Crosslinkage of receptor-bound IgE molecules by antigen (allergen) induces degranulation of basophils and mast cells; as a result, a variety of pharmacologically active mediators in the granules are released, giving rise to allergic manifestations (Figure 4-16). Localized mast-cell degranulation induced by IgE also may release mediators that facilitate a buildup of various cells necessary for antiparasitic defense (see Chapter 16).

Immunoglobulin D (IgD)

IgD was first discovered when a patient developed a multiple myeloma whose myeloma protein failed to react with anti-isotype antisera against the then-known isotypes: IgA, IgM, and IgG. When rabbits were immunized with this myeloma protein, the resulting antisera identified this same class of antibody at low levels in normal human serum. This new class, called IgD, has a serum concentration of 30 μg/ml and constitutes about 0.2% of the total immunoglobulin in serum. IgD, together with IgM, is the major membrane-bound immunoglobulin expressed by mature B cells, and it is thought to function in the activation of B cells by antigen. No biological effector function has been identified for IgD.

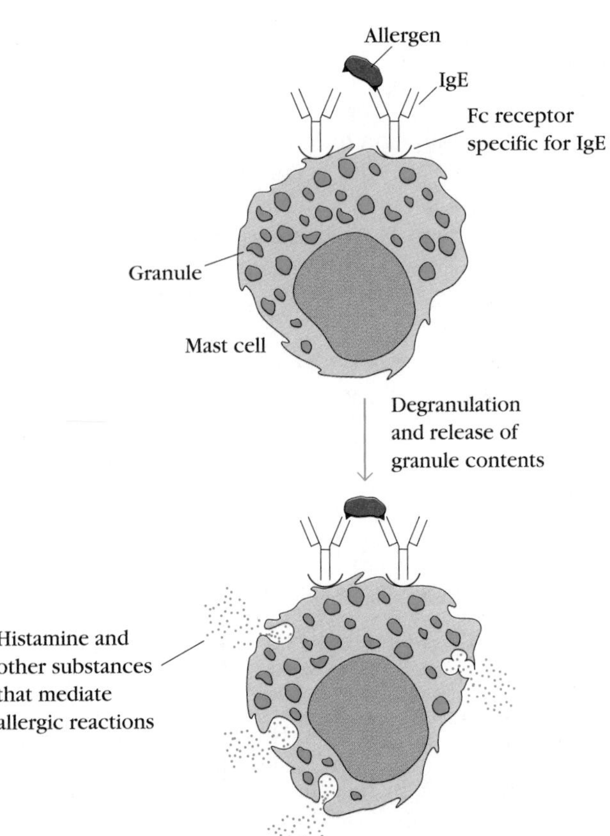

FIGURE 4-16 Allergen cross-linkage of receptor-bound IgE on mast cells induces degranulation, causing release of substances (blue dots) that mediate allergic manifestations.

Antigenic Determinants on Immunoglobulins

Since antibodies are glycoproteins, they can themselves function as potent immunogens to induce an antibody response. Such anti-Ig antibodies are powerful tools for the study of B-cell development and humoral immune responses. The antigenic determinants, or epitopes, on immunoglobulin molecules fall into three major categories: isotypic, allotypic, and idiotypic determinants, which are located in characteristic portions of the molecule (Figure 4-17).

Isotype

Isotypic determinants are constant-region determinants that collectively define each heavy-chain class and subclass and each light-chain type and subtype within a species (see Figure 4-17a). Each isotype is encoded by a separate constant-region gene, and all members of a species carry the same constant-region genes. Within a species, each normal individual will express all isotypes in the serum. Different species inherit different constant-region genes and therefore express different isotypes. Therefore, when an antibody from one species is injected into another species, the isotypic determinants will be recognized as foreign, inducing an antibody response to the isotypic determinants on the foreign antibody. Anti-isotype antibody is routinely used for research purposes to determine the class or subclass of serum antibody produced during an immune response or to characterize the class of membrane-bound antibody present on B cells.

Allotype

Although all members of a species inherit the same set of isotype genes, multiple alleles exist for some of the genes (see Figure 4-17b). These alleles encode subtle amino acid differences, called allotypic determinants, that occur in some, but not all, members of a species. In humans, allotypes have been characterized for all four IgG subclasses, for one IgA subclass, and for the κ light chain. The γ-chain allotypes are referred to as Gm markers. At least 25 different Gm allotypes have been identified; they are designated by the class and subclass followed by the allele number, for example, G1m(1), G2m(23), G3m(11), G4m(4a). Of the two IgA subclasses, only the IgA2 subclass has allotypes, as A2m(1) and A2m(2). The κ light chain has three allotypes, designated κm(1), κm(2), and κm(3). Each of these allotypic determinants represents differences in one to four amino acids that are encoded by different alleles.

Antibody to allotypic determinants can be produced by injecting antibodies from one member of a species into another member of the same species who carries different allotypic determinants. Antibody to allotypic determinants sometimes is produced by a mother during pregnancy in response to paternal allotypic determinants on the fetal immunoglobulins. Antibodies to allotypic determinants can also arise from a blood transfusion.

(a) Isotypic determinants

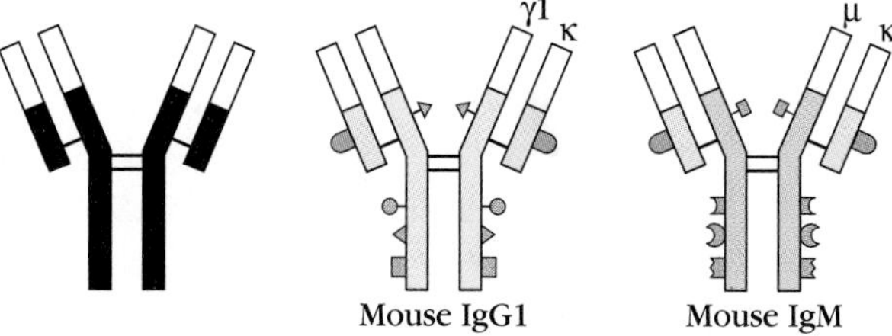

(b) Allotypic determinants

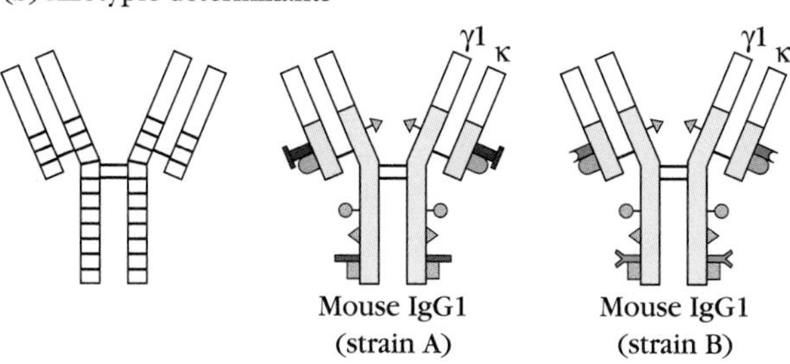

(c) Idiotypic determinants

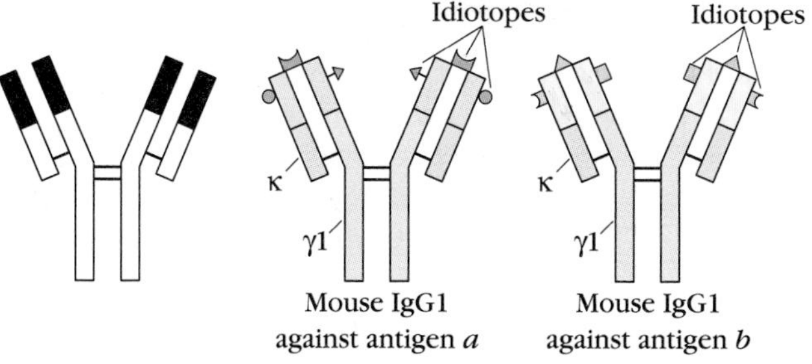

FIGURE 4-17 Antigenic determinants of immunoglobulins. For each type of determinant, the general location of determinants within the antibody molecule is shown (*left*) and two examples are illustrated (*center* and *right*). (a) Isotypic determinants are constant-region determinants that distinguish each Ig class and subclass within a species. (b) Allotypic determinants are subtle amino acid differences encoded by different alleles of isotype genes. Allotypic differences can be detected by comparing the same antibody class among different inbred strains. (c) Idiotypic determinants are generated by the conformation of the amino acid sequences of the heavy- and light-chain variable regions specific for each antigen. Each individual determinant is called an idiotope, and the sum of the individual idiotopes is the idiotype.

Idiotype

The unique amino acid sequence of the V_H and V_L domains of a given antibody can function not only as an antigen-binding site but also as a set of antigenic determinants. The idiotypic determinants are generated by the conformation of the heavy- and light-chain variable regions. Each individual antigenic determinant of the variable region is referred to as an idiotope (see Figure 4-17c). In some cases an idiotope may be the actual antigen-binding site, and in some cases an idiotope may comprise variable-region sequences outside of the antigen-binding site. Each antibody will present multiple idiotopes; the sum of the individual idiotopes is called the idiotype of the antibody.

Because the antibodies produced by individual B cells derived from the same clone have identical variable-region sequences, they all have the same idiotype. Anti-idiotype antibody is produced by injecting antibodies that have minimal variation in their isotypes and allotypes, so that the idiotypic difference can be recognized. Often a homogeneous antibody such as myeloma protein or monoclonal antibody is used. Injection of such an antibody into a syngeneic recipient will result in the formation of anti-idiotype antibody to the idiotypic determinants.

B-Cell Receptor

Immunologists have long been puzzled about how mIg mediates an activating signal after contact with an antigen. The dilemma is that all isotypes of mIg have very short cytoplasmic tails: the mIgM and mIgD cytoplasmic tails contain only 3 amino acids; the mIgA tail, 14 amino acids; and the mIgG and mIgE tails, 28 amino acids. In each case, the cytoplasmic tail is too short to be able to associate with intracellular signaling molecules (e.g., tyrosine kinases and G proteins).

The answer to this puzzle is that mIg does not constitute the entire antigen-binding receptor on B cells. Rather, the **B-cell receptor (BCR)** is a transmembrane protein complex composed of mIg and disulfide-linked heterodimers called Ig-α/Ig-β. Molecules of this heterodimer associate with an mIg molecule to form a single BCR (Figure 4-18). The Ig-α chain has a long cytoplasmic tail containing 61 amino acids; the tail of the Ig-β chain contains 48 amino acids. The tails in both Ig-α and Ig-β are long enough to interact with intracellular signaling molecules. Discovery of the Ig-α/Ig-β heterodimer has substantially furthered understanding of B-cell activation, which is discussed in detail in Chapter 11.

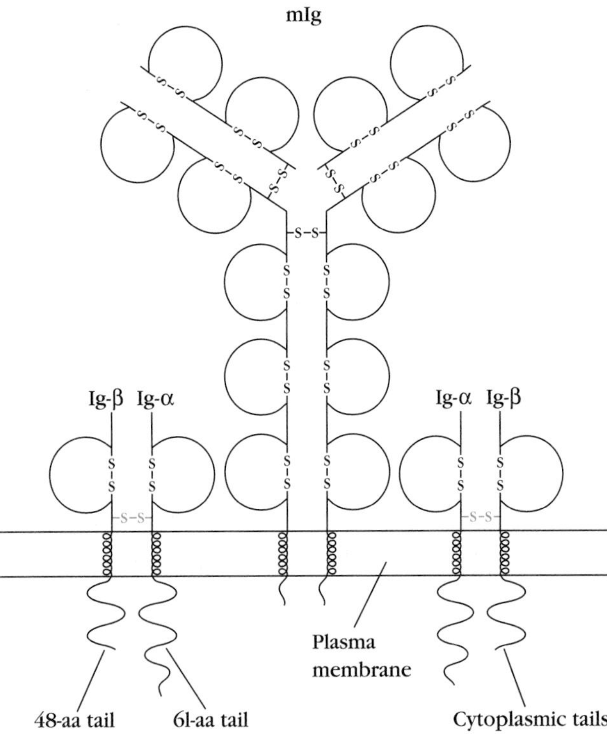

FIGURE 4-18 General structure of the B-cell receptor (BCR). This antigen-binding receptor is composed of membrane-bound immunoglobulin (mIg) and disulfide-linked heterodimers called Ig-α/Ig-β. Each heterodimer contains the immunoglobulin-fold structure and cytoplasmic tails much longer than those of mIg. As depicted, an mIg molecule is thought to be associated with two heterodimer molecules. [Adapted from AD Keegan and WE Paul, 1992, *Immunol. Today* **13:**63, and M Reth, 1992, *Annu. Rev. Immunol.* **10:**97.]

The Immunoglobulin Superfamily

The structures of the various immunoglobulin heavy and light chains described earlier share several features, suggesting that they have a common evolutionary ancestry. In particular, all heavy- and light-chain classes have the immunoglobulin-fold domain structure (see Figure 4-6). The presence of this characteristic structure in all immunoglobulin heavy and light chains suggests that the genes encoding them arose from a common primordial gene encoding a polypeptide of about 110 amino acids. Gene duplication and later divergence could then have generated the various heavy- and light-chain genes.

Large numbers of membrane proteins have been shown to possess one or more regions homologous to an immunoglobulin domain. Each of these membrane proteins is classified as a member of the **immunoglobulin superfamily.** The term *superfamily* is used to denote proteins whose corresponding genes derived from a common primordial gene encoding the basic domain structure. These genes have evolved independently and do not share genetic linkage or function. The following proteins, in addition to the immunoglobulins themselves, are representative members of the immunoglobulin superfamily (Figure 4-19):

- Ig-α/Ig-β heterodimer, part of the B-cell receptor
- Poly-Ig receptor, which contributes the secretory component to secretory IgA and IgM
- T-cell receptor
- T-cell accessory proteins, including CD2, CD4, CD8, CD28, and the γ, δ, and ε chains of CD3
- Class I and class II MHC molecules
- β_2-microglobulin, an invariant protein associated with class I MHC molecules
- Various cell-adhesion molecules, including VCAM-1, ICAM-1, ICAM-2, and LFA-3
- Platelet-derived growth factor

Numerous other proteins, some of them discussed in other chapters, belong to the immunoglobulin superfamily.

X-ray crystallographic analysis has not been accomplished for most members of the immunoglobulin superfamily. Nonetheless, the primary amino acid sequence of these proteins suggests that they all contain typical immunoglobulin-fold domains consisting of about 110 amino acids, arranged in pleated sheets of antiparallel β strands, usually with an invariant intrachain disulfide bond spanning 50–70 residues.

Most members of the immunoglobulin superfamily cannot bind antigen. Thus, the characteristic Ig-fold structure found in so many membrane proteins must have some function other than antigen binding. One possibility is that the immunoglobulin fold may facilitate interactions between membrane proteins. As described earlier, interactions can occur between the faces of β pleated sheets both of homologous immunoglobulin domains (e.g., C_H2/C_H2 interaction) and of nonhomologous domains (e.g., V_H/V_L and C_H1/C_L interactions).

Monoclonal Antibodies

As noted in Chapter 3, most antigens possess multiple epitopes and therefore induce proliferation and differentiation of a variety of B-cell clones, each derived from a B cell that recognizes a particular epitope. The resulting serum antibodies are heterogeneous, comprising a mixture of antibodies, each specific for one epitope (Figure 4-20). Such a **polyclonal antibody** response facilitates the localization, phagocytosis, and complement-mediated lysis of antigen; it thus has clear advantages for the organism in vivo. Unfortunately, the antibody heterogeneity that increases immune protection in vivo often reduces the efficacy of an antiserum for various in vitro uses. For most research, diagnostic, and therapeutic purposes, **monoclonal antibodies,** derived from a single clone and thus specific for a single epitope, are preferable.

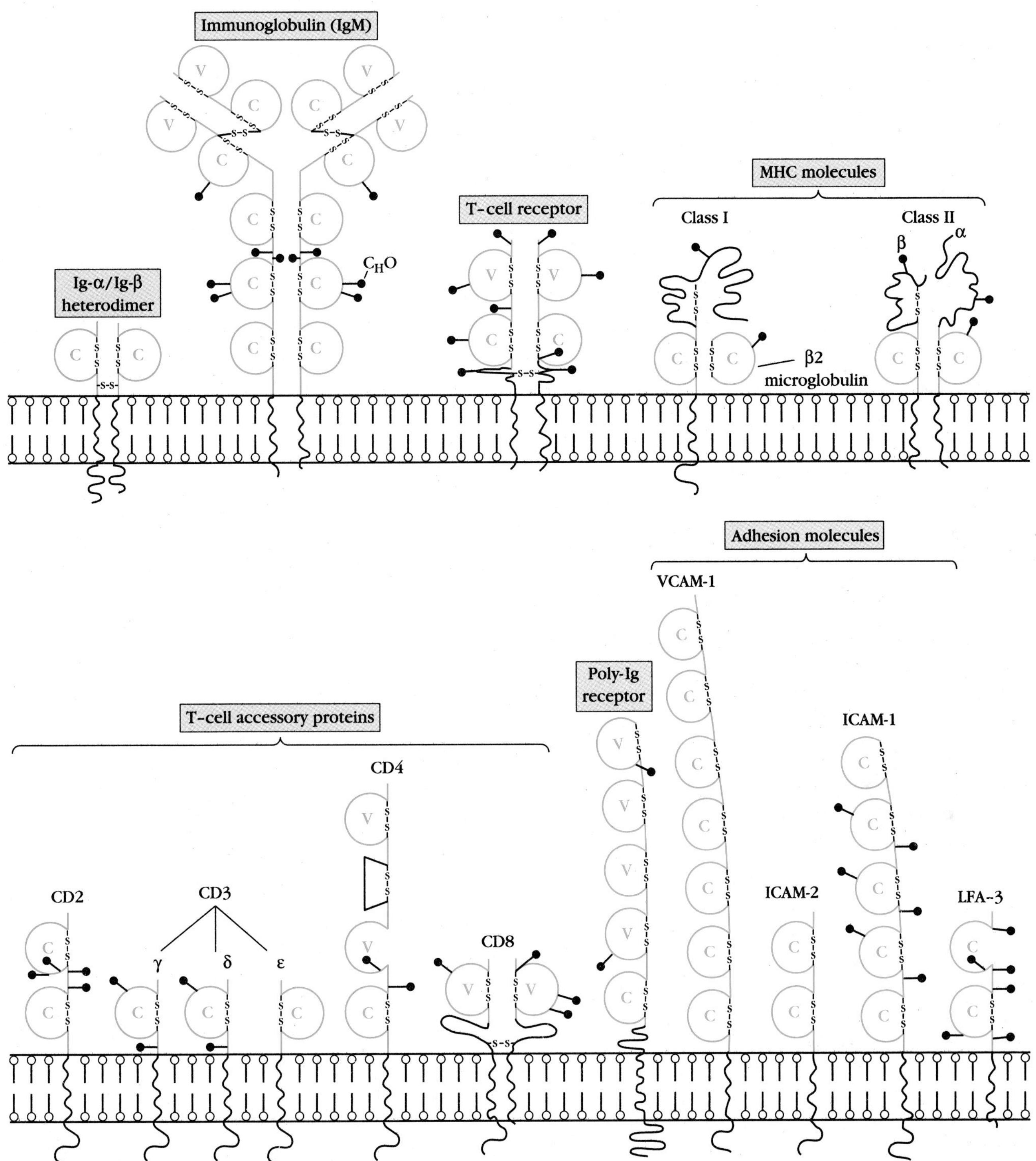

FIGURE 4-19 Some members of the immunoglobulin superfamily, a group of structurally related, usually membrane-bound glycoproteins. The loops shown in blue represent those portions of the molecule with the characteristic Ig-fold structure. In all cases shown here except for β_2-microglobulin, the carboxyl-terminal end of the molecule is anchored in the membrane.

Direct biochemical purification of a monoclonal antibody from a polyclonal antibody preparation is not feasible. In 1975, Georges Köhler and Cesar Milstein devised a method for preparing monoclonal antibody, which quickly became one of immunology's key technologies. By fusing a normal activated, antibody-producing B cell with a myeloma cell (a cancerous plasma cell), they were able to generate a hybrid cell, called a **hybridoma,** that possessed the immortal-growth properties of the myeloma cell and secreted the antibody produced by the B cell (see Figure 4-20).

VISUALIZING CONCEPTS

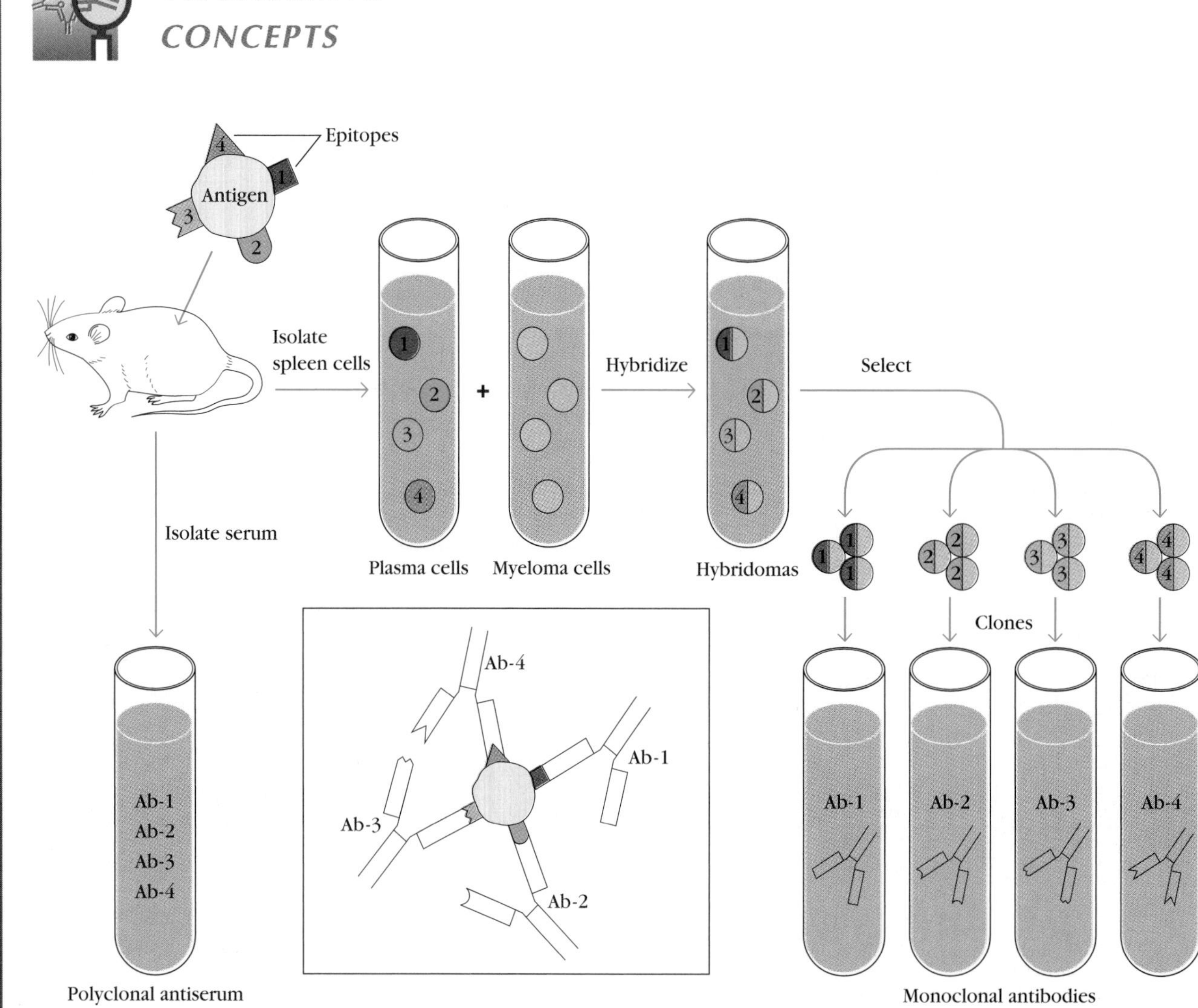

FIGURE 4-20 The conventional polyclonal antiserum produced in response to a complex antigen contains a mixture of antibodies, each specific for one of the four epitopes shown on the antigen. In contrast, a monoclonal antibody, which is derived from a single plasma cell, is specific for one epitope on a complex antigen (inset). The outline of the basic method for obtaining a monoclonal antibody is illustrated here.

The resulting clones of hybridoma cells, which secrete large quantities of monoclonal antibody, can be cultured indefinitely. The development of techniques for producing monoclonal antibody gave immunologists (and molecular biologists in general) a powerful and versatile research tool. The significance of the work by Köhler and Milstein was acknowledged when each was awarded a Nobel Prize in 1984.

Formation and Selection of Hybrid Cells

B-cell hybridomas are produced by using polyethylene glycol to fuse myeloma cells with B cells from animals that have been immunized with the antigen against which one wants to make antibodies. The myeloma cells contribute the immortal growth properties to the fused cells, and the B cells, which are only capable of limited growth in vitro, contribute the genetic information for synthesis of the specific antibody of interest. In practice, not all of the cells fuse, and the procedure gives a complex mixture of unfused myeloma and spleen cells ("parental cells") as well as numbers of fused cells. Among the fused cells, there are three different combinations; unwanted fusions of a B-cell with a B-cell, or of a myeloma cell with a myeloma cell, and the desired fusions of a B cell with a myeloma cell. Thus, the conditions of the procedure must selectively allow the survival and growth of the

B-cell × myeloma hybridomas only. One common method requires the use of myeloma cells that are deficient (because of previously selected mutation) for one of the nucleotide salvage pathways, making them unable to grow in HAT medium (named for its three components—hypoxanthine, aminopterin, and thymidine). If the mixture of hybridomas and unfused parental cells is placed in this medium, the parental myeloma cells cannot survive. The B-cell × myeloma cells can survive because the B cell contributes the missing enzyme for the salvage pathway. Although unfused B cells are able to survive in HAT medium, these cells do not live for extended periods in vitro and thus die out.

HAT selection depends on the fact that mammalian cells can synthesize nucleotides by two different pathways: the de novo and the salvage pathways (Figure 4-21). The de novo pathway, in which a methyl or formyl group is transferred from an activated form of tetrahydrofolate, is blocked by aminopterin, a folic acid analog. When the de novo pathway is blocked, cells utilize the salvage pathway, which bypasses the aminopterin block by converting purines and pyrimidines directly into nucleotides for synthesis of DNA and RNA. The enzymes catalyzing the salvage pathway include hypoxanthine-guanine phosphoribosyl transferase (HGPRT) and thymidine kinase (TK). A mutation in either of these two enzymes blocks the ability of the cell to use the salvage pathway. HAT medium contains aminopterin to block the de novo pathway and hypoxanthine and thymidine to allow growth by the salvage pathway. Therefore, cells that lack either HGPRT or TK will die in HAT medium, because they lack the ability to use the salvage pathway to acquire essential intermediates for the synthesis of nucleic acids.

In hybridoma technology, the myeloma cells used are actually double mutants. As mentioned above, they lack the enzyme HGPRTase and therefore are deselected in HAT. They have also lost the ability to produce immunoglobulin (Ig^- mutants). By using Ig^- mutants one assures that the antibodies produced by the hybridoma are encoded solely by the spleen cell partner and the myeloma cells only contribute immortal growth properties to the fused cells. The other fusion partner is usually a population of spleen cells containing antigen activated $HGPRT^+$ B-cells. These cells contribute the capacity to utilize the salvage pathway for hypoxanthine to the hybridomas, thereby enabling their survival in HAT medium.

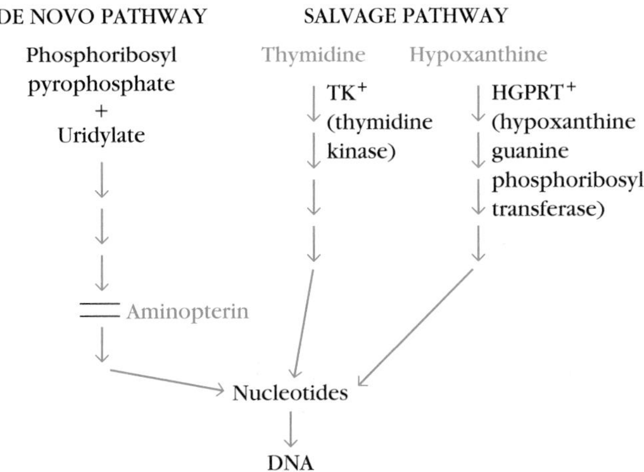

FIGURE 4-21 Aminopterin blocks DNA synthesis by the de novo pathway. It acts as an analog of dihydrofolic acid and binds with a high affinity to dihydrofolate reductase, inhibiting purine synthesis. In the presence of aminopterin, cells must use the salvage pathway to produce DNA.

Production of Monoclonal Antibodies

Monoclonal antibody production is outlined in Figure 4-22. Once antibody-secreting hybridomas are obtained, they must be screened for the desired antigenic specificity. Although some hybridomas will produce antibody specific for the antigen used for immunization, others will be specific for unwanted antigens. Two of the most common screening techniques are ELISA and RIA, which are described in Chapter 6.

Following identification, hybridomas of the desired specificity are recloned to ensure that the culture is truly monoclonal and are then propagated in one of several ways to produce the desired monoclonal antibody. When a hybridoma is grown in tissue-culture flasks, the antibody is secreted into the medium, usually at fairly low concentrations (1–20 μg/ml). A hybridoma can also be propagated in the peritoneal cavity of histocompatible mice, where it secretes the monoclonal antibody into the ascites fluid at much higher concentrations (usually about 1–10 mg/ml); the antibody can be purified from the mouse ascites fluid by chromatography. To meet the increased demand for monoclonal antibodies, in vitro techniques for growth of hybridoma cells at very high densities ($>10^7$/ml) have been developed.

The production of human monoclonal antibodies has been hampered by a number of technical difficulties. The most important of these has been the lack of human myeloma cells that exhibit immortal growth, are susceptible to HAT selection, do not secrete antibody, and support antibody production in the hybridomas made with them. As an alternative to conferring immortality on human B cells by fusion to myeloma cells, normal human B lymphocytes can be transformed with Epstein-Barr virus (EBV). When B lymphocytes are cultured with antigen in the presence of EBV, some of them acquire the immortal-growth properties of a transformed cell while continuing to secrete antibody. Cloning of such primed, transformed cells has permitted production of human monoclonal antibody, but the amounts secreted are generally small.

Another problem is the difficulty of readily obtaining antigen-activated B cells from the human lymphoid tissues equivalent to the mouse spleen. Generally, human hybridomas are

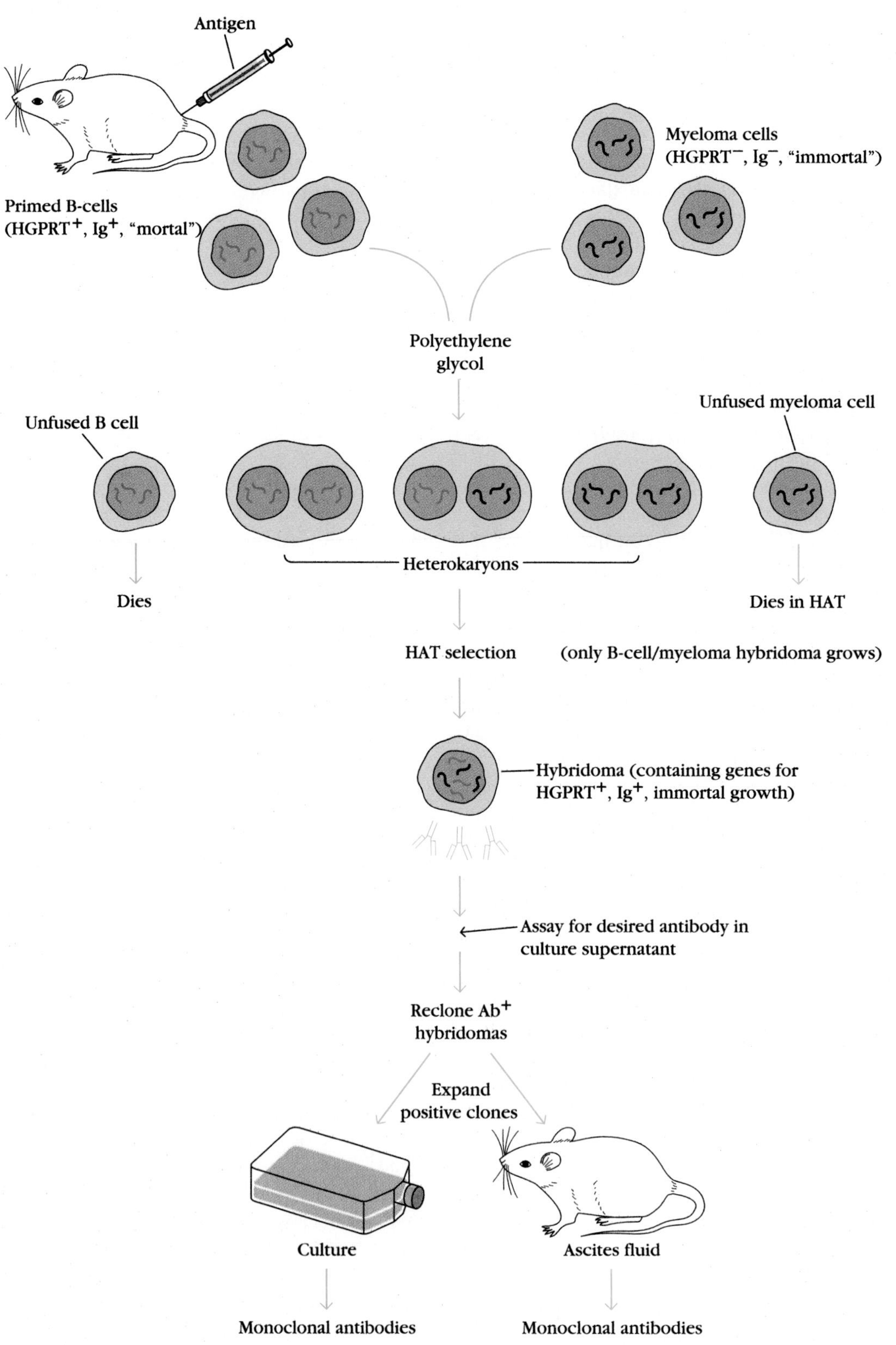

FIGURE 4-22 The procedure for producing monoclonal antibodies specific for a given antigen developed by G. Kohler and C. Milstein. Spleen cells (HGPRT$^+$ and Ig$^+$) from an antigen-primed mouse are fused with mouse myeloma cells (HGPRT$^-$ and Ig$^-$). The spleen cell provides the necessary enzymes for growth on HAT medium, while the myeloma cell provides immortal-growth properties. Unfused myeloma cells or myeloma/myeloma fusions fail to grow because of their lack of HGPRT. Unfused spleen cells have limited growth capabilities in vitro and will die within a few days.

prepared from human peripheral blood, which contains few activated B cells engaged in an immune response. It is possible to obtain B cells that have been activated by antigens present in vaccines that are normally given to people, but human volunteers cannot be immunized with the range of antigens that can be given to mice or other animals. To overcome this difficulty, cultured human cells are sometimes primed with antigen in vitro. However, the in vitro system cannot mimic the normal microenvironment of lymphoid tissue; as a result, the B cells usually produce only low-affinity IgM antibody.

One way to avoid the need for in vitro priming of human B cells is to transplant the cells necessary to support a human immune response from humans into SCID mice. Although normal mice would reject such transplants, they are readily performed in SCID mice, because these animals lack a functional immune system. Consequently, one can make SCID-human mice that contain human B and T cells. Following immunization of these mice, activated human B cells can be isolated from the mouse spleen and used to produce human monoclonal antibodies.

Clinical Uses for Monoclonal Antibodies

Monoclonal antibodies are proving to be very useful as diagnostic, imaging, and therapeutic reagents in clinical medicine. Initially, monoclonal antibodies were used primarily as in vitro diagnostic reagents. Among the many monoclonal antibody diagnostic reagents now available are products for detecting pregnancy, diagnosing numerous pathogenic microorganisms, measuring the blood levels of various drugs, matching histocompatibility antigens, and detecting antigens shed by certain tumors.

Radiolabeled monoclonal antibodies can also be used in vivo for detecting or locating tumor antigens, permitting earlier diagnosis of some primary or metastatic tumors in patients. For example, monoclonal antibody to breast-cancer cells is labeled with iodine-131 and introduced into the blood to detect the spread of a tumor to regional lymph nodes. This monoclonal imaging technique can detect breast-cancer metastases that would be undetected by other, less sensitive scanning techniques.

Immunotoxins composed of tumor-specific monoclonal antibodies coupled to lethal toxins are potentially valuable therapeutic reagents. The toxins used in preparing immunotoxins include ricin, *Shigella* toxin, and diphtheria toxin, all of which inhibit protein synthesis. These toxins are so potent that a single molecule has been shown to kill a cell. Each of these toxins consists of two types of functionally distinct polypeptide components, an inhibitory (toxin) chain and one or more binding chains, which interact with receptors on cell surfaces; without the binding polypeptide(s) the toxin cannot get into cells and therefore is harmless. An immunotoxin is prepared by replacing the binding polypeptide(s) with a monoclonal antibody that is specific for a particular tumor cell (Figure 4-23a). In theory, the attached monoclonal antibody will deliver the toxin chain specifically to tumor cells, where it will cause death by inhibiting protein synthesis (Figure 4-23b). The initial clinical responses to such immunotoxins in patients with leukemia, lymphoma, and some other types of cancer have shown promise, and clinical trails to establish their effectiveness are underway.

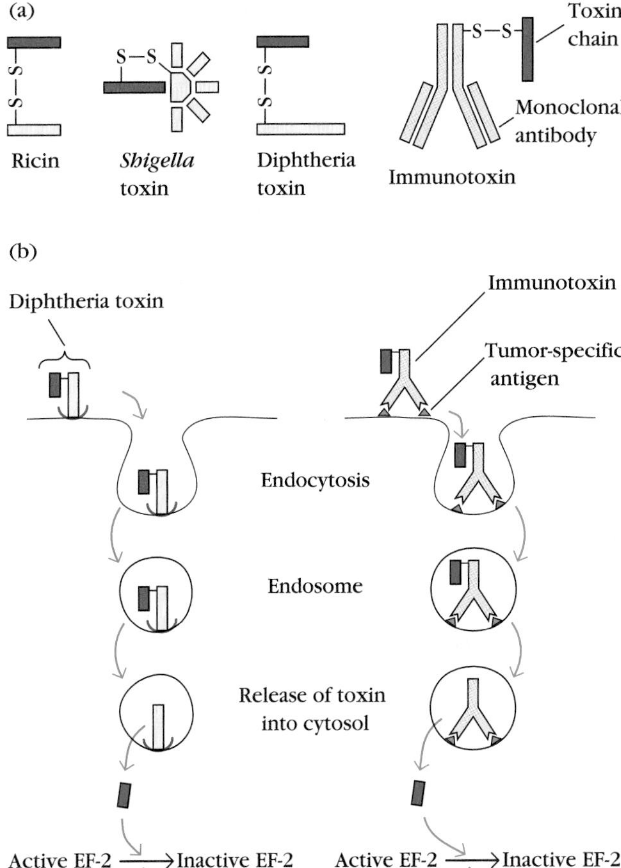

FIGURE 4-23 (a) Toxins used to prepare immunotoxins include ricin, *Shigella* toxin, and diphtheria toxin. Each toxin contains an inhibitory toxin chain (red) and a binding component (yellow). To make an immunotoxin, the binding component of the toxin is replaced with a monoclonal antibody (blue). (b) Diphtheria toxin binds to a cell-membrane receptor (*left*) and a diphtheria-immunotoxin binds to a tumor-associated antigen (*right*). In either case, the toxin is internalized in an endosome. The toxin chain is then released into the cytoplasm, where it inhibits protein synthesis by catalyzing the inactivation of elongation factor 2 (EF-2)

Catalytic Monoclonal Antibodies (Abzymes)

The binding of an antibody to its antigen is similar in many ways to the binding of an enzyme to its substrate. In both cases the binding involves weak, noncovalent interactions and exhibits high specificity and often high affinity. What distinguishes an antibody-antigen interaction from an enzyme-substrate interaction is that the antibody does not alter the antigen, whereas the enzyme catalyzes a chemical change in its substrate. However, like enzymes, antibodies of appropriate specificity can stabilize the transition state of a bound substrate, thus reducing the activation energy for chemical modification of the substrate.

Because of the similarities between antigen-antibody interactions and enzyme-substrate interactions, R. A. Lerner and his colleagues wondered whether some antibodies could behave like enzymes and catalyze chemical reactions. To investigate this possibility, they produced a hapten-carrier complex in which the hapten structurally resembled the transition state of an ester undergoing hydrolysis. Using this conjugate, they generated antihapten monoclonal antibodies. When these monoclonal antibodies were incubated with an ester substrate, some of them accelerated hydrolysis by about 1000-fold; that is, they acted like the enzyme that normally catalyzes the substrate's hydrolysis. The catalytic activity of these antibodies was highly specific; that is, they hydrolyzed only esters whose transition-state structure closely resembled that of the hapten in the immunizing conjugate. These catalytic antibodies have been called **abzymes** in reference to their dual role as antibody and enzyme.

A central goal of catalytic antibody research is the derivation of a battery of abzymes that cut peptide bonds at specific amino acid residues, much as restriction enzymes cut DNA at specific sites. Such abzymes would be invaluable tools in the structural and functional analysis of proteins. Additionally, it may be possible to generate abzymes with the ability to dissolve blood clots or to cleave viral glycoproteins at specific sites, thus blocking viral infectivity. Unfortunately, catalytic antibodies that cleave the peptide bonds of proteins have been exceedingly difficult to derive. Much of the research currently being pursued in this field is devoted to the solution of this important but difficult problem.

Summary

1. The basic structure of an antibody molecule consists of two identical light chains and two identical heavy chains, which are linked by disulfide bonds (see Figure 4-2). The amino-terminal 110 amino acids in each heavy and light chain constitute a variable (V_H and V_L) domain. The remainder of each light chain consists of a single constant domain (C_L); the remainder of each heavy chain contains three or four constant domains (C_H).
2. In any given antibody molecule, the constant region contains one of five basic heavy-chain sequences (μ, γ, δ, α, or ϵ) and one of two basic light-chain sequences (κ or λ). These sequences are called isotypes. The heavy-chain isotypes determine the five classes of antibody (IgM, IgG, IgD, IgA, and IgE) and the effector functions of the molecule (see Figure 4-13 and Tables 4-1 and 4-2).
3. Each of the domains in the immunoglobulin molecule has a characteristic tertiary structure called the immunoglobulin fold (see Figure 4-6). The Ig-fold structure is also present in a large group of membrane proteins (see Figure 4-19). Except for antibodies and T-cell receptors, the members of the immunoglobulin superfamily do not bind antigen. The basic Ig-fold structure may facilitate homologous and nonhomologous interactions between members of this family.
4. Within the amino-terminal variable domain of each heavy and light chain are three hypervariable regions, also called complementarity-determining regions (CDRs). These are formed by some of the loops that connect the β strands of these domains (see Figures 4-6 and 4-7). In the three-dimensional conformation of an antibody molecule, these regions are brought into proximity, forming its antigen-binding site and determining its specificity.
5. Immunoglobulins are expressed in two forms: secreted antibody produced by plasma cells and membrane-bound antibody present on the surface of B cells. Membrane-bound immunoglobulin associates with a heterodimer called Ig-α/Ig-β to form the B-cell receptor (see Figure 4-18). The antigenic specificity of a B cell is determined by the membrane-bound antibody that it expresses. The Ig-α/Ig-β heterodimer of the B-cell receptor mediates the intracellular signals that lead to B-cell activation following interaction with antigen.
6. The five antibody classes differ in their ability to carry out various effector functions, in their average serum concentrations, and in their half-life (see Table 4-2). IgG, the most abundant class in serum, is particularly important for clearing antigen by various mechanisms; it also is the only class that can cross the placenta. Serum IgM exists as a pentamer (see Figure 4-13e); because of its high valency, IgM is more effective than other classes in neutralizing virus, bacterial agglutinating bacteria, and activating complement. IgA is the predominant class in external secretions, including breast milk and mucus. In these secretions, secretory IgA exists as a dimer or tetramer linked by disulfide bonds to the J chain and secretory component (Figure 4-15). IgD and IgE are the two least abundant classes in serum. IgD (along with IgM) is the major membrane-bound antibody on mature B cells, and IgE mediates mast-cell degranulation (see Figure 4-16).
7. There are three major effector functions that enable antibodies to remove antigens and kill pathogens: Opsonization promotes antigen phagocytosis by macrophages and neutrophils. Complement activation by IgM and most human IgG subclasses can activate a pathway that leads to the generation of a collection of proteins that can perforate cell membranes. Antibody-dependent cell-mediated cytotoxicity (ADCC) can cause NK-cell-mediated death of

target cells when antibody bound to the target cells associates with the Fc receptors of NK cells.

8. Unlike polyclonal antibodies, a monoclonal antibody is a homogeneous preparation specific for a single epitope on a complex antigen (see Figure 4-20). In a common procedure for producing monoclonal antibodies, primed splenic B cells ($HGPRT^+$, Ig^+) are fused with mouse myeloma cells ($HGPRT^-$, Ig^-). These hybrid cells, called B-cell hybridomas, continue to secrete the specific antibody of the primed B cell but possess the immortal-growth properties of the myeloma cell (see Figure 4-22).

REFERENCES

Arevalo, JH, MJ Taussig, and IA Wilson. 1993. Molecular basis of crossreactivity and the limits of antibody-antigen complementarity. *Nature* **365:**859.

Branden, C, and J Tooze. 1991. *Introduction to Protein Structure.* New York, Garland.

Carayannopoulos, L, and JD Capra. 1993. Immunoglobulins: structure and function. In *Fundamental Immunology,* 3rd ed., WE Paul, ed., New York, Raven.

Driggers EM, and PG Schultz 1996. Catalytic Antibodies. *Adv. Protein Chem,* **49:**261.

Garcia, KC, et al. 1992. Three-dimensional structure of an angiotensin II-Fab complex at 3 Å: hormone recognition by an anti-idiotypic antibody. *Science* **257:**502.

Greenspan, NS, and CA Bona. 1993. Idiotypes: structure and immunogenicity. *FASEB* **7:**437.

Kohler, G, and C Milstein. 1975. Continuous cultures of fused cells secreting antibody of predefined specificity. *Nature* **256:**495.

Kraehenbuhl, JP, and MR Neutra. 1992. Transepithelial transport and mucosal defence II: secretion of IgA. *Trends Cell Biol.* **2:**134.

Immunology Today, The Immune Receptor Supplement, 2nd ed. 1997. Elsevier Trends Journals, Cambridge, UK (ISSN 1365–1218).

Lerner, RA, and A Tramontano. 1988. Catalytic antibodies. *Sci. Am.* **258**(3):58.

Newman, J. 1995. How breast milk protects newborns. *Sci. Am.* **273**(6):76.

Reth, M. 1995. The B-cell antigen receptor complex and coreceptor. *Immunol. Today* **16:**310.

Stanfield, RL, and IA Wilson. 1995. Protein-peptide interactions. *Curr. Opin. Struc. Biol.* **5:**103.

Underdown, BJ, and JM Schiff. 1986. Immunoglobulin A: strategic defence initiative at the mucosal surface. *Annu. Rev. Immunol.* **4:**389.

Wedemayer, GJ, PA Patten, LH Wang, PG Schultz, and RC Stevens. 1997. Structural insights into the evolution of an antibody combining site. *Science,* **276:**1665.

Wilson, IA, and RL Stanfield. 1994. Antibody-antibody interactions: new structures and new conformational changes. *Curr. Opin. Struc. Biol.* **4:**857.

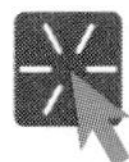

Useful Web Sites

http://immuno.bme.nwu.edu/

The Kabat Database of Sequences of Proteins of Immunological Interest: This site has the amino acid and DNA sequences of many antibodies and other proteins that play important roles in immunology.

http://www.biochem.ucl.ac.uk/~martin/abs

Antibodies—Structure and Sequence: This website summarizes useful information on antibody structure and sequence. It provides general information on antibodies and crystal structures and links to other antibody-related information.

http://www.ncbi.nlm.nih.gov

National Center for Biotechnology Information (NCBI): A unique and comprehensive resource of computerized databases of bibliographic information, nucleic acid sequences, protein sequences, and sequence analysis tools created and maintained by the National Library of Medicine.

http://www.ncbi.nlm.nih.gov/Structure/

The Molecular Modelling Database (MMDB) contains 3-dimensional structures determined by X-ray crystallography and NMR spectroscopy. The data for MMDB are obtained from the Protein Data Bank (PDB). The National Center for Biotechnology Information (NCBI) has crosslinked structural data to bibliographic information, to the databases of protein and nucleic acid sequences, and to the NCBI animal taxonomy database. The NCBI has developed a 3D structure viewer, Cn3D, for easy interactive visualization of molecular structures from within Entrez Med.

STUDY QUESTIONS

1. Indicate whether each of the following statements is true or false. If you think a statement is false, explain why.

a. A rabbit immunized with human IgG3 will produce antibody that reacts with all subclasses of IgG in humans.

b. An $HGPRT^-$ myeloma cell requires hypoxanthine for growth.

c. All immunoglobulin molecules on the surface of a given B cell have the same idiotype.

d. All immunoglobulin molecules on the surface of a given B cell have the same isotype.

e. All myeloma protein molecules derived from a single myeloma clone have the same idiotype and allotype.

f. When a heterokaryon initially is formed, it is multinucleated.

g. The hypervariable regions make significant contact with the epitope.

h. IgG functions more effectively than IgM in bacterial agglutination.

i. Hypoxanthine is added to HAT medium to prevent cell growth by the salvage pathway.

j. All isotypes are normally found in each individual of a species.

k. The heavy-chain variable region (V_H) is twice as long as the light-chain variable region (V_L).

l. An $HGPRT^+$ revertant myeloma cell would be a good fusion

Go to www.whfreeman.com/immunology 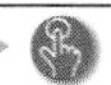 **Self-Test**
Review and quiz of key terms

partner for production of B-cell hybridomas because it would not be able to grow in HAT medium.

2. An energetic immunology student has isolated protein X, which he believes is a new isotype of human immunoglobulin.

a. What structural features would protein X have to have in order to be classified as an immunoglobulin?

b. You prepare rabbit antisera to whole human IgG, human κ chain, and human γ chain. Assuming protein X is, in fact, a new immunoglobulin isotype, to which of these antisera would it bind? Why?

c. Devise an experimental procedure for preparing an antiserum that is specific for protein X.

3. According to the clonal selection theory, all the immunoglobulin molecules on a single B cell have the same antigenic specificity. Explain why the presence of both IgM and IgD on the same B cell does not violate the unispecificity implied by clonal selection.

4. IgG, which contains γ heavy chains, developed much more recently during evolution than IgM, which contains μ heavy chains. Describe two advantages and two disadvantages that IgG has in comparison with IgM.

5. Although the five immunoglobulin isotypes share many common structural features, the differences in their structures affect their biological activities.

a. Draw a schematic diagram of a typical IgG molecule and label each of the following parts: H chains, L chains, interchain disulfide bonds, intrachain disulfide bonds, hinge, Fab, Fc, and all the domains. Indicate which domains are involved in antigen binding.

b. How would you have to modify the diagram of IgG to depict an IgA molecule isolated from saliva?

c. How would you have to modify the diagram of IgG to depict serum IgM?

6. Fill out the accompanying table relating to the properties of IgG molecules and their various parts. Insert a (+) if the molecule or part exhibits the property; a (−) if it does not; and a (+/−) if it does so only weakly.

Property	Whole IgG	H chain	L chain	Fab	$F(ab')_2$	Fc
Binds antigen						
Bivalent antigen binding						
Binds to Fc receptors						
Fixed complement in presence of antigen						
Has V domains						
Has C domains						

7. Because immunoglobulin molecules possess antigenic determinants, they themselves can function as immunogens, inducing formation of antibody. For each of the following immunization scenarios, indicate whether anti-immunoglobulin antibodies would be formed to isotypic (IS), allotypic (AL), or idiotypic (ID) determinants:

a. Anti-DNP antibodies produced in a BALB/c mouse are injected into a C57BL/6 mouse.

b. Anti-BGG monoclonal antibodies from a BALB/c mouse are injected into another BALB/c mouse.

c. Anti-BGG antibodies produced in a BALB/c mouse are injected into a rabbit.

d. Anti-DNP antibodies produced in a BALB/c mouse are injected into an outbred mouse.

e. Anti-BGG antibodies produced in a BALB/c mouse are injected into the same mouse.

8. Write YES or NO in the accompanying table to indicate whether the rabbit antisera listed at the top react with the mouse antibody components listed at the left.

	Rabbit antisera to mouse antibody component				
	γ chain	κ chain	IgG Fab fragment	IgG Fc fragment	J chain
Mouse γ chain					
Mouse κ chain					
Mouse IgM whole					
Mouse IgM Fc fragment					

9. The myeloma cells used in production of B-cell hybridomas have three properties that make them suitable fusion partners. List these properties and explain why they are necessary for the production of hybridomas that secrete B-cell antibodies.

10. The characteristic structure of immunoglobulin domains, termed the immunoglobulin fold, also occurs in the numerous membrane proteins belonging to the immunoglobulin superfamily.

a. Describe the typical features that define the immunoglobulin-fold domain structure.

b. List three membrane proteins that belong to the immunoglobulin superfamily. How might the presence of the immunoglobulin-fold domain structure in these proteins facilitate their function?

11. Where are the hypervariable regions located on an antibody molecule and what are their functions?

12. What would be the consequences if you omitted aminopterin from the HAT medium used to select hybridomas in the standard procedure for producing monoclonal antibodies?

13. You prepare an immunotoxin by conjugating diphtheria toxin with a monoclonal antibody specific for a tumor antigen.

a. If this immunotoxin is injected into an animal, will any normal cells be killed? Explain.

b. If the antibody part of the immunotoxin is degraded so that the toxin is released, will normal cells be killed? Explain.

14. An investigator wanted to make a rabbit antiserum specific for mouse IgG. She injected a rabbit with purified mouse IgG and obtained an antiserum that reacted strongly with mouse IgG. To her dismay, however, the antiserum also reacted with each of the other mouse isotypes. Explain why she got this result. How could she make the rabbit antiserum specific for mouse IgG?

15. You fuse spleen cells having a normal genotype for immunoglobulin heavy chains (H) and light chains (L) with three myeloma-cell preparations differing in their immunoglobulin genotype as follows: (a) H^+, L^+; (b) H^-, L^+; and (c) H^-, L^-. For each hybridoma, predict how many unique antigen-binding sites, composed of one H and one L chain, theoretically could be produced and show the chain structure of the possible antibody molecules. For each possible antibody molecule indicate whether the chains would originate from the spleen (S) or from the myeloma (M) fusion partner (e.g., H_SL_S/H_mL_m).

16. For each immunoglobulin isotype (a–e) select the description(s) listed below (1–12) that are true about that isotype. Each description may be used once, more than once, or not at all; more than one description may apply to some isotypes.

Isotypes

a. _____ IgA c. _____ IgE e. _____ IgM

b. _____ IgD d. _____ IgG

Descriptions

(1) Secreted form is a pentamer of the basic H_2L_2 unit

(2) Binds to Fc receptors on mast cells

(3) Multimeric forms have a J chain

(4) Present on the surface of mature, unprimed B cells

(5) The most abundant isotype in serum

(6) Major antibody in secretions such as saliva, tears, and breast milk

(7) Present on the surface of immature B cells

(8) The first serum antibody made in a primary immune response

(9) Plays an important role in immediate hypersensitivity

(10) Plays primary role in protecting against pathogens that invade through the gut or respiratory mucosa

(11) Multimeric forms may contain a secretory component

(12) Least abundant isotype in serum

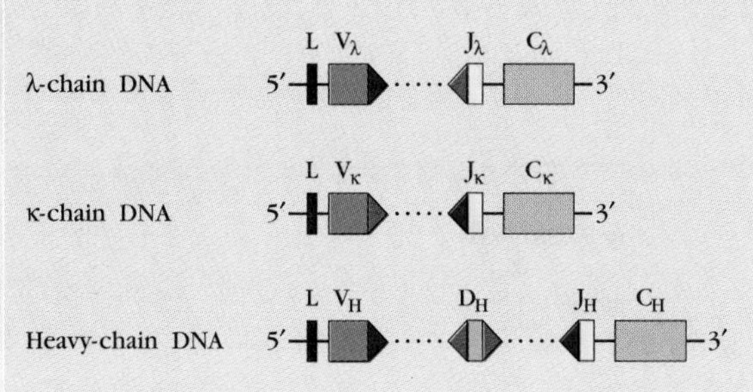

CHAPTER 5

ORGANIZATION AND EXPRESSION OF IMMUNOGLOBULIN GENES

One of the most remarkable features of the vertebrate immune system is its ability to respond to an apparently limitless array of foreign antigens. As immunoglobulin (Ig) sequence data accumulated, virtually every antibody molecule studied was found to contain a unique amino acid sequence in its variable region but only one of a limited number of invariant sequences in its constant region. The genetic basis of such tremendous variation coupled with constancy in a single protein molecule lies in the organization of the immunoglobulin genes.

In germ-line DNA, multiple gene segments encode portions of a single immunoglobulin heavy or light chain. These gene segments are carried in the germ cells but cannot be transcribed and translated into heavy and light chains until they are rearranged into functional genes. During B-cell maturation in the bone marrow, certain of these gene segments are randomly shuffled by a dynamic genetic system capable of generating more than 10^{10} combinations. This process is carefully regulated: the maturation of a progenitor B cell progresses through an ordered sequence of Ig-gene rearrangements. By the end of this process, a mature, immunocompetent B cell will contain a single functional heavy-chain variable-region sequence and a single functional light-chain variable-region sequence, so that the individual B cell is antigenically committed to a specific epitope. After antigenic stimulation of a mature B cell in peripheral lymphoid organs, further rearrangement of constant-region gene segments can generate changes in the isotype expressed, producing changes in the biological effector functions without changing the specificity of the immunoglobulin molecule. Thus, mature B cells contain chromosomal DNA that is no longer identical to germ-line DNA. While we think of genomic DNA as a stable genetic blueprint, the lymphocyte cell lineage does not retain an intact copy of this blueprint. Genomic rearrangement is an essential feature of lymphocyte differentiation, and no other vertebrate cell type has been shown to undergo this process.

This chapter first describes the detailed organization of the immunoglobulin genes, the process of Ig-gene rearrangement, and the mechanisms by which the dynamic immunoglobulin genetic system generates more than 10^{10} different antigenic specificities. Then it describes the mechanism of class switching, the role of differential RNA processing in the expression of immunoglobulin genes, and regulation of Ig-gene transcription. The chapter concludes with the application of our knowledge of the molecular biology of immunoglobulin genes to the engineering of antibody molecules for therapeutic applications. A later chapter, Chapter 11, covers in detail the entire process of B-cell development from the first gene rearrangements in progenitor B cells to final differentiation into memory B cells and antibody-secreting plasma cells. Figure 5-1 outlines the sequential stages in B-cell development, many of which result from critical rearrangements.

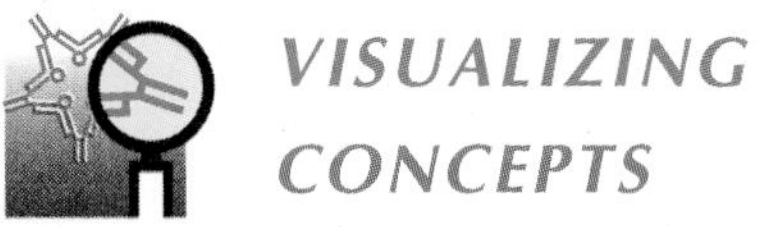

VISUALIZING CONCEPTS

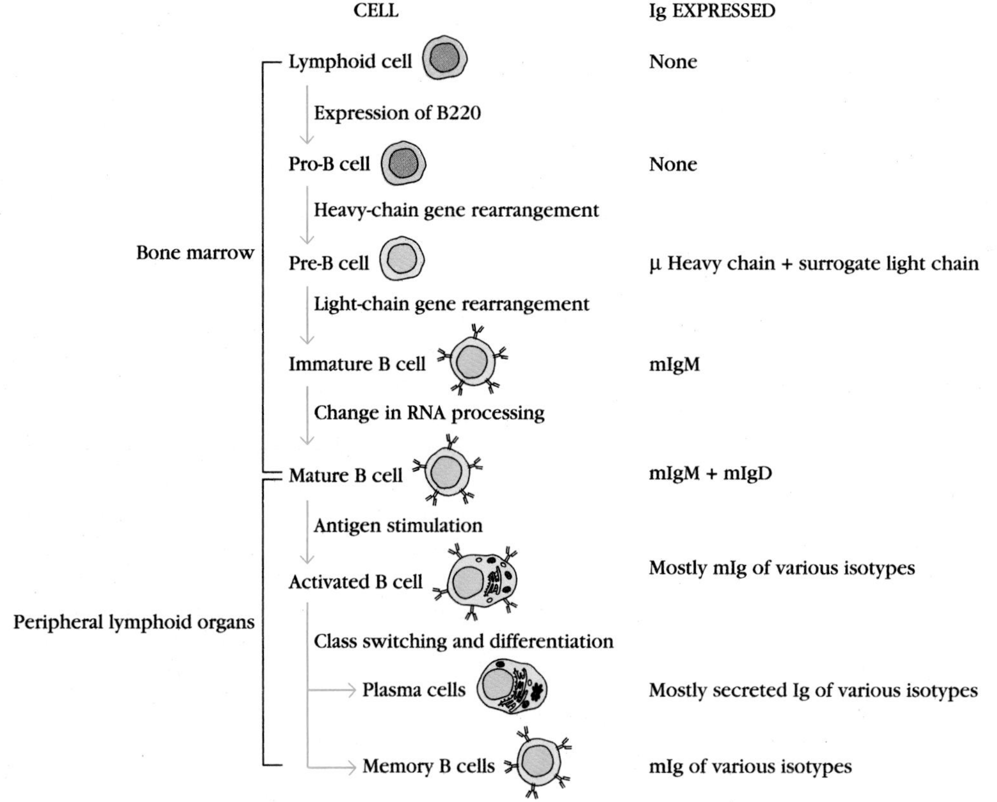

FIGURE 5-1 Overview of B-cell development. The events that occur during maturation in the bone marrow do not require antigen, whereas activation and differentiation of mature B cells in peripheral lymphoid organs require antigen. The labels mIgM, mIgD, and mIgG refer to membrane-associated Igs.

Genetic Model Compatible with Ig Structure

The results of the immunoglobulin-sequencing studies discussed in Chapter 4 revealed a number of features of immunoglobulin structure that were difficult to reconcile with classic genetic models. Any viable model of the immunoglobulin genes had to account for the following properties of antibodies:

- The vast diversity of antibody specificities
- The presence of a variable region at the amino-terminal end and of a constant region at the carboxyl-terminal end of Ig heavy and light chains
- The existence of isotypes with the same antigenic specificity, which result from the association of a given variable region with different heavy-chain constant regions

Germ-Line and Somatic-Variation Models

It has been estimated that the mammalian immune system can generate more than 10^{10} different antibodies, allowing an animal to respond to a vast number of potential antigens. Since antibodies are proteins and proteins are encoded by genes, it follows that this tremendous diversity in antibody structure must arise from a genetic system capable of generating enormous diversity. For several decades, immunologists sought to imagine a genetic mechanism that might generate such diversity. Two very different sets of theories emerged. The **germ-line theories** maintained that the genome contributed by the germ cells, egg and sperm, contains a large repertoire of immunoglobulin genes; thus, these theories invoked no special genetic mechanisms to account for antibody diversity. They argued that the immense survival value of the immune system justified the dedication of the requisite 15% of the genome to the coding of antibodies. In contrast, the **somatic-variation theories** maintained that the genome contains a small number of immunoglobulin genes, from which a large number of antibody specificities are generated in the somatic cells by mutation or recombination.

As the amino acid sequences of more and more immunoglobulins were determined, it became clear that there must be mechanisms not only for generating antibody diversity but also for maintaining constancy. Whether diversity was generated by germ-line or by somatic mechanisms, a paradox remained: How could stability be maintained in the constant (C) region while some kind of diversifying mechanism generated the variable (V) region?

Neither the germ-line nor the somatic variation proponents could offer a reasonable explanation of this central feature of immunoglobulin structure. Germ-line proponents found it difficult to account for an evolutionary mechanism that could generate diversity in the variable part of the many heavy and light chain genes while preserving the constant region of each unchanged. Somatic-variation proponents found it difficult to conceive of a mechanism that could diversify the variable region of a single heavy or light chain gene in the somatic cells without allowing alteration in the amino acid sequence encoded by the constant region.

A third structural feature requiring an explanation emerged when amino acid sequencing of the human myeloma protein called Til revealed that identical variable-region sequences were associated with both γ and μ heavy-chain constant regions. A similar phenomenon was observed in rabbits by C. Todd, who found that a particular allotypic marker in the heavy-chain variable region could be associated with α, γ, and μ heavy-chain constant regions. Considerable additional evidence has confirmed that a single variable-region sequence, defining a particular antigenic specificity, can be associated with multiple heavy-chain constant-region sequences; in other words, different classes, or isotypes, of antibody (e.g., IgG, IgM) can be expressed with identical variable-region sequences.

The Two-Gene Model of Dreyer and Bennett

In an attempt to develop a genetic model consistent with these findings about the structure of immunoglobulins, W. Dreyer and J. Bennett suggested, in their classic theoretical paper of 1965, that two separate genes encode a single immunoglobulin heavy or light chain, one gene for the V region (variable region) and the other for the C region (constant region). They suggested that these two genes must somehow come together at the DNA level to form a continuous message that can be transcribed and translated into a single Ig heavy or light chain. Moreover, they proposed that hundreds or thousands of V-region genes were carried in the germ line, whereas only single copies of C-region class and subclass genes need exist.

The strength of this type of recombinational model (which combined elements of the germ-line and somatic-variation theories) was that it could account for those immunoglobulins in which a single V region was combined with various C regions. By postulating a single constant-region gene for each immunoglobulin class and subclass, the model also could account for the conservation of necessary biological effector functions while allowing for evolutionary diversification of variable-region genes.

At first, support for the Dreyer and Bennett hypothesis was indirect. Early studies of DNA hybridization kinetics using a radioactive constant-region DNA probe indicated that the probe hybridized with only one or two genes, confirming the model's prediction that only one or two copies of each constant-region class and subclass gene existed. Not only was the evidence in support of the Dreyer and Bennett model initially indirect, there was stubborn resistance to their hypothesis in the scientific community. The suggestion that two genes encoded a single polypeptide contradicted the existing one gene–one polypeptide principle and was without precedent in any known biological system.

As so often is the case in science, theoretical and intellectual understanding of Ig-gene organization progressed ahead of the available methodology. Although the Dreyer and Bennett model provided a theoretical framework for reconciling the dilemma between Ig-sequence data and gene organization, actual validation of their hypothesis had to wait for several major technological advances in the field of molecular biology. In time, the Dreyer and Bennett hypothesis was proven to be essentially correct. Indeed, the genetic mechanisms that produce Ig have turned out to be far more complex than could have been imagined when Dreyer and Bennett published their paper.

Verification of the Dreyer and Bennett Hypothesis

In 1976, S. Tonegawa and N. Hozumi found the first direct evidence that separate genes encode the V and C regions of immunoglobulins and that the genes are rearranged in the course of B-cell differentiation. This work changed not only the field of immunology, but all of the biological sciences. In 1987, Tonegawa was awarded the Nobel Prize for this work.

Using various restriction endonucleases, Tonegawa and Hozumi cleaved DNA from embryonic cells and from adult myeloma cells into fragments. These fragments were separated by size and analyzed for their ability to hybridize with

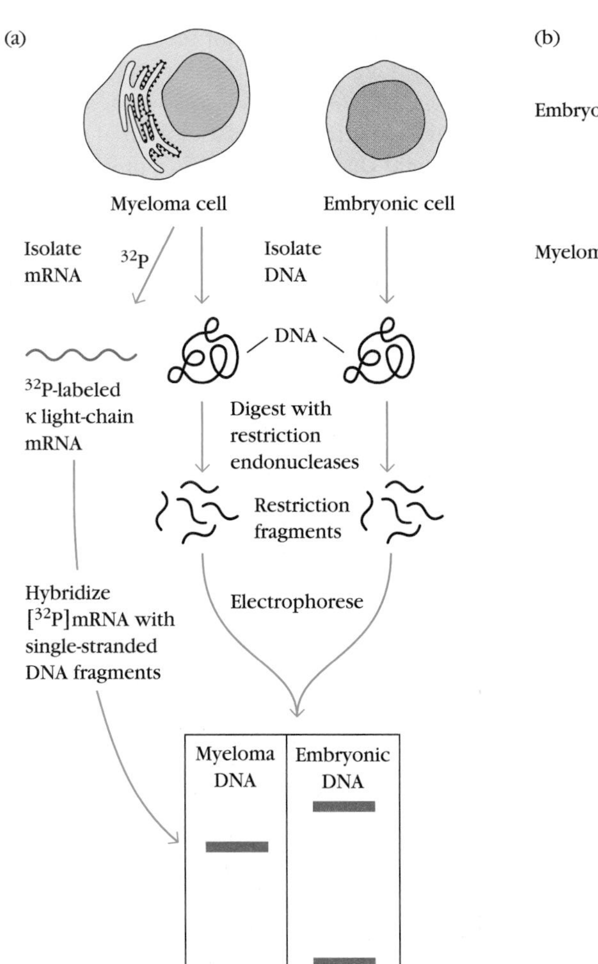

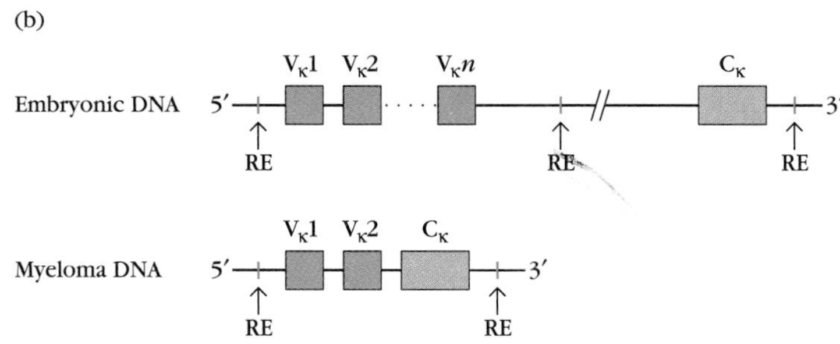

FIGURE 5-2 Experimental demonstration that genes encoding κ light chains are rearranged during B-cell development. (a) DNA from embryonic cells and myeloma cells (equivalent to differentiated plasma cells) was digested with several restriction endonucleases, and the digests were subjected to agarose gel electrophoresis. After the gels were cut into slices and eluted, the eluted samples were treated to denature the double-stranded DNA fragments into single-stranded DNA, and then incubated with ^{32}P-labeled mRNA encoding κ light chains. The mRNA probe hybridized with two bands from the germline embryonic DNA but with only a single band from the differentiated myeloma DNA. (b) Structure of embryonic and myeloma κ light-chain DNA compatible with the experimental results supports the Dreyer and Bennett two-gene model. During development of B cells, κ exons (V_κ and C_κ) are brought closer together and the restriction-endonuclease (RE) site between them is eliminated. [Adapted from N Hozumi and S Tonegawa, 1976, *Proc. Natl. Acad. Sci. USA* **73:**3628.]

a radiolabeled κ-chain mRNA probe. Two separate restriction fragments from the embryonic DNA hybridized with the mRNA, whereas only a single restriction fragment of the myeloma DNA hybridized with the same probe (Figure 5-2a). Tonegawa and Hozumi suggested that during differentiation of lymphocytes from the embryonic state to the fully differentiated plasma-cell stage (represented in their system by myeloma cells), the V and C genes undergo rearrangement. In the embryo, the V and C genes are separated by a large DNA segment that contains a restriction-endonuclease site; during differentiation, the V and C genes are brought closer together and the intervening DNA sequence is eliminated (Figure 5-2b).

Subsequently, researchers took an approach similar to that of Tonegawa and Hozumi but used the newly developed technique of Southern blotting, thus eliminating the need to elute the separated restriction DNA fragments from the gel slices before hybridization. Southern-blot analyses permitted comparisons of the light-chain and heavy-chain gene arrangement in non-B cells (e.g., embryonic cells and liver cells) with the arrangement in myeloma cells, which represent fully differentiated B cells. These results, analogous to those in Figure 5-2, demonstrated that the Dreyer and Bennett two-gene model—one gene encoding the variable region and one gene encoding the constant region—applied to both heavy- and light-chain genes.

Multigene Organization of Ig Genes

As cloning and sequencing of the light- and heavy-chain DNA was accomplished, even greater complexity was revealed than had been predicted by Dreyer and Bennett. The κ and λ light chains and the heavy chains are encoded by separate multigene families situated on different chromosomes (Table 5-1). In germ-line DNA, each of these multigene families contains several coding sequences, called **gene segments,** separated by noncoding regions. During B-cell maturation, these gene segments are rearranged and brought together to form functional immunoglobulin genes.

The κ and λ light-chain families contain **V, J,** and **C gene segments;** the rearranged VJ segments encode the variable

TABLE 5-1 CHROMOSOMAL LOCATIONS OF IMMUNOGLOBULIN GENES IN HUMAN AND MOUSE

	Chromosome	
Gene	Human	Mouse
λ Light chain	22	16
κ Light chain	2	6
Heavy chain	14	12

region of the light chains. The heavy-chain family contains **V, D, J,** and **C gene segments;** the rearranged VDJ gene segments encode the variable region of the heavy chain. In each gene family, C gene segments encode the constant regions. Each V gene segment is preceded at its 5′ end by a small exon that encodes a short **signal** or **leader (L) peptide** that guides the heavy or light chain through the endoplasmic reticulum. The signal peptide is cleaved from the nascent light and heavy chains before assembly of the finished immunoglobulin molecule. Thus, amino acids encoded by this leader sequence do not appear in the immunoglobulin molecule.

λ-Chain Multigene Family

The first evidence appeared that the light-chain variable region was actually encoded by two gene segments when Tonegawa cloned the germ-line DNA that encodes the variable region of mouse λ light chain and determined its complete nucleotide sequence. When the nucleotide sequence was compared with the known amino acid sequence of the λ-chain variable region, an unusual discrepancy was observed. Although the first 97 amino acids of the λ-chain variable region corresponded to the nucleotide codon sequence, the remaining 13 carboxyl-terminal amino acids of the protein's variable region did not correspond to the sequential nucleotide sequence. It turned out that many base pairs away a separate, 39-bp gene segment, called J for *joining,* encoded the remaining 13 amino acids of the λ-chain variable region. Thus, a functional λ variable-region gene contains two coding segments—a 5′ V segment and a 3′ J segment—which are separated by a noncoding DNA sequence in unrearranged germ-line DNA.

The λ multigene family in the mouse germ line contains two V_λ gene segments, four J_λ gene segments, and four C_λ gene segments (Figure 5-3a). The $J_\lambda 4$ and $C_\lambda 4$ gene segments are **pseudogenes,** defective genes that are incapable of encoding protein; these are indicated with the psi symbol (ψ). The V_λ and the three functional J_λ gene segments encode the

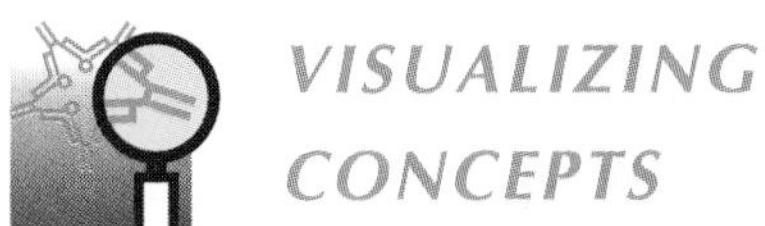

(a) λ-chain DNA

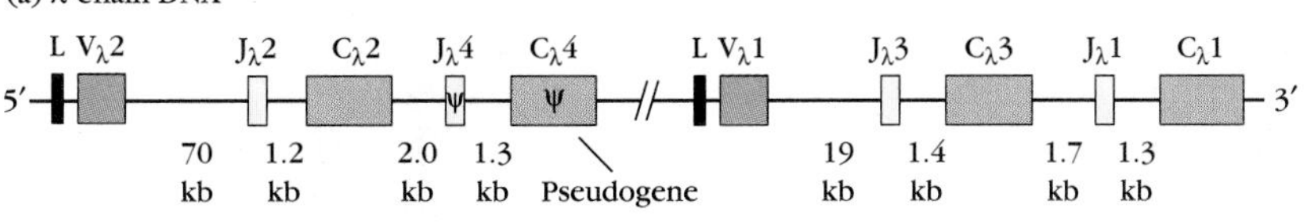

(b) κ-chain DNA

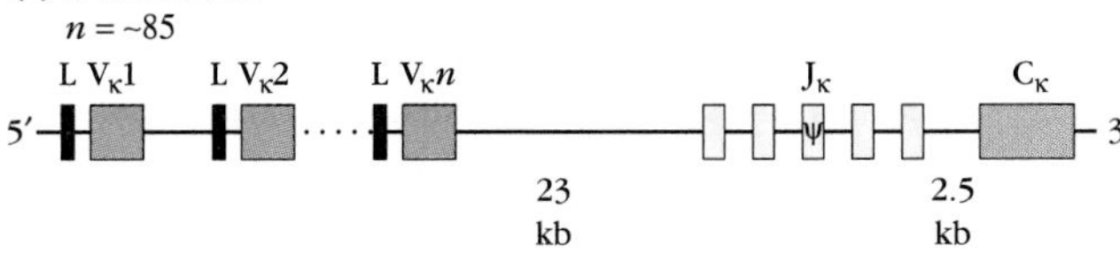

(c) Heavy-chain DNA

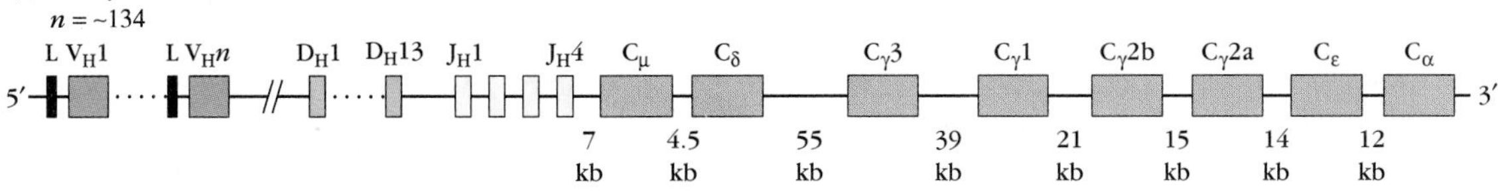

FIGURE 5-3 Organization of immunoglobulin germ-line gene segments in the mouse: (a) λ light chain, (b) κ light chain, and (c) heavy chain. The λ and κ light chains are encoded by V, J, and C gene segments. The heavy chain is encoded by V, D, J, and C gene segments. The distances in kilobases (kb) separating the various gene segments in mouse germ-line DNA are shown below each chain diagram.

variable region of the light chain, and each of the three functional C_λ gene segments encodes the constant region of one of the three λ-chain subtypes (λ1, λ2, and λ3). In humans, there are 30 V_λ gene segments, 4 J_λ segments, and 4 C_λ segments.

κ-Chain Multigene Family

The κ-chain multigene family in the mouse contains approximately 85 V_κ gene segments, each with an adjacent leader sequence a short distance upstream (i.e., on the 5′ side). There are five J_κ gene segments (one of which is a nonfunctional pseudogene) and a single C_κ gene segment (Figure 5-3b). As in the λ multigene family, the V_κ and J_κ gene segments encode the variable region of the κ light chain, and the C_κ gene segment encodes the constant region. Since there is only one C_κ gene segment, there are no subtypes of κ light chains. Comparison of parts *a* and *b* of Figure 5-3 shows that the arrangement of the gene segments is quite different in the κ and λ gene families. The κ-chain multigene family in humans, which is similar to that in the mouse, contains approximately 40 V_κ gene segments, 5 J_κ segments, and a single C_κ segment.

Heavy-Chain Multigene Family

The organization of the immunoglobulin heavy-chain genes is similar to, but more complex than, that of the κ and λ light-chain genes (Figure 5-3c). An additional gene segment encodes part of the heavy-chain variable region. The existence of this gene segment was first proposed by Leroy Hood and his colleagues, who compared the heavy-chain variable-region amino acid sequence with the V_H and J_H nucleotide sequences. The V_H gene segment was found to encode amino acids 1 to 94 and the J_H gene segment was found to encode amino acids 98 to 113; however, neither of these gene segments carried the information to encode amino acids 95 to 97. When the nucleotide sequence was determined for a rearranged myeloma DNA and compared with the germ-line DNA sequence, an additional nucleotide sequence was observed between the V_H and J_H gene segments. This nucleotide sequence corresponded to amino acids 95 to 97 of the heavy chain.

From these results, Hood proposed that a third germ-line gene segment must join with the V_H and J_H gene segments to encode the entire variable region of the heavy chain. This gene segment, which encoded amino acids within the third complementarity-determining region (CDR3), was designated D for *diversity*, because of its contribution to the generation of antibody diversity. Tonegawa and his colleagues located the D gene segments within mouse germ-line DNA with a cDNA D-region probe, which hybridized with a stretch of DNA lying between the V_H and J_H gene segments.

The heavy-chain multigene family on chromosome 14 in the human has been shown by direct sequencing of DNA to contain 51 V_H gene segments located upstream from a cluster of 27 functional D_H gene segments. As with the light-chain genes, each V_H gene segment has a leader sequence a short distance upstream from it. Downstream from the D_H gene segments are six functional J_H gene segments, followed by a series of C_H gene segments. Each C_H gene segment encodes the constant region of an immunoglobulin heavy-chain isotype. The C_H gene segments consist of coding exons and noncoding introns. Each exon encodes a separate domain of the heavy-chain constant region. A similar heavy-chain gene organization is found in the mouse.

The conservation of important biological effector functions of the antibody molecule is maintained by the limited number of heavy-chain constant-region genes. In humans and mice, the C_H gene segments are arranged sequentially in the order C_μ, C_δ, C_γ, C_ϵ, C_α (see Figure 5-3). This sequential arrangement is no accident; it is generally related to the sequential expression of the immunoglobulin classes in the course of B-cell development and the initial IgM response of a B-cell to its first encounter with an antigen.

Variable-Region Gene Rearrangements

The previous sections have shown that functional genes that encode immunoglobulin light and heavy chains are assembled by recombinational events at the DNA level. These events and those involving T receptor genes are the only known site-specific DNA rearrangements in vertebrates. Variable-region gene rearrangements occur in an ordered sequence during B-cell maturation in the bone marrow. The heavy-chain variable-region genes rearrange first, then the light-chain variable-region genes. At the end of this process, each B cell contains a single, functional variable-region DNA sequence for its heavy chain and a single, functional variable-region DNA sequence for its light chain.

This process of variable-region gene rearrangement produces mature, immunocompetent B cells; each such cell is committed to produce antibody with a binding site encoded by the particular sequence of its rearranged V genes. As described in detail later, it is for this reason that even though the rearrangement of heavy-chain constant-region genes generates further changes in the immunoglobulin class (isotype) expressed by a B cell, it does so without changing the cell's antigenic specificity. Although the steps in variable-region gene rearrangement occur in an ordered sequence, they are random events that result in the random determination of B-cell specificity. The order, mechanism, and consequences of these rearrangements are described in this section.

V-J Rearrangements in Light-Chain DNA

Expression of both κ and λ light chains requires rearrangement of the variable-region V and J gene segments. In the

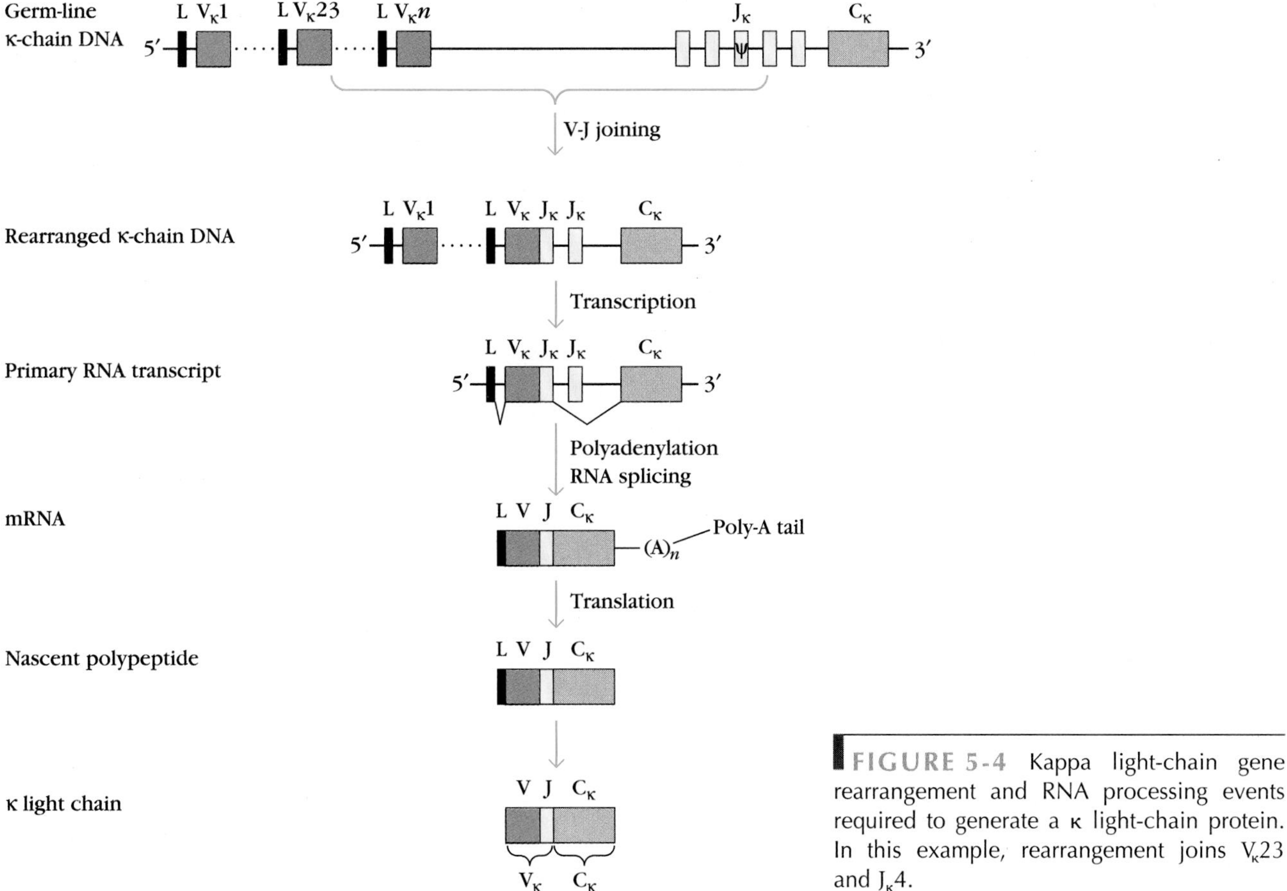

FIGURE 5-4 Kappa light-chain gene rearrangement and RNA processing events required to generate a κ light-chain protein. In this example, rearrangement joins $V_\kappa 23$ and $J_\kappa 4$.

human, any of the functional V_λ genes can combine with any of the four functional J_λ-C_λ combinations. In the mouse, things are slightly more complicated. DNA rearrangement can join the $V_\lambda 1$ gene segment with either the $J_\lambda 1$ or the $J_\lambda 3$ gene segment, or the $V_\lambda 2$ gene segment can be joined with the $J_\lambda 2$ gene segment. In human or mouse κ light-chain DNA, any one of the V_κ gene segments can be joined with any one of the functional J_κ gene segments.

Rearranged κ and λ genes contain the following regions in order from the 5′ to 3′ end: a short leader (L) exon, a noncoding sequence (intron), a joined VJ gene segment, a second intron, and the constant region. Upstream from each leader gene segment is a promoter sequence. The rearranged light-chain sequence is transcribed by RNA polymerase from the L exon through the C segment to the stop signal, generating a light-chain primary RNA transcript (Figure 5-4). The introns in the primary transcript are removed by RNA-processing enzymes, and the resulting light-chain messenger RNA then exits from the nucleus. The light-chain mRNA binds to ribosomes and is translated into the light-chain protein. The leader sequence at the amino terminus pulls the growing polypeptide chain into the lumen of the rough endoplasmic reticulum and is then cleaved, so it is not present in the finished light-chain protein product.

V-D-J Rearrangements in Heavy-Chain DNA

Generation of a functional immunoglobulin heavy-chain gene requires two separate rearrangement events within the variable region. As illustrated in Figure 5-5, a D_H gene segment first joins to a J_H segment; the resulting D_HJ_H segment then moves next to and joins a V_H segment to generate a $V_HD_HJ_H$ unit that encodes the entire variable region. In heavy-chain DNA, variable-region rearrangement produces a rearranged gene consisting of the following sequences, starting from the 5′ end: a short L exon, an intron, a joined VDJ segment, another intron, and a series of C gene segments. As with the light-chain genes, a promoter sequence is located a short distance upstream from each heavy-chain leader sequence.

Once heavy-chain gene rearrangement is accomplished, RNA polymerase can bind to the promoter sequence and transcribe the entire heavy-chain gene, including the introns. Initially, both C_μ and C_δ gene segments are transcribed. Differential polyadenylation and RNA splicing remove the introns and process the primary transcript to generate mRNA including either the C_μ or the C_δ transcript. These two mRNAs then are translated, and the leader peptide of the

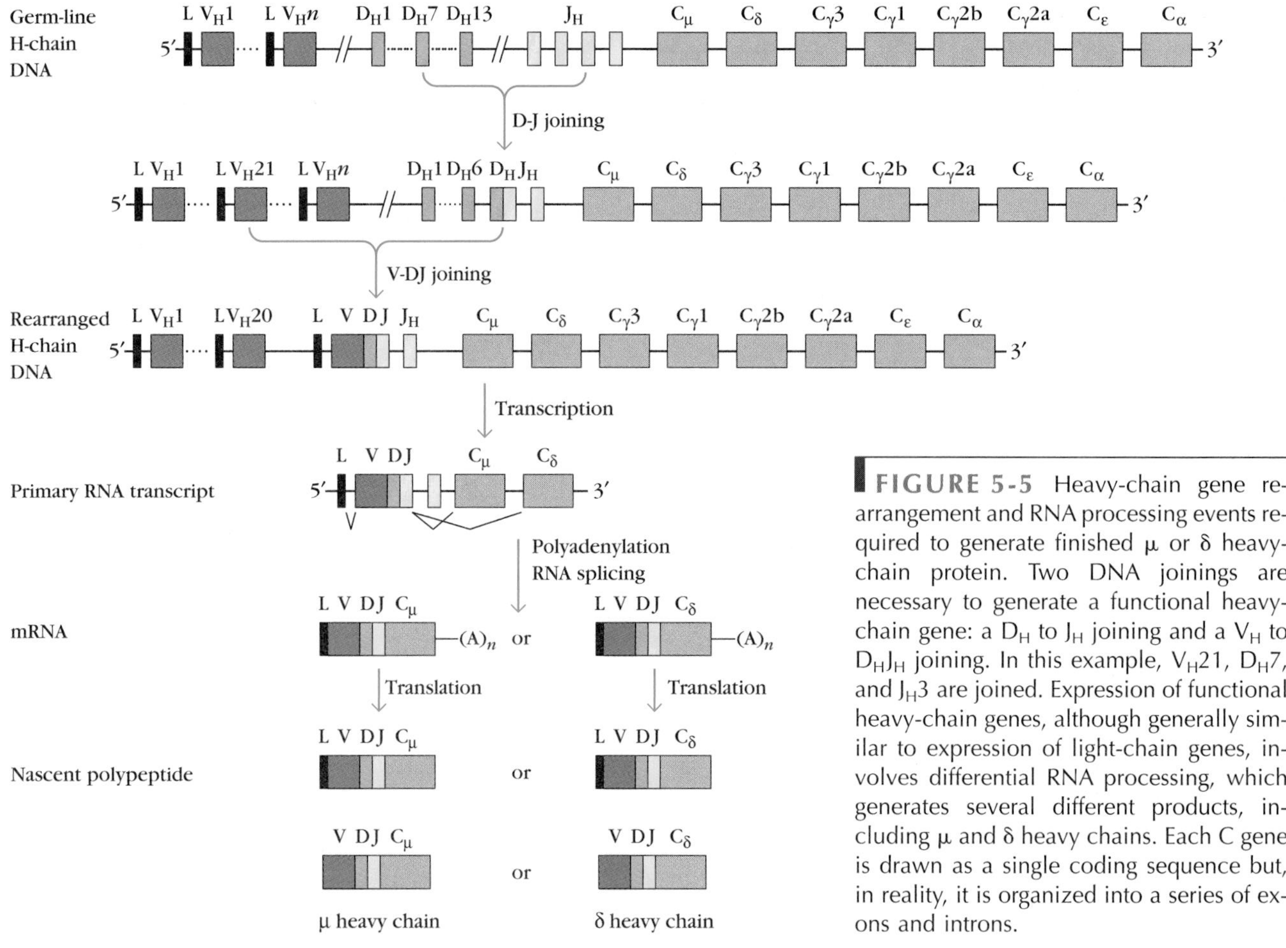

FIGURE 5-5 Heavy-chain gene rearrangement and RNA processing events required to generate finished μ or δ heavy-chain protein. Two DNA joinings are necessary to generate a functional heavy-chain gene: a D_H to J_H joining and a V_H to D_HJ_H joining. In this example, V_H21, D_H7, and J_H3 are joined. Expression of functional heavy-chain genes, although generally similar to expression of light-chain genes, involves differential RNA processing, which generates several different products, including μ and δ heavy chains. Each C gene is drawn as a single coding sequence but, in reality, it is organized into a series of exons and introns.

resulting nascent polypeptide is cleaved, generating finished μ and δ chains. Since two different heavy-chain mRNAs are produced by heavy-chain variable-region gene rearrangement, a mature, immunocompetent B cell expresses both IgM and IgD with identical antigenic specificity on its surface.

Mechanism of Variable-Region DNA Rearrangements

Now that we've seen the results of variable-region gene rearrangements, let's examine in detail how this process occurs during maturation of B cells.

Recombination Signal Sequences

Discovery of two closely related conserved sequences in variable-region germ-line DNA paved the way to fuller understanding of the mechanism of gene rearrangements. DNA sequencing studies revealed the presence of unique **recombination signal sequences (RSSs)** flanking each germ-line V, D, and J gene segment. One RSS is located 3′ to each V gene segment, 5′ to each J gene segment, and on both sides of each D gene segment. These sequences function as signals for the recombination process that rearranges the genes. Each RSS contains a conserved palindromic heptamer and a conserved AT-rich nonamer sequence separated by an intervening sequence of 12 or 23 base pairs (Figure 5-6a). Leroy Hood observed that the intervening 12- and 23-bp sequences correspond, respectively, to one and two turns of the DNA helix; for this reason the sequences are called **one-turn recombination signal sequences** and **two-turn signal sequences.**

The V_κ signal sequence has a one-turn spacer, and the J_κ signal sequence has a two-turn spacer. In λ light-chain DNA, this order is reversed; that is, the V_λ signal sequence has a two-turn spacer, and the J_λ signal sequence has a one-turn spacer. In heavy-chain DNA, the signal sequences of the V_H and J_H gene segments have two-turn spacers, the signals on either side of the D_H gene segment have one-turn spacers (Figure 5-6b). Signal sequences having a one-turn spacer can join only with sequences having a two-turn, spacer (the so-called one-turn/two-turn joining rule). This

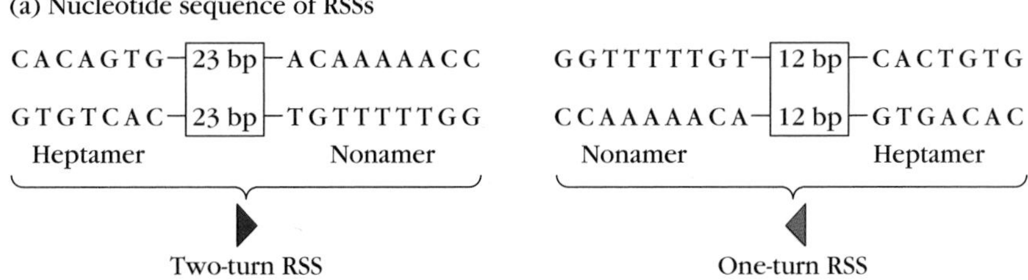

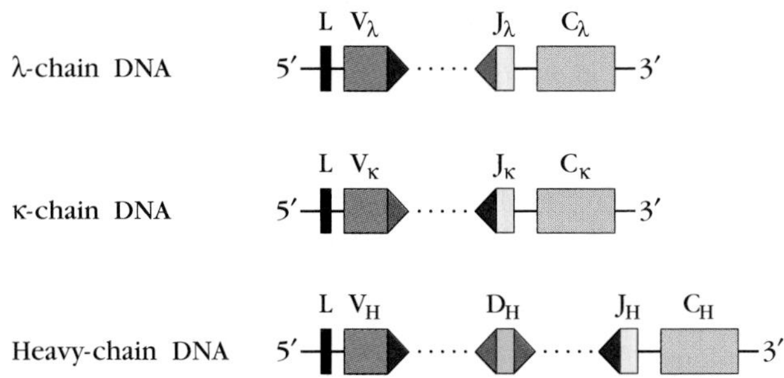

FIGURE 5-6 Two conserved sequences in light-chain and heavy-chain DNA function as recombination signal sequences (RSSs). (a) Both signal sequences consist of a conserved palindromic heptamer and conserved AT-rich nonamer; these are separated by nonconserved spacers of 12 or 23 base pairs. (b) The two types of RSS—designated one-turn RSS and two-turn RSS—have characteristic locations within λ-chain, κ-chain, and heavy-chain germ-line DNA. During DNA rearrangement, gene segments adjacent to the one-turn RSS can join only with segments adjacent to the two-turn RSS.

joining rule ensures, for example, that a V_L segment joins only to a J_L segment and not to another V_L segment; the rule likewise ensures that V_H, D_H, and J_H segments join in proper order and that segments of the same type do not join each other.

Enzymatic Joining of Gene Segments

V-(D)-J recombination, which takes place at the junctions between RSSs and coding sequences, is catalyzed by enzymes collectively called **V(D)J recombinase.**

Identification of the enzymes that catalyze recombination of V, D, and J gene segments began in the late 1980s and is still ongoing. In 1990 David Schatz, Marjorie Oettinger, and David Baltimore first reported identification of two **recombination-activating genes,** designated ***RAG-1*** and ***RAG-2,*** whose encoded proteins act synergistically to mediate V-(D)-J joining. The RAG-1 and RAG-2 proteins and the enzyme **terminal deoxynucleotidyl transferase (TdT)** are the only lymphoid-specific gene products that are required for V-(D)-J rearrangement.

Current evidence suggests that recombination of variable-region gene segments is a multistep process catalyzed by a system of recombinase enzymes (Figure 5-7):

- Recognition of recombination signal sequences (RSSs) by recombinase enzymes, followed by synapsis in which two signal sequences and the adjacent coding sequences (gene segments) are brought into proximity
- Cleavage of one strand of DNA by RAG-1 and RAG-2 at the junctures of the signal sequences and coding sequences
- A reaction catalyzed by RAG-1 and RAG-2 in which the free 3′-OH group on the cut DNA strand attacks the phosphodiester bond linking the opposite strand to the signal sequence, simultaneously producing a hairpin structure at the cut end of the coding sequence and a flush, 5′-phosphorylated, double-strand break at the signal sequence
- Cutting of the hairpin to generate sites for the addition of **P-region nucleotides,** followed by the trimming of a few nucleotides from the coding sequence by a single-strand endonuclease
- Optional addition of up to 15 nucleotides, called **N-region nucleotides,** at the cut ends of the V, D, and J coding sequences of the heavy chain by an enzyme called terminal deoxynucleotidyl transferase (TdT)
- Repair and ligation to join the coding sequences and to join the signal sequences, catalyzed by normal double-strand break repair (DSBR) enzymes

Recombination results in the formation of a **coding joint,** between the coding sequences, and a **signal joint,** between the RSSs. The transcriptional orientation of the gene segments to be joined determines the fate of the signal joint and intervening DNA. When the two gene segments are in the same transcriptional orientation, joining results in deletion of the signal joint and intervening DNA as a circular excision product (Figure 5-8). Less frequently, the two gene segments have opposite orientations. In this case joining occurs by inversion of the DNA, resulting in the retention of both the coding joint and the signal joint (and intervening DNA) on the chromosome. In the human κ locus, about half of the

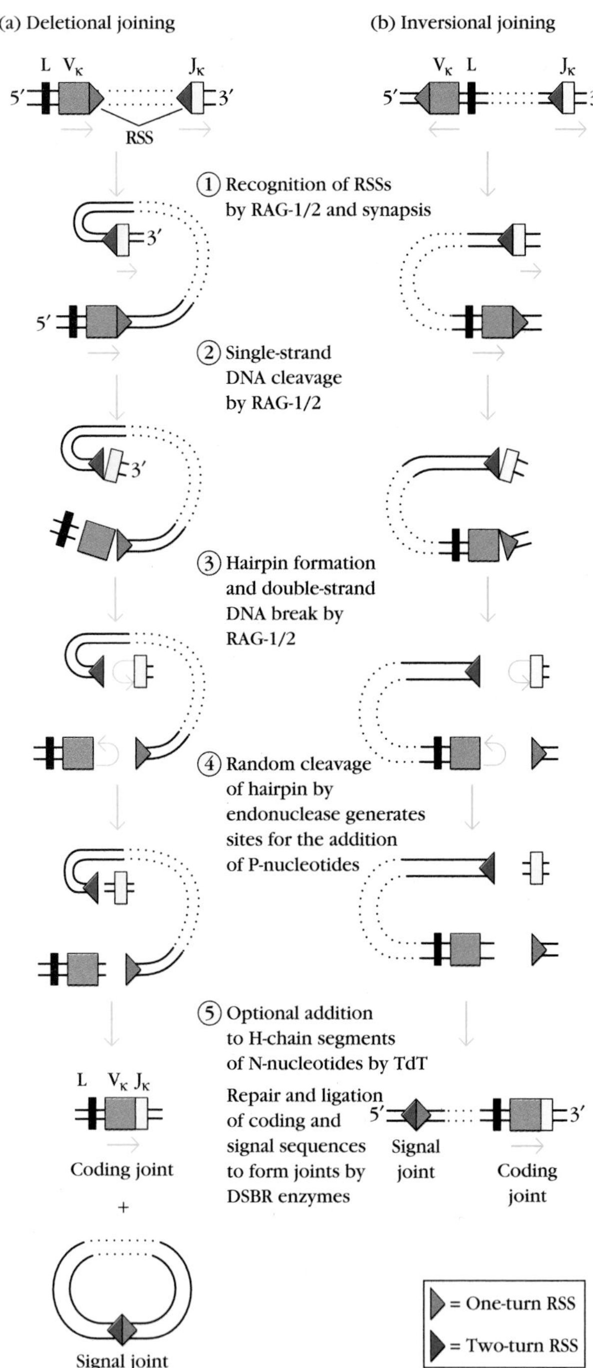

FIGURE 5-7 Model depicting the general process of recombination of immunoglobulin gene segments is illustrated with V_κ and J_κ. (a) Deletional joining occurs when the gene segments to be joined have the same transcriptional orientation (indicated by horizontal blue arrows). This process yields two products: a rearranged VJ unit that includes the coding joint and a circular excision product consisting of the recombination signal sequences (RSSs), signal joint, and intervening DNA. (b) Inversional joining occurs when the gene segments have opposite transcriptional orientations. In this case, the RSSs, signal joint, and intervening DNA are retained, and the orientation of one of the joined segments is inverted. In both types of recombination, a few nucleotides may be deleted from or added to the cut ends of the coding sequences before they are rejoined.

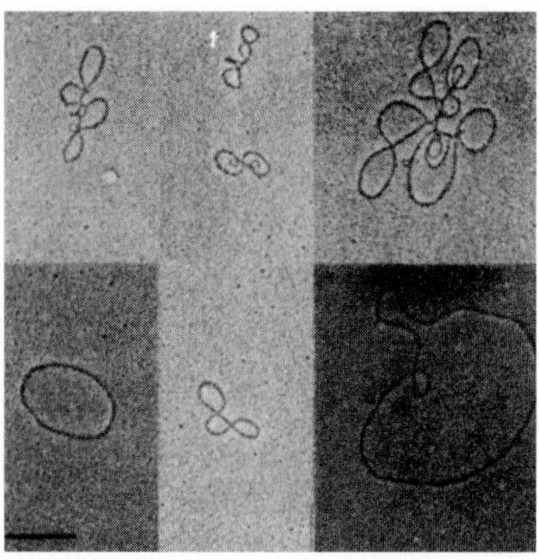

FIGURE 5-8 Circular DNA isolated from thymocytes in which the DNA encoding the chains of the T-cell receptor (TCR) undergoes rearrangement in a process like that involving the immunoglobulin genes. Isolation of this circular excision product is direct evidence for the mechanism of deletional joining shown in Figure 5-7. [From K Okazki et al, 1987, *Cell* **49**:477.]

V_κ gene segments are inverted with respect to J_κ and their joining is thus by inversion.

One of the striking features of gene-segment recombination is the diversity of the coding joints that are formed between any two gene segments. This junctional diversity at the V-J and V-D-J coding joints is generated by a number of mechanisms: variation in cutting of the hairpin to generate P-nucleotides, variation in trimming of the coding sequences, variation in N-nucleotide addition, and flexibility in joining the coding sequences. As will be explained, this variation contributes greatly to the diversity of the CDR3 region of the antigen-binding site.

Experimental Identification of RAG-1 and RAG-2 Genes

When Schatz, Oettinger, and Baltimore set out to identify the *RAG-1* and *RAG-2* genes, they first had to develop an assay system for demonstrating recombination between immunoglobulin gene segments. Their novel approach employed a retroviral construct containing a promoter sequence, V and J gene segments with flanking signal sequences, and a gene that confers resistance to mycophenolic acid (Figure 5-9). The genes were arranged in an unusual way so that the promoter was oriented in the opposite transcriptional orientation from that of the gene for mycophenolic acid resistance. If the V and J gene segments were rearranged by inversional joining, then the orientation of the gene for mycophenolic acid resistance would also be inverted, placing the gene in the correct 5′ to 3′ orientation to be transcribed from the promoter. Cells transfected with this construct thus would acquire resistance to mycophenolic acid if they could rearrange the V and J gene segments, whereas transfected cells that could not rearrange the V and J gene segments would not be resistant to mycophenolic acid.

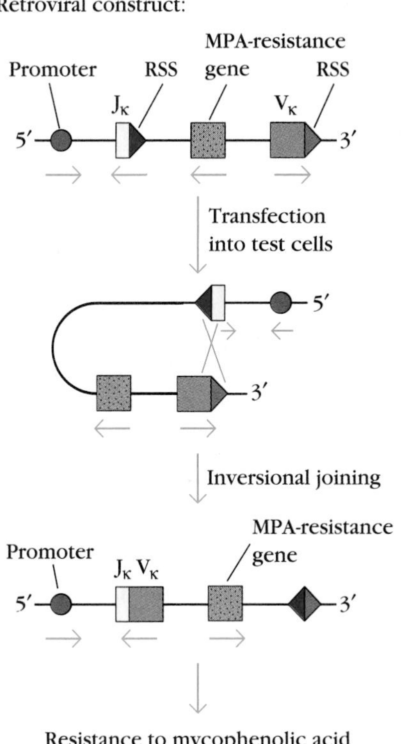

FIGURE 5-9 Assay system for demonstrating recombination of immunoglobulin gene segments. If the test cells possess all the enzymes required for inversional joining, then the transfected cells will be resistant to mycophenolic acid (MPA), as shown. If the test cells lack one or more of these enzymes, the MPA-resistance gene will not be expressed because its transcriptional orientation (horizontal blue arrows) will remain opposite to that of the promoter.

When a variety of cell types were tested in this system, only pre-B cells and pre-T cells were able to rearrange the V and J gene segments. (As is described in Chapter 9, the pre-T cell employs the same recombinase enzymes and signal sequences in rearranging the genes for the T-cell receptor, which is why it also proved to be positive in this assay.) Mature B and T cells were unable to rearrange the retroviral construct, indicating that the recombinase activity is limited to an early stage in the maturation of both B and T cells.

Once these researchers established that the retroviral construct could be rearranged in pre-B cells, they then set out to isolate the recombinase genes. First fibroblasts were transfected with the retroviral construct. Since fibroblasts do not express the recombinase genes, the transfected cells could not rearrange the construct. Assuming that the recombinase genes were located on a single locus, the researchers then transfected genomic DNA from pre-B cells into fibroblasts containing the retroviral construct. The presence of activated recombinase genes in the transfected genomic DNA could be detected by the rearrangement of the retroviral construct, which conferred resistance to mycophenolic acid upon the transfected fibroblasts. With this experimental system, the researchers identified *RAG-1* and *RAG-2*, two closely linked genes, both of which were needed to mediate recombination of the retroviral construct at a high frequency. *RAG-1* and *RAG-2* mRNA was shown to be present in pre-B cells and pre-T cells but absent in mature B and T cell stages.

Defects in Ig-Gene Rearrangements

Several strains of mice with defects in various recombination genes have been developed and are proving valuable in unraveling the various steps in the recombination process. For example, knockout mice lacking either *RAG-1* or *RAG-2* are unable to initiate the recombination process because they cannot introduce double-strand DNA breaks between the recombination signal sequences (RSSs) and coding sequences in germ-line immunoglobulin DNA (Figure 5-10). As a

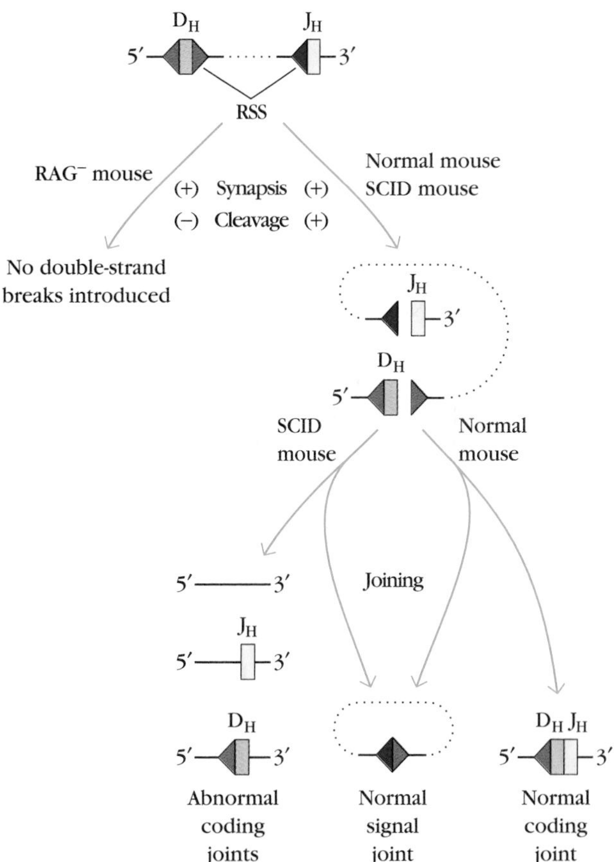

FIGURE 5-10 Recombination defects have been identified in RAG-deficient mice and SCID mice. Mice that lack a functional *RAG-1* or *RAG-2* cannot even start the recombination process. In contrast, SCID mice can carry out synapsis between D_H and J_H gene segments, introduce double-strand breaks to produce normal recombination intermediates, and form a normal signal joint. However, SCID mice cannot properly join the coding sequences. Both types of defective mice lack mature B and T cells and thus exhibit a severe combined immunodeficiency. [Adapted from FW Alt et al, 1992, *Immunol. Today* **13**:306.]

result of this defect, the V, D, and J gene segments remain unrearranged. Since both B and T cells utilize the same recombination machinery, the RAG-1$^-$ and RAG-2$^-$ knockout mice lack mature T and B cells and consequently exhibit a severe combined immunodeficiency (SCID). In humans, mutations in the *RAG* genes, located on chromosome 11, have been linked to several different cases of autosomal SCIDs (see Chapter 19).

Another recombination defect is found in CB-17 SCID mice. These mice have an autosomal recessive mutation that impairs the V-(D)-J recombination process. SCID mice have a general absence of mature functional T and B cells and, like RAG$^-$ mice, manifest a severe combined immunodeficiency. Unlike the *RAG* mutants, SCID mice begin the recombination process normally: synapsis occurs between the D and J gene segments; double-strand DNA breaks are properly introduced at the juncture of the recombination signal sequences and coding sequences; and the signal sequences are then rejoined. Joining of the coding sequences, however, occurs some distance from the D and J gene segments, resulting in deletion of one or both of the coding sequences (see Figure 5-10). These SCID mice have functional RAG-1 and RAG-2 enzymes; their defect is instead in one or more double-strand break repair (DSBR) enzymes that rejoin the cut DNA.

Productive and Nonproductive Rearrangements

Although the double-strand DNA breaks that initiate V-(D)-J rearrangements are introduced precisely at the junctions of signal sequences and coding sequences, the subsequent joining of the coding sequences is imprecise. This imprecision in the joining process helps generate antibody diversity by contributing to the hypervariability of the antigen-binding site. (This phenomenon is covered in more detail in the section on generation of antibody diversity below.)

Another consequence of imprecise joining is that gene segments may be joined out of phase, so that the triplet reading frame for translation is not preserved. In such a **nonproductive rearrangement,** the resulting VJ or VDJ unit will

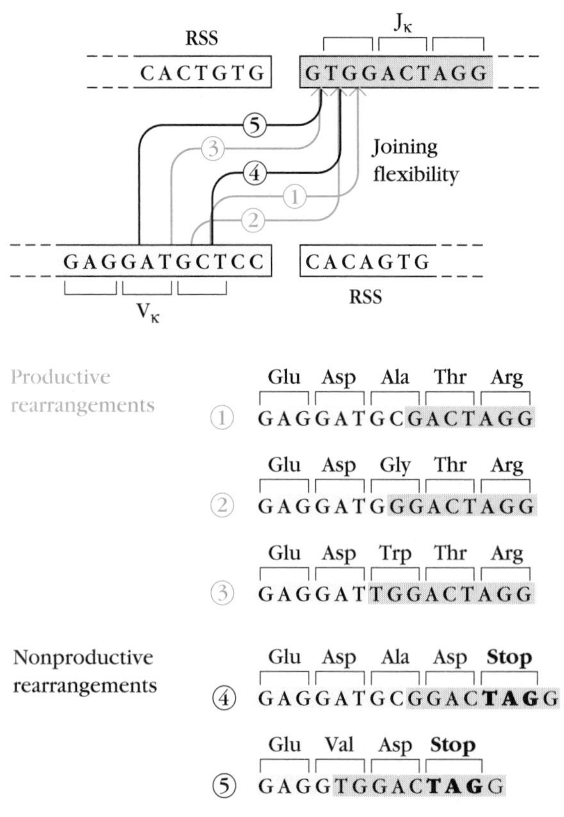

FIGURE 5-11 Junctional flexibility in the joining of immunoglobulin gene segments is illustrated with V_κ and J_κ. In-phase joining (arrows 1, 2, and 3) generates a productive rearrangement, which can be translated into protein. Out-of-phase joining (arrows 4 and 5) leads to a nonproductive rearrangement, which contains stop codons and is not translated into protein.

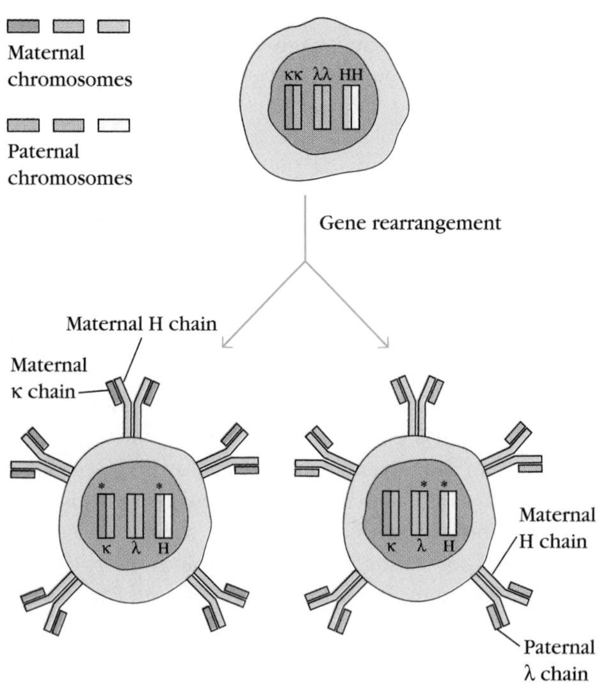

FIGURE 5-12 Because of allelic exclusion, the immunoglobulin heavy- and light-chain genes of only one parental chromosome are expressed per cell. This process ensures that a single B cell will be specific for a given epitope. The selection of which allele of each pair is rearranged to produce a functional gene is random. Thus the expressed immunoglobulin may contain one maternal and one paternal chain or both chains may derive from only one parent. Only B cells and T cells exhibit allelic exclusion. Asterisks (*) indicate the expressed alleles.

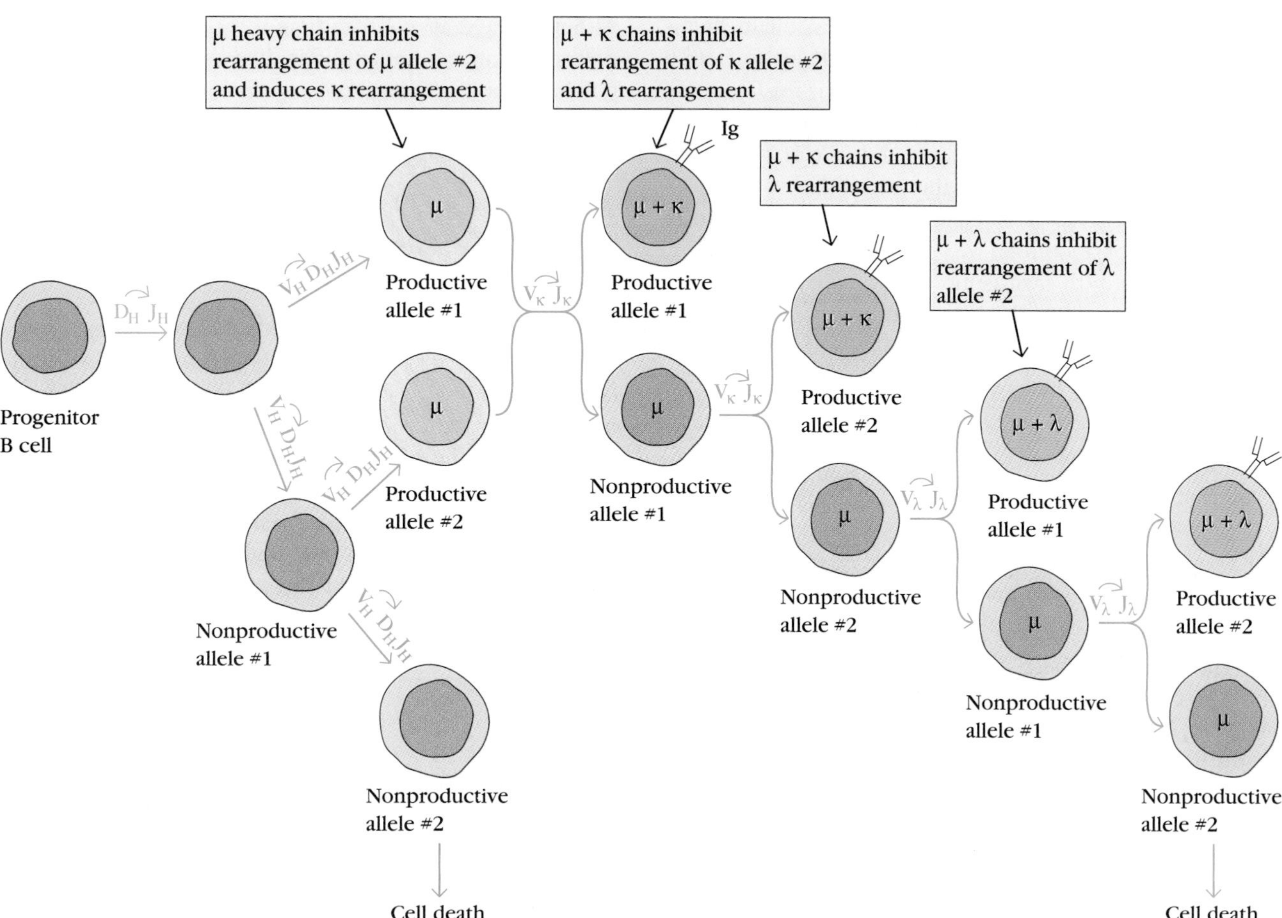

FIGURE 5-13 Model to account for allelic exclusion. Heavy-chain genes rearrange first, and once a productive heavy-chain gene rearrangement occurs, the μ protein product prevents rearrangement of the other heavy-chain allele and initiates light-chain gene rearrangement. In the mouse, rearrangement of κ light-chain genes precedes rearrangement of the λ genes, as shown here. In humans, however, either κ or λ rearrangement can proceed once a productive heavy-chain rearrangement has occurred. Formation of a complete immunoglobulin inhibits further light-chain gene rearrangement. If a nonproductive rearrangement occurs for one allele, then the cell attempts rearrangement of the other allele. [Adapted from GD Yancopoulos and FW Alt, 1986, *Annu. Rev. Immunol.* **4**:339.]

contain numerous stop codons, which interrupt translation (Figure 5-11). When gene segments are joined in phase, the reading frame is maintained. In such a **productive rearrangement,** the resulting VJ or VDJ unit can be translated in its entirety, yielding a complete antibody.

If one allele rearranges nonproductively, a B cell may still be able to rearrange the other allele productively. If an in-phase rearranged heavy-chain and light-chain gene are not produced, the B cell dies by apoptosis. It is estimated that only one in three attempts at V_L-J_L, D_H-J_H, and V_H-D_HJ_H joining are productive. As a result, only about 8% of the pre-B cells in the bone marrow progress to maturity and leave the bone marrow as mature, immunocompetent B cells.

Allelic Exclusion

B cells, like all somatic cells, are diploid and contain both maternal and paternal chromosomes. Even though a B cell is diploid, it expresses the rearranged heavy-chain genes from only one chromosome and the rearranged light-chain genes from only one chromosome. This process, called **allelic exclusion,** ensures that functional B cells never contain more than one $V_HD_HJ_H$ and one V_LJ_L unit (Figure 5-12). This is, of course, essential for the antigenic specificity of the B cell, because the expression of both alleles would render the B cell multispecific. The phenomenon of allelic exclusion suggests that once a productive V_H-D_H-J_H rearrangement and a productive V_L-J_L rearrangement have occurred, the recombination machinery is turned off, so that the heavy- and light-chain genes on the homologous chromosomes are not expressed.

G. D. Yancopoulos and F. W. Alt have proposed a model to account for allelic exclusion (Figure 5-13). They suggest that once a productive rearrangement is attained, its encoded protein is expressed and the presence of this protein acts as a signal to prevent further gene rearrangement. According to their model, the presence of μ heavy chains signals the maturing B cell to turn off rearrangement of the other heavy-chain allele and to turn on rearrangement of the κ light-chain genes. If a productive κ rearrangement occurs, κ light chains are produced and then pair with μ heavy chains to form a complete antibody molecule. The presence of this antibody then turns off further light-chain rearrangement. If κ rearrangement is nonproductive for both κ alleles, rearrangement of the λ-chain genes begins. If neither λ allele rearranges productively, the B cell presumably ceases to mature and soon dies by apoptosis.

Two studies with transgenic mice have supported the hypothesis that the protein products encoded by rearranged heavy- and light-chain genes regulate rearrangement of the remaining alleles. In one study, transgenic mice carrying a rearranged μ heavy-chain transgene were prepared. The μ transgene product was expressed by a large percentage of the B cells, and rearrangement of the endogenous immunoglobulin heavy-chain genes was blocked. Similarly, cells from a transgenic mouse carrying a κ light-chain transgene did not rearrange the endogenous κ-chain genes when the κ transgene was expressed and was associated with a heavy chain to form complete immunoglobulin. These studies suggest that expression of the heavy- and light-chain proteins may indeed prevent gene rearrangement of the remaining alleles and thus account for allelic exclusion.

Generation of Antibody Diversity

As the organization of the immunoglobulin genes was deciphered, the sources of the vast diversity in the variable region began to clarify. The germ-line theory, mentioned earlier, argued that the entire variable-region repertoire is encoded in the germ line of the organism and is transmitted from parent to offspring through the germ cells (egg and sperm). The somatic-variation theory held that the germ line contains a limited number of variable genes, which are diversified in the somatic cells by mutational or recombinational events during development of the immune system. With the cloning and sequencing of the immunoglobulin genes, both models were partly vindicated.

To date, seven means of antibody diversification have been identified in mice and humans:

- Multiple germ-line gene segments
- Combinatorial V-(D)-J joining
- Junctional flexibility
- P-region nucleotide addition (P-addition)
- N-region nucleotide addition (N-addition)
- Somatic hypermutation
- Combinatorial association of light and heavy chains

Although the exact contribution of each of these avenues of diversification to total antibody diversity is not known, the potential number of antibodies of distinct sequences that the mammalian immune system is capable of generating is extremely high and exceeds 10^{10}.

Multiple Germ-Line V, D, and J Gene Segments

As indicated earlier, human germ-line DNA contains 51 V_H, 27 D, 6 J_H, 40 V_κ, 5 J_κ, 30 V_λ, and 4 J_λ gene segments. It should be borne in mind that these numbers were derived in a landmark study by sequencing the DNA of the immunoglobulin loci of a single individual, David Perry. The immunoglobulin loci of other individuals might contain slightly different numbers of particular types of gene segments.

In the mouse, although the numbers are known with less precision than in the human, there appear to be about 85 V_κ gene segments and 134 V_H gene segments, 4 functional J_H, 4 functional J_κ, 3 functional J_λ, and an estimated 13 D_H gene segments, but only two V_λ gene segments. Although the number of germ-line genes found in either humans or mice is far fewer than predicted by early proponents of the germ-line model, multiple germ-line V, D, and J gene segments clearly do contribute to diversity of the antigen-binding sites in antibodies.

Combinatorial V-J and V-D-J Joining

The contribution of multiple germ-line gene segments to antibody diversity is magnified by the random rearrangement of these segments in somatic cells. This combinatorial diversity generated by the gene rearrangements can be calculated (Table 5-2). In humans, the ability of any of the 51 V_H gene segments to combine with any of the 27 D_H segments and any of the 6 J_H segments allows a considerable amount of heavy-chain gene diversity to be generated ($51 \times 27 \times 6 = 8262$ possible combinations). Similarly, 40 V_κ gene segments randomly combining with 5 J_κ segments has the potential of generating 200 possible combinations at the κ locus, while 30 V_λ and 4 J_λ gene segments allow up to 120 possible combinations at the human λ locus. It is important to realize that these are minimal calculations of diversity. Junctional flexibility and P- and N-nucleotide addition, as mentioned above, and, especially, somatic hypermutation, which will be described shortly, together make an enormous contribution to antibody diversity. Although it is not possible to make an exact calculation of their contribution, most workers in this field agree that they raise the potential for antibody combining-site diversity in humans to well over 10^{10} or even 10^{11}. This does not mean that, at any given time, a single individual has a repertoire of 10^{10} different antibody combining sites. These very large numbers describe the set of possible variations, of which any individual carries a much smaller subset.

TABLE 5-2 COMBINATORIAL ANTIBODY DIVERSITY IN HUMANS AND MICE

Multiple germ-line segments	Heavy chain	Light chains κ	Light chains λ
	Estimated number of segments in humans*		
V	51	40	30
D	27	0	0
J	6	5	4
Combinatorial V-D-J and V-J joining (possible number of combinations)	$51 \times 27 \times 6 = 8262$	$40 \times 5 = 200$	$30 \times 4 = 120$
Possible combinatorial associations of heavy and light chains†	$8262 \times (200 + 120) = 2.64 \times 10^6$		
	Estimated number of segments in mice*		
V	134	85	2
D	13	0	0
J	4	4	3
Combinatorial V-D-J and V-J joining (possible number of combinations)	$134 \times 13 \times 4 = 6968$	$85 \times 4 = 340$	$2 \times 3 = 6$
Possible combinatorial associations of heavy and light chains†	$6968 \times (340 + 6) = 2.41 \times 10^6$		

*These numbers have been determined from studies of single subjects; slight differences may be seen among different individuals. Also, in the human case, only the functional gene segments have been listed. The genome contains additional segments that are incapable of rearrangement or contain stop codons or both. In the mouse case, the figures contained in the table are only best estimates, because the locus has not been completely sequenced.

†Because of the diversity contributed by junctional flexibility, P-region nucleotide addition, N-region nucleotide addition, and somatic mutation, the actual potential exceeds these estimates by several orders of magnitude.

Junctional Flexibility

The enormous diversity generated by means of V, D, and J combinations is further augmented by a phenomenon called **junctional flexibility.** As described above, recombination involves both the joining of recombination signal sequences to form a signal joint and the joining of coding sequences to form a coding joint (see Figure 5-7). Although the signal sequences are always joined precisely, joining of the coding sequences often is imprecise. In one study, for example, joining of the $V_\kappa 21$ and $J_\kappa 1$ coding sequences was analyzed in several pre-B cell lines. Sequence analysis of the signal and coding joints revealed precise joining of the signal sequences but flexible joining of the coding sequences (Figure 5-14).

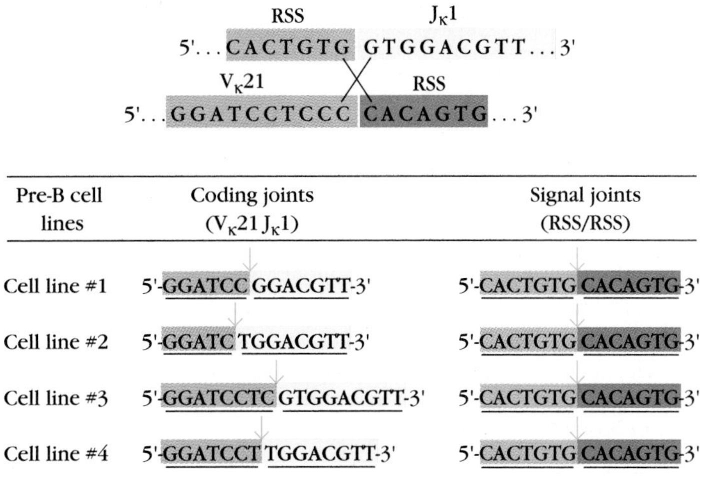

RSS $J_\kappa 1$
5'...CACTGTG GTGGACGTT...3'
$V_\kappa 21$ RSS
5'...GGATCCTCCC CACAGTG...3'

Pre-B cell lines	Coding joints ($V_\kappa 21 J_\kappa 1$)	Signal joints (RSS/RSS)
Cell line #1	5'-GGATCC GGACGTT-3'	5'-CACTGTG CACAGTG-3'
Cell line #2	5'-GGATC TGGACGTT-3'	5'-CACTGTG CACAGTG-3'
Cell line #3	5'-GGATCCTC GTGGACGTT-3'	5'-CACTGTG CACAGTG-3'
Cell line #4	5'-GGATCCT TGGACGTT-3'	5'-CACTGTG CACAGTG-3'

FIGURE 5-14 Experimental evidence for junctional flexibility in immunoglobulin-gene rearrangement. The nucleotide sequences flanking the coding joints between $V_\kappa 21$ and $J_\kappa 1$ and of the corresponding signal joints were determined in four pre-B cell lines. The sequence constancy in the signal joints contrasts with the sequence variability in the coding joints. Pink and yellow shading indicate nucleotides derived from $V_\kappa 21$ and $J_\kappa 1$, respectively, and purple and orange shading indicate nucleotides from the two RSSs.

TABLE 5-3 SOURCES OF SEQUENCE VARIATION IN COMPLEMENTARITY-DETERMINING REGIONS OF IMMUNOGLOBULIN HEAVY- AND LIGHT-CHAIN GENES

Source of variation	CDR1	CDR2	CDR3
Sequence encoded by:	V segment	V segment	V_L-J_L junction; V_H-D_H-J_H junctions
Junctional flexibility	–	–	+
P-nucleotide addition	–	–	+
N-nucleotide addition*	–	–	+
Somatic hypermutation	+	+	+

*N-nucleotide addition occurs only in heavy-chain DNA.

As illustrated previously, this junctional flexibility leads to many nonproductive rearrangements, but it also generates several productive combinations that encode alternative amino acids at each coding joint (see Figure 5-11), thereby increasing antibody diversity. The amino acid sequence variation generated by junctional flexibility in the coding joints has been shown to fall within the third hypervariable region (CDR3) in immunoglobulin heavy-chain and light-chain DNA (Table 5-3). Since CDR3 makes a major contribution to antigen binding by the antibody molecule, amino acid changes generated by junctional flexibility can make a major contribution to antibody diversity.

P-Addition

As described earlier, after the initial single-strand DNA cleavage at the junction of a variable-region gene segment and attached signal sequence, the nucleotides at the end of the coding sequence turn back to form a hairpin structure (see Figure 5-7). This hairpin is later cleaved by an endonuclease. This second cleavage sometimes occurs at a position that leaves a short single strand at the end of the coding sequence. Subsequent addition **(P-addition)** of complementary nucleotides to this strand by repair enzymes generates a palindromic sequence in the coding joint, and so these nucleotides are called **P-nucleotides** (Figure 5-15a). Variation in the position at which the hairpin is cut thus leads to variation in the sequence of the coding joint.

N-Addition

Variable-region coding joints in rearranged heavy-chain genes have been shown to contain short amino acid sequences that are not encoded by the germ-line V, D, or J gene segments. These amino acids are encoded by nucleotides **(N-nucleotides)** that are added during the D-J and V to

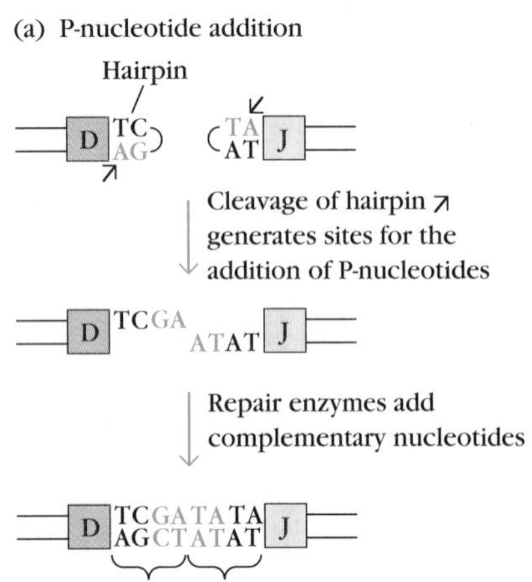

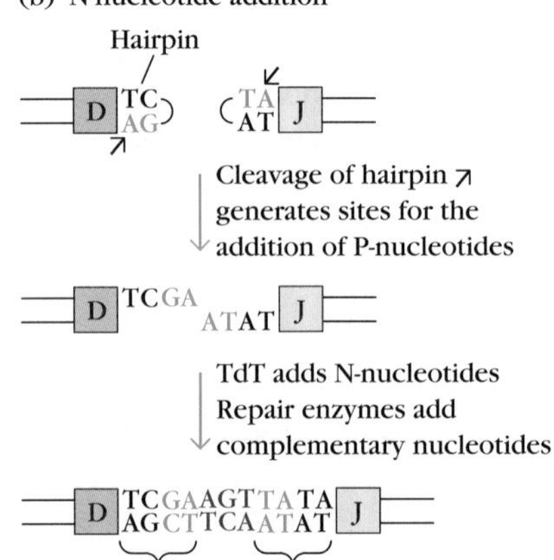

FIGURE 5-15 P-nucleotide and N-nucleotide addition during joining. (a) If cleavage of the hairpin intermediate yields a double-stranded end on the coding sequence, then P-nucleotide addition does not occur. In many cases, however, cleavage yields a single-stranded end. During subsequent repair, complementary nucleotides are added, called P-nucleotides, to produce palindromic sequences (indicated by brackets). In this example, an extra four base pairs (blue) are present in the coding joint as the result of P-nucleotide addition. (b) Besides P-nucleotide addition, addition of random N-nucleotides (light red) by TdT can occur during joining of heavy-chain coding sequences.

D-J joining process by a terminal deoxynucleotidyl transferase (TdT) catalyzed reaction (Figure 5-15b). Evidence that TdT is responsible for N-nucleotide addition has come from transfection studies in fibroblasts. When fibroblasts were transfected with the *RAG-1* and *RAG-2* genes, V-D-J rearrangement occurred but no N-nucleotides were present in the coding joints. However, when the fibroblasts were also transfected with the gene encoding TdT, then V-D-J rearrangement was accompanied by addition of N-nucleotides at the coding joints.

Up to 15 N-nucleotides can be added to both the D_H-J_H and V_H-D_HJ_H joints. Thus, a complete heavy-chain variable region is encoded by a $V_HND_HNJ_H$ unit. The additional heavy-chain diversity generated by N-region nucleotide addition is quite large because N regions appear to consist of wholly random sequences. Since this diversity occurs at V-D-J coding joints, it is localized in the CDR3 of the heavy-chain genes.

Somatic Hypermutation

All the antibody diversity discussed so far stems from mechanisms that operate during formation of specific variable regions by gene rearrangement. The implicit assumption throughout this chapter has been that once a functional variable-region gene unit is formed, it is not altered. This assumption turns out to be false, and additional antibody diversity is generated in rearranged variable-region gene units by a process called **somatic hypermutation.** As a result of somatic hypermutation, individual nucleotides in VJ or VDJ units are replaced with alternatives, thus potentially altering the specificity of the encoded immunoglobulins.

Normally, somatic hypermutation occurs only within germinal centers (see Chapters 2 and 11), structures that form in secondary lymphoid organs within a week or so of immunization with an antigen that activates a T-cell-dependent B-cell response. Somatic hypermutation is targeted to rearranged V-regions located within a DNA sequence containing about 1500 nucleotides, which includes the whole of the VJ or VDJ segment. Somatic hypermutation occurs at a frequency approaching 10^{-3} per base pair per generation. This rate is at least a hundred thousand-fold higher (hence the name *hypermutation*) than the spontaneous mutation rate, about 10^{-8}/bp/generation, in other genes. Since the combined length of the H-chain and L-chain variable-region genes is about 600 bp, then an average of one mutation will be introduced by somatic hypermutation in every one or two cell divisions.

The mechanism of somatic hypermutation has not yet been determined. Most of the mutations are nucleotide substitutions rather than deletions or insertions. Somatic hypermutation introduces these substitutions in a largely, but not completely, random fashion. Recent evidence suggests that certain nucleotide motifs and palindromic sequences within V_H and V_L may be especially susceptible to somatic hypermutation.

Because the process of somatic hypermutation is largely random, it will generate antibodies with varying affinity for antigen. Following exposure to antigen, those B cells with higher-affinity receptors will be preferentially selected for survival because of their greater ability to bind to the antigen. This process, called **affinity maturation,** takes place within germinal centers, and is described more fully in Chapter 11. Although somatic hypermutations occur throughout the VJ or VDJ segment, in mature B cells they are clustered within the CDRs of the V_H and V_L sequences. This clustering reflects the role of antigen in selecting B cells with higher-affinity receptors during affinity maturation. Because the CDRs are directly involved in antigen recognition, mutation within the CDRs is more likely to influence the overall affinity for antigen.

Claudia Berek and Cesar Milstein obtained experimental evidence demonstrating somatic hypermutation during the course of an immune response to a hapten-carrier conjugate. These researchers were able to sequence the mRNA encoding antihapten antibodies produced in response to primary, secondary, or tertiary immunization with a hapten-carrier conjugate. The hapten that they chose was 2-phenyl-5-oxazolone (phOx), coupled to a protein carrier. They chose this hapten because it had previously been shown that the majority of antibodies it induced were encoded by a single germ-line V_H and V_κ gene segment (i.e., antibodies against a single epitope). Berek and Milstein immunized mice with the phOx-carrier conjugate and then used the mouse spleen cells to prepare hybridomas secreting monoclonal antibodies specific for the phOx hapten. The mRNA sequence for the H chain and κ light chain of each hybridoma was then determined to identify deviations from the germ-line sequences.

The results of this experiment are depicted in Figure 5-16. Of the 12 hybridomas obtained from mice seven days after a primary immunization, all used the V_H Ox-1 gene segment and all but one used the V_κ Ox-1 gene segment. Moreover, only a few mutations from the germ-line sequence were present in these hybridomas. By day 14 after primary immunization, analysis of eight hybridomas revealed that six continued to use the germ-line V_H Ox-1 gene segment and all continued to use the V_κ Ox-1 gene segment. Now, however, all of these hybridomas included one or more mutations from the germ-line sequence. Hybridomas analyzed from the secondary and tertiary responses showed a larger percentage utilizing germ-line V_H gene segments other than the V_H Ox-1 gene. In those hybridoma clones that utilized the V_H Ox-1 and V_κ Ox-1 gene segments, most of the mutations were clustered in the CDR1 and CDR2 hypervariable regions. The number of mutations in the anti-phOx hybridomas progressively increased following primary, secondary, and tertiary immunizations, as did the overall affinity of the antibodies for phOx (see Figure 5-16).

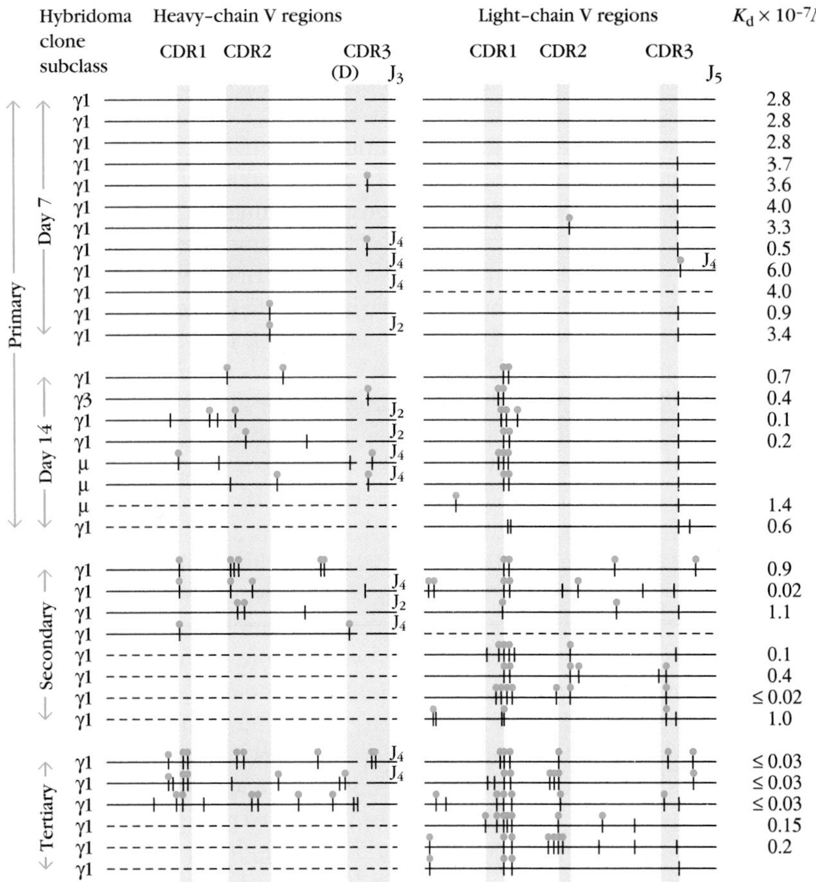

FIGURE 5-16 Experimental evidence for somatic mutation in variable regions of immunoglobulin genes. The diagram compares the mRNA sequences of heavy chains and of light chains from hybridomas specific for the phOx hapten. The horizontal solid lines represent the germ-line V_H and V_κ Ox-1 sequences; dashed lines represent sequences derived from other germ-line genes. Blue shading shows the areas where mutations clustered; the blue circles with vertical lines indicate locations of mutations that encode a different amino acid than the germ-line sequence. These data show that the frequency of mutation (1) increases in the course of the primary response (day 7 vs. day 14) and (2) is higher after secondary and tertiary immunizations than after primary immunization. Moreover, the dissociation constant (K_D) of the anti-phOx antibodies decreases in going from the primary to tertiary response, indicating an increase in the overall affinity of the antibody. Note also that most of the mutations are clustered within CDR1 and CDR2 of both the heavy and the light chains. [Adapted from C Berek and C Milstein, 1987, *Immunol. Rev.* **96**:23.]

Association of Heavy and Light Chains

The final source of antibody diversity is the combinatorial association of heavy and light chains. Because the specificity of an antibody's antigen-binding site is determined by the variable regions in both its heavy and light chains, combinational association of H and L chains also can generate diversity. In humans, there is the potential to generate 8262 heavy-chain genes and 320 light-chain genes as a result of variable-region gene rearrangements. Assuming that any one of the possible heavy-chain and light-chain genes can occur randomly in the same cell, the potential number of heavy- and light-chain combinations is 2,644,240. This number is probably higher than the amount of combinatorial diversity actually generated in an individual, because it is not likely that all V_H and V_L will pair with each other. Furthermore, the recombination process is not completely random; not all V_H, D, or V_L gene segments are used at the same frequency. Some are used often, others only occassionally, and still others almost not at all.

Although the number of different antibody combining sites the immune system can generate may be difficult to calculate with any degree of precision, we know that it is quite high. Because the very large number of new sequences created by junctional flexibility, P-nucleotide addition, and N-nucleotide addition are within the third CDR, they are positioned to influence the structure of the antibody binding site. In addition to these sources of antibody diversity, the phenomenon of somatic hypermutation contributes enormously to the repertoire after antigen stimulation. Taken together with the combinatorial processes mentioned above, these processes push estimates of potential antibody diversity well above 10^{11}.

Class Switching Among Constant-Region Genes

After antigenic stimulation of a B cell, the heavy-chain DNA can undergo a further rearrangement in which the $V_HD_HJ_H$ unit can combine with any C_H gene segment. The exact mechanism of this process, called **class (isotype) switching,** is unclear, but evidence suggests that DNA flanking sequences (called **switch regions**) located 2–3 kb upstream from each C_H segment (except C_δ) are involved. These switch regions, though rather large, are composed of multiple copies of short sequences. One hypothesis is that a series of class-specific recombinase proteins bind to these switch regions and facilitate DNA recombination. The particular immunoglobulin class that is expressed thus may depend on the specificity of the recombinase protein expressed at a given stage of a cell's development.

Various cytokines secreted by activated T_H cells have been shown to induce B cells to class-switch to a particular isotype. Interleukin 4 (IL-4), for example, induces class switching from C_μ to $C_\gamma1$ or C_ϵ. IL-4 induces class switching in a successive manner: first from C_μ to $C_\gamma1$ and then from $C_\gamma1$ to C_ϵ (Figure 5-17). By identifying the circular DNA excision products produced during class switching, the class switch from C_μ to $C_\gamma1$ was shown to generate a circular excision product containing C_μ together with the 5′ end of the γ1 switch region ($S_\gamma1$) and the 3′ end of the μ switch region (S_μ). The switch from $C_\gamma1$ to C_ϵ was shown to generate circular excision products containing $C_\gamma1$ together with portions of the μ, γ, and ϵ switch regions. The role of cytokines in immunoglobulin class switching is described more fully in Chapter 11.

Expression of Ig Genes

As in the expression of other genes, post-transcriptional processing of immunoglobulin primary transcripts is required to produce functional mRNAs (see Figures 5-4 and 5-5). The primary transcripts produced from rearranged heavy-chain and light-chain genes contain intervening DNA sequences, which include noncoding introns and J gene segments not lost during V-(D)-J rearrangement. In addition, as noted earlier, the heavy-chain C-gene segments are organized as a series of coding exons and noncoding introns. Each exon of a C_H gene segment corresponds to a constant-region domain or a hinge region of the heavy-chain polypeptide. The primary transcript must be processed to remove the intervening DNA sequences, and their flanking exons connected, by a process called RNA splicing. Short, moderately conserved splice sequences, or splice sites, which are located at the intron-exon boundaries within a primary transcript, signal

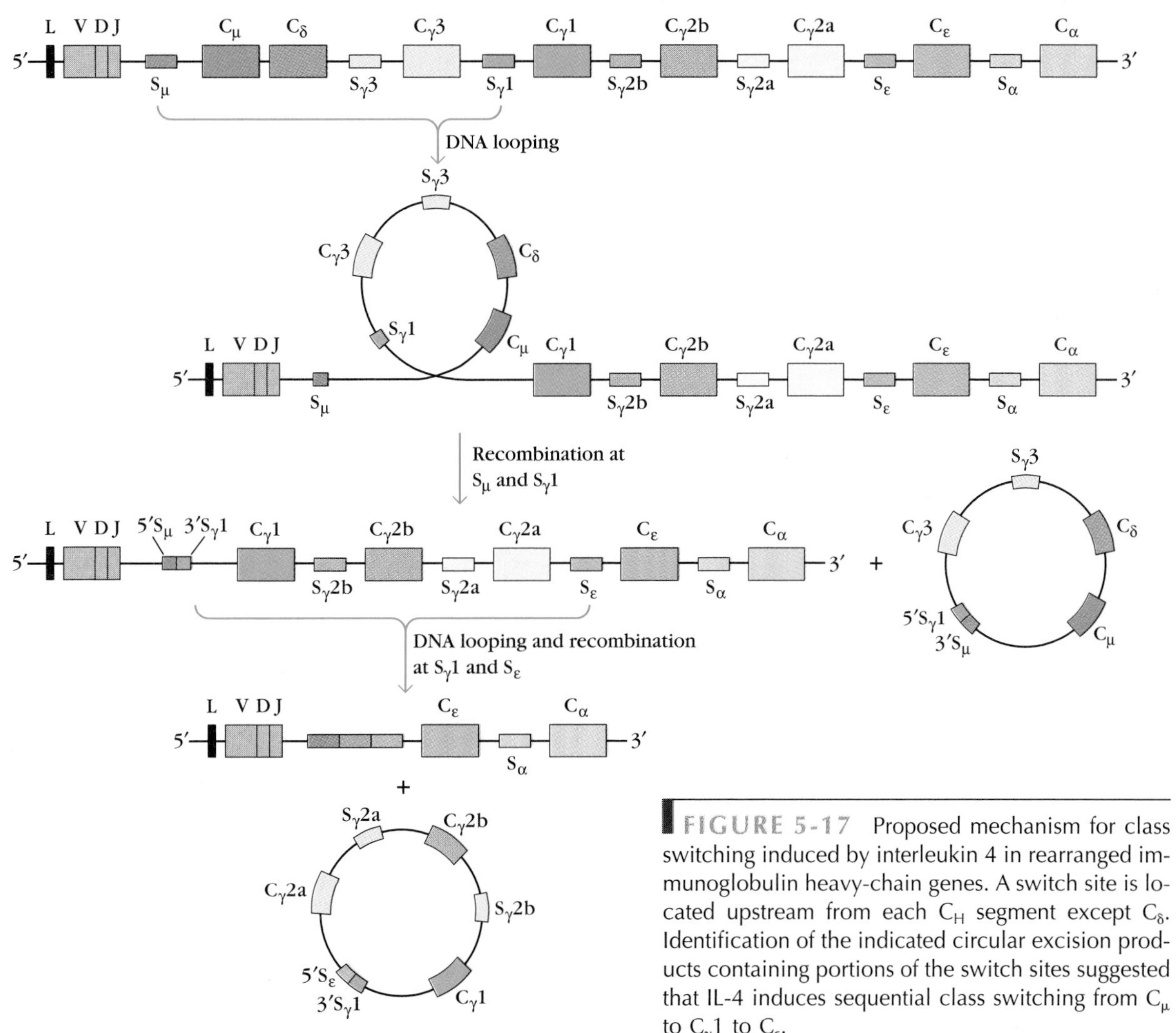

FIGURE 5-17 Proposed mechanism for class switching induced by interleukin 4 in rearranged immunoglobulin heavy-chain genes. A switch site is located upstream from each C_H segment except C_δ. Identification of the indicated circular excision products containing portions of the switch sites suggested that IL-4 induces sequential class switching from C_μ to $C_\gamma1$ to C_ϵ.

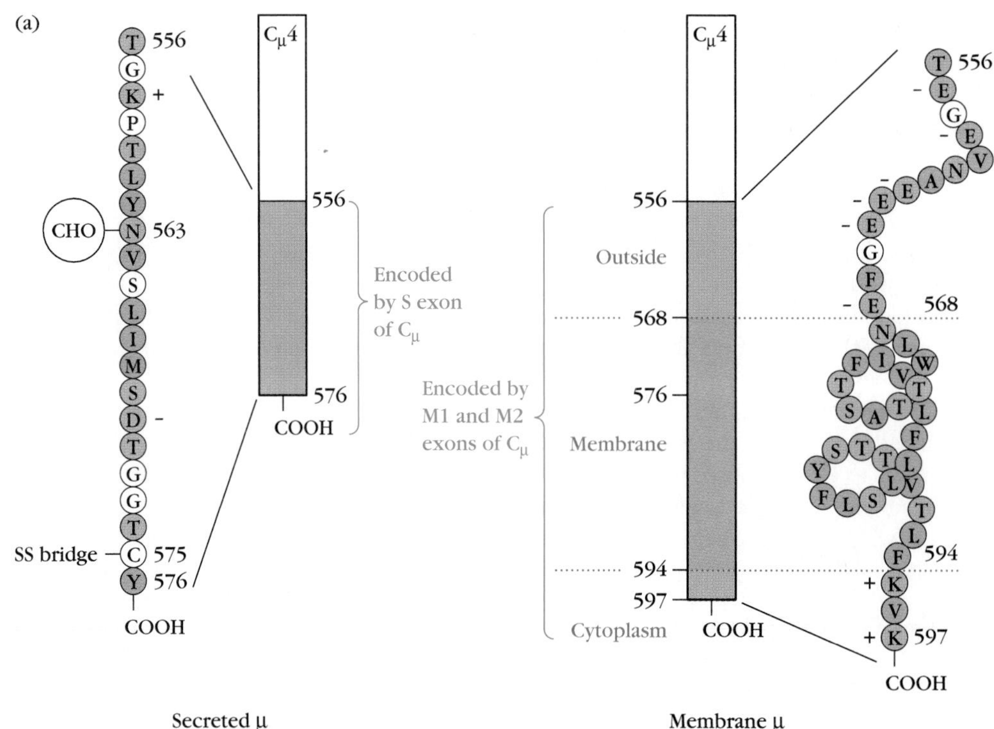

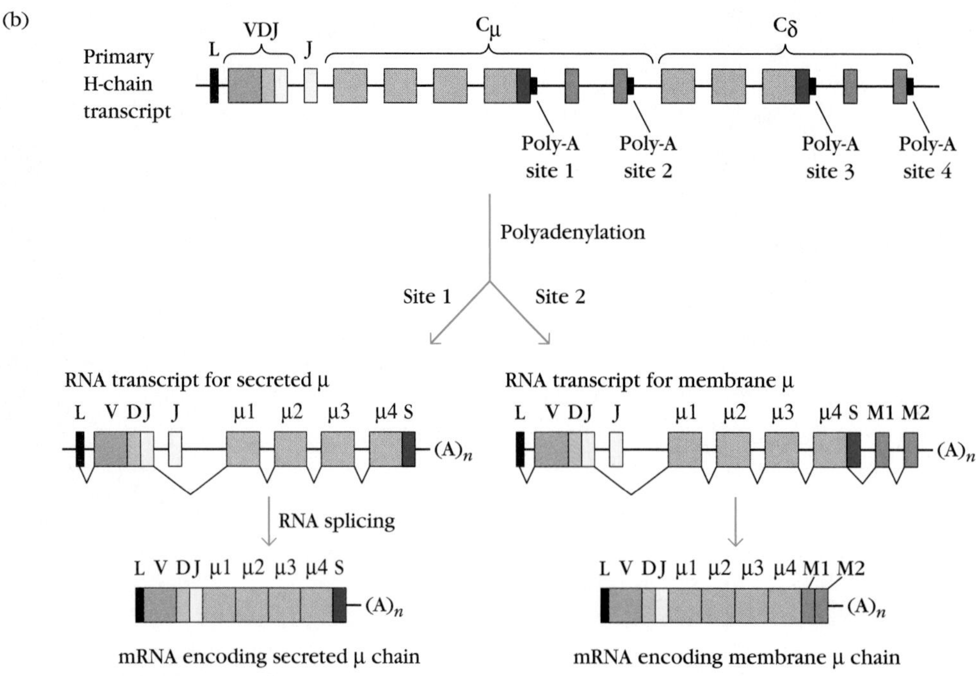

FIGURE 5-18 Expression of secreted and membrane forms of the heavy chain by alternative RNA processing. (a) Amino acid sequence of the carboxyl-terminal end of secreted and membrane μ heavy chains. Residues are indicated by the single-letter amino acid code. Hydrophilic residues and regions are shaded purple; hydrophobic residues and regions are shaded orange. Charged amino acids are indicated with a + or −. The rest of the sequence is identical in both forms. (b) Structure of the primary transcript of a rearranged heavy-chain gene showing the C_μ exons and poly-A sites. Polyadenylation of the primary transcript at either site 1 or site 2 and subsequent splicing (indicated by V-shaped lines) generates mRNAs encoding either secreted or membrane μ chains.

the positions at which splicing occurs. Processing of the primary transcript in the nucleus removes each of these intervening sequences to yield the final mRNA product. The mRNA is then exported from the nucleus and goes to polyribosomes for translation into complete H or L chains.

Differential RNA Processing of Heavy-Chain Primary Transcripts

Processing of an immunoglobulin heavy-chain primary transcript can yield different mRNAs. Such differential RNA processing of heavy-chain transcripts explains the production of secreted or membrane-bound forms of a particular immunoglobulin and the simultaneous expression of IgM and IgD by a single B cell.

Expression of Membrane or Secreted Immunoglobulin

As explained in Chapter 4, a particular immunoglobulin can exist in a membrane-bound form or in a secreted form. The two forms differ in the amino acid sequence of the heavy-chain carboxyl-terminal domains (C_H3/C_H3 in IgA, IgD, and IgG and C_H4/C_H4 in IgE and IgM). The secreted form has a hydrophilic sequence of about 20 amino acids in the carboxyl-terminal domain; this is replaced in the membrane-bound form with a sequence of about 40 amino acids containing a hydrophilic segment that is outside the cell, a hydrophobic transmembrane segment, and a short hydrophilic cytoplasmic segment at the carboxyl terminus (Figure 5-18a). For some time, the existence of these two forms seemed inconsistent with the structure of germ-line heavy-chain DNA, which had been shown to contain a single C_H gene segment corresponding to each class and subclass.

The explanation of this apparent paradox came from DNA sequencing of the C_μ gene segment, which consists of four exons ($C_\mu 1$, $C_\mu 2$, $C_\mu 3$, and $C_\mu 4$) corresponding to the four domains of the IgM molecule. The $C_\mu 4$ exon contains a nucleotide sequence (S) at its 3′ end that encodes the hydrophilic sequence in the C_H4 domain of secreted IgM. Two additional exons called M1 and M2 are located just 1.8 kb downstream from the 3′ end of the $C_\mu 4$ exon. The M1 exon encodes the transmembrane segment, and M2 encodes the cytoplasmic segment of the C_H4 domain in membrane-bound IgM. Later DNA sequencing revealed that all the C_H gene segments have two additional downstream M1 and M2 exons that encode the transmembrane and cytoplasmic segments.

The primary transcript produced by transcription of a rearranged μ heavy-chain gene contains two polyadenylation signal sequences, or poly-A sites. Site 1 is located at the 3′ end of the $C_\mu 4$ exon, and site 2 is at the 3′ end of the M2 exon (Figure 5-18b). If cleavage of the primary transcript and addition of the poly-A tail occurs at site 1, the M1 and M2 exons are lost. Excision of the introns and splicing of the remaining exons then produces mRNA encoding the secreted form of the heavy chain. If cleavage and polyadenylation of the primary transcript occurs instead at site 2, then a different pattern of splicing results. In this case, splicing removes the S sequence at the 3′ end of the $C_\mu 4$ exon, which encodes the hydrophilic carboxyl-terminal end of the secreted form, and joins the remainder of the $C_\mu 4$ exon with the M1 and M2 exons, producing mRNA for the membrane form of the heavy chain.

Production of the secreted or membrane form of an immunoglobulin thus depends on differential processing of a common primary transcript. As noted previously, mature naive B cells produce only membrane-bound antibody, whereas differentiated plasma cells produce secreted antibodies. Presumably, some mechanism exists in naive B cells and in plasma cells that directs RNA processing preferentially toward the production of mRNA encoding either the membrane form or the secreted form of an immunoglobulin.

Simultaneous Expression of IgM and IgD

The phenomenon of differential RNA processing also explains the simultaneous expression of membrane-bound IgM and IgD by mature B cells. As mentioned already, transcription of rearranged heavy-chain genes in mature B cells produces primary transcripts containing both the C_μ and C_δ gene segments. One explanation for this is that the close proximity of C_μ and C_δ, which are only about 5 kb apart, and the lack of a switch site between them permit the entire $VDJC_\mu C_\delta$ region to be transcribed into a long primary RNA transcript, about 15 kb long, which contains four poly-A sites (Figure 5-19a). Sites 1 and 2 are associated with C_μ, as described in the previous section; sites 3 and 4 are located at similar places in the C_δ gene segment.

If the heavy-chain transcript is cleaved and polyadenylated at site 2 after the C_μ exons, then the mRNA will encode the membrane form of the μ heavy chain (Figure 5-19b); if polyadenylation is instead further downstream at site 4, after the C_δ exons, then RNA splicing will remove the intervening C_μ exons and produce mRNA encoding the membrane form of the δ heavy chain (Figure 5-19c). Since the mature B cell expresses both IgM and IgD on its membrane, processing by both pathways must occur simultaneously. Likewise, cleavage and polyadenylation of the primary heavy-chain transcript at poly-A site 1 or 3 in plasma cells and subsequent splicing will yield the secreted form of the μ or δ heavy chains, respectively (see Figure 5-18b).

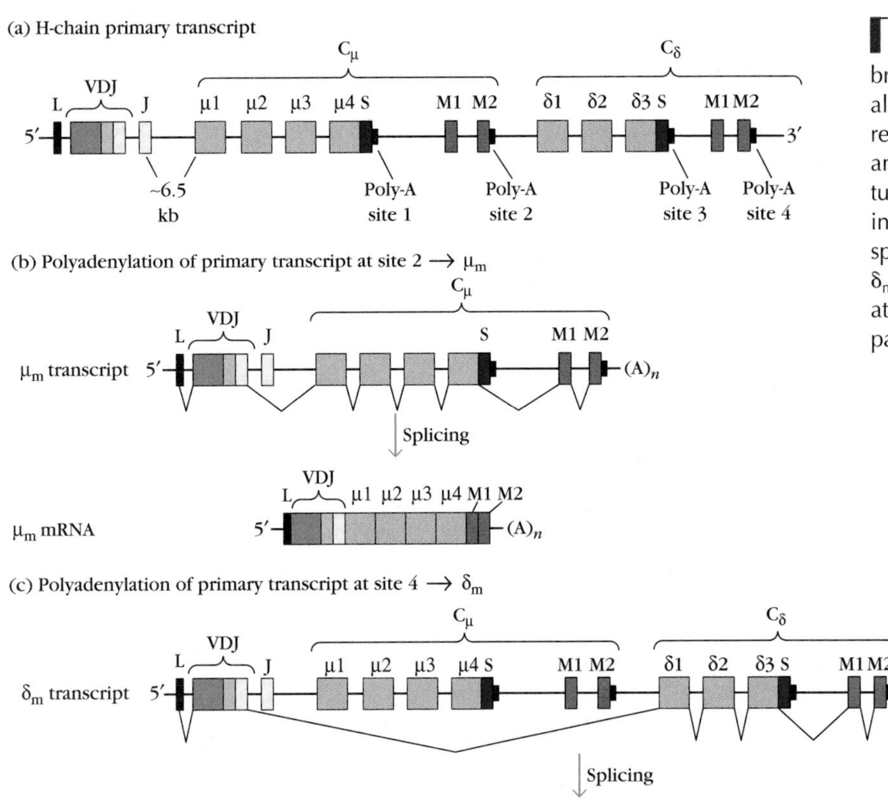

FIGURE 5-19 Expression of membrane forms of μ and δ heavy chains by alternative RNA processing. (a) Structure of rearranged heavy-chain gene showing C_μ and C_δ exons and poly-A sites. (b) Structure of μ_m transcript and μ_m mRNA resulting from polyadenylation at site 2 and splicing. (c) Structure of δ_m transcript and δ_m mRNA resulting from polyadenylation at site 4 and splicing. Both processing pathways can proceed in any given B cell.

Synthesis, Assembly, and Secretion of Immunoglobulins

Immunoglobulin heavy- and light-chain mRNAs are translated on separate polyribosomes of the rough endoplasmic reticulum (RER). Newly synthesized chains contain an amino-terminal leader sequence, which serves to guide the chains into the lumen of the RER, where it is then cleaved off. The assembly of light (L) and heavy (H) chains into the disulfide-linked and glycosylated immunoglobulin molecule occurs as the chains pass through the cisternae of the RER. The complete molecules are transported to the Golgi apparatus and then into secretory vesicles, which fuse with the plasma membrane (Figure 5-20).

The order of chain assembly varies among the immunoglobulin classes. In the case of IgM, the H and L chains assemble within the RER to form half-molecules, and then two half-molecules assemble to form the complete molecule. In the case of IgG, two H chains assemble, then an H_2L intermediate is assembled, and finally the complete H_2L_2 molecule is formed. Interchain disulfide bonds are formed, and the polypeptides are glycosylated as they move through the Golgi apparatus.

If the molecule contains the transmembrane sequence of the membrane form, it becomes anchored in the membrane of a secretory vesicle and is inserted into the plasma membrane as the vesicle fuses with the plasma membrane (see Figure 5-20, insert). If the molecule contains the hydrophilic sequence of secreted immunoglobulins, it is transported as a free molecule in a secretory vesicle and is released from the cell when the vesicle fuses with the plasma membrane.

Regulation of Ig-Gene Transcription

The immunoglobulin genes are expressed only in B-lineage cells, and even within this lineage, the genes are expressed at different rates during different developmental stages. As with other eukaryotic genes, three major classes of cis regulatory sequences in DNA regulate transcription of immunoglobulin genes:

- **Promoters:** relatively short nucleotide sequences, extending about 200 bp upstream from the

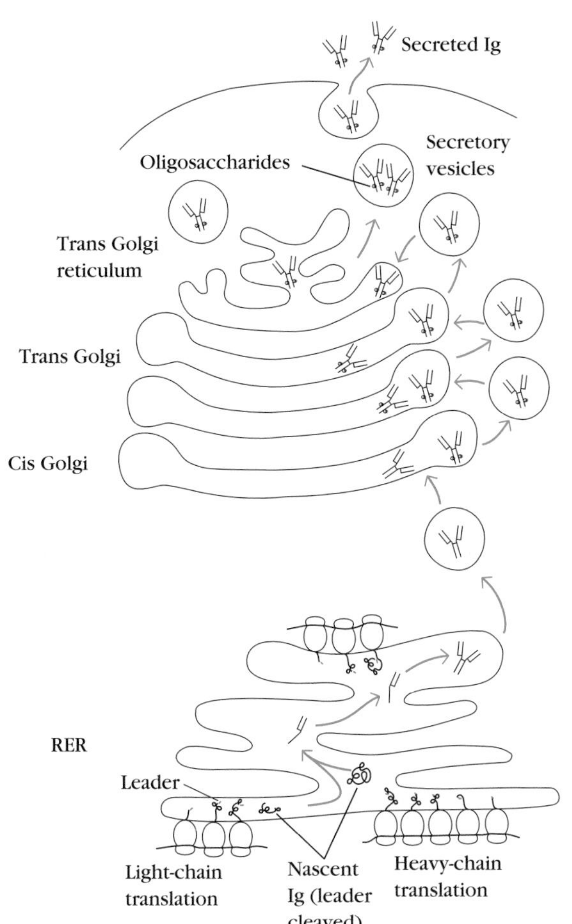

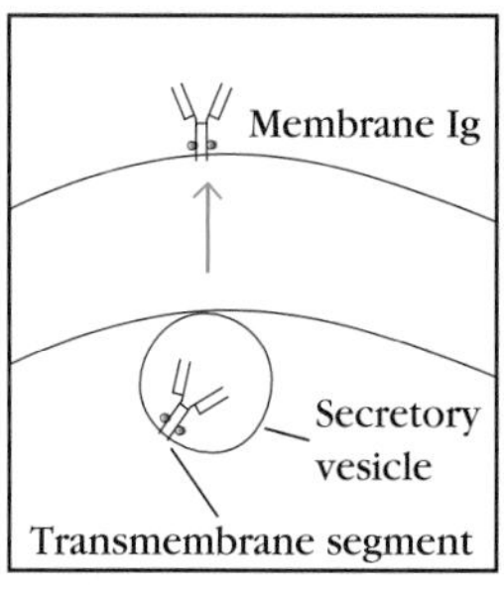

FIGURE 5-20 Synthesis, assembly, and secretion of the immunoglobulin molecule. The heavy and light chains are synthesized on separate polyribosomes (polysomes). The assembly of the chains to form the disulfide-linked and glycosylated immunoglobulin molecule occurs as the chains pass through the cisternae of the rough endoplasmic reticulum (RER) into the Golgi apparatus and then into secretory vesicles. The main figure depicts assembly of a secreted antibody. The inset depicts a membrane-bound antibody, which contains the carboxyl-terminal transmembrane segment. This form becomes anchored in the membrane of secretory vesicles and then is inserted into the cell membrane when the vesicles fuse with the membrane.

transcription initiation site, that promote initiation of RNA transcription in a specific direction

- **Enhancers:** nucleotide sequences situated some distance upstream or downstream from a gene that activate transcription from the promoter sequence in an orientation-independent manner
- **Silencers:** nucleotide sequences that down-regulate transcription, operating in both directions over a distance.

The locations of the three types of regulatory elements in germ-line immunoglobulin DNA are shown in Figure 5-21.

Each V_H and V_L gene segment has a promoter located just upstream from the leader sequence. Like other promoters, the immunoglobulin promoters contain a highly conserved AT-rich sequence called the TATA box, which serves as a site for the binding of a number of proteins that are necessary for the initiation of RNA transcription. The actual process of transcription is performed by RNA polymerase II, which starts transcribing DNA from the initiation site, located about 25 bp downstream of the TATA box.

The mechanism by which enhancers and silencers modulate transcription is still not fully understood. It is thought that DNA-binding factors bound to an enhancer may alter chromatin structure in the vicinity, thereby facilitating the formation of a stable transcription-initiation complex at the promoter site. Similarly, silencer-binding proteins may interact directly with histones, causing the chromatin structure to become inaccessible for transcription.

One heavy-chain enhancer is located within the intron between the last (3′) J gene segment and the first (5′) C gene segment (C_μ), which encodes the μ heavy chain. Because this heavy-chain enhancer (E_μ) is located 5′ of the S_μ switch site near to C_μ, it can continue to function after class switching has occurred. Another heavy-chain enhancer ($3'_\alpha E$) has been detected 3′ of the C_α gene segment. One κ light-chain enhancer (E_κ) is located between the J_κ segment and the C_κ segment, and another enhancer ($3'_\kappa E$) is located 3′ of the C_κ segment. The λ light-chain enhancers are located 3′ of $C_\lambda 4$ and 3′ of $C_\lambda 1$. Silencers have been identified in heavy-chain and κ-chain DNA, adjacent to enhancers, but not in λ-chain DNA.

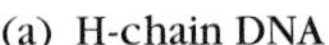

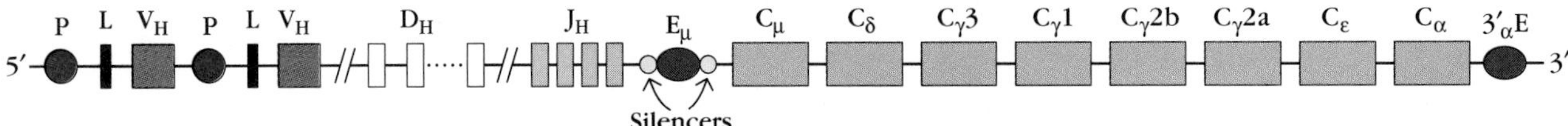

(b) κ-chain DNA

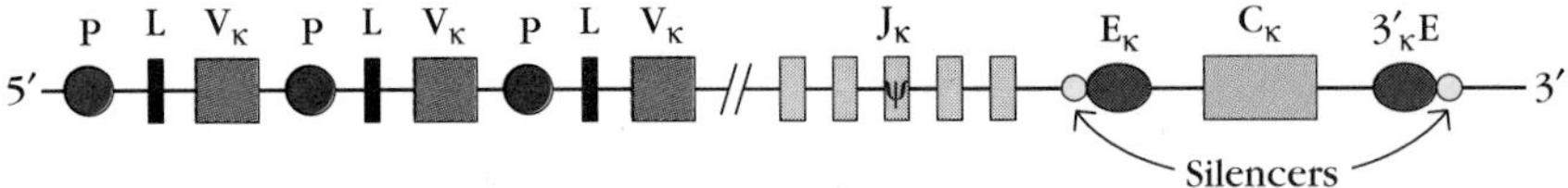

(c) λ-chain DNA

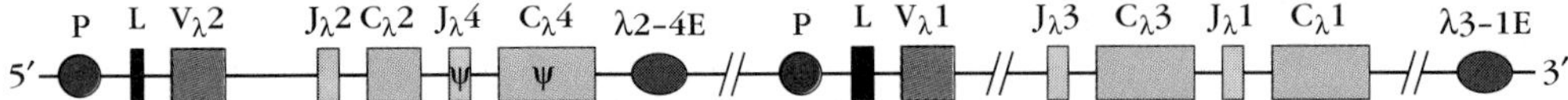

FIGURE 5-21 Location of promoters (dark red), enhancers (green), and silencers (yellow) in mouse heavy-chain, κ light-chain, and λ light-chain germ-line DNA. Variable-region DNA rearrangement moves an enhancer close enough to a promoter that the enhancer can activate transcription from the promoter.

Effect of DNA Rearrangement on Transcription

The promoters associated with the immunoglobulin V gene segments bind RNA polymerase II very weakly. For this reason, the rate of transcription of V_H and V_L coding regions is almost negligible in unrearranged germ-line DNA. In germ-line DNA, the variable-region enhancers are about 250–300 kb away from the promoters. Variable-region gene rearrangement brings a promoter and enhancer within 2 kb of each other, close enough for the enhancer to influence transcription from the nearby promoter. As a result, the rate of transcription of a rearranged V_LJ_L or $V_HD_HJ_H$ unit is as much as 10^4 times the rate of transcription of unrearranged V_L or V_H segments. For example, in one study, B cells transfected with rearranged heavy-chain genes from which the enhancer had been deleted did not transcribe the genes, whereas B cells transfected with similar genes that contained the enhancer transcribed the transfected genes at a high rate. These findings highlight the importance of enhancers in the normal transcription of immunoglobulin genes.

Genes that promote cellular proliferation or prohibit cell death, called cellular **oncogenes,** sometimes translocate to the immunoglobulin heavy- or light-chain loci. Here, under the influence of an immunoglobulin enhancer, the normally silent oncogene is activated, leading to increased expression of the oncogene product. Translocations of the c-*myc* and *bcl*-2 oncogenes have each been associated with malignant B-cell lymphomas. The translocation of c-*myc* leads to constitutive expression of c-Myc and an aggressive B-cell lymphoma called Burkitt's lymphoma. The translocation of *bcl*-2 leads to suspension of programmed cell death in B cells, resulting in follicular B-cell lymphoma. This topic is covered in greater detail in Chapter 22.

Inhibition of Ig-Gene Expression in T Cells

As noted earlier, germ-line DNA encoding the T-cell receptor (TCR) undergoes V-(D)-J rearrangement to generate functional TCR genes. Rearrangement of both immunoglobulin and TCR germ-line DNA occurs by a similar recombination process mediated by RAG-1 and RAG-2 and involving recombination signal sequences with one-turn or two-turn spacers (see Figure 5-7). Despite this common process, complete Ig-gene rearrangement of H and L chains occurs only in B cells and complete TCR-gene rearrangement is limited to T cells.

Hitoshi Sakano and coworkers have obtained results suggesting that a sequence within the κ-chain 3 enhancer 3 $_{\kappa}$E2 serves to regulate the joining of V_κ to J_κ in B and T cells. When a sequence known as the PU.1 binding site within the 3 κ-chain enhancer was mutated, these researchers found that V_κ-J_κ joining occurred in T cells as well as B cells. They propose that binding of a protein expressed by T cells, but not B cells, to the unmutated κ-chain enhancer normally prevents V_κ-J_κ joining in T cells. The nature of this DNA-binding protein in T cells remains to be determined. Similar processes may prevent rearrangement of heavy-chain and λ-chain DNA in T cells.

Antibody Genes and Antibody Engineering

There are many clinical applications in which the exquisitely specific mouse monoclonal antibody would be useful. However, when mouse monoclonal antibodies are introduced into humans they are recognized as foreign and evoke an antibody response. The induced human anti-mouse antibodies (HAMA) quickly reduce the effectiveness of the mouse monoclonal antibody by clearing it from the bloodstream. In addition, circulating complexes of mouse and human antibodies can cause allergic reactions. In some cases, the buildup of these complexes in organs such as the kidney can cause serious and even life-threatening reactions. Clearly, one way to avoid these undesirable reactions is to use human monoclonal antibodies for clinical applications. However, the preparation of human monoclonal antibodies has been hampered by numerous technical problems. Because of the difficulty of producing human monoclonal antibodies and the complications resulting from use of mouse monoclonal antibodies in humans, efforts to engineer monoclonal antibodies and antibody binding sites with recombinant DNA technology have begun.

The growing knowledge of antibody gene structure and regulation has made possible what Cesar Milstein, one of the inventors of monoclonal antibody technology, has called "man-made antibodies." It is now possible to design and construct genes that encode immunoglobulin molecules in which the variable regions come from one species and the constant regions come from another. New genes have been created that link nucleotide sequences that encode nonantibody proteins with nucleotide sequences that encode antibody variable regions specific for particular antigens. This has made it possible to build molecular hybrids or chimeras that can deliver a powerful toxin to a particular antigenic target, such as a tumor cell. Finally, by replacement of the immunoglobulin loci of one species with that of another, animals of one species have been endowed with the capacity to respond to immunization by producing antibodies encoded by the donor's genetically transplanted Ig genes. By capturing a significant sample of all of the immunoglobulin heavy- and light-chain variable-region genes, it has been possible to achieve significant and useful reconstructions of the entire antibody repertoires of individuals. The next few sections describe each of these types of antibody genetic engineering.

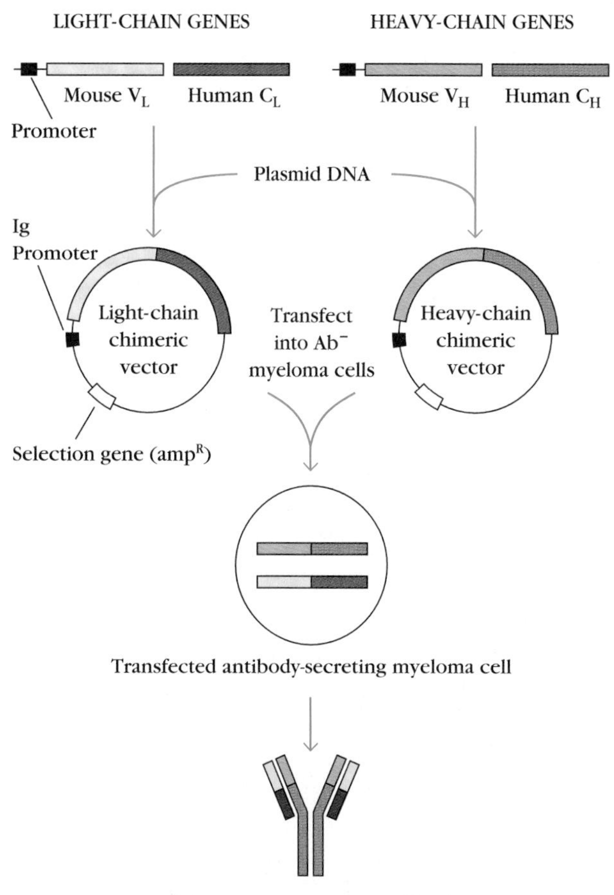

FIGURE 5-22 Production of chimeric mouse-human monoclonal antibodies. Chimeric mouse-human heavy- and light-chain expression vectors are produced. These vectors are transfected into Ab^- myeloma cells. Culture in ampicillin medium selects for transfected myeloma cells which secrete the chimeric antibody. [Adapted from M Verhoeyen and L Reichmann, 1988, *BioEssays* **8:**74.]

Chimeric and Hybrid Monoclonal Antibodies

One approach to engineering an antibody is to clone recombinant DNA containing the promoter, leader, and variable-region sequences from a mouse antibody gene and the constant-region exons from a human antibody gene (Figure 5-22). The antibody encoded by such a recombinant gene is a mouse-human **chimera,** commonly known as a **humanized antibody.** Its antigenic specificity, which is determined by the variable region, is derived from the mouse DNA; its isotype, which is determined by the constant region, is derived from the human DNA. Because their constant regions are encoded by human genes, these chimeric antibodies have fewer mouse antigenic determinants and are far less immunogenic than mouse monoclonal antibodies when administered to humans (Figure 5-23a). The potential for the mouse variable region remaining in these humanized antibodies to induce a useful antibody response in humans has encouraged further exploration of this approach. It is possible to produce chimeric human-mouse antibodies in which only the sequences of the CDRs are of mouse origin (Figure 5-23b). Another advantage of all the humanized chimeric antibodies is that they retain the biological effector functions of human antibody and are more likely to trigger human complement activation or Fc receptor binding. One such chimeric human-mouse antibody has been used to treat patients with B-cell varieties of non-Hodgkin's lymphoma (see Clinical Focus).

Chimeric monoclonal antibodies that function as immunotoxins (see Figure 4-23), can also be prepared. In this case, the terminal constant-region domain in a tumor-specific monoclonal antibody is replaced with toxin chains (Figure 5-23c). Because these immunotoxins lack the terminal Fc domain, they are not able to bind to cells bearing Fc receptors. These immunotoxins can bind only to tumor cells, making them highly specific as therapeutic reagents.

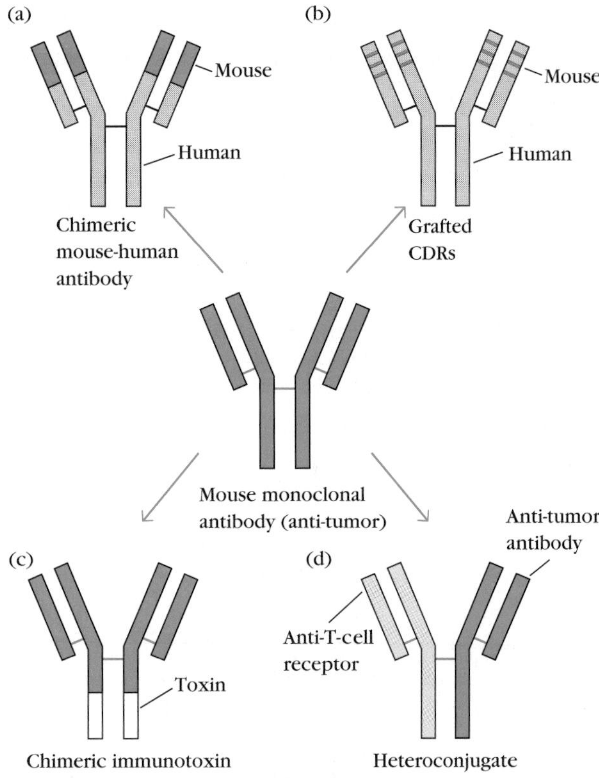

FIGURE 5-23 Chimeric and hybrid monoclonal antibodies engineered by recombinant DNA technology. (a) Chimeric mouse-human monoclonal antibody containing the V_H and V_L domains of a mouse monoclonal antibody (blue) and C_L and C_H domains of a human monoclonal antibody (gray). (b) A chimeric monoclonal antibody containing only the CDRs of a mouse monoclonal antibody (blue bands) grafted within the framework regions of a human monoclonal antibody. (c) A chimeric monoclonal antibody in which the terminal Fc domain is replaced by toxin chains (white). (d) A heteroconjugate in which one-half of the mouse antibody molecule is specific for a tumor antigen and the other half is specific for the CD3/T-cell receptor complex.

Heteroconjugates, or **bispecific antibodies,** are hybrids of two different antibody molecules (Figure 5-23d). They can be constructed by chemically crosslinking two different antibodies or synthesized in hybridomas consisting of two different monoclonal-antibody-producing cell lines that have been fused. Both of these methods generate mixtures of monospecific and bispecific antibodies from which the desired bispecific molecule must be purified, however. Using genetic engineering to construct genes that will encode molecules only with the two desired specificities is a much simpler and more elegant approach. Several bispecific molecules have been designed in which one half of the antibody has specificity for a tumor and the other half has specificity for a surface molecule on an immune effector cell, such as an NK cell, an activated macrophage, or a cytotoxic T lymphocyte (CTL). Such heteroconjugates have been designed to activate the immune effector cell when it is crosslinked to the tumor cell so that it begins to mediate destruction of the tumor cell.

Monoclonal Antibodies Constructed from Ig-Gene Libraries

A quite different approach for generating monoclonal antibodies employs the polymerase chain reaction (PCR) to amplify the DNA that encodes antibody heavy-chain and light-chain Fab fragments from hybridoma cells or plasma cells. A promoter region and *Eco*RI restriction site (see Chapter 23) are added to the amplified sequences, and the resulting constructs are inserted into bacteriophage λ, yielding separate heavy- and light-chain libraries. Cleavage with *Eco*RI and random joining of the heavy- and light-chain genes yield numerous novel heavy-light constructs (Figure 5-24).

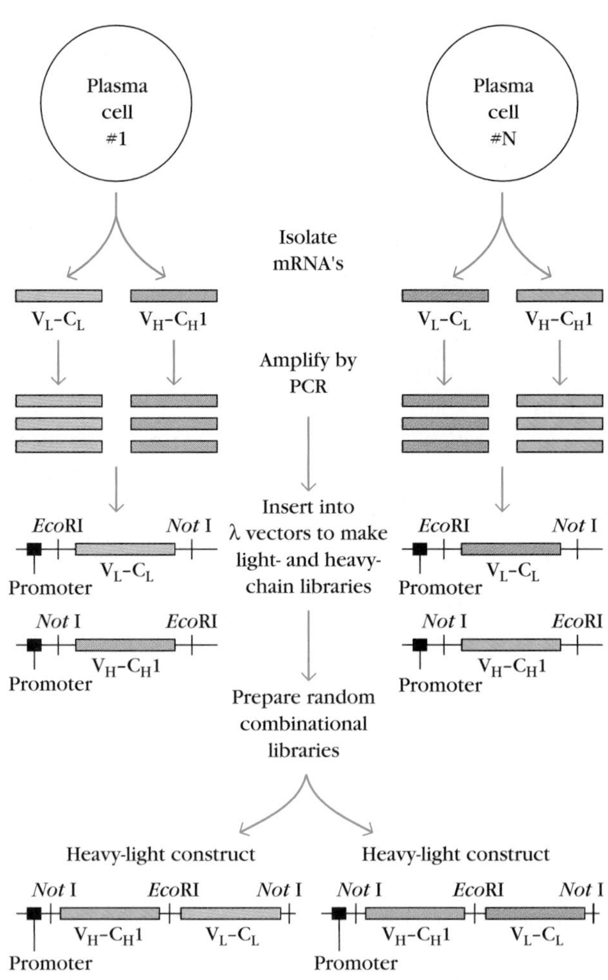

FIGURE 5-24 General procedure for producing gene libraries encoding Fab fragments. In this procedure, isolated mRNA that encodes heavy and light chains is amplified by the polymerase chain reaction (PCR) and cloned in λ vectors. Random combinations of heavy- and light-chain genes generate an enormous number of heavy-light constructs encoding Fab fragments with different antigenic specificity. [Adapted from WD Huse et al, 1989, *Science* **246:**1275.]

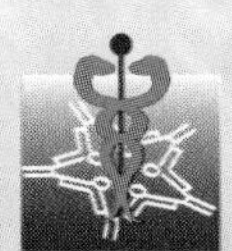

CLINICAL FOCUS

THERAPY FOR NON-HODGKIN'S LYMPHOMA BY A GENETICALLY ENGINEERED ANTIBODY

Lymphomas are cancers of lymphatic tissue in which the tumor cells are of lymphocytic origin. There are two major forms of lymphoma: Hodgkin's lymphoma and non-Hodgkin's lymphoma. The less common form is Hodgkin's lymphoma, named for its discoverer, Thomas Hodgkin, an English physician. This unusually gifted early pathologist, who worked without the benefit of a microscope, recognized this condition in several patients and first described the anatomical features of the disease in 1832. Because many tissue specimens taken from patients Hodgkin suspected of harboring the disease were saved in the Gordon Museum of Guy's Hospital in London, it has been possible for later generations to judge the accuracy of his diagnoses. Hodgkin has fared well. Studies of these preserved tissues confirm that he was right in about 60% of the cases, a surprising achievement, considering the technology of the time. Actually, most lymphoma is non-Hodgkin's type and includes about 10 different types of disease. B-cell lymphomas are an important fraction of these.

For some years now, the major therapies directed against lymphomas have been radiation or chemotherapy or a combination of both. While these therapies benefit large numbers of patients by increasing survival, relapses after treatment are common, and many treated patients experience debilitating and sometimes severe side effects. Such side effects are an expected consequence of these therapies, because the agents used kill or severely damage a broad spectrum of normal cells as well as tumor cells. One of the holy grails of cancer treatment is the discovery or creation of therapies that will affect only the tumor cells and completely spare normal cells. If particular types of cancer cells had antigens that were tumor specific, these antigens would be ideal targets for immune attack. Unfortunately, there are few such molecules known. However, a number of antigens are known that are restricted to the cell lineage in which the tumor originated and are expressed on the tumor cells.

Many cell-lineage-specific antigens have been identified for B lymphocytes and B lymphomas, including immunoglobulin, the hallmark of the B cell, and CD20, a membrane-bound phosphoprotein. CD20 has emerged as an attractive candidate for antibody-mediated immunotherapy, because it is present on B lymphomas and antibody-mediated crosslinking does not cause it to down-regulate or internalize. Indeed, some years ago, mouse monoclonal antibodies were raised against CD20, and one of these has formed the basis for an anti-B-cell lymphoma immunotherapy. This approach appears ready to take its place alongside radiation and chemotherapy, in some cases as an alternative to chemotherapy and radiation, in others as a partner in combined therapies that employ both immunological and cytotoxic drugs. The development of this anti-tumor antibody is an excellent case study of the combined application of immunological insights and molecular biology to engineer a novel therapeutic agent.

The original anti-CD20 antibody was a mouse monoclonal antibody with murine γ heavy chains and κ light chains. The DNA sequences of the light- and heavy-chain variable regions of this antibody were amplified by PCR. Then a chimeric gene was created by replacing the CDR gene sequences of a human γ1 heavy chain with those from the murine heavy chain. In a similar maneuver, CDRs from the mouse κ were ligated into a human κ gene. The chimeric genes thus created were incorporated into vectors that permitted high levels of expression in mammalian cells. When an appropriate cell line was co-transfected with both of these constructs, it produced chimeric antibodies containing CDRs of mouse origin together with human variable-region frameworks and constant regions. After purification, the biological activity of the antibody was evaluated, first in vitro and then in a primate animal model.

The initial results were quite promising. The grafted human constant region supported effector functions such as the complement-mediated lysis or antibody-dependent cytotoxicity (ADCC) of human B lymphoid cells. Furthermore, weekly injections of the antibody into monkeys resulted in the rapid and sustained depletion of B cells from peripheral blood, lymph nodes, and even bone marrow. When the anti-CD20 antibody infusions were stopped, the differentiation of new B cells from progenitor populations allowed B-cell populations eventually to recover and approach normal levels. From these results, the hope grew that this immunologically active chimeric antibody could be used to clear entire B cell populations, including B lymphoma cells, from the body in a way that spared other cell populations. This led to the trial of the antibody in human patients.

The human trials enrolled patients with B-cell lymphoma who had a relapse after chemotherapy or radiation treatment. These trials addressed three important issues: efficacy, safety, and immunogenicity. While not all patients responded to treatment with anti-CD20, close to 50% exhibited full or partial remission. Thus, efficacy was demonstrated, because this level of response is compara-

(continued)

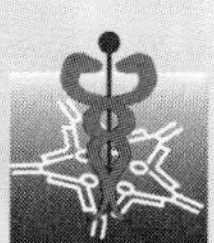

CLINICAL FOCUS (continued)

ble to the success rate with traditional approaches that employ highly cytotoxic drugs or radiation—it offers a truly alternative therapy. Side effects such as nausea, low blood pressure, and shortness of breath were seen in some patients (usually during or shortly after the initiation of therapy); these were, for the most part, not serious or life-threatening. Consequently, treatment with the chimeric anti-CD20 appears safe. Patients who received the antibody have been observed closely for the appearance of human anti-mouse-Ig antibodies (HAMA) and for human anti-chimeric antibody (HACA) responses. Such responses were not observed. Therefore, the antibody was not immunogenic. The absence of such responses demonstrtes that antibodies can be genetically engineered to minimize, or even avoid, untoward immune reactions.

Antibody engineering has also contributed to the therapy of other malignancies such as breast cancer, which is diagnosed in more than 180,000 American women each year. A little more than a quarter of all breast cancer patients have cancers that overexpress a growth factor receptor called HER2 (human epidermal growth factor receptor 2). Many tumors that overexpress HER2 grow faster and pose a more serious threat than those with normal levels of this protein on their surface. A chimeric anti-HER2 monoclonal antibody in which all of the protein except the CDRs are of human origin was created by genetic engineering. Specifically, the DNA sequences for the heavy-chain and light-chain CDRs were taken from cloned mouse genes encoding an anti-HER2 monoclonal antibody. As in the anti-CD20 strategy described above, each of the mouse CDR gene segments were used to replace the corresponding human CDR gene segments in human genes encoding the human IgG_1 heavy chain and the human κ light chain. When this engineered antibody is used in combination with a chemotherapeutic drug, it is highly effective against metastatic breast cancer. The effects on patients who were given only a chemotherapeutic drug were compared with those for patients receiving both the chemotherapeutic drug and the engineered anti-HER2 antibody. The combination anti-HER2/chemotherapy treatment showed significantly reduced rates of tumor progression, a higher percentage of responding patients, and a higher one-year survival rate. Treatment with Herceptin, as this engineered monoclonal antibody is called, has become a part of the standard repertoire of breast cancer therapies.

The development of engineered antibodies for the treatment of other malignancies and other diseases, too, can be expected.

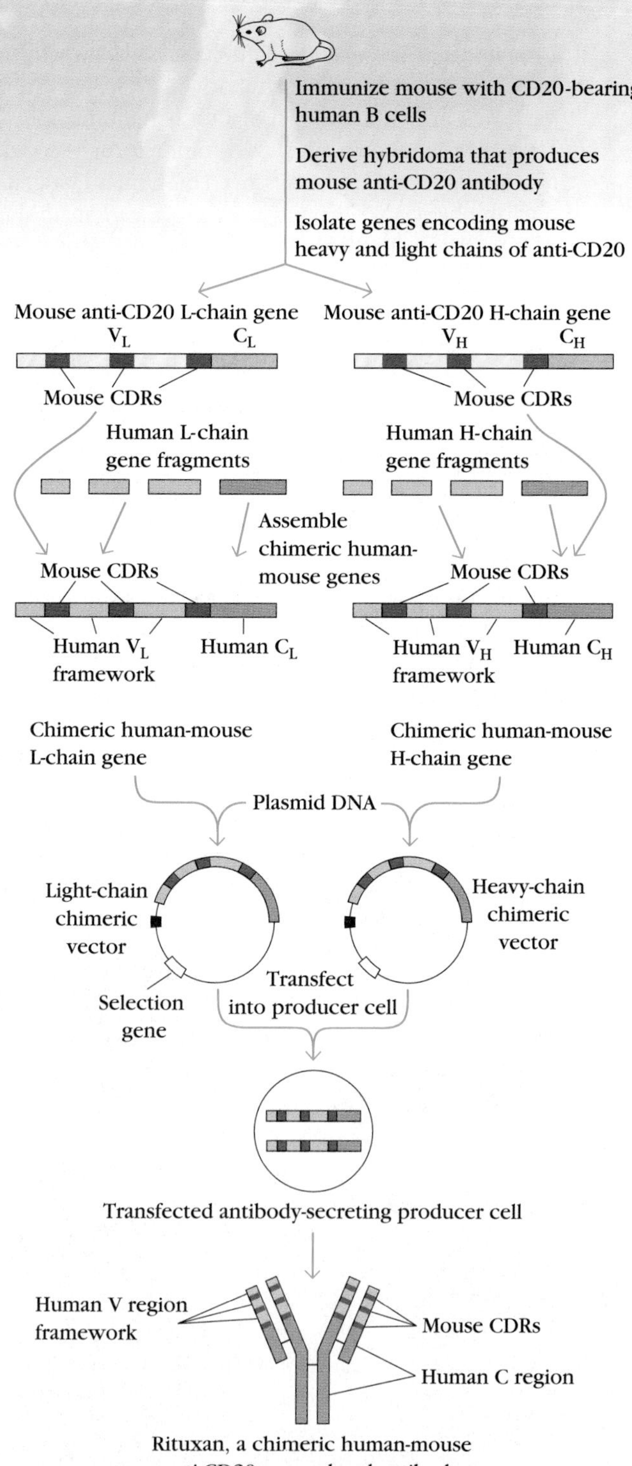

Assembling a chimeric antibody for anti-tumor therapy.

This procedure generates an enormous diversity of antibody specificities; clones containing these random combinations of H + L chains can be rapidly screened for those secreting antibody to a particular antigen. Impressive amounts of diversity have been achieved and libraries with $>10^{10}$ unique members have been obtained. This is a level that is certainly comparable to the human in vivo repertoire, and it is possible to demonstrate that specificities against a wide variety of antigens can be obtained from these libraries. Such a combinatorial library approach opens the possibility of obtaining specific antibodies without any need whatsoever for immunization.

However, the real challenge to bypassing in vivo immunization in the derivation of useful antibodies of high affinity lies in finding ways to mimic the biology of the humoral immune response. As we shall see in Chapter 11, the in vivo evolution of most humoral immune responses produces two desirable outcomes. One is class switching, in which a variety of antibody classes of the same specificity are produced. This is an important consideration because the class switching that occurs during an immune response produces antibodies that have the same specificity but different effector functions and hence, greater biological versatility. The other is the generation of antibodies of higher and higher affinity as the response progresses. A central goal of Ig-gene library approaches is the development of strategies to produce antibodies of appropriate affinity in vitro as readily as they are generated by an in vivo immune response. When the formidable technical obstacles to the achievement of these goals are overcome, combinatorial approaches based on phage libraries will allow the routine and widespread production of useful antibodies from any desired species without the limitations of immunization and hybridoma technology that currently complicate the production of monoclonal antibodies.

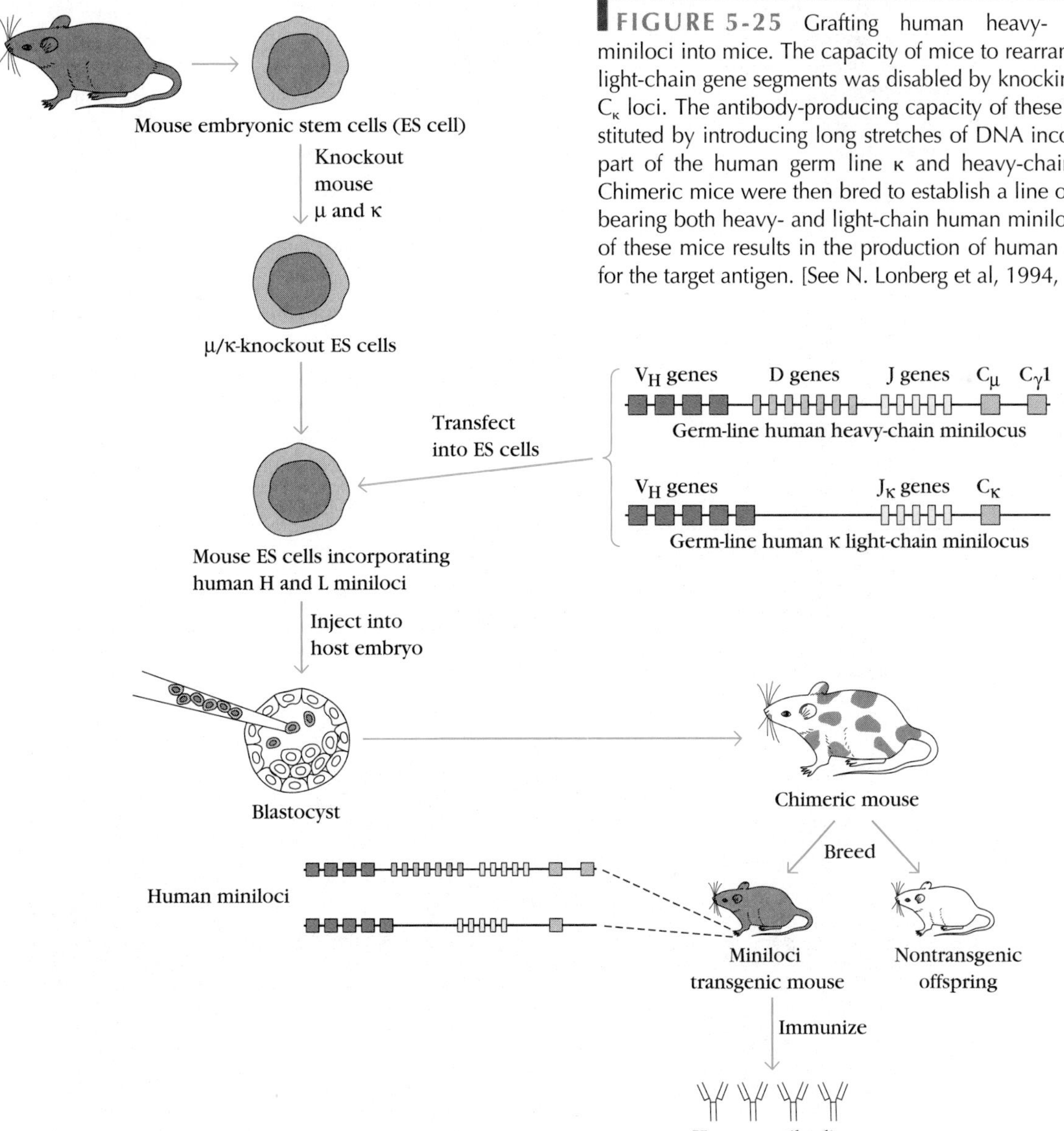

FIGURE 5-25 Grafting human heavy- and light-chain miniloci into mice. The capacity of mice to rearrange Ig heavy- and light-chain gene segments was disabled by knocking out the C_μ and C_κ loci. The antibody-producing capacity of these mice was reconstituted by introducing long stretches of DNA incorporating a large part of the human germ line κ and heavy-chain loci (miniloci). Chimeric mice were then bred to establish a line of transgenic mice bearing both heavy- and light-chain human miniloci. Immunization of these mice results in the production of human antibody specific for the target antigen. [See N. Lonberg et al, 1994, *Nature* 368:856.]

Mice with Human Instead of Mouse Immunoglobulin Loci

It is possible to functionally knockout, or disable, the heavy- and light-chain immunoglobulin loci in mouse embryonic stem (ES) cells. Subsequently, very large DNA sequences (as much as 80 kb) containing human heavy- and light-chain gene segments can be introduced. The DNA sequences inserted are very large and contain constant-region gene segments, J segments, many V-region segments, and in the case of the heavy chain, D_H segments. The ES cells containing these miniature human Ig gene loci (miniloci) are used to derive lines of transgenic mice that respond to antigenic challenge by producing antigen-specific *human* antibodies (Figure 5-25). Because the human heavy- and light-chain miniloci undergo rearrangement, and all the other diversity-generating processes such as N-addition and P-addition and, after antigen challenge, even somatic hypermutation occur in these mice, there is the opportunity for the generation of a great deal of diversity. The presence of human heavy-chain minilocus genes for more than one isotype and their accompanying switch sites allows class switching as well. A strength of this method is that these completely human antibodies are made in cells of the mouse B-cell lineage, from which antibody-secreting hybridomas are readily derived by cell fusion. This approach thus offers a solution to the problem of producing human monoclonal antibodies of any specificity desired.

Summary

1. Immunoglobulin κ and λ light chains and heavy chains are encoded by three separate multigene families located on different chromosomes. In germ-line DNA, each multigene family contains numerous gene segments (see Figure 5-3). The variable-region gene segments are designated V and J in light-chain DNA and V, D, and J in heavy-chain DNA. Multiple constant-region (C) gene segments are also present.
2. Functional light-chain and heavy-chain genes are generated by random rearrangement of the variable-region gene segments in germ-line DNA. Conserved DNA sequences, termed recombination signal sequences, flank each V, D, and J gene segment and direct the joining of segments. Each recombination signal contains a conserved heptamer sequence, a conserved nonamer sequence, and either a 12-bp (one-turn) or 23-bp (two-turn) spacer; the length, but not the nucleotide sequence, of these spacers is conserved (see Figure 5-6). During rearrangement, gene segments flanked by a one-turn spacer join only to segments flanked by a two-turn spacer. This one-turn/two-turn joining rule assures proper V_L-J_L and V_H-D_H-J_H joining. The multistep recombination process is mediated by several enzymes including RAG-1, RAG-2, terminal deoxynucleotidyl transferase (in heavy-chain rearrangement), and double-strand break repair (DSBR) enzymes (see Figure 5-7).
3. Immunoglobulin gene rearrangements occur in sequential order, heavy-chain rearrangements first, followed by light-chain rearrangements (see Figure 5-13). These rearrangements are carefully regulated so that the immunoglobulin DNA of only one parental chromosome is rearranged to form a functional light-chain or heavy-chain gene. This allelic exclusion is necessary to assure that a mature B cell expresses immunoglobulin with a single antigenic specificity.
4. The various mechanisms contributing to antibody diversity are estimated to generate $>10^{10}$ possible combinations in mammals such as humans and mice. Major sources of antibody diversity are the random joining of multiple V, J, and D germ-line gene segments and the random association of a given heavy-chain and light-chain in a particular cell (see Table 5-2). Other mechanisms that augment antibody diversity by a significant but unknown extent are junctional flexibility, P-addition and N-addition (which produce variability in the nucleotide sequences at the coding joints between gene segments), and somatic mutation after antigenic stimulation.
5. After antigenic stimulation of mature B cells, additional rearrangement of their heavy-chain C gene segments can occur (see Figure 5-17). Such class switching results in expression of different classes of antibody (IgG, IgA, and IgE) with the same antigenic specificity.
6. Differential RNA processing of the immunoglobulin heavy-chain primary transcript generates membrane-bound antibody in mature B cells and secreted antibody in plasma cells (see Figure 5-18). Differential processing is also responsible for the simultaneous expression of IgM and IgD by mature B cells (see Figure 5-19).
7. Transcription of immunoglobulin genes is regulated by three types of DNA regulatory sequences: promoters, enhancers, and silencers. A promoter is located just upstream of the leader sequence associated with each V_H and V_L gene segment, whereas enhancers and silencers are located considerable distances from the transcription start site (see Figure 5-21). In germ-line DNA, transcription of V_H and V_L gene segments is negligible; gene rearrangement brings enhancers close to the promoter they influence, greatly increasing the transcription rate of rearranged V_LJ_L and $V_HD_HJ_H$ units.
8. Growing knowledge of the molecular biology of immunoglobulin genes has teamed with recombinant DNA technology in various ways to engineer antibodies for research and therapy. In particular, these techniques have been used to make chimeric antibodies in which the desirable antigen binding properties of an antibody molecule made in one species are genetically grafted onto the constant regions of the antibodies of a different species (see Figures 5-22 and 5-23). This approach has been used

for a number of applications, including the design of antitumor agents (see Clinical Focus). Additional approaches based on recombinant DNA technology include the derivation and use of Ig-gene combinatorial libraries (see Figure 5-24) and the transplantation of extensive segments of entire human Ig loci into mice (see Figure 5-25).

REFERENCES

Arulampalam, V, L Eckhardt, and S Pettersson. 1997. The enhancer shift: a model to explain the developmental control of Ig H gene expression in B-lineage cells. *Immunol. Today* **18:**549

Chen J, Y Shinkai, F Young, and FW Alt. 1994. Probing immune functions in RAG-deficient mice. *Curr. Opin. Immunol.* **6:**313.

Cook, GP, and IM Tomlinson. 1995. The human immunoglobulin V_H repertoire. *Immunol. Today* **16:**237.

Dreyer, WJ and JC Bennett. 1965. The molecular basis of antibody formation. *Proc. Natl. Acad. Sci. USA* **54:**864.

Hagmann, M. 1997. RAGged repair: what's new in V(D)J recombination. *Biol. Chem.* **378:**815.

Harriman, W, et al. 1993. Immunoglobulin class switch recombination. *Annu. Rev. Immunol.* **11:**361.

Hayden, MS, LK Gilliand, and JA Ledbetter. 1997. Antibody engineering. *Curr. Opin. Immunol.* **9:**201.

Hiramatsu, R, et al. 1995. The 3 enhancer region determines the B/T specificity and pro-B/pre-B specificity of immunoglobulin V_κ-J_κ joining. *Cell* **83:**1.

Hozumi, N, and S Tonegawa. 1976. Evidence for somatic rearrangement of immunoglobulin genes coding for variable and constant regions. *Proc. Natl. Acad. Sci. USA* **73:**3628.

Kirschbaum, T, R Jaenichen, and HG Zachau. 1996. The mouse immunoglobulin kappa locus contains about 140 variable gene segments. *European Journal of Immunology* **26:**1613.

Lewis, SM. 1994. The mechanisms of V(D)J rejoining: lessons from molecular, immunological, and comparative analysis. *Adv. Immunol.* **56:**27.

Maloney, DG, et al. 1997. IDEC-C2B8 (Rituximab) anti-CD20 monoclonal antibody therapy in patients with relapsed low-grade non-Hodgkin's lymphoma. *Blood* **90:**2188.

Max, EE. 1993. Immunoglobulins: molecular genetics. In *Fundamental Immunology,* 3rd ed., WE Paul, ed. Raven Press, New York.

Oettinger, MA, et al. 1990. *RAG*-1 and *RAG*-2, adjacent genes that synergistically activate V(D)J recombination. *Science* **248:**1517.

Ramsden, DA, DC van Gent, and M Gellert. 1997. Specificity in V(D)J recombination: new lessons from biochemistry and genetics. *Curr. Opin. Immunol.* **9:**114.

Reth, M. 1992. Antigen receptors on B lymphocytes. *Annu. Rev. Immunol.* **10:**97.

Schatz, DG, and TM Leu. 1996. *RAG*-1 and *RAG*-2: biochemistry and protein interactions. *Curr. Top. Microbiol. Immunol.* **217:**11.

Schatz, DG, MA Oettinger, and MS Schlissel. 1992. V(D)J recombination: molecular biology and regulation. *Annu. Rev. Immunol.* **10:**359.

Storb, U. 1996. The molecular basis of somatic hypermutation of immunoglobulin genes. *Curr. Opin. Immunol.* **8:**206.

Tomlinson, IM, JP Cox, E Gherardi, AM Lesk, and C Chothia. 1995. The structural repertoire of the human V kappa domain. *EMBO J* **1514:**4628.

Tonegawa, S. 1983. Somatic generation of antibody diversity. *Nature* **302:**575.

Van Gent, DC, et al. 1995. Initiation of V(D)J recombination in a cell-free system. *Cell* **81:**925.

Williams, SC, JP Frippiat, IM Tomlinson, O Ignatovich, MP Lefranc, and G Winter. 1996. Sequence and evolution of the human germline V lambda repertoire. *J. Mol. Biol.* **264:**220.

Winter, G, AD Griffiths, RE Hawkins, and HR Hoogenboom. 1994. Making antibodies by phage display technology. *Annu. Rev. Immunol.* **12:**433.

Winter, G, and C Milstein. 1990. Man made antibodies. *Nature* **349:**293.

Yancopoulos, GD, and FW Alt. 1986. Regulation of the assembly and expression of variable-region genes. *Annu. Rev. Immunol.* **4:**339.

Useful Web Sites

http://www.mrc-cpe.cam.ac.uk/imt-doc/public/INTRO.html#maps
V BASE: This data base and informational site is maintained at the MRC Centre for Protein Engineering, in England. It is an excellent and comprehensive directory of information on the human germ-line variable region.

http://www.mgen.uni-heidelberg.de/SD/SDscFvSite.html
The Recombinant Antibody Page: This site has a number of links that provide interesting opportunities to explore the potential of genetic engineering of antibodies.

STUDY QUESTIONS

1. Indicate whether each of the following statements is true or false. If you think a statement is false, explain why.

a. V_κ gene segments sometimes join to C_λ gene segments.

b. Immunoglobulin class switching usually is mediated by DNA rearrangements.

c. Separate exons encode the transmembrane portion of each membrane immunoglobulin.

d. Although each B cell carries two alleles encoding the immunoglobulin heavy and light chains, only one allele is expressed.

e. Primary transcripts are processed into functional mRNA by removal of introns, capping, and addition of a poly-A tail.

f. The primary transcript is an RNA copy of the DNA and includes both introns and exons.

Go to www.whfreeman.com/immunology **Self-Test**
Review and quiz of key terms

2. Explain why a V_H segment cannot join directly with a J_H segment in heavy-chain gene rearrangement.

3. Considering only combinatorial joining of gene segments and association of light and heavy chains, how many different antibody molecules potentially could be generated from germ-line DNA containing 500 V_L and 4 J_L gene segments and 300 V_H, 15 D_H, and 4 J_H gene segments?

4. For each incomplete statement below (a–g), select the phrase(s) that correctly completes the statement. More than one choice may be correct.

a. Recombination of immunoglobulin gene segments serves to

(1) promote Ig diversification

(2) assemble a complete Ig coding sequence

(3) allow changes in coding information during B-cell maturation

(4) increase the affinity of immunoglobulin for antibody

(5) all of the above

b. Somatic mutation of immunoglobulin genes accounts for

(1) allelic exclusion

(2) class switching from IgM to IgG

(3) affinity maturation

(4) all of the above

(5) none of the above

c. The frequency of somatic mutation in Ig genes is greatest during

(1) differentiation of pre-B cells into mature B cells

(2) differentiation of pre-T cells into mature T cells

(3) generation of memory B cells

(4) antibody secretion by plasma cells

(5) none of the above

d. Kappa and lambda light-chain genes

(1) are located on the same chromosome

(2) associate with only one type of heavy chain

(3) can be expressed by the same B cell

(4) all of the above

(5) none of the above

e. Generation of combinatorial diversity among immunoglobulins involves

(1) mRNA splicing

(2) DNA rearrangement

(3) recombination signal sequences

(4) one-turn/two-turn joining rule

(5) switch sites

f. A B cell becomes immunocompetent

(1) following productive rearrangement of variable-region heavy-chain gene segments in germ-line DNA

(2) following productive rearrangement of variable-region heavy-chain and light-chain gene segments in germ-line DNA

(3) following class switching

(4) during affinity maturation

(5) following binding of T_H cytokines to their receptors on the B cell

g. The mechanism that permits immunoglobulins to be synthesized in either a membrane-bound or secreted form is

(1) allelic exclusion

(2) codominant expression

(3) class switching

(4) one-turn/two-turn joining rule

(5) differential RNA processing

5. What mechanisms generate the three hypervariable regions (complementarity-determining regions) of immunoglobulin heavy and light chains? Why is the third hypervariable region (CDR3) more variable than the other two (CDR1 and CDR2)?

6. You have been given a cloned myeloma cell line that secretes IgG with the molecular formula $\gamma_2\lambda_2$. Both the heavy and light chains in this cell line are encoded by genes derived from allele 1. Indicate the form(s) in which each of the genes listed below would occur in this cell line using the following symbols: G = germ-line form; R = productively rearranged form; NP = nonproductively rearranged form. State the reason for your choice in each case.

a. Heavy-chain allele 1

b. Heavy-chain allele 2

c. κ-chain allele 1

d. κ-chain allele 2

e. λ-chain allele 1

f. λ-chain allele 2

7. You have a B-cell lymphoma that has made nonproductive rearrangements for both heavy-chain alleles. What is the arrangement of its κ light-chain DNA? Why?

8. Indicate whether each of the class switches indicated below can occur (Yes) or cannot occur (No).

a. IgM to IgD

b. IgM to IgA

c. IgE to IgG

d. IgA to IgG

e. IgM to IgG

9. Describe one advantage and one disadvantage of N-nucleotide addition during the rearrangement of immunoglobulin heavy-chain gene segments.

10. X-ray crystallographic analyses of over two dozen antibody molecules bound to their respective antigens have revealed that the CDR3 of both the heavy and light chains make contact with the epitope. Moreover, sequence analyses reveal that the variability of CDR3 is greater than that of either CDR1 or CDR2. What mechanisms account for the greater diversity in CDR3?

11. How many chances does a developing B cell have to generate a functional immunoglobulin light-chain gene?

12. Select the description(s) listed below (1–11) that are true about each of the following terms (a–h). Each description may be used once, more than once, or not at all; more than one description may apply to some terms.

Terms

a. ______ RAG-1 and RAG-2

b. ______ Double-strand break repair (DSBR) enzymes

c. ______ Coding joints
d. ______ RSSs
e. ______ P-nucleotides
f. ______ N-nucleotides
g. ______ Promoters
h. ______ Enhancers

Descriptions

(1) Junctions between immunoglobulin gene segments formed during rearrangement

(2) Source of diversity in antibody heavy chains

(3) DNA regulatory sequences

(4) Conserved DNA sequences, located adjacent to V, D, and J segments, that help direct gene rearrangement

(5) Enzymes expressed in developing B cells

(6) Enzymes expressed in mature B cells

(7) Nucleotide sequences located close to each leader segment in immunoglobulin genes to which RNA polymerase binds

(8) Product of endonuclease cleavage of hairpin intermediates in Ig-gene rearrangement

(9) Enzymes that are defective in SCID mouse

(10) Nucleotide sequences that greatly increase the rate of transcription of rearranged immunoglobulin genes compared with germ-line DNA

(11) Nucleotides added by TdT enzyme

13. For each immunoglobulin heavy-chain or light-chain DNA, mRNA, or polypeptide (a–g) described below, select the corresponding schematic diagram (1–9) in the figure below.

a. ______ Heavy-chain DNA in a liver cell
b. ______ λ-Chain DNA in a liver cell
c. ______ Heavy-chain DNA in a mature B cell
d. ______ Primary RNA transcript encoding heavy chain in a mature B cell
e. ______ mRNA encoding light chain in a mature B cell
f. ______ Heavy-chain proteins observed on the membrane of a mature B cell before any class switching
g. ______ Heavy-chain DNA in a plasma cell secreting IgE

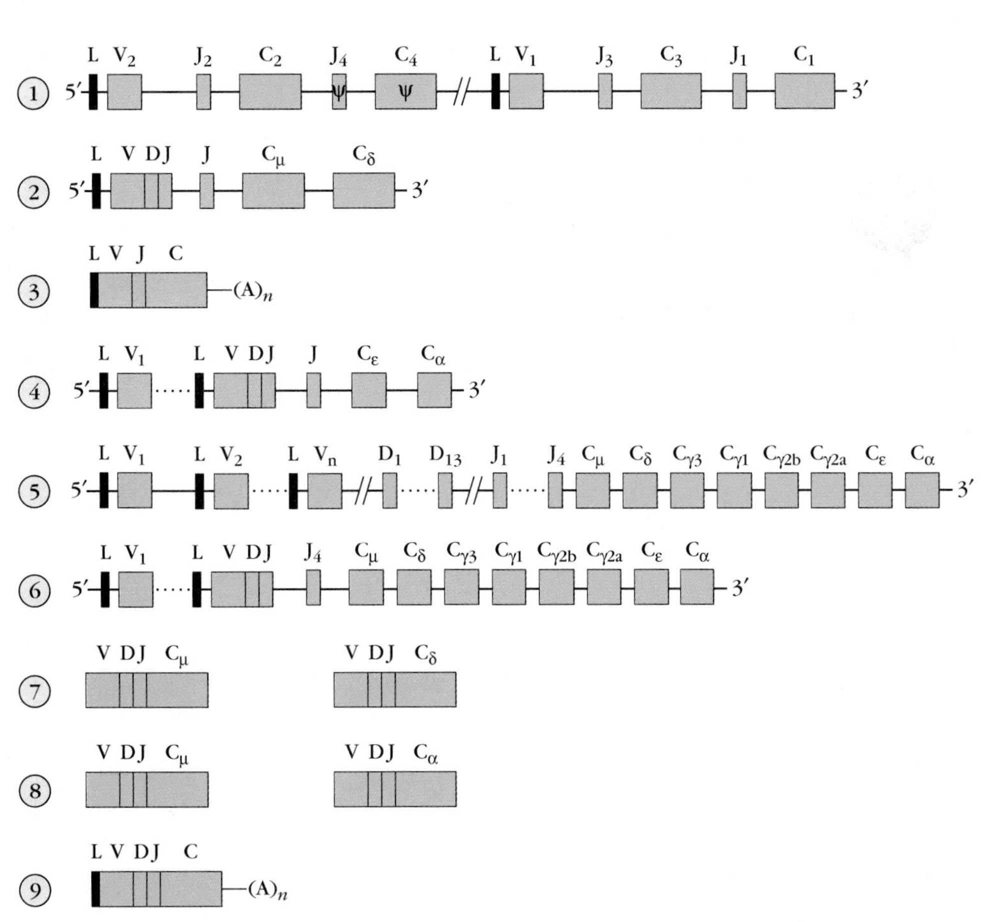

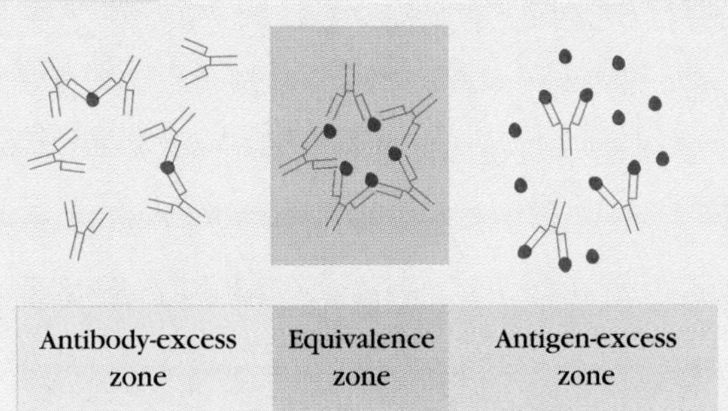

CHAPTER 6

ANTIGEN-ANTIBODY INTERACTIONS

The antigen-antibody interaction is a bimolecular association similar to an enzyme-substrate interaction, with an important distinction: it does not lead to an irreversible chemical alteration in either the antibody or the antigen and therefore is reversible. The interaction between an antibody and an antigen involves various noncovalent interactions between the antigenic determinant, or epitope, of the antigen and the variable-region (V_H/V_L) domain of the antibody molecule, particularly the hypervariable regions, or complementarity-determining regions (CDRs). The exquisite specificity of antigen-antibody interactions has led to the development of a variety of immunologic assays. These assays can be used to detect the presence of either antibody or antigen and have played vital roles in diagnosing diseases, monitoring the level of the humoral immune response, and identifying molecules of biological or medical interest. These assays differ in their speed and their sensitivity; some are strictly qualitative, and others are quantitative. This chapter examines the nature of the antigen-antibody interaction, and it describes various immunologic assays that measure or exploit this interaction.

Strength of Antigen-Antibody Interactions

The noncovalent interactions that form the basis of antigen-antibody (Ag-Ab) binding include hydrogen bonds, ionic bonds, hydrophobic interactions, and van der Waals interactions (Figure 6-1). Because the strength of each of these interactions is weak (compared with that of a covalent bond), a large number of such interactions are required to form a strong Ag-Ab interaction. Furthermore, each of these noncovalent interactions operates over a very small distance, generally about 1×10^{-7} mm (1 angstrom, Å) or a little less; consequently, a strong Ag-Ab interaction depends on a very close fit between the antigen and antibody. Such fits require a high degree of complementarity between antigen and antibody, and this requirement is the basis of the exquisite specificity that characterizes antigen-antibody interactions.

Antibody Affinity

The strength of the total noncovalent interactions between a *single* antigen-binding site on an antibody and a *single* epitope is the **affinity** of the antibody for that epitope. Low-affinity antibodies bind antigen weakly and tend to dissociate readily, whereas high-affinity antibodies bind antigen more tightly and remain bound longer. The association between a binding site on an antibody (Ab) with a monovalent antigen (Ag) can be described by the equation

$$\text{Ag} + \text{Ab} \underset{k_{-1}}{\overset{k_1}{\rightleftharpoons}} \text{Ag-Ab}$$

VISUALIZING CONCEPTS

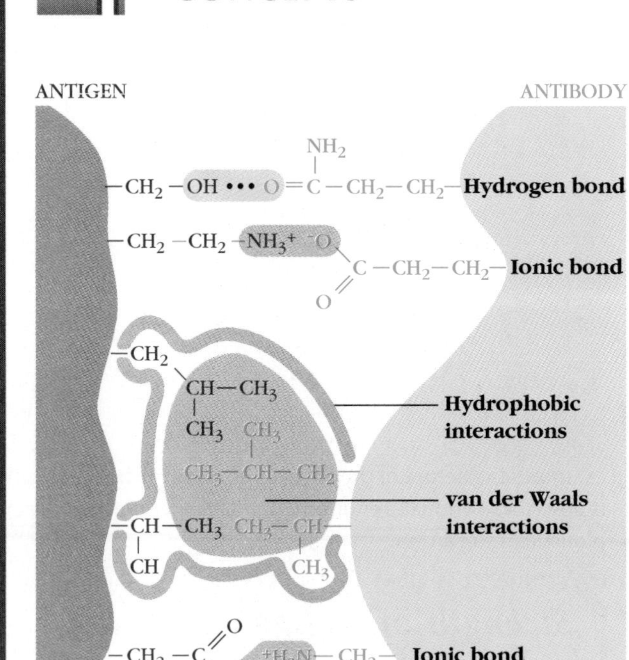

FIGURE 6-1 The interaction between an antibody and an antigen depends on four types of noncovalent forces: (1) hydrogen bonds, in which a hydrogen atom is shared between two electronegative atoms; (2) ionic bonds between oppositely charged residues; (3) hydrophobic interactions, in which water forces hydrophobic groups together; and (4) van der Waals interactions between the outer electron clouds of two or more atoms. In an aqueous environment, noncovalent interactions are extremely weak and depend upon close complementarity of the shapes of antibody and antigen.

where k_1 is the forward (association) rate constant and k_{-1} is the reverse (dissociation) rate constant. The ratio of k_1/k_{-1} is the association constant K_a (i.e., $k_1/k_{-1} = K_a$), a measure of affinity. Because K_a is the equilibrium constant for the above reaction, it can be calculated from the ratio of the molar concentration of bound Ag-Ab complex to the molar concentrations of unbound antigen and antibody at equilibrium as follows:

$$K_a = \frac{[\text{Ag-Ab}]}{[\text{Ab}][\text{Ag}]}$$

The value of K_a varies for different Ag-Ab complexes and depends upon both k_1, which is expressed in units of liters/mole/second (L/mol/s), and k_{-1}, which is expressed in units of 1/second. For small haptens, the forward rate constant can be extremely high; in some cases, k_1 can be as high as 4×10^8 L/mol/s, approaching the theoretical upper limit of diffusion-limited reactions (10^9 L/mol/s). For larger protein antigens, however, k_1 is smaller, with values in the range of 10^5 L/mol/s.

The rate at which bound antigen leaves an antibody's binding site (i.e., the dissociation rate constant, k_{-1}) plays a major role in determining the antibody's affinity for an antigen. Table 6-1 illustrates the role of k_{-1} in determining the association constant K_a for several Ag-Ab interactions. For example, the k_1 for the DNP-L-lysine system is about one fifth that for the fluorescein system, but its k_{-1} is 200 times greater; consequently, the affinity of the antifluorescein antibody K_a for the fluorescein system is about a 1000-fold higher than that of anti-DNP antibody. Low-affinity Ag-Ab complexes have K_a values between 10^4 and 10^5 L/mol; high-affinity complexes can have K_a values as high as 10^{11} L/mol.

For some purposes, the dissociation of the antigen-antibody complex is of interest:

$$\text{Ag-Ab} \rightleftharpoons \text{Ab} + \text{Ag}$$

The equilibrium constant for that reaction is K_d, the reciprocal of K_a:

$$K_d = [\text{Ab}][\text{Ag}]/\text{Ab-Ag} = 1/K_a$$

K_d is a quantitative indicator of the stability of an Ag-Ab complex; very stable complexes have very low values of K_d and less stable ones have higher values.

TABLE 6-1 FORWARD (k_1) AND REVERSE (k_{-1}) RATE CONSTANTS AND ASSOCIATION (K_a) AND DISSOCIATION (K_d) CONSTANTS OF THREE LIGAND-ANTIBODY INTERACTIONS

Antibody	Ligand	k_1	k_{-1}	K_a	K_d
Anti-DNP	ϵ-DNP-L-lysine	8×10^7	1	1×10^8	1×10^{-8}
Anti-fluorescein	Fluorescein	4×10^8	5×10^{-3}	1×10^{11}	1×10^{-11}
Anti-bovine serum albumin (BSA)	Dansyl-BSA	3×10^5	2×10^{-3}	1.7×10^8	5.9×10^{-9}

SOURCE: Adapted from HN Eisen, 1990, *Immunology,* 3rd ed., Harper & Row Publishers.

The association constant, K_a, can be determined by **equilibrium dialysis** or by various newer methods. Because equilibrium dialysis remains for many the standard against which other methods are evaluated, it is described here. This procedure uses a dialysis chamber containing two equal compartments separated by a semipermeable membrane. Antibody is placed in one compartment, and a radioactively labeled ligand that is small enough to pass through the semipermeable membrane is placed in the other compartment (Figure 6-2). Suitable ligands include haptens as well as oligosaccharides and oligopeptides composing the epitope of complex polysaccharide or protein antigens. In the absence of antibody, ligand added to compartment B will equilibrate on both sides of the membrane (Figure 6-2a). In the

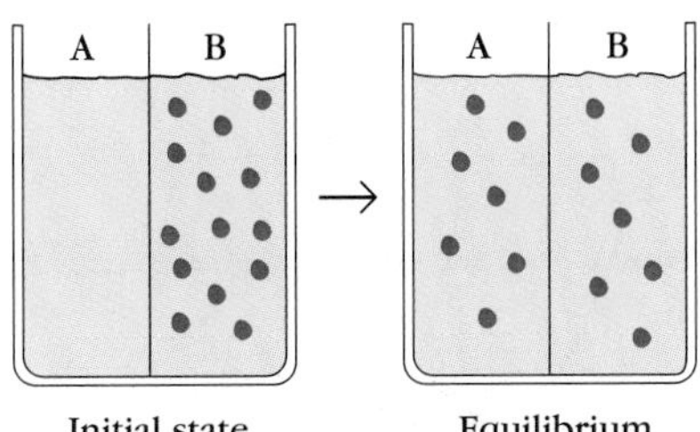

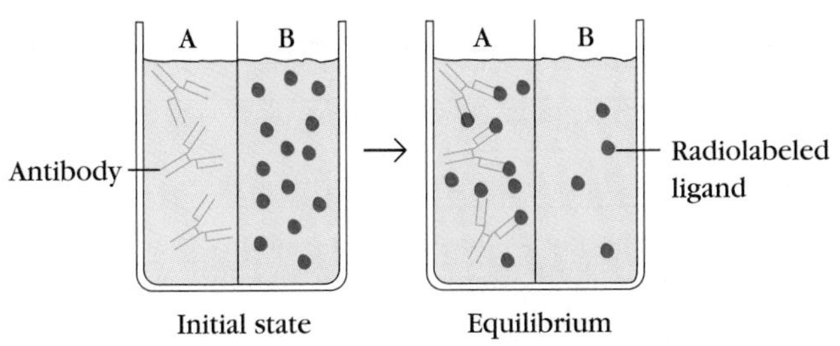

FIGURE 6-2 Determination of antibody affinity by equilibrium dialysis. (a) The dialysis chamber contains two compartments (A and B) separated by a semipermeable membrane. Antibody is added to one compartment and a radiolabeled ligand to another. At equilibrium, the concentration of radioactivity in both compartments is measured. (b) Plot of concentration of ligand in each compartment with time. At equilibrium, the difference in the concentration of radioactive ligand in the two compartments represents the amount of ligand bound to antibody.

presence of antibody, however, part of the labeled ligand will be bound to the antibody at equilibrium, and the unbound ligand will be equally distributed in both compartments. Thus the total concentration of ligand will be greater in the compartment containing antibody (Figure6-2b). The difference in the ligand concentration in the two compartments represents the concentration of ligand bound to the antibody (i.e., the concentration of Ag-Ab complex). The higher the affinity of the antibody, the more ligand is bound.

Since the total concentration of antibody in the equilibrium dialysis chamber is known, the equilibrium equation can be rewritten as:

$$K_a = \frac{[\text{Ab-Ag}]}{[\text{Ab}][\text{Ag}]} = \frac{r}{c(n-r)}$$

where r = the ratio of the concentration of bound ligand to total antibody concentration, c = concentration of free ligand, and n = number of binding sites per antibody molecule. This expression can be rearranged to give the **Scatchard equation:**

$$\frac{r}{c} = K_a n - K_a r$$

Values for r and c can be obtained by repeating the equilibrium dialysis with the same concentration of antibody but with different concentrations of ligand. If K_a is a constant, that is, if all the antibodies within the dialysis chamber have the same affinity for the ligand, then a Scatchard plot of r/c versus r will yield a straight line with a slope of $-K_a$ (Figure 6-3a). As the concentration of unbound ligand c increases, r/c approaches 0, and r approaches n, the **valency.**

Most antibody preparations are polyclonal, and K_a is therefore not a constant because a heterogeneous mixture of antibodies with a range of affinities is present. A Scatchard plot of heterogeneous antibody yields a curved line whose slope is constantly changing, reflecting this antibody heterogeneity (Figure 6-3b). With this type of Scatchard plot, it is possible to determine the average affinity constant, K_0, by determining the value of K_a when half of the antigen-binding sites are filled. This is conveniently done by determining the slope of the curve at the point where half of the antigen binding sites are filled.

Antibody Avidity

The affinity at one binding site does not always reflect the true strength of the antibody-antigen interaction. When complex antigens containing multiple, repeating antigenic determinants are mixed with antibodies containing multiple binding sites, the interaction of an antibody molecule with an antigen molecule at one site will increase the probability of reaction between those two molecules at a second site.

(a) Homogeneous antibody

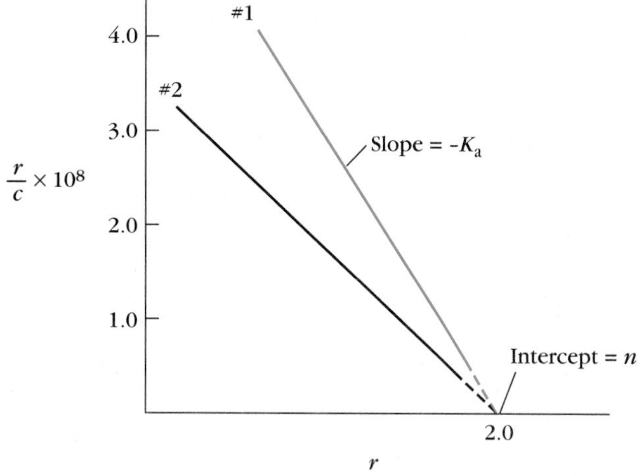

(b) Heterogeneous antibody

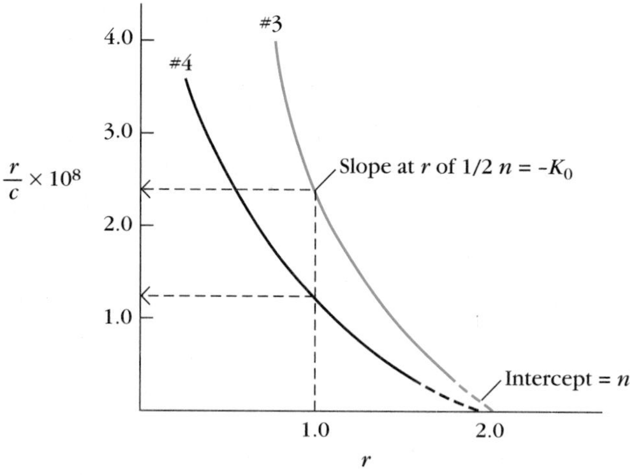

FIGURE 6-3 Scatchard plots are based on repeated equilibrium dialyses with a constant concentration of antibody and varying concentration of ligand. In these plots, r = moles bound ligand/mole antibody and c = free ligand. From a Scatchard plot, both the equilibrium constant (K_a) and the number of binding sites per antibody molecule (n), or its valency, can be obtained. (a) If all antibodies have the same affinity, then a Scatchard plot yields a straight line with a slope of $-K_a$. The x intercept is n, the valence of the antibody, which is 2 for IgG and other divalent Igs. For IgM, which is pentameric, n = 10, and for dimeric IgA, n = 4. In this graph, antibody #1 has a higher affinity than antibody #2. (b) If the antibodies are polyclonal and have a range of affinities, a Scatchard plot yields a curved line, whose slope is constantly changing. The average affinity constant K_0 can be calculated by determining the value of K_a when one half of the binding sites are occupied (i.e., when r = 1 in this example). In this graph, antiserum #3 has a higher affinity ($K_0 = 2.4 \times 10^8$) than antiserum #4 ($K_0 = 1.25 \times 10^8$). Note that the curves shown in (a) and (b) are for divalent antibodies such as IgG. The intercept value, n, for an IgM antibody would be 10.

of reaction between those two molecules at a second site. The strength of such multiple interactions between a multivalent antibody and antigen is called the **avidity.** The avidity of an antibody is a better measure of its binding capacity within biological systems (e.g., the reaction of an antibody with antigenic determinants on a virus or bacterial cell) than the affinity of its individual binding sites. High avidity can compensate for low affinity. For example, secreted pentameric IgM often has a lower affinity than IgG, but the high avidity of IgM, resulting from its higher valence, enables it to bind antigen effectively.

Cross-Reactivity

Although Ag-Ab reactions are highly specific, in some cases antibody elicited by one antigen can cross-react with an unrelated antigen. Such **cross-reactivity** occurs if two different antigens share an identical epitope or if antibodies specific for one epitope also bind to an unrelated epitope possessing similar chemical properties. In the latter case, the antibody's affinity for the cross-reacting epitope is usually less than that for the original epitope.

Cross-reactivity is often observed among polysaccharide antigens that contain similar oligosaccharide residues. The **ABO blood-group antigens,** for example, are glycoproteins expressed on red blood cells. Subtle differences in the terminal sugar residues distinguish the A and B blood-group antigens. An individual lacking one or both of these antigens will have serum antibodies to the missing antigen(s). A type O individual thus has anti-A and anti-B antibodies; a type A individual has anti-B; and a type B individual has anti-A (Table 6-2).

Cross-reactivity is the basis for the presence of these blood-group antibodies, which are induced in an individual not by exposure to red blood cell antigens but by exposure to cross-reacting microbial antigens present on common intestinal bacteria. These cross-reacting microbial antigens induce the formation of antibodies in individuals lacking these antigens on their red blood cells. The blood-group antibodies, although elicited by microbial antigens, will cross-react with similar oligosaccharides on red blood cells.

A number of viruses and bacteria have antigenic determinants identical or similar to normal host-cell components.

TABLE 6-2 ABO BLOOD TYPES

Blood type	Antigens on RBCs	Serum antibodies
A	A	Anti-B
B	B	Anti-A
AB	A and B	Neither
O	Neither	Anti-A and anti-B

In some cases, these microbial antigens have been shown to elicit antibody that cross-reacts with the host-cell components, resulting in a tissue-damaging autoimmune reaction. The bacterium *Streptococcus pyogenes,* for example, expresses cell-wall proteins called M antigens. Antibodies produced to streptococcal M antigens have been shown to cross-react with several myocardial and skeletal muscle proteins and have been implicated in heart and kidney damage following streptococcal infections. The role of other cross-reacting antigens in the development of autoimmune diseases is discussed in Chapter 20.

Some vaccines also exhibit cross-reactivity. For instance, vaccinia virus, which causes cowpox, expresses cross-reacting epitopes with variola virus, the causative agent of smallpox. This cross-reactivity was the basis of Jenner's method of using vaccinia virus to induce immunity to smallpox, as mentioned in Chapter 1.

Precipitation Reactions

The interaction between an antibody and a soluble antigen in aqueous solution forms a lattice that eventually develops into a visible precipitate. Antibodies that thus aggregate soluble antigens are called **precipitins.** Although formation of the soluble Ag-Ab complex occurs within minutes, formation of the visible precipitate occurs more slowly and often takes a day or two to reach completion.

Formation of an Ag-Ab lattice depends on the valency of both the antibody and antigen:

- The antibody must be bivalent; a precipitate will not form with monovalent Fab fragments.
- The antigen must be either bivalent or polyvalent; that is, it must have at least two copies of the same epitope, or have different epitopes that react with different antibodies present in polyclonal antisera.

Myoglobin illustrates the requirement that protein antigens be bivalent or polyvalent for a precipitin reaction to occur. Myoglobin precipitates well with specific polyclonal antisera but fails to precipitate with a specific monoclonal antibody because it contains multiple, distinct epitopes but only a single copy of each epitope (Figure 6-4a). Myoglobin thus can form a crosslinked lattice structure with polyclonal antisera but not with monoclonal antisera. The principles that underlie precipitation reactions will be presented because they are essential for an understanding of commonly used immunological assays. Although various modifications of the precipitation reaction were at one time the major types of assay used in immunology, they have been largely replaced by methods that are faster and require only very small quantities of antigen or antibody because they are far more sensitive. Also, these modern assay methods are not limited to antigen-antibody reactions that produce a

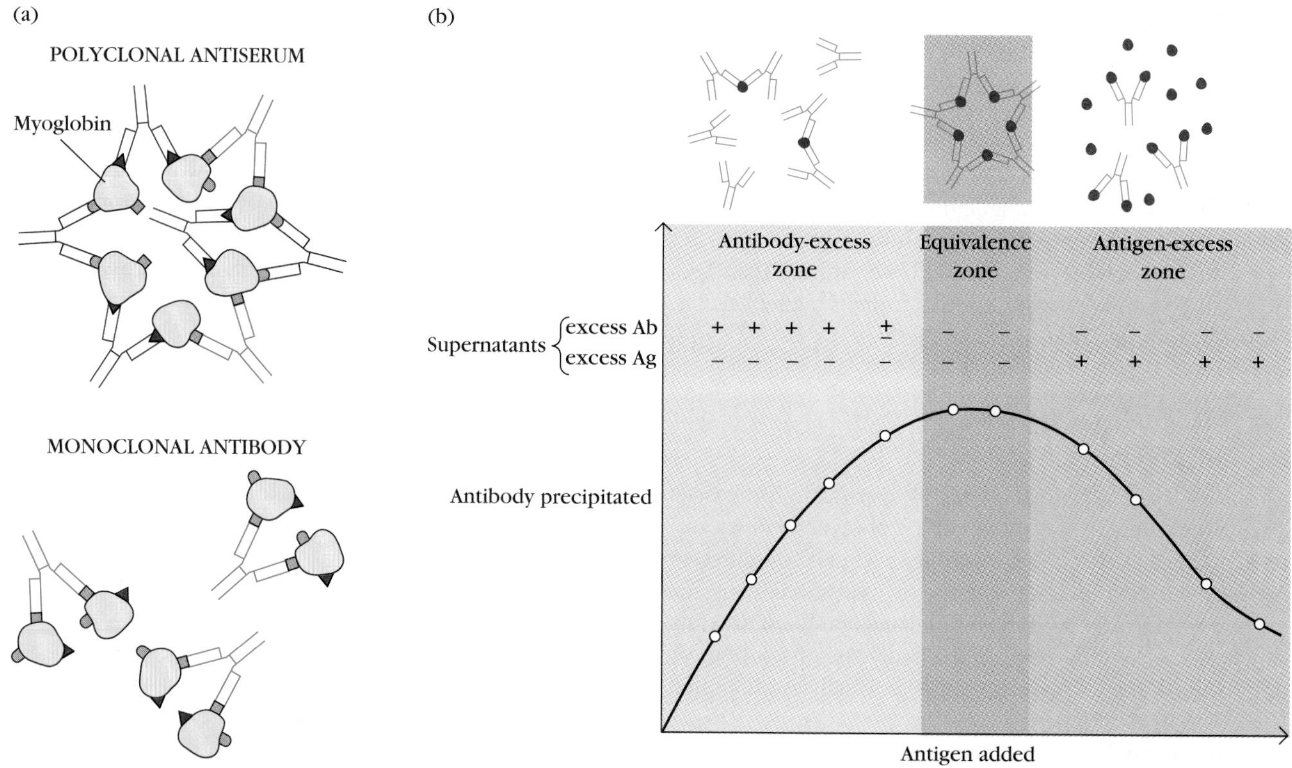

FIGURE 6-4 Precipitation reactions. (a) Polyclonal antibodies can form lattices, or large aggregates, that precipitate out of solution. However, if each antigen molecule contains only a single epitope recognized by a given monoclonal antibody, the antibody can link only two molecules of antigen and no precipitate is formed. (b) A precipitation curve for a system of one antigen and its antibodies. This plot of the amount of antibody precipitated versus increasing antigen concentrations (at constant total antibody) reveals three zones: a zone of antibody excess, in which precipitation is inhibited and antibody not bound to antigen can be detected in the supernatant; an equivalence zone of maximal precipitation in which antibody and antigen form large insoluble complexes and neither antibody nor antigen can be detected in the supernatant; and a zone of antigen excess in which precipitation is inhibited and antigen not bound to antibody can be detected in the supernatant.

ity, or minimum amount of antibody detectable, by a number of immunoassays.

Precipitation Reactions in Fluids

A quantitative precipitation reaction can be performed by placing a constant amount of antibody in a series of tubes and adding increasing amounts of antigen to the tubes. At one time this method was used to measure the amount of antigen or antibody present in a sample of interest. After the precipitate forms, each tube is centrifuged to pellet the precipitate, the supernatant is poured off, and the amount of precipitate is measured. Plotting the amount of precipitate against increasing antigen concentrations yields a precipitin curve. As Figure 6-4b shows, excess of either antibody or antigen interferes with maximal precipitation, which occurs in the so-called **equivalence zone,** when the ratio of antibody to antigen is optimal. As a large multimolecular lattice is formed at equivalence, the complex increases in size and precipitates out of solution. In the region of *antibody excess,* unreacted antibody is found in the supernatant along with small, soluble complexes consisting of multiple molecules of antibody bound to a single molecule of antigen. In the region of *antigen excess,* unreacted antigen can be detected and small, soluble complexes are again observed, this time consisting of one or two molecules of antigen bound to a single molecule of antibody. In either case, extensive lattices cannot be formed and precipitation is inhibited. Although the quantitative precipitation reaction is seldom used experimentally today, the principles of antigen excess, antibody excess, and equivalence apply to many Ag-Ab reactions.

Precipitation Reactions in Gels

Immune precipitates can form not only in solution but also in an agar matrix. When antigen and antibody diffuse toward one another in agar, or when antibody is incorporated into the agar and antigen diffuses into the antibody-containing matrix, a visible line of precipitation will form. As in a precipitation reaction in fluid, visible precipitation occurs in the region of equivalence, whereas no visible precipitate forms in regions of antibody or antigen excess. These

TABLE 6-3 SENSITIVITY OF VARIOUS IMMUNOASSAYS

Assay	Sensitivity* (μg Antibody/ml)
Precipitation reaction in fluids	20–200
Precipitation reactions in gels	
Mancini radial immunodiffusion	10–50
Ouchterlony double immunodiffusion	20–200
Immunoelectrophoresis	20–200
Rocket electrophoresis	2
Agglutination reactions	
Direct	0.3
Passive agglutination	0.006–0.06
Agglutination inhibition	0.006–0.06
Radioimmunoassay	0.0006–0.006
Enzyme-linked immunosorbent assay (ELISA)	6 0.0001–0.01
ELISA using chemiluminescence	0.00001–0.01
Immunofluorescence	1.0
Flow cytometry	0.006–0.06

*The sensitivity depends upon the affinity of the antibody as well as the epitope density and distribution.

SOURCE: Adapted from NR Rose et al, eds., 1986 and 1997 eds., *Manual of Clinical Laboratory Immunology,* American Society for Microbiology, Washington, D.C.

immunodiffusion reactions can be used to determine relative concentrations of antibodies or antigens, to compare antigens, or to determine the relative purity of an antigen preparation. Two immunodiffusion techniques are **radial immunodiffusion** (Mancini method) and **double immunodiffusion** (Ouchterlony method); both are carried out in a semisolid medium such as agar.

Radial Immunodiffusion (Mancini Method)

The relative concentrations of an antigen can be determined by a simple quantitative assay in which an antigen sample is placed in a well and allowed to diffuse into agar containing a suitable dilution of an antiserum. As the antigen diffuses into the agar, the region of equivalence is established and a ring of precipitation, a precipitin ring, forms around the well (Figure 6-5, upper panel). The area of the precipitin ring is proportional to the concentration of antigen. By comparing the area of the precipitin ring with a standard curve (obtained by measuring the precipitin areas of known concentrations of the antigen), the concentration of the antigen sample can be determined.

Double Immunodiffusion (Ouchterlony Method)

In the Ouchterlony method, both antigen and antibody diffuse radially from wells toward each other, thereby establishing a concentration gradient. As equivalence is reached, a visible line of precipitation, a precipitin line, forms (Figure 6-5, lower panel). This simple technique is an effective *qualitative* tool for determining the relationship between antigens and the number of different Ag-Ab systems present. The pattern of the precipitin lines that form when two different antigen preparations are placed in adjacent wells indicates whether they share epitopes:

- **Identity** occurs when two antigens share identical epitopes. As the antiserum forms a single precipitin line with each antigen, the two lines grow toward each other and fuse to give a single curved line of identity (Figure 6-6a).

RADIAL IMMUNODIFFUSION

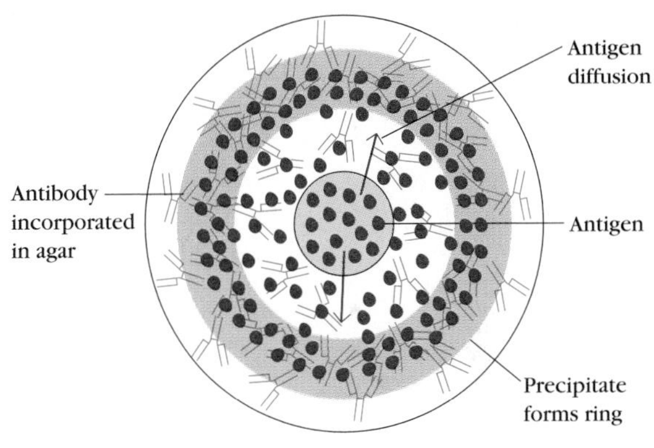

DOUBLE IMMUNODIFFUSION

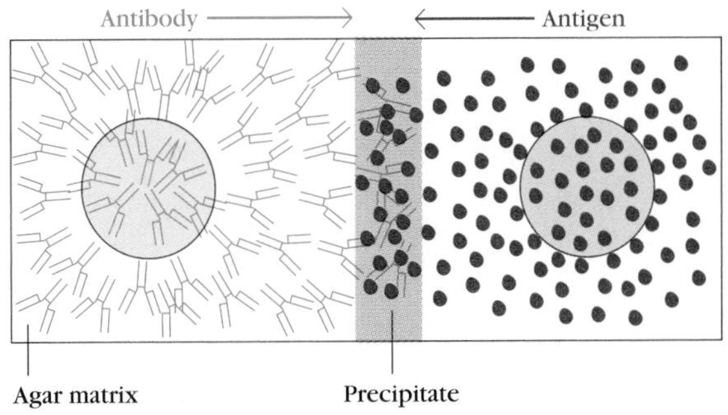

FIGURE 6-5 Diagrammatic representation of radial (Mancini) and double (Ouchterlony) immunodiffusion in a gel. In both cases, large insoluble complexes form in the agar in the zone of equivalence, which are visible as a line of precipitation (purple region). Only the antigen (red) diffuses in radial immunodiffusion, whereas both the antibody (blue) and antigen (red) diffuse in double immunodiffusion.

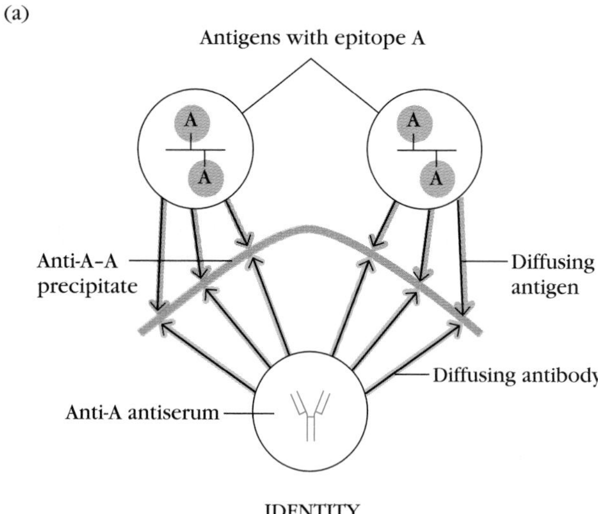

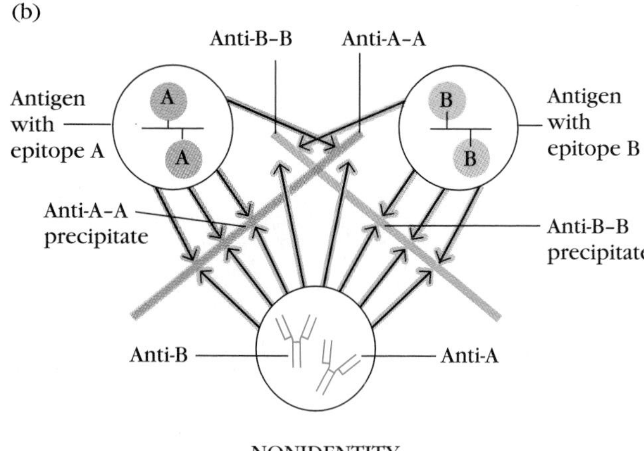

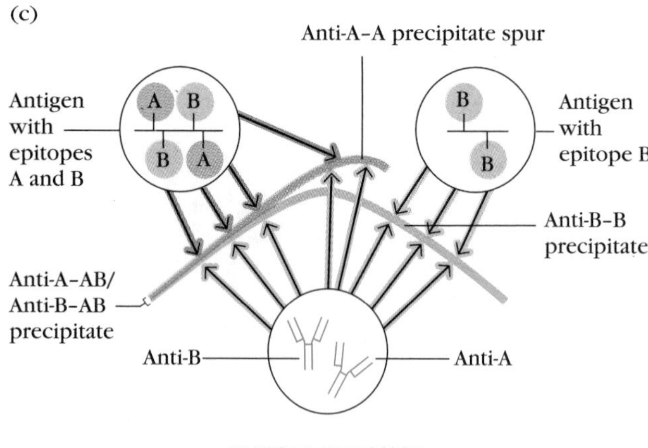

FIGURE 6-6 Diagram of possible precipitin patterns obtained in double immunodiffusion (Ouchterlony method) of antiserum with two different antigen preparations. The pattern of lines indicates whether the two antigens have (a) identical epitopes (identity), (b) no epitopes in common (nonidentity), or (c) partly identical epitopes (partial identity). In (c), diffusion of the antigen that has both epitope A (pink) and epitope B (yellow) is indicated by orange arrows.

- **Nonidentity** occurs when two antigens are unrelated (i.e., share no common epitopes). The antiserum forms an independent precipitin line with each antigen, and the two lines cross (Figure 6-6b).
- **Partial identity** occurs when two antigens share some epitopes but one or the other has a unique epitope(s). The antiserum forms a line of identity with the common epitope(s) and a curved spur with the unique epitope(s) (Figure 6-6c).

Immunoelectrophoresis

The technique of **immunoelectrophoresis** combines separation by electrophoresis with identification by double immunodiffusion (Figure 6-7a). An antigen mixture is first electrophoresed to separate its components by charge. Troughs are then cut into the agar gel parallel to the direction of the electric field, and antiserum is added to the troughs. Antibody and antigen then diffuse toward each other and produce lines of precipitation where they meet in appropriate proportions. Immunoelectrophoresis is used in clinical laboratories to detect the presence or absence of proteins in the serum. A sample of serum is electrophoresed, and the individual serum components are identified with antisera specific for a given protein or immunoglobulin class (Figure 6-7b). This technique is useful in determining whether a patient produces abnormally low amounts of one or more isotypes, characteristic of certain immunodeficiency diseases. It can also show whether a patient overproduces some serum protein, such as albumin, immunoglobulin, or transferrin. The immunoelectrophoretic pattern of serum from patients with multiple myeloma, for example, shows a heavy distorted arc caused by the large amount of myeloma protein, which is monoclonal Ig and therefore uniformly charged.

Immunoelectrophoresis is a strictly *qualitative* technique that can detect relatively high antibody concentrations (greater than several hundred μg/ml). It is useful for detecting quantitative anomalies only when the departure from normal is striking, as in immunodeficiency and immunoproliferative disorders.

A related *quantitative* technique, rocket electrophoresis, does permit measurement of antigen levels. In **rocket electrophoresis,** a negatively charged antigen is electrophoresed in a gel containing antibody. The precipitate formed between antigen and antibody has the shape of a rocket, the height of which is proportional to the concentration of antigen in the well. One limitation of rocket electrophoresis is the need for the antigen to be negatively charged for electrophoretic movement within the agar matrix. Some proteins, such as immunoglobulins, are not sufficiently charged to be quantitatively analyzed by rocket electrophoresis; nor is it possible to measure the amounts of several antigens in a mixture at the same time.

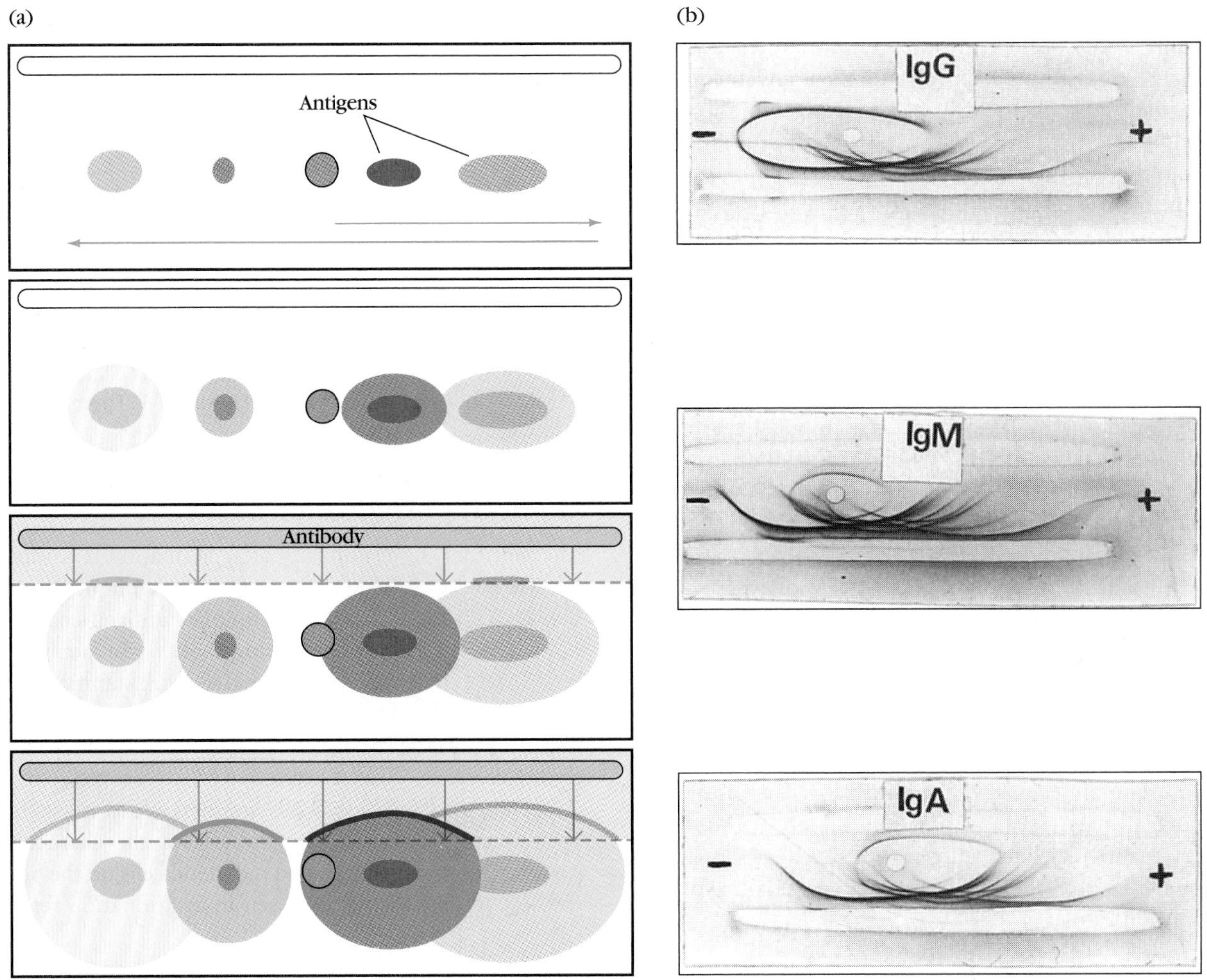

FIGURE 6-7 Immunoelectrophoresis of an antigen mixture. (a) An antigen preparation (orange) is first electrophoresed, which separates the component antigens on the basis of charge. Antiserum (blue) is then added to troughs on one or both sides of the separated antigens and allowed to diffuse; in time, lines of precipitation (colored arcs) form where specific antibody and antigen interact. (b) Immunoelectrophoretic patterns of human serum. Goat antibody to whole human serum was placed in the bottom trough of each slide; goat antibody to human IgG, IgM, or IgA was placed in the top trough of each slide. After electrophoresis, the IgG, IgM, and IgA antibodies form a single line of precipitation with their respective antisera. The position of the human IgG, IgM, and IgA in the electrophoresed whole human serum sample can be determined by comparing the position of the single band at the top of each slide with the complex band pattern of the whole serum sample at the bottom of each slide. [Part (b) JS Garvey et al, 1977, *Methods in Immunology*, 3d ed., W. A. Benjamin Inc., Advanced Book Program.]

Agglutination Reactions

The interaction between antibody and a particulate antigen results in visible clumping called **agglutination.** Antibodies that produce such reactions are called **agglutinins.** Agglutination reactions are similar in principle to precipitation reactions; they depend on the crosslinking of polyvalent antigens. Just as an excess of antibody inhibits precipitation reactions, such excess can also inhibit agglutination reactions; this inhibition is called the **prozone effect.** Because prozone effects can be encountered in many types of immunoassays, understanding the basis of this phenomenon is of general importance.

Several mechanisms can cause the prozone effect. First, at high antibody concentrations, the number of antibody binding sites may greatly exceed the number of epitopes. As a result, antibodies can bind antigen only univalently instead of multivalently. Antibodies that bind univalently cannot crosslink one antigen to another. Prozone effects are readily diagnosed by performing the assay at a variety of antibody (or antigen) concentrations. As one dilutes to an optimum antibody concentration, one sees higher levels of agglutination or whatever parameter is measured in the assay being used. When one is using polyclonal antibodies, the prozone effect can also occur for another reason. The antiserum may contain high concentrations of antibodies that bind to the antigen but do not induce agglutination; these antibodies, called **incomplete antibodies,** are often of the IgG class. At high concentrations of IgG, incomplete antibodies may occupy all of the antigenic sites, thus blocking access by IgM, which is a good agglutinin. This effect is not seen with agglutinating monoclonal antibodies. The lack of agglutinating activity of an incomplete antibody may be due to restricted flexibility in the hinge region, making it difficult for the antibody to assume the required angle for optimal cross-linking of epitopes on two or more particulate antigens. Alternatively, the density of epitope distribution or the location of some epitopes in deep pockets of a particulate antigen may make it difficult for the antibodies specific for these epitopes to agglutinate certain particulate antigens. When feasible, the solution to both of these problems is to try different antibodies that may react with other epitopes of the antigen that do not present these limitations.

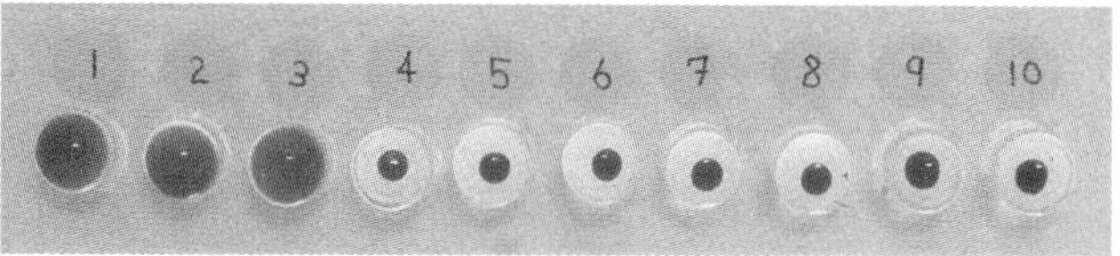

FIGURE 6-8 Demonstration of hemagglutination using antibodies against sheep red blood cells (SRBCs). The control tube (10) contains only SRBCs, which settle into a solid "button." The experimental tubes 1-9 contain a constant number of SRBCs plus serial two-fold dilutions of anti-SRBC serum. The spread pattern in the experimental series indicates positive hemagglutination through tube 3. [Louisiana State University Medical Center/MIP. Courtesy of Harriet CW Thompson.]

Hemagglutination

Agglutination reactions (Figure 6-8) are routinely performed to type red blood cells (RBCs). In typing for the ABO antigens, RBCs are mixed on a slide with antisera to the A or B blood-group antigens. If the antigen is present on the cells, they agglutinate, forming a visible clump on the slide. Determination of which antigens are present on donor and recipient RBCs is the basis for matching blood types for transfusions.

Bacterial Agglutination

A bacterial infection often elicits the production of serum antibodies specific for surface antigens on the bacterial cells. The presence of such antibodies can be detected by bacterial agglutination reactions. Serum from a patient thought to be infected with a given bacterium is serially diluted in a series of tubes to which the bacteria is added. The last tube showing visible agglutination will reflect the serum antibody **titer** of the patient. The agglutinin titer is defined as the reciprocal of the greatest serum dilution that elicits a positive agglutination reaction. For example, if serial twofold dilutions of serum are prepared and if the dilution of 1/640 shows agglutination but the dilution of 1/1280 does not, then the agglutination titer of the patient's serum is 640. In some cases serum can be diluted up to 1/50,000 and still show agglutination of bacteria.

The agglutinin titer of an antiserum can be used to diagnose a bacterial infection. Patients with typhoid fever, for example, show a significant rise in the agglutination titer to *Salmonella typhi.* Agglutination reactions also provide a way to type bacteria. For instance, different species of the bacterium *Salmonella* can be distinguished by agglutination reactions with a panel of typing antisera.

Passive Agglutination

The sensitivity and simplicity of agglutination reactions can be extended to soluble antigens by the technique of passive hemagglutination. In this technique, antigen-coated red blood cells are prepared by mixing a soluble antigen with red blood cells that have been treated with tannic acid or chromium chloride, both of which promote adsorption of the antigen to the surface of the cells. Serum containing antibody is serially diluted into microtiter plate wells, and the antigen-coated red blood cells are then added to each well; agglutination is assessed by the size of the characteristic spread pattern of agglutinated red blood cells on the bottom of the well, like the pattern seen in agglutination reactions (see Figure 6-8).

Over the past several years, there has been a shift away from red blood cells to synthetic particles, such as latex beads, as matrices for agglutination reactions. Once the antigen has been coupled to the latex beads, the preparation can either be used immediately or stored for later use. The use of synthetic beads offers the advantages of consistency, uniformity, and stability. Furthermore, agglutination reactions employing synthetic beads can be read rapidly, often within 3 to 5 minutes of mixing the beads with the test sample. Like hemagglutination reactions, agglutination reactions are simple to perform, do not require expensive equipment, and can detect small amounts of antibody (concentrations as low as nanograms per milliliter).

Agglutination Inhibition

A modification of the agglutination reaction, called **agglutination inhibition,** provides a highly sensitive assay for small quantities of an antigen. For example, one of the early types of home pregnancy test kits included latex particles coated with human chorionic gonadotropin (HCG) and antibody to HCG (Figure 6-9). The addition of urine from a pregnant woman, which contained HCG, inhibited agglutination of the latex particles when the anti-HCG antibody was added; thus the absence of agglutination indicated pregnancy.

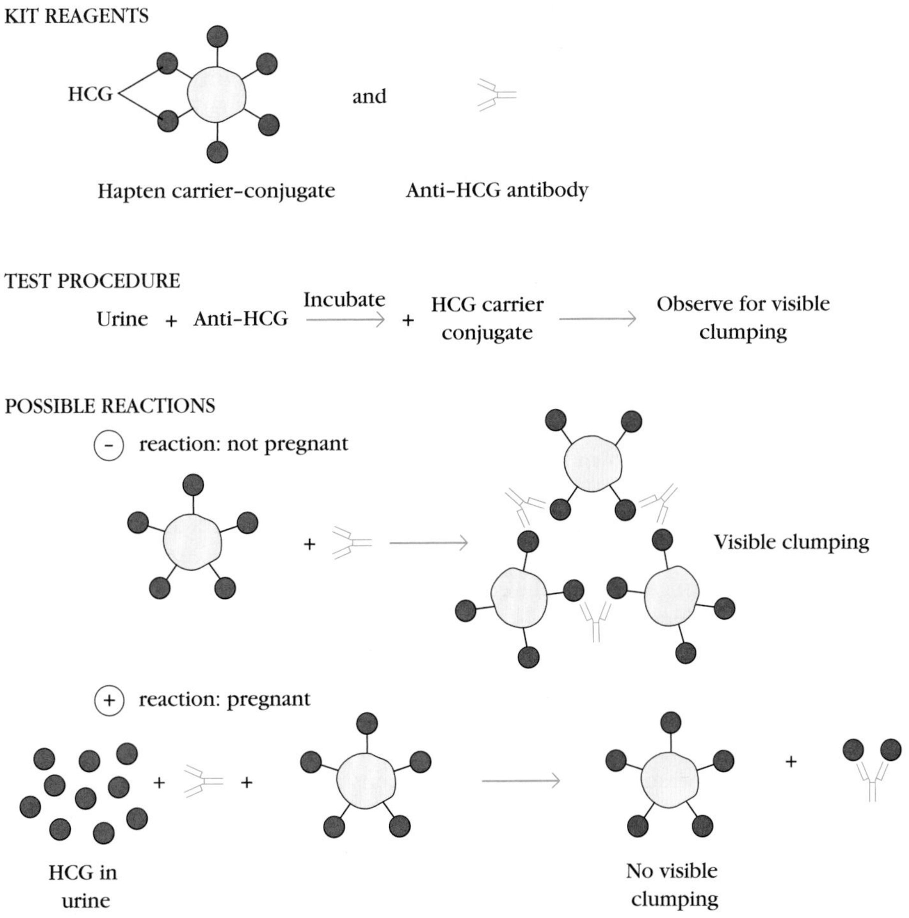

KIT REAGENTS

HCG

and

Hapten carrier-conjugate

Anti-HCG antibody

TEST PROCEDURE

Urine + Anti-HCG $\xrightarrow{\text{Incubate}}$ + HCG carrier conjugate ⟶ Observe for visible clumping

POSSIBLE REACTIONS

(−) reaction: not pregnant

Visible clumping

(+) reaction: pregnant

HCG in urine

No visible clumping

FIGURE 6-9 The early home pregnancy test kit employed hapten inhibition to determine the presence or absence of human chorionic gonadotropin (HCG). The original test kits used the presence or absence of visible clumping to determine whether HCG was present. If a woman was not pregnant, her urine would not contain HCG; in this case, the anti-HCG antibodies and HCG-carrier conjugate in the kit would react, producing visible clumping. If a woman was pregnant, the HCG in her urine would bind to the anti-HCG antibodies, thus inhibiting the subsequent binding of the antibody to the HCG-carrier conjugate. Because of this inhibition, no visible clumping occurred if a woman was pregnant. The kits currently on the market use ELISA-based assays (see Figure 6-11).

Agglutination inhibition assays also can be used to determine if an individual is using certain types of illegal drugs, such as cocaine or heroin. A urine or blood sample is first incubated with antibody specific for the suspected drug. Then red blood cells (or other particles) coated with the drug are added. If the red blood cells are not agglutinated by the antibody, it indicates the sample contained an antigen recognized by the antibody, suggesting that the individual was using the illicit drug. One problem with these tests is that some legal drugs have chemical structures similar to those of illicit drugs, and these legal drugs may thus cross-react with the antibody, giving a false-positive reaction. For this reason a positive reaction must be confirmed by a nonimmunologic method.

Agglutination inhibition assays are widely used in clinical laboratories to determine whether an individual has been exposed to certain types of viruses that cause agglutination of red blood cells. If an individual's serum contains specific antiviral antibodies, then the antibodies will bind to the virus and interfere with hemagglutination by the virus. This technique is commonly used in premarital testing to determine the immune status of women with respect to rubella virus. The reciprocal of the last serum dilution to show inhibition of rubella hemagglutination is the titer of the serum. A titer greater than 10 (1:10 dilution) indicates that a woman is immune to rubella, whereas a titer of less than 10 is indicative of a lack of immunity and the need for immunization with the rubella vaccine.

Radioimmunoassay

One of the most sensitive techniques for detecting antigen or antibody is **radioimmunoassay (RIA).** The technique was first developed by two endocrinologists, S. A. Berson and

Rosalyn Yalow, in 1960 to determine levels of insulin–anti-insulin complexes in diabetics. Although their original attempts to publish a report of this research met with some resistance from immunologists, the technique soon proved its own value for measuring hormones, serum proteins, drugs, and vitamins at concentrations of 0.001 *micrograms* per milliliter or less. In 1977, some years after Berson's death, the significance of the technique was acknowledged by the award of a Nobel Prize to Yalow.

The principle of RIA involves competitive binding of radiolabeled antigen and unlabeled antigen to a high-affinity antibody. The labeled antigen is mixed with antibody at a concentration that saturates the antigen-binding sites of the antibody molecule, and then increasing amounts of the test sample containing unlabeled antigen of unknown concentration are added. The antibody does not distinguish labeled from unlabeled antigen, and so the two kinds of antigen compete for available binding sites on the antibody. With increasing concentrations of unlabeled antigen, more labeled antigen will be displaced from the binding sites.

The antigen is generally labeled with a gamma-emitting isotope such as ^{125}I, but beta-emitting isotopes such as tritium (^{3}H) are also routinely used as labels. The decrease in amount of radiolabeled antigen bound to specific antibody in the presence of the test sample is measured in order to determine the amount of antigen (insulin in the Yalow assay) present in the test sample. The radiolabeled antigen is part of the assay mixture; the test sample may be a complex mixture, such as serum or other body fluids, which contains the unlabeled antigen. The first step in setting up an RIA is to determine the amount of antibody needed to bind 50%–70% of a fixed quantity of radioactive antigen (Ag*) in the assay mixture. This ratio of antibody to Ag* is chosen such that the number of epitopes presented by the labeled antigen always exceeds the total number of antibody binding sites. This insures that any unlabeled antigen added to the sample mixture will compete with radiolabeled antigen for the limited supply of antibody. Even a small amount of unlabeled antigen added to the assay mixture of labeled antigen and antibody will cause a decrease in the amount of radioactive antigen bound, and this decrease will be proportional to the amount of unlabeled antigen added. To determine the amount of labeled antigen bound, the Ag-Ab complex is precipitated to separate it from free antigen (not bound to Ab), and the radioactivity in the precipitate is measured. A standard curve can be generated using unlabeled antigen samples of known concentration (in place of the test sample), and from this plot the amount of antigen in the test mixture may be precisely determined.

Several methods have been developed for separating the bound antigen from the free antigen in RIA. One method involves precipitating the Ag-Ab complex with a secondary anti-isotype antiserum. For example, if the Ag-Ab complex contains rabbit IgG antibody, then goat anti-rabbit IgG will bind to the rabbit IgG and precipitate the complex. Another method makes use of the fact that protein A of *Staphylococcus aureus* has high affinity for IgG. If the Ag-Ab complex contains an IgG antibody, the complex can be precipitated

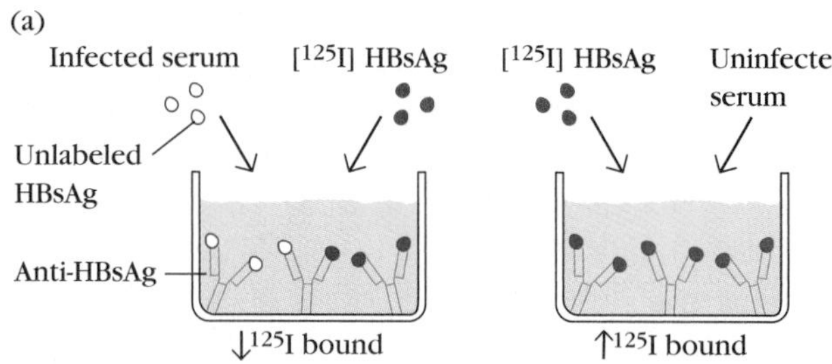

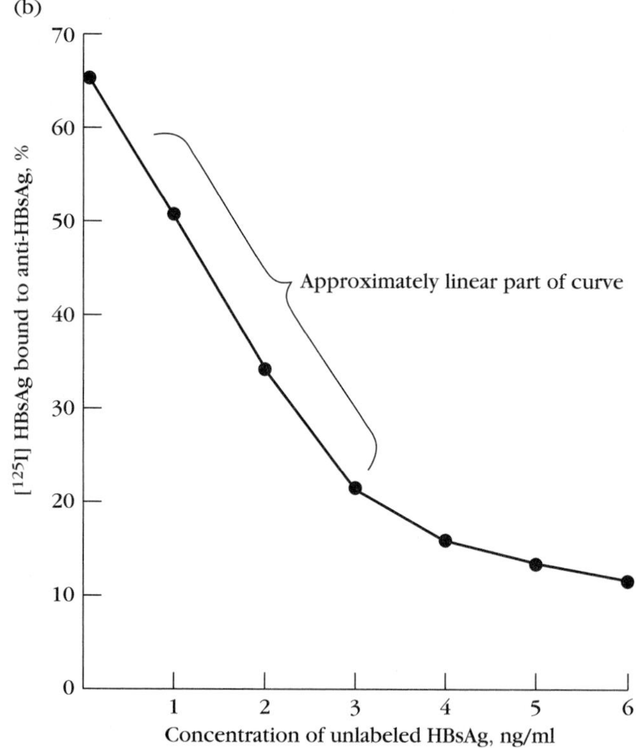

FIGURE 6-10 A solid-phase radioimmunoassay (RIA) to detect hepatitis B virus in blood samples. (a) Microtiter wells are coated with a constant amount of antibody specific for HBsAg, the surface antigen on hepatitis B virions. A serum sample and [^{125}I]HBsAg are then added. After incubation, the supernatant is removed and the amount of radioactivity bound to the antibody is determined. If the sample is infected, the amount of label bound will be less than in controls with uninfected serum. (b) A standard curve is obtained by adding increasing concentrations of unlabeled HBsAg to a fixed quantity of [^{125}I]HBsAg and specific antibody. From the plot of the percentage of labeled antigen bound versus the concentration of unlabeled antigen, the concentration of HBsAg in unknown serum samples can be determined by using the linear part of the curve.

by mixing with formalin-killed *S. aureus.* After removal of the complex by either of these methods, the amount of free labeled antigen remaining in the supernatant can be measured in a radiation counter; subtracting this value from the total amount of labeled antigen added yields the amount of labeled antigen bound.

Various solid-phase RIAs have been developed that make it easier to separate the Ag-Ab complex from the unbound antigen. In some cases, the antibody is covalently cross-linked to Sepharose beads. The amount of radiolabeled antigen bound to the beads can be measured after the beads have been centrifuged and washed. Alternatively, the antibody can be immobilized on polystyrene or polyvinylchloride wells and the amount of free labeled antigen in the supernatant can be determined in a radiation counter. In another approach, the antibody is immobilized on the walls of microtiter wells and the amount of bound antigen determined. This procedure is well suited for determining the concentration of a particular antigen in large numbers of samples. For example, a microtiter RIA has been widely used to screen for the presence of the hepatitis B virus (Figure 6-10). RIA screening of donor blood has sharply reduced the incidence of hepatitis B infections in recipients of blood transfusions.

Enzyme-Linked Immunosorbent Assay

Enzyme-linked immunosorbent assay, commonly known as **ELISA** (or EIA), is similar in principle to RIA but depends on an enzyme rather than a radioactive label. An enzyme conjugated with an antibody reacts with a colorless substrate to generate a colored reaction product. Such a substrate is called a **chromogenic substrate.** A number of enzymes have been employed for ELISA, including alkaline phosphatase, horseradish peroxidase, and β-galactosidase. These assays approach the sensitivity of RIAs and have the advantage of being safer and less costly.

A number of variations of ELISA have been developed, allowing qualitative detection or quantitative measurement of either antigen or antibody. Each type of ELISA can be used qualitatively to detect the presence of antibody or antigen. Alternatively, a standard curve based on known concentrations of antibody or antigen is prepared, from which the unknown concentration of a sample can be determined.

Indirect ELISA

Antibody can be detected or quantitatively determined with an indirect ELISA (Figure 6-11a). Serum or some other sample containing primary antibody (Ab_1) is added to an antigen-coated microtiter well and allowed to react with the antigen attached to the well. After any free Ab_1 is washed away, the presence of antibody bound to the antigen is detected by adding an enzyme-conjugated secondary anti-isotype antibody (Ab_2), which binds to the primary antibody. Any free Ab_2 then is washed away, and a substrate for the enzyme is added. The amount of colored reaction product that forms is measured by specialized spectrophotometric plate readers, which can measure the absorbance of all of the wells of a 96-well plate in less than a few seconds.

Indirect ELISA is the method of choice to detect the presence of serum antibodies against human immunodeficiency virus (HIV), the causative agent of AIDS. In this assay recombinant envelope and core proteins of HIV are adsorbed as solid-phase antigens to microtiter wells. Individuals infected with HIV will produce serum antibodies to epitopes on these viral proteins. Generally, serum antibodies to HIV can be detected by indirect ELISA within 6 weeks of infection.

Sandwich ELISA

Antigen can be detected or measured by a sandwich ELISA (Figure 6-11b). In this technique, the antibody (rather than the antigen) is immobilized on a microtiter well. A sample containing antigen is added and allowed to react with the immobilized antibody. After the well is washed, a second enzyme-linked antibody specific for a different epitope on the antigen is added and allowed to react with the bound antigen. After any free second antibody is removed by washing, substrate is added, and the colored reaction product is measured.

Competitive ELISA

Another variation for measuring amounts of antigen is competitive ELISA (Figure 6-11c). In this technique, antibody is first incubated in solution with a sample containing antigen. The antigen-antibody mixture is then added to an antigen-coated microtiter well. The more antigen present in the sample, the less free antibody will be available to bind to the antigen-coated well. Addition of an enzyme-conjugated secondary antibody (Ab_2) specific for the isotype of the primary antibody can be used to determine the amount of primary antibody bound to the well as in an indirect ELISA. In the competitive assay, however, the higher the concentration of antigen in the original sample, the lower the absorbance.

Chemiluminescence

Measurement of light produced by chemiluminescence during certain chemical reactions provides a convenient and highly sensitive alternative to absorbance measurements in ELISA assays. In versions of the ELISA using chemiluminescence, a luxogenic (light-generating) substrate takes the place of the chromogenic substrate in conventional ELISA reactions. For example, oxidation of the compound luminol by H_2O_2 and the enzyme horseradish peroxidase (HRP) produces light:

$$\text{Ab-HRP} + \text{Ag} \longrightarrow \text{Ab-HRP-Ag} \xrightarrow{\text{luminol} + H_2O_2} \text{light}$$

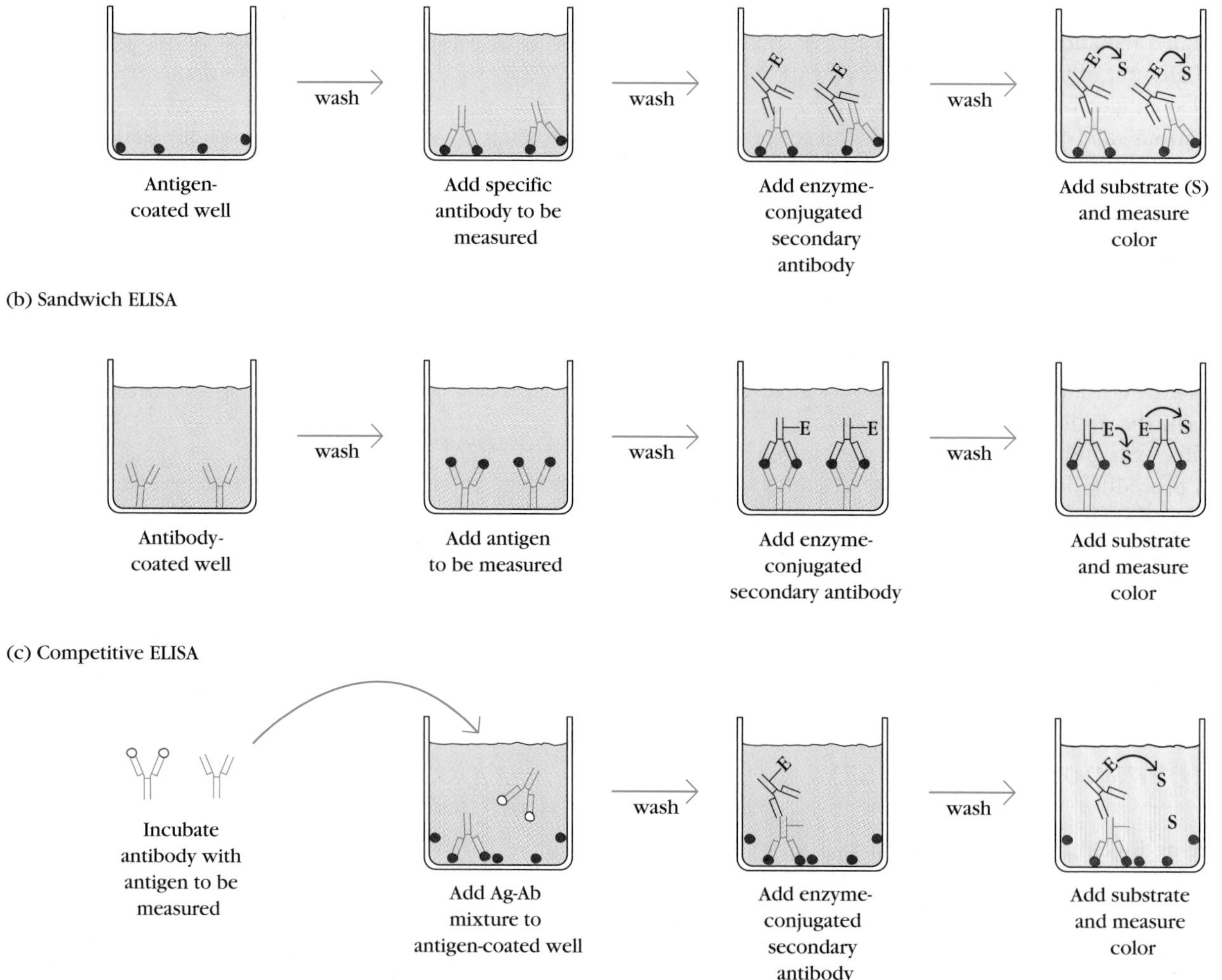

FIGURE 6-11 Variations in the enzyme-linked immunosorbent assay (ELISA) technique allow determination of antibody or antigen. Each assay can be used qualitatively, or quantitatively by comparison with standard curves prepared with known concentrations of antibody or antigen. Antibody can be determined with an indirect ELISA (a), whereas antigen can be determined with a sandwich ELISA (b) or competitive ELISA (c). In the competitive ELISA, which is an inhibition-type assay, the concentration of antigen is inversely proportional to the color produced.

The appeal of chemiluminescence assays over chromogenic ones is enhanced sensitivity. In general, the detection limit can be increased at least ten-fold by switching from a chromogenic to a luxogenic substrate, and with the addition of enhancing agents, more than 200-fold. In fact, under ideal conditions, as little as 5×10^{-18} moles of target antigen have been detected.

ELISPOT Assay

A modification of the ELISA assay called the ELISPOT assay allows the quantitative determination of the number of cells in a population that are producing antibodies specific for a given antigen or an antigen for which one has a specific antibody (Figure 6-12). In this approach, the plates are coated with the antigen (capture antigen) recognized by the antibody of interest or with the antibody (capture antibody) specific for the antigen whose production is being assayed. A suspension of the cell population under investigation is then added to the coated plates and incubated. The cells settle onto the surface of the plate, and secreted molecules reactive with the capture molecules are bound by the capture molecules in the vicinity of the secreting cells, producing a ring of antigen-antibody complexes around each cell that is producing the molecule of interest. The plate is then washed and an enzyme-linked

Go to www.whfreeman.com/immunology Animation
hCG Pregnancy Test (ELISA)

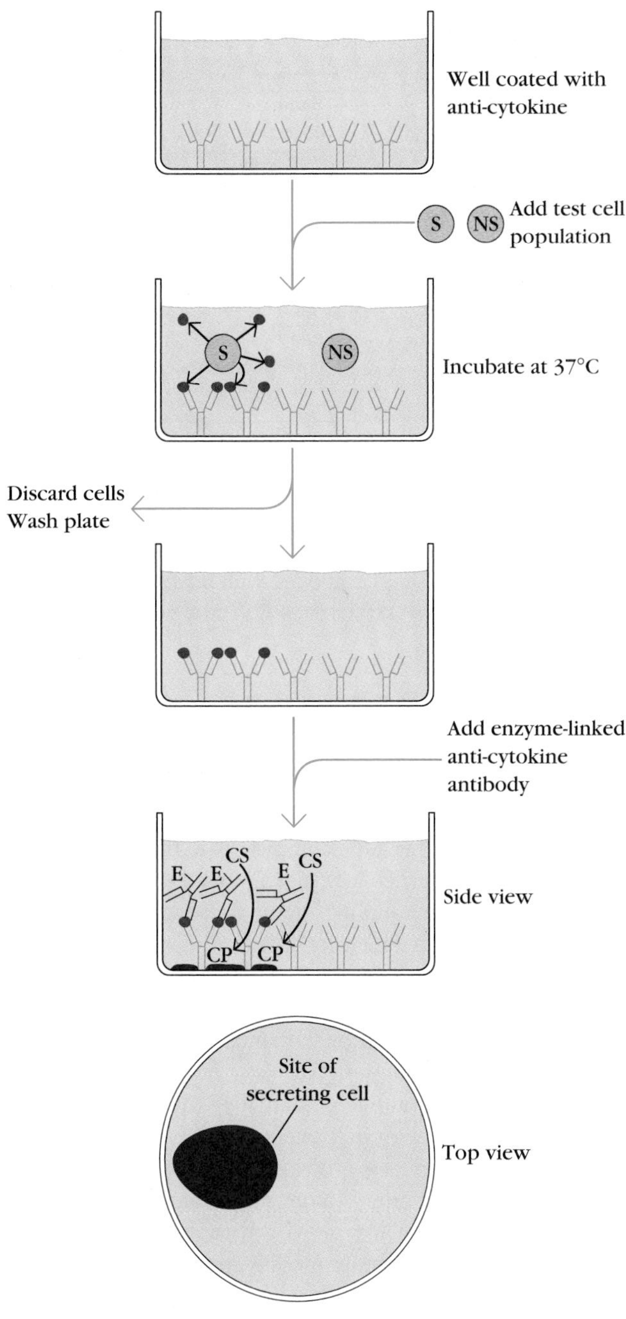

FIGURE 6-12 In the ELISPOT assay, a well is coated with antibody against the antigen of interest, a cytokine in this example, and then a suspension of a cell population thought to contain some members synthesizing and secreting (S) the cytokine and some that are nonsecretors (NS) are layered onto the bottom of the well and incubated. Most of the cytokine molecules secreted by a particular cell react with nearby well-bound antibodies. At the close of the incubation period, the well is washed and an enzyme-labeled anti-cytokine antibody is added. After washing away unbound antibody, a chromogenic substrate (CS) that forms an insoluble colored product (CP) is added. The colored product (purple) precipitates and forms a spot only on the areas of the well where cytokine-secreting cells had been deposited. By counting the number of colored spots, it is possible to determine how many cytokine-secreting cells were present in the added cell suspension.

antibody specific for the secreted antigen or specific for the species (e.g., goat anti-rabbit) of the secreted antibody is added and allowed to bind. Subsequent development of the assay by addition of a suitable chromogenic or chemiluminescence-producing substrate reveals the position of each antibody- or antigen-producing cell as a point of color or light.

Western Blotting

Identification of a specific protein in a complex mixture of proteins can be accomplished by a technique known as **Western blotting,** named for its similarity to Southern blotting, which detects DNA fragments, and Northern blotting, which detects mRNAs. In Western blotting, a protein mixture is electrophoretically separated on an **SDS-polyacrylamide gel (SDS-PAGE)**, a polyacrylamide slab gel infused with sodium dodecyl sulfate (SDS), a dissociating agent. The protein bands are transferred to a nitrocellulose membrane by electrophoresis and the individual protein bands are identified by flooding the nitrocellulose membrane with radiolabeled or enzyme-linked polyclonal or monoclonal antibody specific for the protein of interest. The Ag-Ab complexes that form on the band containing the protein recognized by the antibody can be visualized in a variety of ways. If the protein of interest was bound by a radioactive antibody, its position on the blot can be determined by exposing the membrane to a sheet of x-ray film, a procedure called autoradiography (Figure 6-13). However, the most generally used detection procedures employ enzyme-linked antibodies against the protein. After binding of the enzyme-antibody conjugate, addition of a chromogenic substrate that produces a highly colored and insoluble product causes the appearance of a colored band at the site of the target antigen. The site of the protein of interest can be determined with much higher sensitivity if a chemiluminescent compound along with suitable enhancing agents is used to produce light at the antigen site.

Western blotting can also identify a specific antibody in a mixture. In this case, known antigens of well-defined molecular weight are separated by SDS-PAGE and blotted onto nitrocellulose. The separated bands of known antigens are then probed with the sample suspected of containing antibody

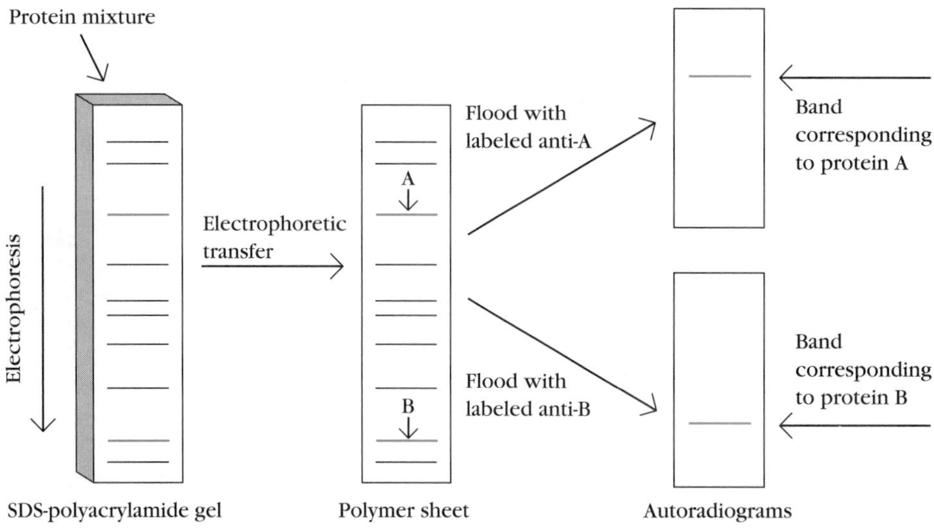

FIGURE 6-13 In Western blotting, a protein mixture is separated by electrophoresis; then the protein bands are transferred by electrophoresis onto a nitrocellulose or other polymer sheet. After the sheet is flooded with radiolabeled specific antibodies, the various protein bands can be visualized by autoradiography.

specific for one or more of these antigens. Reaction of an antibody with a band is detected by using either radiolabeled or enzyme-linked secondary antibody that is specific for the species of the antibodies in the test sample. The most widely used application of this procedure is in confirmatory testing for HIV, where Western blotting is used to determine whether the patient has antibodies that react with one or more viral proteins.

Immunoprecipitation

The immunoprecipitation technique has the advantages of allowing the isolation of the antigen of interest for further analysis. It also provides a sensitive assay for the presence of a particular antigen in a given cell or tissue type. An extract produced by disruption of cells or tissues is mixed with an antibody against the antigen of interest in order to form an antigen-antibody complex that will precipitate. However, if the antigen concentration is low, as it often is in cell and tissue extracts, the assembly of antigen-antibody complexes into precipitates can take hours, even days, and it is difficult to isolate the small amount of immunoprecipitate that forms.

Fortunately, there are a number of ways to avoid these limitations. One of these is to attach the antibody to a solid support, such as a synthetic bead, which allows the antigen-antibody complex to be collected by centrifugation. Another is to add a secondary antibody specific for the primary antibody to bind the antigen-antibody complexes. If the secondary antibody is attached to a bead, the immune complexes can be collected by centrifugation. Alternatively, bead-coupled protein A or bead-coupled protein G can be used to bind the secondary antibody and any antigen-antibody complexes it has bound, and the complexes are then collected by centrifugation. A particularly ingenious version of this procedure involves the coupling of the secondary antibody to magnetic beads. After the secondary antibody binds to the primary antibody, immunoprecipitates are collected by placing a magnet against the side of the tube (Figure 6-14).

When used in conjunction with biosynthetic radioisotope labeling, immunoprecipitation can also be used to determine whether a particular antigen is actually synthesized by a cell or tissue. Radiolabeling of proteins synthesized by cells of interest can be done by growing the cells in cell culture medium containing one or more radiolabeled amino acids. Generally, the amino acids used for this application are those most resistant to metabolic modification, such as leucine, cysteine, or methionine. After growth in the radioactive medium, the cells are lysed and subjected to a primary antibody specific for the antigen of interest. The Ag-Ab complex is collected by immunoprecipitation, washed free of unincorporated radiolabeled amino acid and other impurities, and then analyzed. The complex can be counted in a scintillation counter to obtain a quantitative determination of the amount of the protein synthesized. Further analysis often involves disruption of the complex, usually by use of SDS and heating, so that the identity of the immunoprecipitated antigen can be confirmed by checking that its molecular weight is that expected for the antigen of interest. This is done by separation of the disrupted complex by SDS-PAGE and subsequent autoradiography to determine the position of the radiolabeled antigen on the gel.

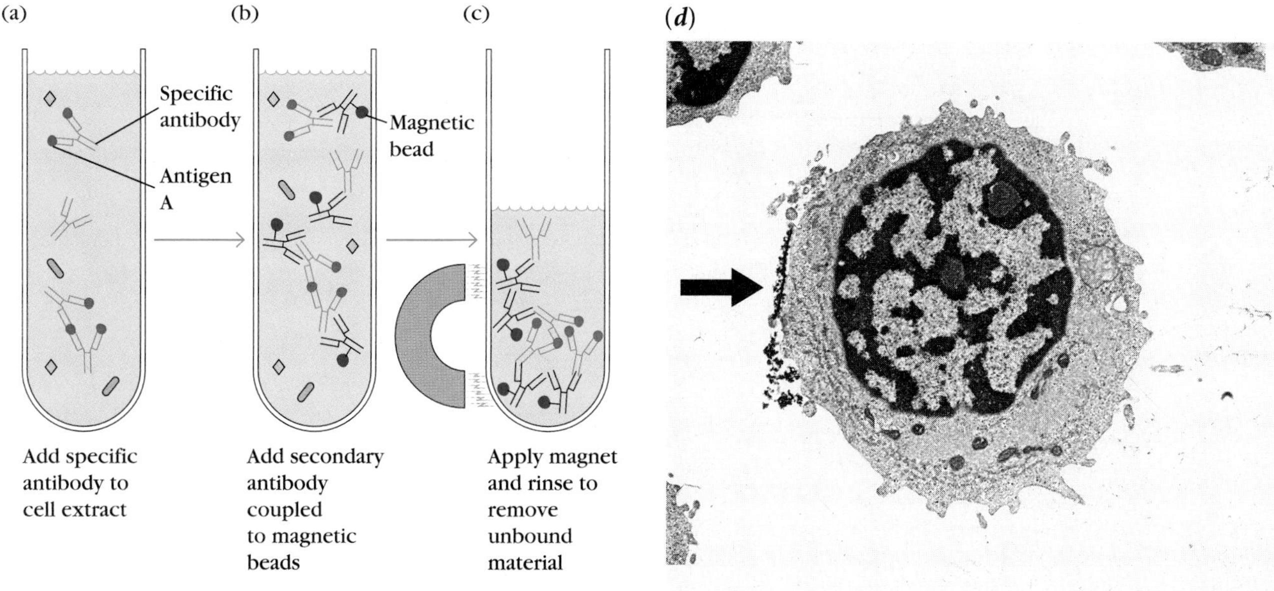

FIGURE 6-14 Immunoprecipitates can be collected using magnetic beads coupled to a secondary antibody. (a) Treatment of a cell extract containing antigen A (red) with a mouse anti-A antibody (blue) results in the formation of antigen-antibody complexes. (b) Addition of magnetic beads to which a rabbit anti-mouse antibody is linked binds the antigen-antibody complexes (and any unreacted mouse Ig). (c) Placing a magnet against the side of the tube allows the rapid collection of the antigen-antibody complexes. After rinsing to remove any unbound material, the antigen-antibody complexes can be dissociated and the antigen studied. (d) An electron micrograph showing a cell with magnetic beads (arrow) attached to its surface via antibodies. [Part (d) P Groscurth, Institute of Anatomy, University of Zurich-Irchel.]

Immunofluorescence

In 1944, Albert Coons showed that antibodies could be labeled with molecules that have the property of fluorescence. Fluorescent molecules absorb light of one wavelength (excitation) and emit light of another wavelength (emission). If antibody molecules are tagged with a fluorescent dye, or **fluorochrome,** immune complexes containing these fluorescently labeled antibodies (FA) can be detected by colored light emission when excited by light of the appropriate wavelength. Antibody molecules bound to antigens in cells or tissue sections can similarly be visualized. The emitted light can be viewed with a fluorescence microscope, which is equipped with a UV light source. In this technique, known as **immunofluorescence,** the most commonly used fluorescent dyes are fluorescein and rhodamine, but other highly fluorescent substances, such as phycoerythrin and phycobiliproteins have also come into use. The dyes can be conjugated to the Fc region of an antibody molecule without affecting the specificity of the antibody. Each of these dyes absorbs light at one wavelength and emits light at a longer wavelength:

- **Fluorescein,** an organic dye that is the most widely used label for immunofluorescence procedures, absorbs blue light (490 nm) and emits an intense yellow-green fluorescence (517 nm).
- **Rhodamine,** another organic dye, absorbs in the yellow-green range (515 nm) and emits a deep red fluorescence (546 nm). Because it emits fluorescence at a longer wavelength than fluorescein, it can be used in two-color immunofluorescence assays. An antibody specific to one determinant is labeled with fluorescein, and an antibody recognizing a different antigen is labeled with rhodamine. The location of the fluorescein-tagged antibody will be visible by its yellow-green color, easy to distinguish from the red color emitted where the rhodamine-tagged antibody has bound. By conjugating fluorescein to one antibody and rhodamine to another antibody, one can visualize simultaneously two different cell membrane antigens on the same cell, for example.
- **Phycoerythrin** and other *phycobiliproteins* are light-gathering proteins that play important roles in photosynthesis in some species of algae. Because they are efficient absorbers of light (~30-fold greater than fluorescein) and brilliant emitters of red fluorescence, these proteins have become widely used labels for immunofluorescence.

Fluorescent-antibody staining of cell membrane molecules or tissue sections can be direct or indirect (Figure 6-15). In **direct staining,** the specific antibody (the primary antibody) is directly conjugated with fluorescein; in **indirect**

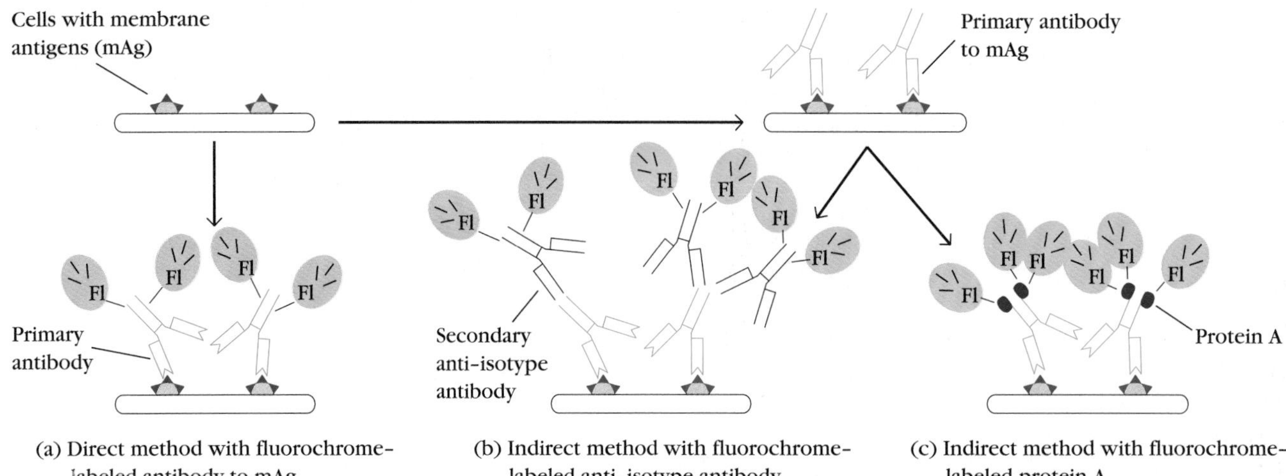

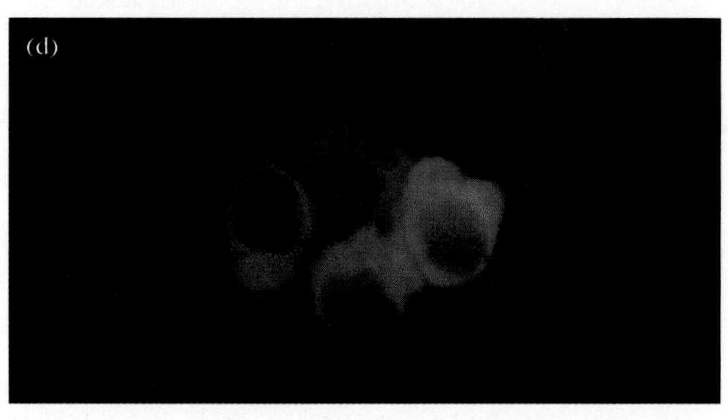

FIGURE 6-15 Direct and indirect immunofluorescence staining of membrane antigen (mAg). Cells are affixed to a microscope slide. In the direct method (a), cells are stained with anti-mAg antibody that is labeled with a fluorochrome (Fl). In the indirect methods (b and c), cells are first incubated with unlabeled anti-mAg antibody and then stained with a fluorochrome-labeled secondary reagent that binds to the primary antibody. Cells are viewed under a fluorescence microscope to see if they have been stained. (d) In this micrograph, antibody molecules bearing μ heavy chains are detected by indirect staining of cells with rhodamine-conjugated second antibody. [Part (d) HA Schreuder et al, 1997, *Nature* **386:**196, courtesy H Schreuder, Hoechst Marion Roussel.]

staining, the primary antibody is unlabeled and is detected with an additional fluorochrome-labeled reagent. A number of reagents have been developed for indirect staining. The most common is a secondary antibody, a *fluorochrome-labeled anti-isotype antibody,* such as fluorescein-labeled goat anti-mouse immunoglobulin. Another reagent is *fluorochrome-labeled protein A* from *Staphylococcus aureus,* which binds with high affinity to the Fc region of IgG antibody molecules. A third indirect approach uses a secondary biotin-conjugated anti-isotype antibody followed by fluorochrome-conjugated avidin, a protein that binds to biotin with extremely high affinity.

Indirect immunofluorescence staining has two advantages over direct staining. First, the primary antibody does not need to be conjugated with a fluorochrome. Because the supply of primary antibody is often a limiting factor, indirect methods avoid the loss of antibody that usually occurs during the conjugation reaction. Second, indirect methods increase the sensitivity of staining because multiple molecules of the fluorochrome reagent bind to each primary antibody molecule, increasing the amount of light emitted at the location of each primary antibody molecule.

Immunofluorescence has been applied to identify a number of subpopulations of lymphocytes, notably the $CD4^+$ and $CD8^+$ T-cell subpopulations. The technique is also suitable for identifying bacterial species, detecting Ag-Ab complexes in autoimmune disease, detecting complement components in tissues, and localizing hormones and other cellular products stained in situ. Indeed, a major application of the fluorescent antibody technique is the localization of antigens in tissue sections or in subcellular compartments. Because it can be used to map the actual location of target antigens, fluorescence microscopy is a powerful tool for relating the molecular architecture of tissues and organs to their overall gross anatomy.

Flow Cytometry and Fluorescence

These fluorescent antibody techniques are extremely valuable qualitative tools, but they do not provide quantitative data. This shortcoming was remedied by development of flow cytometry, a version of which is called the FACS (fluorescence-activated cell sorter), which was designed to automate the analysis and separation of cells stained with fluorescent antibody. The FACS uses a laser beam and light detector to count single intact cells in suspension (Figure 6-16). Every time a cell passes the laser beam in the FACS, the laser light is deflected from the detector, and this inter-

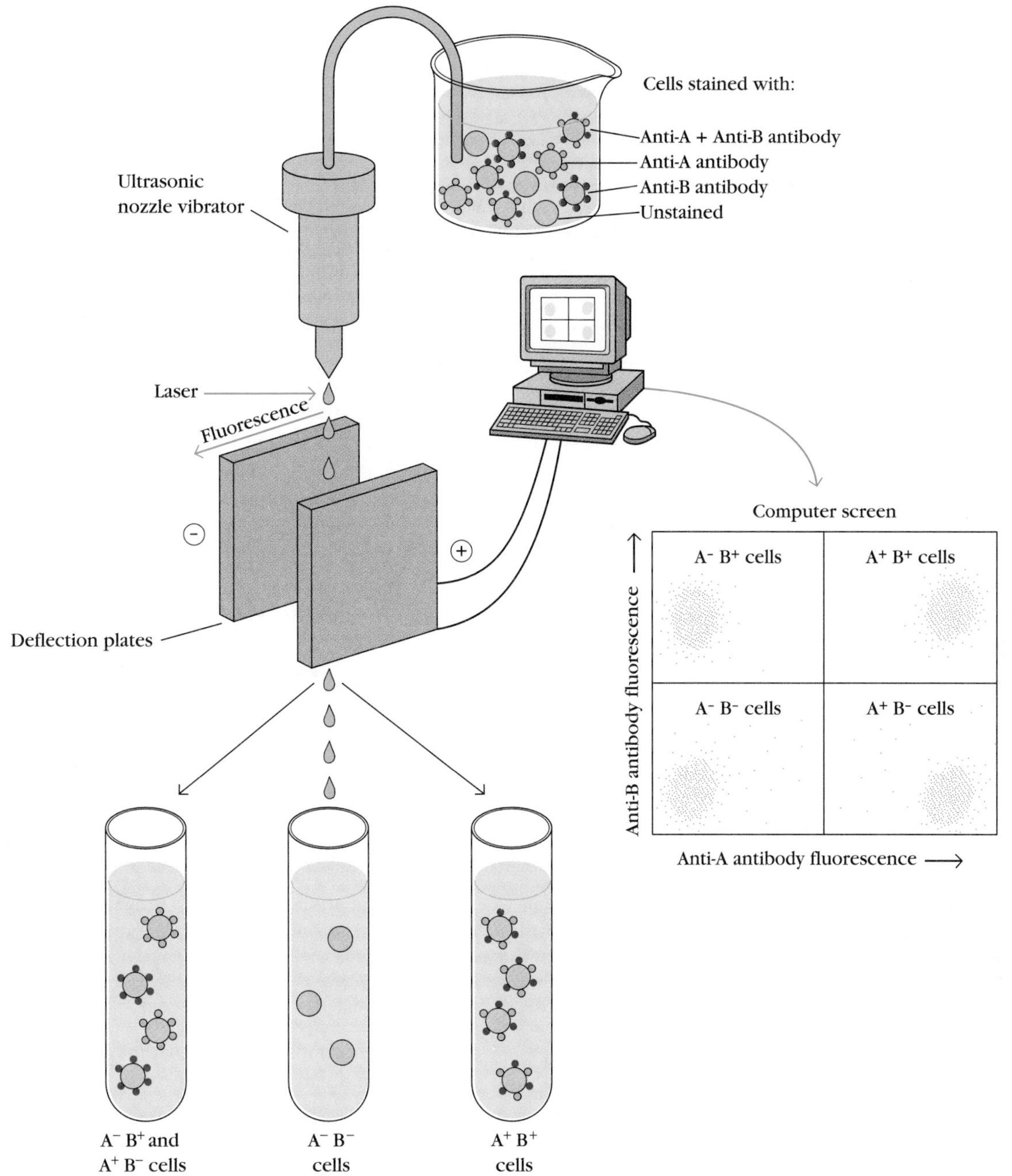

FIGURE 6-16 Separation of fluorochrome-labeled cells with the fluorescence-activated cell sorter (FACS). In the example shown, a mixed cell population is stained with two antibodies, one specific for surface antigen A and the other specific for surface antigen B. The anti-A antibodies are labeled with fluorescein (green) and the anti-B antibodies with rhodamine (red). The stained cells are loaded into the sample chamber of the FACS. The cells are expelled, one at a time, from a small vibrating nozzle that generates microdroplets, each containing no more than a single cell. As it leaves the nozzle, each droplet receives a small electrical charge, and the computer that controls the flow cytometer can detect exactly when a drop generated by the nozzle passes through the beam of laser light that excites the fluorochrome. The intensity of the fluorescence emitted by each droplet that contains a cell is monitored by a detector and displayed on a computer screen. Because the computer tracks the position of each droplet, it is possible to determine when a particular droplet will arrive between the deflection plates. By applying a momentary charge to the deflection plates when a droplet is passing between them, it is possible to deflect the path of a particular droplet into one or another collecting vessel. This allows the sorting of a population of cells into subpopulations having different profiles of surface markers.

In the computer display, each dot represents a cell. Cells that fall into the lower left-hand panel have background levels of fluorescence and are judged not to have reacted with either antibody anti-A or anti-B. Those that appear in the upper left panel reacted with anti-B but not anti-A, and those in the lower right panel reacted with anti-A but not anti-B. The upper right panel contains cells that react with both anti-A and anti-B. In the example shown here, the A^-B^- and the A^+B^+ subpopulations have each been sorted into a separate tube. Staining with anti-A and anti-B fluorescent antibodies allows four subpopulations to be distinguished: A^-B^-, A^+B^+, A^-B^+, and A^+B^-.

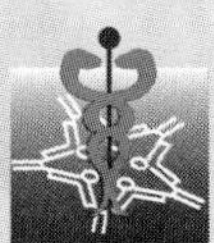

CLINICAL FOCUS

FLOW CYTOMETRY AND LEUKEMIA TYPING

Leukemia is the unlimited and unchecked proliferation of an abnormal clone of hematopoietic cells. Typically, leukemic cells respond poorly or inappropriately to regulatory signals, display aberrant patterns of differentiation, or even fail to differentiate. Furthermore, they sometimes suppress the growth of normal lymphoid and myeloid cells. Leukemia can arise at any maturational stage of any one of the hematopoietic lineages. Lymphocytic leukemias display many characteristics of cells of the lymphoid lineage; another broad group, myelogenous leukemias, have attributes of members of the myeloid lineage. Aside from lineage, many leukemias can be classified as acute or chronic. Some examples are acute lymphocytic leukemia (ALL), the most common childhood leukemia; acute myelogenous leukemia (AML), found more often in adults than in children; and chronic lymphocytic leukemia (CLL), which is rarely seen in children but is the most common form of adult leukemia in the Western world. A fourth type, chronic myelogenous leukemia (CML), occurs much more often in older adults than in children.

The diagnosis of leukemia is made on the basis of two findings. One of these is the detection of abnormal cells in the bloodstream and the other is observation of abnormal cells in the bone marrow. Clinical experience has shown that designing the most appropriate therapy for the patient requires knowing which type of leukemia is present. In this regard, two of the important questions are: (1) What is the lineage of the abnormal cells and (2) What is their maturational stage? A variety of approaches, including cytologic examination of cell morphology and staining characteristics, immunophenotyping, and, in some cases, an analysis of gene rearrangements, are useful in answering these questions. One of the most powerful of these approaches is immunophenotyping, the determination of the profile of selected cell surface markers displayed by the leukemic cell. Although leukemia-specific antigens have not yet been found, profiles of expressed surface antigens often can establish cell lineage, and they are frequently helpful in determining the maturational stages present in leukemic cell populations. For example, an abnormal cell that displays surface immunoglobulin would be assigned to the B cell lineage and its maturational stage would be that of a mature B cell. On the other hand, a cell that had cytoplasmic μ heavy chains, but no surface immunoglobulin, would be a B-lineage leukemic cell but at the maturational stage of a pre-B cell. The most efficient and precise technology for immunophenotyping uses flow cytometry and monoclonal antibodies. The availability of monoclonal antibodies specific for each of the more than 170 antigens found on various types and subtypes of

ruption of the laser signal is recorded. Those cells having a fluorescently tagged antibody bound to their cell surface antigens are excited by the laser and emit light that is recorded by a second detector system located at a right angle to the laser beam. The simplest form of the instrument counts each cell as it passes the laser beam and records the level of fluorescence the cell emits; an attached computer generates plots of the number of cells as the ordinate and their fluorescence intensity as the abscissa. Use of the instrument to determine which and how many members of a cell population bind fluorescently labeled antibodies is called analysis; use of the instrument to place cells having different patterns of reactivity into different containers is called cell sorting.

The FACS has multiple applications to clinical and research problems. A common clinical use is to determine the kind and number of white blood cells in each population in patients' blood samples. By treating appropriately processed blood samples with a fluorescently labeled antibody and performing FACS analysis, one can obtain the following information:

- How many cells express the target antigen as an absolute number and also as a percentage of cells passing the beam. For example, if one uses a fluorescent antibody specific for an antigen present on all T cells, it would be possible to determine the percentage of T cells in the total white blood cell population. Then, using the cell-sorting capabilities of the FACS, it would be possible to isolate the T-cell fraction of the leukocyte population.
- The distribution of cells in a sample population according to antigen densities as determined by fluorescence intensity. It is thus possible to obtain a measure of the distribution of antigen density within the population of cells that possess the antigen. This is a powerful feature of the instrument, since the same type of cell may express different levels of antigen depending upon its developmental or physiological state.
- The size of cells. This information is derived from analysis of the light-scattering properties of members of the cell population under examination.

FACS technology now allows the use of multiple fluorescent antibodies. Highly sophisticated flow cytometers simultaneously analyze cell populations that have been labeled

hematopoietic cells has made it possible to identify patterns of antigen expression that are typical of cell lineages, maturational stages, and a number of different types of leukemia. Most cancer centers are equipped with flow cytometers that are capable of performing and interpreting the multiparameter analyses necessary to provide useful profiles of surface markers on tumor cell populations. Flow cytometric determination of immunophenotypes allows:

- Confirmation of diagnosis
- Diagnosis when no clear judgment can be made based on morphology or patterns of cytochemical staining
- Identification of aberrant antigen profiles that can help identify the return of leukemia during remission
- Improved prediction of the course of the disease

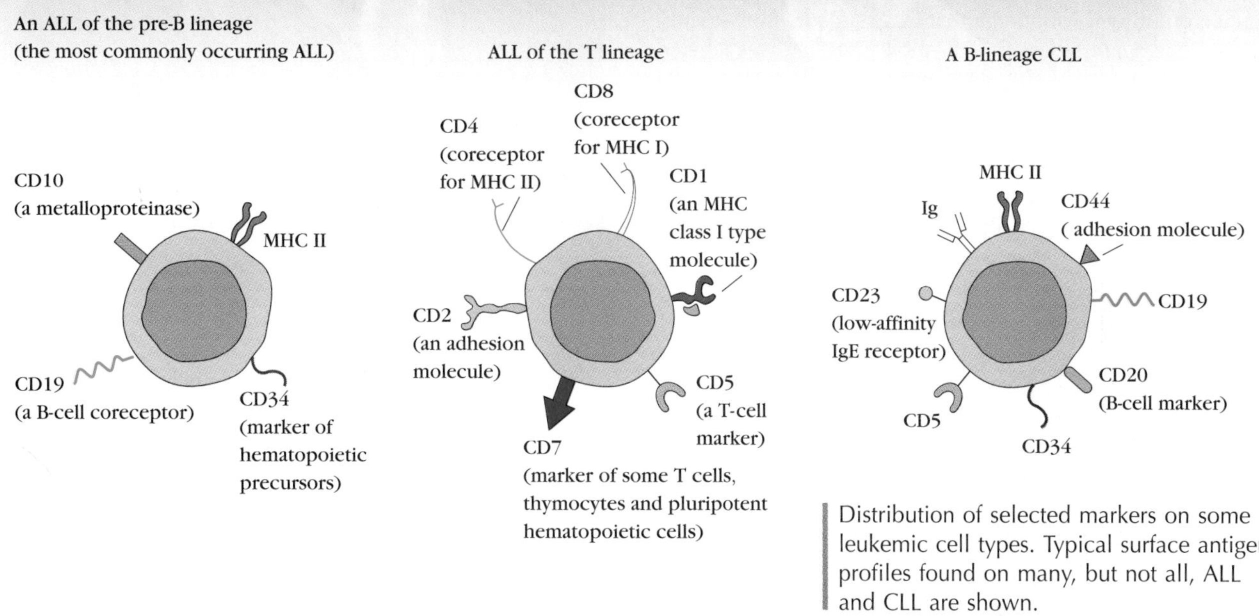

Distribution of selected markers on some leukemic cell types. Typical surface antigen profiles found on many, but not all, ALL and CLL are shown.

with two or even three different fluorescent antibodies. For example, if one reacts a blood sample with a fluorescein-tagged antibody specific for T cells, and also with a phycoerythrin-tagged antibody specific for B cells, the percentages of B and T cells may be determined simultaneously with a single analysis. Numerous variations of such "two-color" analyses are routinely carried out, and "three-color" experiments are not uncommon with modern instruments and sophisticated computer analysis.

Flow cytometry now occupies a key position in immunology and cell biology, and it has become an indispensable clinical tool as well. In many medical centers, the FACS is one of the essential tools for the detection and classification of leukemias (see the Clinical Focus). The choice of treatment for leukemia depends heavily on the cell types involved, making precise identification of the neoplastic cells an essential part of clinical practice. Likewise, the rapid measurement of T-cell subpopulations, an important prognostic indicator in AIDS, is routinely done by FACS analysis. In this procedure, labeled monoclonal antibodies against the major T-cell subtypes bearing the CD4 and CD8 antigens are used to determine their ratios in the patient's blood. When the number of CD4 T cells falls below a certain level, the patient is at high risk for opportunistic infections.

Immunoelectron Microscopy

The fine specificity of antibodies has made them powerful tools for visualizing specific intracellular tissue components by **immunoelectron microscopy.** In this technique, an electron-dense label is either conjugated to the Fc portion of a specific antibody for direct staining or conjugated to an anti-immunoglobulin reagent for indirect staining. A number of electron-dense labels have been employed, including ferritin and colloidal gold. Because the electron-dense label absorbs electrons, it can be visualized with the electron microscope as small black dots. In the case of immunogold labeling, different antibodies can be conjugated with gold particles of different sizes, allowing identification of several antigens within a cell by the different sizes of the electron-dense gold particles attached to the antibodies (Figure 6-17).

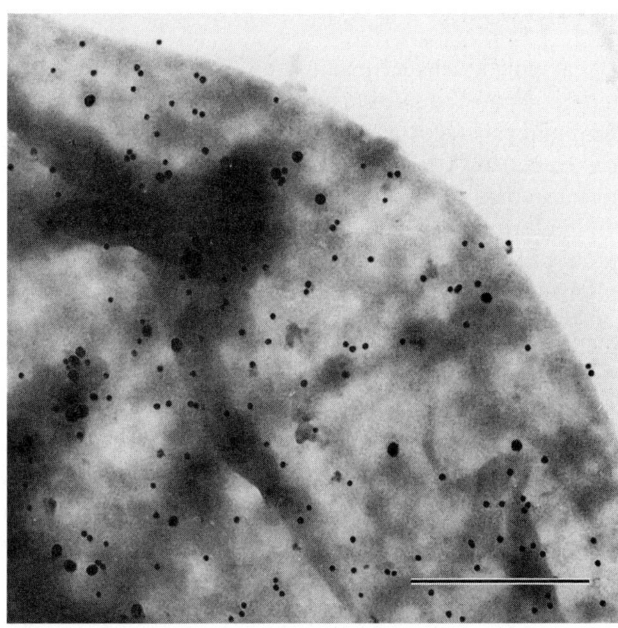

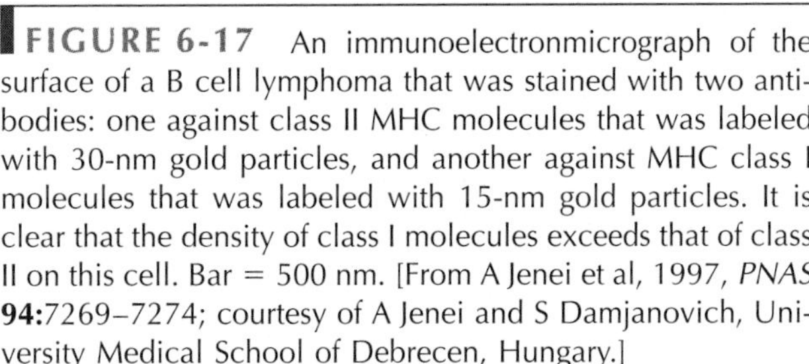

FIGURE 6-17 An immunoelectronmicrograph of the surface of a B cell lymphoma that was stained with two antibodies: one against class II MHC molecules that was labeled with 30-nm gold particles, and another against MHC class I molecules that was labeled with 15-nm gold particles. It is clear that the density of class I molecules exceeds that of class II on this cell. Bar = 500 nm. [From A Jenei et al, 1997, *PNAS* **94:**7269–7274; courtesy of A Jenei and S Damjanovich, University Medical School of Debrecen, Hungary.]

Summary

1. The Ag-Ab interaction depends on noncovalent interactions, including hydrogen bonds, ionic bonds, hydrophobic interactions, and van der Waals interactions (see Figure 6-1). The strength of the Ag-Ab interaction depends on the number of these weak noncovalent interactions between antigen and antibody. The affinity of an antibody for an antigen refers to the strength of the noncovalent interactions between the antibody and antigen at a single binding site, which can be determined by Scatchard analysis (see Figure 6-3). The avidity reflects the overall strength of the interactions between a multivalent antibody molecule and a multivalent antigen molecule at multiple sites.
2. The interaction of a soluble antigen and precipitating antibody (precipitin) forms an Ag-Ab complex that has a lattice structure and precipitates out of solution (see Figure 6-4). Precipitation reactions can be performed in liquids or gels. Most are useful primarily for qualitative comparison of antibodies or antigens (see Figure 6-5). Electrophoresis can be combined with precipitation in gels in a technique called immunoelectrophoresis, and a variety of immunoelectrophoretic techniques have been developed.
3. The interaction between a particulate antigen and agglutinating antibody (agglutinin) produces visible clumping, or agglutination. In some cases, the antigen is a membrane protein on a bacterial cell or red blood cell. In other cases, the antigen may be attached to a latex particle or adsorbed on the surface of a red blood cell. Agglutination reactions are more sensitive and much faster than precipitin reactions and can often detect 100- or 1000-fold lower levels of antigen or antibody than can be detected with a precipitin reaction.
4. Radioimmunoassay (RIA) utilizes radioactively labeled antigen or antibody and is therefore a highly sensitive technique. Liquid-phase RIA is based on the principle of competition between labeled and unlabeled antigen for a limited amount of antibody. In solid-phase RIA, antigen (or antibody) is immobilized on a solid matrix (see Figure 6-10). The main advantage of this technique over liquid-phase RIA is its simplicity of performance and the ease with which bound Ag-Ab complex can be separated from unreacted antigen. Both types of RIA can be used to measure amounts of antibody or antigen.
5. The enzyme-linked immunosorbent assay (ELISA) is based on principles similar to those of RIA but, rather than using a radiolabel, depends on an enzyme-substrate reaction that generates a colored reaction product. An indirect ELISA detects antibody, whereas sandwich ELISA and competitive ELISA detect antigen (see Figure 6-11). ELISA assays that employ chemiluminescence instead of a chromogenic reaction are the most sensitive immunoassays available.
6. In Western blotting, a protein mixture is separated by electrophoresis; then the protein bands are electrophoretically transferred onto nitrocellulose and identified with labeled antibody or labeled antigen (see Figure 6-13).
7. Fluorescent-antibody staining can visualize antigen on cells. Various direct and indirect immunofluorescence

staining techniques have been developed (see Figure 6-15). The fluorescence-activated cell sorter analyzes and sorts cells labeled with fluorescent antibody (see Figure 6-16).

REFERENCES

Berzofsky, JA, IJ Berkower, and SL Epstein. 1991. Antigen-antibody interactions and monoclonal antibodies. In *Fundamental Immunology,* 3rd ed., WE Paul, ed. Raven Press, New York.

Coligan, JE, AM Kruisbeek, DH Margulies, EM Shevach, and W Strober. 1997. *Current Protocols in Immunology.* Wiley, New York.

Rose, NR, EC de Macario, JD Folds, CH Lane, and RM Nakamura. 1997. *Manual of Clinical Laboratory Immunology.* American Society of Microbiology, Washington, D.C.

Stites, DP, C Rodgers, JD Folds, and J Schmitz. 1997. Clinical laboratory detection of antigens and antibodies. In *Medical Immunology,* 9th ed., DP Stites, AI Terr, and TG Parslow, eds., Appelton and Lange, Stamford, CT.

Herzenberg, LA, ed. 1996. *Weir's Handbook of Experimental Immunology,* 5th ed. Oxford, Blackwell Scientific Publications.

Useful Web Sites

http://pathlabsofark.com/flowcyttests.html
Pathology Laboratories of Arkansas is a place to see just what kinds of samples are taken from patients and what markers are used to evaluate lymphocyte populations by flow cytometry.

http://jcsmr.anu.edu.au/facslab/AFCG/standards.html
At the highly informative Australian Flow Cytometry Group Web site, one can find a carefully detailed and illustrated guide to the interpretation of flow cytometric analyses of clinical samples.

http://www.kpl.com
The Kirkegaard & Perry Laboratories Web site contains a subsite, http://www.kpl.com/support/immun/pds/50datasht/54-12-10.html, which allows one to follow a step-by-step procedure for using a chemiluminescent substrate in a sensitive immunoassay.

STUDY QUESTIONS

1. Indicate whether each of the following statements is true or false. If you think a statement is false, explain why.

a. Indirect immunofluorescence is a more sensitive technique than direct immunofluorescence.

b. Most antigens induce a polyclonal response.

c. A papain digest of anti-SRBC antibodies can agglutinate sheep red blood cells (SRBCs).

d. A pepsin digest of anti-SRBC antibodies can agglutinate SRBCs.

e. Indirect immunofluorescence can be performed using a Fab fragment as the primary, nonlabeled antibody.

f. For precipitation to occur, both antigen and antibody must be multivalent.

g. The Ouchterlony technique is a quantitative precipitin technique.

h. Precipitation tests are generally more sensitive than agglutination tests.

2. Briefly outline the ELISA test for HIV infection, indicating which antigen and antibody are used.

3. You have obtained a preparation of purified albumin from normal bovine serum. To determine whether any other serum proteins remain in this preparation of BSA, you decide to use immunoelectrophoresis.

a. What antigen would you use to prepare the antiserum needed to detect impurities in the BSA preparation?

b. Assuming that the BSA preparation is pure, draw the immunoelectrophoretic pattern you would expect if the assay was performed with bovine serum in one well, the BSA sample in a second well, and the antiserum you prepared in (a) in the trough between the wells.

4. The labels from four bottles (A, B, C, and D) of hapten-carrier conjugates were accidentally removed. However, it was known that each bottle contained either hapten 1–carrier 1 (H1-C1), hapten 1–carrier 2 (H1-C2), hapten 2–carrier 1 (H2-C1), or hapten 2–carrier 2 (H2-C2). Double-immuno-diffusion (Ouchterlony) assays with either anti–H1-C2 or anti–H2-C2 were performed. From the precipitin patterns shown below, determine which conjugate is in each bottle.

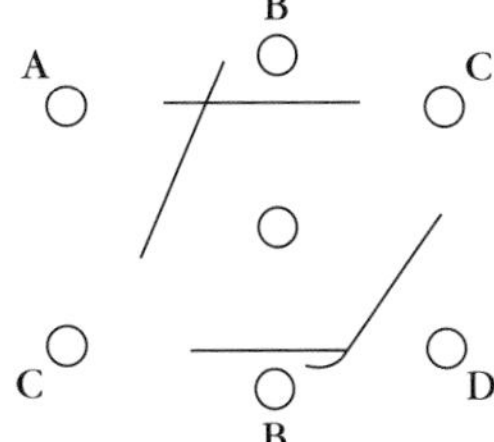

Anti–H1-C2 in central well   Anti–H2-C2 in central well

5. The concentration of a hapten can be determined by which of the following assays: (a) ELISA, (b) Ouchterlony method, (c) rocket electrophoresis, and (d) RIA.

6. You perform an Ouchterlony assay in which the central well contains goat antiserum against the $F(ab')_2$ fragment of pooled mouse IgG, and the surrounding wells (A–F) contain six different test antigens. The resulting precipitin pattern is shown below.

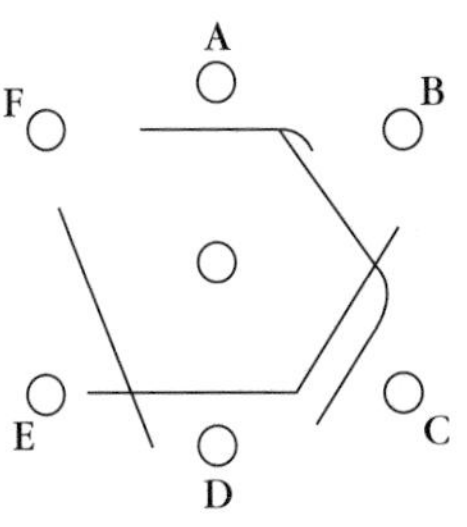

Go to www.whfreeman.com/immunology Self-Test
Review and quiz of key terms

Based on this pattern, indicate which well contains each of the following test antigens:

a. ______ Fab fragment from an IgG myeloma protein ($\gamma_2\kappa_2$)

b. ______ Kappa (κ) light chains

c. ______ Gamma (γ) heavy chains

d. ______ Lambda (λ) light chains

e. ______ Fc fragment from IgG myeloma protein ($\gamma_2\lambda_2$)

f. ______ A mixture of γ heavy chains and κ light chains

7. You have a myeloma protein X whose isotype is unknown and several other myeloma proteins of known isotype (e.g., IgG, IgM, and IgA).

a. How could you produce anti-isotype antibodies that could be used to determine the isotype of myeloma protein X?

b. How could you use this anti-isotype antibody to measure the level of myeloma protein X in normal serum?

8. For each antigen or antibody listed below, indicate an appropriate assay method and the necessary test reagents. Keep in mind the sensitivity of the assay and the expected concentration of each protein.

a. IgG in serum

b. Insulin in serum

c. IgE in serum

d. Complement component C3 on glomerular basement membrane

e. Anti-A antibodies to blood-group antigen A in serum

f. Horsemeat contamination of hamburger

g. Syphilis spirochete in a smear from a chancre

9. Which of the following does *not* participate in the formation of antigen-antibody complexes?

a. Hydrophobic bonds

b. Covalent bonds

c. Electrostatic interactions

d. Hydrogen bonds

e. Van der Waals forces

10. Explain the difference between antibody affinity and antibody avidity. Which of these properties of an antibody better reflects its ability to contribute to the humoral immune response to invading bacteria?

11. You want to develop a sensitive immunoassay for a hormone that occurs in the blood at concentrations around 10^{-7} M. You are offered a choice of three different antisera whose affinities for the hormone have been determined by equilibrium dialysis. The results are shown in the Scatchard plots.

a. What is the value of K_0 for each antiserum?

b. What is the valence of each of the antibodies?

c. Which of the antisera might be a monoclonal antibody?

d. Which of the antisera would you use for your assay? Why?

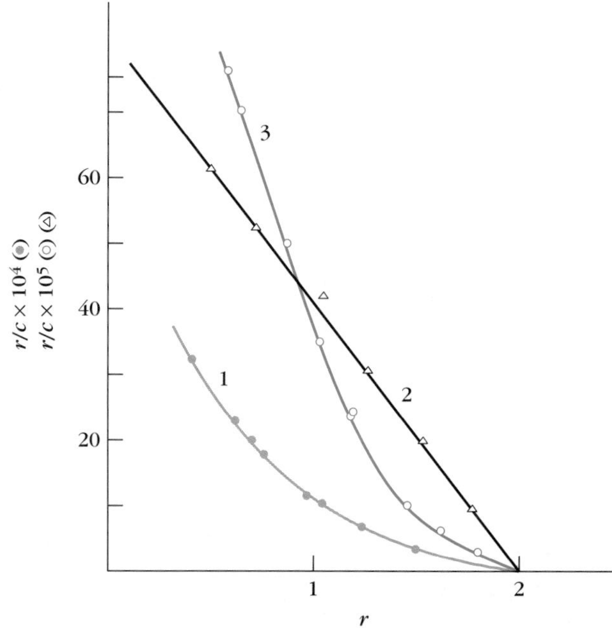

12. In preparing a demonstration for her immunology class, an instructor purified IgG antibodies to sheep red blood cells (SRBCs) and digested some of the antibodies into Fab, Fc, and $F(ab')_2$ fragments. She placed each preparation in a separate tube, labeled the tubes with a water-soluble marker, and left them in an ice bucket. When the instructor returned for her class period, she discovered that the labels had smeared and were unreadable. Determined to salvage the demonstration, she relabeled the tubes 1, 2, 3, and 4 and proceeded. Based on the test results described below, indicate which preparation was contained in each tube and explain why you so identified the contents.

a. The preparation in tube 1 agglutinated SRBCs but did not lyse them in the presence of complement.

b. The preparation in tube 2 did not agglutinate SRBCs or lyse them in the presence of complement. However, when this preparation was added to SRBCs before the addition of whole anti-SRBC, it prevented agglutination of the cells by the whole anti-SRBC antiserum.

c. The preparation in tube 3 agglutinated SRBCs and also lysed the cells in the presence of complement.

d. The preparation in tube 4 did not agglutinate or lyse SRBCs and did not inhibit agglutination of SRBCs by whole anti-SRBC antiserum.

13. You are given two solutions, one containing protein X and the other antibody to this protein. When you add 1 ml of anti-X to 1 ml of protein X, a precipitate forms. But when you dilute the antibody solution 100-fold and then mix 1 ml of the diluted anti-X with 1 ml of protein X, no precipitate forms.

a. Explain why no precipitate formed with the diluted antibody.

b. Which species (protein X or anti-X) would likely be present in the supernatant of the antibody-antigen mixture in each case?

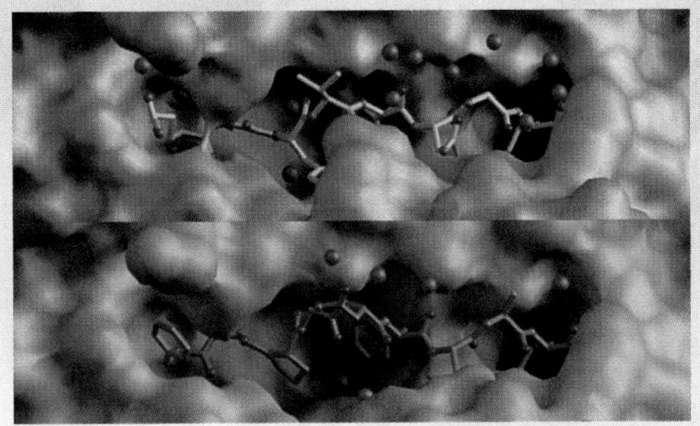

CHAPTER 7
MAJOR HISTOCOMPATIBILITY COMPLEX

Every mammalian species studied to date possesses a tightly linked cluster of genes, the **major histocompatibility complex (MHC)**, whose products play a role in intercellular recognition and in discrimination between self and nonself. The MHC is a region of multiple loci that play major roles in determining whether transplanted tissue is accepted as self (**histocompatible**) or rejected as foreign (**histoincompatible**).

The MHC plays a central role in the development of both humoral and cell-mediated immune responses. While antibodies may react with antigens alone, most T cells recognize antigen only when it is combined with an MHC molecule; thus, MHC molecules play a critical role in antigen recognition by T cells. Because MHC molecules act as antigen-presenting structures, the particular set of MHC molecules expressed by an individual influences the repertoire of antigens to which that individual's T_H cells and T_C cells can respond. For this reason, the MHC partly determines the response of an individual to antigens of infectious organisms and the MHC has, therefore, been implicated in the susceptibility to disease and in the development of autoimmunity. This chapter examines the organization and inheritance of MHC genes, the structure of the MHC molecules, and the central function that these molecules play in producing an immune response.

General Organization and Inheritance of the MHC

The concept that the rejection of foreign tissue is the result of an immune response to cell-surface molecules (now called **histocompatibility antigens**) originated from the work of Peter Gorer in the mid-1930s. Gorer was using inbred strains of mice to identify blood-group antigens. In the course of these studies, he identified four groups of genes, designated I through IV, that encoded blood-cell antigens. Work carried out in the 1940s and 1950s by Gorer and George Snell established that antigens encoded by the genes in the group designated II took part in the rejection of transplanted tumors and other tissue. Snell called these genes "histocompatibility genes"; their current designation as histocompatibility-2 (H-2) genes was in reference to Gorer's group II blood-group antigens. Although Gorer died before his contributions were recognized fully, Snell was awarded the Nobel Prize in 1980 for this work, attesting to the significance of these observations.

Location and Function of MHC Regions

The major histocompatibility complex is a collection of genes arrayed within a long continuous stretch of DNA on chromosome 6 in humans and on chromosome 17 in mice. The MHC is referred to as the **HLA complex** in humans and as the **H-2 complex** in mice. Although the arrangement of genes is somewhat different, in both cases the MHC genes

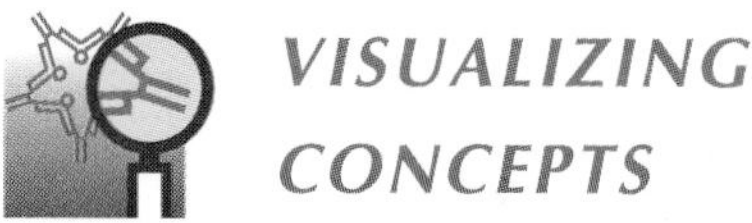

Mouse H-2 complex

Complex	H-2						
MHC class	I	II		III		I	
Region	K	IA	IE	S		D	
Gene products	H-2K	IA $\alpha\beta$	IE $\alpha\beta$	C′ proteins	TNF-α TNF-β	H-2D	H-2L

Human HLA complex

Complex	HLA							
MHC class	II			III		I		
Region	DP	DQ	DR	C4, C2, BF		B	C	A
Gene products	DP $\alpha\beta$	DQ $\alpha\beta$	DR $\alpha\beta$	C′ proteins	TNF-α TNF-β	HLA-B	HLA-C	HLA-A

FIGURE 7-1 Simplified organization of the major histocompatibility complex (MHC) in the mouse and human. The MHC is referred to as the H-2 complex in mice and as the HLA complex in humans. In both species the MHC is organized into a number of regions encoding class I (pink), class II (blue), and class III (green) gene products. The class I and class II gene products shown in this figure are considered to be the classical MHC molecules. The class III gene products include complement (C′) proteins and the tumor necrosis factors (TNF-α and TNF-β.) The IE β gene is actually located in the IA region but for pedagogical reasons is shown in the IE region.

are organized into regions encoding three classes of molecules (Figure 7-1):

- **Class I MHC genes** encode glycoproteins expressed on the surface of nearly all nucleated cells; the major function of the class I gene products is presentation of peptide antigens to T_C cells.
- **Class II MHC genes** encode glycoproteins expressed primarily on antigen-presenting cells (macrophages, dendritic cells, and B cells), where they present processed antigenic peptides to T_H cells.
- **Class III MHC genes** generally encode various secreted proteins that have immune functions, including components of the complement system and molecules involved in inflammation.

Class I MHC molecules encoded by the K and D regions in mice and by the A, B, and C loci in humans, which were the first discovered, are expressed in the widest range of cell types. These are referred to as *classical class I molecules.* Additional genes or groups of genes within the H-2 or HLA complexes, designated Qa and Tla in mice and HLA-E, -F, -G, -H in humans (not shown in Figure 7-1), also encode class I molecules; these are designated *nonclassical class I genes.* Expression of the nonclassical gene products is limited to certain specific cell types. Although functions are not known for all of them, some may have highly specialized roles in immunity. For example, the expression of the class I HLA-G molecules on cytotrophoblasts at the fetal–maternal interface has been implicated in protection of the fetus from being recognized as foreign (this may occur when paternal antigens begin to appear) and being rejected by maternal T_C cells.

The two chains of the class II MHC molecules are encoded by the IA and IE regions in mice and by the DP, DQ, and DR regions in humans. The terminology is somewhat confusing, since the D region in mice encodes class I MHC molecules, whereas the D (DR, DQ, DP) in humans refers to genes encoding class II MHC molecules! Fortunately, the designation D for the general chromosomal location encoding the human class II molecules is seldom used today; the precise chromosomal map of the so-called D region is available so that the more imprecise reference to region is seldom necessary. As with the class I molecules, there are class II molecules in addition to IA and IE and HLA-DP, -DQ, and -DR that have specialized functions in the immune process. The best studied of these nonclassical class II products is HLA-DM, which has an important role in the processing of peptide antigens for presentation to T_H cells.

The class I and II MHC molecules have common structural features and they both have roles in antigen processing. By contrast, the class III MHC region, which is flanked by the class I and II regions, encodes molecules that are critical to immune function but have little in common with class I or II molecules. Class III products include the complement components C4, C2, BF (see Chapter 13) and inflammatory cytokines, including tumor necrosis factor (TNF) and heat-shock proteins.

MHC Haplotypes

As described in more detail later, the loci constituting the MHC are highly **polymorphic**; that is, many alternative forms of the gene, or **alleles**, exist at each locus. The MHC loci are also closely linked; for example, the recombination frequency within the H-2 complex is only 0.5%. For this reason, most individuals inherit the alleles encoded by these closely linked loci as two sets, one from each parent. Each set of alleles is referred to as a **haplotype**. An individual inherits one haplotype from the mother and one haplotype from the father. In outbred populations, the offspring are generally heterozygous at many loci and will express both maternal and paternal MHC alleles. The alleles are *codominantly expressed*; that is, both maternal and paternal gene products are expressed in the same cells. If mice are inbred, however, each H-2 locus will be homozygous because the maternal and paternal haplotypes are identical, and all offspring therefore express identical haplotypes.

Certain inbred mouse strains have been designated as prototype strains, and the MHC haplotype expressed by these strains is designated by an arbitrary italic superscript (e.g., H-2^a, H-2^b, H-2^d, H-2^k). Each designation simply is a way of referring to the entire set of inherited H-2 alleles within a strain without having to refer to each allele individually (Table 7-1). If another inbred strain has inherited the same set of alleles as the prototype strain, its MHC haplotype is the same as the prototype strain. For example, the CBA, AKR, and C3H strains all have the same MHC haplotype (H-2^k). The three strains differ, however, in genes outside the H-2 complex.

If two mice from inbred strains having different MHC haplotypes are bred to one another, the F_1 generation inherits haplotypes from both parental strains and therefore expresses both parental alleles at each MHC locus. For example, if strain C57BL/10 (H-2^b) is crossed with strain CBA (H-2^k), then the F_1 inherits both parental sets of alleles and is said to be H-$2^{b/k}$ (Figure 7-2a). Because such an F_1 expresses the MHC proteins of both parental strains on its cells, it is histocompatible with both strains and able to accept grafts from either parental strain (see example in Figure 7-2b). However, neither of the inbred parental strains can accept a graft from the F_1 mice because half of the MHC molecules will be foreign to the parent.

The inheritance of HLA haplotypes from heterozygous human parents is illustrated in Figure 7-2c. In an outbred population, each individual is generally heterozygous at each locus. The human HLA complex is highly polymorphic and multiple alleles of each class I and class II gene exist. However, as with mice, the human MHC loci are closely linked and usually inherited as a haplotype. When the father and mother have different haplotypes, as in the example shown (Figure 7-2c) there is a one-in-four chance that siblings will inherit the same paternal and maternal haplotypes and therefore be histocompatible with each other; none of the offspring is histocompatible with the parents. The fact that genetic recombinations or crossovers between parental haplotypes occur at a frequency of around 0.5% contributes significantly to the diversity of the HLA loci in the human population. Genetic recombination generates new allelic combinations (Figure 7-2d). Although recombination is

TABLE 7-1 H-2 HAPLOTYPES OF SOME MOUSE STRAINS

			H-2 alleles				
Prototype strain	Other strains with the same haplotype	Haplotype	*K*	*IA*	*IE*	*S*	*D*
CBA	AKR, C3H, B10.BR, C57BR	*k*	*k*	*k*	*k*	*k*	*k*
DBA/2	BALB/c, NZB, SEA, YBR	*d*	*d*	*d*	*d*	*d*	*d*
C57BL/10 (B10)	C57BL/6, C57L, C3H.SW, LP, 129	*b*	*b*	*b*	*b*	*b*	*b*
A	A/He, A/Sn, A/Wy, B10.A	*a*	*k*	*k*	*k*	*d*	*d*
A.SW	B10.S, SJL	*s*	*s*	*s*	*s*	*s*	*s*
A.TL		*t1*	*s*	*k*	*k*	*k*	*d*
DBA/1	STOLI, B10.Q, BDP	*q*	*q*	*q*	*q*	*q*	*q*

(a) Mating of inbred mouse strains with different MHC haplotypes

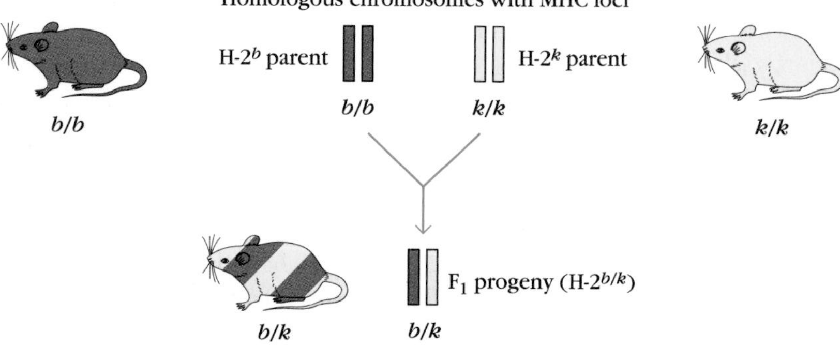

(b) Skin transplantation between inbred mouse strains with same or different MHC haplotypes

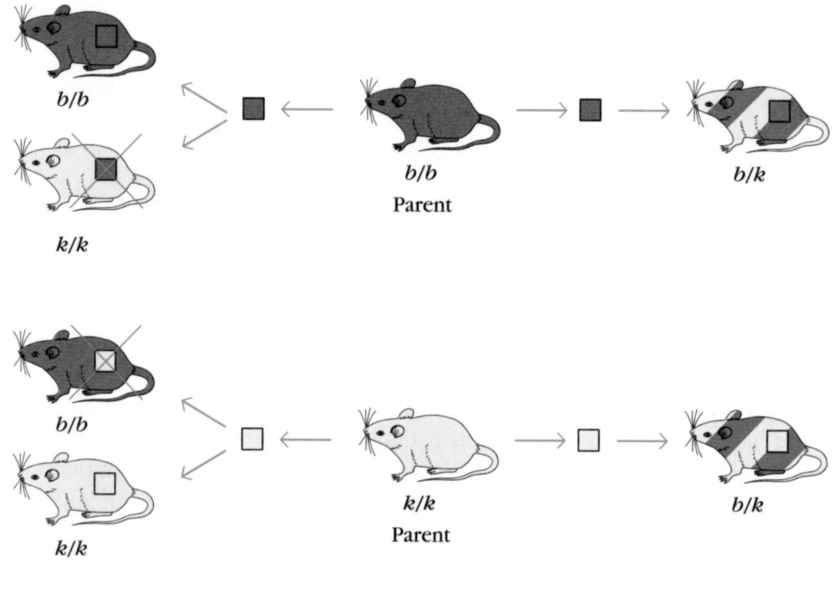

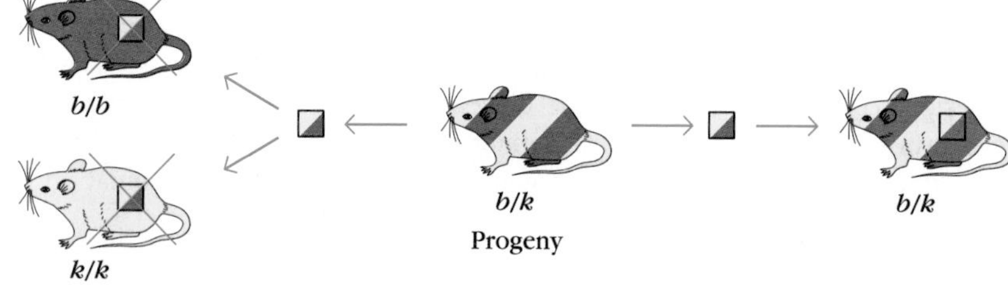

(c) Inheritance of HLA haplotypes in a typical human family

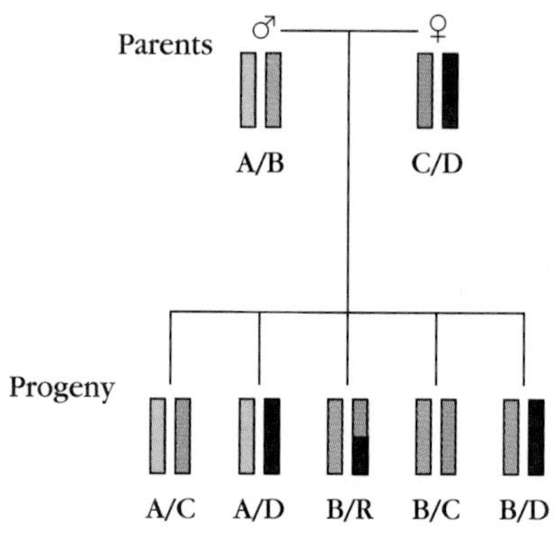

(d) A new haplotype (R) arises from recombination of maternal haplotypes

Haplotypes	HLA Alleles A	B	C	DR	DQ	DP
A	1	7	w3	2	1	1
B	2	8	w2	3	2	2
C	3	44	w4	4	1	3
D	11	35	w1	7	3	4
R	3	44	w4	7	3	4

FIGURE 7-2 (a) Illustration of inheritance of MHC haplotypes in inbred mouse strains. The letters *b/b* designate a mouse homozygous for the H-2^b MHC haplotype, *k/k* homozygous for the H-2^k haplotype, and *b/k* a heterozygote. Because the MHC loci are closely linked and inherited as a set, the MHC haplotype of F_1 progeny from the mating of two different inbred strains can be predicted easily. (b) Acceptance or rejection of skin grafts is controlled by the MHC type of the inbred mice. The progeny of the cross between two inbred strains with different MHC haplotypes (H-2^b and H-2^k) will express both haplotypes (H-2$^{b/k}$) and will accept grafts from either parent and from one another. Neither parent strain will accept grafts from the offspring. (c) Inheritance of HLA haplotypes in a hypothetical human family. In humans, the paternal HLA haplotypes are arbitrarily designated A and B, maternal C and D. Because humans are an outbred species and there are many alleles at each HLA locus, the alleles comprising the haplotypes must be determined by typing parents and progeny. (d) The genes that make up each parental haplotype in the hypothetical family in (c) are shown along with a new haplotype that arose from recombination (R) of maternal haplotypes.

infrequent, the long period of time since the appearance of humans as a species and the high number of intervening generations have allowed extensive recombination, so that it is rare for any two unrelated individuals to have completely matched sets of identical HLA genes.

Congenic MHC Mouse Strains

Detailed analysis of the H-2 complex in mice was made possible by the development of congenic mouse strains. Inbred mouse strains are **syngeneic** or identical at all genetic loci. Two strains are **congenic** if they are genetically identical except at a single genetic locus or region. Any phenotypic differences that can be detected between congenic strains are related to the genetic region that distinguishes the strains. Congenic strains that are identical with each other except at the MHC can be produced by a series of crosses, backcrosses, and selections. Figure 7-3 outlines the steps by which the H-2 complex of homozygous strain B can be introduced into the background genes of homozygous strain A to generate a congenic strain, denoted A.B. The first letter in a congenic strain designation refers to the strain providing the genetic background and the second letter to the strain providing the genetically different MHC region. Thus, strain A.B will be genetically identical to strain A except for the MHC locus or loci contributed by strain B.

During production of congenic mouse strains, a crossover event sometimes occurs within the H-2 complex, yielding a recombinant strain that differs from the parental strains or the congenic strain at one or a few loci within the H-2 complex. Figure 7-4 depicts haplotypes present in several **recombinant congenic** strains that were obtained during production of a B10.A congenic strain. Such recombinant strains have been extremely useful in analyzing the MHC because they permit comparisons of functional differences between strains that differ in only a few genes within the MHC. Furthermore, the generation of new H-2 haplotypes under the experimental conditions of congenic strain development provides an excellent illustration of the means by which the MHC continues to maintain heterogeneity even in populations with limited diversity.

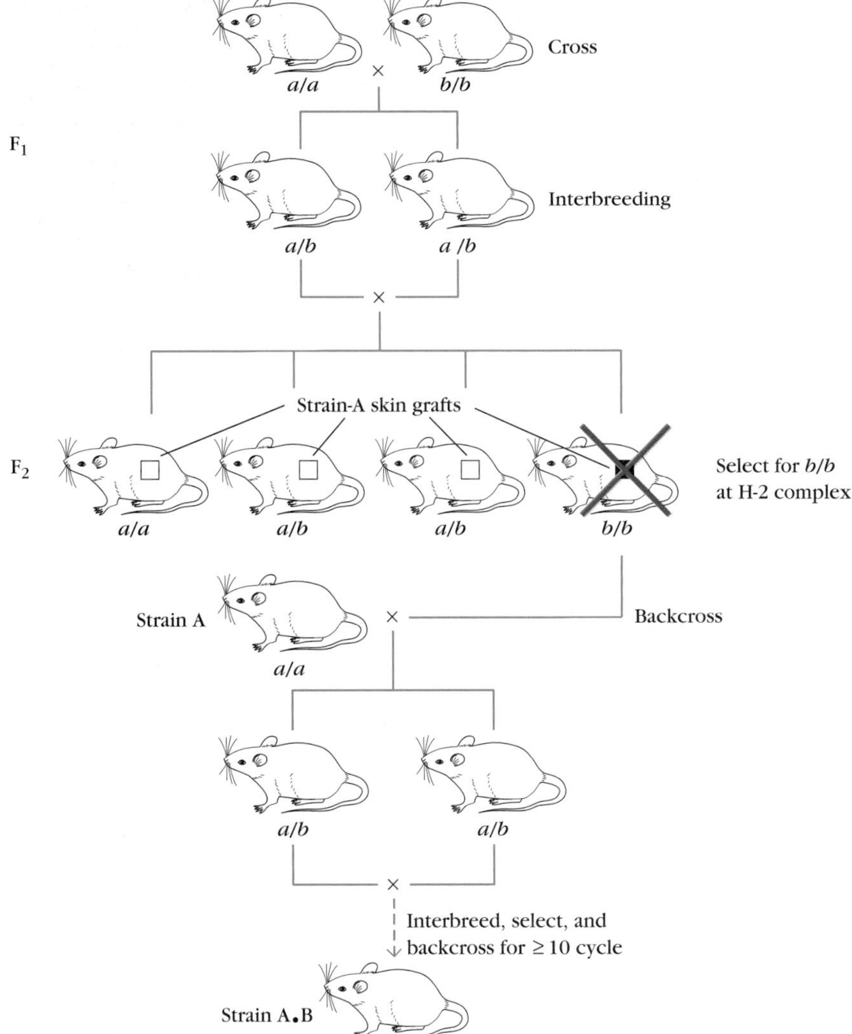

FIGURE 7-3 Production of congenic mouse strain A.B, which has the genetic background of parental strain A but the H-2 complex of strain B. Crossing inbred strain A (H-2^a) with strain B (H-2^b) generates F_1 progeny that are heterozygous (*a/b*) at all H-2 loci. The F_1 progeny are interbred to produce an F_2 generation, which includes *a/a*, *a/b*, and *b/b* individuals. The F_2 progeny homozygous for the B-strain H-2 complex are selected by their ability to reject a skin graft from strain A; any progeny that accept an A-strain graft are eliminated from future breeding. The selected *b/b* homozygous mice are then backcrossed to strain A; the resulting progeny are again interbred and their offspring are again selected for *b/b* homozygosity at the H-2 complex. This process of backcrossing to strain A, intercrossing, and selection for ability to reject an A-strain graft is repeated for at least 12 generations. In this way A-strain homozygosity is restored at all loci except the H-2 locus, which is homozygous for the B strain.

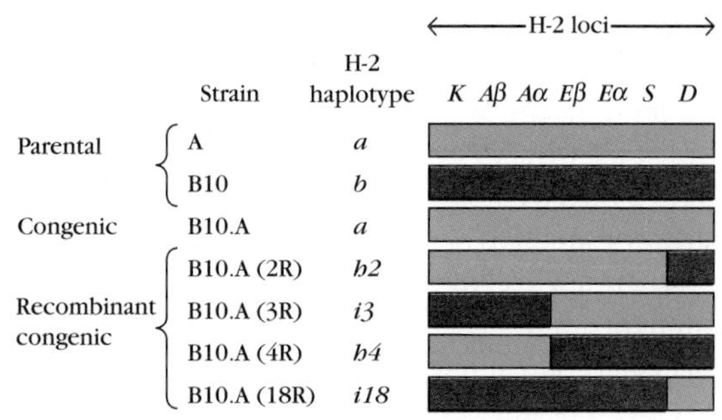

FIGURE 7-4 Examples of recombinant congenic mouse strains generated during production of the B10.A strain from parental strain B10 (H-2^b) and parental strain A (H-2^a). Crossover events within the H-2 complex produce recombinant strains, which have *a*-haplotype alleles (blue) at some H-2 loci and *b*-haplotype alleles (orange) at other loci.

MHC Molecules and Genes

Class I and class II MHC molecules are membrane-bound glycoproteins that are closely related in both structure and function. Both class I and class II MHC molecules have been isolated and purified and the three-dimensional structures of their extracellular domains have been determined by x-ray crystallography. Both types of membrane glycoproteins function as highly specialized antigen-presenting molecules that form unusually stable complexes with antigenic peptides, displaying them on the cell surface for recognition by T cells. In contrast, class III MHC molecules are a group of unrelated proteins that do not share the structural similarity and common function with class I and II molecules. The class III molecules will be examined in more detail in later chapters.

Structure of Class I Molecules

Class I MHC molecules contain a large α chain associated noncovalently with the much smaller **β_2-microglobulin** molecule (see Figure 7-5). The α chain is a polymorphic transmembrane glycoprotein of about 45 kilodaltons (kDa) encoded by genes within the A, B, and C regions of the human HLA complex and within the K and D/L regions of the mouse H-2 complex (see Figure 7-1). β_2-Microglobulin is a protein of about 12 kDa encoded by a gene located on a different chromosome. Association of the α chain with β_2-microglobulin is required for expression of class I molecules on cell membranes. The α chain is anchored in the plasma membrane by its hydrophobic transmembrane segment and hydrophilic cytoplasmic tail.

Amino acid sequence analyses have revealed that the α chain of class I MHC molecules is organized into three ex-

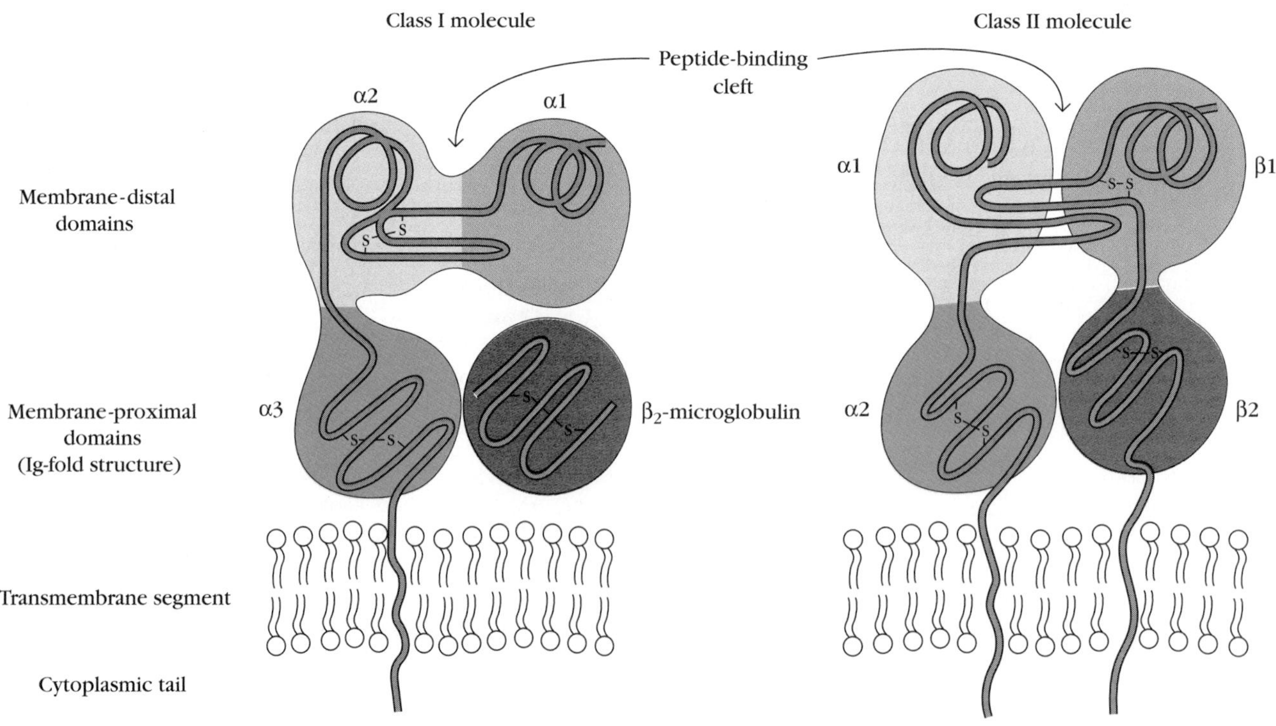

FIGURE 7-5 Schematic diagrams of a class I and class II MHC molecule showing the external domains, transmembrane segment, and cytoplasmic tail. The peptide-binding cleft is formed by the membrane-distal domains in both class I and class II molecules. The membrane-proximal domains possess the basic immunoglobulin-fold structure; thus, class I and class II MHC molecules are classified as members of the immunoglobulin superfamily.

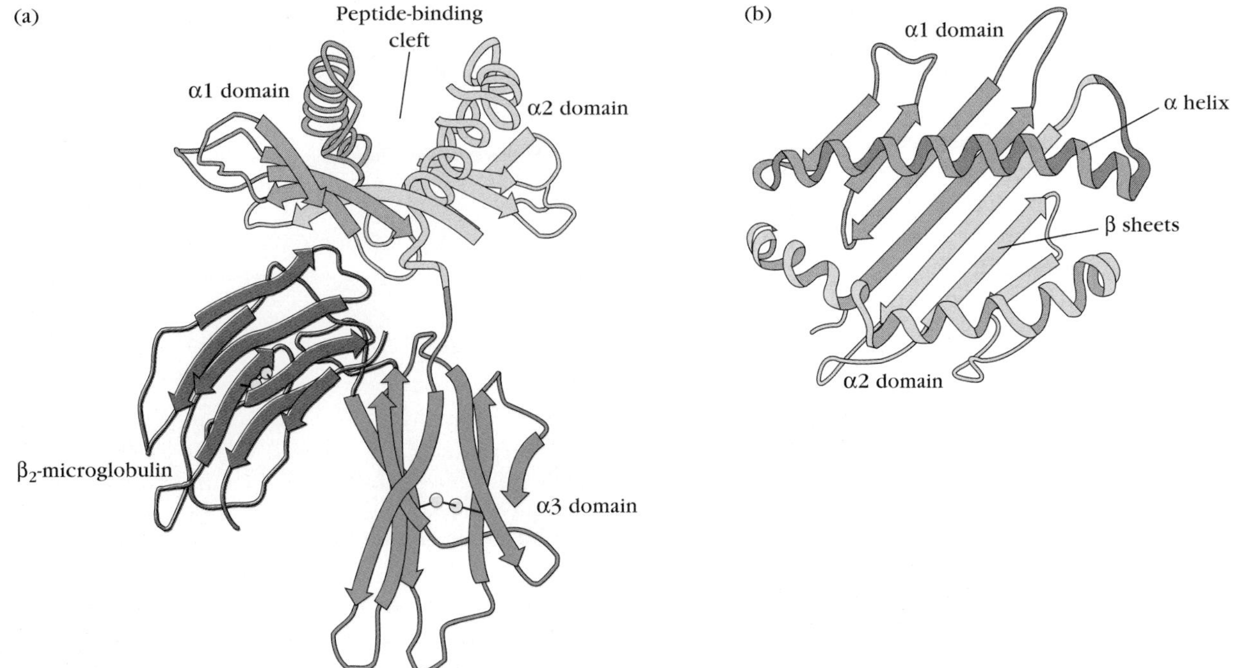

FIGURE 7-6 Representations of the three-dimensional structure of the external domains of a human class I HLA molecule based on x-ray crystallographic analysis. (a) Side view in which the β strands are depicted as thick arrows and the α helices as spiral ribbons. Disulfide bonds are shown as two interconnected spheres. The α1 and α2 domains interact to form the peptide-binding cleft. Note the immunoglobulin-fold structure of the α3 domain and β_2-microglobulin. (b) The α1 and α2 domains as viewed from top, showing the peptide-binding cleft consisting of a base of antiparallel β strands and sides of α helices. This cleft in class I molecules can accommodate peptides containing 8–10 residues.

ternal domains (α1, α2, and α3), each containing approximately 90 amino acids; a transmembrane domain of about 25 hydrophobic amino acids followed by a short stretch of charged (hydrophilic) amino acids; and a cytoplasmic anchor segment of 30 amino acids. In size (about 100 amino acids) and organization, β_2-microglobulin is similar to the α3 external domain; it does not contain a transmembrane region and is noncovalently bound to the class I glycoprotein. Comparison of sequence data has shown that considerable homology exists between the α3 domain, β_2-microglobulin and the constant-region domains in immunoglobulins. The enzyme papain cleaves the α chain just 13 residues proximal to its transmembrane domain, releasing the extracellular portion of the molecule consisting of α1, α2, α3, and β_2-microglobulin. Purification and crystallization of the extracellular portion revealed two pairs of interacting domains: a membrane-distal pair made up of the α1 and α2 domains and a membrane-proximal pair composed of the α3 domain and β_2-microglobulin (Figure 7-6a).

The α1 and α2 domains interact to form a platform of eight antiparallel β strands spanned by two long α-helical regions. The structure forms a deep groove, or cleft, approximately 25 Å × 10 Å × 11 Å, with the long α helices as sides and the β strands of the β sheet as the bottom (Figure 7-6b). This *peptide-binding cleft* is located on the top surface of the class I MHC molecule, and it is large enough to bind a peptide of 8–10 amino acids. The great surprise in the x-ray crystallographic analysis of class I molecules was the finding of small peptides in the cleft that had cocrystallized with the protein. These peptides are, in fact, processed antigen and self-peptides bound to the α1 and α2 domains in this deep groove.

The α3 domain and β_2-microglobulin are organized into two β pleated sheets each formed by antiparallel β strands of amino acids. As described in Chapter 4, this structure, known as the immunoglobulin fold, is characteristic of immunoglobulin domains. Because of this structural similarity, which is not surprising given the considerable sequence homology with the immunoglobulin constant regions, class I MHC molecules and β_2-microglobulin are classified as members of the immunoglobulin superfamily (see Figure 4-19). The α3 domain appears to be highly conserved among class I MHC molecules and contains a sequence that interacts with the CD8 membrane molecule present on T_C cells.

β_2-Microglobulin interacts extensively with the α3 domain and also interacts with amino acids of the α1 and α2 domains. The interaction of β_2-microglobulin and a peptide with a class I α chain is essential for the class I molecule to reach its fully folded conformation. As described in detail in Chapter 8, assembly of class I molecules is believed to occur by the initial interaction of β_2-microglobulin with the folding class I α chain. This metastable "empty" dimer is then stabilized by the binding of an appropriate peptide to form the native trimeric class I structure consisting of the class I α chain, β_2-microglobulin, and a peptide. This complete molecular complex is ultimately transported to the cell surface.

In the absence of β_2-microglobulin, the class I MHC α chain is not expressed on the cell membrane. This is illustrated by Daudi tumor cells, which are unable to synthesize β_2-microglobulin. These tumor cells possess class I MHC genes, which they can transcribe into mRNA. Although the mRNA is translated into protein, the cells do not express class I MHC α chains on the membrane. However, if Daudi cells are transfected with a functional gene encoding β_2-microglobulin, they will begin to express class I molecules on the membrane.

Structure of Class II Molecules

Class II MHC molecules contain two different polypeptide chains, a 33-kDa α chain and a 28-kDa β chain, which associate by noncovalent interactions (see Figure 7-5b). Like class I MHC molecules, class II MHC molecules are membrane-bound glycoproteins that contain external domains, a transmembrane segment, and a cytoplasmic anchor segment. Each chain in a class II molecule contains two external domains: $\alpha 1$ and $\alpha 2$ domains in one chain and $\beta 1$ and $\beta 2$ domains in the other. The membrane-proximal $\alpha 2$ and $\beta 2$ domains, like the membrane-proximal $\alpha 3/\beta_2$-microglobulin domains of class I MHC molecules, bear sequence homology to the immunoglobulin-fold structure; for this reason, class II MHC molecules also are classified in the immunoglobulin superfamily. The membrane-distal portion of a class II molecule is composed of the $\alpha 1$ and $\beta 1$ domains and forms the antigen-binding cleft for processed antigen.

Three-dimensional structures for several human and mouse class II molecules have been determined by x-ray crystallographic analysis. The overall three-dimensional structure of the class II molecules is similar to that of class I molecules. The peptide-binding cleft of HLA-DR1, like that in class I molecules, is composed of a floor of eight antiparallel β strands and sides of antiparallel α helices. Despite some differences in fine structure, which will be explored below, the similarity is such that the class II and class I peptide-binding clefts can be superimposed (Figure 7-7).

A striking difference between crystallized class I and class II molecules was observed for human DR1 in that the latter occurred as a dimer of the $\alpha\beta$ heterodimer, a "dimer of dimers" (Figure 7-8). The dimer is oriented so that the two peptide-binding clefts face in opposite directions. It has not yet been determined whether this dimeric form exists in vivo. A recently reported structure of a human class II molecule crystallized in the presence of the superantigen (see Chapter 10) *Staphylococcus aureus* enterotoxin B occurred as a single $\alpha\beta$ chain pair (Figure 7-8c). Superantigens bind to class II molecules in regions outside of the cleft. This complex included a peptide in the binding site of the class II molecule, suggesting that the $\alpha\beta$ heterodimer is functional.

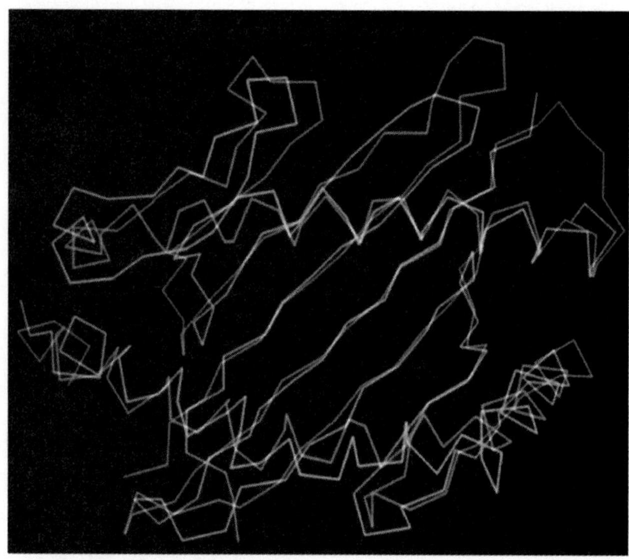

FIGURE 7-7 The membrane-distal, peptide-binding cleft of a human class II MHC molecule, HLA-DR1 (blue), superimposed over the corresponding regions of a human class I MHC molecule, HLA-A2 (red). [From JH Brown et al, 1993, *Nature* **364:**33.]

Organization of Class I and Class II Genes

A number of class I and class II MHC genes have been cloned and sequenced. Comparison of the amino acid sequence of the protein products with the DNA sequences reveals that separate exons encode each region of the proteins (Figure 7-9).

Each of the mouse and human class I genes has a 5′ leader exon encoding a short signal peptide followed by five or six exons encoding the α chain of the class I molecule (see Figure 7-9a). The signal peptide serves to facilitate insertion of the α chain into the endoplasmic reticulum and is removed, after translation is completed, by proteolytic enzymes in the endoplasmic reticulum. The next three exons encode the extracellular $\alpha 1$, $\alpha 2$, and $\alpha 3$ domains. The next downstream exon encodes the transmembrane (T_m) region; finally, one or two 3′-terminal exons encode the cytoplasmic domains (C).

Like class I MHC genes, the class II genes are organized into a series of exons and introns mirroring the domain structure of the α and β chains (see Figure 7-9b). Both the α and the β genes encoding mouse and human class II MHC molecules have a leader exon, an $\alpha 1$ or $\beta 1$ exon, an $\alpha 2$ or $\beta 2$ exon, a transmembrane exon, and one or more cytoplasmic exons.

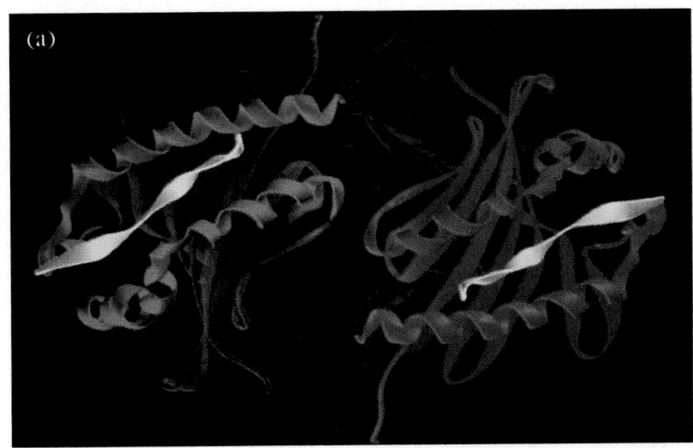

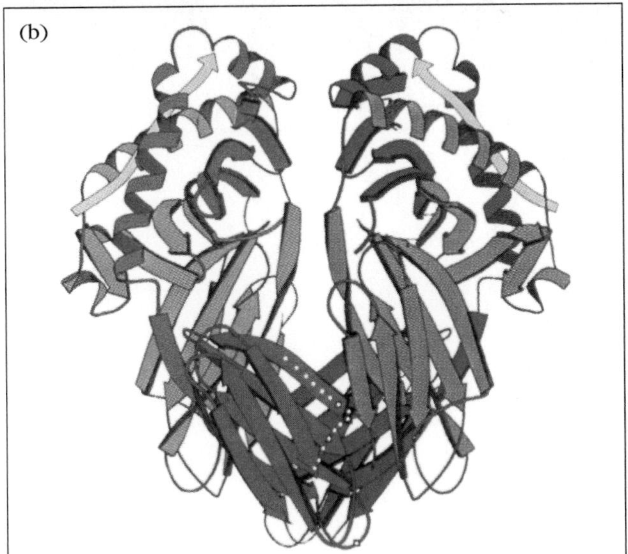

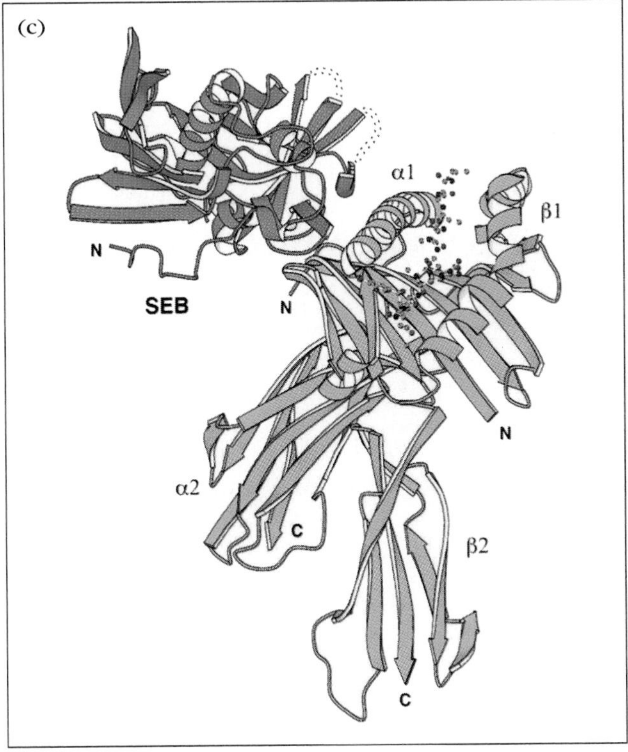

FIGURE 7-8 Antigen-binding cleft of dimeric class II DR1 molecule in (a) top view and (b) side view. This molecule crystallized as a dimer of the αβ heterodimer. The crystallized dimer is shown with one DR1 molecule in red and the other DR1 molecule in blue. The bound peptides are shown in yellow. The two peptide-binding clefts in the dimeric molecule face in opposite directions. (c) Ribbon diagram of HLA-DR4, shown in yellow, complexed outside the MHC antigen-binding cleft with *Staphylococcus* enterotoxin B (SEB), shown in blue. The bound peptide in the antigen-binding cleft is from human collagen II, shown by the large dots. [(a) and (b) From JH Brown et al, 1993, *Nature* **364:**33. (c) From Dessen et al., 1997, *Immunity* **7:**473–481.]

Peptide Binding by MHC Molecules

Several hundred different allelic variants of class I and II MHC molecules have been identified in humans. Any one individual, however, expresses only a small number of these molecules—up to 6 different class I molecules and up to 12 different class II molecules. Yet this limited number of MHC molecules must be able to present an enormous array of different antigenic peptides to T cells, permitting the immune system to respond specifically to a wide variety of antigenic challenges. Thus peptide binding by class I and II molecules does not exhibit the fine specificity characteristic of antigen binding by antibodies and T-cell receptors. Instead, a given MHC molecule can bind numerous different peptides, and some peptides can bind to several different MHC molecules. Because of this broad specificity, the binding between a peptide and an MHC molecule is often referred to as "promiscuous."

Given the similarities in the structure of the peptide-binding cleft in class I and II MHC molecules, it is not surprising that they exhibit some common peptide-binding features (Table 7-2). In both types of MHC molecules, peptide ligands are held in a largely extended conformation that runs the length of the cleft. The peptide-binding cleft in class I molecules is blocked at both ends, whereas the cleft is open in class II molecules (Figure 7-10). As a result of this difference, class I molecules bind peptides that typically contain 8–10 amino acid residues, while the open groove of class II molecules accommodates slightly longer peptides of 13–18 amino acids. Another difference, explained in more detail below, is that class I binding requires that the peptide contain certain amino acid residues, called anchor residues, near the N and C termini; there is no such requirement for class II peptide binding.

The binding affinity of various peptides for MHC molecules has been determined by equilibrium dialysis (see Figure 6-2). In these experiments, a labeled peptide was added to a solubilized class I or class II MHC molecule in a dialysis bag and the amount of labeled peptide bound to the MHC

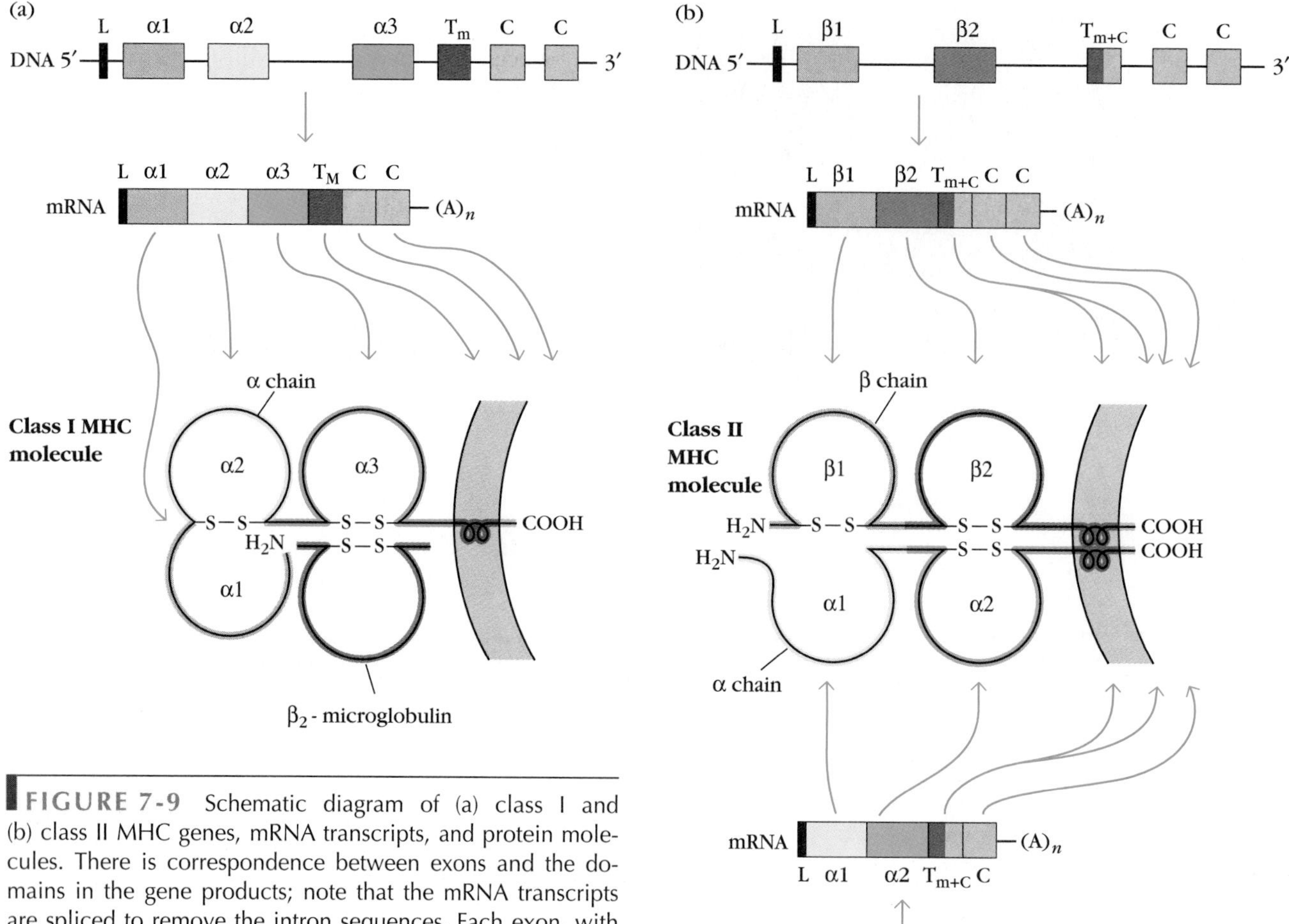

FIGURE 7-9 Schematic diagram of (a) class I and (b) class II MHC genes, mRNA transcripts, and protein molecules. There is correspondence between exons and the domains in the gene products; note that the mRNA transcripts are spliced to remove the intron sequences. Each exon, with the exception of the leader (L) exon, encodes a separate domain of the MHC molecule. The leader peptides are removed in a post-translational reaction before the molecules are expressed on the cell surface. The gene encoding β_2-microglobulin is located on a different chromosome. T_m = transmembrane; C = cytoplasmic.

TABLE 7-2 PEPTIDE BINDING BY CLASS I AND CLASS II MHC MOLECULES

	Class I molecules	Class II molecules
Peptide-binding domain	α1/α2	α1/β1
Nature of peptide-binding cleft	Closed at both ends	Open at both ends
General size of bound peptides	8–10 amino acids	13–18 amino acids
Peptide motifs involved in binding to MHC molecule	Anchor residues at both ends of peptide; generally hydrophobic carboxyl-terminal anchor	Anchor residues distributed along the length of the peptide
Nature of bound peptide	Extended structure in which both ends interact with MHC cleft but middle arches up away from MHC molecule	Extended structure that is held at a constant elevation above the floor of MHC cleft

(a) Class I MHC

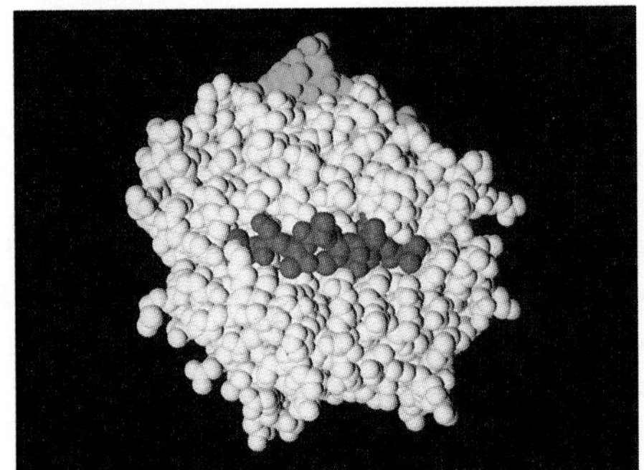

(b) Class II MHC

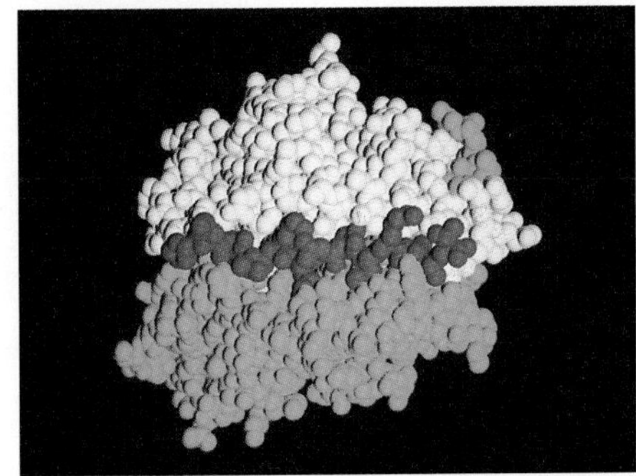

FIGURE 7-10 MHC class I and class II molecules with bound peptides. (a) Space-filling model of human class I molecule HLA-A2 (white) with peptide (brown) from HIV reverse transcriptase (amino acid residues 309–317) in the binding groove. β_2-microglobulin is shown in blue. Sequences above the peptide are from the $\alpha 1$ domain, those below from $\alpha 2$. (b) Space-filling model of human class II molecules HLA-DR1 with the DRα chain shown in white and the DRβ chain in blue. The peptide (brown) in the binding groove is from influenza hemagglutinin (amino acid residues 306–318). [From DA Vignali and J Strominger, 1994, *The Immunologist* **2:**112.]

molecule at equilibrium was determined. Scatchard plots (see Figure 6-3) of the data revealed that the dissociation constant K_D of the peptide–MHC molecule complex is approximately 10^{-6}; the rate of association is slow, but the rate of dissociation is even slower. What this means is that the peptide–MHC molecule association is very stable under physiologic conditions; thus, most of the MHC molecules expressed on the membrane of a cell will be associated with a peptide of self or nonself origin.

Class I MHC–Peptide Interaction

Class I MHC molecules bind peptides and present them to $CD8^+$ T cells. In general, these peptides are derived from endogenous intracellular proteins, which are digested into peptides within the cytosol. These peptides are then transported from the cytosol into the cisternae of the endoplasmic reticulum, where they interact with class I MHC molecules. This process, known as the cytosolic or endogenous processing pathway, is discussed in detail in the next chapter.

Each type of class I MHC molecule (K, D, and L in mice or A, B, and C in humans) binds a unique set of peptides. In addition, each allelic variant of a class I MHC molecule (e.g., H-2K^k and H-2K^d) also binds a distinct set of peptides. Because a single nucleated cell expresses about 10^5 copies of each class I molecule, then many different peptides will be expressed simultaneously on the surface of a nucleated cell by class I MHC molecules.

Various approaches have been used to obtain information about the nature of the interaction between peptide and class I MHC molecules. In one experimental approach, peptide-MHC complexes are isolated from cells, purified, and then denatured to release the bound peptide. In a healthy cell these released peptides have been shown to be various self-peptides derived from common intracellular proteins such as cytochrome *c*, histones, and ribosomal proteins. In an altered self-cell (e.g., a virus-infected cell), some of the self-peptides are replaced with peptides from viral proteins.

In a critical study of peptide binding by MHC molecules, the peptides released from two allelic variants of a class I MHC molecule were analyzed by HPLC mass spectrometry. These two class I MHC molecules were found to bind more than 2000 distinct peptides. Since there are approximately 10^5 copies of each class I allelic variant per cell, it is estimated that each of the 2000 distinct peptides is presented with a frequency of 100–4000 copies per cell. Evidence suggests that as few as 100 peptide-MHC complexes are sufficient to target a cell for recognition and lysis by a cytotoxic T lymphocyte with a receptor specific for this target structure.

The bound peptides isolated from different class I molecules have been found to have two distinguishing features: they are eight to ten amino acids in length, most commonly nine, and they contain specific amino acid residues that appear to be essential for binding to a particular MHC molecule. The finding that the peptides most frequently isolated from class I MHC molecules are nonamers (nine residues) suggests that this peptide length is most compatible with the size of the peptide-binding cleft in class I molecules. As noted earlier, the peptide-binding cleft in class I molecules is closed at both ends (see Figure 7-10a); this structural feature places constraints on the size of the bound peptide. The binding site will accommodate peptides from eight to ten amino acids in length; those of nine amino acids bind most tightly. Indeed, binding studies have shown that nonameric peptides bind to class I molecules with a 100- to 1000-fold higher affinity than do peptides that are either longer or shorter.

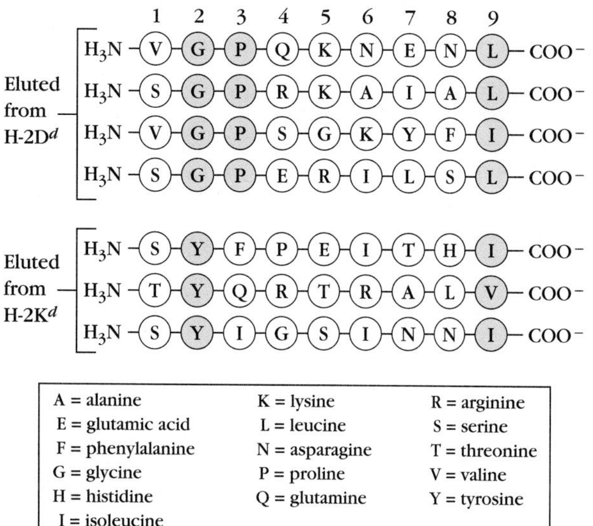

FIGURE 7-11 Examples of anchor residues (blue) in nonameric peptides eluted from two class I MHC molecules. Anchor residues that interact with the class I MHC molecule tend to be hydrophobic amino acids. [Data from VH Engelhard, 1994, *Curr. Opin. Immunol.* **6**:13.]

The ability of an individual class I MHC molecule to bind to a diverse spectrum of peptides is due to the presence of the same or similar amino acid residues at several defined positions along the peptide (Figure 7-11). Because these amino acid residues anchor the peptide into the groove of the MHC molecule, they are called *anchor residues.* The side chains of the anchor residues in the peptide insert into pockets within the binding cleft of the class I MHC molecule. These pockets in the MHC molecule are lined by polymorphic amino acid residues that vary among different class I allelic variants; as a result, the identity of these residues in a particular class I molecule determines the identity of the peptide anchor residues that can interact with the molecule.

All peptides examined to date that bind to class I molecules contain a carboxyl-terminal anchor. These anchors are generally hydrophobic residues (e.g., leucine, isoleucine), although a few charged amino acids have been reported. Besides the anchor residue found at the carboxyl terminus, another anchor is often found at the second or second and third positions at the amino-terminal end of the peptide (see Figure 7-11). In general, any peptide of correct length that contains the same or similar anchor residues will bind to the same class I MHC molecule. The discovery of conserved anchor residues in peptides that bind to various class I MHC molecules may permit prediction of which peptides in a complex antigen will bind to a particular MHC molecule based on the presence or absence of these motifs.

X-ray crystallographic analyses of peptide–class I MHC complexes have revealed how the peptide-binding cleft in a given MHC molecule can interact stably and yet flexibly with a broad spectrum of different peptides. The anchor residues at both ends of the peptide are buried within the binding cleft, thereby holding the peptide firmly in place (Figure 7-12). As noted already, nonameric peptides are bound preferentially; the majority of contacts between class I MHC molecules and peptides involve residue 2 at the amino-terminal end and residue 9 at the carboxyl terminus of the nonameric peptide. The bound peptide, which assumes an extended structure, interacts with the MHC cleft at both ends but arches away from the floor of the cleft in the middle (Figure 7-13). Since the middle of the peptide does not make significant contact with the cleft of the MHC molecule, peptides that are slightly longer or shorter can be accommodated by slight differences in the number of residues that bulge away from the cleft. In addition, peptides that have different middle residues but the correct anchor residues at each end can be bound to the same MHC molecule (see Figure 7-12 for examples). It is thought that the amino acids that arch away from the MHC molecule are more exposed and therefore can interact directly with the T-cell receptor.

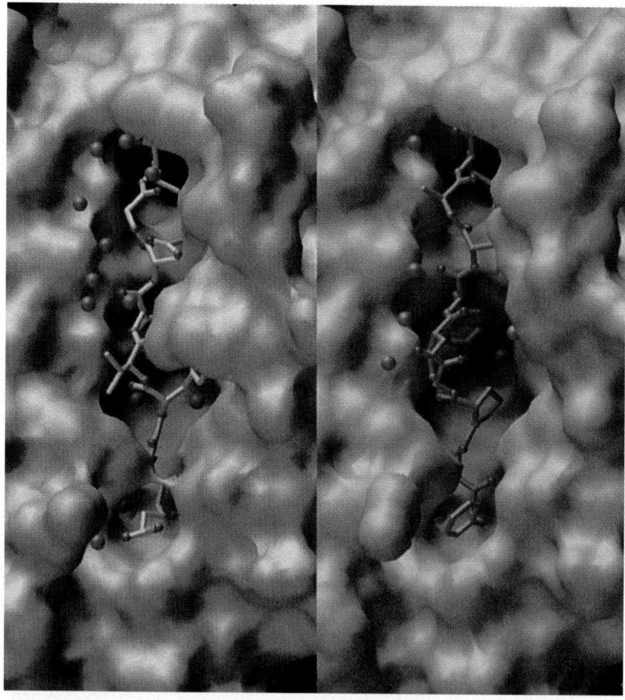

FIGURE 7-12 Model of the solvent-accessible area of class I H-2K^b, depicting the complex formed with a vesicular stomatitis virus (VSV-8) peptide (*left*, yellow backbone) and Sendai virus (SEV-9) nucleoprotein (*right*, blue backbone). Water molecules (blue spheres) interact with the bound peptides. The majority of the surface of both peptides is inaccessible for direct contact with T cells (VSV-8 is 83% buried; SEV-9 is 75% buried). The H-2K^b surface in the two complexes exhibits a small, but potentially significant, conformational variation, especially in the central region of the binding cleft on the right side of the peptides, which corresponds to the α helix in the α2 domain (see Figure 7-6b). [From M Matusumura et al, 1992, *Science* **257**:927.]

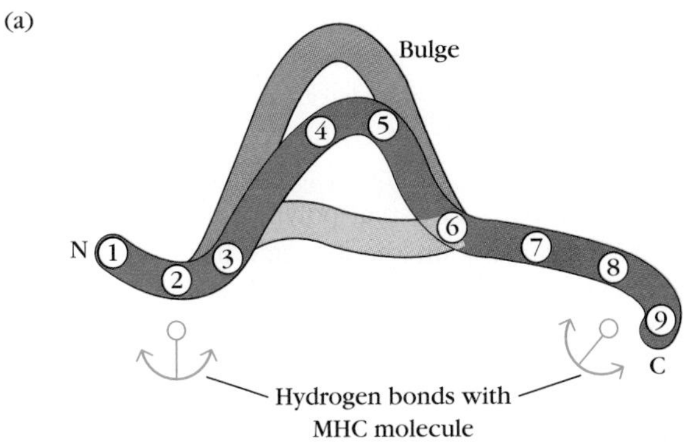

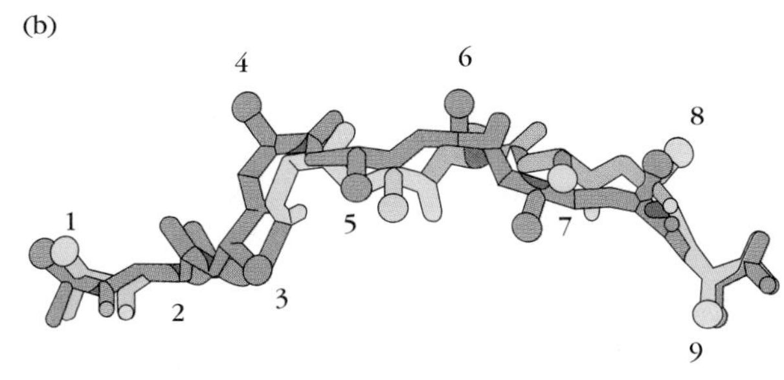

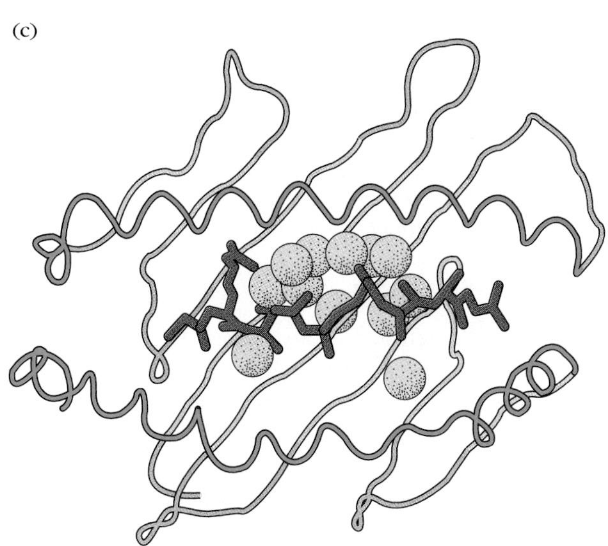

FIGURE 7-13 Conformation of peptides bound to class I MHC molecules. (a) Schematic diagram of conformational difference in bound peptides of different lengths. Longer peptides bulge in the middle, whereas shorter peptides are more extended. Contact with the MHC molecule is by hydrogen bonds to anchor residues 1/2 and 8/9. (b) Molecular models based on crystal structure of an influenza virus antigenic peptide (blue) and an endogenous peptide (purple) bound to a class I MHC molecule. Residues are identified by small numbers corresponding to those in part (a). (c) Representation of α1 and α2 domains of HLA-B27 and a bound antigenic peptide based on x-ray crystallographic analysis of the cocrystallized peptide–HLA molecule. The peptide (maroon) arches up away from the β strands forming the floor of the binding cleft and interacts with twelve water molecules (spheres). [Part (a) adapted from P Parham, 1992, *Nature* **360:**300; part (b) adapted from ML Silver et al, 1992, *Nature* **360:**367; part (c) adapted from DR Madden et al, 1992, *Cell* **70:**1035.]

Class II MHC–Peptide Interaction

Class II MHC molecules bind peptides and present these peptides to $CD4^+$ T cells. Like class I molecules, class II molecules can bind a variety of peptides. In general, these peptides are derived from exogenous proteins (either self or nonself), which are degraded within the endocytic processing pathway (see Chapter 8). Most of the peptides associated with class II MHC molecules are derived from membrane-bound proteins or proteins associated with the vesicles of the endocytic processing pathway. The membrane-bound proteins presumably are internalized by phagocytosis or by receptor-mediated endocytosis and enter the endocytic processing pathway at this point. For instance, peptides derived from digestion of membrane-bound class I MHC molecules often are bound to class II MHC molecules. Other peptides associated with class II MHC molecules are derived from digestion of the invariant chain, which is involved in the intracellular vesicular transport of class II MHC molecules from the endoplasmic reticulum to the endocytic processing pathway. When the invariant chain is digested within the endocytic pathway, the resulting peptides bind to the class II MHC cleft. Almost all class II MHC molecules investigated so far have been shown to bind the same invariant-chain peptide, a good example of promiscuous binding.

In studies similar to those done with class I molecules, peptides have been released and characterized from class II MHC–peptide complexes. The isolated peptides generally contain 13–18 amino acid residues, and thus are slightly longer than the nonameric peptides that most commonly bind to class I molecules. The peptide-binding cleft in class II molecules is open at both ends, allowing a bound peptide to extend beyond the ends, much like a long hot dog in a bun (see Figure 7-10b). This feature enables class II molecules to bind longer peptides than do class I molecules. Peptide binding studies and structural data for class II molecules indicate that a central core of 13 amino acids determines the ability of a peptide to bind class II. Despite the fact that longer peptides are accommodated within the class II cleft, binding characteristics are determined by the central 13 residues. Peptides bound to class II MHC molecules maintain a roughly constant elevation on the floor of the binding cleft, another feature that distinguishes peptide binding to class I and class II molecules.

The peptides that bind to a particular class II molecule often have internal conserved "motifs," but unlike class I–binding peptides, they lack conserved anchor residues at the ends of the peptide. Instead, hydrogen bonds between the backbone of the peptide and the class II molecule are distributed throughout the binding site rather than being clustered predominantly at the ends of the site as for class I–bound peptides. Peptides that bind to class II MHC molecules contain a sequence comprising 7–10 amino acids that provide the major contact points. Generally, this sequence has an aromatic or hydrophobic residue at the amino terminus and three additional hydrophobic residues in the middle portion and carboxyl-terminal end of the peptide. In addition, over 30% of the peptides eluted from class II molecules contain a proline residue at position 2 and another cluster of prolines at the carboxyl-terminal end.

Polymorphism of Class I and Class II Molecules

An enormous diversity is exhibited by the MHC molecules within a species, and there is diversity in individual members of the species as well. However, the source of the diversity of MHC molecules differs from the source for antibodies and T-cell receptors. The diversity of antibodies and T-cell receptors is generated by a continual process of random gene rearrangements and somatic mutation of rearranged genes. Thus, the process is dynamic, changing over time within an individual. By contrast, the MHC molecules expressed by an individual do not change over time. The MHC molecules in one individual may differ significantly from those expressed by another individual of the same species. The diversity of the MHC within a species stems from **polymorphism,** the presence of multiple alleles at a given genetic locus within the species. Diversity of MHC molecules in an individual results not only from having different alleles of each gene but also from the presence of duplicated genes with similar or overlapping functions, not unlike the isotypes of immunoglobulins. Because it includes genes with similar, but not identical structure and function (for example, HLA-A, -B, and -C), the MHC may be said to be **polygenic.**

The MHC possesses an extraordinarily large number of different alleles at each locus and is one of the most polymorphic genetic complexes known in higher vertebrates. These alleles differ in their DNA sequences from one individual to another by 5% to 10%, and consequently the gene products expressed by different individuals have unique structural differences. The number of amino acid differences between MHC alleles can be quite significant, with up to 20 amino acid residues contributing to the unique nature of each allele. Analysis of human HLA class I molecules has revealed approximately 60 A alleles, 110 B alleles, and 40 C alleles. In mice, the polymorphism is equally staggering, with more than 55 alleles now identified at the K locus and 60 alleles identified at the D locus. The human class II molecules are also highly polymorphic and, in some cases, there are different gene numbers in different individuals. The number of HLA-DR beta-chain genes may vary from 2 to 5 in different haplotypes, and 122 alleles of DRB have been reported. Interestingly, the DRA chain is identical in all individuals studied. Current estimates of actual polymorphism in the human MHC is probably on the low side because the most detailed data were obtained in populations of European descent. The fact that many non-European population groups cannot be typed using the MHC serologic typing reagents available suggests that the worldwide diversity of the MHC genes is even greater. Now that MHC genes can be sequenced directly, it is likely that additional alleles will be detected.

This enormous polymorphism results in a tremendous diversity of MHC molecules within a species. Given 100 different alleles for each class I and class II gene in the mouse H-2 complex, for example, the theoretical diversity possible for that species is

$$100(K) \times 100(IA\alpha) \times 100(IA\beta) \times 100(IE\alpha) \times 100(IE\beta) \times 100(D) = 10^{12}$$

Linkage Disequilibrium

In humans the theoretical diversity of the MHC is even larger than in the mouse because humans have more class I and class II genes. Although it may be expected that HLA haplotypes in humans would contain completely random combinations of the multiple alleles, this has not been observed. The actual diversity observed in humans is less than the theoretical calculations predict. The theoretical estimates assume that, given sufficient time, all combinations of MHC alleles will occur in the species and no combination should have a higher frequency than another. The fact that this random distribution does not occur and that certain allelic combinations occur more frequently than predicted is referred to as *linkage disequilibrium.* Briefly, linkage disequilibrium is the difference between the frequency observed for a particular combination of alleles and that expected from the frequencies of the individual alleles. The expected frequency for the combination may be calculated by multiplying the frequencies of the two alleles. For example, if HLA-A1 occurs in 16% of individuals in a population (frequency = 0.16) and HLA-B8 in 9% of that group (frequency = 0.09) it is expected that about 1.4% of the group should have both alleles ($0.16 \times 0.09 = 0.014$). However, the data showed that HLA-A1 and HLA-B8 are found together in 8.8% of individuals studied. This difference is a measure of the linkage disequilibrium between these alleles of class I MHC genes.

Reasons for linkage disequilibrium are not fully understood, but several possible explanations have been advanced. The most simple is that sufficient time, or sufficient numbers of generations, have not elapsed to allow the number of crossovers necessary to reach equilibrium among the alleles present in founders of the population. The haplotypes that are over-represented in the population today would then reflect the combinations of alleles present in the founders. Alternatively, selective effects could also result in the higher frequency of certain allelic combinations. For example, certain combinations of alleles might interact to produce resistance to certain diseases or to generate harmful effects such as susceptibility to autoimmune disorders. Positive effects of allelic combinations would cause them to be favored and thus over-represented, whereas those combinations of alleles with negative consequences would be rarer than predicted. A third hypothesis is that crossovers are more frequent in certain DNA sequence regions than in others and the presence or absence of regions prone to crossover (hotspots) between alleles can dictate the frequency of allelic association. Data in support of this was found in mouse breeding studies that generated new recombinant H-2 types. The points of crossover in the new MHC haplotypes were not randomly distributed throughout the complex. Instead, the same regions of crossover were found in more than one recombinant haplotype. This suggests that hotspots of recombination do exist; these would influence linkage disequilibrium in populations.

Despite linkage disequilibrium, there is still enormous polymorphism in the human MHC and it remains very difficult to match donor and acceptor MHC types for successful organ transplants. The consequences of this major obstacle to the therapeutic use of transplantation are described in Chapter 21.

Functional Relevance of MHC Polymorphism

A comparison of the amino acid sequences of several allelic MHC molecules encoded at a single locus reveals an unusually high degree of sequence divergence. Indeed, the sequence divergence among alleles of the MHC within a species is as great as the divergence observed for the genes encoding some enzymes (e.g., lactate dehydrogenase) across species lines. What is also unusual is that the sequence variation among MHC molecules is not randomly distributed along the entire polypeptide chain but instead is clustered in short stretches, largely within the membrane-distal α1 and α2 domains of class I molecules (Figure 7-14a).

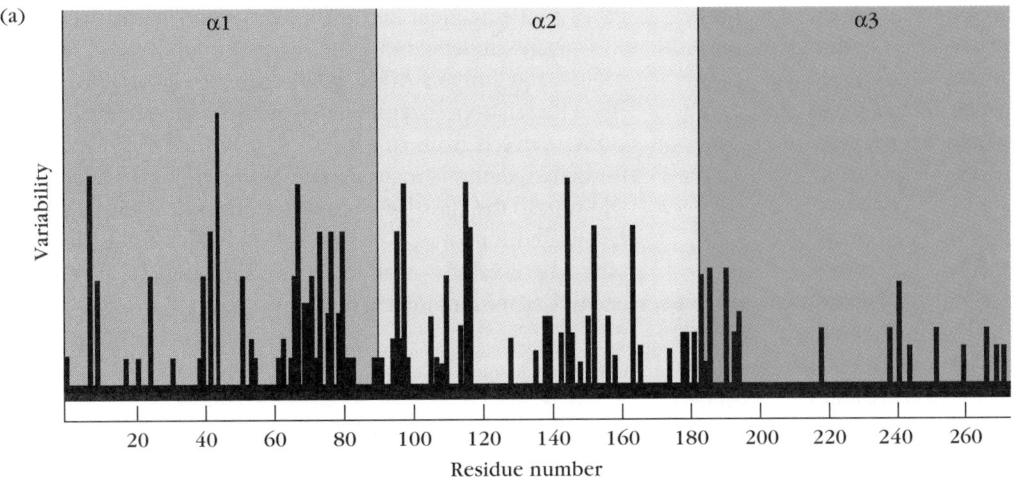

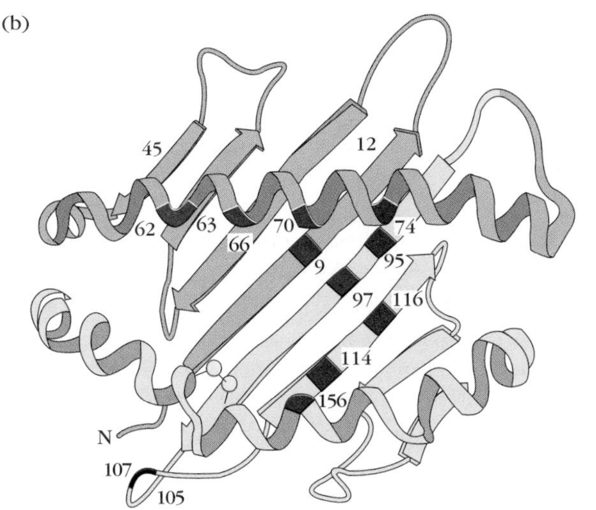

FIGURE 7-14 (a) Plots of variability in the amino acid sequence of allelic class I MHC molecules in humans versus residue position. In the external domains, most of the variable residues are in the membrane-distal α1 and α2 domains. (b) Location of polymorphic amino acid residues (red) in the α 1/α2 domain of a human class I MHC molecule. [Part (a) adapted from R Sodoyer et al, 1984, *EMBO J.* **3:**879; part (b) adapted from P Parham, 1989, *Nature* **342:**617.]

Similar patterns of diversity are observed in the α1 and β2 domains of class II molecules.

Some progress has been made in locating the polymorphic residues within the three-dimensional structure of the membrane-distal domains in class I and class II MHC molecules and in relating allelic differences to functional differences. The polymorphic amino acids of class I MHC molecules are clustered in the membrane-distal α1/α2 domain. High-resolution x-ray crystallographic analyses of several class I molecules has determined the location of the polymorphic residues within the structure of the α1/α2 domain (Figure 7-14b). For example, of 17 amino acids previously shown to display significant polymorphism in the HLA-A2 molecule, 15 were shown by crystallographic analysis to be in the peptide-binding cleft of this molecule. The location of so many polymorphic amino acids within the binding site for processed antigen strongly suggests that allelic differences contribute to the observed differences in the ability of MHC molecules to interact with a given antigenic peptide.

Experiments described later in this chapter show that different class II molecules preferentially bind different labeled peptides. Studies with mutated class II MHC molecules, as well as x-ray crystallographic analyses of class II molecules, have located the peptide-binding cleft in the membrane-distal α1/β1 domain, the very region that displays localized polymorphism. A number of researchers have suggested that such allelic differences in the class II molecules expressed by antigen-presenting cells may influence the cells' ability to recognize a particular peptide.

Class III Molecules

As noted earlier, several structurally and functionally diverse proteins are encoded within the third region of the MHC (see Figure 7-1). These class III molecules include several complement components (C2, C4a, C4b, and factor B), two steroid 21-hydroxylase enzymes (21-OHA and 21-OHB), the inflammatory cytokines, tumor necrosis factors α and β TNF-α and TNF-β), and two heat-shock proteins.

Unlike class I and class II MHC molecules, the class III molecules are not membrane proteins, are not related structurally to class I and II molecules, and have no role in antigen presentation, although most play some role in immune responses. It is not known why the class III genes are situated within the MHC complex. As will be explained below, the observed genetic association of certain MHC alleles with various diseases may in some cases reflect regulatory disorders of genes within the class III region.

The **heat-shock proteins** are an unusual group of highly conserved proteins that are produced by cells in response to various stresses, including heat shock (for which they were named), nutrient deprivation, oxygen radicals, and viral infection. Some heat-shock proteins are thought to bind incompletely or aberrantly folded proteins and may be involved in the intracellular trafficking of proteins necessary for proper presentation of antigen. These proteins have been shown to associate with ribonucleoproteins in the nucleus during heat shock. Evidence suggesting that heat-shock proteins may be linked to certain autoimmune diseases is discussed in Chapter 20.

Detailed Genomic Map of MHC Genes

The MHC, located on chromosome 17 of mice and on chromosome 6 of humans, is now known to contain nearly 100 genes, spanning some 2000 kb of mouse DNA and some 4000 kb of human DNA. Once congenic and recombinant congenic mouse strains became available, mapping of the position and function of the individual genes within the H-2 complex began. Initially, serologic assays were used to assess the gene products encoded by the MHC genes. More recently, cloning of both mouse and human MHC genes has permitted restriction-enzyme mapping of the MHC. Detailed mapping and sequence determination of large DNA stretches within the MHC is progressing at a rapid pace, and additional genes are being identified within this complex each year.

Current understanding of the genomic organization of mouse and human MHC genes is diagrammed in Figure 7-15. Restriction-enzyme mapping and sequence analysis of clones derived from the MHC have refined and expanded the earlier genomic maps derived from serologic analyses. In addition to the class I and class II MHC genes that had been recognized for some time (see Figure 7-1), molecular mapping has revealed a number of so-called nonclassical MHC genes that were not previously known.

Map of Class I MHC

In humans, the class I MHC region is about 2000 kb long and contains approximately 20 genes. In mice, the class I MHC consists of two regions separated by the intervening class II and class III regions. Included within the class I region are the genes encoding the well-characterized classical class I MHC molecules designated HLA-A, HLA-B, and HLA-C in humans and H-2K, H-2D, and H-2L in mice. Many nonclassical class I genes, identified by molecular mapping, also are present in both the mouse and human MHC. In mice, the nonclassical class I genes are located in three regions (*H-2Q*, *T*, and *M*) downstream from the H-2 complex (*M* is not shown in Figure 7-15). In humans, the nonclassical class I genes include the *HLA-E*, *HLA-F*, *HLA-G*, *HLA-H*, *HLA-J*, and *HLA-X* loci as well as a recently discovered family of genes called *MIC*, which includes *MICA* through *MICE*. Some of the nonclassical class I MHC genes are pseudogenes and do not encode a protein product, but others, such as *HLA-G* and *HLA-H*, encode class I-like products with highly specialized functions.

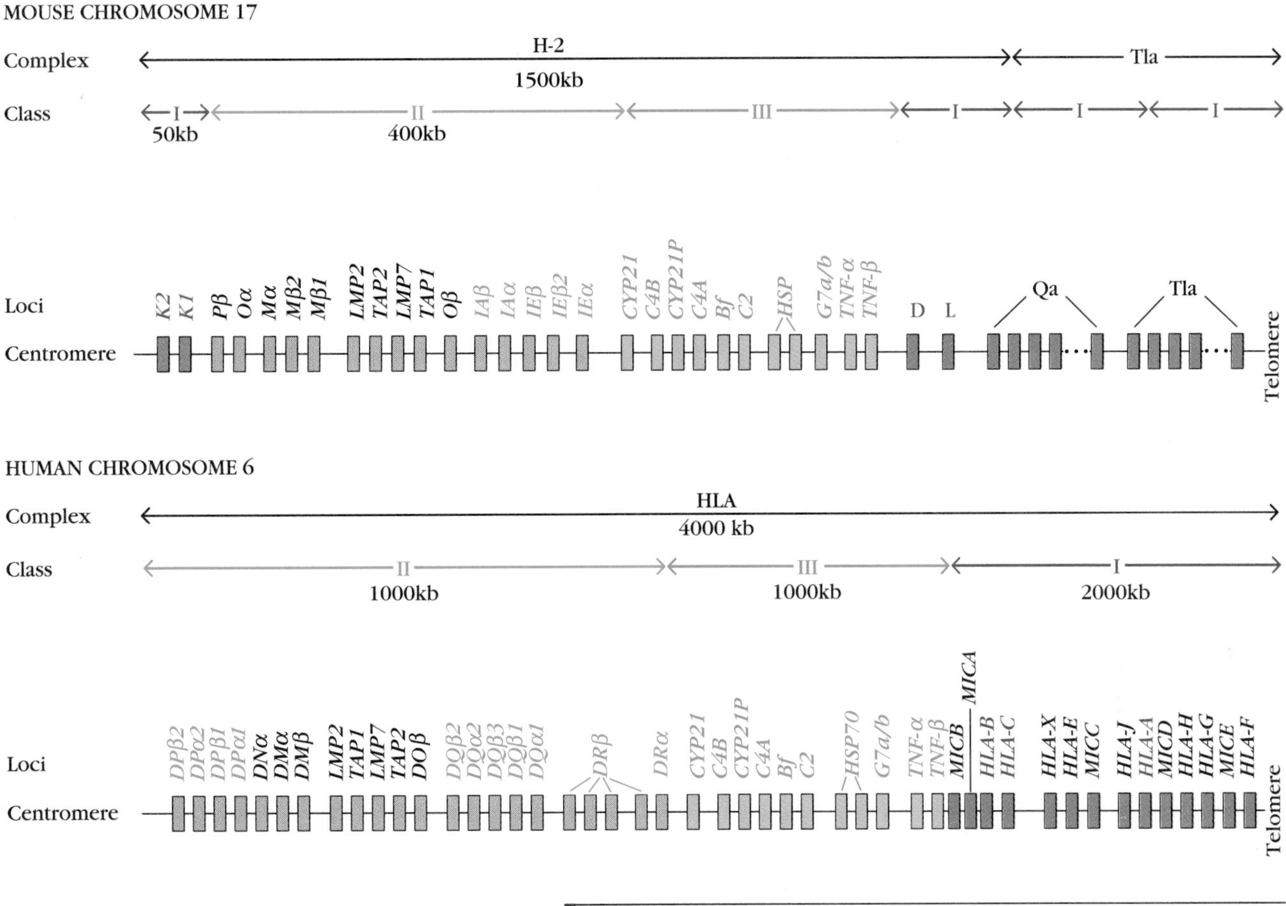

KEY

Gene	Encoded protein
C2, C4A, C4B, Bf	Complement components
CYP21,CYP21P	Steroid 21-hydroxylases
G7a/b	Valyl-tRNA synthetase
HSP	Heat-shock protein
LMP2, LMP7	Proteasome-like subunits
TAP1, TAP2	Peptide-transporter subunits
TNF-α, TNF-β	Tumor necrosis factors α and β

FIGURE 7-15 Detailed genomic map of the mouse and human MHC, including genes encoding classical and nonclassical MHC molecules. The class I MHC genes are colored red, MHC II genes are colored blue, and genes in MHC III are colored green. Classical class I genes are labeled in red, class II in blue, and the nonclassical MHC genes are labeled in black. The concept of classical and nonclassical does not apply to class III. The functions for certain proteins encoded by the nonclassical class I genes are known. In the mouse, there are nonclassical genes located downstream from Tla that are not shown. The nonclassical class II genes encode proteins that function in antigen processing.

Certain of the nonclassical class I MHC gene products are categorized as *class Ib molecules.* Like the classical class I molecules, class Ib molecules generally have an α chain that associates with β_2-microglobulin. However, the class Ib molecules generally are less polymorphic and expressed at lower levels than classical class I MHC molecules. In addition, the tissue distribution of the class Ib proteins usually is more limited than that of classical class I molecules. The Ib molecules have about 70% sequence identity to classical class I molecules. By contrast, the MIC family of class I genes has only 15%–30% sequence identity to classical class I and is highly polymorphic. The MIC gene products are expressed at low levels in epithelial cells and are induced by heat or other stimuli that influence heat shock proteins. Whether they function in antigen presentation remains to be learned.

The functions of the nonclassical class I MHC molecules remain largely unknown, although a few studies suggest that some of these molecules, like the classical class I MHC molecules, may present peptides to T cells. One intriguing finding is that the class Ib molecule encoded by the *H-2M* locus is able to bind a self-peptide derived from a subunit of NADH dehydrogenase, an enzyme encoded by the mitochondrial genome. This particular self-peptide contains an amino-terminal formylated methionine. What is interesting about this finding is that peptides derived from prokaryotic organisms often have formylated amino-terminal methionine residues. This *H-2M*–encoded class I molecule may thus be uniquely suited to present peptides from prokaryotic organisms that are able to grow intracellularly. Such organisms include *Mycobacterium tuberculosis, Listeria monocytogenes,*

Brucella abortus, and *Salmonella typhimurium*. Perhaps the limited polymorphism and unusual tissue distribution of nonclassical class I MHC molecules enables these molecules to present antigens from microorganisms that invade at specific tissue sites or infect specific types of cells.

Up to this point, all description of antigen presentation by class I and class II molecules has been confined to presentation of peptide antigens. As will be seen in the description of antigen presentation (Chapter 8), there are also molecules with structural similarity to class I molecules that present non-peptide antigens, such as glycolipids, to T cells. A major family of such molecules, designated CD1, has been shown to present lipid antigens derived from bacteria. The CD1 molecules are not encoded within the MHC but are on a different chromosome.

Map of Class II MHC

The class II MHC region contains the genes encoding the α and β chains of the classical class II MHC molecules designated HLA-DR, DP, and DQ in humans and H-2IA and IE in mice. Molecular mapping of the class II MHC has revealed multiple β-chain genes in some regions in both mice and humans, as well as multiple α-chain genes in humans (see Figure 7-15). In the human DR region, for example, there are three or four functional β-chain genes. All of the β-chain gene products can be expressed together with the α-chain gene product in a given cell, thereby increasing the number of different antigen-presenting molecules on the cell. Although the human DR region contains just one α-chain gene, the DP and DQ regions each contains two functional α-chain genes.

Genes encoding nonclassical class II MHC molecules also have been identified in both humans and mice. In mice, several class II genes (*Oa, Ob, Ma,* and *Mb*) encode nonclassical MHC molecules that exhibit limited polymorphism and a different pattern of expression than the classical IA and IE class II molecules. In the human class II region, nonclassical genes designated *DM, DN,* and *DO* have been identified. The *DM* genes encode a class II–like molecule (HLA-DM) that facilitates the loading of antigenic peptides into the class II MHC molecules. Class II DO molecules, which have a pattern of expression limited to the thymus and to mature B cells, have been shown to serve as regulators of class II antigen processing. The functions of HLA-DM and HLA-DO will be described further in Chapter 8.

Mapping analysis of the class II MHC region also has revealed the presence, in both mice and humans, of two genes (*LMP2* and *LMP7*) that encode proteasome subunits and of two genes (*TAP1* and *TAP2*) that encode peptide-transporter subunits. As described in Chapter 8, proteasomes that contain the LMP2 and LMP7 products are thought to mediate cytoplasmic degradation of endogenous proteins into peptides, which then are transferred by peptide transporters (TAP1 and TAP2) into the lumen of the endoplasmic reticulum; here the peptides can encounter newly synthesized class I MHC molecules.

Map of Class III MHC

The class III region of the MHC in humans and mice contains a heterogeneous collection of genes (see Figure 7-15). These genes encode several complement components, two steroid 21-hydroxylases, two heat-shock proteins, and two cytokines (TNF-α and TNF-β). Some of these class III MHC gene products play a role in certain diseases. For example, mutations in the genes encoding 21-hydroxylase have been linked to congenital adrenal hyperplasia.

Cellular Distribution of MHC Molecules

In general, the classical class I MHC molecules are expressed on most somatic cells, but the level of class I MHC expression differs among different cell types. The highest levels of class I molecules are expressed by lymphocytes, where they constitute approximately 1% of the total plasma-membrane proteins, or some 5×10^5 molecules per cell. In contrast, fibroblasts, muscle cells, liver hepatocytes, and neural cells express very low levels of class I MHC molecules. The low level of class I MHC molecules on liver cells may reduce the likelihood of graft recognition by T cytotoxic lymphocytes of the recipient, thus contributing to the considerable success of liver transplants. A few cell types (e.g., neurons and sperm cells at certain stages of differentiation) appear to lack class I MHC molecules altogether.

As noted earlier, any particular MHC molecule can bind many different peptides. Since the MHC alleles are codominantly expressed, a heterozygous individual expresses on its cells the gene products encoded by both alleles at each MHC locus. An F_1 mouse, for example, expresses the K, D, and L from each parent (six different class I MHC molecules) on each of its nucleated cells (Figure 7-16). A similar situation occurs in humans; that is, a heterozygous individual expresses the A, B, and C alleles from each parent (six different class I MHC molecules) on the membrane of each nucleated cell. The expression of so many class I MHC molecules allows each cell to display a large number of peptides in the peptide-binding clefts of its MHC molecules. If a cell is a normal healthy cell, its class I molecules will display self-peptides resulting from normal turnover of self proteins. For example, self-peptides derived from cytochrome *c*, histones, and ribosomal protein have been eluted from class I MHC molecules on normal cells.

On the other hand, if a cell has been infected by a virus, then viral peptides, as well as self-peptides, will be displayed by its class I MHC molecules. A single virus-infected cell should be envisioned as having various class I molecules on its membrane, each displaying different sets of viral peptides. Because of individual allelic differences in the peptide-binding clefts of the class I MHC molecules, different individuals within a species will have the ability to bind different sets of viral peptides.

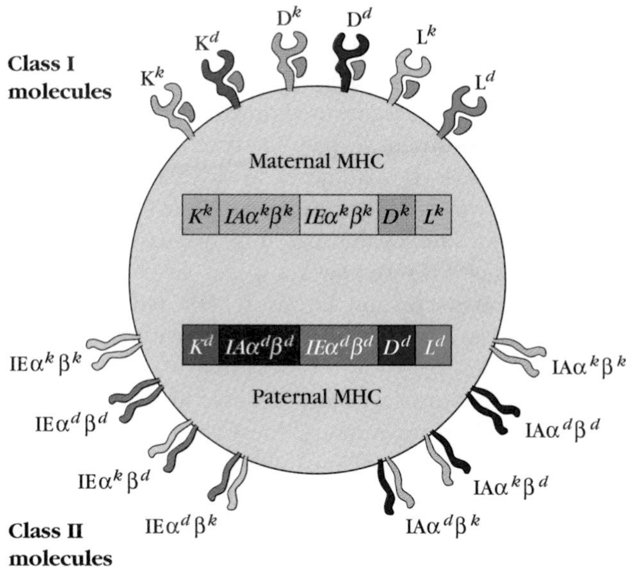

FIGURE 7-16 Diagram illustrating various MHC molecules expressed on antigen-presenting cells of a heterozygous H-$2^{k/d}$ mouse. Both the maternal and paternal MHC genes are expressed. Because the class II molecules are heterodimers, heterologous molecules containing one maternal-derived and one paternal-derived chain are produced. The β_2-microglobulin component of class I molecules (pink) is encoded by a gene on a separate chromosome and may be derived from either parent.

Unlike class I MHC molecules, class II molecules are expressed constitutively only by antigen-presenting cells. The primary antigen-presenting cells are macrophages, dendritic cells, and B cells; thymic epithelial cells and some other cell types can be induced to function and do then express MHC II as antigen-presenting cells under certain conditions and under stimulation of some cytokines (see Chapter 8). Among the various cell types that express class II MHC molecules, marked differences in expression have been observed. In some cases, class II expression depends on the cell's differentiation stage. For example, class II molecules cannot be detected on pre-B cells but are expressed on the membrane of mature B cells. Dendritic cells (including Langerhans cells) and mature B cells constitutively express class II MHC molecules. In contrast, monocytes and macrophages that have not interacted with antigen express only low levels of class II molecules, but these cells increase their expression significantly after they have been activated.

Because each of the classical class II MHC molecules is composed of two different polypeptide chains, which are encoded by different loci, a heterozygous individual expresses not only the parental class II molecules but also molecules containing α and β chains from different chromosomes. For example, an H-2^k mouse expresses IA^k and IE^k class II molecules; similarly, an H-2^d mouse expresses IA^d and IE^d molecules. The F_1 progeny resulting from crosses of mice with these two haplotypes express four parental class II molecules and four molecules containing one parent's α chain and the other parent's β chain (as shown in Figure 7-16). Since the human MHC contains three classical class II genes (*DP, DQ,* and *DR*), a heterozygous individual expresses six parental class II molecules and six molecules containing α and β chain combinations from either parent. The number of different class II molecules expressed by an individual is increased further by the presence of multiple β-chain genes in mice and humans, and in humans by multiple α-chain genes. The diversity generated by these mechanisms presumably increases the number of different antigenic peptides that can be presented and thus is advantageous to the organism.

Regulation of MHC Expression

As the previous section indicates, differential expression of the MHC genes occurs. Class II MHC genes are expressed only in a limited number of cell types, and the level of expression of both class I and class II genes differs among cell types. Certain nonclassical MHC molecules appear on rare cell types. Research on the regulatory mechanisms that control this differential expression is still in its infancy.

Both class I and class II MHC genes are flanked by 5′ promoter sequences, which bind sequence-specific transcription factors. The promoter motifs and transcription factors that bind to these motifs are beginning to be identified. Transcriptional regulation of the MHC is mediated by both positive and negative elements. For example, an MHC II transactivator, called *CIITA*, and another transcription factor, called *RFX*, both have been shown to bind to the promoter region of class II MHC genes. Defects in these transcription factors cause one form of *bare lymphocyte syndrome.* Patients with this disorder lack class II MHC molecules on their cells and as a result suffer a severe immunodeficiency due to the central role of class II MHC molecules in T-cell maturation and activation.

The expression of MHC molecules is also regulated by various cytokines. The interferons (alpha, beta, and gamma) and tumor necrosis factor have each been shown to increase expression of class I MHC molecules on cells. Interferon gamma (IFN-γ), for example, appears to induce the formation of a specific transcription factor that binds to the promoter sequence flanking the class I MHC genes. Binding of this transcription factor to the promoter sequence appears to coordinate the up-regulation of transcription of the genes encoding the class I α chain, β_2-microglobulin, the proteasome subunits (LMP), and the transporter subunits (TAP). IFN-γ also has been shown to induce expression of the class II transactivator (CIITA), thereby indirectly increasing expression of class II MHC molecules on a variety of cells, including non-antigen-presenting cells (e.g., skin keratinocytes, intestinal epithelial cells, vascular endothelium, placental cells, and pancreatic beta cells). Other cytokines influence MHC expression only in certain cell types; for example, IL-4 increases expression of class II molecules by resting B cells. Expression of class II molecules by B cells is down-regulated by IFN-γ; corticosteroids and prostaglandins also decrease expression of class II molecules.

MHC expression is decreased by infection with certain viruses, including human cytomegalovirus (CMV), hepatitis B virus (HBV), and adenovirus 12 (Ad12). In some cases, reduced expression of class I MHC molecules is due to reduction in a component needed for peptide transport or MHC class I assembly rather than in a decrease in transcription as such. In cytomegalovirus infection, for example, a viral protein binds to β_2-microglobulin, preventing assembly of class I MHC molecules and their transport to the plasma membrane. Adenovirus 12 infection causes a pronounced decrease in transcription of the transporter genes (*TAP1* and *TAP2*). As the next chapter describes, the TAP gene products play an important role in peptide transport from the cytoplasm into the rough endoplasmic reticulum. Blocking of *TAP* gene expression inhibits peptide transport; as a result, class I MHC molecules cannot assemble with β_2-microglobulin or be transported to the cell membrane. Decreased expression of class I MHC molecules, by whatever mechanism, is likely to help viruses evade the immune response by reducing the likelihood that virus-infected cells can display MHC–viral peptide complexes and become targets for CTL-mediated destruction.

MHC and Immune Responsiveness

Early studies by B. Benacerraf in which guinea pigs were immunized with simple synthetic antigens first showed that the ability of an animal to mount an immune response, as measured by the production of serum antibodies, is determined by its MHC haplotype. Later experiments by H. McDevitt, M. Sela, and their colleagues used congenic and recombinant congenic mouse strains to map the control of *immune responsiveness* to class II MHC genes. In early reports, the genes responsible for this phenotype were designated Ir or immune response genes, and for this reason mouse class II products are called IA and IE. We now know that the dependence of immune responsiveness on the class II MHC reflects the central role of class II MHC molecules in presenting antigen to T_H cells.

Two explanations have been proposed to account for the variability in immune responsiveness observed among different haplotypes. According to the *determinant-selection model*, different class II MHC molecules differ in their ability to bind processed antigen. According to the alternative *holes-in-the-repertoire model*, T cells bearing receptors that recognize foreign antigens closely resembling self-antigens may be eliminated during thymic processing. Since the T-cell response to an antigen involves a trimolecular complex of the T cell's receptor, an antigenic peptide, and an MHC molecule (see Figure 3-9), both models may be correct. That is, the absence of an MHC molecule that can bind and present a given peptide, or the absence of T-cell receptors that can recognize a given peptide–MHC molecule complex, could result in the absence of immune responsiveness and so account for the observed relationship between MHC haplotype and immune responsiveness to exogenous antigens.

TABLE 7-3 DIFFERENTIAL BINDING OF PEPTIDES TO MOUSE CLASS II MHC MOLECULES AND CORRELATION WITH MHC RESTRICTION

		Percentage of labeled peptide bound to‡			
Labeled peptide*	MHC restriction of responders†	IA^d	IE^d	IA^k	IE^k
Ovalbumin (323–339)	IA^d	**11.8**	0.1	0.2	0.1
Influenza hemagglutinin (130–142)	IA^d	**18.9**	0.6	7.1	0.3
Hen egg-white lysozyme (46–61)	IA^k	0.0	0.0	**35.2**	0.5
Hen egg-white lysozyme (74–86)	IA^k	2.0	2.3	**2.9**	1.7
Hen egg-white lysozyme (81–96)	IE^k	0.4	0.2	0.7	**1.1**
Myoglobin (132–153)	IE^d	0.8	**6.3**	0.5	0.7
Pigeon cytochrome *c* (88–104)	IE^k	0.6	1.2	1.7	**8.7**
λ repressor (12–26)§	$IA^d + IE^k$	1.6	**8.9**	0.3	2.3

*Amino acid residues included in each peptide are indicated by the numbers in parentheses.

†Refers to class II molecule (IA or IE) and haplotype associated with a good response to the indicated peptides.

‡Binding determined by equilibrium dialysis. Bold-faced values indicate binding was significantly greater ($p < 0.05$) than that of the other three class II molecules tested.

§The λ repressor is an exception to the rule that high binding correlates with the MHC restriction of high-responder strains. In this case, the T_H cell specific for the λ peptide–IE^d complex has been deleted; this is an example of the hole-in-the-repertoire mechanism.

SOURCE: Adapted from S Buus et al, 1987, *Science* **235**:1353.

The determinant-selection model assumes that the structure of a particular MHC molecule determines the strength of its association with any given antigen. Animals that respond, for example, to antigen A must express at least one class II MHC molecule whose structure facilitates interaction with antigen A, whereas animals that do not respond must express class II MHC molecules that do not interact effectively with antigen A. According to this model, the MHC polymorphism within a species will generate different patterns of responsiveness and nonresponsiveness to different antigens. If this model is correct, then class II MHC molecules from mouse strains that respond to a particular antigen and those that do not should show differential binding of that antigen. Table 7-3 presents data on the binding of various radiolabeled peptides to class II IA and IE molecules with the H-2^d or H-2^k haplotype. Each of the listed peptides binds significantly to only one of the IA or IE molecules. Furthermore, in all but one case, the haplotype of the class II molecule showing the highest affinity for a particular peptide is the same as the haplotype of responder strains for that peptide, as the determinant-selection model predicts.

The single exception to the general pattern in Table 7-3 (residues 12–26 of the λ repressor protein) gives evidence that the influence on immune responsiveness can also be caused by absence of functional T cells (holes-in-the-repertoire model) capable of recognizing a given antigen–MHC molecule complex. The λ repressor peptide binds best in vitro to IE^d, yet the MHC restriction for response to this peptide is known to be associated not with IE^d but instead with IA^d and IE^k. This suggests that T cells recognizing this repressor peptide in association with IE^d may have been eliminated by negative selection in the thymus, leaving a hole in the T-cell repertoire.

MHC and Disease Susceptibility

An extensive body of information links certain HLA alleles to susceptibility to certain diseases. A number of different diseases have been associated with particular MHC alleles. Among them are some autoimmune diseases, certain viral diseases, disorders of the complement system, some neurologic disorders, and several different allergies. Researchers have shown that some HLA alleles occur at a much higher frequency among those suffering from certain diseases than in the general population. This association between HLA alleles and a given disease may be quantified by typing the HLA alleles expressed by individuals with the disease and the HLA alleles of the general population. By comparing the frequency of that allele in the patients with the allele frequency in the general population, the **relative risk** may be calculated (see Table 7-4). A relative risk value of 1 means that the HLA allele is expressed with the same frequency in the patient and

TABLE 7-4 SOME SIGNIFICANT ASSOCIATIONS OF HLA ALLELES WITH INCREASED RISK FOR VARIOUS DISEASES

Disease	Associated HLA allele	Relative risk*
Ankylosing spondylitis	*B27*	90
Goodpasture's syndrome	*DR2*	16
Gluten-sensitive enteropathy	*DR3*	12
Hereditary hemochromatosis	*A3*	9.3
	B14	2.3
	A3/B14	90
Insulin-dependent diabetes mellitus	*DR4/DR3*	20
Multiple sclerosis	*DR2*	5
Myasthenia gravis	*DR3*	10
Narcolepsy	*DR2*	130
Reactive arthritis (*Yersinia, Salmonella, Gonococcus*)	*B27*	18
Reiter's syndrome	*B27*	37
Rheumatoid arthritis	*DR4*	10
Sjogren's syndrome	*Dw3*	6
Systemic lupus erythematosus	*DR3*	5

*Relative risk is calculated by dividing the frequency of the HLA allele in the patient population by the frequency in the general population:

$$RR = \frac{(Ag^+/Ag^-)\text{ disease}}{(Ag^+/Ag^-)\text{ control}}$$

SOURCE: *SAM CD: A Comprehensive Knowledge Base of Internal Medicine,* DC Dale and DD Federman, eds., 1997, Scientific American, New York.

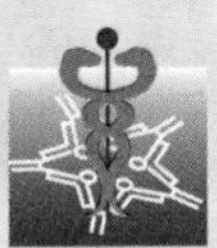

CLINICAL FOCUS

HLA-H AND HEREDITARY HEMOCHROMATOSIS

Hereditary hemochromatosis (HH) is a disease in which there is defective regulation of dietary iron absorption, which leads to increased levels of iron. HH (which in earlier reports may be referred to as *idiopathic* or *primary* hemochromatosis) is the most common known autosomal recessive genetic disorder in North Americans of European descent, with a frequency of 3–4 cases per 1000 persons. Recent studies show that this disease is associated with a mutation in the nonclassical class I gene *HLA-H,* which lies to the telomeric side of *HLA-A*. The association of the *HLA-H* gene with HH is an example of how potentially life-saving clinical information was obtained by studying the connection of HLA genes with disease.

The total iron content of a normal human adult is 3 to 4 grams; the average dietary intake of iron is about 10 to 20 milligrams per day; of this, only 1 to 2 mg is absorbed. The iron balance is maintained by control of its absorption from digested food in the intestinal tract. The primary defect in HH is increased gastrointestinal uptake of iron and, as a result of this, patients with HH may throughout their lives accumulate 15 to 35 grams of iron instead of the normal 3 to 4 grams. The iron overload results in pathologic accumulation of iron in cells of many organs, including the heart and liver. Although a severe form of HH may result in heart disease in children, the clinical manifestations of the disease are not usually seen until 40 to 50 years of age. Males are affected eight times more frequently than females. Early symptoms of HH are rather nonspecific and include weakness, lethargy, abdominal pain, diabetes, impotency, and severe joint pain. Physical examination of HH sufferers reveals liver damage, skin pigmentation, arthritis, enlarged spleen, jaundice, and peripheral edema. If untreated, HH results in hepatic cancer, liver failure, severe diabetes, and heart disease. Exactly how the increase in iron content results in these diseases is not known, but repeated phlebotomy (taking blood) is an effective treatment if the disease is recognized before there is extensive damage to organs. Phlebotomy does not reverse damage already done. Phlebotomy (called blood letting) was used as treatment for many conditions in former times; HH may be one of the rare instances in which the treatment has a positive rather than a harmful effect on the patient.

Prior to appearance of the recognized signs of the disease, such as the characteristic skin pigmentation or liver dysfunction, diagnosis is difficult unless for some reason (such as family history of the disease) HH is suspected and specific tests for iron metabolism are performed. A reliable genetic test for HH would allow treatment to commence prior to disease manifestation and irreversible organ damage.

Because it is a common disease, the HLA association with HH was studied; a significant association with the *HLA-A3* allele was found (RR of 9.3). This association is well documented, but the relatively high frequency of the *HLA-A3* allele (present in 20% of the North American population) makes this an inadequate marker; the majority of individuals with *HLA-A3* will not have HH. Further studies showed a greatly increased relative risk in individuals with the combination of *HLA-A3* and *HLA-B14*; homozygotes for these two alleles carried a relative risk for HH of 90. Detailed studies in several populations in the

general populations; therefore, the allele confers no increased risk for the disease. By contrast, a relative risk value substantially above 1 indicates an association between the HLA allele and the disease, implying that persons with that allele are more likely to acquire the disease. So relative risk is a measure of the increased susceptibility of an individual with the allele over those lacking the allele. For example, individuals with DR4 have a ten times greater chance of acquiring rheumatoid arthritis than do those in the same population who lack DR4.

Table 7-4 lists some diseases for which association between a particular MHC allele and disease susceptibility has been demonstrated. As seen in the table, the relative risk established for the listed diseases associated with the identified allele varies considerably. For example, a strong association exists between the HLA-B27 allele and the autoimmune disease *ankylosing spondylitis*, an inflammatory disease of vertebral joints characterized by destruction of cartilage. Individuals who have HLA-B27 have a 90 times greater likelihood (relative risk of 90) of developing ankylosing spondylitis than do individuals with a different HLA-B allele. However, the existence of such an association should not be interpreted to imply that the expression of a particular MHC allele has caused the disease, because the relationship between MHC alleles and development of disease is complex. For example, it has been suggested that because of the close linkage of the TNF-α and

US and in France with high incidence of HH revealed a mutation in the nonclassical HLA class I gene *HLA-H* in 83%–100% of patients with HH. *HLA-H,* which lies close to the *HLA-A* locus, was shown in several independent studies to carry a characteristic mutation at position 283 in HH patients. In the patients there was substitution of a tyrosine residue for a cysteine normally found at this position. This substitution precludes formation of the disulfide link between cysteines in the $\alpha3$ domain, which is necessary for association of the MHC α chain with β_2-microglobulin and for expression on the cell surface. HLA-H molecules are normally expressed on the surface of cells in the stomach, intestines, and liver. There is evidence suggesting that HLA-H plays a role in the ability of these organs to regulate iron uptake from the circulation.

There are several possible reasons for why this defect continues to be so common in our population. Factors that favor the spread of the defective *HLA-H* gene would include the fact that this is a recessive trait, so that only homozygotes are affected; the gene is silent in carriers. In addition, even in homozygotes who are affected with HH, the disease does not manifest itself until later in life and so may have minimal influence on the breeding success of the HH sufferer.

Studies of knockout mice that lack the gene for β_2-microglobulin give evidence for the need of MHC class I products on cell surfaces to maintain normal iron metabolism. These mice, which are unable to express any of their class I molecules on the cell surfaces, suffer from iron overload with disease consequences similar to HH. Studies are in progress to determine how the *HLA-H* mutation leads to increased iron uptake and to the defective regulation of iron storage that so often causes serious illness. Such studies may lead to more rapid diagnosis of HH in children, allowing treatment to begin before there is severe damage to major organs. It is possible that, in the more distant future, HH may be treatable by gene therapy if the single defect in *HLA-H* is confirmed to be the sole causative factor.

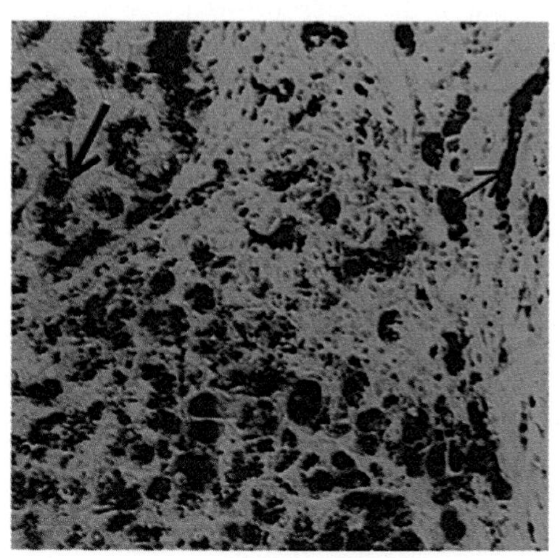

High-magnification iron stain of liver cells from HH patient. This high-magnification iron stain of the liver cells confirms the presence of iron in both parenchymal cells (thick arrow) and bile duct cells (thin arrow). This woman with hemochromatosis required removal of 72 units (9 gallons) of blood during one and a half years to render her liver free of excess iron. [Source: *SAM CD: A Comprehensive Knowledge Base of Internal Medicine,* DC Dale and DD Federman, eds., 1997, Scientific American, New York.]

TNF-β genes with the HLA-B locus, these cytokines may be involved in the destruction of cartilage. An association of HLA class I genes A3 and B14 with the disease hereditary hemochromatosis is discussed in the Clinical Focus.

In weak associations between MHC and disease, reflected by low relative risk values, it is likely that multiple genes, of which only one is in the MHC, influence susceptibility. That these diseases are not inherited by simple mendelian segregation of MHC alleles can be seen in identical twins; both inherit the MHC risk factor, but sometimes only one develops the disease. This finding suggests that multiple genetic and environmental factors have roles in the development of disease, especially autoimmune diseases, with the MHC playing an important but not exclusive role. An additional difficulty in associating a particular MHC product with disease is the genetic phenomenon of linkage disequilibrium, which we described above. The fact that some of the class I MHC alleles were in linkage disequilibrium with the class II MHC alleles made their contribution to disease susceptibility appear more pronounced than it actually was. If, for example, DR4 were the causative gene, and it occurs frequently in combination with A3 because of linkage disequilibrium, then A3 would incorrectly appear to be associated with the disease. Improved genomic mapping techniques make it possible to analyze the linkage between the MHC and various diseases more fully and to assess the contributions from other loci.

A number of hypotheses have been offered to account for the role of the MHC in disease susceptibility. Susceptibility to a given pathogen may reflect the role of particular MHC alleles in responsiveness or nonresponsiveness to the pathogen. This may result from variations in antigen presentation by different MHC alleles, which determine the effectiveness of the immune response to a pathogen. If major epitopes on a given pathogen mimic certain self-MHC molecules, it is possible that an animal may lack functional T cells specific for those epitopes. Allelic forms of MHC genes may encode molecules that serve as receptors for viruses or bacterial toxins. As will be explained in Chapter 16, the genetic analysis of disease must consider the possibility that genes at multiple loci and complex interactions among them may be involved.

Some evidence suggests that a reduction in MHC polymorphism within a species may predispose that species to infectious disease. Cheetahs, for example, have been shown to be far more susceptible to viral disease than are other big cats. Because the present cheetah population (Figure 7-17) arose from a limited breeding stock, the species suffers from a loss of MHC diversity. The increased susceptibility of cheetahs to various viral diseases may result from a reduction in the number of different MHC molecules available to the species as a whole and a corresponding limitation on the range of processed antigens with which these MHC molecules can interact. Thus, the high level of MHC polymorphism that has been observed in various species may provide the advantage of a broad range of antigen-presenting MHC molecules. Although some individuals within a species probably will not be able to develop an immune response to any given pathogen and therefore will be susceptible to infection by it, this extreme polymorphism ensures that at least some members of a species will be able to respond and will be resistant. In this way, MHC diversity appears to protect a species from a wide range of infectious diseases.

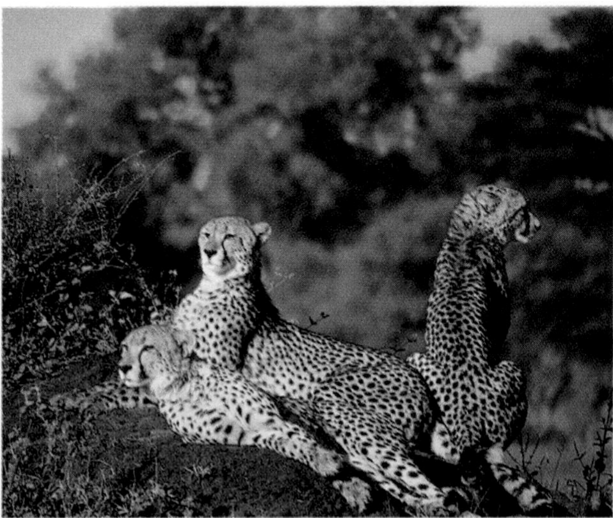

FIGURE 7-17 Cheetah female with two nearly full grown cubs. Polymorphism in MHC genes of the cheetah is very limited, presumably because of a bottleneck in breeding that occurred in the not too distant past. It is assumed that all cheetahs alive today are descents of a very small breeding pool. [Photograph taken in the Okavango Delta, Botswana, by TJ Kindt.]

Summary

1. The major histocompatibility complex (MHC) comprises a stretch of tightly linked genes that encode proteins associated with intercellular recognition and antigen presentation to T lymphocytes. The MHC, called the H-2 complex in mice and the HLA complex in humans, is organized into three regions based on the type of molecules encoded (see Figure 7-1). Class I molecules are encoded by the K and D regions in mice and the A, B, and C regions in humans. Class II molecules are encoded by the IA and IE regions in mice and the DP, DQ, and DR regions in humans. Class III molecules in both humans and mice are encoded in the region between class I and II. Many alleles exist for each class I and class II MHC gene; the entire set of MHC alleles on a chromosome is referred to as its haplotype.
2. Class I MHC molecules consist of a large glycoprotein α chain, encoded by the class I MHC genes, and a much smaller molecule of β_2-microglobulin, encoded by a gene outside of the MHC (see Figure 7-5). The α chain contains three external domains ($\alpha1$, $\alpha2$, and $\alpha3$), a hydrophobic transmembrane segment, and a cytoplasmic tail. The latter two domains anchor the α chain to the plasma membrane, and the $\alpha1$ and $\alpha2$ domains interact to form a cleft that binds antigenic peptides. Class II MHC molecules are heterodimers composed of two noncovalently associated glycoproteins, the α and β chain, which are encoded by separate class II genes (see Figure 7-5). Each chain contains two external domains, a transmembrane segment, and a cytoplasmic tail. The genes encoding the class I α chain and class II α and β chains are organized as a series of exons and introns, with each exon encoding a separate region of the polypeptide chain (see Figure 7-9).
3. X-ray crystallographic analysis has been accomplished for several class I and class II MHC molecules. These analyses have revealed that the peptide-binding region in both class I and class II molecules is a deep cleft with eight antiparallel β strands forming the floor and two antiparallel α helices forming the sides (see Figure 7-6). Certain class II molecules that have been crystallized did so as dimers of the $\alpha\beta$ heterodimer, although others have been crystallized as a single $\alpha\beta$ pair (see Figure 7-8).
4. Because portions of both class I and class II MHC molecules exhibit the immunoglobulin-fold structure, these

molecules are considered members of the immunoglobulin superfamily. Both class I and class II MHC molecules present antigen to T cells. Class I molecules, which appear on the surface of nearly all nucleated cells, present processed endogenous antigen to $CD8^+$ T cells. Class II molecules, which are expressed on a limited number of antigen-presenting cells (macrophages, dendritic cells, B cells), present processed exogenous antigen to $CD4^+$ T cells.

5. The interactions between class I and II MHC molecules and peptides have been studied with several different experimental approaches. Elution experiments and binding experiments have demonstrated that peptide length and the presence or absence of certain conserved motifs in peptides influence their ability to interact with class I and class II MHC molecules (see Table 7-2). Studies with hybrid and mutated genes have demonstrated that both membrane-distal domains in class I and class II MHC molecules are necessary for antigen presentation. Direct evidence of the interaction between a peptide and the cleft formed by the two membrane-distal domains in class I and class II molecules has been obtained from x-ray crystallographic analyses of peptide–MHC molecule complexes (see Figure 7-10).
6. The class III region of the MHC encodes molecules that include a diverse group of nonmembrane proteins that play no role in antigen presentation. Disturbances in the expression of some class III molecules (e.g., certain complement components, tumor necrosis factors, and heat-shock proteins) may be associated with certain autoimmune diseases.
7. Genomic mapping analyses of the MHC have supplemented earlier results obtained by serologic analyses (see Figure 7-15). The detailed genomic map of the MHC developed to date includes a number of "nonclassical" class I and class II genes. Some of these are pseudogenes, but others encode protein products with highly specific functions. Nonclassical genes within the class II region in both mice and humans encode proteasome subunits and peptide-transporter subunits; these proteins function in the cytosolic pathway for processing endogenous proteins.
8. Studies with congenic and recombinant congenic mouse strains have shown that MHC haplotype influences immune responsiveness and the ability to present antigen. The variation in amino acid sequences (i.e., the polymorphism) that gives rise to different haplotypes occurs primarily in the membrane-distal domains of class I and class II MHC molecules (see Figure 7-14). The polymorphic residues in class I MHC molecules have been shown to be localized primarily in the peptide-binding cleft.
9. Increased susceptibility to a number of diseases, predominantly but not exclusively of an autoimmune nature, has been linked to certain MHC alleles (see Table 7-4). There is a large range of risk carried by the MHC alleles; in all cases, other hereditary and environmental factors determine whether an individual will be afflicted. In certain cases, the MHC genes appear to act in concert with other, non-MHC, genes to influence risk of disease, while some variations in other MHC genes have been more directly linked to disease.

REFERENCES

Bahram, S, and T Spies. 1996. The MIC gene family. *Res. Immunol.* **147:**328.

Bjorkman, PJ, and WP Burmeister. 1994. Structures of two classes of MHC molecules elucidated: crucial differences and similarities. *Curr. Opin. Struc. Biol.* **4:**852.

Borot, N, et al. 1997. Mutations in the MHC class I–like candidate gene for hemochromatosis in French patients. *Immunogenetics* **45:**320.

Brown, JH, et al. 1993. Three-dimensional structure of the human class II histocompatibility antigen HLA-DR1. *Nature* **364:**33.

Dessen, A, et al. 1997. X-ray crystal structure of HLA-DR4 (DRA*0101, DRB1*0401) complexed with a peptide from human collagen II. *Immunity* **7:**473.

Engelhard, VH. 1994. Structure of peptides associated with MHC class I molecules. *Curr. Opin. Immunol.* **6:**13.

Gao, GF, et al. 1997. Crystal structure of the complex between human CD8 alpha alpha and HLA-A2. *Nature* **387:**630.

Garboczi, DN, et al. 1996. Structure of the complex between human T-cell receptor, viral peptide and HLA-A2 . *Nature* **384:**134.

Ghosh, P, et al. 1995. The structure of an intermediate in class II MHC maturation: CLIP bound to HLA-DR3. *Nature* **378:**457.

Guo, HC, et al. 1992. Different length peptides bind to HLA-Aw68 similarly at their ends but bulge out in the middle. *Nature* **360:**364.

Gruen, JR, and SM Weissman. 1997. Evolving views of the Major Histocompatibility Complex. *Blood* **90:**4252.

Hedrick, SM. 1992. Dawn of the hunt for nonclassical MHC function. *Cell* **70:**177.

Hughes, AL, M Yeager, and M Carrington. 1996. Peptide binding function and the paradox of HLA disease associations. *Immunol. Cell Biol.* **74:**444.

Jardetzky, TS, et al. 1996. Crystallographic analysis of endogenous peptides associated with HLA-DR1 suggests a common, polyproline II-like conformation for bound peptides. *Proc. Natl. Acad. Sci. USA* **93:**734.

Jazwinska, EC, and LW Powell. 1997. Hemochromatosis and "HLA-H": definite! *Hepatology* **25:**495.

Jouanolle, AM, et al. 1997. A candidate gene for hemochromatosis: frequency of the C282Y and H63D mutations. *Hum. Genet.* **100:**544.

Kim, J, et al. 1994. Toxic shock syndrome toxin-1 complexed with a class II MHC major histocompatibility molecule HLA-DR-1. *Science* **266:**1870.

Madden, DR. 1995. The three-dimensional structure of peptide-MHC complexes. *Annu. Rev. Immunol.* **13:**587.

Madden, DR, et al. 1992. The three dimensional structure of HLA-B27 at 2.1 Å resolution suggests a general mechanism for tight peptide binding to MHC. *Cell* **70:**1035.

Nepon, GT. 1995. Class II antigens and disease susceptibility. *Annu. Rev. Med.* **46:**17.

Parham, P. 1992. Deconstructing the MHC. *Nature* **360:**300.

Parham P. 1996. Presentation of HLA class I-derived peptides: potential involvement in allorecognition and HLA-B27-associated arthritis. *Immunol. Rev.* **154:**137.

Rothenberg, BE, and JR Voland. 1996. Beta 2 knockout mice develop parenchymal iron overload: A putative role for class I genes of the major histocompatibility complex in iron metabolism. *Proc. Natl. Acad. Sci. USA* **93:**1529.

Rotzschke, O, and K Falk. 1994. Origin, structure and motifs of naturally processed MHC class II ligands. *Curr. Opin. Immunol.* **6:**45.

Rouas-Freiss, N, et al. 1997. Direct evidence to support the role of HLA-G in protecting the fetus from maternal uterine natural killer cytolysis. *Proc. Natl. Acad. Sci. USA* **94:**11520.

Silver, ML, et al. 1992. Atomic structure of a human MHC molecule presenting an influenza virus peptide. *Nature* **360:**367.

Stroynowski, I, and J Forman. 1995. Novel molecules related to MHC antigens. *Curr. Opin. Immunol.* **7:**97.

Vyse, TJ, and JA Todd. 1996. Genetic analysis of autoimmune disease. *Cell* **85:**311.

Useful Web Sites

http://www.bioscience.org/knockout/b2micrgl.htm for beta-2 microglobulin KO

http://www.bioscience.org/knockout/mhci.htm for MHC class I KO

http://www.bioscience.org/knockout/mhcii.htm for KO of an MHC class II chain

http://www.bioscience.org/knockout/mhc2inva.htm for KO of the invariant chain

This series of destinations in the Bioscience Web site provide updated information on studies of the consequences of targeted disruption of MHC molecules and other component molecules including β2 microglobulin and the class II invariant chain.

STUDY QUESTIONS

1. Indicate whether each of the following statements is true or false. If you think a statement is false, explain why.

a. A monoclonal antibody specific for β_2-microglobulin can be used to detect both class I MHC K and D molecules on the surface of cells.

b. Antigen-presenting cells express both class I and class II MHC molecules on their membranes.

c. Class III MHC genes encode membrane-bound proteins.

d. In outbred populations, an individual is more likely to be histocompatible with one of its parents than with its siblings.

e. Class II MHC molecules typically bind to longer peptides than do class I molecules.

f. All cells express class I MHC molecules.

g. The majority of the peptides displayed by class I and class II MHC molecules on cells are derived from self-proteins.

2. You wish to produce a syngeneic and a congenic mouse strain. Indicate whether each of the following characteristics applies to production of syngeneic (S), congenic (C), or both (S and C) mice.

a. Requires the greatest number of generations

b. Requires backcrosses

c. Yields mice that are genetically identical

d. Requires selection for homozygosity

e. Requires sibling crosses

f. Can be started with outbred mice

g. Yields progeny that are genetically identical to the parent except for a single genetic region

3. You have generated a congenic A.B mouse strain that has been selected for the MHC. The haplotype of strain A was *a/a* and of strain B was *b/b.*

a. Which strain provides the genetic background of this mouse?

b. Which strain provides the haplotype of the MHC of this mouse?

c. To produce this congenic strain, the F_1 progeny are always backcrossed to which strain?

d. Why was backcrossing to one of the parents performed?

e. Why was interbreeding of the F_1 and F_2 progeny performed?

f. Why was selection necessary and what kind of selection was performed?

4. You cross a BALB/c (H-2^d) mouse with a CBA (H-2^k) mouse. What MHC molecules will the F_1 progeny express on (a) its liver cells and (b) its macrophages?

5. To carry out studies on the structure and function of the class I MHC molecule K^b and the class II MHC molecule IA^b, you decide to transfect the genes encoding these proteins into a mouse fibroblast cell line (L cell) derived from the C3H strain (H-2^k). L cells do not normally function as antigen-presenting cells. In the following table, indicate which of the listed MHC molecules will (+) or will not (−) be expressed on the membrane of the transfected L cells.

	MHC molecules expressed on the membrane of the transfected L cells					
Transfected gene	D^k	D^b	K^k	K^b	IA^k	IA^b
None						
K^b						
$IA\alpha^b$						
$IA\beta^b$						
$IA\alpha^b$ and $IA\beta^b$						

Go to www.whfreeman.com/immunology Self-Test
Review and quiz of key terms

6. The SJL mouse strain, which has the H-2^k haplotype, has a deletion of the *IEα* locus.

a. List the classical MHC molecules that are expressed on the membrane of macrophages from SJL mice.

b. If the class II *IEα* and *IEβ* genes from an H-2^s strain are transfected into SJL macrophages, what additional classical MHC molecules would be expressed on the transfected macrophages?

7. Draw diagrams illustrating the general structure, including the domains, of class I MHC molecules, class II MHC molecules, and membrane-bound antibody on B cells. Label each chain and the domains within it, the antigen-binding regions, and regions that have the immunoglobulin-fold structure.

8. One of the characteristic features of the MHC is the large number of different alleles at each locus.

a. Where are most of the polymorphic amino acid residues located in MHC molecules? What is the significance of this location?

b. How is MHC polymorphism thought to be generated?

9. As a student in an immunology laboratory class, you have been given spleen cells from a mouse immunized with the LCM virus. You determine the antigen-specific functional activity of these cells with two different assays. In assay 1, the spleen cells are incubated with macrophages that have been briefly exposed to the LCM virus; the production of interleukin 2 (IL-2) is a positive response. In assay 2, the spleen cells are incubated with LCM-infected target cells; lysis of the target cells represents a positive response in this assay. The results of the assays using macrophages and target cells of different haplotypes are presented in the table below. Note that the experiment has been set up in a way to exclude alloreactive responses.

a. The activity of which cell population is detected in each of the two assays?

b. The functional activity of which MHC molecules is detected in each of the two assays?

c. From the results of this experiment, which MHC molecules are required, in addition to the LCM virus, for specific reactivity of the spleen cells in each of the two assays?

d. What additional experiments could you perform to unambiguously confirm the MHC molecules required for antigen-specific reactivity of the spleen cells?

e. Which of the mouse strains listed in the table below could have been the source of the immunized spleen cells tested in the functional assays? Give your reasons.

10. A T_C-cell clone recognizes a particular measles virus peptide when it is presented by H-$2D^b$. Another MHC molecule has an identical peptide-binding cleft as H-$2D^b$ but differs from H-$2D^b$ at several other amino acids in the α1β1 domain. Predict whether the second MHC molecule could present this measles virus peptide to the T_C-cell clone. Briefly explain your answer.

11. How can you determine if two different inbred mouse strains have identical MHC haplotypes?

12. Human red blood cells are not nucleated and do not express any MHC molecules. Why is this property fortuitous for blood transfusions?

13. The hypothetical allelic combination *HLA-A99* and *HLA-B276* carries a relative risk of 200 for a rare, and yet unnamed, disease that is fatal to pre-adolescent children.

a. Will every individual with *A99/B276* contract the disease?

b. Will everyone with the disease have the *A99/B276* combination?

c. How frequently will the *A99/B276* allelic combination be observed in the general population? Do you think that this combination will be more or less frequent than predicted by the frequency of the two individual alleles? Why?

For use with Question 9.

Mouse strain used as source of macrophages and target cells	MHC haplotype of macrophages and virus-infected target cells				Response of spleen cells	
	K	IA	IE	D	IL-2 production in response to LCM-pulsed macrophages (assay 1)	Lysis of LCM-infected cells (assay 2)
C3H	*k*	*k*	*k*	*k*	+	–
BALB/c	*d*	*d*	*d*	*d*	–	+
(BALB/c × B10.A)F_1	*d/k*	*d/k*	*d/k*	*d/d*	+	+
A.TL	*s*	*k*	*k*	*d*	+	+
B10.A (3R)	*b*	*b*	*b*	*d*	–	+
B10.A (4R)	*k*	*k*	–	*b*	+	–

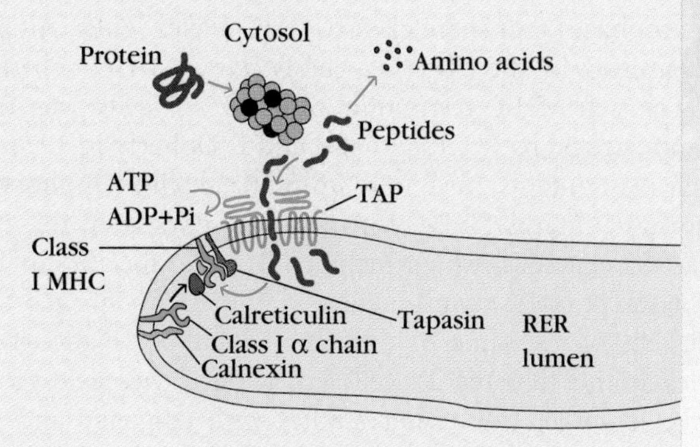

CHAPTER 8

ANTIGEN PROCESSING AND PRESENTATION

Self-MHC Restriction of T Cells

Role of Antigen-Presenting Cells

Evidence for Two Processing and Presentation Pathways

Endogenous Antigens: The Cytosolic Pathway

Exogenous Antigens: The Endocytic Pathway

Presentation of Nonpeptide Bacterial Antigens

Recognition of foreign antigen by a T cell requires that peptides derived from the antigen be displayed within the cleft of an MHC molecule on the membrane of a cell. The formation of these peptide-MHC complexes requires that a protein antigen be degraded into peptides by a sequence of events called **antigen processing.** The degraded peptides then associate with MHC molecules within the cell interior, and the peptide-MHC complexes are transported to the membrane, where they are displayed **(antigen presentation).**

As described briefly in Chapter 1, class I and class II MHC molecules associate with peptides that have been processed in different intracellular compartments. Class I MHC molecules bind peptides derived from **endogenous antigens** that have been processed within the cytoplasm of the cell (e.g., normal cellular proteins, tumor proteins, or viral and bacterial proteins produced within infected cells). Class II MHC molecules bind peptides derived from **exogenous antigens** that are internalized by phagocytosis or endocytosis and processed within the endocytic pathway. This chapter examines in more detail the mechanism of antigen processing and the means by which processed antigen and MHC molecules are combined within different intracellular compartments for presentation. In addition, the chapter describes recent data indicating the existence of a third pathway for the presentation of nonpeptide antigens derived from bacterial pathogens.

Self-MHC Restriction of T Cells

Both $CD4^+$ and $CD8^+$ T cells can recognize antigen only when it is presented with a self-MHC molecule on the membrane of another. This attribute, called *self-MHC restriction,* distinguishes recognition of antigen by T cells from that by B cells. Self-MHC restriction was first discovered in experiments in which T cells from one inbred strain were mixed with macrophages, B cells, or virus-infected cells from another inbred strain. In each experiment, T cells responded to the antigen only if they shared MHC alleles with the other cells in the mixture.

Beginning in the mid-1970s, experiments conducted by a number of researchers demonstrated self-MHC restriction in T-cell recognition. A. Rosenthal and E. Shevach, for example, showed that antigen-specific proliferation of T_H cells occurred only in response to antigen presented by macrophages of the same MHC haplotype. In their experimental system, guinea pig macrophages from strain 2 initially were incubated with an antigen, which allowed the macrophages to process the antigen and subsequently present it on their surface. These "antigen-pulsed" macrophages then were mixed with T cells from the same strain (strain 2), a different strain (strain 13), or (2×13) F_1 animals, and the magnitude of T-cell proliferation in response to the antigen-pulsed macrophages was measured.

The results of these experiments, outlined in Figure 8-1, showed that strain-2 antigen-pulsed macrophages activated strain-2 and F_1 T cells but not strain-13 T cells. Similarly, strain-13 antigen-pulsed macrophages activated strain-13 and F_1 T cells but not strain-2 T cells. Subsequently, congenic and recombinant congenic strains of mice, which differed from each other only in selected regions of the H-2 complex, were used as the source of macrophages and T cells. These experiments confirmed that the $CD4^+$ T_H cell is activated and proliferates only in the presence of antigen-pulsed

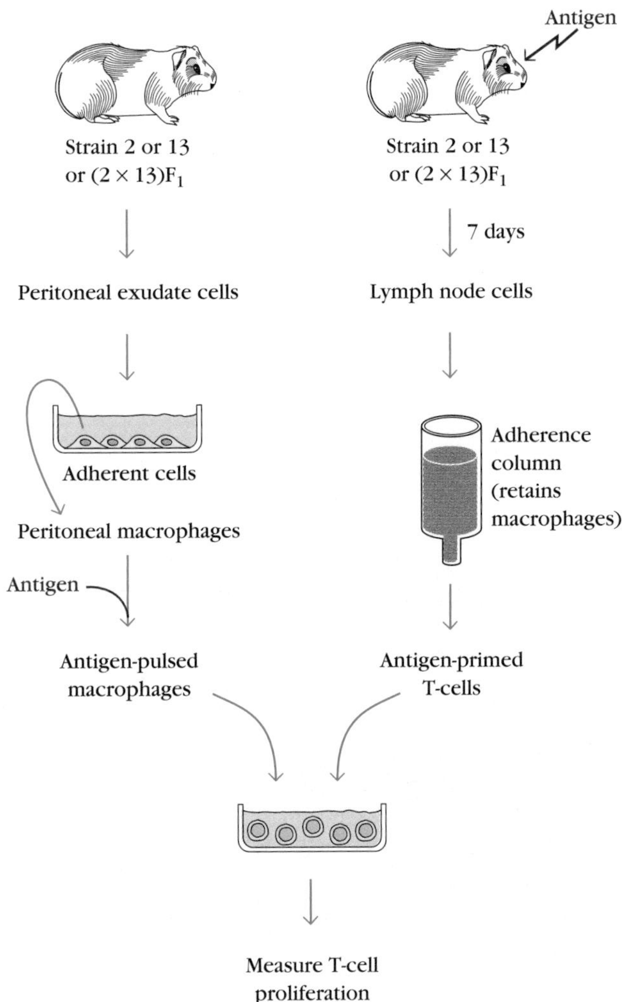

Antigen-primed T cell	Antigen-pulsed macrophages		
	Strain 2	Strain 13	$(2 \times 13)F_1$
Strain 2	+	–	+
Strain 13	–	+	+
$(2 \times 13)F_1$	+	+	+

FIGURE 8-1 Experimental demonstration of self-MHC restriction of T_H cells. Peritoneal exudate cells from strain 2, strain 13, or (2 × 13) F_1 guinea pigs were incubated in plastic Petri dishes, allowing enrichment of macrophages, which are adherent cells. The peritoneal macrophages were then incubated with antigen, generating "antigen-pulsed macrophages." These antigen-pulsed macrophages were incubated in vitro with T cells from strain 2, strain 13, or (2 × 13) F_1 guinea pigs, and the degree of T-cell proliferation was assessed. The results indicated that T_H cells could proliferate only in response to antigen presented by macrophages that shared MHC alleles. [Adapted from A Rosenthal and E Shevach, 1974, *J. Exp. Med.* **138:**1194).]

macrophages that share class II MHC alleles. Thus, antigen recognition by the $CD4^+$ T_H cell is *class II MHC restricted.*

The self-MHC restriction of $CD8^+$ T cells was first demonstrated by R. Zinkernagel and P. Doherty in 1974. In their experiments, mice were immunized with lymphocytic choriomeningitis (LCM) virus; several days later, the animals' spleen cells, which included T_C cells specific for the virus, were isolated and incubated with LCM-infected target cells of the same or different haplotype (Figure 8-2). They found that the T_C cells killed only syngeneic virus-infected target cells. Later studies with congenic and recombinant congenic strains showed that the T_C cell and the virus-infected target cell must share class I molecules encoded by the K or D regions of the MHC. Thus, antigen

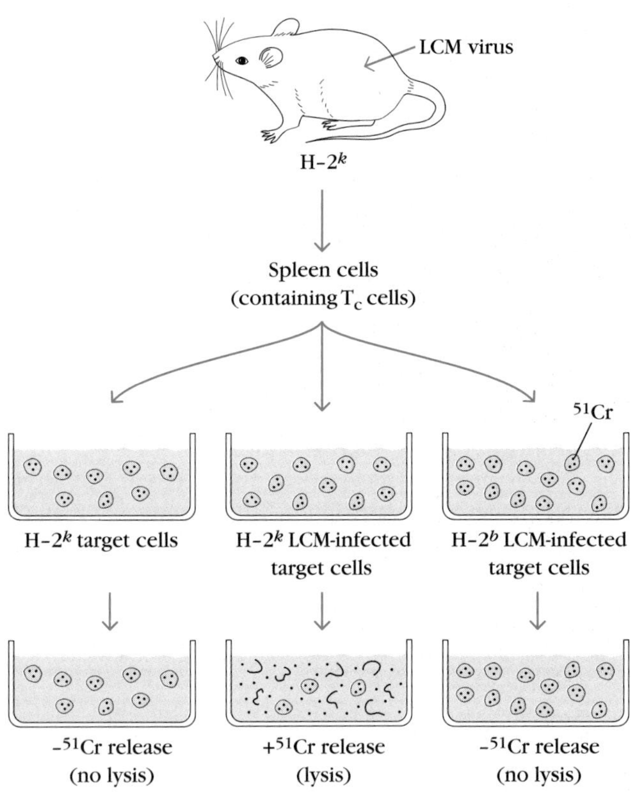

FIGURE 8-2 Classic experiment of Zinkernagel and Doherty demonstrating that antigen recognition by T_C cells exhibits MHC restriction. H-2^k mice were primed with the lymphocytic choriomeningitis (LCM) virus to induce cytotoxic T lymphocytes (CTLs) specific for the virus. Spleen cells from this LCM-primed mouse were then added to target cells of different H-2 haplotypes that were intracellularly labeled with ^{51}Cr (black dots) and either infected or not with the LCM virus. CTL-mediated killing of the target cells, as measured by the release of ^{51}Cr into the culture supernatant, occurred only if the target cells were infected with LCM and had the same MHC haplotype as the CTLs. [Adapted from PC Doherty and RM Zinkernagel 1975. *J Exp. Med.* **141:**502.]

recognition by $CD8^+$ T_C cells is *class I MHC restricted.* In 1996, Doherty and Zinkernagel were awarded the Nobel Prize for their major contribution to the understanding of cell-mediated immunity.

Role of Antigen-Presenting Cells

As early as 1959, immunologists were confronted with data suggesting that T cells and B cells recognized antigen by different mechanisms. The dogma of the time, which persisted until the 1980s, was that cells of the immune system recognize the entire protein in its native conformation. However, the experiments by P. G. H. Gell and B. Benacerraf mentioned in Chapter 3 demonstrated that when a primary antibody response and cell-mediated response were induced by a protein in its native conformation, a secondary antibody response (mediated by B cells) could be induced only by native antigen, whereas a secondary cell-mediated response could be induced by either the native or the denatured antigen (see Table 3-4). These findings were viewed as an interesting enigma, but their implications were completely overlooked until the early 1980s.

Early Evidence for the Necessity of Antigen Processing

The results obtained by K. Ziegler and E. R. Unanuae were among those that contradicted the prevailing dogma that antigen recognition by B and T cells was basically similar. These researchers observed that T_H-cell activation by bacterial protein antigens was prevented by treating the antigen-presenting cells with paraformaldehyde prior to antigen exposure. However, if the antigen-presenting cells were allowed to ingest the antigen and were fixed with paraformaldehyde 1–3 h later, T_H-cell activation still occurred (Figure 8-3a,b).

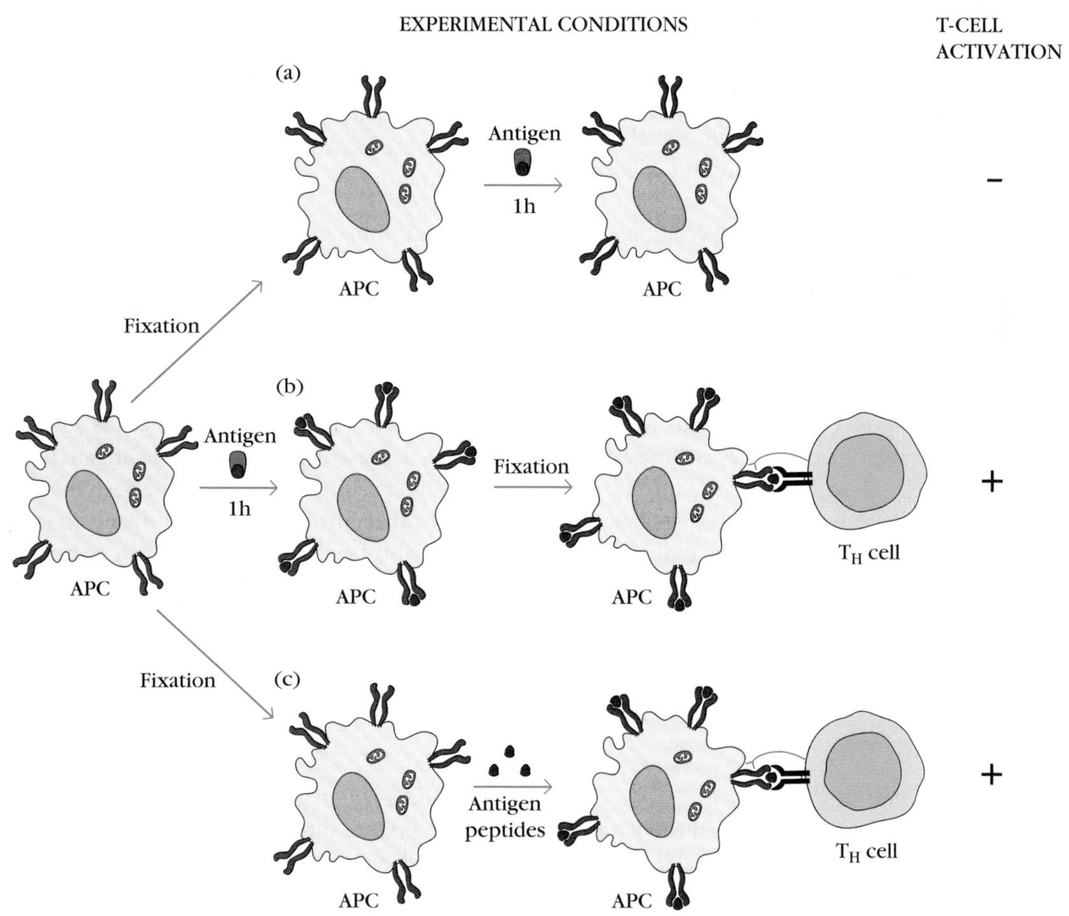

FIGURE 8-3 Experimental demonstration that antigen processing is necessary for T_H-cell activation. (a) When antigen-presenting cells (APCs) are fixed before exposure to antigen, they are unable to activate T_H cells. (b) In contrast, APCs fixed at least 1 h after antigen exposure can activate T_H cells. (c) When APCs are fixed before antigen exposure and incubated with peptide digests of the antigen (rather than native antigen), they also can activate T_H cells. T_H-cell activation is determined by measuring a specific T_H-cell response (e.g., cytokine secretion).

TABLE 8-1 ANTIGEN-PRESENTING CELLS

Professional antigen-presenting cells	Nonprofessional antigen-presenting cells	
Dendritic cells (several types)	Fibroblasts (skin)	Thymic epithelial cells
Macrophages	Glial cells (brain)	Thyroid epithelial cells
B cells	Pancreatic beta cells	Vascular endothelial cells

During that interval of 1–3 h, the antigen-presenting cells had processed the antigen and had displayed it on the membrane in a form able to activate T cells.

Subsequent experiments by R. P. Shimonkevitz showed that internalization and processing could be bypassed if antigen-presenting cells were exposed to peptide digests of an antigen instead of the native antigen (Figure 8-3c). In these experiments, antigen-presenting cells were treated with glutaraldehyde and then incubated with native ovalbumin or with ovalbumin that had been subjected to partial enzymatic digestion. The digested ovalbumin was able to interact with the glutaraldehyde-fixed antigen-presenting cells, thereby activating ovalbumin-specific T_H cells, whereas the native ovalbumin failed to do so. These results suggest that antigen processing involves the digestion of the protein into peptides that are recognized by the ovalbumin-specific T_H cells.

At about the same time, A. Townsend and his colleagues began to identify the proteins of influenza virus that were recognized by T_C cells. Contrary to their expectations, they found that internal proteins of the virus, such as matrix and nucleocapsid proteins, were often recognized by T_C cells better than the more exposed envelope proteins. Moreover, Townsend's work revealed that T_C cells recognized short linear peptide sequences of the influenza protein. In fact, when noninfected target cells were incubated in vitro with synthetic peptides corresponding to sequences of internal influenza proteins, these cells could be recognized by T_C cells and subsequently lysed just as well as target cells that had been infected with live influenza virus. These findings along with those presented in Figure 8-3 suggest that antigen processing is a metabolic process that digests proteins into peptides, which can then be displayed on the cell membrane together with a class I or class II MHC molecule.

Cells That Function in Antigen Presentation

Since all cells expressing either class I or class II MHC molecules can present peptides to T cells, strictly speaking they all could be designated as antigen-presenting cells. However, by convention, cells that display peptides associated with class I MHC molecules to $CD8^+$ T_C cells are referred to as *target cells;* cells that display peptides associated with class II MHC molecules to $CD4^+$ T_H cells are called **antigen-presenting cells (APCs).** This convention is followed throughout this text.

A variety of cells can function as antigen-presenting cells. The distinguishing feature of these cells is their ability to express class II MHC molecules and to deliver a co-stimulatory signal. Three cell types are classified as *professional* antigen-presenting cells: dendritic cells, macrophages, and B lymphocytes. These cells differ in their mechanisms of antigen uptake, in whether they constitutively express class II MHC molecules, and in their co-stimulatory activity:

- Dendritic cells are the most effective of the antigen-presenting cells. Because these cells constitutively express a high level of class II MHC molecules and co-stimulatory activity, they can activate naive T_H cells.
- Macrophages must be activated by phagocytoses of microorganisms before they express class II MHC molecules or the co-stimulatory B7 membrane molecule.
- B cells constitutively express class II MHC molecules but must be activated before they express the co-stimulatory B7 molecule.

Several other cell types, classified as *nonprofessional* antigen-presenting cells, can be induced to express class II MHC molecules or a co-stimulatory signal (Table 8-1). Many of these cells function in antigen presentation only for short periods of time during a sustained inflammatory response.

Because nearly all nucleated cells express class I MHC molecules, virtually any nucleated cell is able to function as a target cell presenting endogenous antigens to T_C cells. Most often, target cells are cells that have been infected by a virus or some other intracellular microorganism. However, target cells can also be altered self-cells such as cancer cells, aging body cells, or allogeneic cells from a graft.

Evidence for Two Processing and Presentation Pathways

Intracellular (endogenous) and extracellular (exogenous) antigens present different challenges to the immune system. Extracellular antigens are eliminated by secreted antibody, whereas intracellular antigens are most effectively eliminated by cytotoxic T lymphocytes (CTLs). To mediate these responses, the immune system uses two different antigen-presenting pathways: endogenous antigens are processed in the *cytosolic pathway* and presented on the membrane with class I MHC molecules; exogenous antigens are processed in the *endocytic pathway* and presented on the membrane with class II MHC molecules (Figure 8-4).

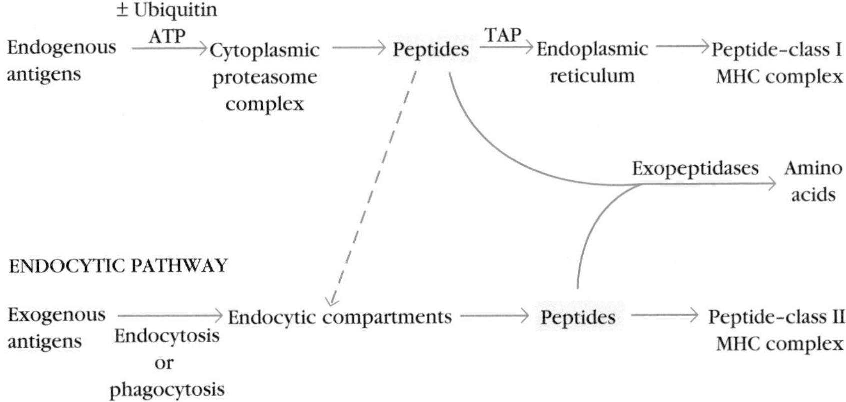

FIGURE 8-4 Overview of cytosolic and endocytic pathways for processing antigen. The proteasome complex contains enzymes that cleave peptide bonds, converting proteins into peptides. The antigenic peptides from proteasome cleavage and those from endocytic compartments associate with class I or class II MHC molecules, and the peptide-MHC complexes then are transported to the cell membrane. TAP (transporter of antigenic peptides) transports the peptides to the endoplasmic reticulum. It should be pointed out that the ultimate fate of most peptides in the cell is neither of these pathways, but rather to be degraded completely into amino acids.

Early evidence suggesting that class I and class II MHC molecules present antigenic peptides derived from different processing pathways was obtained from experiments carried by L. A. Morrison and T. J. Braciale with two clones of T_C cells specific for influenza virus. One clone was a typical T_C line that recognized influenza hemagglutinin (HA) associated with a class I MHC molecule and the other an atypical T_C line that recognized influenza HA associated with a class II MHC molecule. The existence of these clones, as well as those reported by others, provides evidence that the association between T-cell function and MHC restriction is not absolute. An increasing number of reports describe cross-functional T-cell lines—that is, $CD4^+$, class II–restricted T_C clones, and $CD8^+$, class I–restricted T_H clones.

Morrison and Braciale used the cytotoxic T cells recognizing the same influenza antigen to determine whether antigen is processed along different pathways for association with class I or class II MHC molecules. In one set of experiments, target cells that expressed both class I and class II MHC molecules were incubated with infectious influenza virus or with UV-inactivated influenza virus. (The inactivated virus retained its antigenic properties but was no longer capable of replicating within the target cells.) The target cells were then incubated with the class I–restricted or class II–restricted T_C cells and subsequent lysis of the target cells was determined. The results of their experiments, presented in Table 8-2, show that the class II–restricted T_C cells responded to target cells treated with infectious or noninfectious influenza virions.

TABLE 8-2 EFFECT OF ANTIGEN PRESENTATION ON ACTIVATION OF CLASS I AND CLASS II MHC-RESTRICTED T_C CELLS

	CTL activity†	
Treatment of target cells*	Class I restricted	Class II restricted
Infectious virus	+	+
UV-inactivated virus (noninfectious)	−	+
Infectious virus + emetine	−	+
Infectious virus + chloroquine	+	−

*Target cells, which expressed both class I and class II MHC molecules, were treated with the indicated preparations of influenza virus and other agents. Emetine inhibits viral protein synthesis, and chloroquine inhibits the endocytic processing pathway.

†Determined by lysis (+) and no lysis (−) of the target cells.

SOURCE: Adapted from TJ Braciale et al., 1987, *Immunol. Rev.* **98**:95.

The class I–restricted T_C cells also responded to target cells treated with infectious virions but not to target cells treated with noninfectious virions. Similarly, target cells that had been treated with infectious influenza virions in the presence of emetine, which inhibits viral protein synthesis, stimulated the class II–restricted T_C cells but not the class I–restricted T_C cells. Conversely, target cells that had been treated with infectious virions in the presence of chloroquine, a drug that blocks the endocytic processing pathway, stimulated class I but not class II–restricted T_C cells.

These results support the distinction between exogenous and endogenous antigens and the preferential association of exogenous antigens with class II MHC molecules and of endogenous antigens with class I MHC molecules. In other words, the mode of antigen entry into cells and its subsequent processing within either the endocytic processing pathway (exogenous antigens) or cytosolic pathway (endogenous antigens) determine whether the resulting antigenic peptides will associate with class I or class II MHC molecules. In the Morrison and Braciale experiments, association of viral antigen with class II MHC molecules did not require viral replication or protein synthesis. On the other hand, association of viral antigen with class I MHC molecules required replication of the influenza virus and viral protein synthesis within the target cells. These findings provided early evidence to suggest separate routing of class I and class II MHC molecules to separate intracellular compartments. This separate routing dictates whether the class I and II MHC molecules interact with peptides derived from cytosolic degradation of endogenously synthesized proteins or with peptides derived from endocytic degradation of exogenous antigens. In the next two sections, we shall examine each of these pathways in detail.

Endogenous Antigens: The Cytosolic Pathway

Endogenous antigens, such as those produced by a virus replicating within a cell, are degraded within the cytoplasm into peptides that can associate with class I MHC molecules. Soluble protein antigens that are experimentally delivered into the cytoplasm of a cell also have been shown to be degraded into peptides that can be presented to T_C cells by class I MHC molecules. (One way to deliver soluble protein antigens into the cytoplasm is to load them inside membrane liposomes; as these fuse with the plasma membrane, the antigen is released into the cytoplasm.) The pathway by which endogenous antigens are degraded for presentation with class I MHC molecules utilizes pathways involved in the normal turnover of intracellular proteins.

Peptide Generation by Proteasomes

In eukaryotic cells, protein levels are carefully regulated. Every protein is subject to continuous turnover and is degraded at a rate that is generally expressed in terms of its half-life. Some proteins (e.g., transcription factors, cyclins, and key metabolic enzymes) have very short half-lives; denatured, misfolded, or otherwise abnormal proteins also are degraded rapidly. Intracellular proteins are degraded into short peptides by a cytosolic proteolytic system present in all cells. Those proteins targeted for proteolysis often have a small protein, called *ubiquitin,* attached to them (Figure 8-5a). Ubiquitin-protein conjugates can be degraded by a multifunctional protease complex called a **proteasome.** Each proteasome is a large (26S), cylindrical particle consisting of four rings of protein subunits with a central channel of 10–50 Å. A proteasome can cleave peptide bonds between 2 or 3 different amino acid combinations in an ATP-dependent process (Figure 8-5b). Degradation of ubiquitin-protein complexes is thought to occur within the central hollow of the proteasome, thereby preventing lysis of other proteins within the cytoplasm.

(a)

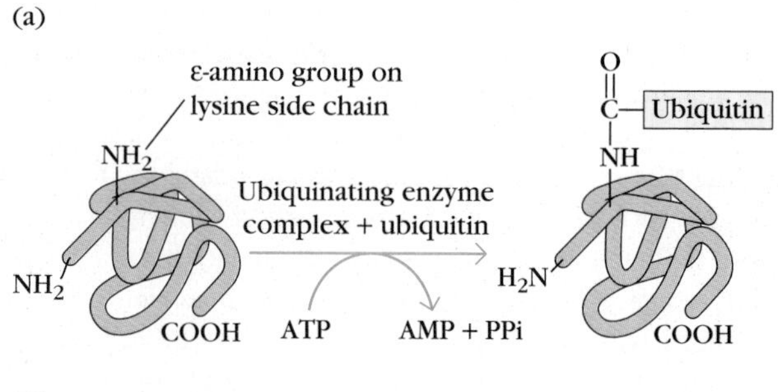

(b)

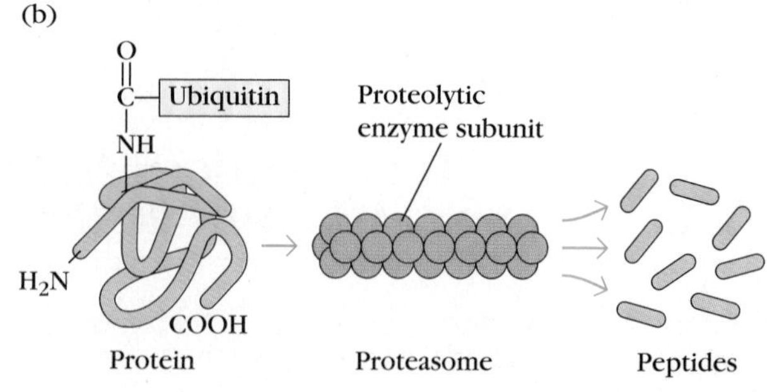

FIGURE 8-5 Cytosolic proteolytic system for degradation of intracellular proteins. (a) Proteins to be degraded often are covalently linked to a small protein called ubiquitin. In this reaction, which requires ATP, a ubiquinating enzyme complex links several ubiquitin molecules to a lysine-amino group near the amino terminus of the protein. (b) Degradation of ubiquitin-protein complexes occurs within the central channel of proteasomes, generating a variety of peptides. Proteasomes are large cylindrical particles whose subunits catalyze cleavage of peptide bonds.

Experimental evidence indicates that the immune system utilizes this general pathway of protein degradation to produce small peptides for presentation with class I MHC molecules. The immune system appears to modify the proteasome by the addition of two subunits to the proteasome: LMP2 and LMP7. These subunits are encoded within the MHC gene cluster and are induced by increased levels of IFN-γ. An additional modifier that is added to the proteasome is also induced by IFN-γ but is not MHC encoded. This modifier was originally designated MECL-1 but has also been called LMP10. The peptidase activities of proteasomes containing LMP2, LMP7, and LMP10 preferentially generate peptides that bind to MHC class I molecules. Such proteasomes, for example, show increased hydrolysis of peptide bonds that follow basic and/or hydrophobic residues. As described in Chapter 7, peptides that bind to class I MHC molecules terminate almost exclusively with hydrophobic or basic residues.

Peptide Transport from the Cytosol to the Rough Endoplasmic Reticulum (RER)

Insight into the role that peptide transport, the delivery of peptides to the MHC molecule, plays in the cytosolic processing pathway came from studies of cell lines with defects in peptide presentation by class I MHC molecules. One such mutant cell line, called RMA-S, expresses about 5% of the normal levels of class I MHC molecules on its membrane. Although RMA-S cells synthesize normal levels of class I α chains and β_2-microglobulin, both molecules remain intracellular instead of appearing on the membrane. A clue to the mutation in the RMA-S cell line was the discovery by A. Townsend and his colleagues that "feeding" these cells peptides restored their level of membrane-associated class I MHC molecules to normal. These investigators suggested that peptides might be required to stabilize the interaction between the class I α chain and β_2-microglobulin. This led them to speculate that the RMA-S cell line might have a defect in peptide transport. The ability to restore expression of class I MHC molecules on the membrane by feeding the cells predigested peptides would be compatible with this type of defect.

Subsequent experiments with the RMA-S cell line showed that the defect in these cells is in the protein that transports peptides from the cytoplasm to the RER, where class I molecules are synthesized. When RMA-S cells were transfected with a functional gene encoding the transporter protein, the cells began to express class I molecules on the membrane. The transporter protein, designated **TAP** (for **transporters associated with antigen processing**) is a membrane-spanning heterodimer consisting of two proteins: TAP1 and TAP2 (Figure 8-6a). In addition to their multiple transmembrane segments, the TAP1 and TAP2 proteins each have one hydrophobic domain, which is thought to project through the membrane into the lumen of the RER, and one ATP-binding domain, which projects into the cytosol. Both TAP1 and TAP2 belong to the family of ATP-binding cassette proteins found in the membranes of many cells, including bacteria; these proteins mediate ATP-dependent transport of amino acids, sugars, ions, and peptides.

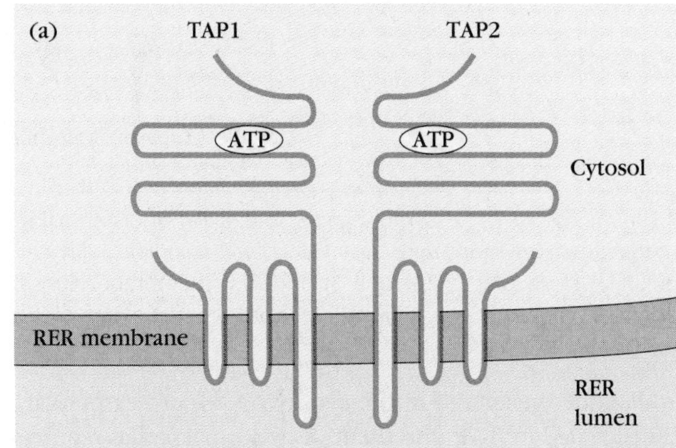

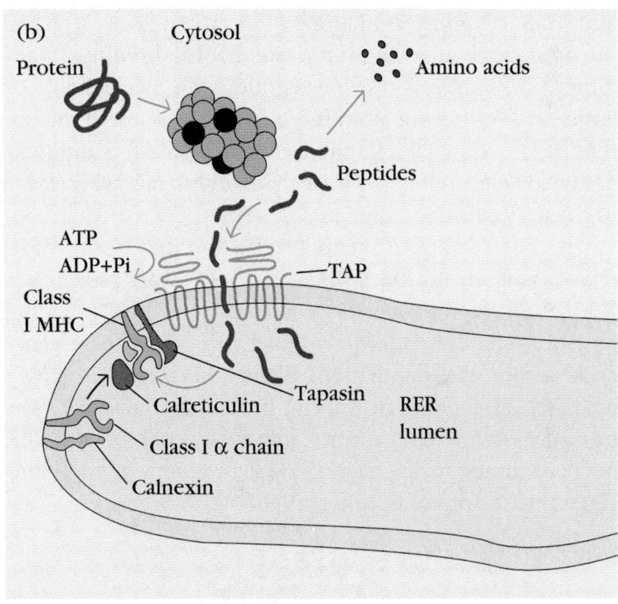

FIGURE 8-6 Generation of antigenic peptide–class I MHC complexes in the cytosolic pathway. (a) Schematic diagram of TAP (transporters associated with antigen processing), a heterodimer anchored in the membrane of the rough endoplasmic reticulum (RER). The two chains are encoded by *TAP1* and *TAP2*. The cytosolic domain in each TAP subunit contains an ATP-binding site, and peptide transport depends on the hydrolysis of ATP. (b) In the cytosol, association of LMP2, LMP7, and LMP10 (black spheres) with a proteasome changes its catalytic specificity to favor production of peptides that bind to class I MHC molecules. Within the RER membrane, newly synthesized class I α chain associates with calnexin until β_2-microglobulin binds to the α chain. The class I α chain–β_2-microglobulin heterodimer then binds to calreticulin and the TAP-associated protein tapasin. When a peptide delivered by TAP is bound to the class I molecule, folding of MHC class I is complete and it is released from the RER and transported through the Golgi to the surface of the cell.

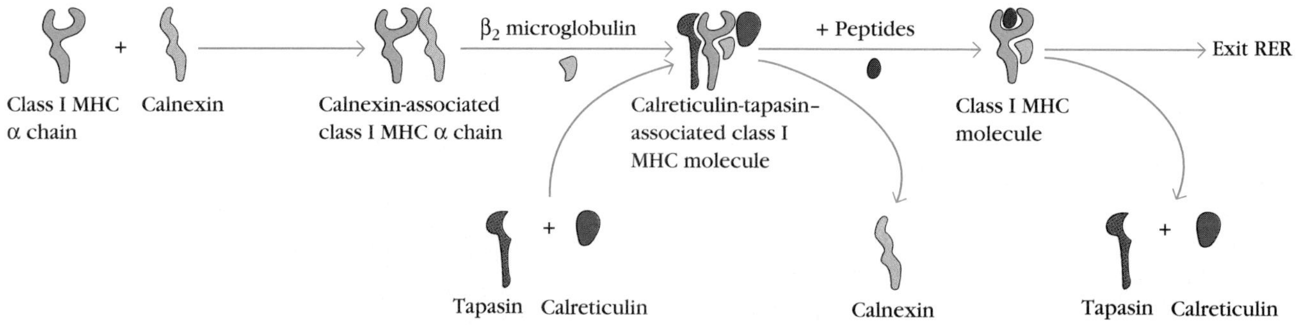

FIGURE 8-7 Assembly and stabilization of class I MHC molecules. Newly formed class I α chains associate with calnexin, a molecular chaperone, in the RER membrane. Subsequent binding to β_2-microglobulin releases calnexin and allows binding to the chaperonin calreticulin and to tapasin, which is associated with the peptide transporter TAP. This association promotes binding of an antigenic peptide, which stabilizes the class I molecule–peptide complex, allowing its release from the RER.

Peptides generated in the cytosol by the proteasome are translocated by TAP into the RER by a process that requires the hydrolysis of ATP (Figure 8-6b). TAP has the highest affinity for peptides containing 8–13 amino acids, which is the optimal peptide length for class I MHC binding. In addition, TAP appears to favor peptides with hydrophobic or basic carboxyl-terminal amino acids, the preferred anchor residues for class I MHC molecules. Thus, TAP is uniquely designed to transport peptides that will interact with class I MHC molecules.

The *TAP1* and *TAP2* genes map within the class II MHC region, adjacent to the *LMP2* and *LMP7* genes (see Figure 7-15). Both the transporter genes and these *LMP* genes are polymorphic; that is, different allelic forms of these genes exist within the population. Allelic differences in LMP-mediated proteolytic cleavage of protein antigens or in the transport of different peptides from the cytosol into the RER may contribute to the observed variation among individuals in their response to different endogenous antigens.

Assembly of Peptides with Class I MHC Molecules

Like other proteins, the α chain and β_2-microglobulin components of the class I MHC molecule are synthesized on polysomes along the rough endoplasmic reticulum (RER). Assembly of these components into a stable class I MHC molecular complex that can exit the RER requires the presence of a peptide in the binding groove of the class I molecule. The assembly process leading to a stable class I MHC molecule takes place in several steps and involves the participation of *molecular chaperones,* which facilitate the folding of polypeptides. The molecular chaperone first involved in class I MHC assembly is *calnexin,* a resident membrane protein of the endoplasmic reticulum. Calnexin associates with the free class I α chain and promotes its folding. When β_2-microglobulin binds to the α chain, calnexin is released and the class I molecule associates with the chaperonin *calreticulin* and with *tapasin.* Tapasin (TAP-associated protein) brings the TAP transporter into proximity with the class I molecule and allows it to acquire an antigenic peptide (Figure 8-7). The physical association of the α chain–β_2-microglobulin heterodimer with the TAP protein (see Figure 8-6b) promotes peptide capture by the class I molecule before the peptides are exposed to the luminal environment of the RER. Peptides not bound by class I molecules are rapidly degraded. As a consequence of peptide binding, the class I molecule displays increased stability and can dissociate from calreticulin and tapasin, exit from the RER, and proceed to the cell surface via the Golgi. Recently, an additional protein, ERp57, has been observed in association with the class I–tapasin–calreticulin complexes. Because the role of this resident endoplasmic reticulum protein in the class I peptide assembly and loading process has not yet been defined, ERp57 is not shown in Figures 8-6 and 8-7.

Overview of the Class I Endogenous Pathway

The current model of the pathway by which endogenous antigens are processed and presented is shown on the left side of Figure 8-8. As mentioned earlier, endogenous antigens are thought to be degraded within the cytoplasm by the proteasome complex. Peptides are then transported across the membrane of the RER by an ATP-binding transporter called TAP. The calnexin-associated class I MHC α chain binds to β_2-microglobulin, dissociates from calnexin, and binds to calreticulin and to tapasin, which is associated with the transmembrane TAP protein (ERp57 may be involved also at this step). This class I MHC complex then captures an antigenic peptide, which allows dissociation of the MHC-peptide complex from the chaperones. Finally, the class I MHC molecule–peptide is transported from the RER through the Golgi complex to the plasma membrane.

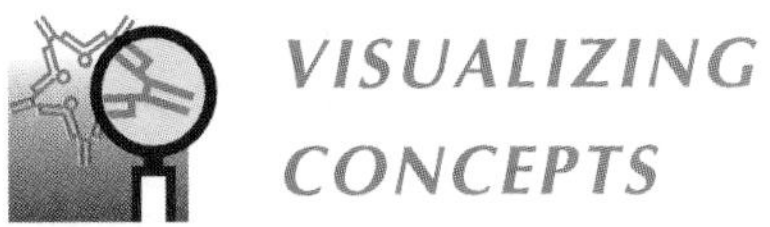

VISUALIZING CONCEPTS

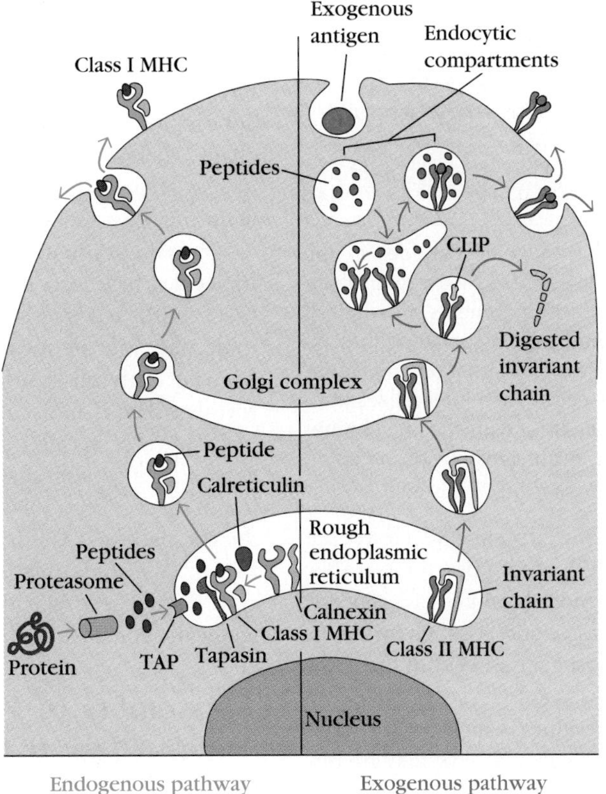

FIGURE 8-8 Model of separate antigen-presenting pathways for endogenous (green) and exogenous (red) antigens. The mode of antigen entry into cells and the site of antigen processing appear to determine whether antigenic peptides associate with class I MHC molecules in the rough endoplasmic reticulum or with class II molecules in endocytic compartments.

Exogenous Antigens: The Endocytic Pathway

Antigen-presenting cells can internalize antigen by phagocytosis, endocytosis, or both. Macrophages internalize antigen by both processes, whereas most other APCs are not phagocytic or are poorly phagocytic and therefore internalize exogenous antigen only by endocytosis (either receptor-mediated endocytosis or pinocytosis). B cells, for example, internalize antigen very effectively by receptor-mediated endocytosis using antigen-specific membrane antibody as the receptor.

Peptide Generation in Endocytic Vesicles

Once an antigen is internalized, it is degraded into peptides within compartments of the endocytic processing pathway. As the experiment shown in Figure 8-3 demonstrated, internalized antigen takes 1–3 h to transverse the endocytic pathway and appear at the cell surface in the form of peptide–class II MHC complexes. The endocytic pathway appears to involve three increasingly acidic compartments: early endosomes (pH 6.0–6.5); late endosomes, or endolysosomes (pH 5.0–6.0); and lysosomes (pH 4.5–5.0). Internalized antigen moves from early to late endosomes and finally to

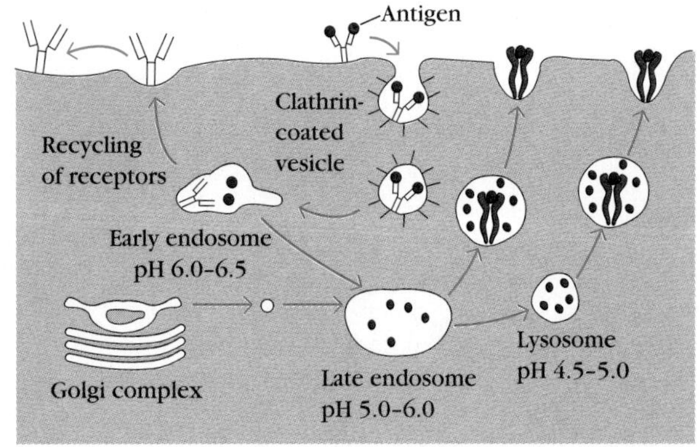

FIGURE 8-9 Generation of antigenic peptides in the endocytic processing pathway. Internalized exogenous antigen moves through several acidic compartments, in which it is degraded into peptides that ultimately associate with class II MHC molecules transported in vesicles from the Golgi complex. The cell shown here is a B cell, which internalizes antigen by receptor-mediated endocytosis, with the membrane-bound antibody functioning as an antigen-specific receptor.

lysosomes, encountering hydrolytic enzymes and a lower pH in each compartment (Figure 8-9). Lysosomes, for example, contain a unique collection of more than 40 acid-dependent hydrolases, including proteases, nucleases, glycosidases, lipases, phospholipases, and phosphatases. Within the compartments of the endocytic pathway, antigen is degraded into oligopeptides of about 13–18 residues, which bind to class II MHC molecules. Because the hydrolytic enzymes are optimally active under acidic conditions (low pH), antigen processing can be inhibited by chemical agents that increase the pH of the compartments (e.g., chloroquine) as well as by protease inhibitors (e.g., leupeptin).

The mechanism by which internalized antigen moves from one endocytic compartment to the next has not been conclusively demonstrated. Some have suggested that early endosomes from the periphery move inward to become late endosomes and finally lysosomes. Others have suggested that small transport vesicles carry antigens from one compartment to the next, in a manner similar to the way in which small transport vesicles carry proteins from one compartment of the Golgi complex to the next. Eventually the endocytic compartments, or portions of them, return to the cell periphery, where they fuse with the plasma membrane. In this way, the surface receptors may be recycled.

Transport of Class II MHC Molecules to Endocytic Vesicles

Since antigen-presenting cells express both class I and class II MHC molecules, some mechanism must exist to prevent class II MHC molecules from binding to the same set of antigenic peptides as the class I molecules. When a class II MHC molecule is synthesized within the RER, it associates with another protein called the **invariant (Ii) chain.** Three pairs of the class II αβ chains associate with a preassembled invariant chain trimer. This trimeric protein interacts with the peptide-binding cleft of the class II molecule, preventing any endogenously derived peptides from binding to the cleft while the class II molecule is within the RER (see right side of Figure 8-8). In addition to its role in preventing peptide binding to class II MHC molecules, the invariant chain also appears to be involved in the folding of the class II α and β chains, their exit from the RER, and the subsequent routing of class II molecules to the endocytic processing pathway from the trans-Golgi network.

The role of the invariant chain in the routing of class II molecules has been demonstrated in transfection experiments with cells that lack the genes encoding class II MHC molecules and the invariant chain. Immunofluorescent labeling of such cells transfected only with class II MHC genes revealed class II molecules localized within the Golgi complex. However, in cells transfected with both the class II MHC genes and invariant-chain gene, the class II molecules were localized in the cytoplasmic vesicular structures of the endocytic pathway. The invariant chain contains sorting signals in its cytoplasmic tail that directs the transport of the class II MHC complex from the trans-Golgi network to the endocytic compartments.

Assembly of Peptides with Class II MHC Molecules

Recent experiments indicate that most class II MHC–invariant chain complexes are transported from the RER, where they are formed, through the Golgi complex and trans-Golgi network to early endosomes. Here, within the endocytic pathway, these complexes move from early endosomes to late endosomes, and finally to lysosomes. As the proteolytic activity increases in each successive compartment, the invariant chain is gradually degraded. However, a short fragment of the invariant chain termed *CLIP* (for *class II–associated invariant chain peptide*) remains bound to the class II molecule after the invariant chain has been cleaved within the endosomal compartment. CLIP physically occupies the peptide-binding groove of the class II MHC molecule, presumably preventing any premature binding of antigenic peptide (see Figure 8-8).

A nonclassical class II MHC molecule, called *HLA-DM*, plays a role in the removal of CLIP and in the subsequent loading of class II molecules with antigenic peptides. HLA-DM is required to catalyze the exchange of CLIP with antigenic peptides (Figure 8-10a). The reaction between HLA-DM and the class II CLIP complex facilitating exchange of CLIP for another peptide is inhibited in the presence of HLA-DO, which binds to HLA-DM and blocks the exchange reaction.

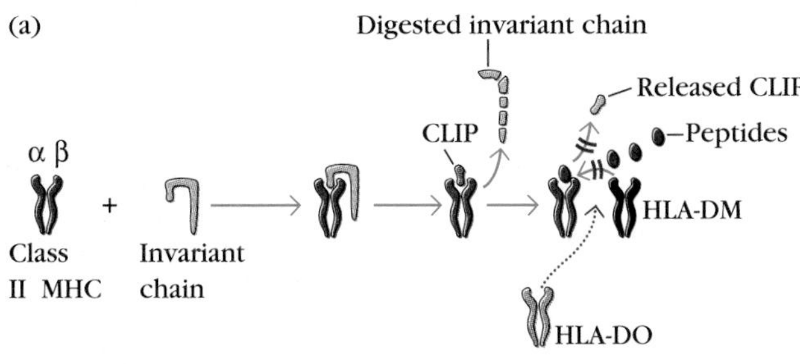

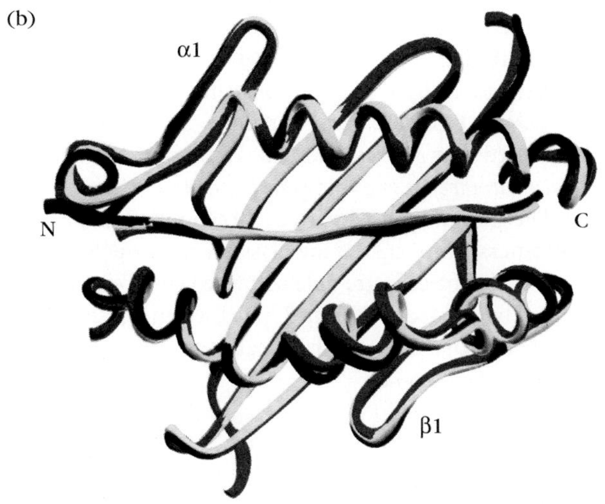

FIGURE 8-10 (a) Assembly of class II MHC molecules. Within the rough endoplasmic reticulum, a newly synthesized class II MHC molecule binds an invariant chain. The bound invariant chain prevents premature binding of peptides to the class II molecule and helps to direct the complex to endocytic compartments containing peptides derived from exogenous antigens. Digestion of the invariant chain leaves CLIP, a small fragment remaining in the binding groove of the class II MHC molecule. HLA-DM, a nonclassical MHC class II molecule expressed within endosomal compartments, mediates exchange of antigenic peptides for CLIP. The nonclassical class II molecule HLA-DO may act as a negative regulator of class II antigen processing by binding to HLA-DM and inhibiting its role in the dissociation of CLIP from class II molecules. (b) Comparison of three-dimensional structures showing the binding groove of HLA class II molecules (α1 and β1) containing different antigenic peptides or CLIP. The red lines show DR4 complexed with collagen II peptide, yellow lines are DR1 with influenza hemagglutinin peptide, and blue lines are DR3 associated with CLIP. (N indicates the amino terminus and C the carboxyl terminus of the peptides.) No major differences in the structures of the class II molecules or in the conformation of the bound peptides are seen. This comparison shows that CLIP binds the class II molecule in a manner identical to that of antigenic peptides. [From Dessen et al, 1997. *Immunity.* **7**:473–481. Courtesy of Don Wiley, Harvard University.]

MHC class II genes encoding HLA-DM have been identified in the mouse and rabbit, indicating that HLA-DM is widely conserved among mammalian species. Like other class II MHC molecules, HLA-DM is a heterodimer of α and β chains. However, unlike other class II molecules, HLA-DM is not polymorphic and is not expressed at the cell membrane but is found predominantly within the endosomal compartment. The *DMα* and *DMβ* genes are located near the *TAP* and *LMP* genes in the MHC complex of humans. HLA-DO, like HLA-DM, is a nonclassical and nonpolymorphic class II molecule that is also found in the MHC of other species. DO differs from DM in that it is expressed only by B cells and the thymus.

Earlier descriptions of the class II processing pathway suggested that CLIP did not bind to HLA class II molecules in a stable fashion, and that this instability fostered its replacement by another peptide. Recent structural evidence makes this mechanism unlikely. An HLA-DR3 molecule associated with CLIP was isolated from a cell line that did not express HLA-DM and was therefore defective in antigen processing. This complex of HLA-DR3–CLIP was crystallized and its three-dimensional structure determined. Comparison of the class II CLIP complex with other DR molecules bound to antigenic peptides shows that CLIP binds to class II in the same manner as do antigenic peptides that form a stable complex (Figure 8-10b).

As with class I MHC molecules, peptide binding is required to maintain the structure and stability of class II MHC molecules. Once a peptide has bound, the peptide–class II complex is transported to the plasma membrane, where the neutral pH appears to enable the complex to assume a compact, stable form. Peptide is bound so strongly in this compact form that it is difficult to replace a class II–bound peptide on the membrane with another peptide at physiologic conditions.

Overview of the Class II Exogenous Pathway

The current model of the pathway for processing and presenting exogenous antigens is summarized in the right side of Figure 8-8. As described above, newly synthesized class II α and β chains associate with an invariant chain within the RER. This association precludes binding of class II MHC molecules with peptides derived from endogenous antigens or other intracellular proteins. Class II molecules, together with the associated invariant chains, are thought to be routed from the RER through the Golgi complex to the endocytic pathway. Once inside an endocytic compartment, the invariant chain is degraded by proteolytic enzymes, leaving the CLIP fragment bound to the peptide-binding cleft of the class II molecules. Within the acidic endocytic compartments, CLIP associated with the class II molecule is replaced with an antigenic peptide, a process catalyzed by HLA-DM. The resulting class II MHC–peptide complexes move to the plasma membrane.

Presentation of Nonpeptide Bacterial Antigens

Although it is well known that nonprotein antigens are recognized by the immune system, we have so far limited the discussion to peptide antigens and their presentation by classical class I and II MHC molecules. At present little is known about the mechanisms used for the processing and presentation of antigens that are not peptides. Some recent progress has been made in this area. It has been shown that antigenic lipid and glycolipid molecules derived from pathogenic bacteria such as *Mycobacterium tuberculosis* are presented by members of the CD1 family of nonclassical class I molecules.

The CD1 family of molecules associates with β_2- microglobulin and has general structural similarity to class I MHC molecules. CD1 gene products are found on antigen-presenting cells. There are five genes encoding human CD1 molecules (*CD1a–e*), which are not located within the MHC but on a different chromosome. These genes have been identified in all mammalian species studied. Sequence identity of CD1 with classical class I is considerably lower than that among the class I molecules. For example, the $\alpha3$ domain of CD1 molecules is closer in sequence to β_2-microglobulin than to the $\alpha3$ of MHC class I. CD1 molecules are recognized by T cells in the absence of foreign antigens, and self restriction can be demonstrated in these reactions.

Examination of antigens presented by CD1 molecules revealed them to be lipid components (mycolic acid) of the *M. tuberculosis* cell wall. Further studies of CD1 presentation indicated that a glycolipid (lipoarabinomannan) from *Mycobacterium leprae* could also be presented by these molecules. The pathway by which the CD1 molecules process antigen differs from that of the classical class I pathway in that TAP-deficient cells are able to present CD1-associated antigens. The data concerning CD1 antigen presentation point out the existence of a third pathway for the process-

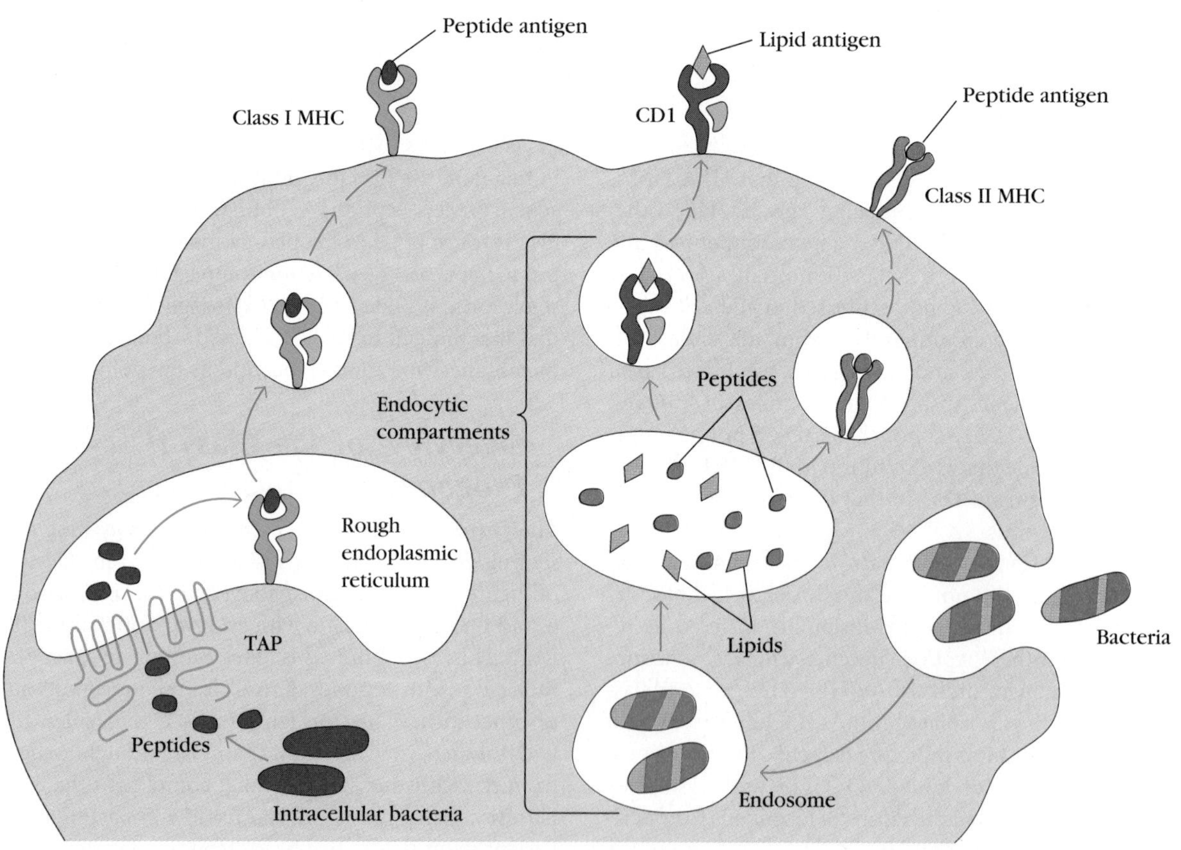

FIGURE 8-11 A role for the class I–like CD1 molecules in presentation of nonpeptide antigens from bacteria. CD1 molecules, which are not encoded within the MHC, have been shown to present lipid and glycolipid antigens from *Mycobacterium tuberculosis* and *Mycobacterium leprae.* A proposed scheme for the action of CD1 comparable to class I and II presentation of peptides is shown. Details of the CD1 pathway remain obscure. [Adapted from Melian et al. 1996. *Curr. Opin. Immunol.* **8:**82–88.]

ing of antigens, a pathway with distinct intracellular steps that do not involve the molecules found to facilitate class I antigen processing. Exactly how the CD1 pathway complements the better understood class I and class II pathways and if and where it intersects with them remain in question (Figure 8-11).

Summary

1. T-cell recognition of antigen requires that antigenic peptides be displayed within the cleft of a self-MHC molecule on the membrane of a cell. This requirement is called self-MHC restriction. In general, $CD4^+$ T_H cells are class II MHC restricted, whereas $CD8^+$ T_C cells are class I MHC restricted.
2. Complexes between antigenic peptides and MHC molecules are formed by degradation of a protein antigen in one of two different antigen-processing pathways. Those cells that process and present peptides associated with class II MHC molecules are called antigen-presenting cells (APCs); those that process and present peptides associated with class I MHC molecules are called target cells.
3. Endogenous antigens are degraded into peptides within the cytosol by a large enzyme complex called the proteasome, which has several types of peptidase activity. The resulting antigenic peptides are transported into the lumen of the RER by TAP, an ATP-dependent heterodimeric protein located in the RER membrane (see Figure 8-6). Within the RER, the peptides assemble with class I MHC molecules (see Figure 8-7); binding of peptide stabilizes the association between the class I α chain and β_2-microglobulin. Peptide–class I complexes then are transported from the RER through the Golgi complex to the plasma membrane (see Figure 8-8, *left*).
4. Exogenous antigens, internalized by phagocytosis or endocytosis, are degraded by various hydrolytic enzymes within the acidic endocytic compartments (see Figure 8-9). Within the RER, newly formed class II MHC molecules associate with the invariant chain, which blocks binding of peptides. Class II molecules with the associated invariant chain are routed to endocytic compartments, where the invariant chain is degraded by proteolytic enzymes, leaving the CLIP fragment in the peptide-binding cleft (see Figure 8-10a). A reaction catalyzed by HLA-DM allows antigenic peptides to displace CLIP. This reaction of HLA-DM may be inhibited by HLA-DO. The peptide–class II complexes are then transported to the plasma membrane (see Figure 8-8, *right*).
5. A third pathway for the processing and presentation of nonpeptide antigens derived from bacteria involves the class I–like CD1 molecules. CD1 molecules mediate restricted responses to lipid and glycolipid antigens by a pathway different from that used by the classical class I molecules (see Figure 8-11). How this third pathway interacts with the other two remains unclear.

REFERENCES

Benichou, G, et al. 1998. The presentation of self and allogeneic MHC peptides to T lymphocytes. *Hum. Immunol.* **59:**540.

Ciechanover, A. 1994. The ubiquitin-proteasome proteolytic pathway. *Cell* **79:**13.

Denzin, LK, et al. 1997. Negative regulation of MHC class II-restricted antigen processing. *Science* **278:**106.

Doherty, PC, and RM Zinkernagel. 1975. H-2 compatibility is required for T-cell mediated lysis of target cells infected with lymphocytic choriomeningitis virus. *J. Exp. Med.* **141:**502.

Ghosh P, M Amaya, E Mellins, and DC Wiley. 1995. The structure of an intermediate in class II MHC maturation: CLIP bound to HLA-DR3. *Nature* **378:**457.

Lehner, PJ, and J Trowsdale. 1998. Antigen presentation: coming out gracefully. *Curr. Biol.* **8:**R605.

Li, H, A Llera, and RA Mariuzza. 1998. Structure-function studies of T-cell receptor-superantigen interactions. *Immunol. Rev.* **163:**177.

Melian, A, et al. 1996. Antigen presentation by CD1 and MHC-encoded class I-like molecules. *Curr. Opin. Immunol.* **8:**82.

Mellman, I, SJ Turley, and RM Steinman. 1998. Antigen processing for amateurs and professionals. *Trends Cell. Biol.* **8:**231.

Niedermann, G, et al. 1995. Contribution of proteasome-mediated proteolysis to the hierarchy of epitopes presented by major histocompatibility complex class I molecules. *Immunity* **2:**289.

Ortmann B, et al. 1997. A critical role for tapasin in the assembly and function of multimeric MHC class I-TAP complexes. *Science* **277:**1306.

Oxenius, A, RN Zinkernagel, and H Hengartner. 1998. $CD4^+$ T-cell induction and effector functions: a comparison of immunity against soluble antigens and viral infections. *Adv. Immunol.* **70:**313.

Pamer, E, and P Cresswell. 1998. Mechanisms of MHC class I–restricted antigen processing. *Annu. Rev. Immunol.* **16:**323.

Park, SH, et al. 1998. Innate and adaptive functions of the CD1 pathway of antigen presentation. *Semin. Immunol.* **10:**391.

Romish, K. 1994. Peptide traffic across the ER membrane: TAPs and other conduits. *Trends Cell. Biol.* **4:**311.

Shastri, N, T Serwold, and P Paz. 1998. Reading within the lines: naturally processed peptides displayed by MHC class I molecules. *Curr. Opin. Immunol.* **10:**137.

Solheim, JC, BM Carreno, and TH Hansen. 1997. Are transporters associated with antigen processing (TAP) and tapasin class I MHC chaperones? *J. Immunol.* **158:**541.

van Ham, SM, et al. 1997. HLA-DO is a negative modulator of HLA-DM-mediated MHC class II peptide loading. *Current Biology* **7:**950.

Yewdell, JW, et al. 1999. Mechanisms of exogenous antigen presentation by MHC class I molecules in vitro and in vivo: implications for generating $CD8^+$ T-cell responses to infectious agents, tumors, transplants, and vaccines. *Advances in Immunol.* **73:** in press.

STUDY QUESTIONS

1. Explain the difference between the terms *antigen-presenting cell* and *target cell,* as they are commonly used in immunology.

2. Define the following terms:

a. Self-MHC restriction

b. Antigen processing

c. Endogenous antigen

d. Exogenous antigen

3. L. A. Morrison and T. J. Braciale conducted an experiment to determine whether antigens presented by class I or II MHC molecules are processed in different pathways. Their results are summarized in Table 8-2.

a. Explain why the class I–restricted T_C cells did not respond to target cells infected with UV-inactivated influenza virus.

b. Explain why chloroquine inhibited the response of the class II–restricted T_C cells to live virus.

c. Explain why emetine inhibited the response of class I–restricted but not class II–restricted T_C cells to live virus.

4. For each of the following cell components or processes, indicate whether it is involved in the processing and presentation of exogenous antigens (EX), endogenous antigens (EN), or both (B). Briefly explain the function of each item.

a. ______ Class I MHC molecules

b. ______ Class II MHC molecules

c. ______ Invariant (Ii) chains

d. ______ Lysosomal hydrolases

e. ______ TAP1 and TAP2 proteins

f. ______ Transport of vesicles from the RER to the Golgi complex

g. ______ Proteasomes

h. ______ Phagocytosis or endocytosis

i. ______ Calnexin

j. ______ CLIP

k. ______ Tapasin

5. Antigen-presenting cells have been shown to present lysozyme peptide 46–61 together with the class II IA^k molecule. When $CD4^+$ T_H cells are incubated with APCs and native lysozyme or the synthetic lysozyme peptide 46–61, T_H-cell activation occurs.

a. If chloroquine is added to the incubation mixture, presentation of the native protein is inhibited, but the peptide continues to induce T_H-cell activation. Explain why this occurs.

b. If chloroquine addition is delayed for 3 h, presentation of the native protein is not inhibited. Explain why this occurs.

6. Cells that can present antigen to T_H cells have been classified into two groups—professional and nonprofessional APCs.

a. Name the three types of professional APCs. For each type indicate whether it expresses class II MHC molecules and a co-stimulatory signal constitutively or must be activated before doing so.

b. Give three examples of nonprofessional APCs. When are these cells most likely to function in antigen presentation?

7. Predict whether T_H-cell proliferation or CTL-mediated cytolysis of target cells will occur with the following mixtures of cells. The $CD4^+$ T_H cells are from lysozyme-primed mice, and the $CD8^+$ CTLs are from influenza-infected mice. Use R to indicate a response and NR to indicate no response.

a. ______ $H\text{-}2^k$ T_H cells + lysozyme-pulsed $H\text{-}2^k$ macrophages

b. ______ $H\text{-}2^k$ T_H cells + lysozyme-pulsed $H\text{-}2^{b/k}$ macrophages

c. ______ $H\text{-}2^k$ T_H cells + lysozyme-primed $H\text{-}2^d$ macrophages

d. ______ $H\text{-}2^k$ CTLs + influenza-infected $H\text{-}2^k$ macrophages

e. ______ $H\text{-}2^k$ CTLs + influenza-infected $H\text{-}2^d$ macrophages

f. ______ $H\text{-}2^d$ CTLs + influenza-infected $H\text{-}2^{d/k}$ macrophages

8. Molecules of the CD1 family were recently shown to present nonpeptide antigens.

a. What is a major source of nonpeptide antigens?

b. Why are CD1 molecules not classified as members of the MHC family even though they associate with β_2-microglobulin?

c. What evidence is there that the CD1 pathway is different from that utilized by classical class I MHC molecules?

Go to www.whfreeman.com/immunology Self-Test
Review and quiz of key terms

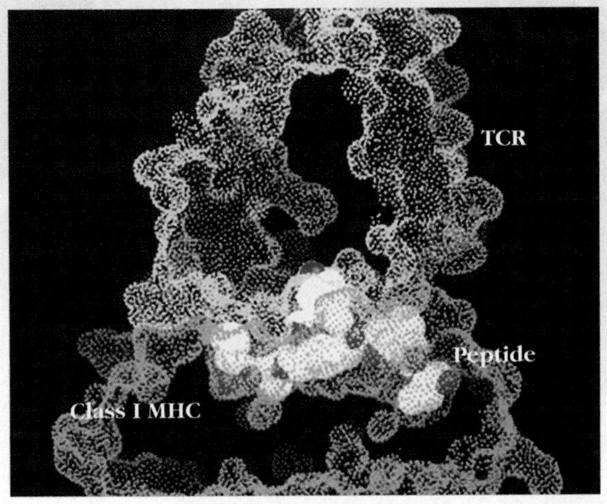

CHAPTER 9

T-CELL RECEPTOR

Although the antigen-specific nature of T-cell responses clearly implies that T cells possess an antigen-specific and clonally restricted receptor, the nature of this receptor remained unknown long after the B-cell receptor (immunoglobulin molecule) had been identified. Relevant experimental results were contradictory and difficult to conceptualize within a single model because the T-cell receptor (TCR) differs from the B-cell antigen-binding receptor in two important ways. First, the T-cell receptor is membrane bound and does not appear in a soluble form as the B cell receptor does; therefore, assessment of its structure by biochemical methods was complicated, and complex cellular assays were necessary to determine its specificity. Second, the T-cell receptor is specific not for antigen alone but for antigen combined with a molecule encoded by the major histocompatibility complex (MHC). This property precludes purification of the T-cell receptor by simple antigen-binding techniques and adds complexity to any experimental system designed to investigate the receptor.

A combination of immunologic, biochemical, and molecular-biological manipulations has determined the nature of antigen recognition by T-cells and the structure of the T-cell receptor. The molecule responsible for T-cell specificity was found to be a heterodimer composed of either α and β or γ and δ chains. The genomic organization and how the diversity of the component chains is generated were found to resemble those of the B-cell receptor chains. It is not surprising that the mechanisms that generate the enormous hypervariability of the immunoglobulin family are used for the equally diverse family of T-cell receptors. Further, the T-cell receptor is associated on the membrane with a signal-transducing complex called CD3; this signal-transducing complex has a function similar to that of the Ig-α/Ig-β complex of the B-cell receptor. X-ray crystallography has been used to determine the structure of the T-cell receptor bound in a ternary complex to an MHC molecule and a peptide; progress in these studies gives new insight into the nature of T-cell recognition. The preceding chapters have outlined the nature of the MHC molecules that take part in antigen presentation and the processes that result in antigens bound to the MHC molecules. This chapter will explore the nature of the T-cell receptor molecules that specifically recognize these MHC-antigen complexes.

Early Studies of the T-Cell Receptor

By the early 1980s, investigators had learned much about T-cell function but were thwarted in their attempts to identify and isolate its antigen-binding receptor. The fact that the receptor is membrane bound and recognizes a complex of MHC and antigenic peptides made classic approaches to isolate it and determine its structure difficult or impossible. Because of this complexity, many blind alleys were explored. The obvious parallels between the recognition functions of T cells and B cells stimulated a great deal of experimental effort to take advantage of the presumed structural similarities between immunoglobulins and T-cell receptors. Reports published in the 1970s claimed discovery of immunoglobulin isotypes associated exclusively with T cells (IgT) and of antisera that recognize variable-region markers (idiotypes) common to antibodies and T-cell receptors with similar specificity. These experiments could not be reproduced; they were proven to be incorrect when it was demonstrated that the T-cell receptor and immunoglobulins do not have common recognition elements and are encoded by separate gene families. As the following sections will show, it would require a series of well-designed experiments that used cutting-edge technology to correctly answer questions about the structure of the T-cell receptor, the genes that encode it, and the manner in which it recognizes antigen.

Self-MHC Restriction of the T-Cell Receptor

By the early 1970s, immunologists had learned to generate cytotoxic T lymphocytes (CTLs) specific for virus-infected target cells. For example, when mice were infected with lymphocytic choriomenigitis (LCM) virus, they would produce CTLs that could lyse LCM-infected target cells in vitro. Yet these same CTLs failed to bind free LCM virus or viral antigens. This finding suggested that antigen recognition by T cells was fundamentally different from that of B cells. Why didn't the CTLs bind the virus or viral antigens directly as immunoglobulins did? The answer began to emerge in the classic experiments of R. M. Zinkernagel and P. C. Doherty in 1974 (see Figure 8-2). These studies demonstrated that antigen recognition by T cells is specific not only for viral antigen but also for an MHC molecule (Figure 9-1). T cells were shown to recognize antigen only when presented on the membrane of a cell by a self-MHC molecule. This attribute, called *self-MHC restriction,* distinguishes recognition of antigen by T cells from that by B cells. In 1996, Doherty and Zinkernagel were awarded the Nobel Prize for this work.

Two models were proposed to explain the MHC restriction of the T-cell receptor. The *dual-receptor model* envisioned a T cell with two separate receptors, one for antigen and one for class I or class II MHC molecules. The *altered-self model* proposed that there was a single receptor capable of recognizing foreign antigen bound to a self-MHC molecule. Unlike the dual-receptor model, in which an antigen and MHC molecule are recognized separately, the altered-self model predicts that a single receptor recognizes an alteration in self-MHC molecules induced by their association with foreign antigens.

FIGURE 9-1 Self-MHC restriction of the T-cell receptor (TCR). A particular TCR is specific for both an antigenic peptide and a self-MHC molecule. In this example, the H-2^k CTL is specific for viral peptide A presented on an H-2^k target cell (a). Antigen recognition does not occur when peptide B is displayed on an H-2^k target cell (b) nor when peptide A is displayed on an H-2^d target cell (c).

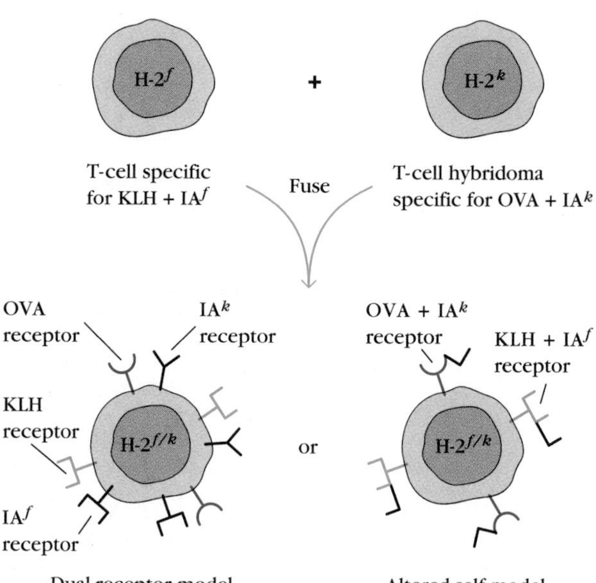

Response of fused cells				
		Expected response		
Antigen	MHC on APCs	Dual-receptor model	Altered-self model	Actual response
OVA	IA^k	+	+	+
OVA	IA^f	+	–	–
KLH	IA^k	+	–	–
KLH	IA^f	+	+	+

FIGURE 9-2 Experimental test of the dual-receptor and altered-self models of T-cell antigen recognition. T cells with two different specificities were fused, and the hybrid cells then were tested for their ability to recognize various antigen-MHC complexes. One fusion partner was specific for ovalbumin (OVA) + the class II MHC molecule IA^k on antigen-presenting cells (APCs), and the other was specific for keyhole limpet hemocyanin (KLH) + IA^f. Comparison of the expected responses of the fused cells, assuming the dual-receptor or altered-self model to be correct, with the actual responses supports the altered-self model. [Based on J Kappler et al, 1981, *J. Exp. Med.* **153:**1198.]

The debate between proponents of these two models was waged for a number of years, until an elegant experiment by J. Kappler and P. Marrack succeeded in testing each model. Two preparations of T cells specific for different complexes of antigen with class II MHC molecules were used for the experiment: one preparation was a T-cell hybridoma specific for ovalbumin (OVA) in the context of an H-2^k class II MHC molecule; the other preparation was a normal T cell reactive to keyhole limpet hemocyanin (KLH) in the context of an H-2^f class II MHC molecule. The experimenters fused these two cells to produce a T-cell hybridoma expressing the receptors of both fusion partners (Figure 9-2). If the dual-receptor model were correct, then the hybrid cells should express separate receptors for each antigen and separate receptors for each class II MHC molecule; therefore, the hybrid cells should respond to both antigens presented by either H-2^k or H-2^f antigen-presenting cells. In fact, Kappler and Marrack found that the hybrid cells continued to respond only to OVA presented by H-2^k cells and to KLH presented by H-2^f cells. In other words, the original specificity for antigen and MHC haplotype appeared to segregate together in the membrane of these hybrid cells. This finding provided early support for the altered-self model.

Isolation of T-Cell Receptors

Identification and isolation of the T-cell receptor finally was accomplished by producing large numbers of monoclonal antibodies to various T-cell clones and then screening these monoclonal antibodies to find one that was clone specific, or *clonotypic*. This approach was based on the assumption that, since the T-cell receptor is specific for both an antigen and an MHC molecule, there should be significant structural differences in the receptor from clone to clone; each T-cell clone should have an antigenic marker similar to the idiotype markers that characterize monoclonal antibodies. The T-cell receptor was first identified by J. P. Allison in 1982, using this approach; other researchers soon isolated the receptor and found that it was a heterodimer consisting of α and β chains.

Using αβ heterodimers isolated from membranes of various T-cell clones, Allison showed that some antisera bound to αβ heterodimers from all the clones, whereas other antisera were clone specific. This finding suggested that the amino acid sequences of the TCR α and β chains, like those of the immunoglobulin heavy and light chains, have constant and variable regions. Later, a second type of TCR heterodimer consisting of δ and γ chains was identified. The majority of T cells express the αβ heterodimer; the remaining express the γδ heterodimer; the exact proportion of T cells expressing αβ or γδ TCR differs in various organs and from species to species, but αβ T cells normally predominate. A cell that expresses TCR has approximately 10^5 TCR molecules on its surface.

Structure of T-Cell Receptors

Amino acid sequencing of the αβ and γδ TCR heterodimers revealed a domain structure that is strikingly similar to that of the immunoglobulins; thus, they are classified as members of the immunoglobulin superfamily (see Figure 4-19). Each chain in a TCR has two domains containing an intrachain disulfide bond that spans 60–75 amino acids. The amino-terminal domain in both chains exhibits marked sequence variation, but the sequences of the remainder of each chain are conserved. Thus the TCR domains—one variable (V) and one constant (C)—are structurally homologous to the V and C domains of immunoglobulins, and the TCR molecule resembles an Fab fragment (Figure 9-3). The TCR

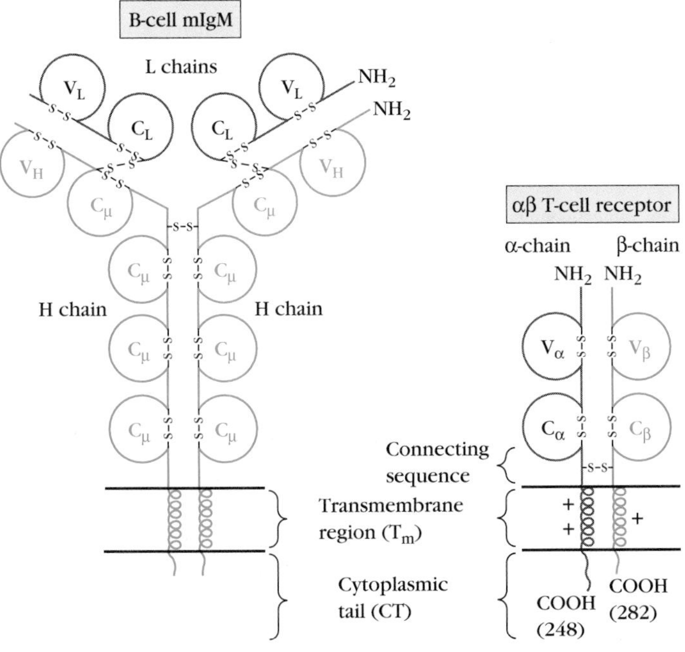

FIGURE 9-3 Schematic diagram illustrating the structural similarity between the αβ T-cell receptor and membrane-bound IgM on B cells. The TCR α and β chain each contain two domains with the immunoglobulin-fold structure. The amino-terminal domains (V_α andV_β) exhibit sequence variation and contain three hypervariable regions equivalent to the CDRs in antibodies. The sequence of the constant domains (C_α and C_β) does not vary. The two TCR chains are connected by a disulfide bond between their constant sequences; the IgM H chains are connected to one another by a disulfide bond in the hinge region of the H chain, and the L chains are connected to the H chains by disulfide links between the C termini of the L chains and the C_μ region. TCR molecules interact with CD3 via positively charged amino acid residues (indicated by +) in their transmembrane regions. The structure of the γδ T-cell receptor is similar. Numbers indicate the length of the chains in the TCR molecule. Unlike the antibody molecule, which is bivalent, the TCR is monovalent.

variable domains have three hypervariable regions, which appear to be equivalent to the complementarity determining regions (CDRs) in immunoglobulin light and heavy chains. There is an additional area of hypervariability (HV4) in the β chain that does not normally contact antigen and therefore is not considered a CDR.

In addition to the constant domain, each TCR chain contains a short connecting sequence, in which a cysteine residue forms a disulfide link with the other chain. Following the connecting region is a transmembrane region of 21 or 22 amino acids, which anchors each chain in the plasma membrane. The transmembrane domains of both chains are unusual in that they contain positively charged amino acid residues. These positively charged residues enable the chains of the TCR heterodimer to interact with chains of the signal-transducing CD3 complex. Finally, each TCR chain contains a short cytoplasmic tail of 5–12 amino acids at the carboxyl-terminal end.

Because both the αβ and γδ T-cell receptors are transmembrane proteins, it is difficult to isolate sufficient quantities for x-ray crystallography; in addition, the chains are not soluble in the absence of detergent. These difficulties have been circumvented to a great extent by expressing the protein in in vitro systems. The clones used for expressing the TCR molecules are engineered to contain premature in-frame stop codons that preclude translation of the membrane-binding sequence that makes the molecule insoluble. As shown later in this chapter, the crystal structure of the TCR shows homology with the Fab portion of immunoglobulins. The three CDRs are oriented in the V domain to form the antigen-binding site. CDR3 is in the center of the site and plays a significant role in contacting the antigenic peptide held in the cleft of the MHC molecule.

Organization and Rearrangement of TCR Genes

The genes that encode the αβ and γδ T-cell receptors are expressed only in cells of the T-cell lineage. The four TCR loci α, β, γ, and δ) have a germ-line organization that is remarkably similar to the multigene organization of the immunoglobulin (Ig) genes. As with the Ig genes, separate V, D, and J gene segments rearrange during T-cell maturation to form functional genes that encode the T-cell receptor.

Identifying and Cloning the TCR Genes

In order to identify and isolate the TCR genes, S. M. Hedrick and M. M. Davis sought to isolate mRNA that encodes the α and β chains from a T_H-cell clone. This was no easy task. Because the T cell does not secrete its antigen-binding receptor, the receptor mRNA represents a minor fraction of the total cell mRNA. By contrast, in the plasma cell, immunoglobulin is a major secreted cell product, and mRNAs encoding the heavy and light chains are abundant and easy to purify. The successful scheme of Hedrick and Davis for isolating TCR genes depended on a number of well-thought-out assumptions, which proved to be correct.

Hedrick and Davis reasoned that the TCR mRNA—like the mRNAs that encode other integral membrane proteins—would be associated with membrane-bound polyribosomes rather than with free cytoplasmic ribosomes. They therefore isolated the membrane-bound polyribosomal mRNA from a T_H-cell clone and used reverse transcriptase to synthesize ^{32}P-labeled cDNA probes (Figure 9-4). Because only 3% of lymphocyte mRNA is in the membrane-bound polyribosomal fraction, this step eliminated the 97% of the mRNA that did not encode any integral membrane protein.

Hedrick and Davis next used a technique called *DNA subtractive hybridization* to remove from their preparation the [^{32}P]cDNA that was not unique to T cells. Their rationale for this step was that, since T cells and B cells are derived from a common progenitor cell, they should express many genes in common. Earlier measurements by Davis had shown that 98% of the genes expressed in lymphocytes are common to B cells and T cells. Hedrick and Davis sought to enrich for the 2% of the expressed genes that are unique to T cells, which should include the genes encoding the T-cell receptor. Therefore, by hybridizing B-cell mRNA with their T_H-cell [^{32}P]cDNA, they were able to remove, or subtract, all the cDNA that was common to B cells and T cells. The unhybridized [^{32}P]cDNA remaining after this step presumably represented the expressed polyribosomal mRNA that was unique to the T_H-cell clone, including the mRNA encoding its T-cell receptor.

Cloning of the unhybridized [^{32}P]cDNA generated a library from which 10 different cDNA clones were identified. To determine which of these T-cell–specific cDNA clones might represent the T-cell receptor, Hedrick and Davis used these clones as probes to look for genes on the genomic DNA that rearranged in mature T cells. This approach was based on the assumption that, since the αβ T-cell receptor appeared to have constant and variable regions, its genes should undergo DNA rearrangements like those observed in the Ig genes of B cells. The two investigators isolated genomic DNA from T cells, B cells, liver cells, and macrophages, cleaved it with restriction endonucleases, and subjected each DNA sample to Southern-blot analysis using the 10 [^{32}P]cDNA probes to identify unique T-cell genomic DNA sequences. They looked for bands that showed DNA rearrangement in T cells but not in liver cells, B cells, or macrophages. One cDNA probe showed the same Southern-blot patterns for DNA isolated from liver cells, B cells, and macrophages but six different patterns for the DNA from six different mature T-cell lines (see Figure 9-4 inset, upper panel). These different patterns presumably represented rearranged TCR genes. Such results would be expected if rearranged TCR genes oc-

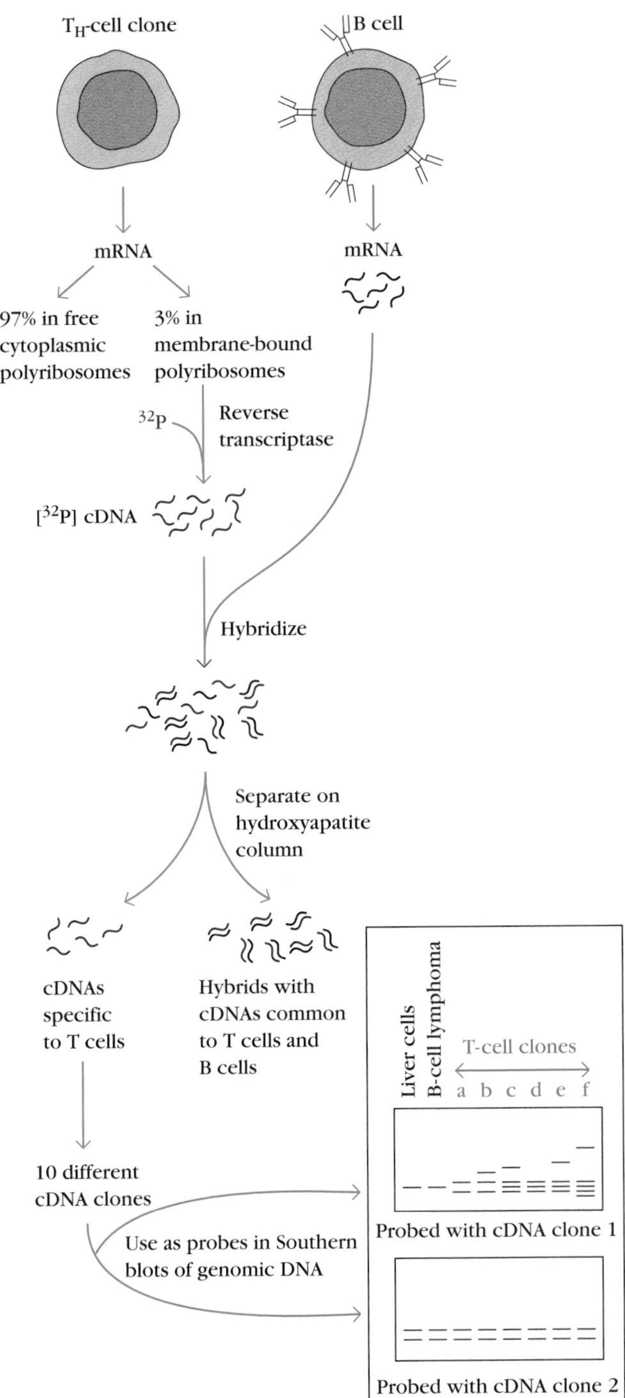

FIGURE 9-4 Production and identification of a cDNA clone encoding the T-cell receptor. The flow chart outlines the procedure used by S. Hedrick and M. Davis to obtain [^{32}P]cDNA clones corresponding to T-cell–specific mRNAs. The technique of DNA subtractive hybridization enabled them to isolate [^{32}P]cDNA unique to the T cell. The labeled T_H-cell cDNA clones were used as probes (*inset*) in Southern-blot analyses of genomic DNA from liver cells, B-lymphoma cells, and six different T_H-cell clones (a–f). Probing with cDNA clone 1 produced a distinct blot pattern for each T-cell clone, whereas probing with cDNA clone 2 did not. Assuming that liver cells and B cells contained unrearranged germ-line TCR DNA, and that each of the T-cell clones contained different rearranged TCR genes, the results using cDNA clone 1 as the probe identified clone 1 as the T-cell receptor gene. The cDNA of clone 2 identified the gene for another T-cell membrane molecule encoded by DNA that does not undergo rearrangement. [Based on S Hedrick et al, 1984, *Nature* **308:**149.]

cur only in mature T cells. The observation that each of the six T-cell lines showed different Southern-blot patterns was consistent with the expected differences in TCR specificity in each T-cell line.

The cDNA clone 1 identified by the Southern-blot analyses shown in Figure 9-4 has all the hallmarks of a putative TCR gene: it represents a gene sequence that rearranges, is expressed as a membrane-bound protein, and is expressed only in T cells. This cDNA clone was found to encode the β chain of the T-cell receptor. Later, cDNA clones were identified encoding the α chain, the γ chain, and finally the δ chain.

TCR Multigene Families

Germ-line DNA contains four TCR multigene families, each encoding one of the receptor chains (Figure 9-5). As in the case of Ig genes, functional TCR genes are produced by rearrangements of V and J segments in the α-chain and γ-chain families and V, D, and J segments in the β-chain and δ-chain families. In the mouse, the α-, β-, and γ-chain gene segments are located on chromosomes 14, 6, and 13, respectively. The δ-chain gene segments are located on chromosome 14 between the V_α and J_α segments. This location of the δ-chain gene family is significant: a productive rearrangement of the α-chain gene segments deletes C_δ, so that, in a given T cell, the αβ TCR receptor cannot be coexpressed with the γδ receptor.

Mouse germ-line DNA contains about 100 V_α and 50 J_α gene segments and a single C_α segment. The δ-chain gene family contains about 10 V gene segments, which are largely distinct from the V_α gene segments, although some sharing of V segments has been observed in rearranged α- and δ-chain genes. Two D_δ and two J_δ gene segments and one C_δ segment have also been identified. The β-chain gene family has 20–30 V gene segments and two almost identical repeats of D, J, and C segments, each repeat consisting of one D_β, six J_β, and one C_β. The γ-chain gene family consists of seven V_γ segments and three different functional J_γ-C_γ repeats. The organization of the TCR multigene families in humans is generally similar to that in mice, although the number of segments differs (Table 9-1).

Mouse TCR α-chain and δ-chain DNA (chromosome 14)

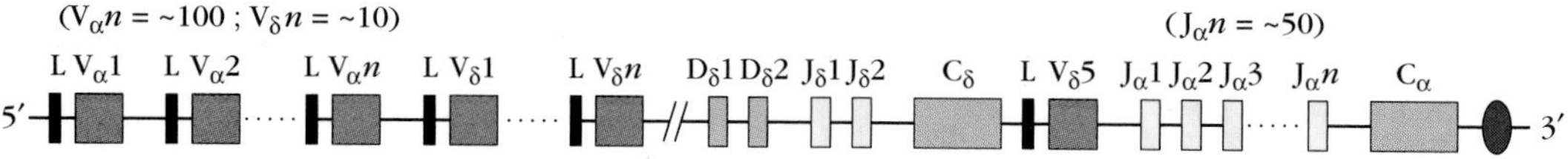

Mouse TCR β-chain DNA (chromosome 6)

(Vβn = 20 – 30)
L Vβ1 L Vβ2 L Vβn Dβ1 —Jβ1.1–Jβ1.7— Cβ1 Dβ2 —Jβ2.1–Jβ2.7— Cβ2 LVβ14
5′
3′

Mouse TCR γ-chain DNA (chromosome 13)

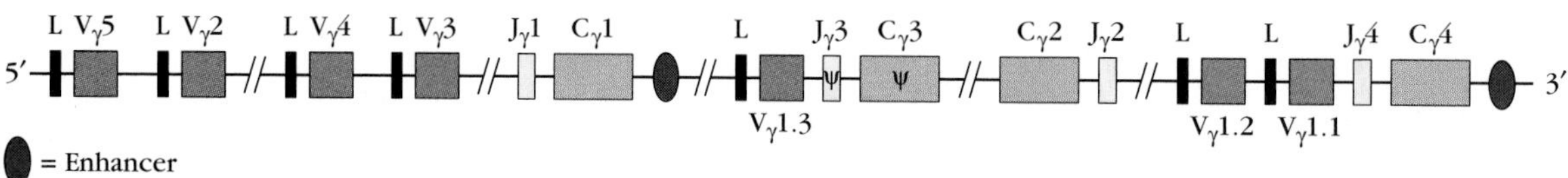

= Enhancer

ψ = pseudogene

FIGURE 9-5 Germ-line organization of the mouse TCR α-, β-, γ-, and δ-chain gene segments. Each C gene segment is composed of a series of exons and introns, which are not shown. The organization of TCR gene segments in humans is similar, although the number of the various gene segments differs in some cases (see Table 9-1). [Adapted from D Raulet, 1989, *Annu. Rev. Immunol.* **7**:175, and M Davis, 1990, *Annu. Rev. Biochem.* **59**:475.]

TABLE 9-1 TCR MULTIGENE FAMILIES IN HUMANS

Gene	Chromosome location	No. of gene segments			
		V	D	J	C
α Chain	14	50		70	1
δ Chain*	14	3	3	3	1
β Chain†	7	57	2	13	2
γ Chain‡	7	14		5	2

*The δ-chain gene segments are located between the V_α and J_α segments.
†There are two repeats, each containing 1 D_β, 6 or 7 J_β, and 1 C_β.
‡There are two repeats, each containing 2 or 3 J_γ and 1 C_γ.

SOURCE: Data from PAH Moss et al, 1992, *Annu. Rev. Immunol.* **10**:71.

Variable-Region Gene Rearrangements

The organization of the gene segments in the germ-line DNA encoding the α and β chains of the T-cell receptor is generally analogous to that of the immunoglobulin germ-line DNA. The α chain, like the immunoglobulin L chain, is encoded by V, J, and C gene segments. The β chain, like the immunoglobulin H chain, is encoded by V, D, J, and C gene segments. Rearrangement of the TCR α- and β-chain gene segments results in VJ joining for the α chain and VDJ joining for the β chain (Figure 9-6).

After transcription of the rearranged TCR genes, RNA processing, and translation, the α and β chains are expressed as a disulfide-linked heterodimer on the membrane of the T cell. Unlike immunoglobulins, which can be membrane bound or secreted, the αβ heterodimer is expressed only in a membrane-bound form; thus, no differential RNA processing is required to produce membrane and secreted forms. Each TCR constant region includes a connecting sequence, a transmembrane sequence, and a cytoplasmic sequence. Also, the constant-region germ-line DNA encoding the TCR α and β chains is much simpler than the immunoglobulin heavy-chain germ-line DNA, which has multiple C gene segments encoding distinct isotypes with different effector functions. TCR α-chain DNA has only a single C gene segment; the β-chain DNA has two C gene segments, but their protein products differ by only a few amino acids and have no known functional differences.

Mechanism of TCR DNA Rearrangements

The mechanisms by which TCR germ-line DNA is rearranged to form functional receptor genes appear to be similar to the mechanisms of Ig-gene rearrangements. For example, conserved heptamer and nonamer recognition signal sequences (RSSs), containing either 12-bp (one-turn) or 23-bp (two-turn) spacer sequences, have been identified flanking each V, D, and J gene segment in TCR germ-line DNA. The recognition signals in T cells have similar heptamer and nonamer sequences as those in B cells (see Figure 5-6). All of the TCR-gene rearrangements follow the one-turn/two-turn joining rule observed for the Ig genes.

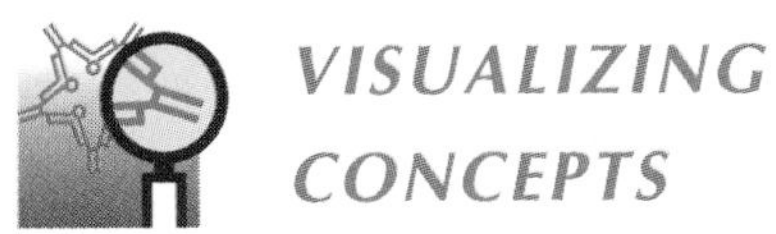

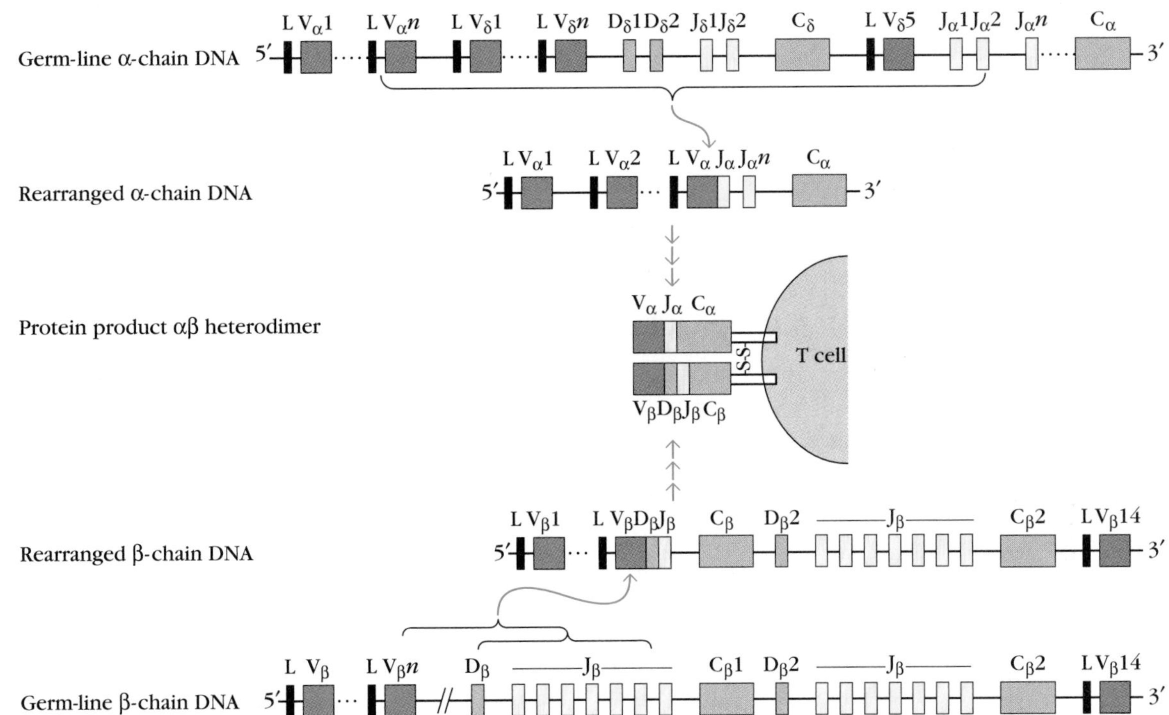

FIGURE 9-6 Example of gene rearrangements that yield a functional gene encoding the αβ T-cell receptor. The α-chain DNA, analogous to immunoglobulin light-chain DNA, undergoes a variable-region V_α-J_α joining. The β-chain DNA, analogous to immunoglobulin heavy-chain DNA, undergoes two variable-region joinings: first D_β to J_β and then V_β to $D_\beta J_\beta$ Transcription of the rearranged genes yields primary transcripts, which are processed to give mRNAs encoding the α and β chains of the membrane-bound TCR. The leader sequence is cleaved from the nascent polypeptide chain and is not present in the finished protein. As no secreted TCR is produced, differential processing of the primary transcripts does not occur. Although the β-chain DNA contains two C genes, the gene products of these two C genes exhibit no known functional differences. The C genes are composed of several exons and introns, which are not individually shown here (see Figure 9-7).

Like the pre-B cell, the pre-T cell expresses the recombination-activating genes (*RAG-1* and *RAG-2*). The RAG-1/2 recombinase enzyme recognizes the heptamer and nonamer recognition signals and catalyzes V-J and V-D-J joining during TCR-gene rearrangement by the same deletional or inversional mechanisms that occur in the Ig genes (see Figure 5-7). As described in Chapter 5 for the immunoglobulin genes, RAG-1/2 introduces a nick on one DNA strand between the coding and signal sequences. The recombinase then catalyzes a transesterification reaction that results in the formation of a hairpin at the coding sequence and a flush 5′ phosphorylated double-strand break at the signal sequence. Circular excision products thought to be generated by looping-out and deletion during TCR-gene rearrangement have been identified in thymocytes (see Figure 5-8).

Studies with SCID mice, which lack functional T and B cells, provide evidence for the similarity in the mechanisms of Ig-gene and TCR-gene rearrangements. As explained in Chapter 19, SCID mice have a defect in a gene required for the repair of double-stranded DNA breaks. As a result of this defect, D and J gene segments are not joined during rearrangement of either Ig or TCR DNA (see Figure 5-10). This finding suggests that the same double-stranded break-repair enzymes are involved in V-D-J rearrangements in B cells and in T cells.

Although B cells and T cells use very similar mechanisms for variable-region gene rearrangements, the Ig genes are not normally rearranged in T cells and the TCR genes are not rearranged in B cells. Presumably, the recombinase enzyme system is regulated in each cell lineage, so that only rearrangement of the correct receptor DNA occurs. As described at the end of Chapter 5, a region within the κ chain 3′ enhancer recently has been shown to suppress the rearrangement of κ L-chain genes in T cells. It is proposed that a protein present in T cells, but not in B cells, binds to this enhancer, thereby preventing the joining of V_κ to J_κ. Deletion of this region in the 3′ enhancer allows V_κ to J_κ joining to occur in T cells as well as in B cells.

The rearrangement of gene segments in a T or B cell creates a DNA sequence unique to that cell and its progeny. The large number of possible configurations of the rearranged genes makes this new sequence a marker that is specific for each T-cell clone. These unique DNA sequences have been used to aid in diagnoses and in treatment of lymphoid leukemias and lymphomas, cancers that involve clonal proliferation of T or B cells (see Clinical Focus).

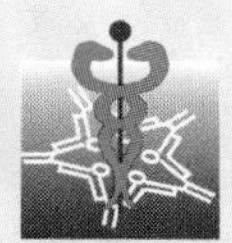

CLINICAL FOCUS

T-CELL REARRANGEMENTS AS MARKERS FOR CANCEROUS CELLS

T-cell cancers, which include leukemia and lymphoma, involve the uncontrolled proliferation of a clonal population of T cells. Successful treatment requires quick and certain diagnosis, in order to apply the most effective treatment, as well as reliable tests to determine whether treatment regimens are successful. In principle, because T-cell cancers are clonal in nature, the cell population that is cancerous could be identified and monitored by the expression of its unique T-cell receptor molecules. However, this approach is rarely practical because detection of a specific TCR molecule requires the tedious and lengthy preparation of a specific antibody directed against its variable region (an anti-idiotype antibody). In addition, because the surface expression of the TCR molecule occurs somewhat late in the development of the T cell, cancers stemming from T cells that have not progressed beyond an early stage of development will not display a TCR molecule and will not be detected by the antibody. An alternative means of identifying a clonal population of T cells is to look at their DNA rather than protein products. The pattern resulting from rearrangement of the TCR genes can provide a unique marker for the cancerous T cell. Because rearrangement of the TCR genes in the T cells occurs before the product molecule is expressed, T cells in early stages of development can be detected. The unique gene fragments that result from TCR gene rearrangement can be detected by simple molecular-biological techniques, and so they provide a true fingerprint for a clonal cell population.

DNA patterns that result from rearrangement of the genes in the TCR β region are used most frequently as markers. There are approximately 50 V_β gene segments that can rearrange to one of two D-region gene segments and subsequently to one of 12 J gene segments (see Figure 9-6). Because each of the 50 or so V-region genes is flanked by unique sequences, this process creates new DNA sequences that are unique to each cell that undergoes the rearrangement; these new sequences may be detected and followed by Southern-blot techniques or by PCR (polymerase chain reaction). Since the entire sequence of the D, J, and C region of the TCR gene β complex is known, the appropriate probes and restriction enzymes are easily chosen for Southern blotting (see diagram).

Detection of rearranged TCR DNA may be used as a diagnostic tool when abnormally enlarged lymph nodes persist; this condition could result either from inflammation due to chronic infection or from proliferation of a cancerous lymphoid cell. If inflammation is the cause, the cells would come from a variety of clones, and the DNA isolated from them would be a mixture of many different TCR sequences resulting from multiple rearrangements; no unique fragments would be detected. If the persistent enlargement of the nodes represents a clonal proliferation, there would be a detectable DNA fragment, because the cancerous cells would all contain the same TCR DNA sequence produced by DNA rearrangement in the parent cell. Thus the question whether the observed enlargement was due to the cancerous growth of T cells could be answered by the presence of a single new gene fragment in the DNA from the cell population. Because Ig genes rearrange in the same fashion as the TCR genes, similar techniques use Ig probes to detect clonal B cell populations by their unique DNA patterns. The technique, therefore, has value for a wide range of lymphoid-cell cancers.

Although the detection of a unique DNA fragment resulting from rearranged TCR or Ig genes indicates clonal proliferation and possible malignancy of T or B cells, the absence of such a fragment does not rule out cancer of a population of lymphoid cells. The cell involved may not contain rearranged TCR or Ig genes that can be detected by the method used, either because of its developmental stage or because it is of another lineage (γδ T cells, for example).

If the DNA fragment test, and other diagnostic criteria, indicate that the unfortunate patient has a lymphoid cell cancer, treatment by radiation therapy or chemother-

Allelic Exclusion of TCR Genes

As with the Ig genes, rearrangement of the TCR β-chain genes exhibits allelic exclusion. The organization of the β-chain gene segments into two clusters means that, if a nonproductive rearrangement occurs, the thymocyte can attempt a second rearrangement. This increases the likelihood of a productive rearrangement for the β chain. Once a productive rearrangement occurs for one β-chain allele, the rearrangement of the other β allele is inhibited.

Allelic exclusion appears to be less stringent for the TCR α-chain genes. For example, analyses of T-cell clones that express a functional αβ T-cell receptor revealed a number of clones with productive rearrangements of both α-chain alleles. Furthermore, when an immature T-cell lymphoma that expressed a particular αβ T-cell receptor was subcloned, several

apy would follow. The success of this treatment could be monitored by probing DNA from the patient for the unique sequence found in the cancerous cell. If the treatment regimen is successful, the number of cancerous cells will decline greatly. If the number of cancerous cells falls below 1% or 2% of the total T-cell population, analysis by Southern blot may no longer detect the unique fragment. In this case, a more sensitive technique, PCR, may be used. (With PCR it is possible to amplify, or synthesize multiple copies of, a specific DNA sequence in a sample; primers can hybridize to the two ends of that specific sequence and thus direct a DNA polymerase to copy it; see Figure 23-13 for details.) To detect a portion of the rearranged TCR DNA, amplification using a sequence from the rearranged V region as one primer and a sequence from the β chain C region as the other primer will yield a rearranged TCR DNA fragment of predicted size in sufficient quantity to be detected by electrophoresis (see red arrow in the diagram). Recently, quantitative PCR methods have been used to follow patients who are in remission in order to make decisions about resuming treatment if the number of cancerous cells, as estimated by these techniques, has risen above a certain level. Therefore, the presence of the rearranged DNA in the clonal population of T cells gives the clinician a valuable tool for diagnosing lymphoid-cell cancer and for monitoring the progress of treatment.

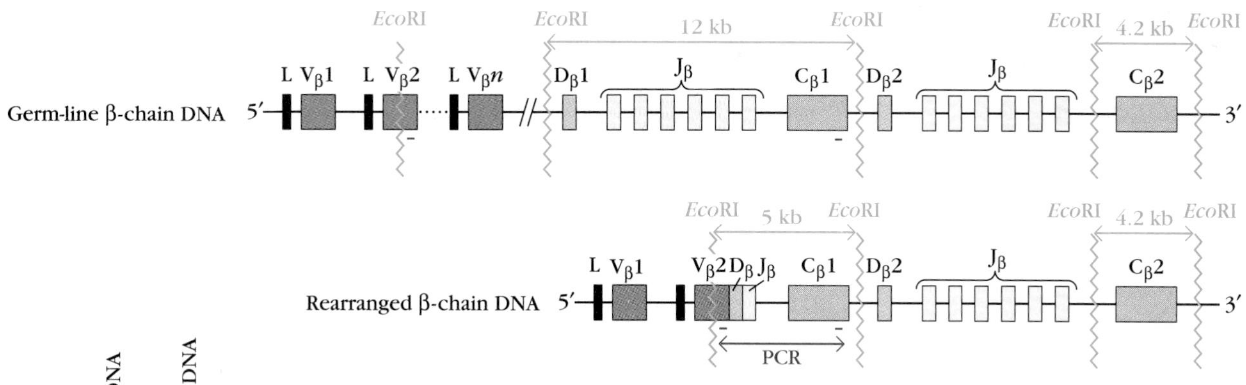

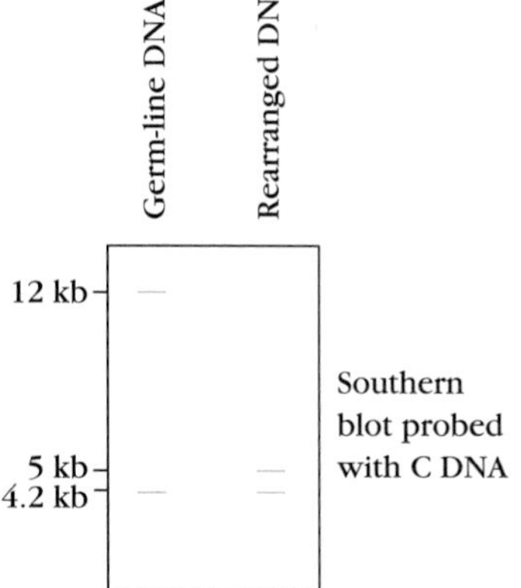

Digestion of human TCR β-chain DNA in a germ-line (nonrearranged) configuration with *Eco*RI and then probing with a C-region sequence will detect the indicated C-containing fragments by Southern blotting. When the DNA has rearranged, a 5′ restriction site will be excised. Digestion with *Eco*RI will yield a different fragment unique to the specific V_β and J_β region gene segments incorporated into the rearranged gene, as indicated in this hypothetical example. The technique used for this analysis derives from that first used by S. M. Hedrick and his coworkers to detect unique TCR β genes in a series of mouse T-cell clones (see inset to Figure 9-4). For highly sensitive detection of the rearranged TCR sequence, the polymerase chain reaction (PCR) is used. The sequence of the 5′ primer (red bar) is based on a unique sequence in the (V_β) gene segment used by the cancerous clone ($V_\beta2$ in this example) and the 3′ primer (red bar) is a constant region sequence. For chromosomes on which this V gene is not rearranged, the fragment will be absent because it is too large to be efficiently amplified.

subclones were obtained that expressed the same β-chain allele but an α-chain allele different from the one expressed by the original parent clone. Studies with transgenic mice also indicate that allelic exclusion is less stringent for TCR α-chain genes than for β-chain genes. Mice that carry a productively rearranged αβ-TCR transgene do not rearrange and express the endogenous β-chain genes. However, the endogenous α-chain genes sometimes are expressed at various levels in place of the already rearranged α-chain transgene.

Since allelic exclusion is not complete for the TCR α chain, there are rare occasions when more than one α chain is expressed on the membrane of a given T cell. The obvious question is how do the rare T cells that express two αβ T-cell receptors maintain a single antigen-binding specificity? One possibility, suggested by some researchers, is that when a T cell expresses two different αβ T-cell receptors, only one is likely to be self-MHC restricted and therefore functional.

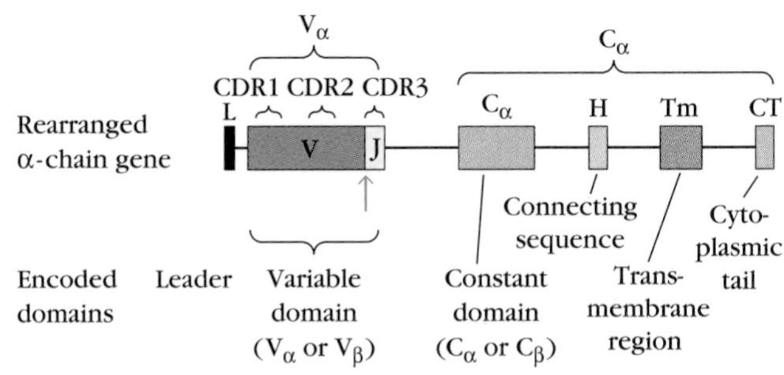

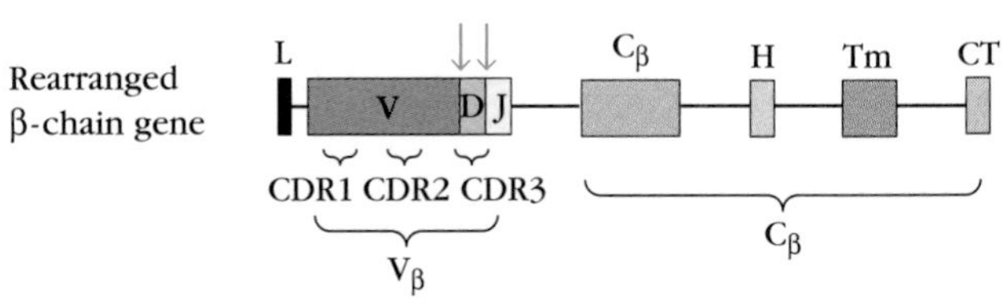

FIGURE 9-7 Schematic diagram of rearranged αβ-TCR genes showing the exons that encode the various domains of the αβ T-cell receptor and approximate position of the CDRs. Junctional diversity (vertical arrows) generates CDR3 (see Figure 9-8). The structures of the rearranged γ- and δ-chain genes are similar, although additional junctional diversity can occur in δ-chain genes.

Structure of Rearranged TCR Genes

The general structure of rearranged TCR genes is shown in Figure 9-7. The variable regions of T-cell receptors are, of course, encoded by rearranged VDJ and VJ sequences. In TCR genes, combinatorial joining of V gene segments appears to generate CDR1 and CDR2, whereas junctional flexibility and N-region nucleotide addition generate CDR3. Rearranged TCR genes also contain a short leader (L) exon

TABLE 9-2 SOURCES OF POSSIBLE DIVERSITY IN MOUSE IMMUNOGLOBULIN AND TCR GENES

	Immunoglobulins		αβ T-cell receptor		γδ T-cell receptor	
Mechanism of diversity	H Chain	κ Chain	α Chain	β Chain	γ Chain	δ Chain
	Estimated number of segments					
Multiple germ-line gene segments						
V	134	85	100	25	7	10
D	13	0	0	2	0	2
J	4	4	50	12	3	2
	Possible number of combinations*					
Combinatorial V-J and V-D-J joining	134 × 13 × 4 = 7 × 10^3	85 × 4 = 3.4 × 10^2	100 × 50 = 5 × 10^3	25 × 2 × 12 = 6 × 10^2	7 × 3 = 21	10 × 2 × 2 = 40
Alternative joining of D gene segments	−	−	−	+ (some)	−	+ (often)
Junctional flexibility	+	+	+	+	+	+
N-region nucleotide addition†	+	−	+	+	+	+
P-region nucleotide addition	+	+	+	+	+	+
Somatic mutation	+	+	−	−	−	−
Combinatorial association of chains	+		+		+	

*A plus sign (+) indicates mechanism makes a significant contribution to diversity but to an unknown extent.
A minus sign (−) indicates mechanism does not operate.
†See Figure 9-8d for theoretical number of combinations generated by N-region addition.

upstream of the joined VJ or VDJ sequences. The amino acids encoded by the leader exon are cleaved as the nascent polypeptide enters the endoplasmic reticulum.

The constant region of each TCR chain is encoded by a C gene segment that has multiple exons (see Figure 9-7) which correspond to the structural domains in the protein (see Figure 9-3). The first exon in the C gene segment encodes most of the C domain of the corresponding chain. Next is a short exon that encodes the connecting sequence, followed by exons that encode the transmembrane region and the cytoplasmic tail.

Generation of TCR Diversity

Although TCR germ-line DNA contains far fewer V gene segments than Ig germ-line DNA does, several mechanisms that operate during TCR gene rearrangements contribute to a high degree of diversity among T-cell receptors. Table 9-2 and Figure 9-8 compare the generation of diversity among antibody molecules and TCR molecules.

Combinatorial joining of variable-region gene segments generates a large number of random gene combinations for

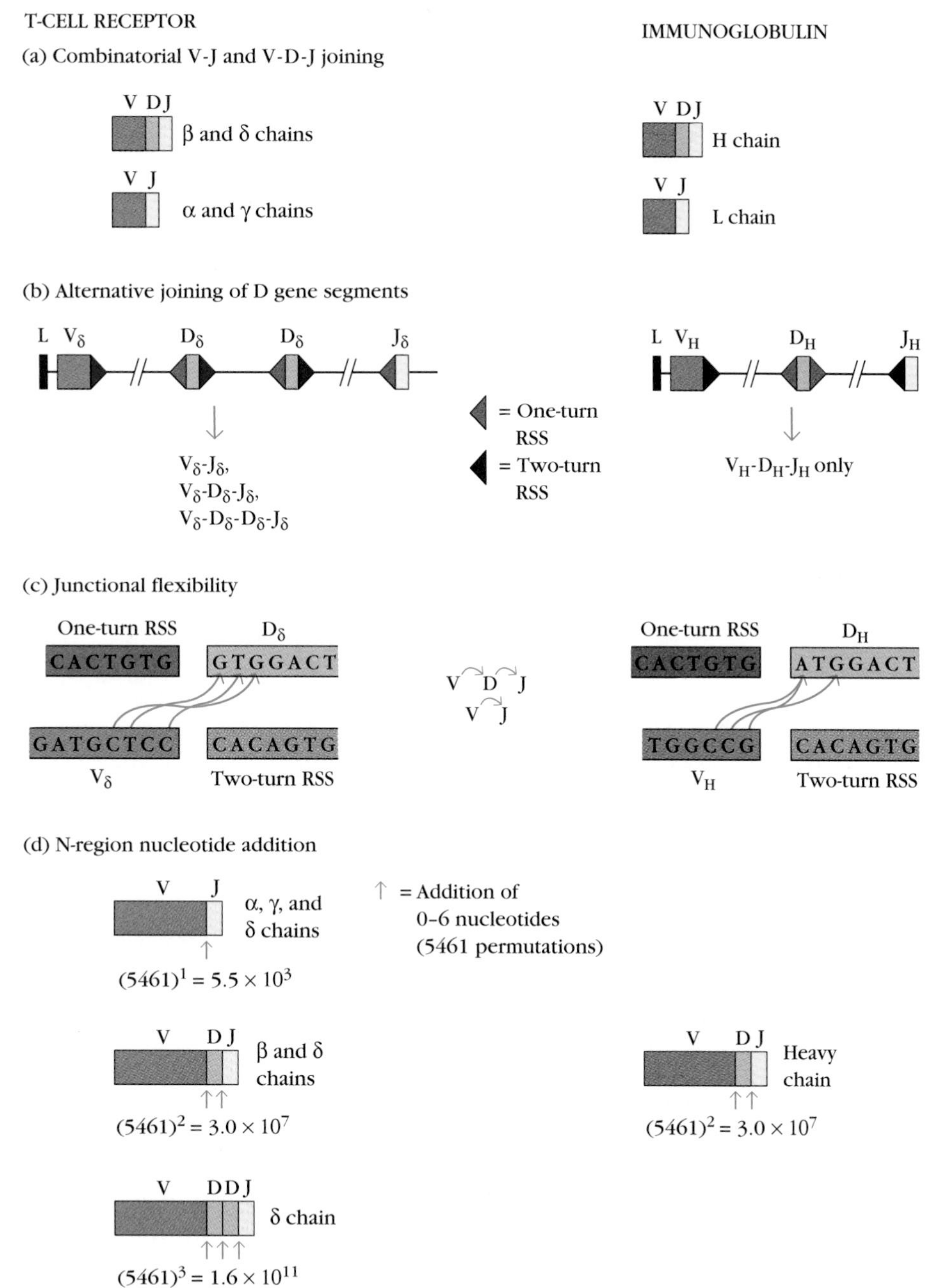

FIGURE 9-8 Comparison of mechanisms for generating diversity in TCR genes and immunoglobulin genes. In addition to the mechanisms shown, P-region nucleotide addition occurs in both TCR and Ig genes, and somatic mutation occurs in Ig genes. Combinatorial association of the expressed chains generates additional diversity among both TCR and Ig molecules.

all the TCR chains, as it does for the Ig heavy- and light-chain genes. For example, 100 V_α and 50 J_α gene segments can generate 5×10^3 possible VJ combinations for the TCR a chain. Similarly, 25 V_β, 2 D_β, and 12 J_β gene segments can give 6×10^2 possible combinations. Although there are fewer TCR V_α and V_β gene segments than immunoglobulin V_H and V_κ segments, this difference is offset by the greater number of J segments in TCR germ-line DNA. Assuming that the antigen-binding specificity of a given T-cell receptor depends upon the variable region in both chains, random association of 5×10^3 V_α combinations with 6×10^2 V_β combinations can generate 3×10^6 possible combinations for the αβ T-cell receptor. As described below, there are additional means to generate diversity in the TCR V genes, so that the 3×10^6 combinations represent a minimum estimate.

As illustrated in Figure 9-8b, the location of one-turn (12-bp) and two-turn (23-bp) recognition signal sequences in TCR β- and δ-chain DNA differs from that in Ig heavy-chain DNA. Because of the arrangement of the recognition signal sequences in TCR germ-line DNA, alternative joining of D gene segments can occur while the one-turn/two-turn joining rule is observed. Thus, it is possible for a V_β gene segment to join directly with a J_β or a D_β gene segment, generating a $(VJ)_\beta$ or $(VDJ)_\beta$ unit. *Alternative joining of δ-chain gene segments* generates similar units; in addition, one D_δ can join with another, yielding $(VDDJ)_\delta$ and, in humans, $(VDDDJ)_\delta$. This mechanism, which cannot operate in Ig heavy-chain DNA, generates considerable additional diversity in TCR genes.

The joining of gene segments during TCR-gene rearrangement exhibits **junctional flexibility.** As with the Ig genes, this flexibility can generate many nonproductive rearrangements, but it also increases diversity by encoding several alternative amino acids at each junction (see Figure 9-8c). In both Ig and TCR genes, nucleotides may be added at the junctions between some gene segments during rearrangement (see Figure 5-15). Variation in endonuclease cleavage leads to the addition of further nucleotides that are palindromic. Such **P-region nucleotide addition** can occur in the genes encoding all the TCR and Ig chains. Addition of **N-region nucleotides,** catalyzed by a terminal deoxynucleotidyl transferase, generates additional junctional diversity. Whereas the addition of N-region nucleotides occurs only in the Ig heavy-chain genes, it occurs in the genes encoding all the TCR chains. As many as six nucleotides can be added by this mechanism at each junction, generating up to 5461 possible combinations, assuming random selection of nucleotides (see Figure 9-8d). Some of these combinations, however, lead to nonproductive rearrangements. This is because certain rearrangements lead to creation of in-frame stop codons that prematurely terminate the TCR chain, and others lead to substitutions of amino acids that render the product nonfunctional. Although each junctional region in a TCR gene encodes only 10–20 amino acids, enormous diversity can be generated in these regions. Estimates suggest that the combined effects of P- and N-region nucleotide addition and joining flexibility can generate as many as 10^{13} possible amino acid sequences in the TCR junctional regions alone.

The T-cell receptor must recognize both a very large number of different processed antigens as well as a smaller number of self-MHC molecules. The way that diversity is generated for the TCR must allow the receptor to have the necessary variability needed to recognize diverse peptides while restricting its MHC-recognition diversity. TCR DNA has far fewer V gene segments than Ig DNA does (see Table 9-2). It has been postulated that the smaller number of V gene segments in TCR DNA have been selected to encode a limited number of CDR1 and CDR2 regions with affinity for regions of the α helices of MHC molecules. Although this is an attractive idea, recent data on the structure of the TCR-peptide-MHC complex show contact between peptide and CDR1 as well as CDR3 (see Figure 9-14). Therefore the TCR residues that bind to peptide versus those that bind MHC are not confined solely to the highly variable CDR3 region.

In contrast to the limited diversity of CDR1 and CDR2, the CDR3 of the TCR has even greater diversity than that seen in immunoglobulins. Diversity in the CDR3 region of the TCR is generated by junctional diversity in the joining of V, D, and J segments, joining of multiple D gene segments, and the introduction of P and N nucleotides at the V-D-J and V-J junctions (see Figure 9-7).

Unlike the Ig genes, the TCR genes do not appear to undergo extensive somatic mutation. That is, the functional TCR genes generated by gene rearrangements during T-cell maturation in the thymus have the same sequences as those found in the mature peripheral T-cell population. The absence of somatic mutation in T cells ensures that T-cell specificity does not change after thymic selection and therefore reduces the possibility that random mutation might generate a self-reactive T cell. Although a few experiments have provided evidence for somatic mutation of receptor genes in T cells in the germinal center, this appears to be the exception and not the rule.

T-Cell Receptor Complex: TCR-CD3

As discussed in Chapter 4, membrane-bound immunoglobulin on B cells associates with another membrane protein, the Ig-α/Ig-β heterodimer, to form the B-cell antigen receptor (see Figure 4-18). Similarly, the T-cell receptor associates with **CD3,** forming the TCR-CD3 membrane complex. In both cases, the accessory molecule participates in signal transduction after interaction of a B or T cell with antigen; it does not influence interaction with antigen.

The first evidence suggesting that the T-cell receptor is associated with another membrane molecule came from experiments in which fluorescent antibody to the receptor was shown to cause aggregation of another membrane protein designated CD3. Later experiments by J. P. Allison and L. Lanier demonstrated that the T-cell receptor and CD3 are located quite close together in the T-cell membrane. These researchers first treated a T-cell membrane preparation with a protein crosslinking agent that spans 12 Å and then precipitated the T-cell receptor with anti-TCR monoclonal antibody. Analysis of the precipitated T-cell receptors showed that they were crosslinked to CD3 molecules, indicating that the two proteins must be within 12 Å of each other in the membrane.

Subsequent experiments demonstrated not only that CD3 is closely associated with the αβ heterodimer but also that its expression is required for membrane expression of αβ and γδ T-cell receptors. Thus each heterodimer forms a complex with CD3 on the T-cell membrane. Loss of the genes encoding either CD3 or the TCR chains results in loss of the entire molecular complex from the membrane.

CD3 is a complex of five invariant polypeptide chains that associate to form three dimers: a heterodimer of gamma and epsilon chains (γϵ), a heterodimer of delta and epsilon chains (δϵ), and a homodimer of two zeta chains (ζζ) or a heterodimer of zeta and eta chains (ζη) (Figure 9-9). The ζ and η chains, which are encoded by the same gene, differ in their carboxyl-terminal ends because of differences in RNA splicing of the primary transcript. About 90% of the CD3 complexes examined to date incorporate the (ζζ) homodimer; the remainder have the (ζη) heterodimer. The T-cell receptor complex can thus be envisioned as four dimers: the αβ or γδ TCR heterodimer determines the ligand-binding specificity, whereas the CD3 dimers (γϵ, δϵ, and ζζ or ζη) are required for expression of the T-cell receptor and for signal transduction.

The γ, δ, and ϵ chains of CD3 are members of the immunoglobulin superfamily, each containing an immunoglobulin-like extracellular domain followed by a transmembrane region and a cytoplasmic domain of more than 40 amino acids. The ζ and η chains have a distinctly different structure: both have a very short external region of only 9 amino acids, a transmembrane region, and a long cytoplasmic tail containing 113 amino acids in ζ and 155 amino acids in η. The transmembrane region of all the CD3 polypeptide chains contains a negatively charged aspartic acid residue. These negatively charged groups enable the CD3 complex to interact with one or two positively charged amino acids in the transmembrane region of each TCR chain.

The cytoplasmic tails of the CD3 chains contain a motif called the **immunoreceptor tyrosine-based activation motif (ITAM).** This motif is found in a number of other receptors,

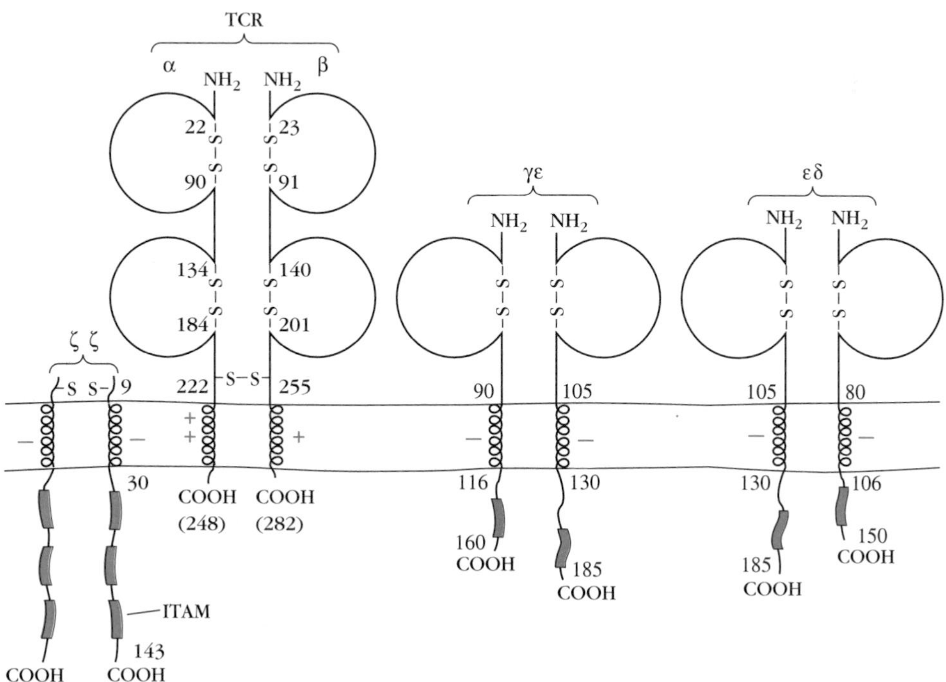

FIGURE 9-9 Schematic diagram of the TCR-CD3 complex, which constitutes the T-cell antigen-binding receptor. The CD3 complex consists of the ζζ homodimer (alternately, a γη heterodimer) plus γϵ and δϵ heterodimers. The external domains of the γ, δ, and ϵ chains of CD3 are similar to the immunoglobulin fold, which facilitates their interaction with the T-cell receptor and each other. Ionic interactions also may occur between the oppositely charged transmembrane regions in the TCR and CD3 chains. The long cytoplasmic tails of the CD3 chains contain a common sequence, the immunoreceptor tyrosine-based activation motif (ITAM), which functions in signal transduction.

including the Ig-α/Ig-β heterodimer of the B-cell receptor complex and the Fc receptors for IgE and IgG. The ITAM sites have been shown to interact with tyrosine kinases and to play an important role in signal transduction. In CD3, the γ, δ, and ε chains each contain a single copy of ITAM, whereas the ζ and η chains contain three copies (see Figure 9-9). The function of CD3 in signal transduction is described more fully in Chapter 10.

T-Cell Accessory Membrane Molecules

Although recognition of antigen-MHC complexes is mediated solely by the TCR-CD3 complex, various other membrane molecules play an important accessory role in antigen recognition and T-cell activation (Table 9-3). Some of these molecules strengthen the interaction between T cells and antigen-presenting cells or target cells; some act in signal transduction; and some do both.

CD4 and CD8 Coreceptors

T cells can be subdivided into two populations according to their expression of CD4 or CD8 membrane molecules. As was described in preceding chapters, $CD4^+$ T cells recognize antigen that is combined with class II MHC molecules and function largely as helper cells, whereas $CD8^+$ T cells recognize antigen that is combined with class I MHC molecules. They function largely as cytotoxic cells. CD4 is a 55-kDa monomeric membrane glycoprotein that contains four extracellular immunoglobulin-like domains (D_1–D_4) a hydrophobic transmembrane region, and a long cytoplasmic tail containing three serine residues, which can be phosphorylated (Figure 9-10). CD8 generally takes the form of a disulfide-linked αβ heterodimer or of an αα homodimer. Both the α and β chains of CD8 are small glycoproteins of approximately 30–38 kDa. Each chain consists of a single extracellular immunoglobulin-like domain, a hydrophobic transmembrane region, and a cytoplasmic tail containing 25–27 residues, several of which can be phosphorylated (see Figure 9-10).

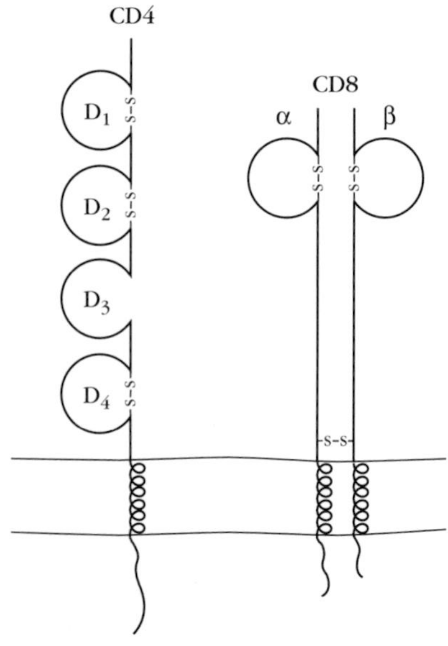

FIGURE 9-10 General structure of the CD4 and CD8 coreceptors. CD8 may take the form of an αβ heterodimer, or an αα homodimer. The monomeric CD4 molecule contains four Ig-fold domains, whereas each chain in the CD8 molecule contains one Ig-fold domain.

Both CD4 and CD8 have two key abilities that allow these membrane molecules to be classified as *coreceptors:* recognition of the peptide-MHC complex and signal transduction. The extracellular domains of CD4 and CD8 bind to the membrane-proximal domains of MHC molecules on antigen-presenting cells (APCs) or target cells: CD4 binds to the β2

TABLE 9-3 SELECTED T-CELL ACCESSORY MOLECULES

		Function		
Name	Ligand	Adhesion	Signal transduction	Member of Ig superfamily
CD4	Class II MHC	+	+	+
CD8	Class I MHC	+	+	+
CD2 (LFA-2)	CD58 (LFA-3)	+	+	+
LFA-1 (CD11a/CD18)	ICAM-1 (CD54)	+	?	+/(−)
CD28	B7	?	+	+
CTLA-4	B7	?	+	−
CD45R	CD22	+	+	+
CD5	CD72	?	+	−

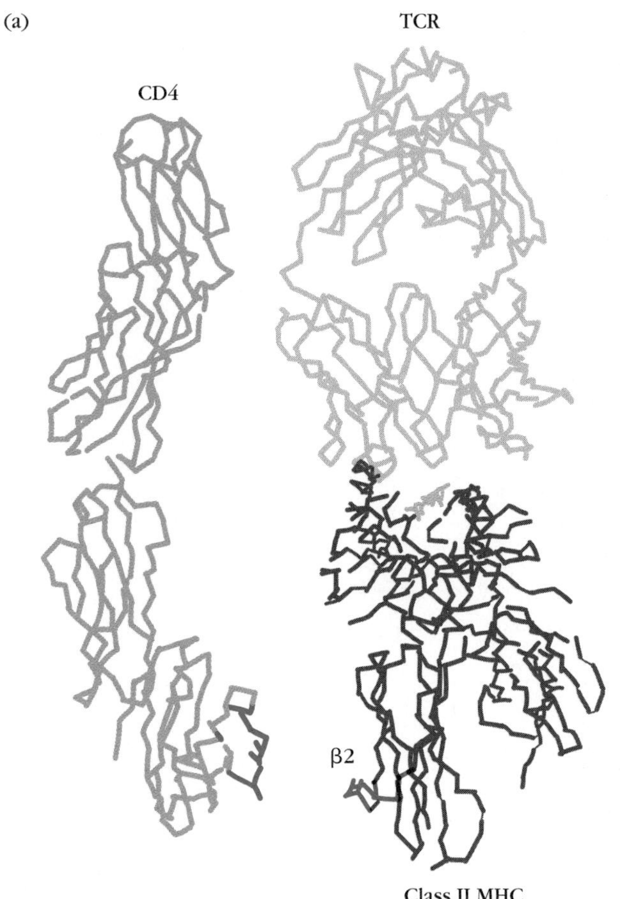

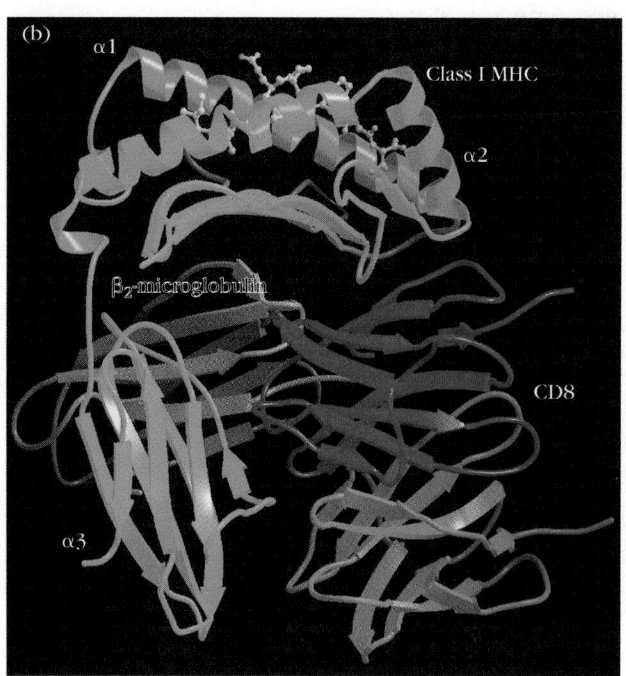

FIGURE 9-11 Interactions of coreceptors with TCR and MHC molecules. (a) Model of the external domains of CD4 (orange), T-cell receptor (blue), and class II MHC molecule (green) showing their orientation to each other. The top of the CD4 and TCR models in this figure would be anchored in the T-cell membrane; the bottom of the class II MHC molecule would be anchored in the membrane of an antigen-presenting cell. Interaction between CD4 and the β2 domain in the class II molecule is mediated by the residues in red. The antigenic peptide is pink. (b) Ribbon diagram showing three-dimensional structure of an HLA-A2 MHC class I molecule bound to a CD8 αα homodimer. The HLA-A2 heavy chain is shown in green, β_2-microglobulin in gold, the CD8 α1 in red, the CD8 α2 in blue, and the bound peptide in white. A flexible loop of the α3 domain (residues 223–229) is in contact with the two CD8 subunits. In this model, the right side of CD8 would be anchored in the T-cell membrane, and the lower left end of the class I MHC molecule (the α3 domain) is attached to the surface of the target cell. [Part (a) from SJ Davis and PA van der Merwe, 1996, *Immunol. Today* **17**(4):181; (b) from GF Gao et al, 1997, *Nature* **387:**630–634, courtesy of EY Jones, University of Oxford.]

domain of class II MHC molecules (Figure 9-11a). Crystallographic studies of a complex composed of the class I MHC molecule HLA-A2, an antigenic peptide, and a CD8 αα homodimer indicate that CD8 binds to class I molecules by contacting the MHC class I α2 and α3 domains as well as having some contact with β_2-microglobulin (Figure 9-11b). The orientation of the class I α3 domain changes slightly upon binding to CD8. This structure is consistent with a single MHC molecule binding to CD8; no evidence for the possibility of multimeric class I–CD8 complexes was observed.

In contrast to the data for CD8–class I binding, which indicates interaction of single units, there is evidence to suggest that, during antigen recognition by a T_H cell, a TCR molecule first binds to a dimer of the class II MHC molecule (that has a bound peptide). The membrane-distal domain of CD4 then binds to the β2 domain of the class II MHC molecule, forming a complex of TCR, CD4, and MHC (Figure 9-12a). Once bound to the MHC molecule, the CD4 molecule is thought to undergo a conformational change, enabling its membrane-proximal domains to interact with the membrane-proximal domains of a second, adjacent CD4 molecule that has complexed in a similar manner with a TCR and MHC molecule. Eventually, tetrameric structures consisting of four of the class II dimers with attached CD4 will be formed on the membrane. As the CD4 molecules contact other such complexes, larger oligomers may form (Figure 9-12b). This crosslinkage of the TCRs on a T cell, forming a lattice-type structure, may be necessary for transmembrane signaling events. Further studies on the structure of the class II–CD4 complex are needed for clarification of the stoichiometry of binding between these molecules.

The interactions of MHC class II molecules with CD4 apparently increase the avidity of the binding of a T-cell

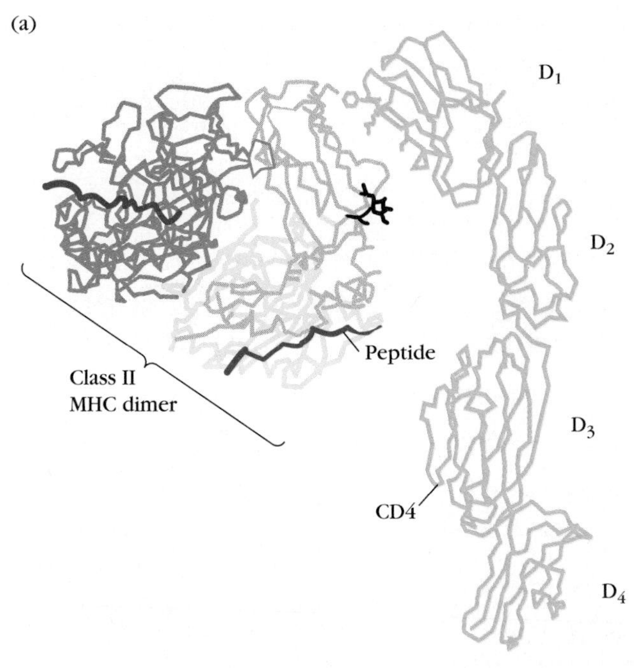

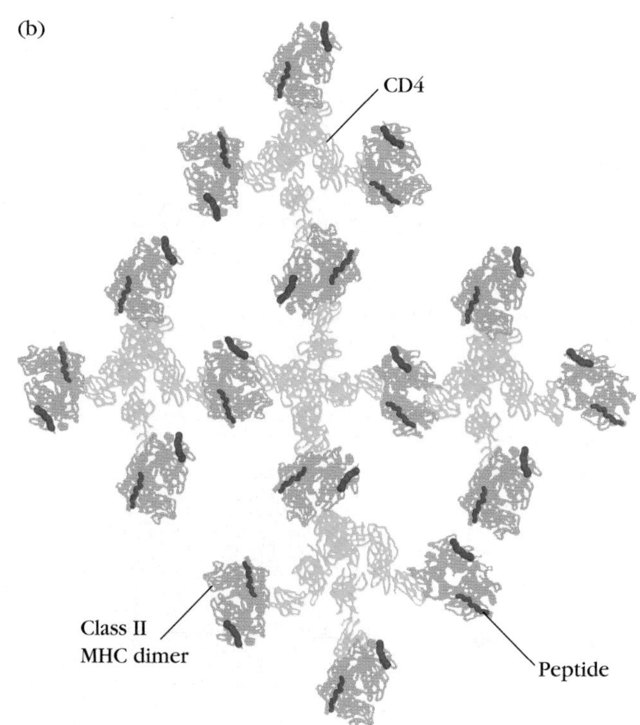

FIGURE 9-12 Possible models of interaction between CD4 and class II MHC molecule during antigen recognition. (a) After binding of a T-cell receptor (not shown) to the dimer form of a class II MHC molecule (pink and blue), the membrane-distal D_1 domain of CD4 (green) interacts with the β2 domain (blue) of the MHC molecule. (b) A lattice-type structure is formed by interaction of the membrane-proximal domains of CD4 with adjacent CD4 molecules that also are complexed with a TCR and MHC molecule. The peptide is represented by the red ribbons.

receptor to a peptide-MHC complex. The binding affinity for T-cell receptors to peptide-class II MHC complexes has been shown to increase about 100-fold when CD4 is present on the membrane. Whether there are differences between the roles played by the CD4 and CD8 coreceptors remains open to speculation. Despite the similarities in structure, recall that the nature of the binding of peptide to class I and class II molecules differs in that class I has a closed groove that binds a short peptide with a higher degree of specificity. The class II molecule has an open groove and specificity is conferred by the N and C termini of the peptide. The differences in the function of the CD4 and CD8 coreceptors may be due to this difference in binding requirements. For example, CD4 may enhance the avidity of the binding of class II to TCR to allow for more flexibility in the peptide structure recognized. As will be explained in Chapter 10, binding of the CD4 and CD8 molecules serves to transmit stimulatory signals to the T cells; the signal-transduction properties of both CD4 and CD8 are mediated through their cytoplasmic domains.

Affinity of TCR for Peptide-MHC Complexes

The affinity of T-cell receptors for peptide-MHC complexes is low to moderate, with K_d values ranging from 10^{-4} to 10^{-7} M. Thus, this interaction is weak compared with antigen-antibody interactions, which generally have K_d values ranging from 10^{-6} to 10^{-10} M (Figure 9-13a). The low affinity of the T-cell receptor for antigenic peptide–MHC complexes suggests that other molecules are needed to enhance the binding of a T-cell to a peptide-MHC complex on an antigen-presenting cell or target cell. T-cell interactions do not depend solely on binding by the TCR; cell-adhesion molecules strengthen the bond between a T cell and an antigen-presenting cell or a target cell.

In addition to CD4 and CD8 coreceptors, which interact with the MHC class II and class I molecules and serve to increase the affinity of the bond between TCR and the MHC-peptide complex, T cells have several accessory membrane molecules, including CD2, LFA-1, CD28, and CD45R. Unlike the CD4 and CD8 coreceptors, these other molecules do not interact with the peptide-MHC complex; rather, they bind independently to other ligands on antigen-presenting cells or target cells (see Table 9-3 and Figure 9-13b). Once cell-to-cell contact has been made by the adhesion molecules, the T-cell receptor may scan the membrane for peptide-MHC complexes. During activation of a T cell by a particular peptide-MHC complex, there is a transient increase in the expression of accessory membrane molecules (e.g., CD2, LFA-1), causing closer contact between the interacting cells, which allows cytokines or cytotoxic substances to be transferred more effectively. Soon after activation, the degree of adhesion declines and the T cell detaches from the antigen-presenting cell or target cell. Like CD4 and CD8, some of these other molecules also function as signal-transducers. Their important role is demonstrated by the ability of monoclonal antibodies specific for them to block T-cell activation.

The discovery of CD3, CD4, CD8, and the other accessory molecules associated with the TCR raised the possibility that they might be necessary for antigen recognition by T cells. The experiment of Kappler and Marrack described above (see Figure 9-2) had supported the notion that a single receptor on the T cell recognizes peptide complexed with a self-MHC molecule. However, that experiment did not rule out the possibility that another membrane molecule (coreceptor) associated with the T-cell receptor might contribute to recognition of either the peptide or the MHC molecule. As the next section shows, a recent demonstration of TCR binding using isolated components of the TCR–peptide-MHC complex provides definitive proof that no other molecule is required for recognition, at least not for binding of TCR to a peptide–class I complex. While the accessory molecules discussed above may enhance that binding, they are not necessary for it.

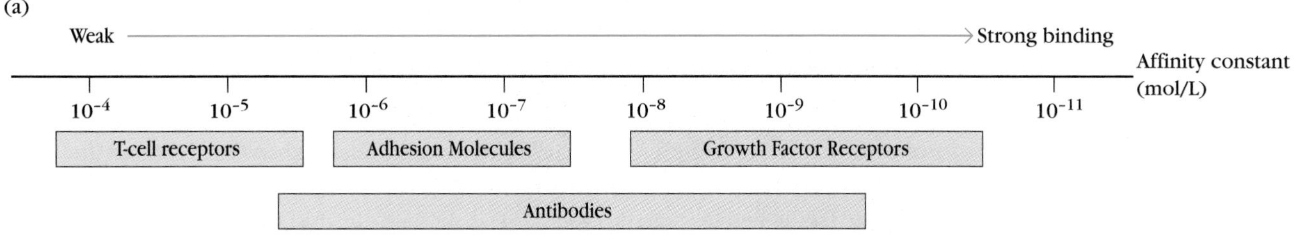

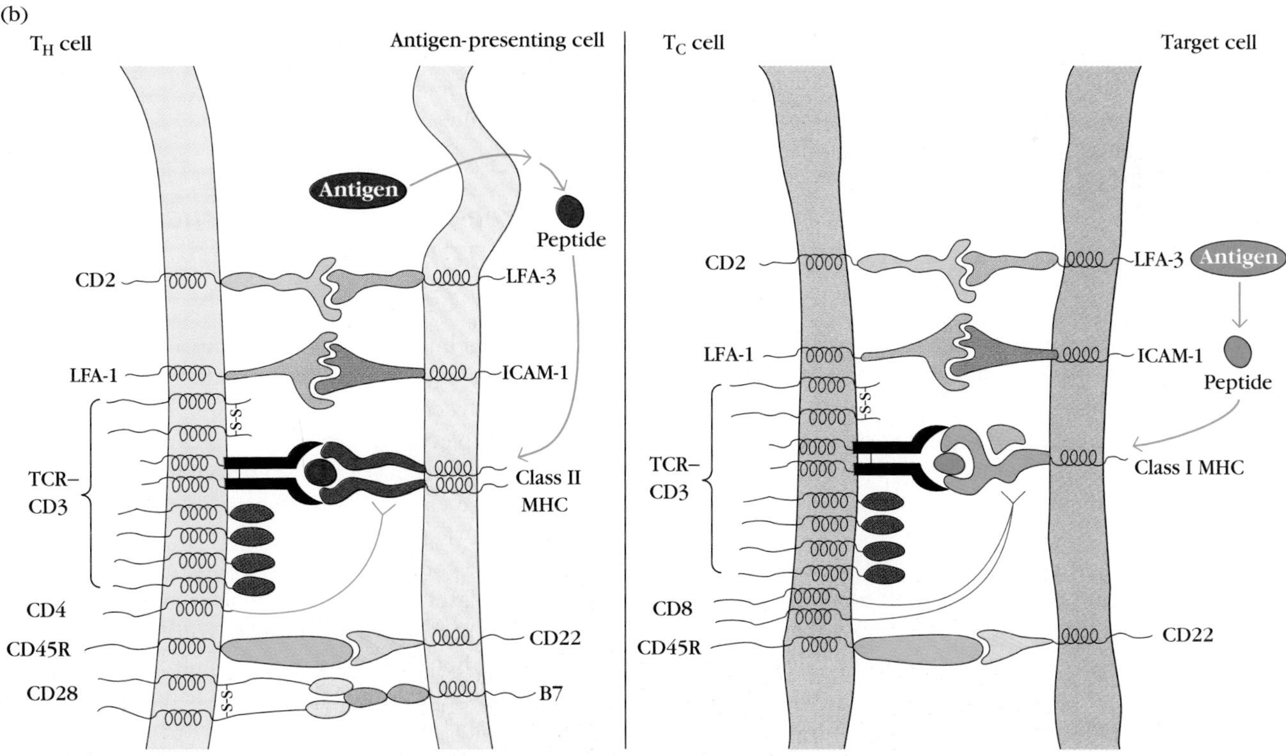

FIGURE 9-13 Role of coreceptors in TCR binding affinity. (a) Affinity constants for various biologic systems. (b) Schematic diagram of the interactions between the T-cell receptor and the peptide-MHC complex and of various accessory molecules with their ligands on an antigen-presenting cell (*left*) or target cell (*right*). Binding of the coreceptors CD4 and CD8 and the other accessory molecules to their ligands strengthens the bond between the interacting cells and/or aids in the signal transduction that leads to activation of the T cell.

Ternary TCR–Peptide-MHC Complex

The interaction between the T-cell receptor and an antigen bound to an MHC molecule is central to both humoral and cell-mediated responses. The molecular elements of this interaction have now been described in detail for TCR molecules binding to peptide–MHC class I complexes in both the human and mouse systems. By x-ray crystallography, a three-dimensional structure has been determined for the trimolecular complex, including TCR α and β chains and an HLA-A2 molecule to which an antigenic peptide is bound. A separate study has described a mouse TCR molecule bound to peptide complexed with the mouse class I molecule H-2K^{b}.

Preparation of the TCR–Peptide–MHC Ternary Complex

As mentioned above, there are formidable obstacles to the direct study of the TCR and its binding to MHC-antigen. In a series of biochemical experiments that overcame these obstacles, D. Garboczi, D. Wiley, and their colleagues demonstrated binding between an isolated human TCR molecule and an MHC class I–peptide complex by in vitro methods. This ternary TCR–peptide-MHC complex was then crystallized and its three-dimensional structure determined. The biochemical experiments showed that the components of the crystal were responsible for recognition of the peptide by the T cell that was the source of the TCR.

The system that Garboczi and Wiley used was the TCR–peptide-MHC complex derived from a T cell with specificity for a viral peptide from human T-cell leukemia virus I (HTLV-I). HTLV-I is a human retrovirus associated with an aggressive leukemia or a chronic neurologic disease. The T cell was specific for a peptide that is part of the HTLV-I protein Tax, a regulatory protein. Patients with the HTLV-I–associated chronic progressive neurologic disease (HTLV-I–associated myelopathy/tropical spastic paraparesis, or HAM-TSP) have large numbers of circulating CD8^{+} T_C cells that react with Tax peptides.

In order to prepare the component proteins needed for the crystal structure, RNA for the TCR α and β chains was isolated from a patient's T cells; cDNA was then prepared and cloned into a plasmid vector that could be expressed in the bacterium *Escherichia coli.* The clones had been engineered with in-frame stop codons after the extracellular portion of each chain so the TCR chains translated from these clones would lack the transmembrane sequences. Complete TCR chains with transmembrane regions are insoluble unless there is detergent in the buffer solution, but engineered TCR chains lacking the hydrophobic transmembrane region are soluble in solutions that mimic physiologic conditions and may be manipulated by standard techniques. Clones for the α and β chains were expressed separately in *E. coli,* and the isolated α and β chains that were synthesized were then mixed under conditions that allowed them to reassociate. The TCR αβ heterodimer reconstituted itself in vitro as a soluble version of the TCR.

The HLA-A2 molecule and β_2-microglobulin were expressed in a similar fashion. The A2 α chain was expressed in a truncated form that lacked the transmembrane sequence that makes the natural protein insoluble. This alteration was not necessary for β_2-microglobulin, which has no membrane-binding sequence and is soluble in its native state. The A2 α chain was combined with the β_2-microglobulin and with the antigenic peptide to form a stable peptide–MHC-class I complex.

Once the TCR αβ and the MHC-peptide complexes had been isolated, the investigators demonstrated binding between them by mixing them in various combinations and analyzing the mixtures by electrophoresis in a system that separates proteins by molecular size. Mixtures containing the TCR chains and the HLA-A2 molecule with the Tax peptide associated to form an aggregation of the appropriate size for a ternary complex. This binding between TCR and the MHC was shown to be specific for the antigen recognized by the original T cell, because no association between TCR and HLA-A2 was seen when the antigenic peptide was omitted from the assay or when other peptides were used in place of the antigenic peptide. This experiment using soluble components provides direct evidence that the TCR by itself can recognize and bind the specific antigen presented by the MHC class I molecule.

A Three-Dimensional Structure of the TCR–Peptide-MHC Ternary Complex

The complex of human TCR and the HLA-A2–peptide crystallized and its three-dimensional structure has been determined. The structure of a ternary complex between the mouse TCR molecule and an antigenic peptide bound to an H-2 class I molecule has also been determined, by methods similar to those used to obtain the components of the human structure (Figure 9-14). The structures of the human and the mouse complexes are very similar. Examination of the two complexes allows certain conclusions to be drawn.

The TCR–peptide-MHC complex consists of a single TCR molecule bound to a single MHC molecule and its peptide. The TCR contacts the MHC molecule through the TCR variable domains (Figure 9-14 a,b). Although the structures of the constant region of the TCR α chain and the MHC α3 domain were not clearly established by studies of the crystallized human complexes (see Figure 9-14a), the overall area of contact and the structure of the complete TCR variable regions were clear. The constant regions were established by studies of the mouse complex, which showed the orientation proposed for the human models (see Figure 9-14b).

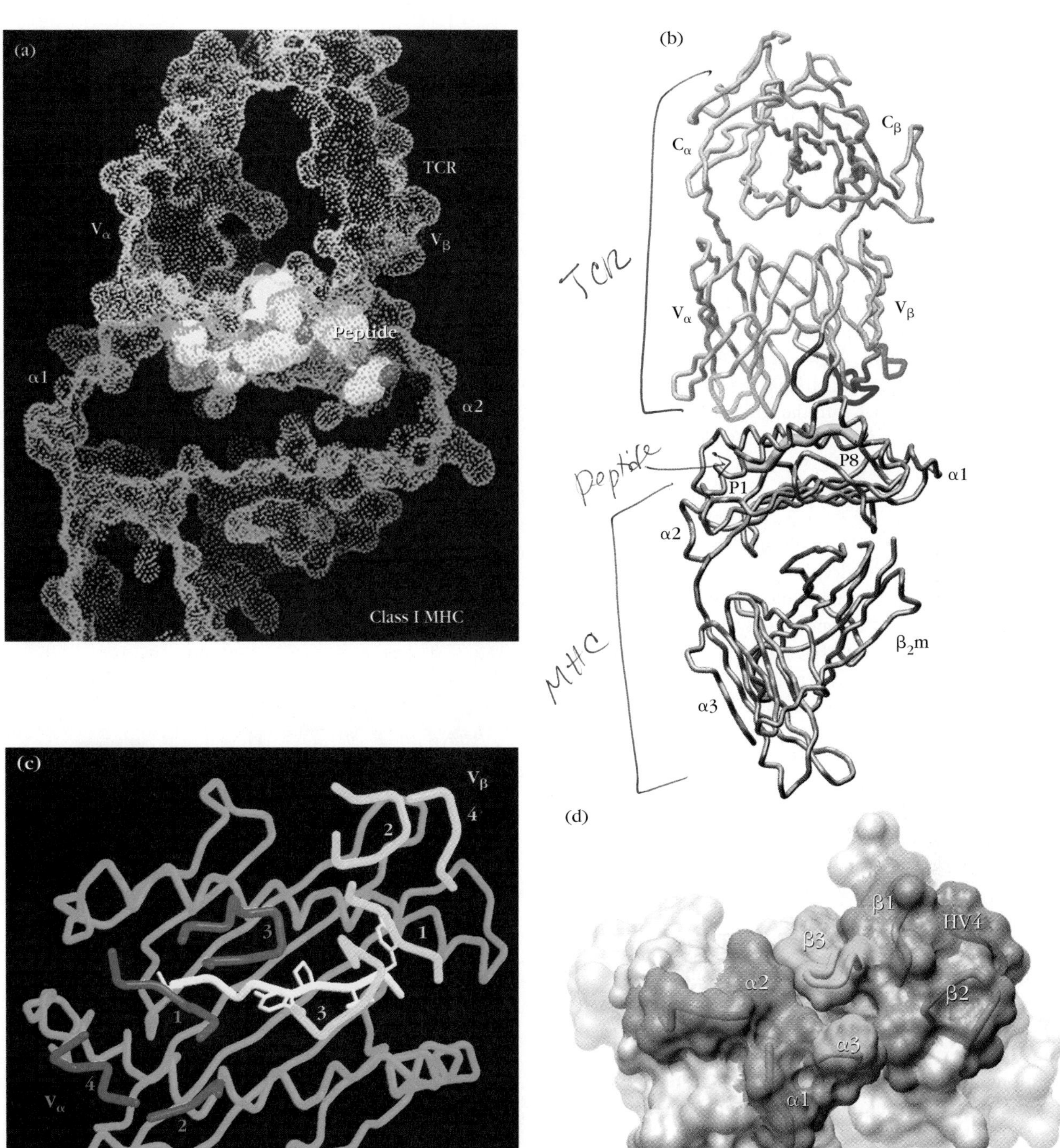

FIGURE 9-14 Three-dimensional structures for the TCR-MHC-peptide complex. (a) Model showing the interaction between the human TCR (top, yellow) and the HLA-A2 class I MHC molecule (bottom, blue) with bound HTLV-I Tax peptide (white and red). (b) Backbone tube diagram of the ternary complex of mouse TCR bound to the class I MHC H-2K^b molecule and peptide (green tube numbered P1–P8). CDR1 and 2 of the TCR α-chain variable domain (V_α) are colored pink; CDR 1 and 2 of the β-chain variable domain (V_β) are blue, and the CDR3s of both chains are green. The HV4 of the β chain is orange. (c) MHC molecule viewed from above (i.e., from top of part (a), with the hypervariable loops (1–4) of the human TCR α (red) and β (yellow) variable chains superimposed on the Tax peptide (white) and the α1 and α2 domains of the HLA-A2 MHC class I molecule (blue). (d) CDR regions of mouse TCR α and β chains viewed from above, showing the surface that is involved in binding the MHC-peptide complex. The CDRs are labeled according to their origin (for example, α1 is CDR1 from the α chain). HV4 is the fourth hypervariable region of the β chain. [Parts (a) and (c) from DN Garboczi et al, 1996, *Nature* **384:**134–141, courtesy of DC Wiley, Harvard University; (b) and (d) from C Garcia et al, 1996, *Science* **274:**209, courtesy of C Garcia, Scripps Research Institute.]

Viewing the MHC molecule with its bound peptide from above, we can see that the TCR is situated across it diagonally, relative to the long dimension of the peptide (Figure 9-14c). The CDR3 loops of the TCR α and β chains meet in the center of the peptide; and the CDR1 loop of the TCR α chain is at the N terminus of the peptide, while CDR1 of the β chain is at the C terminus of the peptide. The CDR2 loops are in contact with the MHC molecule; CDR2α is over the α2 domain alpha helix and CDR2β over the α1 domain alpha helix (Figure 9-14c). A space-filling model of the binding site viewed from above (looking down into the MHC cleft) indicates that the peptide is buried beneath the TCR and therefore is not seen from this angle (Figure 9-14d). The data also show that the fourth hypervariable regions of the α and β chains are not in contact with the antigenic peptide.

As predicted from data for immunoglobulins, the recognition of the peptide-MHC complex occurs through the variable loops in the TCR structure. CDR1 and CDR3 from both the TCR α and the TCR β chain contact the peptide and a large area of the MHC molecule. The peptide is buried (see Figure 9-14d) more deeply in the MHC molecule than it is in the TCR, and the TCR molecule fits across the MHC molecule, contacting it through a flat surface of the TCR at the "high points" on the MHC molecule. The fact that the CDR1 region contacts both peptide and MHC suggests that regions other than CDR3 are involved in peptide binding. Likewise, the use of the terms **epitope** for the part of the peptide that reacts with the TCR and **agretope** for the part that reacts with MHC (see Figure 3-9) may need reexamination in light of the evidence that CDR1 of the TCR β chain may contact the same part of the peptide that the MHC does.

Whether the conclusions drawn from the three-dimensional structure of the TCR–class I-peptide complex may be extrapolated to interactions of TCR with class II-peptide complexes needs to be resolved by analyses of TCR molecules with class II molecules and their specific antigens. The structures of the peptide-binding regions in class I and class II molecules are similar. In particular, the fact that class I and class II MHC molecules have similar three-dimensional orientations of their respective α1 and α2 alpha helices suggests that the model here may have features common to both class I and class II TCR interactions.

The similarity of the TCR to immunoglobulin (see Figure 9-3) is confirmed by examination of the three-dimensional structure of the TCR molecule (Figure 9-15). The α and β chains of the TCR fold into a quaternary structure that resembles the Fab region of an antibody (see Figures 4-5 and 4-6). The TCR domains are similar to Ig domains. The CDRs orient to form a binding site like those of an immunoglobulin. The overall size of the mouse TCR is 61 × 56 × 33 Å; the size of an Fab is about 65 × 46 × 30 Å.

Alloreactivity of T Cells

The preceding section has focused on the role of MHC molecules in the presentation of antigen to T cells. However, as noted in Chapter 7, MHC molecules were first identified because of their role in rejection of foreign tissue. Graft-rejection reactions result from the direct response of T cells to MHC molecules, which function as **histocompatibility antigens.** Because of the extreme polymorphism of the MHC, most individuals of the same species have unique sets of MHC molecules, or histocompatibility antigens, and are

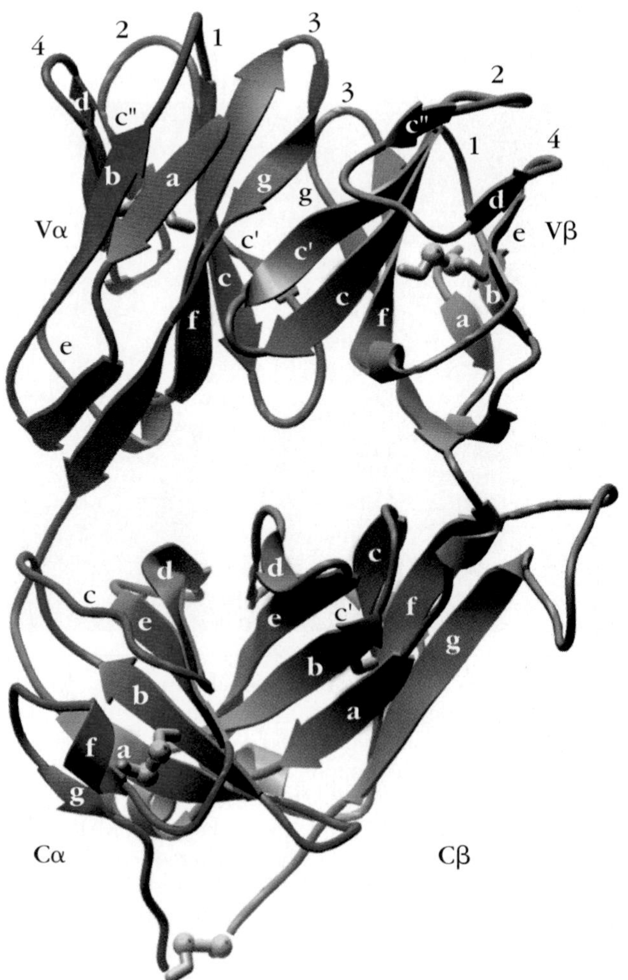

FIGURE 9-15 Structure of mouse TCR molecule as ribbon diagram showing the β chain in blue and the α chain in pink. Disulfide bridges are indicated by yellow balls. Positions of hypervariable regions are shown by numbers 1 through 4. [From C Garcia et al., 1996, *Science* **274:**211, courtesy of C Garcia, Scripps Research Institute.]

considered to be **allogeneic,** a term used to describe genetically different individuals of the same species (see Chapter 21). Therefore, T cells respond even to **allografts** (alloreactivity), and MHC molecules are considered *alloantigens.* Generally, $CD4^+$ T cells respond to class II alloantigens, and $CD8^+$ T cells respond to class I alloantigens.

The alloreactivity of T cells is troubling for two reasons. First, the ability of T cells to respond to allogeneic histocompatibility antigens alone appears to contradict all the evidence indicating that T cells can respond only to foreign antigen plus self-MHC molecules. In responding to allogeneic grafts, however, T cells recognize a foreign MHC molecule directly, instead of responding to an antigen that has been processed and presented together with a self-MHC molecule. A second problem posed by the T-cell response to allogeneic MHC molecules is that the frequency of alloreactive T cells is quite high; it has been estimated that 1%–5% of all T cells are alloreactive, which is far higher than the frequency of T cells reactive with any particular foreign antigenic peptide plus self-MHC molecule. This finding is troubling because the high frequency of alloreactive T cells appears to contradict the basic tenet of clonal selection. If 1 T cell in 20 reacts with a given alloantigen and if one assumes there are on the order of 100 distinct H-2 haplotypes in mice, then there are not enough distinct T-cell specificities to cover all the unique H-2 alloantigens, let alone foreign antigens displayed by self-MHC molecules.

One possible biologically satisfying explanation for the high frequency of alloreactive T cells is that a particular T-cell receptor is not only specific for a foreign antigenic peptide plus a self-MHC molecule but also can cross-react with certain allogeneic MHC molecules. In other words, if an allogeneic MHC molecule plus allogeneic peptide structurally resembles a processed foreign peptide plus self-MHC molecule, the same T-cell receptor may recognize both peptide-MHC complexes (Figure 9-16). Since allogeneic cells express on the order of 10^5 class I MHC molecules per cell, T cells bearing low-affinity cross-reactive receptors might be able to bind by virtue of the high density of membrane alloantigen. Foreign antigen, on the other hand, would be sparsely displayed on the membrane of an antigen-presenting cell or altered self-cell associated with class I or class II MHC molecules, limiting responsiveness to only those T cells bearing high-affinity receptors.

Experimental evidence that antigen-specific T cells can also be alloreactive has come from studies with a number of T-cell clones. For example, after immunizing an H-2^a haplotype mouse with DNP-OVA, B. Sredni and R. H. Schwarz were able to obtain a T-cell clone that responded to DNP-OVA associated with a class II IA^a molecule. This same clone, however, also responded to allogeneic cells bearing IA^s but not DNP-OVA. To determine the frequency of such antigen-specific and alloreactive T cells, Sredni and Schwarz immunized three congenic strains (B10.A, B10, and B10.S) with DNP-OVA and then isolated 20–40 antigen-specific clones from each strain. Each antigen-specific clone was then tested for alloreactivity against cells expressing different MHC haplotypes in the absence of the specific antigen. Between 19% and 44% of the antigen-specific clones were able to respond to allogeneic cells. These findings support the hypothesis that the high percentage of alloreactive T cells reflects the existence of antigen-specific T cells whose receptor recognizes antigen plus a self-MHC molecule but can cross-react with various allogeneic MHC molecules.

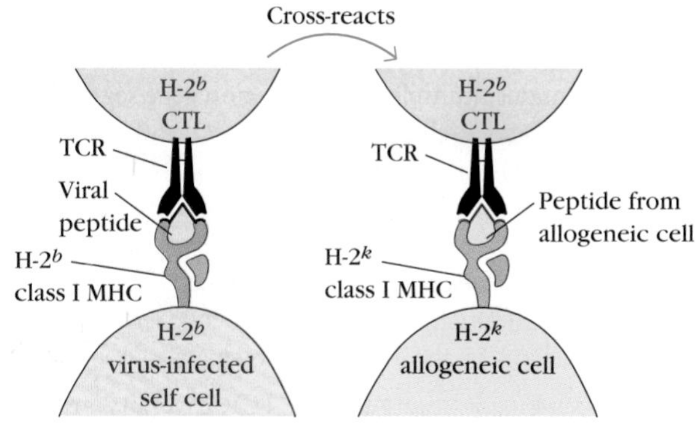

FIGURE 9-16 Possible mechanism of T-cell cross-reactivity that would explain the observed high incidence of alloreactive T cells. As schematically illustrated, a T-cell receptor specific for an H-2^b class I MHC molecule plus viral peptide (*left*) cross-reacts with an allogeneic H-2^k class I molecule plus an allogeneic peptide (*right*). According to this model, the conformation of the allogeneic peptide–MHC complex and the foreign peptide–self-MHC complex is sufficiently similar that the same TCR recognizes both complexes.

Summary

1. T-cell receptors, unlike antibodies, do not react with soluble antigen but rather with processed antigen bound to a self-MHC molecule on an antigen-presenting cell or a target cell. Kappler and Marrack demonstrated that a single TCR molecule interacts with both an antigenic peptide and MHC molecule (see Figure 9-2). T-cell receptors, first isolated by means of clonotypic monoclonal antibodies, are heterodimers consisting of an α and β chain or a γ and δ chain.
2. The membrane-bound T-cell receptor chains are organized into variable and constant domains, which have structures similar to those of immunoglobulins (see Figure 9-3). The TCR variable-region domains contain three hypervariable complementarity-determining regions (CDRs) analogous to those of immunoglobulins. Each chain in a TCR molecule also contains a short membrane-proximal connecting region, a hydrophobic transmembrane segment, and a short cytoplasmic tail.

3. TCR germ-line DNA is organized into multigene families corresponding to the α, β, γ, and δ chains. Each multigene family contains multiple variable-region gene segments (V and J in α- and γ-chain DNA, and V, D, and J in β- and δ-chain DNA) and one or more constant-region C gene segments (see Figure 9-5). By mechanisms similar to those used by B cells to rearrange immunoglobulin germ-line DNA, T cells rearrange the variable-region TCR gene segments to form functional genes that encode either the TCR α and β chains or the TCR γ and δ chains.
4. The mechanisms that generate TCR diversity are generally similar to those that generate antibody diversity (see Table 9-2 and Figure 9-8). However, during rearrangement of TCR β- and δ-chain gene segments, alternative joining of V, D, and J segments can occur, and random N-region nucleotides can be added at the junctions between gene segments that encode all the chains. Because of these mechanisms, the potential diversity of TCR genes is significantly greater than that of immunoglobulin genes, even though somatic mutation does not occur in TCR genes, as it does in immunoglobulin genes.
5. The T-cell receptor is closely associated with CD3, a complex of five different polypeptide chains that associate to form three dimers (see Figure 9-9). The T-cell receptor and CD3 are coexpressed on the membrane of T cells. The cytoplasmic tail of each CD3 chain contains a common sequence known as the immunoreceptor tyrosine-based activation motif (ITAM); this motif is involved in signal transduction after interaction of a T-cell receptor with a peptide-MHC complex. ITAM is also present in the Ig-α/Ig-β heterodimer on B cells and in Fc receptors for IgE and IgG.
6. T cells have several other membrane molecules that play accessory roles in the interaction between T cells and antigen-presenting or target cells; some of these accessory molecules also function in signal transduction (see Table 9-3). The coreceptors CD4 and CD8 bind to the membrane-proximal domains of MHC molecules, thereby strengthening the relatively weak interaction between the T-cell receptor and peptide-MHC complex. CD4 and CD8 also participate in signal transduction via their long cytoplasmic tails. Each of the other accessory membrane molecules (e.g., CD2, LFA-1, CD28, and CD45R) interacts with its own ligand on antigen-presenting cells or target cells (see Figure 9-13).
7. Formation of the ternary complex TCR-antigen-MHC, which is essential for an immune response, requires binding of a peptide to the MHC molecule and recognition of this MHC-peptide complex by the TCR through its complementarity determining regions (CDRs) (see Figure 9-14). The antigen binding by the T-cell receptor involves interaction of CDR3 and CDR1 of the α and β chains with the antigenic peptide in the MHC binding groove. CDR2 of the T-cell receptor α and β chains interacts with the alpha-helical regions of the α1 and α2 domains of the MHC molecule.
8. T cells respond not only to complexes of a foreign antigenic peptide plus self-MHC molecule but also to foreign MHC molecules (histocompatibility antigens) alone. This T-cell response leads to rejection of allogeneic grafts. Some evidence suggests that this alloreactivity results from the ability of T cells specific for an antigenic peptide plus self-MHC molecule to cross-react with various allogeneic peptide–allogeneic MHC complexes (see Figure 9-16).

REFERENCES

Bentley, GA, et al. 1995. Crystal structure of the β chain of a T cell antigen receptor. *Science* **267:**1984.

Davis, MM, and Y Chien. 1995. Issues concerning the nature of antigen recognition by αβ and γδ T-cell receptors. *Immunol. Today* **16:**316.

Fields, BA, et al. 1995. Crystal structure of the V_α domain of a T cell antigen receptor. *Science* **270:**1821.

Gao, GF, et al. 1997. Crystal structure of the complex between human CD8αα and HLA-A2. *Nature* **387:**630.

Garboczi, DN, et al. 1996. Structure of the complex between human T-cell receptor, viral peptide, and HLA-A2. *Nature* **384:**134.

Garboczi, DN, et al. 1996. Assembly, specific binding, and crystallization of a human TCR αβ with an antigenic Tax peptide from human T Lymphotropic Virus Type 1 and the class I MHC molecule HLA-A2. *J. Immunol.* **157:**5403.

Garcia, KC, et al. 1996. An αβ T-cell receptor structure at 2.5 Å and its orientation in the TCR-MHC complex. *Science* **274:**209.

Garcia, KC, et al. 1998. T-cell receptor peptide–MHC interactions: biological lessons from structural studies. *Curr. Opinions in Biotech.* **9:**338.

Hedrick, SM, et al. 1984. Isolation of cDNA clones encoding T cell–specific membrane-associated proteins. *Nature* **308:**149.

Hong, SC, et al. 1992. An MHC interaction site maps to the amino-terminal half of the T-cell receptor α chain variable domain. *Cell* **69:**999.

Janeway, CA. 1995. Ligands for the T-cell receptor: hard times for avidity models. *Immunol. Today* **16:**223.

Jardetzky, T. 1997. Not just another Fab: the crystal structure of a TCR-MHC-peptide complex. *Structure.* **5:**159.

Moss, PAH, WMC Rosenberg, and JI Bell. 1993. The human T-cell receptor in health and disease. *Annu. Rev. Immunol.* **10:**71.

Rockman, SP. 1997. Determination of clonality in patients who present with diagnostic dilemmas: a laboratory experience and review of the literature. *Leukemia* **11:**852.

Sakihama, T, A Smolyar, and EL Reinherz. 1995. Molecular

recognition of antigen between CD4, MHC class II, and TCR molecules. *Immunol. Today* **16:**581.

Sklar, J, et al. 1988. Applications of antigen receptor gene rearrangements to the diagnosis and characterization of lymphoid neoplasms. *Ann. Rev. Med.* **39:**315.

Tanaka, Y, et al. 1995. Natural and synthetic non-peptide antigens recognized by human $\gamma\delta$ T cells. *Nature* **375:**155.

Vignali, DAA, and JL Strominger. 1994. Coreceptor function and the characteristics of MHC-bound peptides: a common link? *The Immunologist* **2:**112.

Yanagi, Y, et al. 1984. A human T-cell specific cDNA clone encodes a protein having extensive homology to immunoglobulin chains. *Nature* **308:**145.

Zamoyska, R. 1998. CD4 and CD8: modulators of T cell recognition of antigen and of immune response. *Curr. Opin. Immunol.* **10:**82.

Zhu, C, and DB Roth. 1995. Characterization of coding ends in thymocytes of SCID mice: implications for the mechanism of V(D)J recombination. *Immunity* **2:**101.

Zinkernagel, RM, and PC Doherty. 1974. Immunological surveillance against altered self-components by sensitized T lymphocytes in lymphocytic choriomeningitis. *Nature* **251:**547.

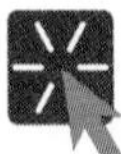

Useful Web Sites

http://imgt.cnusc.fr:8104/home.html
A comprehensive database of genetic information on TCRs, MHC molecules, and immunoglobulins, from the International Immunogenetics Database, University of Montpelier, France.

http://www.bioscience.org/knockout/tcrab.htm
This location presents a brief summary of the effects of TCR knockouts.

STUDY QUESTIONS

1. Indicate whether each of the following statements is true or false. If you think a statement is false, explain why.

a. Monoclonal antibody specific for CD4 will coprecipitate the T-cell receptor along with CD4.

b. Subtractive hybridization can be used to enrich for mRNA that is present in one cell type but absent in another cell type within the same species.

c. Clonotypic monoclonal antibody was used to isolate the T-cell receptor.

d. The T cell uses the same set of V, D, and J gene segments as the B cell but uses different C gene segments.

e. The $\alpha\beta$ TCR is bivalent and has two antigen-binding sites.

f. Each $\alpha\beta$ T cell expresses only one β-chain and one α-chain allele.

g. Mechanisms for generation of diversity of T-cell receptors are identical to those used by immunoglobulins.

h. The Ig-α/Ig-β heterodimer and CD3 serve analogous functions in the B-cell receptor and T-cell receptor, respectively.

2. Describe the critical experiment that proved that the $\alpha\beta$ T-cell receptor alone recognizes both antigen and MHC molecules.

3. Draw the basic structure of the $\alpha\beta$ T-cell receptor and compare it with the basic structure of membrane-bound immunoglobulin.

4. Several membrane molecules, in addition to the T-cell receptor, are involved in antigen recognition and T-cell activation. Describe the properties and distinct functions of the following T-cell membrane molecules: (a) CD3, (b) CD4 and CD8, and (c) CD2.

5. Indicate whether each of the properties listed below applies to the T-cell receptor (TCR), B-cell immunoglobulin (Ig), or both (TCR/Ig).

a. ______ Is associated with CD3

b. ______ Is monovalent

c. ______ Exists in membrane-bound and secreted forms

d. ______ Contains domains with the immunoglobulin-fold structure

e. ______ Is MHC restricted

f. ______ Exhibits diversity generated by imprecise joining of gene segments

g. Exhibits diversity generated by somatic mutation

6. A major obstacle to identifying and cloning TCR genes is the low level of TCR mRNA in T cells.

a. To overcome this obstacle, Hedrick and Davis made three important assumptions that proved to be correct. Describe each assumption and how it facilitated identification of the genes that encode the T-cell receptor.

b. Suppose, instead, that Hedrick and Davis wanted to identify the genes that encode IL-4. What changes in the three assumptions should they make?

7. Hedrick and Davis used the technique of subtractive hybridization to isolate cDNA clones that encode the T-cell receptor. You wish to use this technique to isolate cDNA clones that encode several gene products and have available clones of various cell types to use as the source of cDNA or mRNA for hybridization. For each gene product listed in the left column of the table below, select the most appropriate

Gene product	cDNA source	mRNA source
IL-2		
CD8		
J chain		
IL-1		
CD3		

Go to www.whfreeman.com/immunology Self-Test
Review and quiz of key terms

cDNA and mRNA source clones from the following cell types: T_H1 cell line (A); T_H2 cell line (B); T_C cell line (C); macrophage (D); IgA-secreting myeloma cell (E); IgG-secreting myeloma cell (F); myeloid progenitor cell (G); and B-cell line (H). More than one cell type may be correct in some cases.

8. Mice from different inbred strains listed in the left column of the accompanying table were infected with LCM virus. Spleen cells derived from these LCM-infected mice then were tested for their ability to lyse LCM-infected ^{51}Cr-labeled target cells from the strains listed across the top of the table. Indicate with (+) or (−) whether you would expect to see ^{51}Cr released from the labeled target cells.

Source of spleen cells from LCM-infected mice	Release of ^{51}Cr from LCM-infected target cells			
	B10.D2 (H-2^d)	B10 (H-2^b)	B10.BR (H-2^k)	(BALB/c × B10) F_1 (H-$2^{b/d}$)
B10.D2 (H-2^d)				
B10 (H-2^b)				
BALB/c (H-2^d)				
BALB/b (H-2^b)				

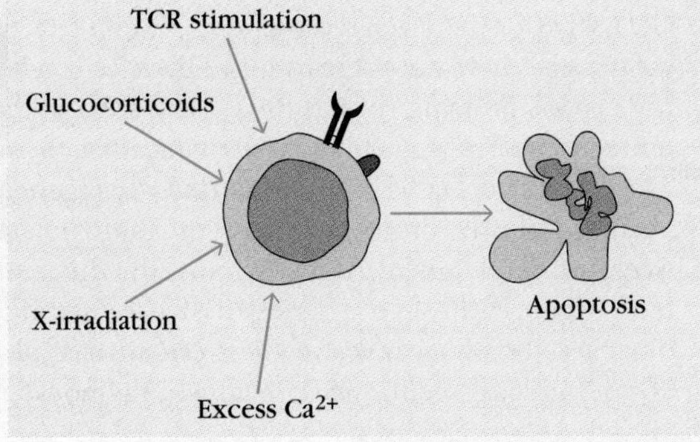

CHAPTER 10

T-CELL MATURATION, ACTIVATION, AND DIFFERENTIATION

The attribute that distinguishes antigen recognition by T cells from recognition by B cells is MHC restriction. In most cases, both the maturation of progenitor T cells in the thymus and the activation of mature T cells in the periphery are influenced by the involvement of MHC molecules. The potential antigenic diversity of the T-cell population is reduced during maturation by a selection process that allows only MHC-restricted and nonself-reactive T cells to mature. The final stages in the maturation of most T cells proceed along two different developmental pathways, which generate functionally distinct $CD4^+$ and $CD8^+$ subpopulations that exhibit class II and class I MHC restriction, respectively.

Activation of mature peripheral T cells begins with the interaction of the T-cell receptor with an antigenic peptide displayed in the groove of an MHC molecule. Although the specificity of this interaction is governed by the TCR, its low avidity necessitates the involvement of coreceptors and other accessory membrane molecules that strengthen the TCR-antigen-MHC interaction and transduce the activating signal. Activation leads to the proliferation and differentiation of T cells into various types of effector cells and memory T cells. Because the vast majority of thymocytes and peripheral T cells express the αβ T-cell receptor rather than the γδ T-cell receptor, all references to the T-cell receptor in this chapter denote the αβ receptor unless otherwise indicated. Similarly, all references to T cells denote those αβ receptor-bearing T cells that undergo MHC restriction.

T-Cell Maturation and the Thymus

Progenitor T cells from the early sites of hematopoiesis begin to migrate to the thymus at about day 11 of gestation in mice and in the eighth or ninth week of gestation in humans. In a manner similar to B-cell maturation in the bone marrow, T-cell maturation involves rearrangements of the germline TCR genes and the expression of various membrane markers. However, B-cell development appears to follow only two developmental pathways, in the thymus, developing T cells, known as **thymocytes**, proliferate and differentiate along several different developmental pathways, which generate functionally distinct subpopulations of mature T cells.

As indicated in Chapter 2, the thymus occupies a central role in T-cell biology. Aside from being the main source of all T cells, it is where T cells diversify and then are shaped into an effective primary T-cell repertoire by an extraordinary pair of selection processes. One of these, **positive selection**, permits the survival of only those T cells whose TCRs recognize self-MHC molecules. It is thus responsible for the creation of a self-MHC-restricted repertoire of T cells. The other, **negative selection,** eliminates T cells that react too strongly with self-MHC or with self-MHC plus self-peptides. These processes generate a primary T-cell repertoire that is self-tolerant.

Various features have been used to characterize the pathway of T-cell development in the thymus:

- Timing of TCR-gene rearrangement
- Activity of genes, such as *RAG-1* and *RAG-2,* that are involved in TCR rearrangement

- Display of surface antigens specific for T-cell differentiation. The overall process can be divided into an early phase when the cells do not express TCRs or the surface molecules characteristic of T cells, such as CD4 or CD8, and a later phase in which further maturation depends upon the expression of a T-cell receptor (Figure 10-1).

When they arrive at the thymus, progenitor T cells do not express surface molecules characteristic of T cells, such as CD4, CD8, or the T-cell receptor complex. In fact, these progenitor cells have not yet rearranged their TCR genes and do not express proteins, such as RAG-1 and RAG-2, that are required for rearrangement. After arriving at the thymus, these T-cell precursors enter the outer cortex (see Figure 2-14) and begin to slowly proliferate. During approximately three weeks of development in the thymus, the differentiating T cells progress through a series of stages that are marked by characteristic changes in their cell-surface phenotype. For example, as mentioned previously, thymocytes early in

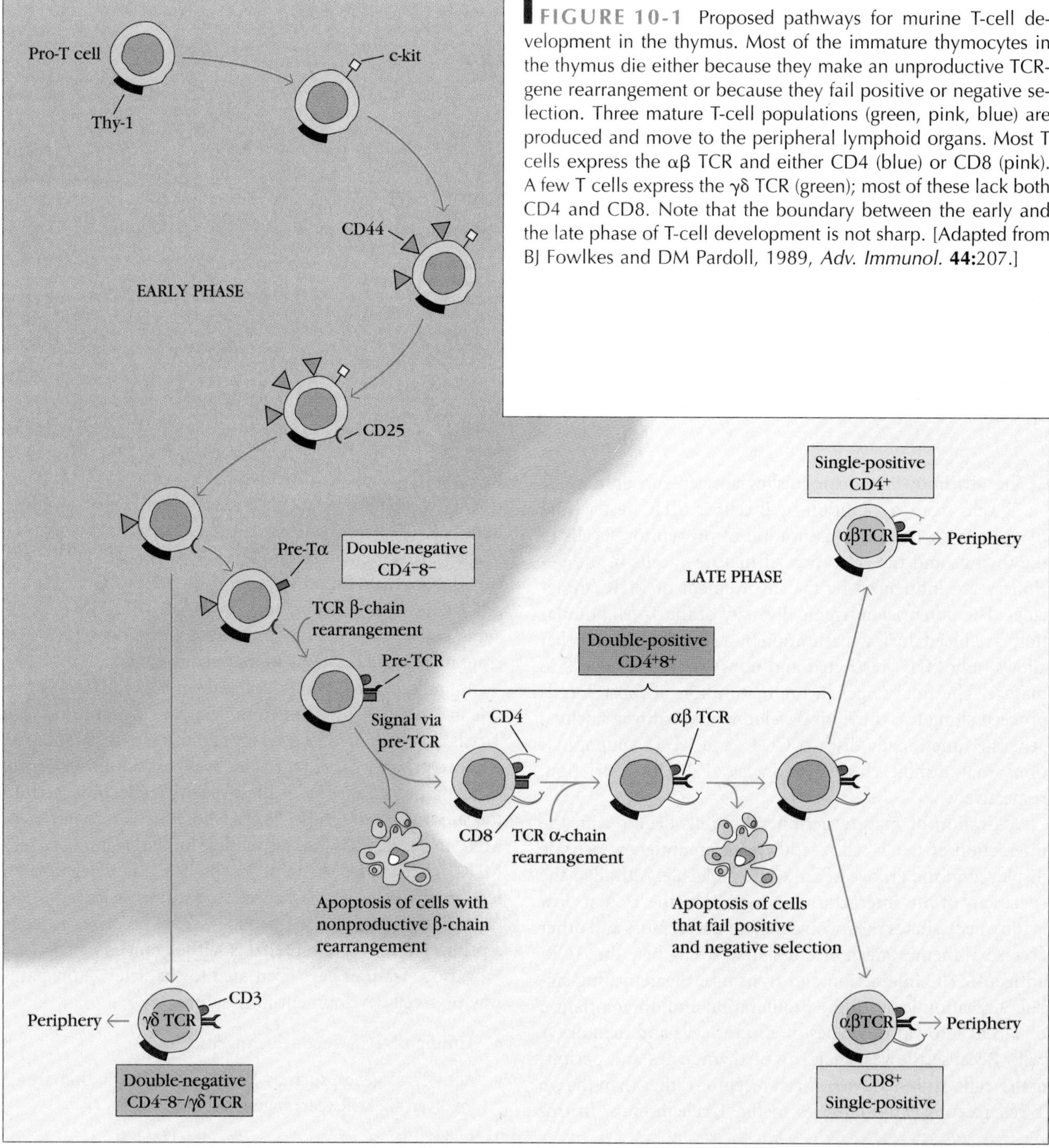

FIGURE 10-1 Proposed pathways for murine T-cell development in the thymus. Most of the immature thymocytes in the thymus die either because they make an unproductive TCR-gene rearrangement or because they fail positive or negative selection. Three mature T-cell populations (green, pink, blue) are produced and move to the peripheral lymphoid organs. Most T cells express the αβ TCR and either CD4 (blue) or CD8 (pink). A few T cells express the γδ TCR (green); most of these lack both CD4 and CD8. Note that the boundary between the early and the late phase of T-cell development is not sharp. [Adapted from BJ Fowlkes and DM Pardoll, 1989, *Adv. Immunol.* **44:**207.]

development lack detectable CD4 and CD8. Because these cells are $CD4^-CD8^-$, they are referred to as **double-negative (DN)** cells.

Even though these coreceptors are not expressed in the early phase, the expression of other cell surface molecules, particularly c-Kit, CD44, and CD25, marks the developmental progression of the DN population. The initial thymocyte population displays c-Kit, the receptor for stem-cell growth factor, and subsequently expresses CD44, an adhesion molecule, and then CD25, the α-chain of the IL-2 receptor. During this period, the cells are proliferating but the TCR genes remain unrearranged. Then the cells stop expressing c-Kit, markedly reduce CD44 expression, and begin to rearrange their TCR genes. Those thymocytes that make productive rearrangements of both the γ- and δ-chain genes develop into double-negative $CD3^+$ γδ T cells, which account for only a small percentage (<5%) of thymocytes in adults. In mice, this thymocyte subpopulation can be detected by day 14 of gestation, reaches maximal numbers between days 17 and 18, and then declines until birth (Figure 10-2).

Most double-negative thymocytes progress down a different developmental pathway. They stop proliferating and begin to rearrange the TCR β-chain genes and express the β chain. Those cells of the αβ lineage that fail to productively rearrange and express β chains die. Newly synthesized β chains combine with a 33-kDa gylcoprotein known as the pre-Tα chain and associate with the CD3 group to form a novel complex called the **pre–T-cell receptor (pre-TCR)**. As illustrated in Figure 10-3, the pre-TCR consists of a complex of the first receptor chain to be expressed (the β chain) complexed with a unique chain (pre-Tα). Thus far, no pre-T analogous to the pre-B in developing B cells has been discovered for the pre-TCR, although its existence has been hypothesized. The pre-TCR is thought to recognize some intrathymic ligand and transmit a signal through the CD3 complex that activates Lck, a protein tyrosine kinase. Signal transduction through the pre-TCR has several effects:

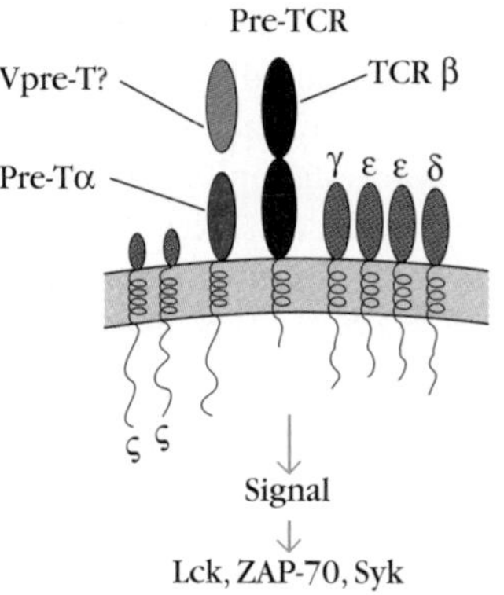

FIGURE 10-3 General structure of the pre–T-cell receptor (pre-TCR) and effects of activating it. Binding of unknown ligands to the pre-TCR is thought to generate intracellular signals leading to generation of pre-T cells ($CD4^+8^+$ thymocytes).

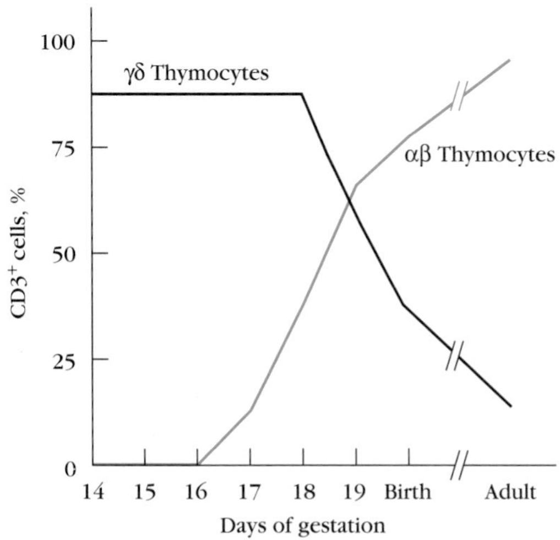

FIGURE 10-2 Time course of appearance of γδ thymocytes and αβ thymocytes during mouse fetal development. The graph shows the percentage of $CD3^+$ cells in the thymus that are double-negative ($CD4^-8^-$) and bear the γδ T-cell receptor (black) or are double-positive ($CD4^+8^+$) and bear the αβ T-cell receptor (blue).

- Indicates that a productive TCR β-chain rearrangement has been made and selects those thymocytes expressing the β chain for further expansion and maturation
- Suppresses further rearrangement of TCR β-chain genes, resulting in allelic exclusion of the β chain
- Enhances rearrangement of the TCR α chain
- Induces developmental progression to the $CD4^+8^+$ *double-positive* state

Once a signal has been transmitted through the pre-TCR, it halts further β-chain gene rearrangement and induces expression of both CD4 and CD8. The thymocytes at this stage are called **double-positive (DP)**, or $CD4^+8^+$, cells. These double-positive thymocytes begin to proliferate. During this proliferative phase, TCR α-chain gene rearrangement does not occur even though both the *RAG-1* and *RAG-2* genes are transcriptionally active. Rearrangement of the α-chain genes cannot take place at this stage because the RAG-2 protein is rapidly degraded in proliferating cells. For this reason, α-chain gene rearrangement does not begin until the double-positive thymocytes stop proliferating and RAG-2 protein levels increase. This proliferative phase contributes to T-cell diversity by generating a clone of cells with a single TCR β-chain rearrangement. Each of the cells within this clone can then rearrange different α-chain genes, allowing for greater diversity. The TCR α-chain genes are not expressed until day 16 or 17 of gestation; double-positive cells expressing both CD3 and the αβ T-cell receptor begin to appear at day 17 and reach maximal levels about the time of birth (see Figure 10-2). By the time in differentiation that a T cell has rearranged and begun to express the α chain of the TCR, the DP cells no longer express such early markers as CD44 and CD25. The possession of a TCR enables DP thymocytes to undergo the rigors of positive and negative selection guided by self-MHC and self-MHC + peptide, as discussed in the next section.

An estimated 98% of all thymocytes do not mature—they die by apoptosis within the thymus either because they fail to make a productive TCR-gene rearrangement or because they fail to survive thymic selection. Double-positive thymocytes that express the αβ TCR-CD3 complex and survive thymic selection develop into either **single-positive CD4$^+$** thymocytes or **single-positive CD8$^+$** thymocytes. These single-positive cells migrate to the periphery of the thymus (see Figure 10-1). An additional small population of double-negative thymocytes expressing the TCR-CD3 complex can also be detected in the thymus. These cells appear late in development, usually within 5 days following birth. The developmental pathway that leads to this population is uncertain.

Thymic Selection of the T-Cell Repertoire

Random gene rearrangement within TCR germ-line DNA combined with junctional diversity can generate an enormous TCR repertoire, with an estimated potential diversity exceeding 10^{15} for the αβ receptor and 10^{18} for the γδ receptor. The gene products encoded by the rearranged TCR genes have no inherent affinity for foreign antigen plus a self-MHC molecule; they theoretically should be capable of recognizing soluble antigen (either foreign or self), self-MHC molecules, or antigen plus a nonself-MHC molecule. Nonetheless, the most distinctive property of mature T cells is that they recognize only foreign antigen combined with self-MHC molecules.

Clearly, from the standpoint of efficiency it would be best if thymocytes that undergo productive TCR-gene rearrangement were "selected" in some way, so that only those thymocytes whose receptors exhibit self-MHC restriction are permitted to mature. Otherwise, left to chance, only a few members of the T-cell population would be able to interact with self-MHC molecules. Most would be unable to recognize and interact with these molecules and therefore would be useless in the defense of the host. By processes described in detail later, *positive selection* ensures that the αβ TCRs expressed on the mature T cells of a given individual will bind to self-MHC. Cells that fail positive selection are eliminated within the thymus by apoptosis. Also eliminated, by *negative selection*, are thymocytes bearing a high-affinity receptor for self-MHC molecules alone or self-antigen plus self-MHC molecules; such thymocytes would pose the threat of an autoimmune response if they matured. As noted already, some 98% or more of all thymocytes die by apoptosis within the thymus. A significant number of these deaths are traceable to negative selection; however, the bulk of this high death rate appears to reflect a weeding out of thymocytes that fail positive selection because their receptors do not specifically recognize foreign antigen plus self-MHC molecules.

Early evidence for the role of the thymus in selection of the T-cell repertoire came from chimeric mouse experiments by R. M. Zinkernagel and his colleagues (Figure 10-4). These researchers implanted thymectomized and lethally irradiated (A × B) F_1 mice with a B-type thymus and then reconstituted the animal's immune system with an intravenous infusion of F_1 bone-marrow cells. To be certain that the thymus graft did not contain any mature T cells, it was irradiated before being transplanted. In such an experimental system, T-cell progenitors from the (A × B) F_1 bone-marrow transplant mature within a thymus that expresses only B-haplotype MHC molecules on its stromal cells. Would these (A × B) F_1 T cells now be MHC-restricted for the haplotype of the thymus? To answer this question, the chimeric mice were infected with LCM virus and the immature T cells were then tested for their ability to kill LCM-infected target cells from the strain A or strain B mice. As shown in Figure 10-4, T_C cells from the chimeric mice could lyse only LCM-infected target cells from the strain B mice, which bear the same MHC haplotype as the implanted B-type thymus. Apparently the implanted thymus had selected for maturation only T cells having receptors capable of recognizing antigen combined with the MHC haplotype of the thymus in which the selection occurred.

As noted above, thymocytes are thought to undergo two selection processes in the thymus (Table 10–1):

- Positive selection of thymocytes bearing receptors capable of binding self-MHC molecules, which results in **MHC restriction**
- Negative selection by elimination of thymocytes bearing high-affinity receptors for self-MHC molecules alone or self-antigen presented by self-MHC, which results in **self-tolerance**

Both processes are necessary to generate mature T cells that are self-MHC restricted and self-tolerant.

Thymic stromal cells, including epithelial cells, macrophages, and dendritic cells, play essential roles in positive and negative selection. These thymic stromal cells express class I MHC molecules and can display high levels of class II MHC also. The interaction of immature thymocytes that express the TCR-CD3 complex with popula-

EXPERIMENT

(A × B)F$_1$ (H-2$^{a/b}$)

① Thymectomy

② Lethal x-irradiation

Strain-B thymus graft (H-2^b)

(A × B)F$_1$ hematopoietic stem cells (H-2$^{a/b}$)

Infect with LCM virus

Spleen cells

LCM-infected strain-A cells — No killing

LCM-infected strain-B cells — Killing

CONTROL

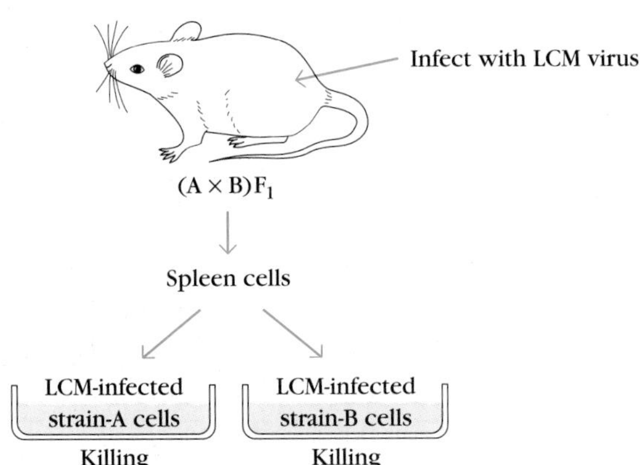

FIGURE 10-4 Experimental demonstration that the thymus selects for maturation only those T cells whose T-cell receptors recognize antigen presented on target cells with the haplotype of the thymus. Thymectomized and lethally irradiated (A × B) F$_1$ mice were grafted with a strain-B thymus and reconstituted with (A × B) F$_1$ bone-marrow cells. After infection with the LCM virus, the CTL cells were assayed for their ability to kill ^{51}Cr-labeled strain-A or strain-B target cells infected with the LCM virus. Only strain-B target cells were lysed, suggesting that the H-2^b grafted thymus had selected for maturation only those T cells that could recognize antigen combined with H-2^b MHC molecules.

tions of thymic stromal cells results in positive and negative selection by mechanisms that are under intense investigation. First, we'll examine the details of each selection process and then we'll consider some of the experimental evidence that supports the existence of these processes.

Positive Selection

Positive selection takes place in the cortical region of the thymus and involves the interaction of immature thymocytes with cortical epithelial cells (Figure 10-5). Electron micrographs reveal close contact between thymocytes and epithelial cells within the thymic cortex, and there is evidence that the T-cell receptors tend to cluster with MHC molecules at sites of contact. Some researchers have suggested that the interaction of immature CD4$^+$8$^+$ thymocytes with thymic epithelial cells, mediated by MHC-restricted T-cell receptors, allows the cells to receive a protective signal that prevents them from undergoing cell death; cells whose receptors are not MHC restricted and therefore not able to bind MHC molecules would not interact with the thymic epithelial cells and consequently would not receive the protective signal, leading to their death by apoptosis (see Figure 10-5).

TABLE 10-1 CHARACTERISTICS OF T-CELL SELECTION IN THE THYMUS

Property	Positive selection	Negative selection
Site	Cortex	Medulla
Stromal cells involved	Epithelial cells	Macrophages and dendritic cells
Selection mechanism	Survival of thymocytes bearing receptors for self-MHC	Elimination of thymocytes bearing high-affinity receptors for self-MHC alone or self-antigen + self-MHC
Immune consequence	Self-MHC restriction	Self-tolerance

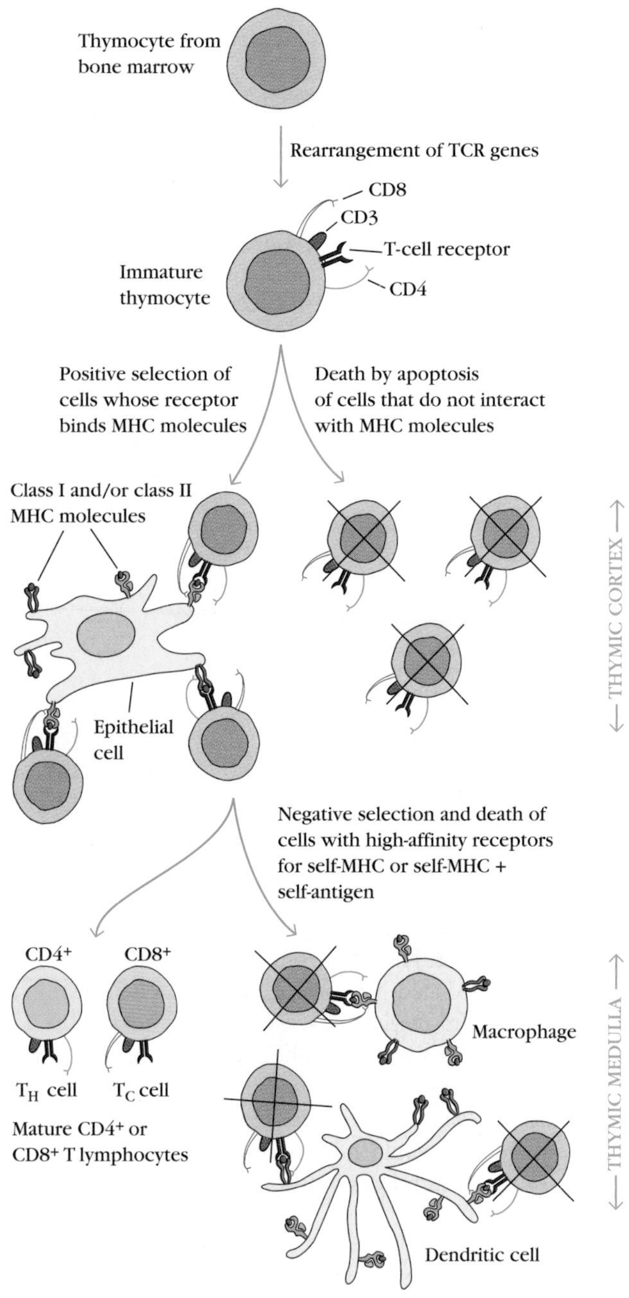

FIGURE 10-5 Positive and negative selection of thymocytes in the thymus. Because of thymic selection, which involves thymic stromal cells (epithelial cells, dendritic cells, and macrophages), mature T cells are both self-MHC restricted and self-tolerant.

During positive selection, the RAG-1, RAG-2, and TdT proteins required for gene rearrangement and modification continue to be expressed. Thus the immature thymocytes in a clone expressing a given β chain continue to rearrange TCR α-chain genes, and the resulting TCRs are then selected for self-MHC recognition. Only those cells whose αβ TCR heterodimer recognizes a self-MHC molecule are selected for survival. Consequently, the capacity to try more than one combination of αβ TCR chains is important because it gives the thymocyte opportunities to "retake" the test for positive selection. If by chance, the cell manages to rearrange an α chain that allows the resulting αβ TCR to recognize self-MHC, the cell is spared; if not, the cell will die by apoptosis within 3 to 4 days.

Negative Selection

The population of MHC-restricted thymocytes that survive positive selection comprises some cells with low-affinity receptors for self-antigen presented by self-MHC molecules and other cells with high-affinity receptors. The latter thymocytes undergo negative selection by an interaction with bone-marrow–derived APCs (dendritic cells and macrophages) in the medulla. During negative selection, dendritic cells and macrophages bearing class I and class II MHC molecules interact with thymocytes bearing high-affinity receptors for self-antigen plus self-MHC molecules or for self-MHC molecules alone (see Figure 10-5). The interaction involves the TCR of the thymocyte that is undergoing selection and MHC molecules on the cells mediating negative selection, but the precise details of the process are not yet known. Cells that experience negative selection are observed to undergo death by apoptosis. Tolerance to self-antigens is thereby achieved by eliminating T cells that are self-reactive and allowing maturation only of T cells specific for foreign antigen plus self-MHC molecules **(altered self).**

Experimental Evidence for Positive Selection

Early experiments by Ada Kruisbeek suggested that binding of thymocytes to class I or class II MHC molecules within the thymus leads to positive selection of MHC-restricted T cells. In her experiments, mouse fetal thymic tissue was grown in tissue-culture media containing high concentrations of monoclonal antibody either to the class I or to the class II MHC molecules expressed by the thymic cells (Figure 10-6). Analysis of the T cells from these fetal thymic organ cultures revealed the absence of $CD4^+$ T cells in cultures grown with anti-class II monoclonal antibody and the absence of $CD8^+$ T cells in cultures grown with anti-class I monoclonal antibody. The results of these experiments suggest that if the class I or class II MHC molecules are blocked by antibody, developing thymocytes cannot bind to the self-MHC molecules on the thymic stromal cells and positive selection cannot occur.

Further evidence that binding of thymocytes to class I or class II MHC molecules is required for positive selection in the thymus came from subsequent experimental studies with knockout mice incapable of producing functional class I or class II MHC molecules (Table 10–2). Class I–deficient mice were found to have a normal distribution of double-negative, double-positive, and $CD4^+$ thymocytes but failed to produce $CD8^+$ thymocytes. Class II–deficient mice had

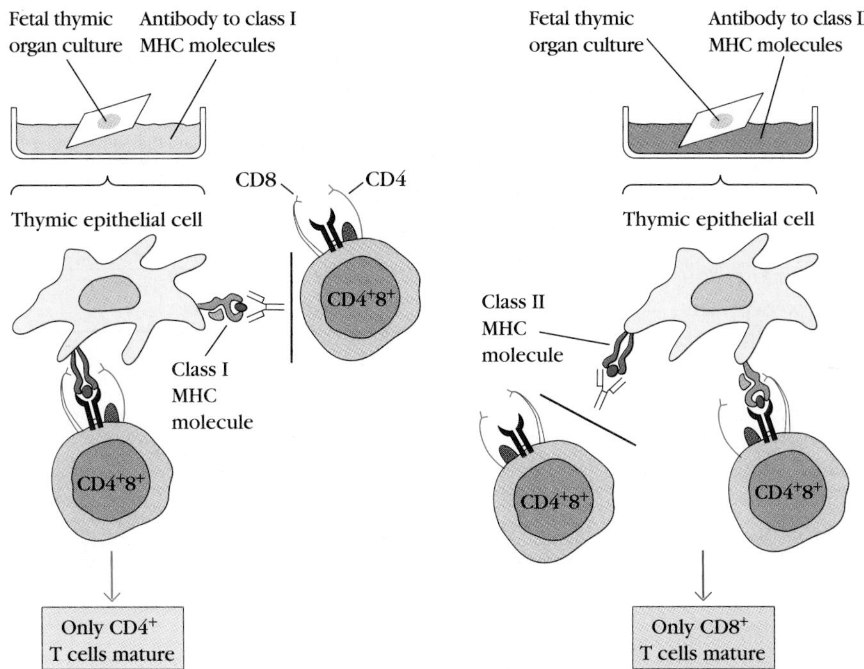

FIGURE 10-6 Experimental demonstration that acquisition of MHC restriction depends on interaction of immature thymocytes with class I or class II MHC molecules on thymic epithelial cells.

TABLE 10-2 EFFECT OF CLASS I OR II MHC DEFICIENCY ON THYMOCYTE POPULATIONS*

		Knockout mice	
Cell type	Control mice	Class I deficient	Class II deficient
$CD4^-8^-$	+	+	+
$CD4^+8^+$	+	+	+
$CD4^+$	+	+	−
$CD8^+$	+	−	+

*Plus sign indicates normal distribution of indicated cell types in thymus. Minus sign indicates absence of cell type.

double-negative, double-positive, and $CD8^+$ thymocytes but lacked $CD4^+$ thymocytes. Not surprisingly, the lymph nodes of these class II–deficient mice lacked $CD4^+$ T cells. Thus the absence of class I or II MHC molecules prevents positive selection of $CD8^+$ or $CD4^+$ T cells, respectively.

Experiments with transgenic mice provided additional evidence that interaction with MHC molecules plays a role in positive selection. In these experiments, rearranged αβ-TCR genes derived from a $CD8^+$ T-cell clone specific for influenza antigen plus H-2^k class I MHC molecules were injected into fertilized eggs from two different mouse strains, one with the H-2^k haplotype and one with the H-2^d haplotype (Figure 10-7).

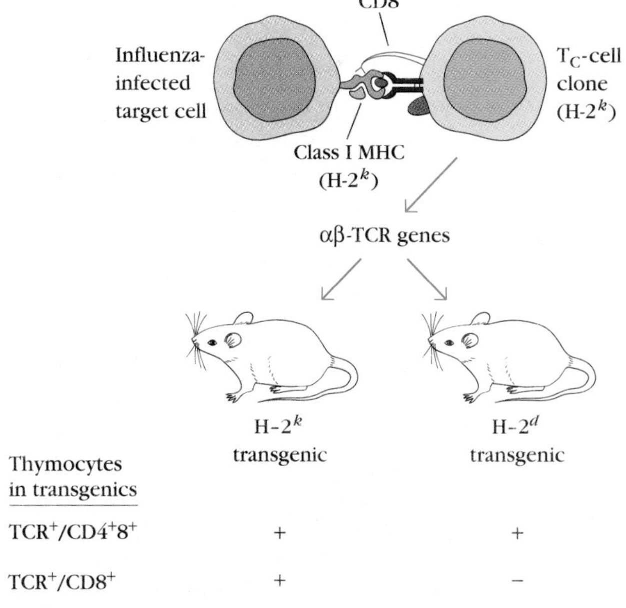

Thymocytes in transgenics	H-2^k transgenic	H-2^d transgenic
$TCR^+/CD4^+8^+$	+	+
$TCR^+/CD8^+$	+	−

FIGURE 10-7 Effect of host haplotype on T-cell maturation in mice carrying transgenes encoding an H-2^b class I–restricted T-cell receptor specific for influenza virus. The presence of the rearranged TCR transgenes suppressed other gene rearrangements in the transgenics; therefore, most of the thymocytes in the transgenics expressed the αβ T-cell receptor encoded by the transgene. Immature double-positive thymocytes matured into $CD8^+$ T cells only in transgenics with the haplotype (H-2^k) corresponding to the MHC restriction of the TCR transgene.

Since the receptor transgenes were already rearranged, other TCR-gene rearrangements were suppressed in the transgenic mice; therefore, a high percentage of the thymocytes in the transgenic mice expressed the T-cell receptor encoded by the transgene. Thymocytes expressing the TCR transgene were found to mature into $CD8^+$ T cells only in the transgenic mice with the H-2^k class I MHC haplotype (i.e., the haplotype for which the transgene receptor was restricted). In transgenic mice with a different MHC haplotype H-2^d), immature, double-positive thymocytes expressing the transgene were present, but these thymocytes failed to mature into $CD8^+$ T cells. These findings suggest that interaction between T-cell receptors on immature thymocytes and self-MHC molecules is required for positive selection. In the absence of self-MHC molecules, as in the H-2^d transgenic mice, positive selection and subsequent maturation do not occur.

Finally, an experiment using knockout mice and transgenesis provides direct evidence that cells of the thymic cortical epithelium play a central role in positive selection. We have already seen that positive selection of class II–restricted T cells does not occur in mice deficient in class II MHC molecules (Table 10–2). However, such mice may be used to produce a line of mice that are transgenic for a class II gene with a promoter that restricts its expression to cortical epithelial cells. Unlike their parents these mice do have class II MHC receptors, but only on their cortical epithelial cells; development of $CD4^+$ T cells proceeded in them normally.

Experimental Evidence for Negative Selection

Evidence for deletion of thymocytes reactive with self-antigen plus MHC molecules has been accumulating in a number of diverse experimental systems. In one system, thymocyte maturation was analyzed in transgenic mice bearing an αβ TCR transgene specific for the H-Y antigen plus class I D^bMHC molecules. The H-Y antigen is encoded on the Y chromosome and therefore is expressed in male mice but not in female mice. Thus, H-Y antigen is a self-molecule only in the male mice. In this experiment, the MHC haplotype of the transgenic mice was H-2^b, the same as the MHC restriction of the transgene-encoded receptor. Therefore any differences in the selection of thymocytes in male and female transgenics would be related to the presence or absence of H-Y antigen.

Analysis of thymocytes in the transgenic mice revealed that female mice contained thymocytes expressing the H-Y–specific TCR transgene, but male mice did not (Figure 10-8). In other words, H-Y–reactive thymocytes were self-reactive in the male mice and were eliminated. However, in the female transgenics, which did not express the H-Y antigen, these cells were not self-reactive and thus were not eliminated. When thymocytes from these male transgenic mice were cultured in vitro with antigen-presenting cells expressing the H-Y antigen, the thymocytes were observed to undergo apoptosis, providing a striking example of negative selection.

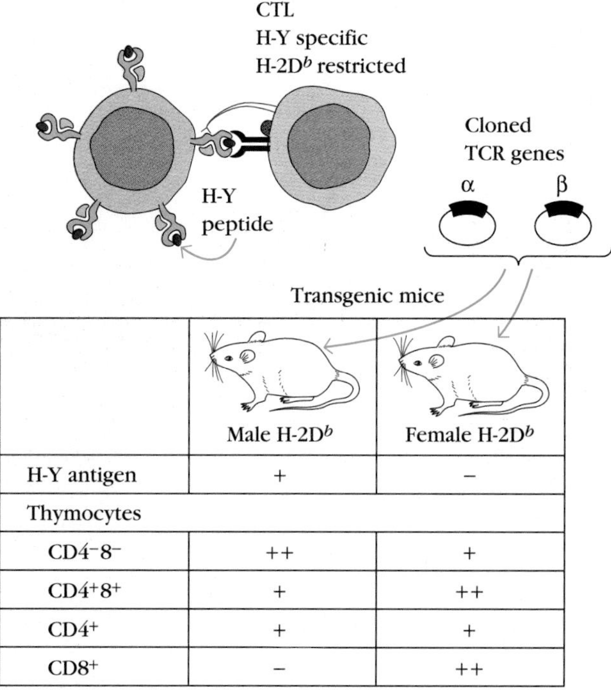

	Male H-2D^b	Female H-2D^b
H-Y antigen	+	–
Thymocytes		
$CD4^-8^-$	++	+
$CD4^+8^+$	+	++
$CD4^+$	+	+
$CD8^+$	–	++

FIGURE 10-8 Experimental demonstration that negative selection of thymocytes requires self-antigen plus self-MHC. In this experiment, H-2^b male and female transgenics were prepared carrying TCR transgenes specific for H-Y antigen plus the D^b molecule. This antigen is expressed only in males. FACS analysis of thymocytes from the transgenics showed that mature $CD8^+$ T cells expressing the transgene were absent in the male mice but present in the female mice, suggesting that thymocytes reactive with a self-antigen (in this case, H-Y antigen in the male mice) are deleted during thymic selection. [Adapted from H von Boehmer and P Kisielow, 1990, *Science* **248:**1370.]

Some Central Issues in Thymic Selection

Although a great deal has been learned about the developmental processes that generate mature $CD4^+$ and $CD8^+$ T cells, important unresolved issues still remain. *What determines whether a cell will undergo positive or negative selection?* A large and persuasive body of evidence demonstrates that positive selection allows thymocytes reactive with self-MHC molecules to survive and allows those that do not recognize self-MHC to die by apoptosis. An equally impressive body of evidence leads to the conclusion that negative selection eliminates the self-MHC–reactive thymocytes. If both positive and negative selection use identical criteria and respond to identical signals, they would be futile activities. Positive selection would select for survival a population of T cells that recognize self-MHC, negative selection would then kill all of them, and no T cells would be allowed to mature. Since this is not the outcome of T-cell development, clearly, other factors operate to prevent these two processes from eliminating the entire repertoire of MHC-restricted T cells. Two hypotheses have emerged to resolve the paradox of MHC-dependent positive and negative selection.

One proposal, called the *avidity hypothesis*, is a quantitative model. It asserts that differences in the strength of the signal received by the thymocyte during interactions between its TCRs and the MHC-peptide complexes of antigen-presenting cells determine the outcome of positive and negative selection. Signal strength is determined by the avidity of MHC-peptide–TCR interactions, and avidity depends upon both the affinity of the interaction between the TCR and MHC-peptide complexes and the density of the relevant peptide-MHC complexes on the antigen-presenting cell. High-avidity interactions result in strong signals, and those of low avidity send weak ones. According to this hypothesis, all thymocytes with TCRs that bind to the diverse collection of peptide-MHC complexes present in the selective environments of the thymus are selected for survival and escape the apoptotic death to which they would otherwise default. On the other hand, thymocytes bearing receptors that react strongly with peptide-MHC complexes are induced to die by apoptosis. The overall result of this process is that only thymocytes whose TCRs bind weakly self-MHC–peptide complexes on antigen-presenting cells in the thymus both undergo positive selection and avoid negative selection, eventually leaving the thymus as mature T cells with self-MHC–restricted receptors.

An alternative model, the *differential-signaling hypothesis*, is a qualitative one and emphasizes the nature of the signal delivered by the TCR rather than its strength. At the core of this model is the suggestion that some MHC-peptide complexes can deliver only a weak or partly activating signal while others can deliver a complete signal. In this model, positive selection takes place when the TCRs of developing thymocytes encounter MHC-peptide complexes that deliver weak or partial signals to their receptors, and negative selection results when the signal is complete.

Experimental evidence for both hypotheses has come from studies in *fetal thymic organ culture (FTOC)*, a model that has been used to analyze thymocyte selection and the role that peptides play in this process. In this system, mouse thymic lobes are excised at a gestational age of day 16 and placed in culture. At this time, the lobes consist predominantly of $CD4^-8^-$ thymocytes. Because these immature, double-negative thymocytes continue to develop in the organ culture, thymic selection can be studied under conditions that permit a range of informative experiments.

Such studies of the role of peptides in thymic selection are facilitated greatly by the use of genetically modified mice as donors. Recall that β_2-microglobulin is required for the stabilization and efficient export of class I MHC molecules from the ER to the plasma membrane. Particular use has been made of knockout mice lacking β_2-microglobulin or the peptide transporter TAP-1. In the absence of β_2-microglobulin or TAP-1, only low levels of MHC class I α chains, without bound peptide, are expressed on the stromal cells, and the development of $CD8^+$ thymocytes is blocked. However, when exogenous peptides and β_2-microglobulin are added to these organ cultures, then class I MHC molecules bearing the peptides are expressed on the surface of the thymic stromal cells, and development of $CD8^+$ T cells is restored. When a diverse peptide mixture is added, the extent of $CD8^+$ T-cell restoration is greater than when a single peptide is added. This would suggest that the role of the peptide is not simply to induce stable MHC expression but also to be recognized itself in the selection process. Use of this system has led to several insights into the role played by peptides in positive and negative selection, and some of the more significant ones are summarized below.

Addition of one peptide or a mixture of only a few peptides can support the selection of a large repertoire of $CD8^+$ T cells with a wide diversity of TCRs. Furthermore, many of the selected cells have TCRs that do not have a high affinity for the peptides used. This observation indicates that peptides play an important but not highly specific role in positive selection.

Fetal thymic organ cultures from mice that lacked the peptide transporter TAP-1 and were transgenic for a single TCR specificity, for a particular peptide bound to class I MHC molecules expressed by the FTOC, were used to investigate the effects of the avidity of the TCR–MHC-peptide interaction on positive and negative selection. The avidity of the interaction was varied by use of different concentrations of peptide. At low peptide concentrations, few MHC molecules bound peptide and the avidity of the TCR-MHC interaction was low. As peptide concentrations were raised, the number of peptide-MHC complexes displayed increased and so did the avidity of the interaction. In this experiment, very few $CD8^+$ cells appeared when peptide was not added, but even low concentrations of the relevant peptide resulted in the appearance of significant numbers of $CD8^+$ T cells bearing the transgenic TCR receptor. However, at higher concentrations of peptide, the numbers of $CD8^+$ T cells produced declined steeply. The results of these experiments support the avidity model, because low avidity was sufficient to produce positive selection and high avidity produced negative selection.

The differential expression of the coreceptor CD8 also can affect thymic selection. In an experiment in which CD8 expression was experimentally raised to twice its normal level, the concentration of mature $CD8^+$ cells in the thymus was one-thirteenth of the concentration in control mice bearing normal levels of CD8 on their surface. Since the interaction of T cells with class I MHC molecules is strengthened by participation of CD8, perhaps the increased expression of CD8 would increase the avidity of thymocytes for class I molecules, possibly making their negative selection more likely.

In another set of FTOC experiments using fetal thymus taken from TCR transgenic mice that lacked TAP-1, the effect on positive and negative selection of an antagonist peptide, one whose MHC-peptide complex yields only a partial signal (antagonist) was compared with the effect of an agonist whose MHC-peptide complex delivers an activating signal to the TCR. The response of FTOCs to three different conditions was informative. The conditions were FTOC + no peptide, FTOC + antagonist peptide, and FTOC + agonist peptide. The MHC of the FTOC matched the MHC-restriction of the transgenic TCR, and the transgenic TCR was specific for the peptides used. As expected, if no peptide was added, no $CD8^+$ T cells bearing the transgenically encoded TCR were found. Addition of the antagonist peptide, whose MHC-peptide complexes are incapable of fully activating their target T cells, resulted in the positive selection of T cells bearing the transgenic TCR. In contrast, addition of the agonist peptide to the FTOC caused the death of thymocytes bearing the transgenic TCR. This experiment supports the differential-signaling hypothesis, because even though MHC complexes of the agonist and antagonist peptides interact with the same TCR, the outcomes are quite different.

It is clear that peptides play an important and central role in both positive and negative selection. Evidence exists for the avidity model, the differential-signaling model, as well as for other variations on these models we have not described here. It is quite possible that in some cases, one of these models applies to the complete exclusion of the other. It is also quite possible that no single mechanism accounts for all the cellular interactions in positive and negative selection and that the T-cell repertoire that emerges from the thymus results from the operation of a combination of mechanisms. Further work will clarify this matter.

How do double-positive thymocytes decide to become $CD4^+8^-$ or $CD4^-8^+$ T cells? Selection of $CD4^+8^+$ thymocytes gives rise to class I MHC–restricted $CD8^+$ T cells and class II–restricted $CD4^+$ T cells. Two models have been proposed to explain the transformation of a double-positive precursor into one of two different single-positive lineages (Figure 10-9). The *instructional model* postulates that the multiple interactions between the TCR, $CD8^+$ or $CD4^+$ coreceptors, and class I or class II MHC molecules instruct the cells to differentiate into either $CD8^+$ or $CD4^+$ single-positive cells, respectively. This model would predict that a class I MHC–specific TCR together with the CD8 coreceptor would generate a signal that is different from the signal induced by a class II MHC–specific TCR together with the CD4 coreceptor. The second model, called the *stochastic model,* suggests that CD4 or CD8 expression is switched off randomly with no relation to the specificity of the TCR. Only those thymocytes whose TCR and remaining coreceptor recognize the same class of MHC molecule will mature. At present, evidence exists in support of both models.

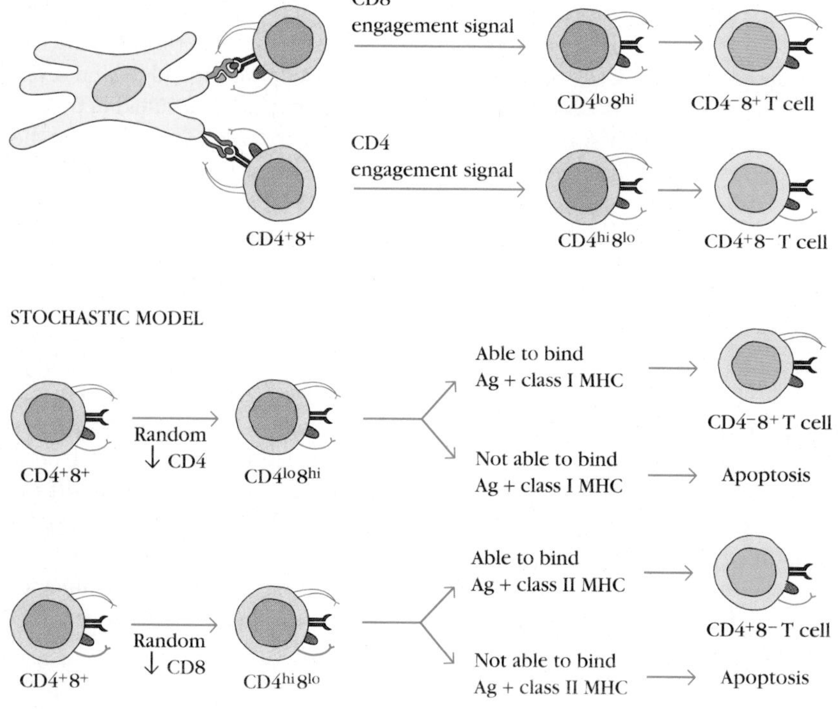

FIGURE 10-9 Proposed models of the role of the CD4 and CD8 coreceptors in thymic selection of double-positive thymocytes leading to single-positive T cells. According to the instructive model, interaction of one coreceptor with MHC molecules on stromal cells results in down-regulation of the other coreceptor. According to the stochastic model, down-regulation of CD4 or CD8 is a random process.

T_H-Cell Activation

The central event in the generation of both humoral and cell-mediated immune responses is the activation and clonal expansion of T_H cells. (Activation of T_C cells, which is generally similar to T_H-cell activation, is described in Chapter 14.) T_H-cell activation is initiated by interaction of the TCR-CD3 complex with a processed antigenic peptide bound to a class II MHC molecule on the surface of an antigen-presenting cell. This interaction and the resulting activating signals also involve various accessory membrane molecules on the T_H cell and the antigen-presenting cell. Interaction of a T_H cell with antigen initiates a cascade of biochemical events that induces the resting T_H cell to enter the cell cycle (G_0-to-G_1 transition). The activated T_H cell progresses through the cell cycle, proliferating and differentiating into memory cells or effector cells. After T_H cells interact with antigen, numerous genes are activated. The gene products that appear can be grouped into three categories depending on how early they can be detected after antigen recognition (Table 10–3):

- *Immediate genes:* expressed within half an hour of antigen recognition; encode a number of transcription factors, including c-Fos, c-Myc, c-Jun, NF-AT, and NF-κB
- *Early genes:* expressed within 1–2 h of antigen recognition; encode IL-2, IL-2R (IL-2 receptor), IL-3, IL-6, IFN-γ, and numerous other proteins
- *Late genes:* expressed more than 2 days after antigen recognition; encode various adhesion molecules

These profound changes are the result of signal-transduction pathways that are activated by the encounter between the TCR and MHC-peptide complexes. An overview of some of the basic strategies of cellular signaling will be useful background for appreciating the specific signaling pathways used by T cells.

TABLE 10-3 TIME COURSE OF GENE EXPRESSION BY T_H CELLS FOLLOWING INTERACTION WITH ANTIGEN

Gene product	Function	Time mRNA expression begins	Location	Ratio of activated to nonactivated cells
		Immediate		
c-Fos	Protooncogene; nuclear-binding protein	15 min	Nucleus	> 100
c-Jun	Cellular oncogene; transcription factor	15–20 min	Nucleus	?
NF-AT	Transcription factor	20 min	Nucleus	50
c-Myc	Cellular oncogene	30 min	Nucleus	20
NF-κB	Transcription factor	30 min	Nucleus	> 10
		Early		
IFN-γ	Cytokine	30 min	Secreted	> 100
IL-2	Cytokine	45 min	Secreted	> 1000
Insulin receptor	Hormone receptor	1 h	Cel! membrane	3
IL-3	Cytokine	1–2 h	Secreted	> 100
TGF-β	Cytokine	<2 h	Secreted	> 10
IL-2 receptor (p55)	Cytokine receptor	2 h	Cell membrane	> 50
TNF-β	Cytokine	1–3 h	Secreted	> 100
Cyclin	Cell-cycle protein	4–6 h	Cytoplasmic	> 10
IL-4	Cytokine	<6 h	Secreted	> 100
IL-5	Cytokine	<6 h	Secreted	> 100
IL-6	Cytokine	<6 h	Secreted	> 100
c-Myb	Protooncogene	16 h	Nucleus	100
GM-CSF	Cytokine	20 h	Secreted	?
		Late		
HLA-DR	Class II MHC molecule	3–5 days	Cell membrane	10
VLA-4	Adhesion molecule	4 days	Cell membrane	> 100
VLA-1, VLA-2, VLA-3, VLA-5	Adhesion molecules	7–14 days	Cell membrane	> 100, ?, ?, ?

SOURCE: Adapted from G Crabtree, *Science* **243:**357.

Some Common Themes in Signal Transduction

The detection and interpretation of signals from the environment is an indispensable feature of all cells, including those of the immune system. Signals take many forms. Among them are physical stimuli, such as radiation, and various chemical stimuli: gases (nitric oxide), small ions (Ca^{2+}), soluble proteins (IL-2), membrane ligands (MHC-peptide complexes), and lipoidal agents (steroid hormones). All signal-transduction pathways begin with receptors that detect the arrival of the signal. Interaction of the receptor and the signal produces changes that set in motion a precisely ordered chain of events that ultimately modifies the targeted process. Although there are an enormous number of different signal-transduction pathways, some common themes are typical of these crucial integrative processes:

- *The involvement of a receptor.* Typically, membrane-impermeable ligands, which are unable to traverse the membrane, bind to the extracellular domains of transmembrane receptors. Many such ligands are water-soluble molecules that arrive in solution. However, membrane-bound ligands (MHC-peptide complexes, for example) are an important class of exceptions. Hydrophobic lipoidal signals, such as steroids, which can freely diffuse through the cell membrane, are bound by intracellular receptors.
- *The generation of second messengers.* The interaction of a signal with a receptor often leads to the generation within the cell of a "second messenger," a molecule or ion that can diffuse to other sites in the cell and evoke changes. There are many such second messengers, including cyclic nucleotides (cAMP, cGMP), calcium ion (Ca^{2+}), and membrane phospholipid derivatives such as diacylglycerol (DAG) and inositol triphosphate (IP_3).
- *The action of protein kinases and protein phosphatases.* These enzymes catalyze the phosphorylation and dephosphorylation of tyrosine, serine, or threonine residues in protein elements of many signal-transduction pathways. The addition or removal of phosphate from key proteins is a major feature in many signal-transduction pathways of immunological interest.
- *The induced assembly of critical components of a signal-transduction pathway.* An early step in many signal-transduction pathways is the induced assembly of essential components of the pathway, sometimes from different cellular compartments. Molecules known as adaptor proteins play central roles in the signal-induced assembly of receptors in key signaling pathways. Adaptor molecules such as Shc or Grb2 have two types of sites, SH2 domains and SH3 domains, that enable them to specifically link two different molecules. SH2 domains are docking sites that allow the adaptor to bind to the phophotyrosines of its target molecules. Typical targets are phosphotyrosines of membrane receptors whose phosphorylation was induced by ligand binding. The SH3 domains of adaptor molecules bind to proline-rich motifs in other molecules. Thus, adaptors can promote the assembly of membrane receptors and other cytoplasmic molecules.
- *Cascades.* Small signals that trigger signal-transduction pathways are often amplified by enzyme cascades. Also, cascades of several steps in which each step depends upon the step that preceded it offer many opportunities to influence the rate and intensity of signal transduction or even to terminate it.
- *The involvement of large and small G proteins.* **G proteins** are polypeptides or polypeptide complexes that are activated when guanosine triphosphate (GTP) is bound to them and are inactive when guanosine diphosphate (GDP) is bound. Consequently, these two forms of guanosine nucleotides act as molecular switches: one form, GTP, turns on the signaling capacities of the G protein; the other form, GDP, which is either exchanged for GTP or results from the hydrolysis of the bound GTP, turns off the signal by returning the G protein to an inactive form. Small G proteins consist of a single polypeptide chain of about 21 kDa, and their release of GDP and binding of GTP is catalyzed by proteins known as *guanine nucleotide exchange factors.* A small G protein, Ras, is a key participant in the activation of an important proliferation-inducing signal-transduction cascade triggered by binding of ligands to their receptor tyrosine kinases. In addition to small G proteins, large G proteins, which are more complex and composed of an α, β, and γ subunit, are critically involved in many processes, including vision, olfaction, the epinephrine-signaled release of glucose from glycogen, and phenomena of immunological interest such as leukocyte chemotaxis.
- *The default setting for signal-transduction pathways is OFF.* In the absence of an appropriately presented signal, transmission through the pathway does not take place.

TCR-Coupled Signaling Pathways

The events that link antigen recognition by the T-cell receptor to gene activation echo many of the themes just reviewed. These events include the generation of DAG and IP_3, which act as second messengers, the adaptor-mediated assembly of components of the signaling pathway, and the activation of Ras-dependent pathways that involve cascades of protein kinases. TCR-mediated signaling is quickly manifested, and within seconds after stimulation one sees an increase in the intracellular Ca^{2+} concentration (Figure 10-10). The key

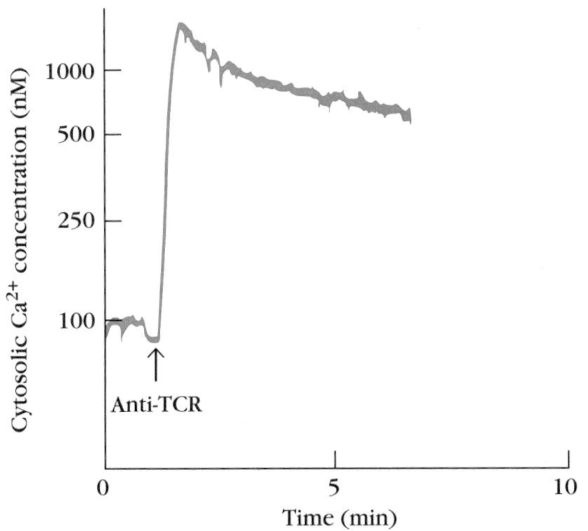

FIGURE 10-10 Calcium uptake following crosslinking of the T-cell receptor by a monoclonal anti-TCR antibody. Within a short time of T-cell stimulation, there is an abrupt and sharp rise in the concentration of Ca^{2+} in the cytosol. [Adapted from A Weiss, 1993, "T-cell activation," in *Fundamental Immunology,* 3rd ed., Raven, New York]

element in the initiation of T-cell activation is the recognition by the TCR of MHC-peptide complexes on antigen-presenting cells. The TCR consists of a mostly extracellular heterodimeric ligand-binding unit, the α and β chains of αβ TCRs, and a predominantly intracellular signaling unit. The signaling unit associated with each ligand-binding unit is composed of three different chains, CD3γ, CD3δ, and CD3ε, collectively known as the CD3 complex. In addition to the CD3 complex, a homodimer of ζ chains completes the intracellular signaling unit. The heterodimeric antigen-receptor part of the complex binds to MHC-peptide complexes but has short cytoplasmic domains, which are unable to mediate signal transduction. Experiments with knockout mice have shown that all of these components are essential for signal transduction. Further knockout experiments have shown that all three components of the CD3 complex and the ζ chain are required as well for surface expression of the TCR. Zeta (ζ) chain knockouts also fail to transmit signal efficiently and show reduced expression of the TCR complex in the cell membrane.

The signaling process is initiated when crosslinking of the TCR occurs by engagement with MHC-peptide complexes (Figure 10-11). This clustering brings Fyn, a protein tyrosine kinase, into association with the cytoplasmic tails of the TCR complex. It also causes the translocation of the coreceptors (CD4 in class II-restricted T cells or CD8 in class-I restricted T cells) to the near neighborhood of the TCR. This is significant because it brings Lck, a protein tyrosine kinase that is bound to the intracellular domain of the coreceptor, into association with the cytoplasmic tails of

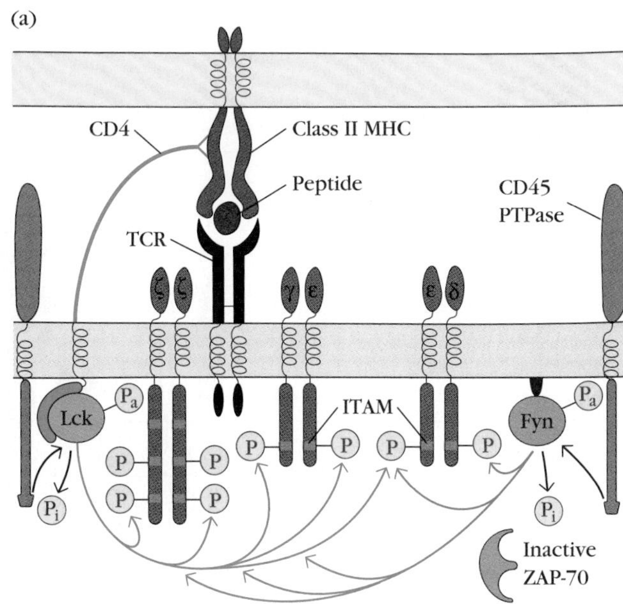

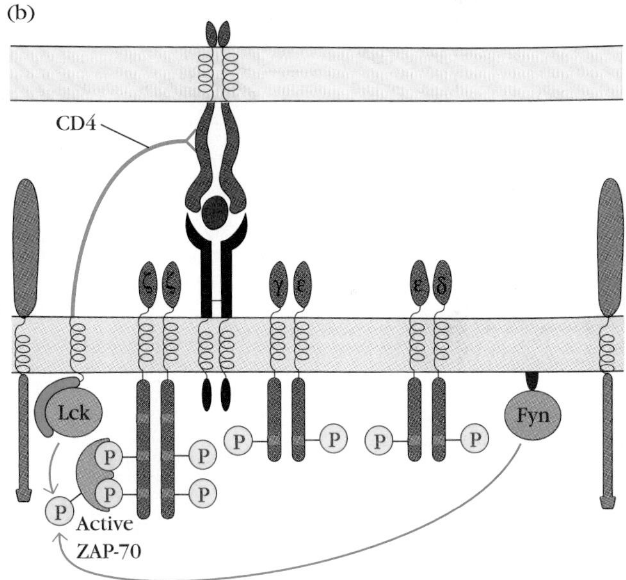

FIGURE 10-11 Initial steps in T_H-cell activation. (a) after TCR-MHC-peptide interaction between the T cell (blue) and the antigen-presenting cell (yellow), the protein tyrosine kinases Fyn and Lck are activated by removal of an inhibitory phosphate (P_i) by the phosphatase activity of an intracellular domain of CD45 and the addition of a phosphate (P_a) by a yet uncharacterized protein tyrosine kinase. Once activated, Fyn and Lck phosphorylate tyrosine residues in the ITAMs of the ε, γ, δ, and ζ chains of the TCR complex. Although T_H-cell activation is shown, very similar events occur in T_C cells, except that Lck is brought to the area of antigen recognition by CD8. The phosphorylation of ITAMs on ζ chains provides docking sites that are occupied by SH groups of ZAP-70, another protein kinase present in inactive form in the cytoplasm. Phosphorylation of ζ-chain–bound ZAP-70 by Fyn and Lck activate this essential element in the further transmission of signals from the TCR complex.

VISUALIZING CONCEPTS

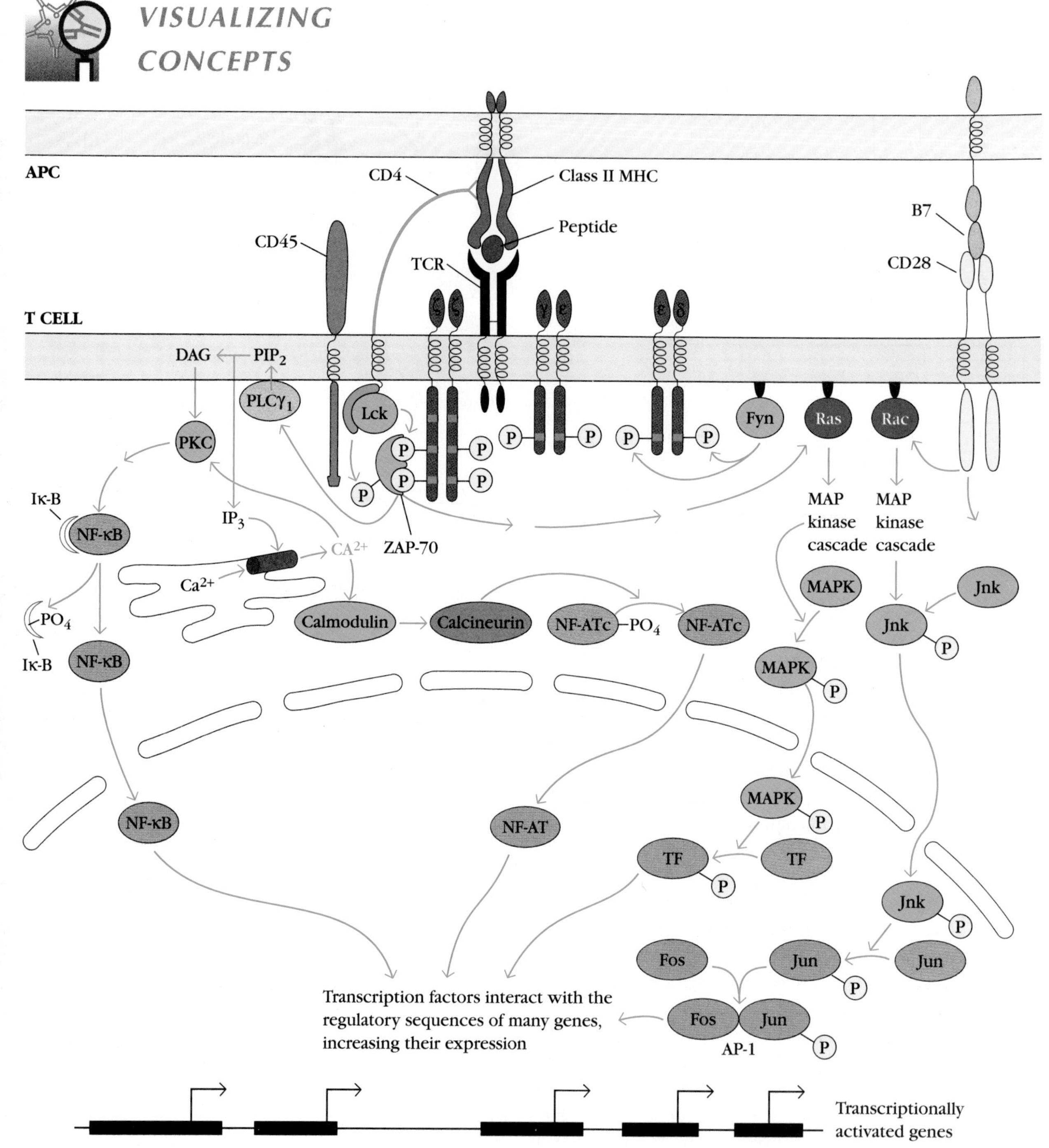

FIGURE 10-12 Overview of signal transduction during T-cell activation. The TCR-mediated signal results in the activation of various signal-transduction pathways, which lead to the formation of several products, including NF-κB, NF-AT, and activated MAPK, three key molecules that have important influences on transcription. In one pathway, ZAP-70 activates PLCγ_1 by tyrosine phosphorylation. Activated PLCγ_1 hydrolyzes PIP_2, a membrane phospholipid, to produce the potent second messengers DAG and IP_3. DAG, together with Ca^{2+} released by the action of IP_3, collaboratively activate the PKC, which phosphorylates Iκ-B, causing the release of the transcription factor NF-κB. Ca^{2+}, acting with calmodulin, activates calcineurin, a phosphatase, which removes a phosphate from cytoplasmic NF-AT, which then translocates to the nucleus, where it acts as a potent transcription factor for a number of genes. In another pathway, ZAP-70 initiates a sequence of events that activates the Ras pathway. Ras initiates a cascade of phosphorylations known as a MAP kinase cascade, which culminates in the activation of MAPK, which translocates into the nucleus and

the TCR. These protein tyrosine kinases are required for the phosphorylation of the **immunoreceptor tyrosine-based activation motif (ITAM)** sequences on the cytoplasmic domains of the CD3 complex. These ITAMs interact with protein tyrosine kinases and possibly other molecules during signal transduction.

Phosphorylation of tyrosines in the ITAMs by Fyn and Lck is an early consequence of crosslinking the TCR, and it sets in motion the initial processes of signal transmission from this receptor complex. However, the activity of Fyn and Lck, like that of many critical components of signal transduction pathways is regulated by phosphorylation. Fyn and Lck are regulated by tyrosine phosphorylation at two key sites. Phosphorylation at an inhibitory site turns off enzyme activity, and phosphorylation at an activation site is necessary for activity. However, even after the activation site has been phosphorylated, enzyme activity is not possible until the inhibitory phosphate has been removed. The removal of phosphate from the inhibitory site of Fyn and Lck is performed by CD45, a transmembrane tyrosine phosphatase found in all leukocytes (the **leukocyte common antigen**). Thus activated, Fyn and Lck proceed to phosphorylate critical tyrosines in the ITAMs of the CD3 complex. The phosphorylation of the ζ chain creates phosphotyrosine docking sites for SH2 sites of the next member of the signaling complex, **ZAP-70, zeta associated protein** (a 70-kDa polypeptide). Once ZAP-70 binds to the ITAMs of the ζ chain, the protein tyrosine kinase activity of ZAP-70 is activated by tyrosine phosphorylation catalyzed by Lck or Fyn.

The activation of the ZAP-70 protein tyrosine kinase leads to the activation of many pathways (Figure 10-12), some of which are initiated by the phosphorylation of phospholipase $C\gamma_1$ ($PLC\gamma$), a member of the phospholipase C group of enzymes. Once activated, $PLC\gamma_1$ hydrolyzes phosphatidylinositol 4,5-bisphosphate (PIP_2), a membrane phospholipid, into two products, inositol 1,4,5-trisphosphate (IP_3) and diacylglycerol (DAG). These second messengers initiate two signaling pathways that are important for T-cell activation. In one pathway, IP_3 triggers an increase in intracellular cytosolic Ca^{2+} and the subsequent activation of a calmodulin-dependent phosphatase called **calcineurin**, which dephosphorylates the inactive cytosolic form of the T-cell–specific nuclear factor NF-AT. In the other pathway, DAG activates protein kinase C (PKC), which then phosphorylates various cellular substrates and mediates release of the nuclear factor NF-κB. Both nuclear factors enter the nucleus, where they participate in activation of various genes, including the IL-2 gene.

The importance of the role played by IP_3 and DAG can be appreciated by noting that T cells can be fully activated if one bypasses crosslinking TCR and directly mimics the effects of these second messengers. Ca^{2+} levels can be raised by treating the cells with a calcium ionophore, an agent that allows Ca^{2+} from the outside medium to enter the cell. Protein kinase C can be activated by any one of a group of chemicals known as phorbol esters, which resemble DAG. Treatment of resting T cells with PMA (phorbol myristic acetate), a phorbol ester, and the calcium ionophore ionomycin causes them to enter the cell cycle, induces secretion of cytokines such as IL-2 and can cause activation-induced cell death.

In addition to the generation of IP_3 and DAG, crosslinking of the T-cell receptor activates the small G protein Ras. Within a minute of TCR crosslinking, inactive Ras has exchanged its bound GDP for GTP to become the active signal-transducing form. Activated Ras causes the initiation of the MAP kinase (mitogen-activated protein kinase) pathway, a series of phosphorylations by a cascade of protein kinases that results in the phosphorylation of members of the Fos and Jun families of transcription factors and their formation of AP1 heterodimers, which promote the transcription of genes required for cell proliferation and IL-2 production.

Of the DNA-binding proteins involved in T_H-cell activation, only NF-AT is T-cell specific; the others are found in many types of cells. After recognition of antigen by T_H cells, NF-ATc-PO_4, the phosphorylated cytosolic form of NF-AT, is dephosphorylated by calcineurin. NF-ATc then translocates to the nucleus where it dimerizes with AP1; the resulting complex then binds to the IL-2 enhancer. If dephosphorylation of NF-ATc-PO_4 is inhibited, as it is by cyclosporin A and FK506, then T_H-cell activation is blocked and the

activates a transcription factor that up-regulates transcription of the gene encoding Fos. Fos joins with Jun to form a key transcription factor known as AP-1. The engagement of the co-stimulatory molecule CD28 by B7 also induces the activation of signal-transduction pathways, one of which is the MAP kinase cascade initiated by the small G protein Rac. The end result of this pathway is the phosphorylation of Jun kinase (Junk or Jnk). Activated Jnk then translocates to the nucleus, where it activates Jun by phosphorylation. Activated Jun joins Fos in AP-1. The collective effect of the several activated transcription factors generated by these signal-transduction pathways is to increase the expression of several genes and to induce the expression of others, including the gene that encodes the T-cell growth-promoting cytokine IL-2. $PLC\gamma_1$ = phospholipase $C\gamma_1$; PKC = protein kinase C; PIP_2 = phosphatidylinositol 4,5-bisphosphate; IP_3 = inositol 1,4,5-trisphosphate; DAG = diacylglycerol; MAPK = mitogen-activated protein kinase; Ras = a small G protein; Rac = a small G protein; TF = transcription factor; I-κB = inhibitor NF-κB; NF-AT = nuclear factor of activated T cells.

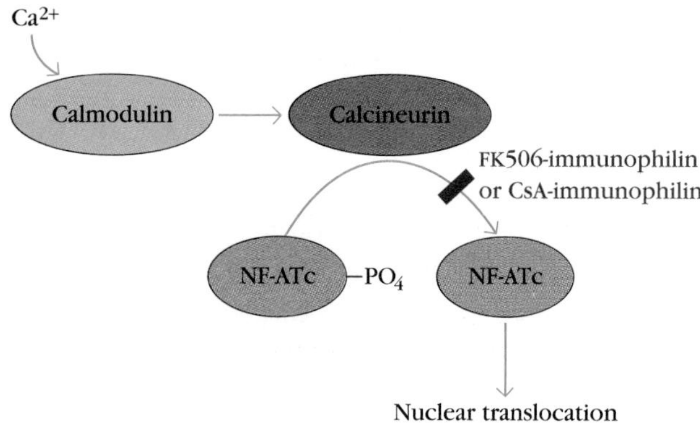

FIGURE 10-13 Mechanism of immunosuppression by cyclosporin A (CsA) and FK506, both of which bind to cytosolic proteins called immunophilins. The complex blocks the phosphatase activity of calcineurin, thereby preventing production of NF-ATc, which is necessary for T-cell activation. The immunophilins are *cis-trans* peptidyl-prolyl isomerase enzymes. CsA binds to an immunophilin called cyclophilin, and FK506 binds to one called FKBP.

immune response is reduced (Figure 10-13). Because of their potent immunosuppressive capabilities, cyclosporin A and FK506 have proven to be extremely effective in prolonging graft survival in transplant recipients (see Chapter 21).

The Co-Stimulatory Signal

T-cell activation by contact with antigen displayed on the membrane of an APC results from the dynamic interaction of multiple membrane molecules generating the necessary intracellular signals. The TCR dictates the antigen specificity of the response and plays a central role in initiating activation. However, this interaction, by itself, is not sufficient to fully activate naive T cells. It is now widely believed that naive T cells require two distinct signals for activation and subsequent proliferation into effector cells:

- The initial signal (signal 1) is generated by interaction of an antigenic peptide with the TCR-CD3 complex.
- A subsequent antigen-nonspecific co-stimulatory signal (signal 2) is provided primarily by interactions between CD28 on the T cell and members of the B7 family on the APC.

B7 molecules are members of the immunoglobulin superfamily; they have a single V-like domain and a single C-like domain. There are two related forms of B7, B7-1 and B7-2 (Figure 10-14). Both molecules have a similar organization of extracellular domains but markedly different cytosolic domains. Both B7 molecules are constitutively expressed on dendritic cells and induced on activated macrophages and activated B cells. The ligands for B7 are CD28 and CTLA-4 (also known as CD152), both of which are expressed on the T-cell membrane as disulfide-linked homodimers; like B7, they are members of the immunoglobulin superfamily. Though structurally similar glycoproteins, CD28 and CTLA-4 act antagonistically. Signaling through CD28 delivers a positive co-stimulatory signal to the T cell, but signaling through CTLA-4 is inhibitory and down-regulates the activation of the T cell. CD28 is expressed by both resting and activated T cells, but CTLA-4 is virtually undetectable on resting cells. Typically, engagement of the TCR causes the induction of CTLA-4 expression, and CTLA-4 is readily detectable within 24 hours of stimulation, with maximal expression within 2 or 3 days post-stimulation. Even though the peak surface levels of CTLA-4 are lower than those of CD28, it still competes favorably for B7 molecules because it has a significantly higher avidity for these molecules than CD28 does. Interestingly, the level of CTLA-4 expression is increased by CD28-generated co-stimulatory signals. This provides a regulatory feedback that effectively applies the CTLA-4 braking in proportion to the acceleration received from CD28. Some of the importance of CTLA-4 in the regulation of lymphocyte activation and proliferation is revealed by experiments with CTLA-4 knockouts, mice that

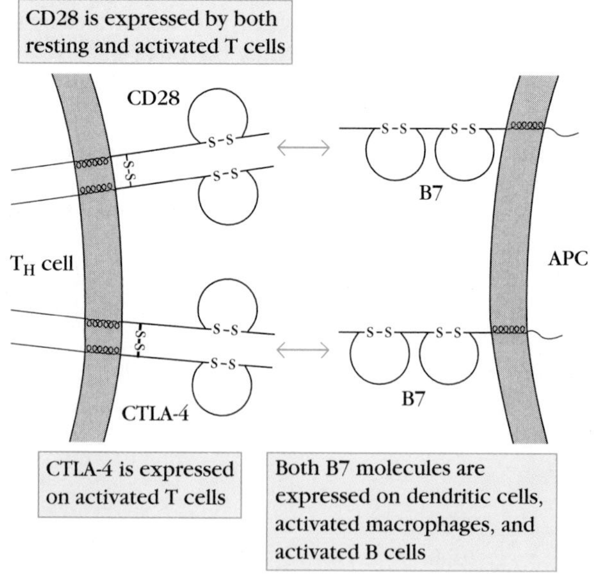

FIGURE 10-14 T_H-cell activation requires a co-stimulatory signal provided by antigen-presenting cells (APCs). Interaction of B7 family members on APCs with CD28 delivers the co-stimulatory signal. Engagement of the closely related CTLA-4 molecule with B7 produces an inhibitory signal. All of these molecules contain at least one immunoglobulin-like domain and thus belong to the immunoglobulin superfamily. [Adapted from PS Linsley and JA Ledbetter, 1993, *Annu. Rev. Immunol.* **11**:191.]

are homozygous for null mutations in the CTLA-4 gene. In these knockout mice, T cells proliferate massively, which leads to lymphadenopathy, splenomegaly, and death at 3 to 4 weeks after birth. Clearly, the production of inhibitory signals by engagement of CTLA-4 is important in lymphocyte homeostasis.

As described later in this chapter, T cells can be activated experimentally in such a way that only the TCR-coupled signaling pathways operate. This kind of activation results in very little production of IL-2 compared with normal activation, in which the CD28-B7 co-stimulatory signal also operates. The co-stimulatory signal appears to synergize with the TCR-coupled signals to augment IL-2 production and T-cell proliferation. An understanding of these effects depends critically upon a knowledge of the signal-transduction pathways involved and the nature of their interactions. The signal-transduction pathways employed by CD28 and CTLA-4 are now being investigated intensely, and there are still many uncertainties about the exact pathways involved and the precise molecular targets of co-stimulation.

Clonal Expansion Versus Clonal Anergy

T_H-cell recognition of an antigenic peptide–MHC complex on an antigen-presenting cell results either in activation and clonal expansion or in a state of nonresponsiveness called **clonal anergy**. Anergy is a state of inactivation marked by the inability of cells to proliferate in response to a peptide-MHC complex. Whether clonal expansion or clonal anergy ensues is determined by the presence or absence of a co-stimulatory signal (signal 2), such as that produced by interaction of CD28 on T_H cells with B7 on antigen-presenting cells. Experiments with cultured cells show that, if a resting T_H cell receives the TCR-mediated signal (signal 1) in the absence of a suitable co-stimulatory signal, then the T_H cell will become anergic. Specifically, if resting T_H cells are incubated with glutaraldehyde-fixed APCs, which do not express B7 (Figure 10-15a), the fixed APCs are able to present peptides together with class II MHC molecules, thereby providing signal 1, but they are unable to provide

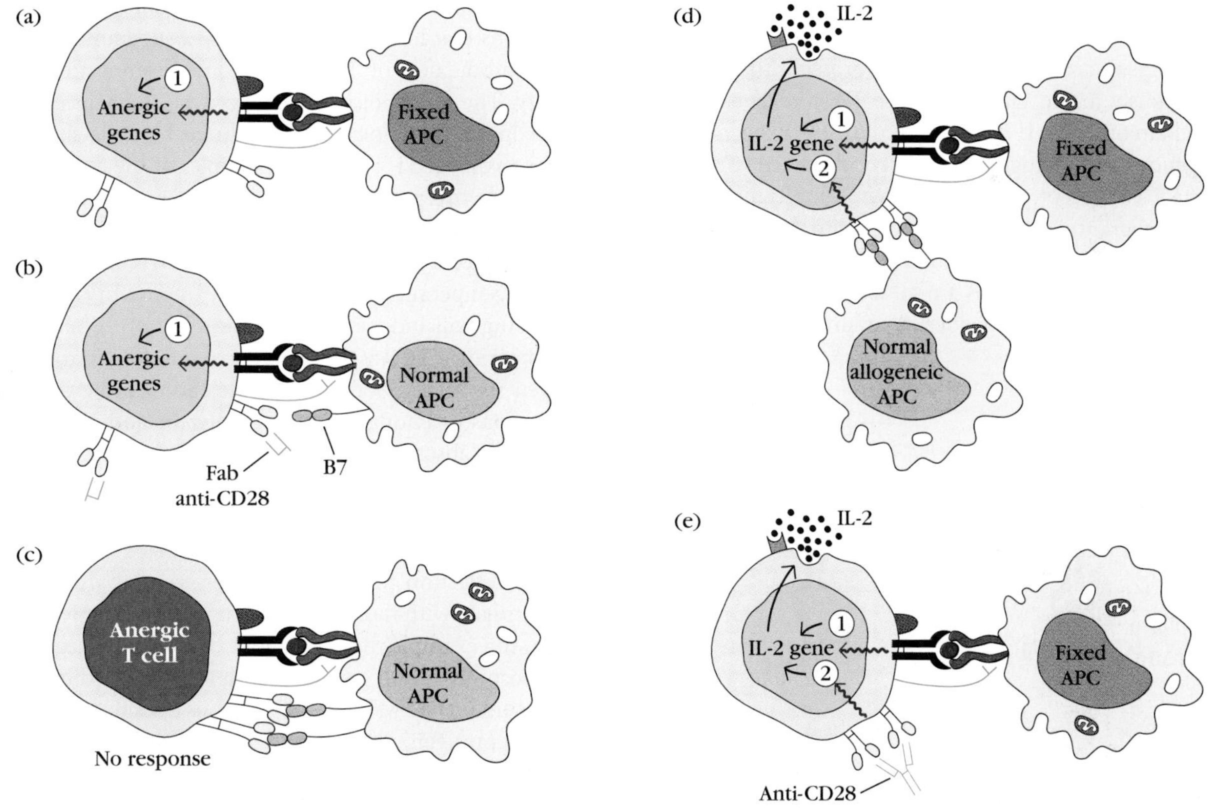

FIGURE 10-15 Experimental demonstration of clonal anergy versus clonal expansion. (a,b) Only signal 1 is generated when resting T_H cells are incubated with glutaraldehyde-fixed antigen-presenting cells (APCs) or with normal APCs in the presence of the Fab portion of anti-CD28. (c) The resulting anergic T cells cannot respond to normal APCs. (d,e) In the presence of normal allogeneic APCs or anti-CD28, both of which produce the co-stimulatory signal 2, T cells are activated by fixed APCs.

the necessary co-stimulatory signal 2. In the absence of a co-stimulatory signal, there is minimal production of cytokines, especially of IL-2. Anergy can also be induced by incubating T_H cells with normal APCs in the presence of the Fab portion of anti-CD28, which blocks the interaction of CD28 with B7 (Figure 10-15b).

Two different control experiments demonstrate that fixed APCs bearing appropriate peptide-MHC complexes can deliver an effective signal mediated by T-cell receptors. In one experiment, T cells are incubated both with fixed APCs bearing peptide-MHC complexes recognized by the TCR of the T cells and with normal APCs, which express B7 (Figure 10-15d). The fixed APCs engage the TCRs of the T cells, and the B7 molecules on the surface of the normal APCs crosslink the CD28 of the T cell. These T cells thus receive both signals and undergo activation. The addition of bivalent anti-CD28 to mixtures of fixed APCs and T cells also provides effective co-stimulation by crosslinking CD28 (Figure 10-15e). Well-controlled systems for studying anergy in vitro have stimulated considerate interest in this phenomenon. However, more work is needed to develop good animal systems for establishing anergy and studying its role in vivo.

Superantigen-Induced T-Cell Activation

Superantigens are viral or bacterial proteins that bind simultaneously to the V_β domain of a T-cell receptor and to the α chain of a class II MHC molecule. Both exogenous and endogenous superantigens have been identified. Crosslinkage of a T-cell receptor and class II MHC molecule by either type of superantigen produces an activating signal that induces T-cell activation and proliferation (Figure 10-16).

Exogenous superantigens are soluble proteins secreted by bacteria. Among the exogenous superantigens are a variety of **exotoxins** secreted by gram-positive bacteria, such as staphylococcal enterotoxins, toxic-shock-syndrome toxin, and exfoliative-dermatitis toxin; mycoplasma-arthritidis supernatant; and streptococcal pyrogenic exotoxins. Each of these exogenous superantigens binds particular V_β sequences in T-cell receptors (Table 10-4) and crosslinks the TCR to a class II MHC molecule.

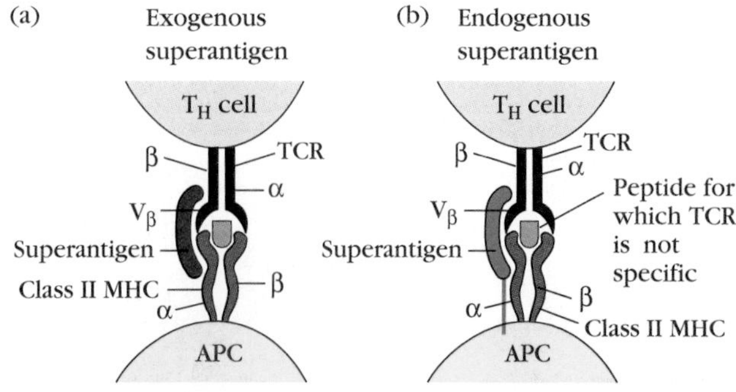

FIGURE 10-16 Superantigen-mediated crosslinkage of T-cell receptor and class II MHC molecules. A superantigen binds to all TCRs bearing a particular V_β sequence regardless of their antigenic specificity. (a) Exogenous superantigens are soluble secreted bacterial proteins, including various exotoxins. (b) Endogenous superantigens are membrane-embedded proteins produced by certain viruses; they include Mls antigens encoded by mouse mammary tumor virus.

Endogenous superantigens are cell-membrane proteins encoded by certain viruses that infect mammalian cells. One group of endogenous superantigens is encoded by mouse mammary tumor virus (MTV). This retrovirus can integrate into the DNA of certain inbred mouse strains; after integration, retroviral proteins are expressed on the membrane of the infected cells. These viral proteins, called **minor lymphocyte stimulating (Mls)** determinants, bind particular V_β sequences in T-cell receptors and crosslink the TCR to a class II MHC molecule. Four Mls superantigens, originating in different MTV strains, have been identified. These superantigens exhibit different V_β specificity, and the four *Mls* loci are located on different chromosomes (Table 10–5).

Because superantigens bind outside of the TCR antigen-binding cleft, any T cell expressing a particular V_β sequence will be activated by a corresponding superantigen. Hence, the activation is polyclonal and can affect a significant percentage (5% is not unusual) of the total T_H population. The massive activations that follow crosslinkage by a superantigen results in overproduction of T_H-cell cytokines, leading to systemic toxicity. The food poisoning induced by staphylococcal enterotoxins and the toxic shock induced by toxic-shock-syndrome toxin (TSST-1) are two examples of the consequences of cytokine overproduction induced by superantigens.

Superantigens not only induce T-cell activation, but also can influence T-cell maturation in the thymus. This occurs because a superantigen present in the thymus during thymic processing will induce the negative selection of all thymocytes bearing a TCR V_β domain corresponding to the superantigen specificity. Such massive deletion can be caused by exogeneous or endogenous superantigens and is characterized by the absence of all T cells whose receptors possess V_β domains targeted by the superantigen.

The effect of expression of an endogeneous superantigen is dramatically demonstrated by comparing the effects of negative selection in animals that possess a particular Mls superantigen with those that do not. The inbred AKR mouse strain, for example, has MTV-7, a retrovirus, integrated in chromosome 1 and expresses Mls1, whereas the B10.BR strain contains no MTV strain and thus does not express any Mls superantigen. Since the Mls1 superantigen binds to the $V_\beta6$, $V_\beta7$, $V_\beta8.1$, and $V_\beta9$ domains in T-cell receptors, negative selection during thymic processing would be expected to eliminate T cells expressing receptors with these V_β domains in AKR mice but not in B10.BR mice. As shown in Table 10-6, both mouse strains have immature thymocytes expressing the V_β domains to which Mls1 binds, but only B10.BR mice contain mature thymocytes bearing T-cell receptors with these V_β domains. Thus, negative selection, me-

TABLE 10-4 EXOGENOUS SUPERANTIGENS AND THEIR V_β SPECIFICITY

Superantigen	Disease*	V_β specificity	
		Mouse	Human
Staphylococcal enterotoxins			
SEA	Food poisoning	1, 3, 10, 11, 12, 17	nd
SEB	Food poisoning	3, 8.1, 8.2, 8.3	3, 12, 14, 15, 17, 20
SEC1	Food poisoning	7, 8.2, 8.3, 11	12
SEC2	Food poisoning	8.2, 10	12, 13, 14, 15, 17, 20
SEC3	Food poisoning	7, 8.2	5, 12
SED	Food poisoning	3, 7, 8.3, 11, 17	5, 12
SEE	Food poisoning	11, 15, 17	5.1, 6.1–6.3, 8, 18
Toxic-shock-syndrome toxin (TSST1)	Toxic-shock syndrome	15, 16	2
Exfoliative-dermatitis toxin (ExFT)	Scalded-skin syndrome	10, 11, 15	2
Mycoplasma-arthritidis supernatant (MAS)	Arthritis, shock	6, 8.1–8.3	nd
Streptococcal pyrogenic exotoxins (SPE-A, B, C, D)	Rheumatic fever, shock	nd	nd

*Disease results from infection by bacteria that produce the indicated superantigens.

TABLE 10-5 PROPERTIES OF Mls ENDOGENOUS SUPERANTIGENS

Mls allele	Retroviral carrier	Chromosome location	V_β specificity
Mls1	MTV-7	1	6, 7, 8.1, 9
Mls2	MTV-13	4	3
Mls3	MTV-6	16	3, 5
Mls4	MTV-1	7	3

TABLE 10-6 NEGATIVE SELECTION OF THYMOCYTES MEDIATED BY MLS1, AN ENDOGENOUS SUPERANTIGEN*

Strain	Mls1	Expression of					
		$V_\beta 3$	$V_\beta 5$	$V_\beta 6$	$V_\beta 7$	$V_\beta 8.1$	$V_\beta 9$
		Immature αβ thymocytes					
AKR	Present	+	+	+	+	+	+
B10.BR	Absent	+	+	+	+	+	+
		Mature peripheral αβ T cells					
AKR	Present	+	+	–	–	–	–
B10.BR	Absent	+	+	+	+	+	+

*Chromosome 1 of the AKR strain carries the MTV-7 genome, which encodes Mls1. This superantigen is specific for $V_\beta 6$, $V_\beta 7$, $V_\beta 8.1$, and $V_\beta 9$. The B10.BR strain does not carry MTV.

diated by the Mls1 superantigen, eliminates T cells bearing the $V_\beta6$, $V_\beta7$, $V_\beta8.1$, or $V_\beta9$ domain in the AKR strain. Note in Table 10-6 that the presence of Mls1 had no effect on thymocytes bearing the $V_\beta3$ or $V_\beta5$ domains, to which Mls1 does not bind.

T-Cell Differentiation

An estimated 90%–95% of peripheral T cells express the αβ T-cell receptor–CD3 complex. There are about twice as many $CD4^+$ T cells as $CD8^+$ T cells in the periphery. In general, $CD4^+$ cells function as T helper cells, and $CD8^+$ cells function as cytotoxic cells. Since both populations express the αβ T-cell receptor, some researchers have proposed that T_H and T_C cells may express different V_α and V_β gene segments. The available evidence, however, seems to suggest that both populations can use the same pool of V_α and V_β gene segments. In one study, for example, the same V_β gene product was identified on both class I MHC–restricted T_C cells and class II MHC–restricted T_H cells.

$CD4^+$ and $CD8^+$ T cells leave the thymus and enter the circulation as resting cells in the G_0 stage of the cell cycle. These naive T cells, which have not yet encountered antigen, are characterized by condensed chromatin, very little cytoplasm, and little transcriptional activity. Naive T cells continually recirculate between the blood and lymph systems. During recirculation, naive T cells reside in secondary lymphoid tissues such as lymph nodes. If a naive cell does not encounter antigen in a lymph node, it exits through the efferent lymphatics, ultimately draining into the thoracic duct and rejoining the blood. It is estimated that each naive T cell recirculates from the blood to the lymph nodes and back again every 12–24 hours. Because only about 1 in 10^5 naive T cells is specific for any given antigen, this large-scale recirculation increases the chances that a naive T cell will encounter appropriate antigen. Naive T cells have generally been thought to survive only about 5–7 weeks in the absence of antigen-stimulated activation, but recent evidence suggests they may have a considerably longer life span.

Generation of Effector and Memory T Cells

If a naive T cell recognizes an antigen-MHC complex on an appropriate antigen-presenting cell or target cell, it will be activated, initiating a *primary response*. About 48 hours after activation, the naive T cell enlarges into a blast cell and begins undergoing repeated rounds of cell division. As described earlier, activation depends on a signal induced by engagement of the TCR complex and a co-stimulatory signal induced by the CD28-B7 interaction (see Figure 10-14). These signals trigger entry of the T cell into the G_1 phase of the cell cycle and, at the same time, induce transcription of the gene for IL-2 and the α chain of the high-affinity IL-2 receptor. In addition, the co-stimulatory signal increases the half-life of the IL-2 mRNA. The increase in IL-2 transcription, together with stabilization of the IL-2 mRNA, increases IL-2 production by 100-fold in the activated T cell. Secretion of IL-2 and its subsequent binding to the high-affinity IL-2 receptor induces the activated naive T cell to proliferate and differentiate (Figure 10-17). T cells activated in this way divide 2–3 times per day for 4–5 days, generating a large clone of progeny cells, which differentiate into memory or effector T-cell populations.

The various *effector T cells* carry out specialized functions such as cytokine secretion and B-cell help (activated $CD4^+$ T_H cells) and cytotoxic killing activity ($CD8^+$ CTLs). The generation and activity of CTL cells are described in detail in Chapter 14. Effector cells are derived from both naive and memory cells after antigen activation. Effector cells are short-lived cells, whose life spans range from a few days to a few weeks. The effector and naive populations express different cell-membrane molecules, which contribute to differences in the recirculation patterns of these two groups of cells.

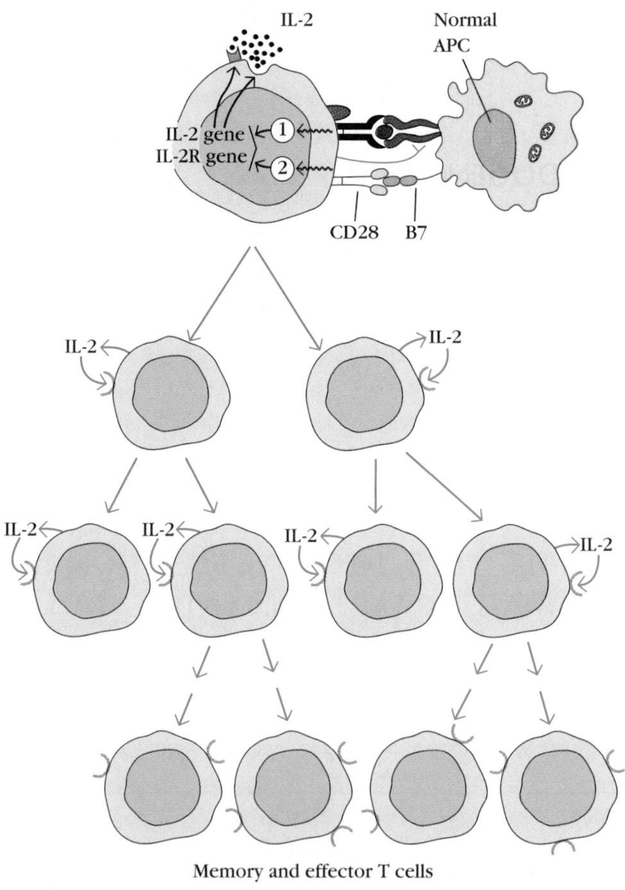

FIGURE 10-17 Activation of a T_H cell by both signal 1 and co-stimulatory signal 2 up-regulates expression of IL-2 and the high-affinity IL-2 receptor, leading to proliferation and differentiation.

As described in more detail in Chapter 12, $CD4^+$ effector T cells form two subpopulations distinguished by the different panels of cytokines they secrete. One population, called the **T_H1 subset,** secretes IL-2, IFN-γ, and TNF-β. The T_H1 subset is responsible for classic cell-mediated functions, such as delayed-type hypersensitivity and the activation of cytotoxic T lymphocytes. The other subset, called the **T_H2 subset**, secretes IL-4, IL-5, IL-6, and IL-10. This subset functions more effectively as a helper for B-cell activation.

The *memory T-cell* population is derived from both naive T cells and from effector cells after they have encountered antigen. Memory T cells are generally thought to be long-lived, antigen-activated T cells that respond with heightened reactivity to a subsequent challenge with the same antigen, generating a *secondary response.* Recent evidence suggests, however, that some memory T cells may be short-lived cells maintained in the population by continued activation by persisting antigen. An expanded population of memory T cells appears to remain long after the population of effector T cells has declined. In general, memory T cells express the same membrane molecules as effector cells.

Like naive T cells, most memory T cells are resting cells in the G_0 stage of the cell cycle, but they appear to have less stringent requirements for activation than naive T cells do. For example, naive T_H cells are activated only by dendritic cells, whereas memory T_H cells can be activated by macrophages, dendritic cells, and B cells. It is thought that the expression of high levels of numerous adhesion molecules by memory T_H cells enables these cells to adhere to a broad spectrum of antigen-presenting cells. Memory cells also display differences in their recirculation patterns that distinguish them from naive or effector T cells.

Co-Stimulatory Differences Among Antigen-Presenting Cells

Only professional antigen-presenting cells (dendritic cells, macrophages, and B cells) are able to present antigen together with class II MHC molecules and deliver the co-stimulatory signal necessary for complete T-cell activation that leads to proliferation and differentiation. The principal co-stimulatory molecules expressed on antigen-presenting cells are the glycoproteins B7-1 and B7-2 (see Figure 10-14). The professional antigen-presenting cells differ in their ability to display antigen and also differ in their ability to deliver the co-stimulatory signal (Figure 10-18).

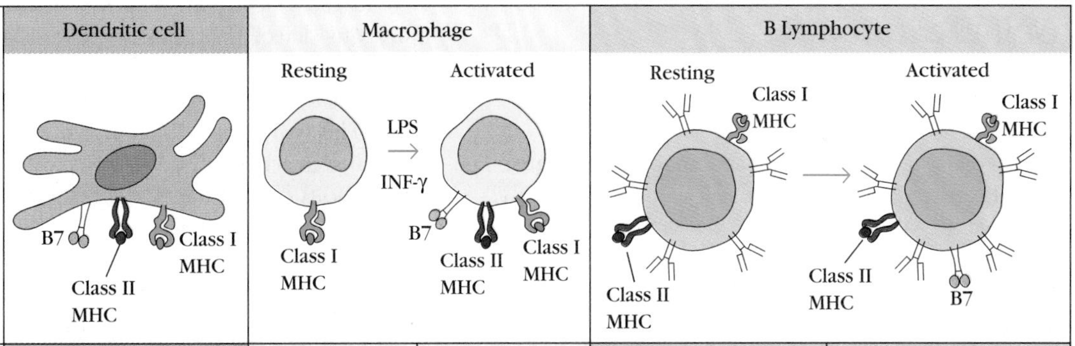

	Dendritic cell	Macrophage		B Lymphocyte	
		Resting	Activated	Resting	Activated
	B7; Class II MHC; Class I MHC	Class I MHC; LPS → INF-γ	B7; Class II MHC; Class I MHC	Class I MHC; Class II MHC	Class I MHC; Class II MHC; B7
Antigen uptake	Endocytosis phagocytosis (by Langerhans cells)	Phagocytosis	Phagocytosis	Receptor-mediated endocytosis	Receptor-mediated endocytosis
Class II MHC expression	Constitutive (+++)	Inducible (–)	Inducible (++)	Constitutive (++)	Constitutive (+++)
Co-stimulatory activity	Constitutive B7 (+++)	Inducible B7 (–)	Inducible B7 (++)	Inducible B7 (–)	Inducible B7 (++)
T-cell activation	Naive T cells Effector T cells Memory T cells	(–)	Effector T cells Memory T cells	Effector T cells Memory T cells	Naive T cells Effector T cells Memory T cells

FIGURE 10-18 Differences in the properties of professional antigen-presenting cells affect their ability to present antigen and induce T-cell activation. Note that activation of effector and memory T cells does not require the co-stimulatory B7 molecule.

Dendritic cells constitutively express high levels of class I and class II MHC molecules as well as high levels of B7-1 and B7-2. For this reason, dendritic cells are very potent activators of naive, memory, and effector T cells. In contrast, all other professional APCs require activation for expression of co-stimulatory B7 molecules on their membranes; consequently, resting macrophages are not able to activate naive T cells and are poor activators of memory and effector T cells. Macrophages can be activated by phagocytosis of bacteria or by bacterial products such as LPS or by IFN-γ, a T_H1-derived cytokine. Activated macrophages up-regulate their expression of class II MHC molecules and co-stimulatory B7 molecules. Thus, activated macrophages are common activators of memory and effector T cells, but their effectiveness in activating naive T cells is considered minimal.

B cells also serve as antigen-presenting cells in T-cell activation. Resting B cells express class II MHC molecules but fail to express co-stimulatory B7 molecules. Consequently, resting B cells cannot activate naive T cells, although they can activate the effector and memory T-cell populations. Upon activation, B cells up-regulate their expression of class II MHC molecules and begin expressing B7. These activated B cells can now activate naive T cells as well as the memory and effector populations.

Cell Death and T-Cell Populations

In recent years, the antigen-signaled apoptotic death of T cells has been recognized as a central feature of normal T-cell biology. It is a key element in the shaping of the T-cell repertoire during development in the thymus and in the regulation of mature T-cell populations. We have seen that apoptosis during T-cell development purges the repertoire of cells unable to interact with self-MHC and eliminates those that are potentially self-reactive. Activation of mature T cells in the periphery causes them to proliferate and differentiate into effector-cell populations. These populations of effector cells no longer benefit the host once the immune response has eliminated the pathogen, and apoptosis also acts to remove the expanded T-cell population and eliminate activated T_H cells. The death of these activated T_H cells is useful because it eliminates cells that are producing high levels of cytokines that are no longer needed and are even potentially deleterious to the host.

Like all apoptotic cell death, TCR-mediated death can be divided into two phases, an inductive phase and an effector phase. The effector phase, which Douglas Green and others have loosely called an "execution" phase, includes a sequence of steps that are common to apoptosis in many cell types and, if not interrupted, will lead to the death of the cell. Much has been learned about the mechanism of the effector phase of apoptosis, and a current picture of these developments is presented in Chapter 14. The induction phase, which often requires the expression of new genes, consists of the set of signals that activate the effector phase.

Go to www.whfreeman.com/immunology Animation
Cell Death

A variety of signals may initiate an induction pathway to cell death, and T cells illustrate well just how diverse these triggering pathways can be. In the thymus, strong engagement of T-cell receptors, glucocorticoids, ionizing radiation, and other agents can cause the death of T cells (Figure 10-19). Typically, each of these agents uses a different induction pathway to trigger a common effector pathway. Often the product of one or more genes is uniquely required for a particular induction pathway. For example, the induction of TCR-mediated apoptosis in thymocytes requires the expression of members of the Nur77/Nor-1 family of genes.

Outside the thymus, most, if not all, of the TCR-mediated apoptosis of mature T cells, sometimes referred to as activation-induced cell death (AICD), is induced through the Fas pathway, which requires the Fas protein and its ligand. The engagement of Fas on the membrane of a cell by Fas ligand (FasL) triggers the death of the Fas-bearing cell (Figure 10-20). Fas belongs to the tumor necrosis factor receptor (TNFR) family of proteins, and FasL is a membrane-resident molecule that is closely related to the cytokine tumor necrosis factor α (TNF α). The mechanism of Fas-FasL–mediated cell death is reviewed in Chapter 14. The importance of Fas in activation-induced apoptosis is readily demonstrated in the lpr strain of mice, which carry a homozygous defect (Fas^-/Fas^-) in the Fas gene. This defect causes a marked lymphoproliferative disorder that results in grossly swollen lymph nodes and the early death of these animals. The symptoms and course of the disease are readily duplicated in artificially created Fas-knockout mice that have homozygous disruptions in the Fas gene. Defects in the Fas-FasL system have also been shown to be associated with similar disease syndromes in humans (see Clinical Focus). Finally, while Fas and FasL are the most important mediators

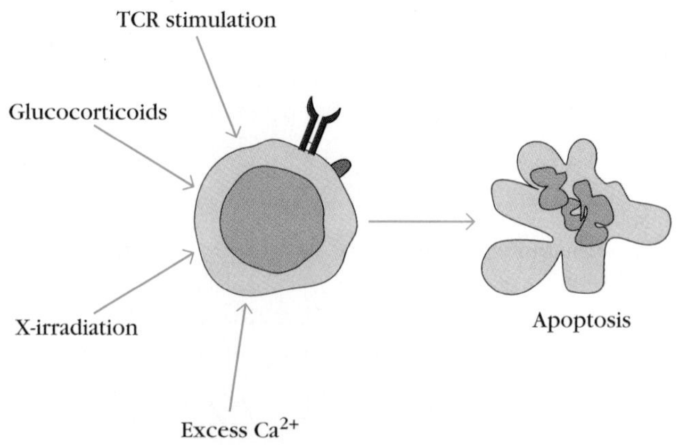

FIGURE 10-19 The death of T cells can be triggered by many different induction pathways: crosslinking of the T-cell receptor by antigen or artifical stimuli, treatment with glucocorticoids, exposure to x-rays, or a rise in cytosolic Ca^{2+} levels.

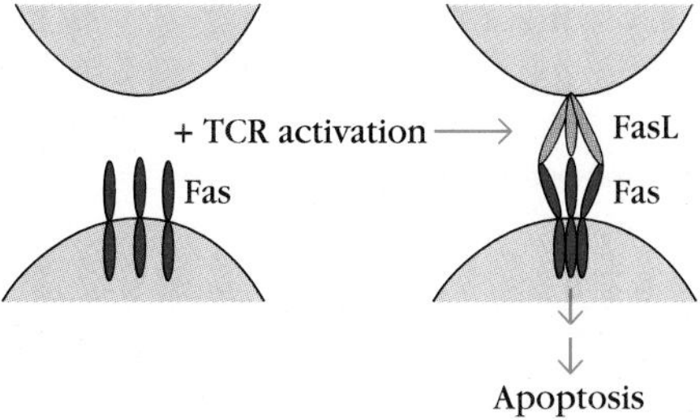

FIGURE 10-20 Fas-induced cell death. Fas is found as monomers on the surface of resting T cells. Activation though the T cell receptor (TCR) induces expression of Fas ligand (FasL). The expression of FasL on either a neighboring cell or on the Fas-bearing cell induces trimerization of Fas, which initiates a signal-transduction cascade that leads to apoptosis of the Fas-bearing cell.

of the activation-induced cell death of mature T cells, the interactions of other members of the TNFR family with ligands belonging to the TNF family have also been shown to account for some TCR-mediated death.

Peripheral γδ T Cells

In 1986, a small population of peripheral-blood T cells was discovered that expressed CD3 but failed to stain with monoclonal antibody specific for the αβ T-cell receptor, indicating an absence of the αβ heterodimer. Many of these cells eventually were found to express the γδ receptor.

Distribution of γδ T Cells

In humans, less than 5% of T cells bear the γδ heterodimer, and the percentage of γδ T cells in the lymphoid organs of mice has been reported to range from 1% to 3%. But, surprisingly, they appear to represent a major T-cell population in the skin, intestinal epithelium, and pulmonary epithelium. Up to 1% of the epidermal cells in the skin of mice are γδ T cells. These cells, called **intraepidermal lymphocytes**, express Thy-1(a T-cell marker found on mouse and rat but not human T cells) and the γδ TCR–CD3 complex, but fail to express either CD4 or CD8. A second population of γδ T cells has been identified in the intestinal epithelium of the mouse; these are called "intestinal epithelial lymphocytes," or **intraepithelial lymphocytes (IELs).** These cells express the γδ TCR–CD3 complex but, unlike intraepidermal lymphocytes of skin, they also express CD8.

Unlike αβ T cells, which recirculate extensively, γδ T cells in these epithelial tissues appear not to circulate and instead remain fixed in these tissue sites. The γδ T cells in different epithelial tissue sites appear to express different V_γ and V_δ gene segments. Comparison of clonal populations of these T cells, for example, has revealed an unusual limitation in TCR diversity. Many of these clones express TCRs of identical sequence and display little or no junctional or N diversity. The intraepithelial-lymphocyte populations found in the intestine are also monospecific, and lack junctional or N diversity, but have a sequence different from that of γδ T cells in the skin. Although there is no convincing evidence that this is the case, some immunologists suggest that this selective expression of different V gene segments in different epithelial tissues may reflect a specialization of these T cells to respond to certain types of antigens that tend to be found at these sites.

Ligands Recognized by γδ T Cells

Both the nature of the antigens recognized by γδ T cells and the functions of these cells have remained elusive. In 1994, several startling findings began to cause another paradigm in immunology to crumble—namely, that all T cells are self-MHC restricted and recognize only peptide antigens displayed in the cleft of the self-MHC molecule. Indeed, Chapters 2 and 8 describe αβ TCR-bearing T cells (NK1-T cells and CD1-restricted T cells) that are not restricted by conventional MHC molecules. In one study, a γδ T-cell clone was found to bind directly to a herpes-virus protein without requiring antigen processing and presentation together with MHC. Also γδ T cells have been reported that bind to some mycobacterial nonpeptide antigens; one such ligand is isopentenyl pyrophosphate. This finding suggests that some γδ T cells bind to epitopes in much the same way that antibodies do.

Function of γδ T cells

Although the limited gene-segment repertoire and unusual ligand recognition exhibited by the γδ heterodimer suggest that γδ T cells may play a unique role in immunity, they have yet to be identified with a clear-cut function. However, several observations have stimulated considerable speculation. The finding that γδ T cells can mediate tumor-cell lysis in a non-MHC-restricted manner indicates that they may function like natural killer cells. The ability of γδ T cells to respond to a mycobacterial antigen called purified protein derivative (PPD) may be an important clue to their function. The PPD antigen belongs to a group of highly conserved proteins, found in all organisms, called heat-shock proteins. These proteins, as their name implies, are produced by cells in response to sudden increases in temperature or other environmental stresses. But heat-shock proteins are also induced by internal stresses such as inflammatory responses and viral infections. Mycobacterial PPD exhibits sequence homology with a mammalian heat-shock protein that is a normal component of the mitochondrial matrix. This observation has led to the proposal that γδ T cells may be uniquely suited to respond to mammalian heat-shock proteins and may have evolved to eliminate damaged cells as well as microbial invaders.

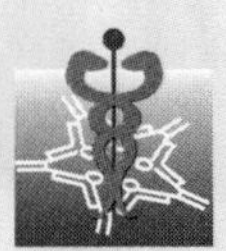

CLINICAL FOCUS

FAILURE OF APOPTOSIS CAUSES DEFECTIVE LYMPHOCYTE HOMEOSTASIS

The maintenance of appropriate numbers of various types of lymphocytes is extremely important to an effective immune system. Consequently, regulation of the size of lymphocyte populations is an essential feature of homeostasis. One of the most important elements in this regulation is apoptosis mediated by the Fas-FasL ligand system. The following excerpts from medical histories show what can happen when this key regulatory mechanism fails.

Patient A A woman, now 43, has had a long history of immunologic imbalances and other medical problems. By age 2, she was diagnosed with the Canale-Smith syndrome (CSS), a severe enlargement of such lymphoid tissues as lymph nodes (lymphadenopathy) and spleen (splenomegaly). Biopsy of lymph nodes showed that, in common with many other CSS patients, she had greatly increased numbers of lymphocytes. She had reduced numbers of platelets (thrombocytopenia) and, because her red blood cells were being lysed, she was anemic (hemolytic anemia). The reduction in numbers of platelets and the lysis of red blood cells could be traced to the action of circulating antibodies (auto-antibodies) that reacted with these host components. At age 21, she was diagnosed with grossly enlarged pelvic lymph nodes that had to be removed. Ten years later, she was again found to have an enlarged abdominal mass, which on surgical removal turned out to be a half-pound lymph-node aggregate. She has continued to have mild lymphadenopathy and, typical of these patients, the lymphocyte populations of enlarged nodes had elevated numbers of T cells (87% as opposed to a normal range of 48%–67% T cells). Examination of these cells by flow cytometry and fluorescent antibody staining revealed an excess of double-negative T cells (see illustration below) Also, like many patients with Canale-Smith syndrome, she has had cancer, breast cancer at age 22 and skin cancer at age 22 and 41.

Patient B A man who was eventually diagnosed with Canale-Smith syndrome had severe lymphadenopathy and splenomegaly as an infant and child. He was treated from age 4 to age 12 with corticosteroids and the immunosuppressive drug, mercaptopurine. These appeared to help, and the swelling of lymphoid tissues became milder during adolescence and adulthood. At age 42, he died of liver cancer.

Patient C An 8-year-old boy, the son of patient B, was also afflicted with Canale-Smith syndrome and showed elevated T cell counts and severe lymphadenopathy at the age of seven months. At age 2 his spleen became so enlarged that it had to be removed. He also developed hemolytic anemia and thrombocytopenia. However, although he continued to have elevated T-cell counts, the severity of his hemolytic anemia and thrombocytopenia have so far been controlled by treatment with methotrexate, a DNA-synthesis-inhibiting drug that is used for immunosuppression and also finds applications in chemotherapy for cancer.

Recognition of the serious consequences of a failure to regulate the number of lymphocytes, as exemplified by these case histories, emerged from detailed study of several children whose enlarged lymphoid tissues attracted medical attention. In each of these cases of Canale-Smith syndrome, examination revealed grossly enlarged lymph nodes that were 1–2 cm in girth and sometimes large enough to distort the local anatomy. In four of a group of five children who were studied intensively, the spleens were so massive that they had to be removed.

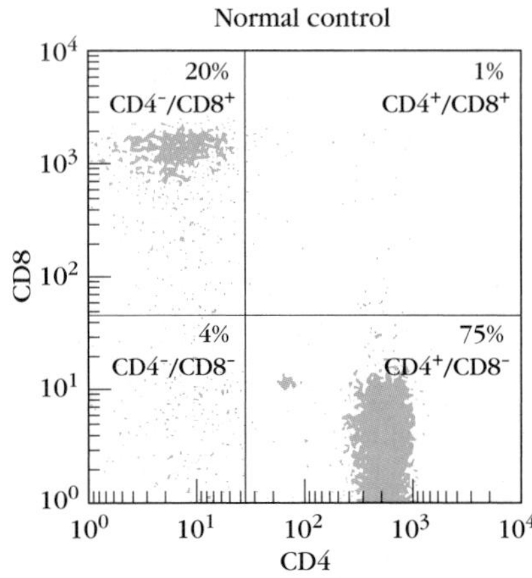

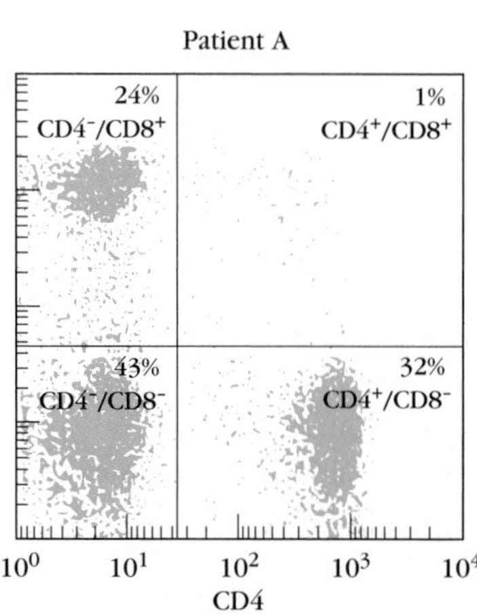

Flow cytometric analysis of T cells in the blood of Patient A and a control subject. The relative staining by an anti-CD8 antibody is shown on the *y* axis and the relative staining by an anti-CD4 antibody appears on the *x* axis. Mature T cells are either $CD4^+$ or $CD8^+$. While almost all of the T cells in the control subject are $CD4^+$ or $CD8^+$, the CSS patient shows high numbers of double-negative T cells (43%), which express neither CD4 nor CD8. The percentage of each category of T cells is indicated in the quadrants. [Adapted from Drappa et al., 1996, *New England Journal of Medicine* **335:**1643.]

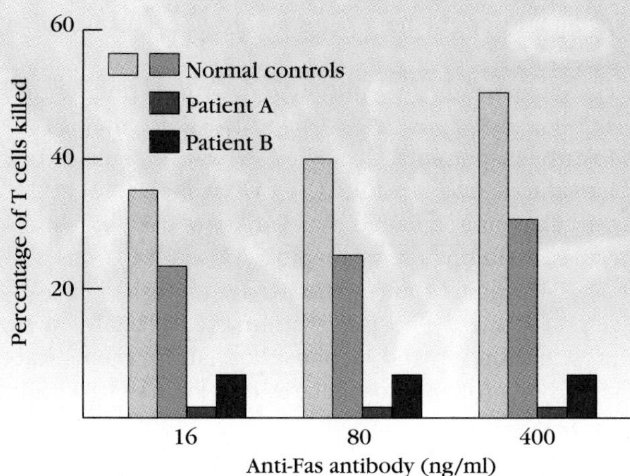

Fas-mediated killing takes place when Fas is crosslinked by FasL, its normal ligand, or by treatment with anti-Fas antibody, which artificially crosslinks Fas molecules. This experiment shows the reduction in numbers of T cells after induction of apoptosis in T cells from patients and controls by crosslinking Fas with increasing amounts of an anti-Fas monoclonal antibody. T cells from the Canale-Smith patients (A and C) are resistant to Fas-mediated death. [Adapted from Drappa et al, 1996, *New England Journal of Medicine* **335:**1643.]

Even though the clinical picture in Canale-Smith syndrome can vary from person to person, with some individuals suffering severe chronic affliction and others only sporadic episodes of illness, there is a common feature, a failure of activated lymphocytes to undergo Fas-mediated apoptosis. Isolation and sequencing of Fas genes from a number of patients and more than 100 controls reveals that CSS patients are heterozygous ($fas^{+/-}$) at the *fas* locus and thus carry one copy of a defective *fas* gene. A comparison of Fas-mediated cell death in T cells from normal controls who do not carry mutant Fas genes with death induced in T cells from CSS patients, shows a marked defect in Fas-induced death (see illustration above). Characterization of the Fas genes so far seen in CSS patients reveals that they have mutations in or around the region encoding the death-inducing domain (the "death domain") of this protein (see illustration below). Such mutations result in the production of Fas protein that lacks biological activity but still competes with normal Fas molecules for interactions with essential components of the Fas-mediated death pathway. Consequently, these mutant Fas molecules inhibit the action of normal Fas molecules. In addition to those mutations in and around the Fas death domain, other mutations have been found in the extracellular domain of Fas. These mutations in the extracellular domain are often associated with milder forms of CSS or no disease at all.

A number of research groups have conducted detailed clinical studies of CSS patients, and the following general observations have been made:

- The cell populations of the blood and lymphoid tissues of CSS patients show dramatic elevations (5-fold to as much as 20-fold) in the numbers of lymphocytes of all sorts, including T cells, B cells, and NK cells.
- Most of the patients have elevated levels of one or more classes of immunoglobulin (hypergammaglobulinemia).
- Immune hyperactivity is responsible for such autoimmune phenomena as the production of autoantibodies against red blood cells, resulting in hemolytic anemia, and a depression in platelet counts due to the activity of anti-platelet auto-antibodies.

These observations establish the importance of the death-mediated regulation of lymphocyte populations in lymphocyte homeostasis. Such death is necessary because the immune response to antigen results in a sudden and dramatic increase in the populations of responding clones of lymphocytes and temporarily distorts the representation of these clones in the repertoire. In the absence of cell death, the periodic stimulation of lymphocytes that occurs in the normal course of life would result in progressively increasing, and ultimately unsustainable, lymphocyte levels. As the Canale-Smith syndrome demonstrates, without the essential culling of lymphocytes by apoptosis, severe and life-threatening disease can result.

Map of *fas* locus. The *fas* gene is composed of 9 exons separated by 8 introns. Exons 1–5 encode the extracellular part of the protein, exon 6 encodes the transmembrane region, and exons 7–9 encode the intracellular region of the molecule. Much of exon 9 is responsible for encoding the critical death domain. [Adapted from GH Fisher et al, 1995, *Cell* **81:**935.]

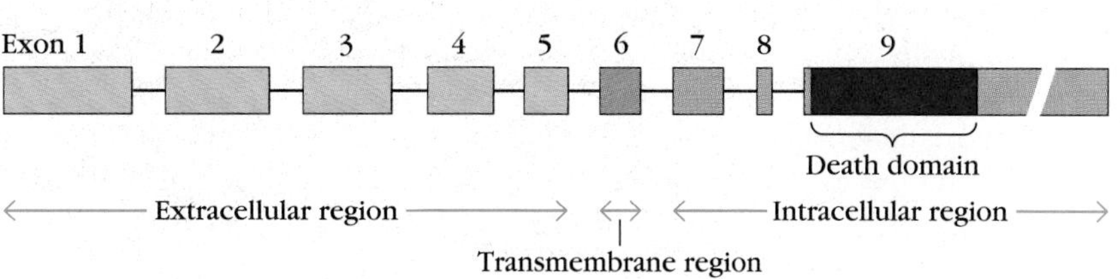

The localization of γδ T cells at epithelial sites, suggests that they are especially suited to combat epidermal or intestinal antigens and thus form a surveillance system that monitors the external milieu of the epithelial cells. These cells may be able to recognize heat-shock proteins or alterations caused by ultraviolet irradiation in the outer epidermal layer. Such a system might protect the epithelial-cell surfaces, preventing the spread of infection or cancer across the basement membrane into the internal milieu. Further study is needed to evaluate the validity of these hypotheses.

Summary

1. T-cell maturation occurs in the thymus as progenitor T cells from the bone marrow enter the thymus and rearrange their TCR genes. The earliest thymocytes lack detectable CD4 and CD8 and are referred to as double-negative cells. These double-negative thymocytes differentiate along two developmental pathways (see Figure 10-1). Those thymocytes that make a productive rearrangement of the γδ TCR genes develop into $CD4^-$, $CD8^-$, $CD3^+$ γδ T cells, which account for only a small minority of thymocytes. The majority of double-negative thymocytes rearrange the αβ TCR genes and develop into $CD4^+$, $CD3^+$ αβ T cells or $CD8^+$, $CD3^+$ αβ T cells. Immature thymocytes in the αβ pathway express a pre–T-cell receptor (see Figure 10-3).
2. Rearrangement of germ-line TCR genes during T-cell maturation in the thymus produces many functional genes encoding receptors that do not recognize self-MHC molecules or are potentially autoreactive. A repertoire of thymocytes with appropriate TCR specificities is shaped by two critical selection processes (see Figure 10-5). One of these is the positive selection of all thymocytes bearing receptors that can bind a self-MHC molecule. This is the basis of MHC-restriction and eliminates T cells that are unable to recognize self-MHC. The second is negative selection, which eliminates thymocytes bearing high-affinity receptors for self-MHC molecules alone or self-antigen plus self-MHC. This process selects the repertoire for self-tolerance. Cells that fail positive or negative selection are eliminated by apoptosis. As a result of these apoptosis-mediated selective processes, only thymocytes that are both self-MHC restricted and tolerant of antigens encountered during thymic development survive to become mature T cells.
3. Signal-transduction pathways allow signals arising outside or inside of the cell to initiate or modify key cellular processes. Some common themes seen in many signal-transduction pathways, including those involved in T cell activation, are the involvement of a receptor, the generation of second messengers, the action of protein kinases and protein phosphatases, the induced assembly of components of the pathway, the activation of enzyme cascades, the involvement of G proteins, and the turning off of signal-transduction pathways in the absence of a signal.
4. T_H-cell activation is initiated by interaction of the TCR-CD3 complex with a peptide-MHC complex on an antigen-presenting cell. The activating signal is not transduced solely by the TCR-CD3 complex but also is mediated and regulated by a variety of accessory molecules, including the coreceptors CD4 and CD8, as well as CD45. Signal transduction is accomplished by a series of protein phosphorylation events catalyzed by protein kinases and dephosphorylation events catalyzed by protein phosphatases (see Figures 10-11 and 10-12).
5. In addition to the signals mediated by the T-cell receptor and its associated accessory molecules (signal 1), activation of the T_H cell requires a co-stimulatory signal (signal 2) provided by the antigen-presenting cell. The co-stimulatory signal is commonly induced by interaction between molecules of the B7 family on the membrane of the APC with CD28 on the membrane of the T_H cell (see Figure 10-14). On the other hand, engagement of CTLA-4, a close relative of CD28, by B7 inhibits T-cell activation.
6. T_H-cell recognition of an antigenic peptide–MHC complex on an antigen-presenting cell results either in activation and clonal expansion or in a state of nonresponsiveness called clonal anergy. The presence or absence of the co-stimulatory signal (signal 2) determines whether activation results in clonal expansion or clonal anergy (see Figure 10-15).
7. More than 95% of peripheral T cells express the αβ T-cell receptor. Those T cells that express CD4 recognize antigen combined with a class II MHC molecule and generally function as T_H cells; those T cells that express CD8 recognize antigen combined with a class I MHC molecule and generally function as T_C cells. Naive T cells are resting cells (G_0) that have not encountered antigen. Activation of naive cells initiates a primary response that leads to the generation of effector and memory T cells (see Figure 10-17). Memory T cells, which are more easily activated than naive cells, are responsible for the secondary response. Effector cells, which are short lived, perform helper, cytotoxic, or delayed-type hypersensitivity functions. The professional antigen-presenting cells—dendritic cells, macrophages, and B cells—differ in their ability to display antigen and activate different T-cell populations (see Figure 10-18).
8. T cells that express the γδ T-cell receptor constitute only a small percentage of the total T-cell population. The γδ T cells are concentrated in several epithelial tissues and may represent a cell-mediated immune system that evolved to protect the integrity of external epithelial surfaces.

REFERENCES

Alberola-Ila, J, S Takaki, JD Kerner, and RM Perlmutter. 1997. Differential signaling by lymphocyte antigen receptors. *Annu. Rev. Immunol.* **15:**125.

Ashton-Rickhardt, PG, A Bandeira, JR Delaney, L Van Kaer, HP Pircher, RM Zinkernagel, and S Tonegawa. 1994. Evidence for a differential avidity model of T-cell selection in the thymus. *Cell* **74:**577.

Boise, L, et al. 1995. CD28 co-stimulation can promote T-cell survival by enhancing the expression of Bcl-X_L. *Immunity* **3:**87.

Cantrell, D. 1996. T-cell antigen receptor signal-transduction pathways. *Annu. Rev. Immunol.* **14:**259.

Chambers, CA, JP Allison. 1997. Co-stimulation in T-cell response. *Curr. Opin. Immunol.* **9:**396.

Chien, Y-H, R Jores, MP Crowley. 1996. Recognition by gamma/delta T cells. *Annu. Rev. Immunol.* **14:**511.

Clipstone, NA, and GR Crabtree. 1992. Identification of calcineurin as a key signaling enzyme in T-lymphocyte activation. *Nature* **357:**695.

Dorshkind, K. 1994. Transcriptional control points during lymphopoiesis. *Cell* **79:**751.

Drappa, MD, AK Vaishnaw, KE Sullivan, BS Chu, and KB Elkon. 1996. *Fas* gene mutations in the Canale-Smith syndrome, an inherited lymphoproliferative disorder associated with autoimmunity. *New England Journal of Medicine* **335:**1643.

Dutton, RW, LM Bradley, and SL Swain. 1998. T-cell memory. *Annu. Rev. Immunol.* **16:**201.

Fowlkes, BJ, and E Schweighoffer. 1995. Positive selection of T cells. *Curr. Opin. Immunol.* **7:**188.

Hatada, MH, et al. 1995. Molecular basis for interaction of the protein tyrosine kinase ZAP-70 with the T-cell receptor. *Nature* **377:**32.

Herman, A, JW Kappler, P Marrack, and AM Pullen. 1991. Superantigens: mechanism of T-cell stimulation and role in immune responses. *Annu. Rev. Immunol.* **9:**745.

Hoquist, KA, SC Jameson, WR Heath, JL Howard, MJ Bevan, and FR Carbane. 1994. T-cell receptor antagonist peptides induce positive selection. *Cell* **76:**17.

Jameson, SC, and MJ Bevan. 1995. T-cell receptor antagonists and partial agonists. *Immunity* **2:**1.

Lanzavecchia, A, G Lezzi, and A Viola. 1999. From TCR engagement to T-cell activation: a kinetic view of T-cell behavior. *Cell* **96:**1.

Neel, BG. 1997. Role of phosphatases in lymphocyte activation. *Curr. Opin. Immunol.* **9:**405.

O'Keefe, SJ, et al. 1992. FK506- and CsA-sensitive activation of the interleukin-2 promoter by calcineurin. *Nature* **357:**692.

Okumura, M, and M Thomas. 1995. Regulation of immune function by protein tyrosine phosphatases. *Curr. Opin. Immunol.* **7:**312.

Osborne, BA. 1996. Apoptosis and maintenance of homeostasis in the immune system. *Curr. Opin. Immunol.* **8:**245.

Owen, JJT, and NC Moore. 1995. Thymocyte–stromal-cell interactions and T-cell selection. *Immunol. Today* **16:**336.

Saito, T. 1998. Negative regulation of T-cell activation. *Curr. Opin. Immunol.* **10:**313.

Schreiber, SL, and GR Crabtree. 1992. The mechanism of action of cyclosporin A and FK506. *Immunol. Today* **13:**136.

Shortman, K, and L Wu. 1996. Early lymphocyte progenitors. *Annu. Rev. Immunol.* **14:**29.

Sigal, NH, and FJ Dumont. 1992. Cyclosporin A, FK506, and rapamycin: pharmacologic probes of lymphocyte signal transduction. *Annu. Rev. Immunol.* **10:**519.

Sloan-Lancaster, J, and PM Allen. 1995. Significance of T-cell stimulation by altered peptide ligands in T-cell biology. *Curr. Opin. Immunol.* **7:**103.

Sprent, J. 1997. Immunological memory. *Curr. Opin. Immunol.* **9:**371.

Sprent, J, and SR Webb. 1995. Intrathymic and extrathymic clonal deletion of T cells. *Curr. Opin. Immunol.* **7:**196.

Vaishnaw, AK, JR Orlinick, JL Chu, PH Krammer, MV Chao, and KB Elkon. 1999. The molecular basis for apoptotic defects in patients with CD95 (Fas/Apo-1) mutations. *Journal of Clinical Investigation* **103:**355.

Von Boehmer, H. 1994. Positive selection of lymphocytes. *Cell* **76:**219.

Webb, SR, and NRJ Gascoigne. 1994. T-cell activation by superantigens. *Curr. Opin. Immunol.* **6:**467.

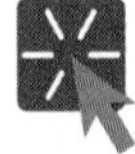

Useful Web Sites

<http://www.ncbi.nlm.nih.gov/Omim/>
<http://www.ncbi.nlm.nih.gov/htbinpost/Omim/getmim>
The Online Mendelian Inheritance in Man Web site contains a subsite that lists ten different inherited diseases that are associated with defects in the TCR complex or associated proteins. Any one of those listed may be studied in detail by following the links in this database.

<http://www.ultranet.com/~jkimball/BiologyPages/A/Apoptosis.html>
<http://www.ultranet.com/~jkimball/BiologyPages/B/B_and_Tcells.html>
These subsites of John Kimball's Biology Pages Web site provide a clear introduction to the bare fundamentals of T-cell biology and a good basic discussion of apoptosis.

<http://www.bioscience.org/knockout/knochome.htm>
Within the Frontiers in Bioscience Database of Gene Knockouts, one can find information on the effects of knockouts of many genes of significance to the development and function of cells of the T lineage.

STUDY QUESTIONS

1. You have a $CD8^+$ CTL clone (from an H-2^k mouse) that has a T-cell receptor specific for the H-Y antigen. You clone the αβ TCR genes from this clone and use them to prepare transgenic mice with the H-2^k or H-2^d haplotype.

Go to www.whfreeman.com/immunology **Self-Test**
Review and quiz of key terms

a. How can you distinguish the immature thymocytes from the mature CD8$^+$ thymocytes in the transgenic mice?

b. For each transgenic mouse listed in the table below, indicate whether the mouse would (+) or would not (−) have immature double-positive and mature CD8$^+$ thymocytes bearing the transgenic T-cell receptor.

Transgenic mouse	Immature thymocytes	Mature CD8$^+$ thymocytes
H-2^k female		
H-2^k male		
H-2^d female		
H-2^d male		

c. Explain your answers for the H-2^k transgenics.

d. Explain your answers for the H-2^d transgenics.

2. Cyclosporin A is a powerful immunosuppressive drug that now is given to transplant recipients. Describe how this drug suppresses the immune response.

3. Antigenic activation of T_H cells leads to the release or induction of various nuclear factors that activate gene transcription.

a. Which two transcription factors required for proliferation of activated T_H cells are present in the cytoplasm of resting T_H cells in inactive forms?

b. Once in the nucleus, what might these transcription factors do?

4. You have fluorescein-labeled anti-CD4 and rhodamine-labeled anti-CD8. You use these antibodies to stain thymocytes and lymph-node cells from normal mice and from RAG-1 knockout mice. In the diagrams below, draw the FACS plots that you would expect.

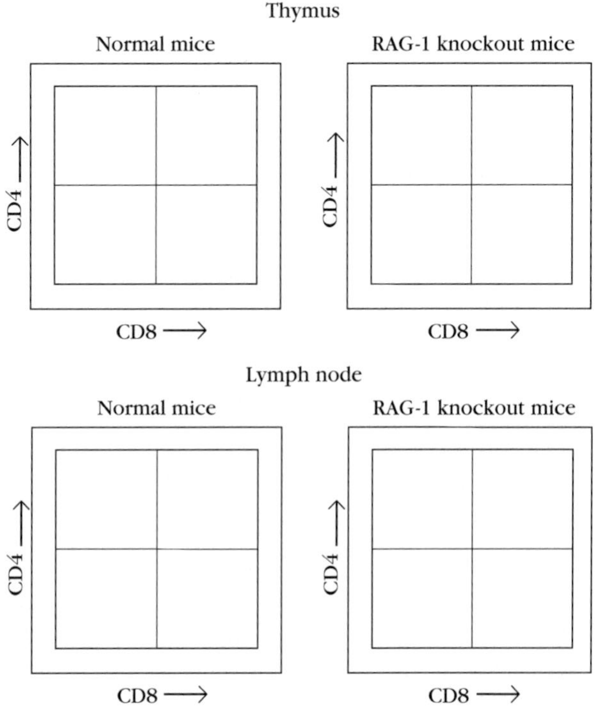

5. In order to demonstrate positive thymic selection experimentally, researchers analyzed the thymocytes from H-2^b mice, which have a deletion of the class II *IE* gene, and from H-2^b mice in which the class II *IA* gene had been knocked out.

a. What MHC molecules would you find on antigen-presenting cells from the normal H-2^b mice?

b. What MHC molecules would you find on antigen-presenting cells from the IA knockout H-2^b mice?

c. Would you expect to find CD4$^+$ T cells, CD8$^+$ T cells, or both in each type of mouse? Why?

6. In his classic chimeric-mouse experiments, Zinkernagel took bone marrow from mouse 1 and a thymus from mouse 2 and transplanted them into mouse 3, which was thymectomized and lethally irradiated. He then challenged the reconstituted mouse with LCM virus and removed its spleen cells. These spleen cells were then incubated with LCM-infected target cells with different MHC haplotypes, and the lysis of the target cells was monitored. The results of two such experiments using H-2^b strain C57BL/6 mice and H-2^d strain BALB/c mice are shown in the table on the facing page.

a. What was the haplotype of the thymus-donor strain in experiment A and experiment B?

b. Why were the H-2^b target cells not lysed in experiment A but were lysed in experiment B?

c. Why were the H-2^k target cells not lysed in either experiment?

7. Fill in the blank(s) in each statement below (a–k) with the most appropriate term(s) from the following list. Terms may be used once, more than once, or not at all.

protein phosphatase(s)	CD8	Class I MHC	CD45
protein kinase(s)	CD4	Class II MHC	B7
phospholipase(s)	CD28	IL-2	IL-6

a. Fyn and ZAP-70 are ___________ .

b. ___________ is a T-cell membrane protein that has cytosolic domains with phosphatase activity.

c. Dendritic cells express ___________ constitutively, whereas B cells must be activated before they express this membrane molecule.

d. Calcineurin, a ___________, is involved in generating the active form of the transcription factor NF-AT.

e. Activation of T_H cells results in secretion of ___________ and expression of its receptor, leading to proliferation and differentiation.

f. The co-stimulatory signal needed for complete T_H-cell activation is triggered by interaction of ___________ on the T cell and ___________ on the APC.

g. Knockout mice lacking class I MHC molecules fail to produce thymocytes bearing ___________ .

h. Macrophages must be activated before they express ___________ molecules and ___________ molecules.

i. T cells bearing ___________ are absent from the lymph nodes of knockout mice lacking class II MHC molecules.

j. PIP_2 is split by a ___________ to yield DAG and IP_3.

For use with Question 6:

Experiment	Bone-marrow donor	Thymectomized, x-irradiated recipient	Lysis of LCM-infected target cells		
			$H\text{-}2^d$	$H\text{-}2^k$	$H\text{-}2^b$
A	C57BL/6 × BALB/c	C57BL/6 × BALB/c	+	–	–
B	C57BL/6 × BALB/c	C57BL/6 × BALB/c	–	–	+

k. In activated T_H cells, DAG activates a ____________, which acts to generate the transcription factor NF-κB.

8. You wish to determine the percentage of various types of thymocytes in a sample of cells from mouse thymus using the indirect immunofluorescence method.

a. You first stain the sample with goat anti-CD3 (primary antibody) and then with rabbit FITC-labeled anti-goat Ig (secondary antibody), which emits a green color. Analysis of the stained sample by flow cytometry indicates that 70% of the cells are stained. Based on this result, how many of the thymus cells in your sample are expressing antigen-binding receptors on their surface? Explain your answer. What are the remaining unstained cells likely to be?

b. You then separate the $CD3^+$ cells with the fluorescent-activated cell sorter (FACS) and restain them. In this case, the primary antibody is hamster anti-CD4 and the secondary antibody is rabbit PE-labeled anti-hamster-Ig, which emits a red color. Analysis of the stained $CD3^+$ cells shows that 80% of them are stained. From this result, can you determine how many T_C cells are present in this sample? If you can, then how many T_C cells are there? If you cannot, what additional experiment would you perform in order to determine the number of T_C cells that are present?

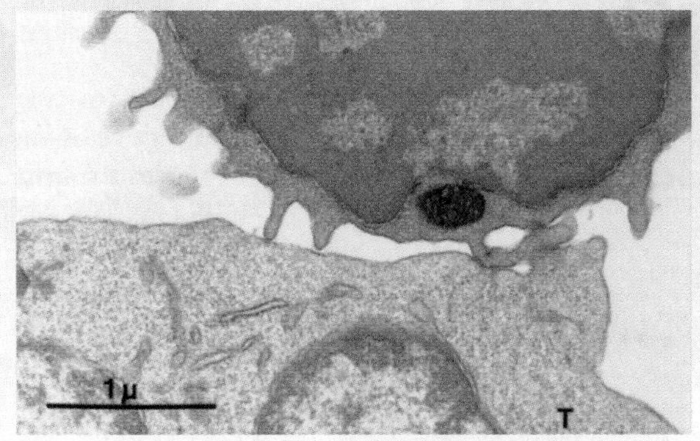

CHAPTER 11
B-CELL GENERATION, ACTIVATION, AND DIFFERENTIATION

The developmental process that results in production of plasma cells and memory B cells can be divided into three broad stages: generation of mature, immunocompetent B cells (maturation), activation of mature B cells when they interact with antigen, and differentiation of activated B cells into plasma cells and memory B cells. In many vertebrates, including humans and mice, the bone marrow generates B cells. This process is an orderly sequence of Ig-gene rearrangements, which progresses in the absence of antigen. This is the antigen-independent phase of B-cell development.

A mature B cell leaves the bone marrow expressing membrane-bound immunoglobulin (mIgM and mIgD) with a single antigenic specificity. These **naive B cells**, which have not encountered antigen, circulate in the blood and lymph and are carried to the secondary lymphoid organs, most notably the spleen and lymph nodes (see Chapter 2). If a B cell is activated by the antigen specific to its membrane-bound antibody, the cell proliferates (clonal expansion) and differentiates to generate a population of antibody-secreting plasma cells and memory B cells. In this activation stage, **affinity maturation** is the progressive increase in the average affinity of the antibodies produced and **class switching** is the change in the isotype of the antibody produced by the B cell from μ to γ, α, or ϵ. Since B cell activation and differentiation in the periphery require antigen, this stage comprises the antigen-dependent phase of B-cell development.

Many B cells are produced in the bone marrow throughout life, but very few of these cells mature. In mice, the size of the recirculating pool of B cells is about 2×10^8 cells. Most of these cells circulate as naive B cells, which have short life spans (half lives of less than 3 days to about 8 weeks) if they fail to encounter antigen. Given that the immune system is able to generate a total antibody diversity that approaches 10^{11}, clearly only a small fraction of this potential repertoire is displayed at any time by membrane immunoglobulin on recirculating B cells. Indeed, throughout the life span of an animal, only a small fraction of the possible antibody diversity is ever generated.

Some aspects of B-cell developmental processes have been described in previous chapters. The overall pathway, beginning with the earliest distinctive B-lineage cell, is described in sequence in this chapter. Figure 11-1 presents an overview of the major events in humans and mice. Most of this chapter applies to humans and mice, but important departures from these developmental pathways may occur in some other vertebrates. Finally, this chapter will consider recent evidence concerning the regulation of B-cell development at various stages.

B-Cell Maturation

The generation of mature B cells first occurs in the embryo and continues throughout life. Before birth, the yolk sac, fetal liver, and fetal bone marrow are the major sites of B-cell maturation; after birth, generation of mature B cells occurs in the bone marrow.

VISUALIZING CONCEPTS

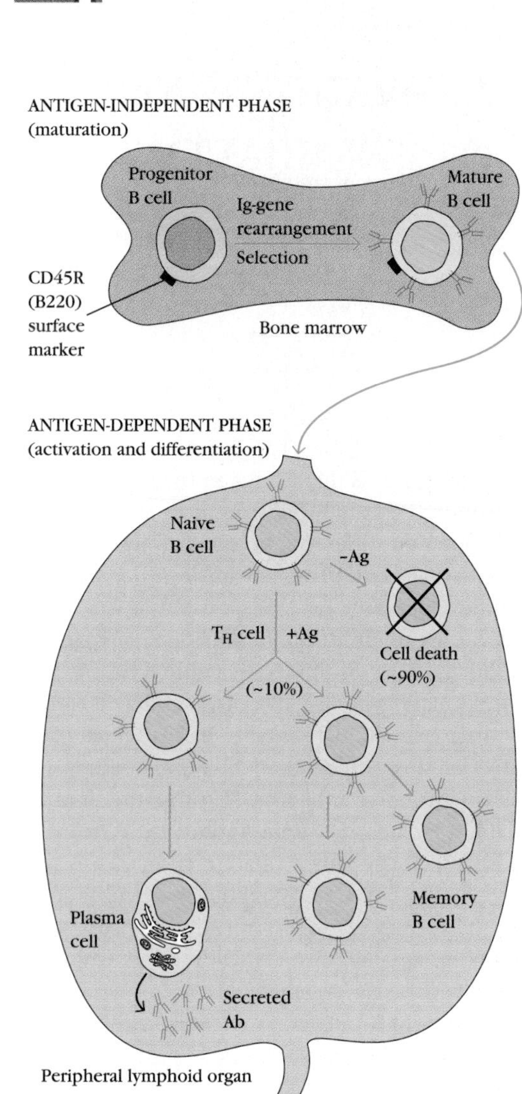

FIGURE 11-1 Overview of B-cell development. During the antigen-independent maturation phase, immunocompetent B cells expressing membrane IgM and IgD are generated in the bone marrow. Only about 10% of the potential B cells reach maturity and exit the bone marrow. In the absence of antigen-induced activation, naive B cells in the periphery die within a few days. In the presence of soluble protein antigen and activated T_H cells, B cells are activated and proliferate within secondary lymphoid organs. Those bearing high-affinity mIg differentiate into plasma cells and memory B cells, which may express different isotypes because of class switching. The numbers cited refer to B-cell development in the mouse, but the overall principles apply to humans as well.

Bone-Marrow Environment

B-cell development begins as lymphoid stem cells differentiate into the earliest distinctive B-lineage cell—the **progenitor B cell (pro-B cell)**—which expresses a transmembrane tyrosine phosphatase called CD45R (sometimes called B220 in mice). Pro-B cells proliferate within the bone marrow, filling the extravascular spaces between large sinusoids in the shaft of a bone. Proliferation and differentiation of pro-B cells into **precursor B cells (pre-B cells)** requires the microenvironment provided by the bone-marrow stromal cells. If pro-B cells are removed from the bone marrow and cultured in vitro, they will not progress to more mature B-cell stages unless stromal cells are present. The stromal cells play two important roles: they interact directly with pro-B and pre-B cells, and they secrete various cytokines, notably, IL-7, that support the developmental process.

At the earliest developmental stage, pro-B cells require direct contact with stromal cells in the bone marrow. This interaction is mediated by several cell-adhesion molecules, including VLA-4 on the pro-B cell and its ligand, VCAM-1, on the stromal cell (Figure 11-2). After initial contact is made, a receptor on the pro-B cell, called c-Kit, interacts with a stromal-cell surface molecule known as stem-cell factor (SCF). This interaction activates c-Kit, which is a tyrosine kinase, and the pro-B cell begins to divide and differentiate into a pre-B cell and begins expressing a receptor for IL-7. The IL-7 secreted by the stromal cells drives the maturation process, eventually inducing down-regulation of the adhesion molecules on the pre-B cells, so that the proliferating cells can detach from the stromal cells. At this stage, pre-B cells no longer require direct contact with stromal cells but continue to require IL-7 for growth and maturation.

Ig-Gene Rearrangements

B-cell maturation depends on rearrangement of the immunoglobulin DNA in early progenitor cells. The mechanisms of Ig-gene rearrangement were described in Chapter 5. First to occur in the pro-B cell stage is a heavy-chain D_H to J_H gene rearrangement; this is followed by a V_H to D_HJ_H rearrangement (Figure 11-3). If the first heavy-chain rearrangement is not productive, then V_H-D_H-J_H rearrangement continues on the other chromosome. Upon completion of heavy-chain rearrangement the cell is classified as a pre-B cell. Continued development of a pre-B cell into an immature B cell requires a productive light-chain gene rearrangement. Because of allelic exclusion, only one light-chain isotype is expressed on the membrane of a B cell. Completion of a productive light-chain rearrangement commits the now immature B cell to a particular antigenic specificity determined by the cell's heavy-chain VDJ sequence and light-chain VJ sequence. Immature B cells express mIgM (membrane IgM) on the cell surface.

As would be expected, the recombinase enzymes RAG-1 and RAG-2, which are required for both heavy-chain and

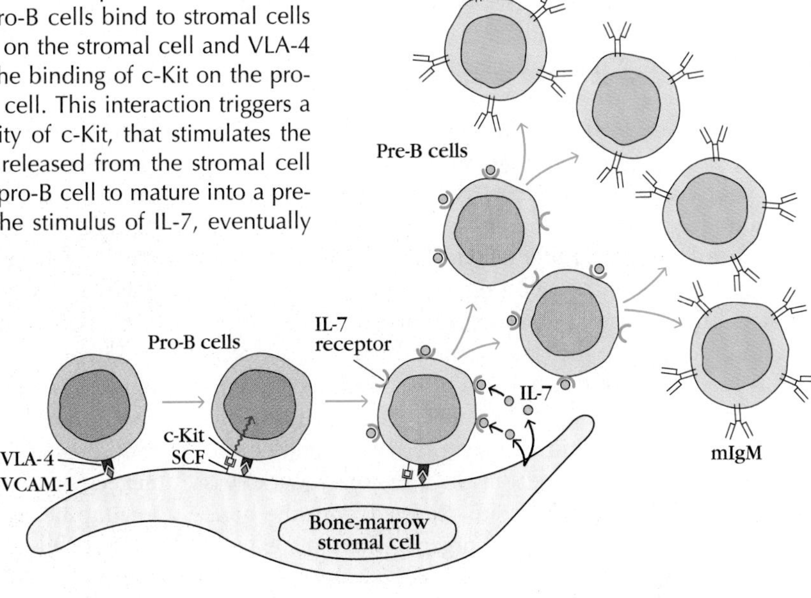

FIGURE 11-2 Bone-marrow stromal cells are required for maturation of progenitor B cells into precursor B cells. Pro-B cells bind to stromal cells by means of an interaction between VCAM-1 on the stromal cell and VLA-4 on the pro-B cell. This interaction promotes the binding of c-Kit on the pro-B cell to stem cell factor (SCF) on the stromal cell. This interaction triggers a signal, mediated by the tyrosine kinase activity of c-Kit, that stimulates the pro-B cell to express receptors for IL-7. IL-7 released from the stromal cell then binds to the IL-7 receptors, inducing the pro-B cell to mature into a pre-B cell. Pre-B cells begin proliferating under the stimulus of IL-7, eventually differentiating into immature B cells.

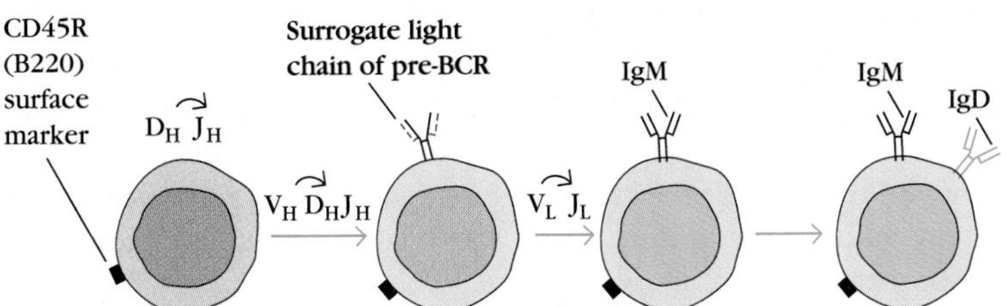

	PRO-B CELL	PRE-B CELL	IMMATURE B CELL	MATURE B CELL
H-chain genes	D_HJ_H	$V_HD_HJ_H$	$V_HD_HJ_H$	$V_HD_HJ_H$
L-chain genes	Surrogate Vpre-B and λ5 Germ-line κ and λ	Surrogate Vpre-B and λ5 Germ-line κ and λ	V_LJ_L	V_LJ_L
RAG-1/2	+	+	–	–
TdT	+	–	–	–
Membrane Ig				
Heavy chain	–	μ	μ	μ + δ
Light chain	Surrogate light chain	Surrogate light chain	κ or λ	κ or λ
Transcription factors	BSAP, E2A, EBF Sox-4	BSAP, EBF, Sox-4	BSAP, Sox-4	BSAP
Surface markers	CD19, HSA (CD24), CD43, CD45R, cKit, Ig-α:Ig-β	CD19, HSA (CD24), CD25, CD45R, Ig-α:Ig-β, pre-BCR	CD19, HSA (CD24), CD45R, Ig-α:Ig-β, mIgM	CD19, CD23, HSA (CD24), CD45R, Ig-α:Ig-β, mIgD, mIgM

FIGURE 11-3 Sequence of events and characteristics of the stages in B-cell maturation in the bone marrow. The pre-B cell expresses a membrane immunoglobulin consisting of a heavy (H) chain and surrogate light chains, Vpre-B and λ5. Changes in the RNA processing of heavy-chain transcripts following the pre-B cell stage lead to synthesis of both membrane-bound IgM and IgD by mature B cells. RAG-1/2 = two enzymes encoded by recombination-activating genes; TdT = terminal deoxyribonucleotidyl transferase. A number of transcription factors are important at various stages of B-cell development, some of which are indicated here.

light-chain gene rearrangements, are expressed during the pro-B and pre-B cell stages (see Figure 11-3). The enzyme terminal deoxyribonucleotidyl transferase (TdT), which catalyzes insertion of N-nucleotides at the D_H-J_H and V_H-D_H-J_H coding joints, is active during the pro-B cell stage and ceases to be active early in the pre–B-cell stage. Because TdT expression is turned off during the part of the pre–B-cell stage when light-chain rearrangement occurs, N-nucleotides are not found in the V_L-J_L coding joints.

Further development of immature B cells leads to the coexpression of IgD and IgM on the membrane, which characterizes mature B cells. This progression involves a change in RNA processing of the heavy-chain primary transcript to permit production of two mRNAs, one encoding the membrane form of the μ chain and the other encoding the membrane form of the δ chain (see Figure 5-19). In addition to IgM, the earliest mature cells in the bone marrow express low levels of IgD. These cells are exported from the bone marrow to peripheral lymphoid organs, where the expression of membrane IgD increases.

Pre–B-Cell Receptor

As we saw in Chapter 10, during one stage in T-cell development, the β chain of the T-cell receptor associates with pre-Tα to form the pre–T-cell receptor (see Figure 10-1). A parallel situation occurs during B-cell development. In the pre-B cell the membrane μ chain is associated with an unusual light-chain complex called the **surrogate light chain.** This complex consists of two proteins: a V-like sequence called **Vpre-B** and a C-like sequence called **λ5,** which associate noncovalently to form a light-chain–like structure. The genes encoding Vpre-B and λ5 are located at an unknown distance from the λ light-chain genes in mouse and human DNA.

The surrogate light chain appears on the pre-B cell as a complex consisting of the membrane-bound μ heavy chain and surrogate light chain associated with the Ig-α/Ig-β heterodimer to form the **pre–B-cell receptor** (Figure 11-4). Only pre-B cells that are able to express membrane-bound μ heavy chains in association with surrogate light chains are able to proceed along the maturation pathway.

There is speculation that the pre–B-cell receptor recognizes a not-yet-identified ligand on the stromal-cell membrane, thereby transmitting a signal to the pre-B cell that prevents V_H to D_HJ_H rearrangement of the other heavy-chain allele, thus leading to allelic exclusion. Following the establishment of an effective pre-B cell receptor, each pre-B cell undergoes multiple cell divisions, producing 32 to 64 descendants. Each of these progeny pre-B cells may then rearrange different light-chain gene segments, thereby increasing the overall diversity of the antibody repertoire.

The critical role of the pre-B cell receptor was demonstrated with knockout mice in which the gene encoding the λ5 protein of the receptor was disrupted. B-cell development in these mice was shown to be blocked at the pre-B stage, which suggests that a signal generated through the receptor is necessary for pre-B cells to proceed to the immature B-cell stage.

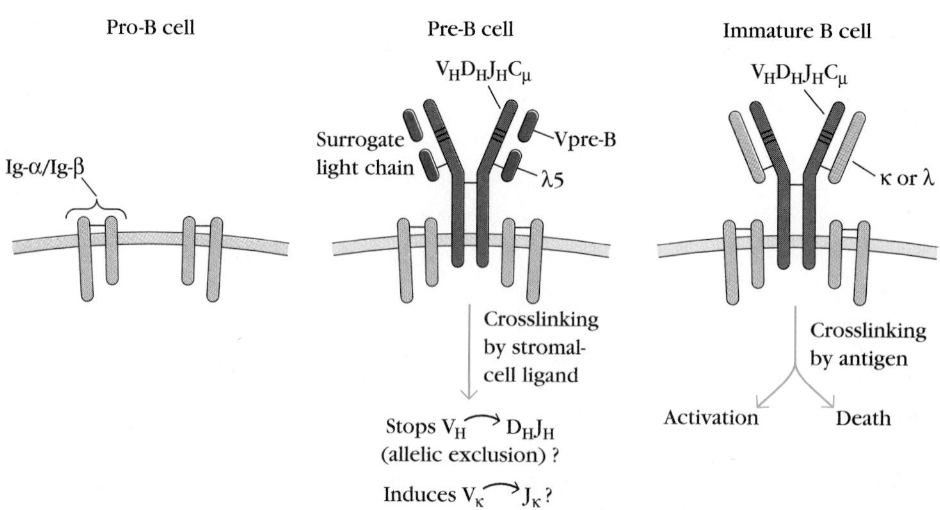

FIGURE 11-4 Schematic diagram of sequential expression of membrane immunoglobulin and surrogate light chain at different stages of B-cell differentiation in the bone marrow. The pre–B-cell receptor contains a surrogate light chain consisting of a Vpre-B polypeptide and a λ5 polypeptide, which are noncovalently associated. The immature B cell no longer expresses the surrogate light chain and instead expresses the κ or λ light chain together with the μ heavy chain.

Transcription-Factor Activity

As we have seen in Chapter 2, many different transcription factors act in the development of hematopoietic cells. Nearly a dozen of them have so far been shown to play roles in B-cell development. Experiments in which particular transcription factors are "knocked out" by gene disruption have shown that four such factors, **E2A, early B-cell factor (EBF), B-cell-specific activator protein (BSAP),** and **Sox-4** are particularly important for B-cell development (see Figure 11-3). Mice that lack E2A do not express RAG-1, are unable to make D_HJ_H rearrangements, and fail to express λ5, a critical component of the surrogate light chain. A similar pattern is seen in EBF-deficient mice. These findings point to important roles for both of these transcription factors early in B-cell development, and they may play essential roles in the early stages of commitment to the B-cell lineage. Knocking out the ***Pax-5*** gene, whose product is the transcription factor BSAP, also results in the arrest of B-cell development at an early stage. Binding sites for BSAP are found in the promoter regions of a number of B-cell-specific genes, including *Vpre-B* and *λ5*, in a number of Ig switch regions, and in the Ig heavy-chain enhancer. This indicates that BSAP plays a role beyond the early stages of B-cell development. This factor is also expressed in the central nervous system, and its absence results in severe defects in mid-brain development. Although the exact site of action of Sox-4 is not known, it affects early stages of B cell activation. While Figure 11-3 shows that all of these transcription factors affect development at an early stage, some of them are active at later stages too.

Cell-Surface Markers

The developmental progression from progenitor to mature B cell is typified by a changing pattern of surface markers (see Figure 11-3). At the pro-B stage, the cells do not display the heavy or light chains of antibody but they do express CD45R, which is a form of the protein tyrosine phophatase found on leukocytes, and the signal-transducing molecules Ig-α and Ig-β, which are found in association with the membrane forms of antibody in later stages of B-cell development. Pro-B cells also express CD19 (part of the B-cell coreceptor), CD43 (leukosialin), and CD24, a molecule also known as heat-stable antigen (HSA) on the surface. At this stage, c-Kit, a receptor for a growth-factor-promoting ligand present on stromal cells, is also found on the surface of pro-B cells. As cells progress from the pro-B to the pre-B stage, they express many of the same markers that were present during the pro-B stage; however, they cease to express c-Kit and CD43 and begin to express CD25, the α chain of the IL-2 receptor. The display of the pre–B-cell receptor (pre-BCR) is a salient feature of the pre-B cell stage. After rearrangement of the light chain, surface immunoglobulin containing both heavy and light chains appears, and the cells, now classified as immature B cells, lose the pre-BCR and no longer express CD25. The developmental process that produces naive mature B cells for export to the periphery is completed when the IgD class of Ig joins IgM on the cell surface. Since there are monoclonal antibodies available that can recognize all of these antigenic markers, it is possible to recognize the various stages of B-cell development by the techniques of immunohistology and flow cytometry described in Chapter 6. In fact, with the capacity of flow cytometers to sort cells with different fluorescent characteristics, it is possible even to isolate B-cell populations at specific stages of differentiation.

B-1 and B-2 β Cells

There is a subset of B cells, called B-1 B cells, that arise before B-2 B cells, the major group of B cells in humans and mice. In humans and mice, B-1 B cells appear during fetal life, express surface IgM but little or no IgD and are marked by the display of CD5. However, CD5 is apparently not an indispensable component of the B-1 lineage, it does not appear on the B-1 cells of rats, and mice that lack a functional CD5 gene still produce B-1 cells. In animals whose B-2 B cells are the major B-cell population, B-1 cells are minor populations in such secondary tissues as lymph nodes and spleen. Despite their scarcity in many lymphoid sites, they are the major B-cell type found in the peritoneum.

Although there is not a great deal of definitive information on the function of B-1 cells, several features set them apart from the B-2 B cells of humans and mice. During fetal life, B-1 cells arise from stem cells in bone marrow. However, in postnatal life this population renews itself by the proliferation of some B-1 cells in sites outside the bone marrow to form additional naive B-1 cells. The B-1 population responds poorly to protein antigens but much better to carbohydrate ones. Most of its members are IgM-bearing cells, and this population undergoes much less somatic hypermutation and class switching than the B-2 set of B cells does. Consequently, the antibodies produced by a high proportion of B-1 cells are of rather low affinity. Finally, many chronic lymphocytic leukemias (CLLs) arise from the B-1 subset. The reasons for this are not known.

Selection of Immature Self-Reactive B Cells

It is estimated that in mice the bone marrow produces about 5×10^7 B cells/day but only 5×10^6 (or about 10%) actually are recruited into the recirculating B-cell pool. This means that 90% of the B cells produced each day die without ever leaving the bone marrow. Some of this loss is attributable to **negative selection** and subsequent elimination **(clonal deletion)** of immature B cells that express auto-antibodies against self-antigens in the bone marrow.

Negative Selection

It has long been established that the crosslinkage of mIgM on immature B cells can cause the cells to die within the bone marrow. This has been demonstrated experimentally by treating immature B cells with antibody against the μ constant region. This treatment causes crosslinking of mIgM molecules and results in the death of the immature B cells by apoptosis. A similar process is thought to occur in vivo when immature B cells that express self-reactive mIgM bind to self-antigens in the bone marrow.

Experiments with transgenic mice have revealed that, when immature B cells encounter self-antigens within the bone marrow, they die, presumably by apoptosis. For example, D. A. Nemazee and K. Burki introduced a transgene encoding the heavy and light chains of an IgM antibody specific for K^k, an H-2^k class I MHC molecule, into H-2^d and into H-$2^{d/k}$ mice (Figure 11-5a,b). Since class I MHC mol-

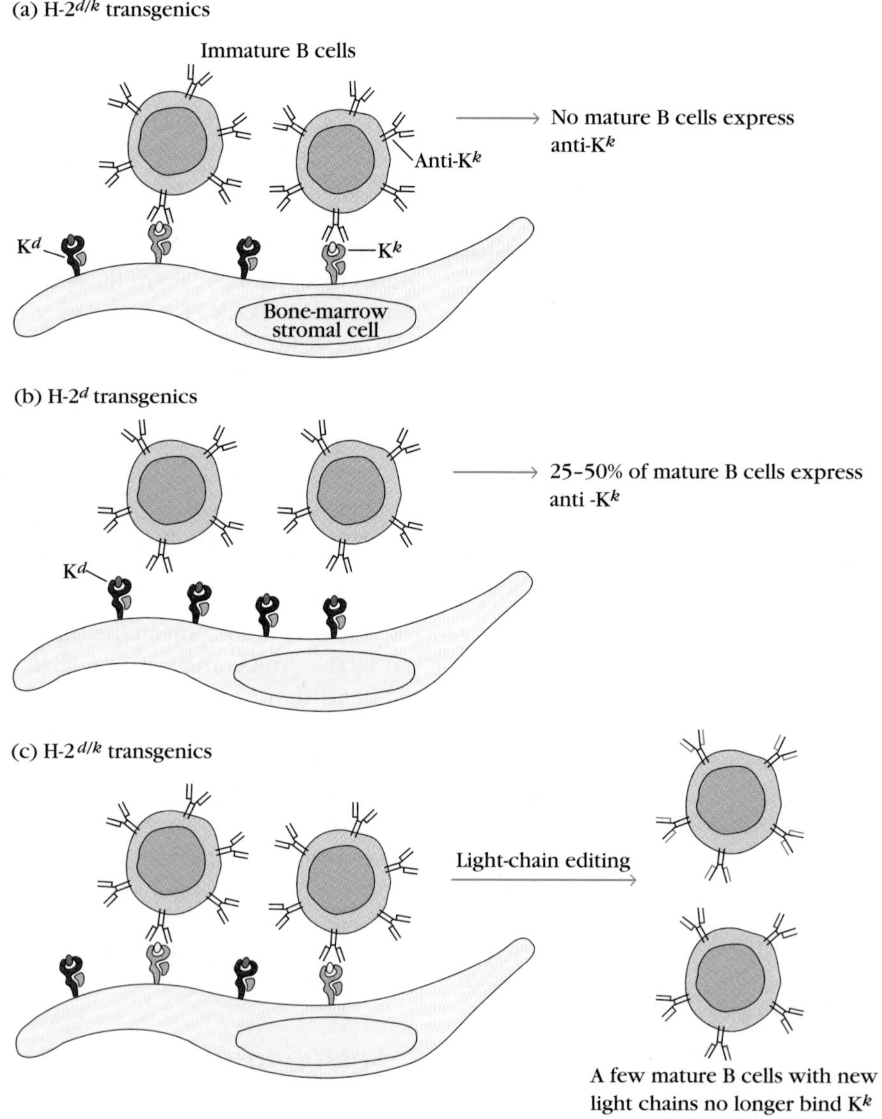

FIGURE 11-5 Experimental evidence for negative selection (clonal deletion) of self-reactive B cells during maturation in the bone marrow. The presence or absence of mature peripheral B cells expressing a transgene-encoded IgM against the H-2 class I molecule K^k was determined in H-$2^{d/k}$ mice (a) and H-2^d mice (b). In the H-$2^{d/k}$ transgenics, the immature B cells recognized the self-antigen K^k and were deleted by negative selection. In the H-2^d transgenics, the immature B cells did not bind to a self-antigen and consequently went on to mature, so that 25%–50% of the splenic B cells expressed the transgene-encoded anti-K^k as membrane Ig. More detailed analysis of the H-$2^{d/k}$ transgenics revealed a few peripheral B cells that expressed the transgene-encoded μ chain but a different light chain (c). Apparently, a few immature B cells underwent light-chain editing, so they no longer bound the K^k molecule and consequently escaped negative selection. [Adapted from DA Nemazee and K Burki, 1989, *Nature* **337:** 562; SL Tiegs et al, 1993, *JEM* **177:**1009.]

TABLE 11-1 EXPRESSION OF TRANSGENE ENCODING IgM ANTIBODY TO H-2^k CLASS I MHC MOLECULES

Experimental animal	Number of animals tested	Expression of transgene	
		As membrane Ab	As secreted Ab (μg/ml)
Nontransgenics	13	(−)	<0.3
H-2^d transgenics	7	(+)	93.0
H-2$^{d/k}$ transgenics	6	(−)	<0.3

SOURCE: Adapted from DA Nemazee and K Burki, 1989, *Nature* **337**:562.

ecules are expressed on the membrane of all nucleated cells, the endogenous H-2^k and H-2^d class I MHC molecules would be present on bone-marrow stromal cells in the transgenic mice. In the H-2^d mice, which do not express K^k, 25%–50% of the mature, peripheral B cells expressed the transgene-encoded anti-K^k both as a membrane antibody and as secreted antibody. In contrast, in the H-2$^{d/k}$ mice, which express K^k, no mature, peripheral B cells expressed the transgene-encoded antibody to H-2^k (Table 11-1). These results suggest that there is negative selection against any immature B cells expressing auto-antibodies on their membranes because these antibodies react with self-antigen (e.g., the K^k molecule in H-2$^{d/k}$ transgenics) present on stromal cells, leading to crosslinking of the antibodies and subsequent death of the immature B cells.

Rescue by Editing of Light-Chain Genes

Later work using the transgenic system described by Nemazee and Burki showed that negative selection of immature B cells does not always result in their immediate deletion (Figure 11-5c). Instead, maturation of the self-reactive cell is arrested while the B cell "edits" its receptor. In this case, the H-2$^{d/k}$ transgenics produced a few mature B cells expressing mIgM containing transgene-encoded μ chains but different, endogenous light chains. This experimental finding suggests that a change in the expression of the light chain can convert self-reactive immature B cells into nonself-reactive cells, thereby rescuing the cells from programmed cell death.

One explanation for these results is that when some immature B cells bind a self-antigen, maturation is arrested; the cells up-regulate RAG-1 and RAG-2 expression and begin further rearrangement of their endogenous light-chain DNA. Some of these cells succeed in replacing the κ light chain of the self-antigen reactive antibody with a λ chain encoded by endogenous λ-chain gene segments. As a result, these cells will begin to express an "edited" mIgM with a different light chain and a specificity that is not self-reactive. Because these cells are no longer self-reactive, they will escape negative selection and leave the bone marrow as mature B cells bearing the edited, nonself-reactive mIgM.

B-Cell Activation and Proliferation

After export of mature B cells from the bone marrow, the subsequent steps in B-cell development—activation, proliferation, and differentiation—occur in the periphery and require antigen. Antigen-driven activation and clonal selection of naive B cells leads to generation of plasma cells and memory B cells. In the absence of antigen-induced activation, naive B cells in the periphery have a short life span, dying within a few weeks by apoptosis (see Figure 11-1).

Thymus-Dependent and Thymus-Independent Antigens

Depending on the nature of the antigen, B-cell activation proceeds by two different routes: one that is dependent upon T_H cells and one that is independent of T_H cells. The B-cell response to **thymus-dependent (TD) antigens** requires direct contact with T_H cells, not simply exposure to T_H-derived cytokines. Antigens that can activate B cells in the absence of this kind of direct participation by T_H cells are known as **thymus-independent (TI) antigens.** TI antigens can be divided into two types, type 1 and type 2, which activate B cells by different mechanisms. Some bacterial cell-wall components, including lipopolysaccharide (LPS), function as *type 1 thymus-independent (TI-1) antigens. Type 2 thymus-independent (TI-2) antigens* are highly repetitious molecules such as polymeric proteins (e.g., bacterial flagellin) or bacterial cell-wall polysaccharides with repeating polysaccharide units.

Most TI-1 antigens are polyclonal B-cell activators (**mitogens);** that is, they are able to activate B cells regardless of their antigenic specificity. At high concentrations, some TI-1 antigens will stimulate proliferation and antibody secretion by as many as one third of all B cells. The mechanism by which TI-1 antigens activate B cells is not understood well. When B cells are exposed to lower concentrations of TI-1 antigens, only those B cells specific for epitopes of the antigen will be activated. These antigens can stimulate antibody production in nude mice (which lack a thymus and

TABLE 11-2 PROPERTIES OF THYMUS-DEPENDENT AND THYMUS-INDEPENDENT ANTIGENS

Property	TD antigens	TI antigens	
		Type 1	Type 2
Chemical nature	Soluble protein	Bacterial cell-wall components (e.g., LPS)	Polymeric protein antigens; capsular polysaccharides
Humoral response			
Isotype switching	Yes	No	Limited
Affinity maturation	Yes	No	No
Immunologic memory	Yes	No	No
Polyclonal activation	No	Yes (high doses)	No

thus are greatly deficient in T cells) and the responses are not greatly augmented by transferring T cells into these athymic mice. Thus, TI-1 antigens are truly T-cell independent. The prototypic TI-1 antigen is **lipopolysaccharide (LPS),** a major component of the cell walls of gram-negative bacteria. At low concentrations, LPS stimulates the production of antibodies specific for LPS. At high concentrations, it is a polyclonal B-cell activator.

TI-2 antigens activate B cells by extensively crosslinking the mIg receptor. However, TI-2 antigens differ from TI-1 antigens in three important respects. First, they are not B-cell mitogens and so do not act as polyclonal activators. Second, TI-1 antigens will activate both mature and immature B cells, but TI-2 antigens activate mature B cells and inactivate immature B cells. Third, although the B-cell response to TI-2 antigens does not require direct involvement of T_H cells, cytokines derived from T_H cells are required for efficient B-cell proliferation and for class switching to isotypes other than IgM. This can be shown by comparing the effect of TI-2 antigens in mice made T-cell-deficient in various ways. In nude mice, which lack thymus-derived T cells but do contain a few T cells that arise from other sites that probably lie in the intestine, TI-2 antigens do elicit B-cell responses. TI-2 antigens do not induce antibody production in mice that cannot express either $\alpha\beta$ or $\gamma\delta$ TCRs because the genes encoding the TCR β and δ chains have been knocked out. Administration of a few T cells to these TCR-knockout mice restores their ability to elicit B-cell responses to TI-2 antigens.

The humoral response to thymus-independent antigens is different from the response to thymus-dependent antigens (Table 11-2). The response to TI antigens is generally weaker, no memory cells are formed, and IgM is the predominant antibody secreted, reflecting a low level of class switching. These differences highlight the important role played by T_H cells in generating memory B cells, affinity maturation, and class switching to other isotypes.

Origin of Activating Signals

Naive, or resting, B cells are nondividing cells in the G_0 stage of the cell cycle. Activation drives the resting cell into the cell cycle, progressing through G_1 into the S phase, in which DNA is replicated. The transition from G_1 to S is a critical restriction point in the cell cycle. Once a cell has reached S, it completes the cell cycle, moving through G_2 and into mitosis (M).

After analyzing the events in the progression of lymphocytes from G_0 to the S phase, Ken Ichi Arai noted a number of similarities with events that had been identified in fibroblast cells. He grouped these events into two categories, competence and progression signals. Competence signals are envisioned as events that drive the B cell from G_0 into early G_1, rendering the cell competent to receive the next level of signals. Progression signals then drive the cell from G_1 into S and ultimately to cell division and differentiation. Competence is not achieved by a single signaling event but rather requires at least two distinct events, which are designated *signal 1* and *signal 2.* These signaling events are generated by different pathways with thymus-independent antigens and thymus-dependent antigens, but both pathways include signals generated when multivalent antigen binds and crosslinks mIg (Figure 11-6). Once the B cell has acquired an effective competence signal in early activation, the interaction of cytokines and possibly other ligands with the B-cell membrane receptors provides progression signals.

Transduction of Activating Signals

For many years, immunologists questioned how engagement of the Ig receptor by antigen could activate intracellular signaling pathways. All isotypes of mIg have very short cytoplasmic tails. Both mIgM and mIgD on B cells extend into the cytoplasm by only three amino acids; the mIgA tail consists of 14 amino acids; and the mIgG and mIgE tails contains 28 amino acids. In each case, the cytoplasmic tail is too short to be able to generate a signal by associating with in-

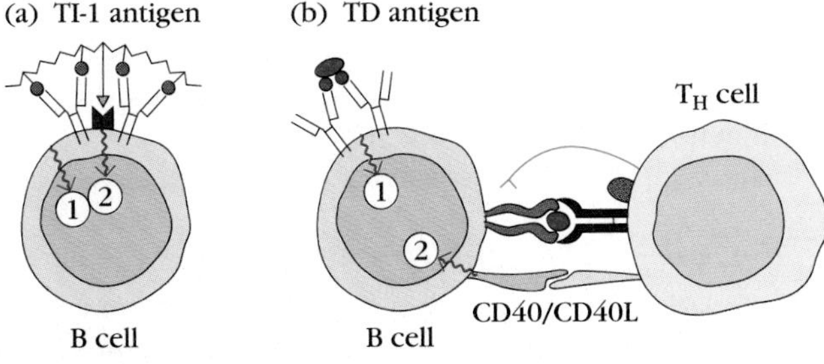

FIGURE 11-6 An effective signal for B-cell activation involves two distinct signals induced by membrane events. Binding of a type 1 thymus-independent (TI-1) antigen to a B cell provides both signals. A thymus-dependent (TD) antigen provides signal 1 by crosslinking mIg, but a separate interaction between CD40 on the B cell and CD40L on an activated T_H cell is required to generate signal 2.

tracellular signaling molecules (e.g., tyrosine kinases and G proteins). The discovery that membrane Ig is associated with the disulfide-linked heterodimer Ig-α/Ig-β, forming the **B-cell receptor (BCR)** solved this longstanding puzzle. Two molecules of the Ig-α/Ig-β heterodimer associate with one mIg to form a single BCR (Figure 11-7). Thus the BCR is functionally divided into the ligand-binding immunoglobulin molecule and the signal-transducing Ig-α/Ig-β heterodimer. A similar functional division marks the pre-BCR, a signal-transduction–capable complex of two Ig-α/Ig-β molecules and μ heavy chains with the Vpre-B/λ5 combination that constitutes the surrogate light chain (see Figure 11-4). The Ig-α chain has a long cytoplasmic tail containing 61 amino acids; the tail of the Ig-β chain contains 48 amino acids. The cytoplasmic tails of both Ig-α and Ig-β contain the 18-residue motif termed the **immunoreceptor tyrosine-based activation motif (ITAM;** see Figure 11-7) which has already been described in several molecules of the T-cell receptor complex (see Figure 10-11). The cytoplasmic tails of Ig-α/Ig-β transduce the stimulus produced by crosslinking of mIg molecules into an effective intracellular signal.

In the BCR and the TCR, as well as in a number of receptors for the Fc regions of particular Ig classes (FcεRI for IgE; FcγRIIA, FcγRIIC, FcγRIIIA for IgG), ligand binding and signal transduction are mediated by a multimeric complex of proteins that is functionally compartmentalized. The ligand-binding portions of these complexes (mIg in the case of the BCR) is on the surface of the cell, and the signal-transducing portion is mostly or wholly within the cell. As is true of the TCR, signaling from the BCR is mediated by protein tyrosine kinases (PTKs). Furthermore, like the TCR, the BCR itself has no PTK activity; this activity is acquired by

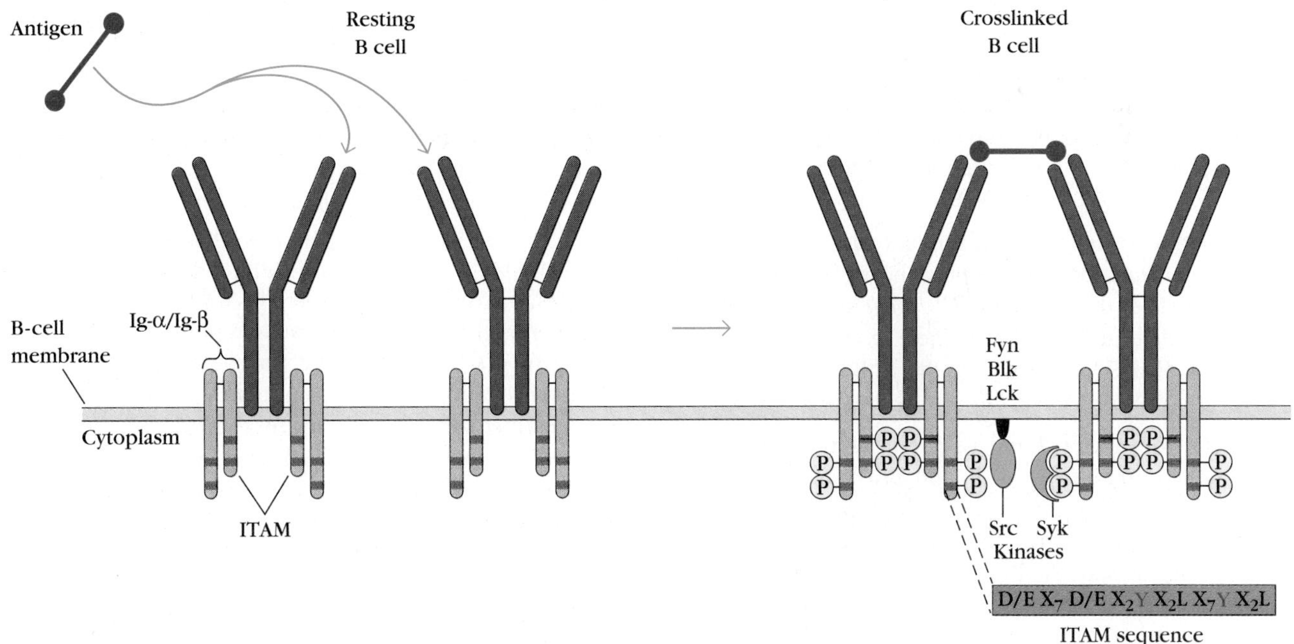

FIGURE 11-7 The initial stages of signal transduction by an activated B-cell receptor (BCR). The BCR comprises an antigen-binding mIg and two signal-transducing Ig-α/Ig-β heterodimers. Following antigen crosslinkage of the BCR, the immunoreceptor tyrosine-based activation motifs (ITAMs) interact with several members of the Src family of tyrosine kinases (Fyn, Blk, and Lck), activating the kinases. The activated enzymes phosphorylate tyrosine residues on the cytoplasmic tails of the Ig-α/Ig-β heterodimer, creating docking sites for Syk kinase, which is then also activated. The highly conserved sequence motif of ITAMs is shown with the tyrosines (Y) in blue. D/E indicates that an aspartate or a glutamate can appear at the indicated position, and X indicates that the position can be occupied by any amino acid.

recruitment of a number of different kinases, from nearby locations within the cell, to the cytoplasmic tails of the signal. Phosphorylation of tyrosines within the ITAM of BCRs is among the earliest events in B-cell activation and plays a central role in bringing critical PTKs to the BCR. With their association, the BCR is able to initiate a number of signaling cascades that ultimately result in the cell's responses to the crosslinking of its surface immunoglobulin by antigen. Figure 11-8 shows some of the important changes that take place within the B cell after the crosslinking of its membrane Ig.

Figure 11-8 shows many parallels between B-cell and T-cell activation. These include:

- *Compartmentalization of function within receptor subunits:* Both the B-cell and T-cell pathways begin with multimeric receptors containing antigen-specific (idiotypic) polypeptides that bind ligand and separate polypeptides that convey signals to the interior. The ligand-binding polypeptide chains have short cytoplasmic tails, but the signaling polypeptides have long cytoplasmic domains that are the signal transducers.
- *Activation by membrane-associated Src protein tyrosine kinases:* The Src PTKs, Lck in T cells and, usually, Lyn in B cells, perform phosphorylations during the early stages of signal transduction that are essential to the formation of a functional receptor signaling complex.
- *Dephosphorylation of key Src protein tyrosine kinases by CD45:* This tyrosine phosphatase performs the important function of removing an inhibitory phosphate from a tyrosine in the C-terminal regions of Lck, Lyn, and other PTKs.
- *Assembly of a large signaling complex with protein-tyrosine-kinase activity:* The phosphorylated tyrosines in the ITAMs of the BCR and TCR provide docking sites for the molecules that endow these receptors with PTK activity; ZAP-70 in T cells and Syk in B cells.
- *The recruitment of other signal-transduction pathways:* Signals from the BCR and TCR result in the production of the second messengers IP_3 and DAG. One of these, IP_3, causes the release of Ca^{2+} from intracellular stores, and the other, DAG, activates PKC. A third important signaling pathway, the Ras pathway, is also activated by signals received through the TCR or BCR.
- *Changes in gene expression:* One of the important outcomes of many signal-transduction processes set in motion with engagement of the BCR or the TCR is the generation of active transcription factors, which stimulate or inhibit the transcription of specific genes in the nucleus. For those transcription factors that reside in the cytoplasm until they are activated, the activation step includes translocation to the nucleus.

Go to www.whfreeman.com/immunology Animation
Signal Transduction

Failures in signal transduction can have severe consequences for the immune system. The Clinical Focus on X-linked agammaglobulinemia describes the effect of defective signal transduction on the development of B cells.

B-Cell–Coreceptor Complex

An emerging theme in immunology is that the consequences of stimulation through antigen receptors can be modified significantly by signals through coreceptors. Recall that co-stimulation through CD28 is an essential feature of effective positive stimulation of T lymphocytes, while signaling through CTLA-4 inhibits the response of the T cell. In B cells a component of the B-cell membrane, called the **B-cell coreceptor,** provides stimulatory modifying signals.

The B-cell coreceptor is a complex of three proteins: CD19, CR2 (CD21), and TAPA-1 (CD81) (Figure 11-9). CD19, a member of the immunoglobulin superfamily, has a long cytoplasmic tail and three extracellular Ig-fold domains. The CR2 component is a receptor of C3d, a breakdown product of the complement system; it also functions as a receptor for a membrane molecule and TAPA-1, a transmembrane protein that spans the membrane four times. In addition to the stimulatory coreceptor, another molecule, CD22, which is constitutively associated with the B-cell receptor in resting B cells, delivers a negative signal that makes B-cells more difficult to activate. As shown in Figure 11-9, the CR2 component of the coreceptor complex binds to complement-coated antigen that has been captured by the mIg on the B cell. This crosslinks the coreceptor to the BCR and allows the CD19 component of the coreceptor to interact with the Ig-α/Ig-β component of the BCR. CD19 contains six tyrosine residues in its long cytoplasmic tail and is a major substrate of the protein tyrosine kinase activity that is mediated by crosslinkage of the BCR. Phosphorylation of CD19 permits it to bind a number of signaling molecules, including the protein tyrosine kinase Lyn. The delivery of these signaling molecules to the BCR complex contributes to the activation process, and the coreceptor complex serves to amplify the activating signal transmitted through the BCR. In one experimental in vitro system, for example, 10^4 molecules of mIgM had to be engaged by antigen for B-cell activation to occur when the coreceptor was not involved. But when CD19/CD2/TAPA-1 coreceptor was crosslinked to the BCR, only 10^2 molecules of mIgM had to be engaged for B-cell activation. In a striking experiment, immunization with a hybrid protein in which genetic engineering was used to join hen's egg lysozyme to C3d, highlighted the role played by the complement receptor CR2 in the co-stimulation by the CD19/CD2/TAPA-1 complex. The fusion protein bearing 2 or 3 copies of C3d produced anti-lysozyme responses that were 1000 to 10,000 times greater than those to lysozyme alone. Perhaps coreceptor phenomena such as these and others help explain how naive B cells that often express mIg with low affinity for antigen are able to respond to low

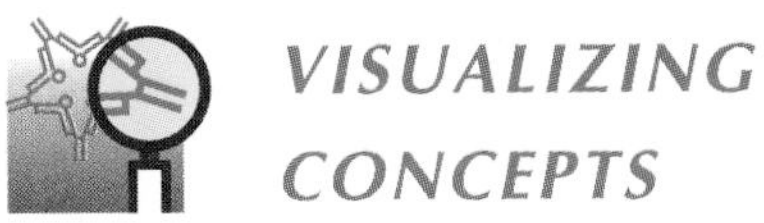

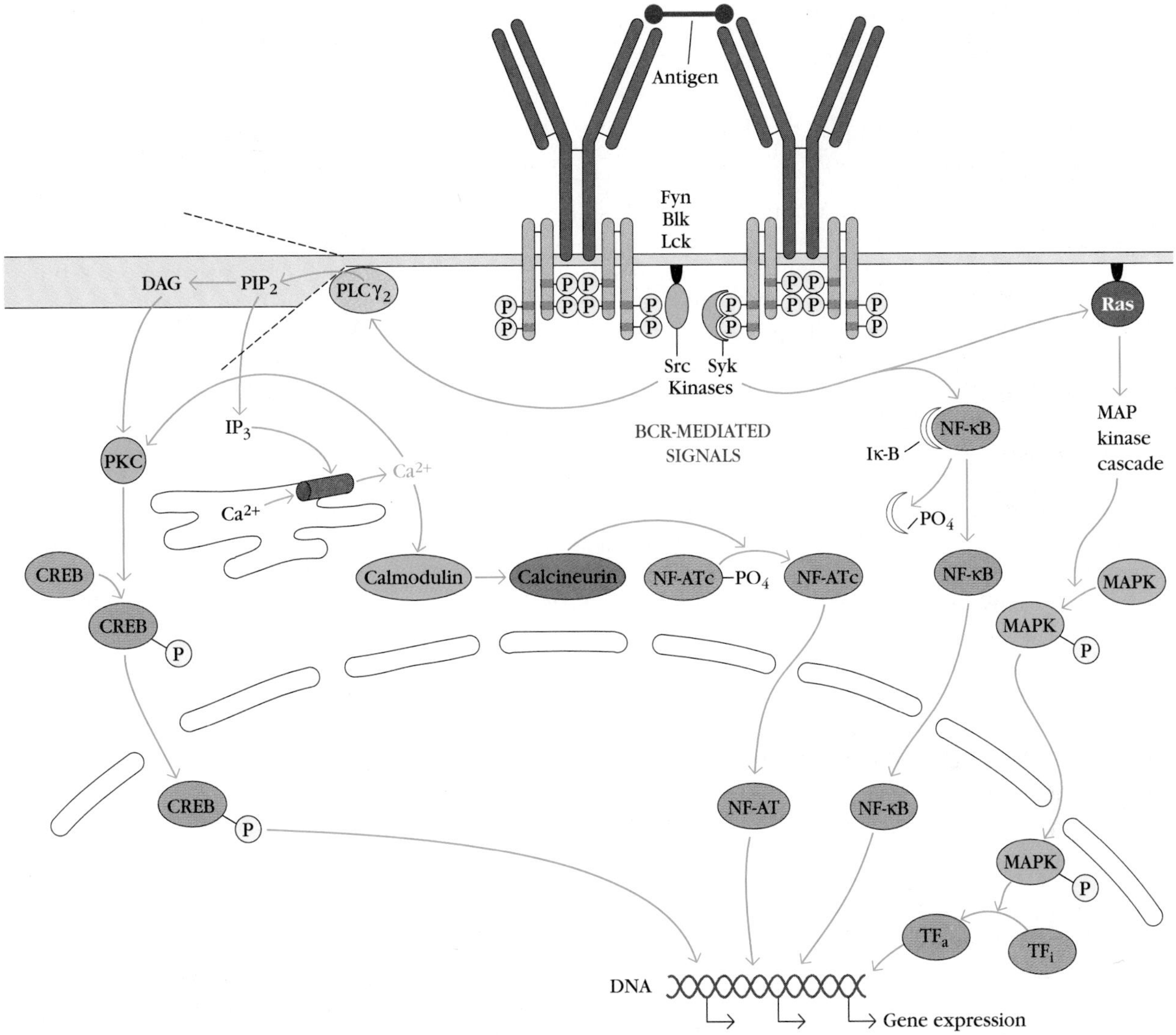

FIGURE 11-8 Some of the many signal-transduction pathways activated by the BCR. In one pathway, Syk activates PLCγ_2 by tyrosine phosphorylation. PLCγ_2 then hydrolyzes PIP_2, a membrane phospholipid, to produce the second messengers DAG and IP_3. DAG and Ca^{2+} released by the action of IP_3 collaboratively activate the PKC, which induces additional signal-transduction pathways, including the one shown here that activates the nuclear transcription factor CREB. Signals from the activated BCR complex also cause the phosphorylation of IκB, resulting in the release of the transcription factor NF-κB. The activated receptor complex also generates signals that initiate a sequence of events that results in the activation of the Ras pathway. Activated Ras initiates a cascade of phosphorylations known as a MAP kinase (MAPK) cascade, which culminates in the activation of MAPK, which translocates into the nucleus, where it activates certain transcription factors (TF). In the nucleus, NF-AT, NF-κB, CREB, and MAPK-activated transcription factors act at a number of sites in the genome to induce the expression of various genes, including such key transcription factors as Fos and Jun. These factors in turn up-regulate the expression of many genes. PLCγ_2 = phospholipase C; PKC = protein kinase C; PIP_2 = phosphatidylinositol 4,5-bisphosphate; IP_3 = inositol 1,4,5-trisphosphate; DAG = diacylglycerol; MAPK = mitogen-activated protein kinase; Ras = a small G protein; TF = transcription factor; IκB = inhibitor of NF-κB; NF-AT = nuclear factor of activated T cells (also in B cells); CREB cyclic-AMP response element/B cell. [Adapted from A Defranco, 1999, p. 239, *Fundamental Immunology,* 4th ed., edited by WE Paul, Lippincott-Raven, Philadelphia and New York.]

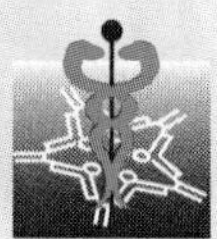

CLINICAL FOCUS

X-LINKED AGAMMAGLOBULINEMIA : A FAILURE IN SIGNAL TRANSDUCTION AND B-CELL DEVELOPMENT

X-linked agammaglobulinemia is a genetically determined immunodeficiency disease that is characterized by the inability to synthesize all classes of antibody. It was discovered in 1952 by O. C. Bruton in what is still regarded as an outstanding example of research in clinical immunology. Bruton's investigation involved a patient, a young boy, who had mumps 3 times and experienced 19 different episodes of serious bacterial infections during a period of just over 4 years. Because pneumococcus bacteria were isolated from the child's blood during 10 of the episodes of bacterial infection, attempts were made to induce immunity to pneumococcus by immunization with pneumococcus vaccine. The failure of these efforts to induce antibody responses prompted Bruton to determine whether the patient could mount antibody responses when challenged with other antigens. Surprisingly, immunization with diphtheria and typhoid vaccine preparations did not raise humoral responses in this patient. The inability to make humoral responses to diphtheria toxoid or typhoid vaccine led Bruton to examine the patient's serum. Electrophoretic analysis of the serum revealed that although normal amounts of albumin and other typical serum proteins were present, gamma globulin, the major antibody fraction of serum, was absent. Having traced the immunodeficiency to a lack of antibody, Bruton tried what was a bold new treatment at the time. He administered monthly doses of human immune serum globulin. The patient's experience of a fourteen-month period free of bacterial sepsis indicated the usefulness of the immunoglobulin replacement for the treatment of immunodeficiency. During this insightful clinical study, Bruton's pioneering efforts established the dose and treatment intervals that were to become standard in the use of human immune serum globulin for the treatment of antibody-deficiency diseases.

Though initially called Bruton's agammaglobulinemia, this hereditary immunodeficiency disease was renamed X-linked agammaglobulinemia, or X-LA, after the discovery that the responsible gene lies on the X chromosome. The disease has the following clinical features:

- Because this defect is X-linked, almost all afflicted individuals are male.

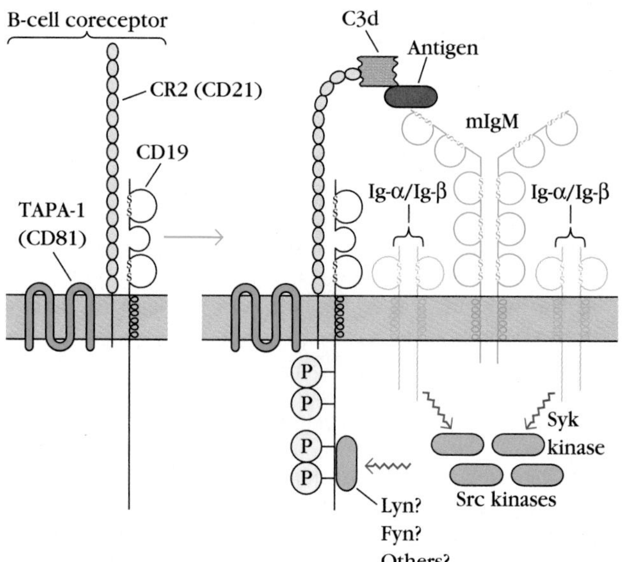

FIGURE 11-9 The B-cell coreceptor is a complex of three cell membrane molecules: TAPA-1(CD81), CR2 (CD21), and CD19. Binding of the CR2 component to complement-derived C3d that has coated antigen captured by mIg results in the phosphorylation of CD19. The Src-family tyrosine kinase Lyn binds to phosphorylated CD19. The resulting activated Lyn and Fyn can trigger the signal-transduction pathways that begin with phospholipase C that are shown in Figure 11-8.

- The first signs of immunodeficiency may appear as early as 9 months after birth, when the supply of maternal antibody acquired in utero has decreased below protective levels.
- There is a high frequency of infection by *Streptococcus pneumoniae* and *Hemophilus influenzae*; bacterial pneumonia, sinusitis, meningitis, or septicemia are often seen in these patients.
- Although infection by many viruses is no more severe in these patients than in normal individuals, long-term antiviral immunity is usually not induced.
- Analysis by fluorescence microscopy or flow cytometry shows few or no mature B cells in the bloodstream.

Studies of this disease at the cellular and molecular level have revealed the basic nature of the disorder and provide insights into the workings of the immune system. A scarcity of B cells in the periphery explained the inability of X-LA patients to make antibody. Studies of the cell populations in bone marrow showed that the lack of B cells can be traced to failures in B-cell development. The samples displayed a ratio of pro-B cells to pre-B cells 10 times normal, suggesting inhibition of the transition from the pro– to the pre–B-cell stage. The presence of very few mature B cells in the marrow indicated a more profound blockade in the development of B cells from pre-B cells.

Pursuit of the problem at the molecular level precisely identified the defect responsible for X-LA. During the early 1990s, the gene responsible for X-LA was cloned. The normal counterpart of this gene encodes a protein tyrosine kinase that has been named Bruton's tyrosine kinase (Btk) in honor of the resourceful and insightful physician who discovered X-LA. Btk has turned out to play important roles in B-cell signaling. For example, crosslinking of the B-cell receptor results in the phosphorylation of a tyrosine residue in the catalytic domain of Btk. This activates the protein-tyrosine-kinase activity of Btk, which then phosphorylates phospholipase C-γ_2 (PLC-γ_2). This activation is important because in vitro studies of cell cultures in which Btk has been knocked out show compromised PLC-γ_2 activation. Once activated, PLC-γ_2 hydrolyzes membrane phospholipids, thereby liberating the potent second messengers, IP_3 and DAG. As mentioned earlier, IP_3 causes a rise in intracellular Ca^{2+}, and DAG is an activator of protein kinase C (PKC). Because Btk plays a pivotal role in activating an important network of intracellular signals, Btk has emerged as a critical participant in the intracellular signaling that is vital to the function of mature B cells and earlier members of the B-cell lineage. Its recognition is an example of how the pursuit of fundamental mechanisms underlying disease can lead to discoveries of general importance to understanding the workings of normal cells.

---

concentrations of antigen in a primary response. Such responses, even though initially of low affinity, can play a significant role in the ultimate generation of high-affinity antibody. As described later in this chapter, response to an antigen can lead to affinity maturation, resulting in higher average affinity of the B-cell population. Finally, note that the involvement of a breakdown product of the complement system in the pathway for coreceptor activity points to ways in which different arms of the immune system interact with each other.

Role of T_H Cells in Humoral Responses

As noted already, activation of B cells by soluble protein antigens requires involvement of T_H cells. In this case, binding of antigen to the mIg does not induce an effective competence signal, and additional interaction with membrane molecules on the T_H cell is needed to induce B-cell activation. In addition, a cytokine-mediated progression is required for B-cell proliferation. Figure 11-10 outlines the probable sequence of events in B-cell activation by a TD antigen. This process is considerably more complex than activation induced by TI antigens.

Formation of T-B Conjugate

After binding of antigen by mIg on B cells, the antigen is internalized by receptor-mediated endocytosis and processed within the endocytic pathway into peptides. Antigen binding also initiates signaling through the BCR that induces the B cell to up-regulate a number of cell-membrane molecules, including class II MHC molecules and the co-stimulatory ligand B7 (see Figure 11-10a). Increased expression of both of these membrane proteins enhances the ability of the B cell to function as an antigen-presenting cell in T_H-cell activation, which was described in detail in Chapter 10. The antigenic peptides produced within the endocytic processing pathway

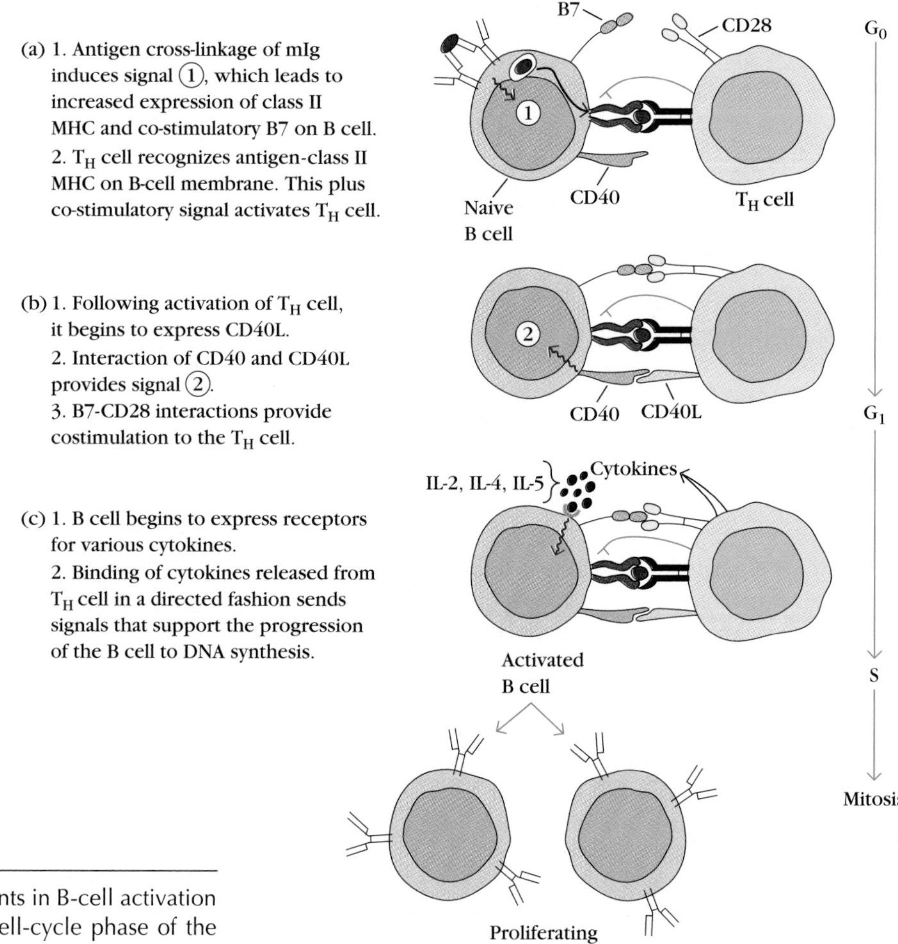

FIGURE 11-10 Sequence of events in B-cell activation by a thymus-dependent antigen. The cell-cycle phase of the B cell is indicated on the right.

associate with class II MHC molecules and are presented on the B-cell membrane to the T_H cell, inducing its activation. It generally takes 30–60 min after internalization of antigen for processed antigenic peptides to be displayed on the B-cell membrane in association with class II MHC molecules. Presumably, this is the time required for antigen processing and association with MHC molecules within B cells.

Because a B cell recognizes and internalizes antigen specifically, by way of its membrane-bound Ig, a B cell is able to present antigen to T_H cells at antigen concentrations that are 100 to 10,000 times lower than what is required for presentation by macrophages or dendritic cells. When antigen concentrations are high, macrophages and dendritic cells serve as effective antigen-presenting cells, but, as antigen levels drop, B cells take over as the major presenter of antigen to T_H cells.

Once a T_H cell recognizes a processed antigenic peptide displayed by a class II MHC molecule on the membrane of a B cell, the two cells interact to form a **T-B conjugate** (Figure 11-11). Micrographs of T-B conjugates reveal that the T_H cells in antigen-specific conjugates have reorganized the Golgi apparatus and the microtubular-organizing center toward the junction with the B cell. This reorganization of the Golgi apparatus may facilitate the release of cytokines toward the antigen-specific B cell. Formation of a T-B conjugate not only leads to the directional release of T_H-cell cytokines, but also to the up-regulation of CD40L (CD154), a T_H-cell membrane protein that then interacts with CD40 on B cells to provide an essential signal for T-cell-dependent B-cell activation.

Contact-Dependent Help Mediated by CD40/CD40L Interaction

Naive B cells express the membrane glycoprotein CD40, which belongs to the tumor necrosis factor (TNF) family of cell-surface proteins and soluble cytokines that regulate cell proliferation and programmed cell death by apoptosis. The CD40L that is up-regulated after the activation of T_H cells belongs to the tumor necrosis factor receptor (TNFR) family. Interaction of CD40L with CD40 on the B cell delivers a signal (signal 2) to the B cell that, in concert with the signal generated by mIg crosslinkage (signal 1), drives the B cell into G_1 (see Figure 11-10b). The signals from CD40 are transduced by a number of intracellular signaling pathways, ultimately resulting in changes in gene expression. Studies have shown that although CD40 does not have kinase activity, its crosslinking is followed by the activation of such protein tyrosine kinases as Lyn and Syk. Crosslinking of CD40 also results in the activation of phospholipase C and the subsequent generation of the second messengers IP_3 and DAG and the activation of a number of transcription factors. Ligation of CD40 also results in its association with members of the TNFR-associated factor (TRAF) family. A consequence of this interaction is the activation of the transcription factor NF-κB.

The role of an inducible T_H-cell membrane protein, CD40L, in B-cell activation initially was revealed by experiments in which naive B cells were incubated with antigen and plasma membranes prepared either from activated T_H-cell clones or from resting T_H-cell clones. Only the membranes from the activated T_H cells induced B-cell proliferation, suggesting that one or more molecules expressed on the membrane of an activated T_H cell engage receptors on the B cell to provide contact-dependent help.

Several lines of evidence have identified the CD40/CD40L interaction as the one involved in contact-dependent help. For example, when antigen-stimulated B cells are treated with anti-CD40 monoclonal antibodies in the absence of T_H cells, they become activated and proliferate. Thus, engagement of CD40, whether by antibodies to CD40 or by CD40L, is critical in providing signal 2 to the B cell. If appropriate cytokines also are added to this experimental system, then the proliferating B cells will differentiate into plasma cells. Conversely, antibodies to CD40L have been shown to block B-cell activation by blocking the CD40/CD40L interaction.

Signals Provided by T_H-Cell Cytokines

Although B cells stimulated with membrane proteins from activated T_H cells are able to proliferate, they fail to differentiate unless cytokines also are present; this finding suggests that both a membrane-contact signal and cytokine signals are necessary to induce B-cell proliferation and differentiation. As noted already, electron micrographs of T-B conjugates reveal that the antigen-specific interaction between a T_H and a B cell induces a redistribution of T_H-cell membrane proteins and cytoskeletal elements that may result in the polarized release of cytokines toward the interacting B cell.

In a simple, yet ingenious experiment, W. J. Poo and C. A. Janeway sought to determine whether cytokines are released from T_H cells in a directional manner. They worked with a T_H-cell clone that secreted IL-4 in response to binding of a clonotypic monoclonal antibody specific for the idiotype of the T-cell receptor. This T_H clone was centrifuged onto a Nucleopore membrane having 3 μ pores. Since the cells were larger than 3 μ, they completely plugged the pores. The cell-packed membrane was then suspended between two chambers, and the anti-TCR monoclonal antibody was

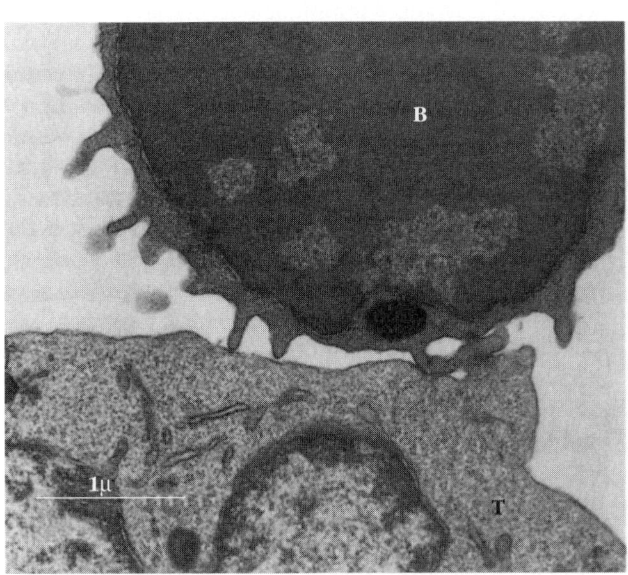

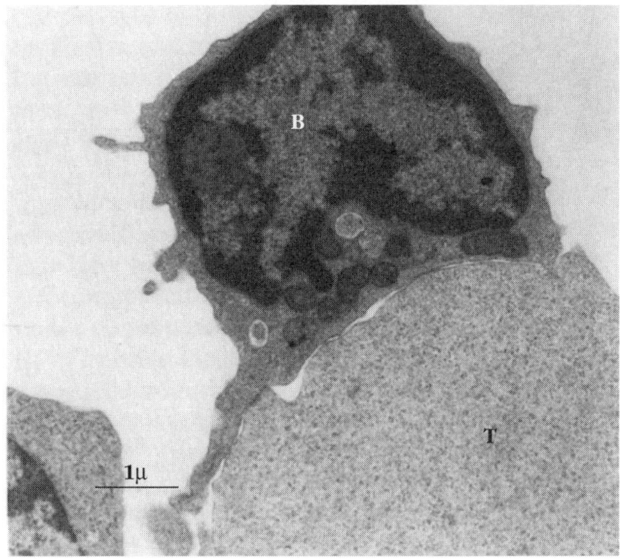

FIGURE 11-11 Transmission electron micrographs of initial contact between a T cell and B cell (*left*) and of a T-B conjugate (*right*). Note the broad area of membrane contact between the cells after formation of the conjugate. The bar = 1μm. [From VM Sanders et al, 1986, *J. Immunol.* **137**:2395.]

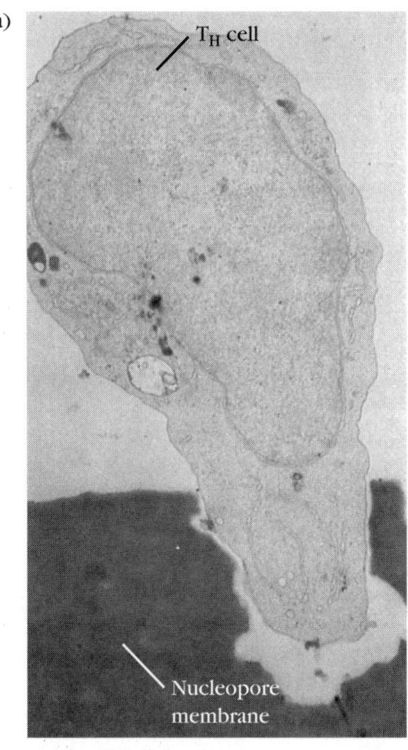

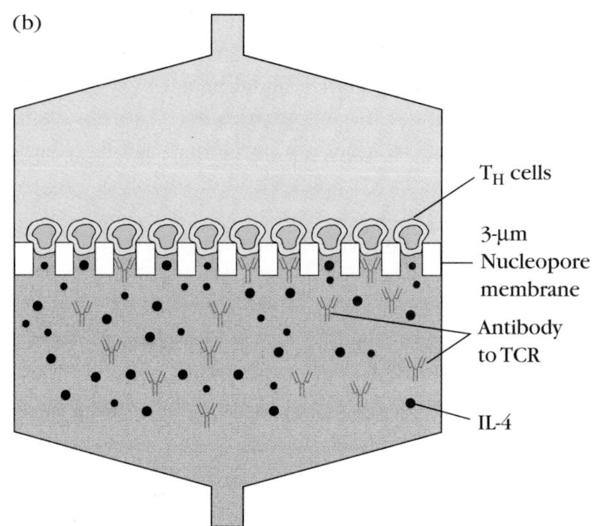

FIGURE 11-12 Experimental demonstration of directional release of cytokines from activated T_H cells. (a) Electron micrograph of a T_H cell centrifuged onto Nucleopore membrane. Note how the cell completely blocks the pore (b) Diagram of culture system. Addition of monoclonal antibody specific for the idiotype of the T-cell receptors resulted in T_H-cell activation and release of IL-4 on one side of the membrane only. [From WJ Poo et al, 1988, *Nature* **332:**378.]

added to one chamber (Figure 11-12). Measurement of IL-4 in both chambers showed that IL-4 was released toward the chamber containing the activating monoclonal antibody. These findings suggest that formation of specific T-B conjugates results in directional release of cytokines toward the interacting B cell.

Once activated, the B cell begins to express membrane receptors for various cytokines, such as IL-2, IL-4, IL-5, and others. These receptors then bind the cytokines produced by the interacting T_H cell. The signals produced by these cytokine-receptor interactions support B-cell proliferation and can induce differentiation. Among these differentiation events are formation of plasma cells and memory B cells, class switching, and affinity maturation. Each of these events is described in a later section.

Negative Selection of Mature Self-Reactive B Cells

Because some self-antigens do not have access to the bone marrow, B cells expressing mIgM specific for such antigens cannot be eliminated by the negative-selection process in the bone marrow described earlier. To avoid autoimmune responses from such mature self-reactive B cells, some process for deleting them or rendering them inactive must occur in peripheral lymphoid tissue.

A transgenic system developed by C. Goodnow and his coworkers has served to clarify the process of negative selection of mature B cells in the periphery. Goodnow's experimental system included two groups of transgenic mice (Figure 11-13a). One group carried a hen egg-white lysozyme (HEL) transgene linked to a metallothionine promoter, which placed transcription of the HEL gene under the control of zinc levels. The other group of transgenic mice carried rearranged immunoglobulin heavy- and light-chain transgenes encoding anti-HEL antibody; in normal mice, the frequency of HEL-reactive B cells is on the order of 1 in 10^3, but in these transgenic mice the rearranged anti-HEL transgene is expressed by 60%–90% of the mature peripheral B cells. Goodnow mated the two groups of transgenics to produce "double-transgenic" offspring carrying both the HEL and anti-HEL transgenes. The question Goodnow then asked was what effect HEL, which is expressed in the periphery but not in the bone marrow, would have upon the development of B cells expressing the anti-HEL transgene.

The Goodnow double-transgenic system has yielded several interesting findings concerning negative selection of B cells (Table 11-3). He found that double-transgenic mice expressing high levels of HEL (10^{-9} M) continued to have mature, peripheral B cells bearing anti-HEL membrane antibody, but these B cells were functionally nonresponsive; that is, they were **anergic.** When these mice were given an immunizing dose of HEL, few anti-HEL plasma cells were induced and the serum anti-HEL titer was low. The endogenous concentration of HEL in these double-transgenic mice

(a)

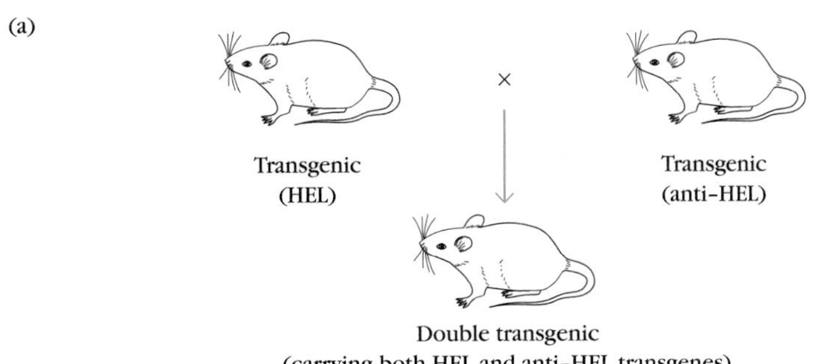

(b)

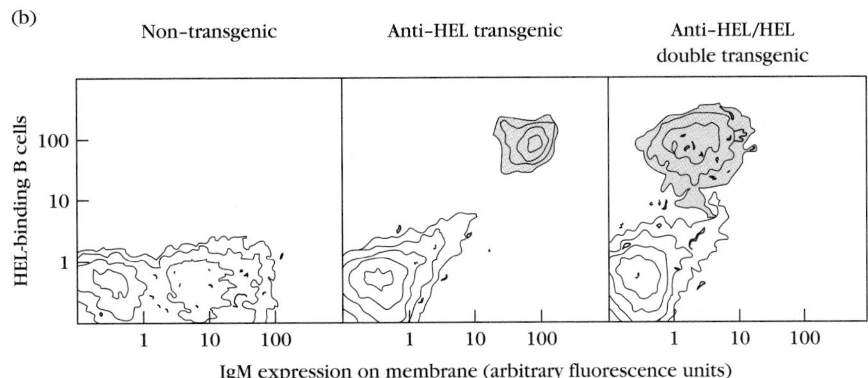

FIGURE 11-13 Goodnow's experimental system for demonstrating clonal anergy in mature peripheral B cells. (a) Production of double-transgenic mice carrying transgenes encoding HEL (hen egg-white lysozyme) and anti-HEL antibody. (b) FACS analysis of peripheral B cells that bind HEL compared with membrane IgM levels. The number of B cells binding HEL was measured by determining how many cells bound fluorescently labeled HEL. Levels of membrane IgM were determined by incubating the cells with anti-mouse IgM antibody labeled with a fluorescent label different from that used to label HEL. Measurement of the fluorescence emitted from this label indicated the level of membrane IgM expressed by the B cells. The nontransgenics (*left*) had many B cells that expressed high levels of surface IgM but almost no B cells that bound HEL above the background level of 1. Both anti-HEL transgenics (*middle*) and anti-HEL/HEL double transgenics (*right*) had large numbers of B cells that bound HEL (blue), although the level of membrane IgM was about twentyfold lower in the double transgenics. The data in Table 11-3 indicate that the B cells expressing anti-HEL in the double transgenics cannot mount a humoral response to HEL.

TABLE 11-3 EXPRESSION OF ANTI-HEL TRANSGENE BY MATURE PERIPHERAL B CELLS IN SINGLE AND DOUBLE-TRANSGENIC MICE

Experimental group	HEL level	Membrane anti-HEL	Anti-HEL PFC/spleen*	Anti-HEL serum titer*
Anti-HEL single transgenics	None	+	High	High
Anti-HEL/HEL double transgenics (Group 1)	10^{-9} M	+	Low	Low

*Experimental animals were immunized with hen egg-white lysozyme (HEL). Several days layer, hemolytic plaque assays for the number of plasma cells secreting anti-HEL antibody were performed and the serum anti-HEL titers were determined. PFC = plaque-forming cells; see Figure 23-1 for a description of the plaque assay.

SOURCE: Adapted from CC Goodnow, 1992, *Annu. Rev. Immunol.* **10:**489.

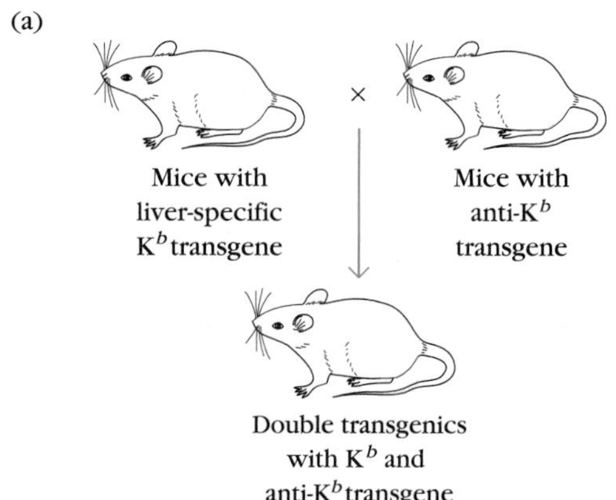

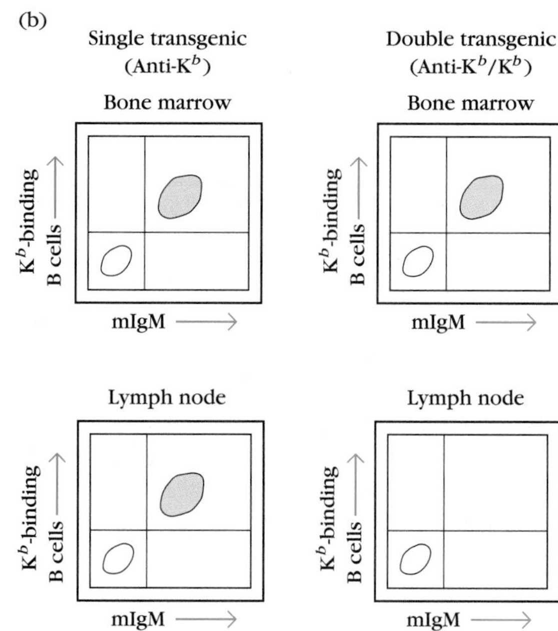

FIGURE 11-14 Experimental demonstration of clonal deletion of self-reactive mature peripheral B cells by Nemazee and Burki. (a) Production of double-transgenic mice expressing the class I K^b molecule and anti-K^b antibody. Because the K^b transgene contained a liver-specific promoter, K^b was not expressed in the bone marrow in the transgenics. (b) FACS analysis of bone marrow and peripheral (lymph node) B cells for K^b binding versus membrane IgM (mIgM). In the double transgenics, B cells expressing anti-K^b (blue) were present in the bone marrow but were absent in the lymph nodes, indicating that mature self-reactive B cells were deleted in the periphery.

before immunization was estimated to be sufficient to occupy 45% of the anti-HEL antibodies on the B cells. A second group of double transgenics, expressing ten times lower levels of HEL (10^{-10} M) was also obtained from the matings. In this case, HEL occupied less than 5% of the anti-HEL antibodies on the B cells; under these conditions, the B cells were shown to be functionally active. Thus the concentration of HEL and mIg occupancy appeared to determine whether the peripheral HEL-reactive B cells became anergic or not. To determine whether the mature HEL-reactive B cells in the low-HEL double transgenics could later be rendered anergic, Goodnow fed the mice zinc water to elevate the serum HEL concentration. Within 4 days, the previously responsive mature anti-HEL B cells became functionally anergic. Thus, clonal anergy could be restored in low-HEL animals by elevating the level of HEL.

Analysis of B cells from the double transgenics showed that the anergic anti-HEL cells expressed about twenty-fold lower levels of membrane IgM than reactive cells did but about the same levels of membrane IgD. Goodnow has suggested that reduction in the mIgM level might cause quantitative differences in signal transduction, leading to the anergic state. The observation that the anergic B cells in this system express both IgM and IgD indicates that anergy is being induced in mature B cells rather than in immature B cells.

To study what would happen if a class I MHC self-antigen were expressed only in the periphery, Nemazee and Burki modified the transgenic system used in the experiments on negative selection in the bone marrow described previously. To achieve this, they produced a transgene consisting of the class I K^b gene linked to a liver-specific promoter, so that the class I K^b molecule could be expressed only in the liver. Transgenic mice expressing an anti-K^b antibody on their B cells also were produced, and the two groups of transgenic mice were then mated (Figure 11-14a). In the resulting double-transgenic mice, the immature B cells expressing anti-K^b mIgM would not encounter class I K^b molecules in the bone marrow. FACS analysis of the B cells in the double transgenics showed that immature B cells expressing the transgene-encoded anti-K^b were present in the bone marrow but not in the peripheral lymphoid organs (Figure 11-14b). In the previous experiments of Nemazee and Burki, the class I MHC self-antigen ($H\text{-}2^k$) was expressed on all nucleated cells; in this system, immature B cells expressing the transgene-encoded antibody to this class I molecule were selected and deleted in the bone marrow (see Figure 11-5a). In their second system, however, the class I self-antigen (K^b) was expressed only in the liver, so that negative selection and deletion occurred at the mature B-cell stage in the periphery.

The Humoral Response

This section considers the differences between the primary and secondary humoral response and the use of hapten-carrier conjugates in studying the humoral response.

Primary and Secondary Responses

The kinetics and other characteristics of the humoral response differ considerably depending on whether they result from activation of naive lymphocytes (primary response) or memory lymphocytes (secondary response). In both cases, activation leads to production of secreted antibodies of various isotypes, which differ in their ability to mediate specific effector functions (see Table 4-2).

The first contact of an exogenous antigen with an individual generates a primary humoral response, characterized by the production of antibody-secreting plasma cells and memory B cells. As Chapter 3 showed, the kinetics of the primary response, as measured by serum antibody level, depend on the nature of the antigen, the route of antigen administration, the presence or absence of adjuvants, and the species or strain being immunized.

In all cases, however, a primary response to antigen is characterized by a lag phase, during which naive B cells undergo clonal selection, subsequent clonal expansion, and differentiation into memory cells or plasma cells (Figure 11-15). The lag phase is followed by a logarithmic increase in serum antibody level, which reaches a peak, plateaus for a variable time, and then declines. The duration of the lag phase varies with the nature of the antigen. Immunization of mice with an antigen such as sheep red blood cells (SRBCs) typically results in a lag phase of 3–4 days. Eight or nine successive cell divisions of activated B cells during days 4 and 5 then generate plasma and memory cells. Peak plasma-cell levels are attained at day 4–5; peak serum antibody levels are attained by around day 7–10. For soluble protein antigens, the lag phase is a little longer, often lasting about a week, peak plasma-cell levels are attained by 9–10 days, and peak serum titers are present by around 14 days. During a primary humoral response, IgM is secreted initially, often followed by a switch to an increasing proportion of IgG. Depending on the persistence of the antigen, a primary response can last for various periods, from only a few days to several weeks.

The memory B cells formed during a primary response stop dividing and enter the G_0 phase of the cell cycle. These cells have variable life spans, and some persist for the life of the individual. The capacity to develop a secondary humoral response (see Figure 11-15) depends on the existence of this population of memory B cells as well as memory T cells. Activation of these memory cells by antigen results in a secondary antibody response that can be distinguished from the primary response in several ways (Table 11-4). The secondary response has a shorter lag period and thus is more rapid, reaches a greater magnitude, and lasts longer. The secondary response is also characterized by secretion of antibody with a higher affinity for the antigen, and isotypes other than IgM predominate.

A major factor in the more rapid onset and greater magnitude of secondary responses is the fact that the population of memory B cells specific for a given antigen is considerably larger than the population of corresponding naive B cells. Another significant factor is the fact that memory cells are more easily activated than naive B cells are. The processes of affinity maturation and class switching are responsible for the higher affinity and different isotypes exhibited in a secondary response. The higher levels of antibody coupled with

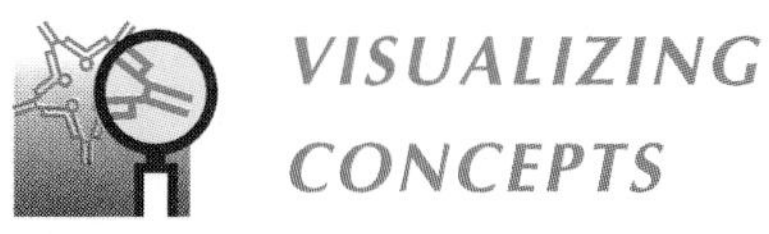

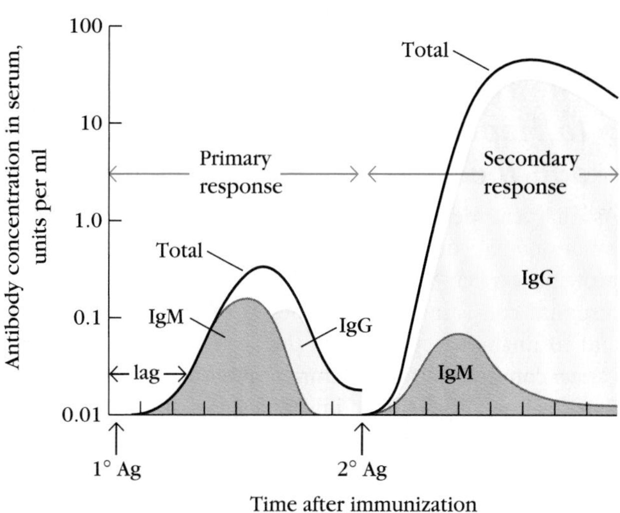

FIGURE 11-15 Concentration and isotype of serum antibody following primary (1°) and secondary (2°) immunization with antigen. The antibody concentrations are plotted on a logarithmic scale. The time units are not specified because the kinetics differ somewhat with type of antigen, administration route, presence or absence of adjuvant, and the species or strain of animal.

TABLE 11-4 COMPARISON OF PRIMARY AND SECONDARY ANTIBODY RESPONSES

Property	Primary response	Secondary response
Responding B cell	Naive (virgin) B cell	Memory B cell
Lag period following antigen administration	Generally 4–7 days	Generally 1–3 days
Time of peak response	7–10 days	3–5 days
Magnitude of peak antibody response	Varies depending on antigen	Generally 100–1000 times higher primary response
Isotype produced	IgM predominates early in the response	IgG predominates
Antigens	Thymus-dependent and thymus-independent	Thymus-dependent
Antibody affinity	Lower	Higher

the overall higher affinity provide an effective host defense against reinfection. The change in isotype provides antibodies whose effector functions are particularly suited to a given pathogen.

The existence of long-lived memory B cells accounts for a phenomenon called "original antigenic sin," which was first observed when the antibody response to influenza vaccines was monitored in adults. Monitoring revealed that immunization with an influenza vaccine of one strain elicited an antibody response to that strain but, paradoxically, also elicited an antibody response of greater magnitude to another influenza strain that the individual had been exposed to during childhood. It was as if the memory of the first antigen exposure had left a life-long imprint on the immune system. This phenomenon can be explained by the presence of a memory-cell population, elicited by the influenza strain encountered in childhood, that is activated by cross-reacting epitopes on the vaccine strain encountered later. This process then generates a secondary response, characterized by antibodies with higher affinity for the earlier viral strain.

The Humoral Response to Hapten-Carrier Conjugates and the Role of Helper T Cells

As Chapter 3 described, when animals are immunized with small organic compounds (haptens) conjugated with large proteins (carriers), the conjugate induces a humoral immune response consisting of antibodies both to hapten epitopes and to unaltered epitopes on the carrier protein. Hapten-carrier conjugates provided immunologists with an ideal system for studying cellular interactions of the humoral response, and such studies demonstrated that the generation of a humoral antibody response requires recognition of the antigen by both T_H cells and B cells, each recognizing different epitopes on the same antigen. A variety of different hapten-carrier conjugates have been used in immunologic research (Table 11-5).

One of the earliest findings with hapten-carrier conjugates was that a hapten had to be chemically coupled to a larger carrier molecule to induce a humoral response to the hapten. If an animal was immunized with both hapten and carrier separately, very little or no hapten-specific antibody was generated. A second important observation was that, in order to generate a secondary antibody response to a hapten, the animal had to be again immunized with the same hapten-carrier conjugate used for the primary immunization. If the secondary immunization was with the same hapten but conjugated to a different, unrelated carrier, no secondary anti-hapten response occurred. This phenomenon, called the **carrier effect**, could be circumvented by priming the animal separately with the unrelated carrier.

TABLE 11-5 COMMON HAPTEN-CARRIER CONJUGATES USED IN IMMUNOLOGIC RESEARCH

Hapten-carrier acronym	Hapten	Carrier protein
DNP-BGG	Dinitrophenol	Bovine gamma globulin
TNP-BSA	Trinitrophenyl	Bovine serum albumin
NIP-KLH	5-Nitrophenyl acetic acid	Keyhole limpet hemocyanin
ARS-OVA	Azophenylarsonate	Ovalbumin
LAC-HGG	Phenyllactoside	Human gamma globulin

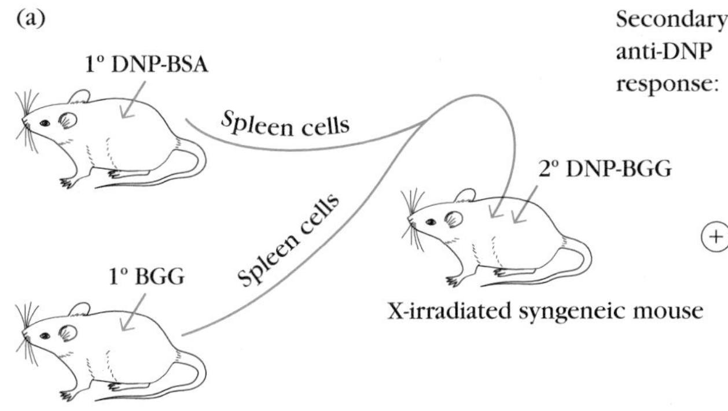

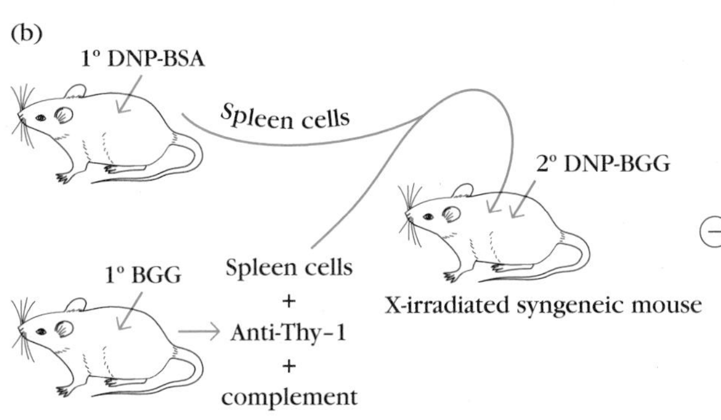

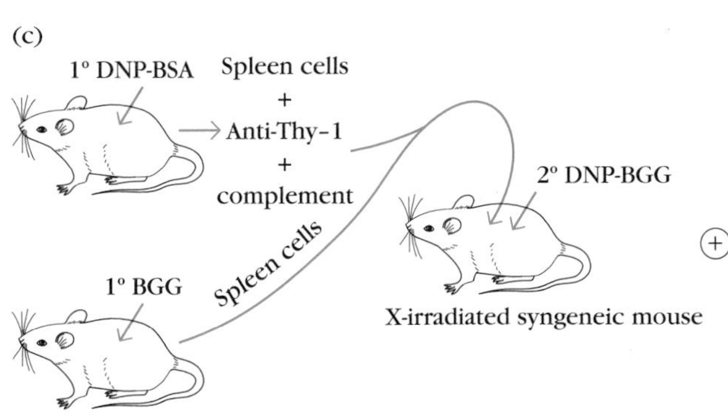

FIGURE 11-16 Adoptive-transfer experiments demonstrating that hapten-primed and carrier-primed cells are separate populations. (a) X-irradiated syngeneic mice reconstituted with spleen cells from both DNP-BSA–primed mice and BGG-primed mice and challenged with DNP-BGG generated a secondary anti-DNP response. (b) Removal of T cells from the BGG-primed spleen cells, by treatment with anti-Thy-1 antiserum, abolished the secondary anti-DNP response. (c) Removal of T cells from the DNP-BSA–primed spleen cells had no effect on the secondary response to DNP. These experiments show that carrier-primed cells are T cells and hapten-primed cells are B cells.

Similar experiments conducted with an **adoptive-transfer** system showed that hapten-primed (hapten immunized) cells and carrier-primed (immunized against the carrier) cells were distinct populations. In these studies, one mouse was primed with the DNP-BSA conjugate and another was primed with the unrelated carrier BGG, which was not conjugated to the hapten. In one experiment, spleen cells from both mice were mixed and injected into a lethally irradiated syngeneic recipient. When this mouse was challenged with DNP conjugated to the unrelated carrier BGG, there was a secondary anti-hapten response to DNP (Figure 11-16a). In a second experiment, spleen cells from the BGG-immunized mice were treated with anti-T-cell antiserum (anti-Thy-1) and complement to lyse the T cells. When this T-cell–depleted sample was mixed with the DNP-BSA–primed spleen cells and injected into an irradiated mouse, no secondary anti-hapten response was observed upon immunizing with DNP-BGG (Figure 11-16b). However, similar treatment of the DNP-BSA–primed spleen cells with anti-Thy-1 and complement did not abolish the secondary anti-hapten response to DNP-BGG (Figure 11-16c). Later experiments, in which antisera were used to specifically deplete $CD4^+$ or $CD8^+$ T cells, showed that the $CD4^+$ T-cell subpopulation was responsible for the carrier effect. These experiments demonstrate that the response of hapten-primed B cells to the hapten-carrier conjugate requires the presence of carrier-primed $CD4^+$ T_H cells specific for carrier epitopes. (It is important to keep in mind that the B-cell response is not limited to the hapten determinant; in fact some B cells do react to epitopes on the carrier; however, the assay can be conducted in such a manner as to detect only anti-hapten responses.)

The experiments with hapten-carrier conjugates revealed that both T_H cells and B cells must recognize antigenic determinants on the same molecule for B-cell activation to occur. This feature of the T- and B-cell interaction in the humoral response is called associative, or linked, recognition. The conclusions drawn from hapten-carrier experiments apply to the humoral response to antigens in general and support the requirement for T-cell help in B-cell activation described earlier in this chapter.

In Vivo Sites for Induction of Humoral Response

In vivo activation and differentiation of B cells occurs in defined anatomic sites whose structure places certain restrictions on the kinds of cellular interactions that can take place. When an antigen is introduced into the body, it becomes concentrated in various peripheral lymphoid organs. Blood-borne antigen is filtered by the spleen, whereas antigen from tissue spaces drained by the lymphatic system is filtered by regional lymph nodes or lymph nodules. The following description focuses on the generation of the humoral response in lymph nodes.

A lymph node is an extremely efficient filter capable of trapping more than 90% of any antigen carried into it by the afferent lymphatics. As antigen percolates through the cellular architecture of a node, it will encounter one of three types of antigen-presenting cells: interdigitating dendritic cells in the paracortex, macrophages scattered throughout the node, or specialized follicular dendritic cells in the follicles and germinal centers. Antigenic challenge leading to a humoral immune response involves a complex series of events, which take place in distinct microenvironments within a lymph node (Figure 11-17). Slightly different pathways may operate during a primary and secondary response because much of the tissue antigen is complexed with circulating antibody in a secondary response.

Antigen or antigen-antibody complexes enter the lymph nodes through afferent lymphatic vessels, either alone or associated with antigen-transporting cells (e.g., Langerhans cells or dendritic cells) and macrophages. Lymphocytes enter the lymph nodes either through the afferent lymphatics or from the blood by extravasation through high-endothelial cells in the postcapillary venules (see Figure 2-18). The initial activation of both B and T cells is thought to take place in the paracortex. This region is heavily populated with T cells, macrophages, and interdigitating dendritic cells. The interdigitating dendritic cells in the paracortex express high levels of class II MHC molecules and have long extensions that have been shown to contact upwards of 200 T_H cells.

Within 1–2 days of antigenic challenge, the antigen is presented by macrophages and interdigitating dendritic cells to naive T cells, resulting in extensive T_H-cell activation and proliferation within the paracortex. In addition, naive B cells

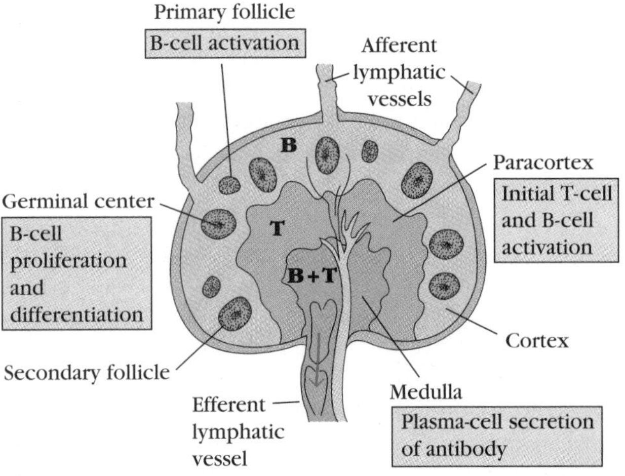

FIGURE 11-17 Schematic diagram of a peripheral lymph node showing anatomic sites at which various steps in B-cell activation, proliferation, and differentiation occur. The cortex is rich in B cells and the paracortex in T cells; both B and T cells are present in large numbers in the medulla. A secondary follicle contains the follicular mantle and a germinal center.

from the B-cell–rich cortex migrate to the T-cell–rich zone of the lymph node. B cells that have bound antigen by mIg will internalize the antigen and present it in association with class II MHC molecules. On entering the T-cell zone, a B cell that is presenting antigen can interact with a T_H cell specific for the displayed antigenic peptide and form a T-B conjugate, thereby inducing initial B-cell activation as described earlier. Once B-cell activation takes place, small foci of proliferating B cells form at the edges of the T-cell–rich zone and reach a maximum size within 3–4 days of antigen challenge. The B cells within these foci differentiate into plasma cells secreting IgM and IgG isotypes. Most of the antibody produced during a primary response comes from plasma cells in these foci. (A similar sequence of events takes place in the spleen, where initial B-cell activation takes place in the T-cell–rich periarterial lymphatic sheath, PALS; see Figure 2-19).

A few days after the formation of foci within lymph nodes, a few activated B cells, together with a few T_H cells, are thought to migrate from the foci to primary follicles. These follicles then develop into secondary follicles, which provide a specialized microenvironment favorable for interactions between B cells, activated T_H cells, and follicular dendritic cells. Note that although they share the highly branched morphology of dendritic cells derived from bone marrow, follicular dendritic cells do not arise in bone marrow, do not express class II MHC molecules, and do not present antigen to $CD4^+$ T cells. Follicular dendritic cells have long extensions, along which are arrayed Fc receptors that bind antigen-antibody complexes by the Fc portion of the antibodies and retain the complexes for long periods of time, even for months, on the cell membrane. Because follicular dendritic cells bind antigen that has been complexed to antibody, they are thought to be particularly important in the secondary response, when circulating antibody levels are significant. The periodicity of these immune complexes along the long dendritic extensions of these cells is thought to provide an optimal display of antigen for the activation of B cells. This interaction is believed to contribute to the activating signal, facilitating further B-cell activation.

Follicular dendritic cells release small membrane-derived particles, 0.3–0.4 μ in diameter, which appear to originate from the beaded structures of the dendritic extensions. These particles, which are heavily coated with immune complexes, are called **iccosomes**, for **immune-complex coated bodies**. Especially during a secondary response, iccosomes released from follicular dendritic cells are bound by mIg on B cells bearing antibody with specificity for antigen in the immune complexes and endocytosed. The endocytosed antigen is then processed and presented on class II MHC molecules, allowing the B cells to function as effective antigen-presenting cells for activated T_H cells. Formation of T-B conjugates may follow, resulting in B-cell activation and in proliferation of both the B cell and the T_H cell.

As cell proliferation continues, the activated B cells (together with some activated T_H cells) may migrate towards the center of the secondary follicle, forming the germinal center (see Figure 2-18). Development of germinal centers

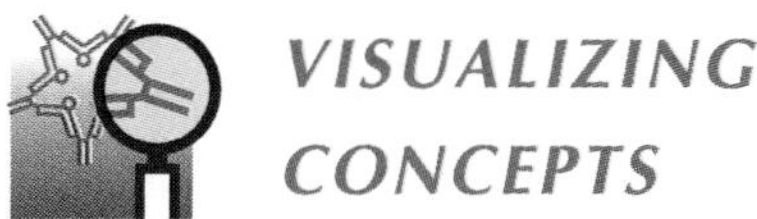

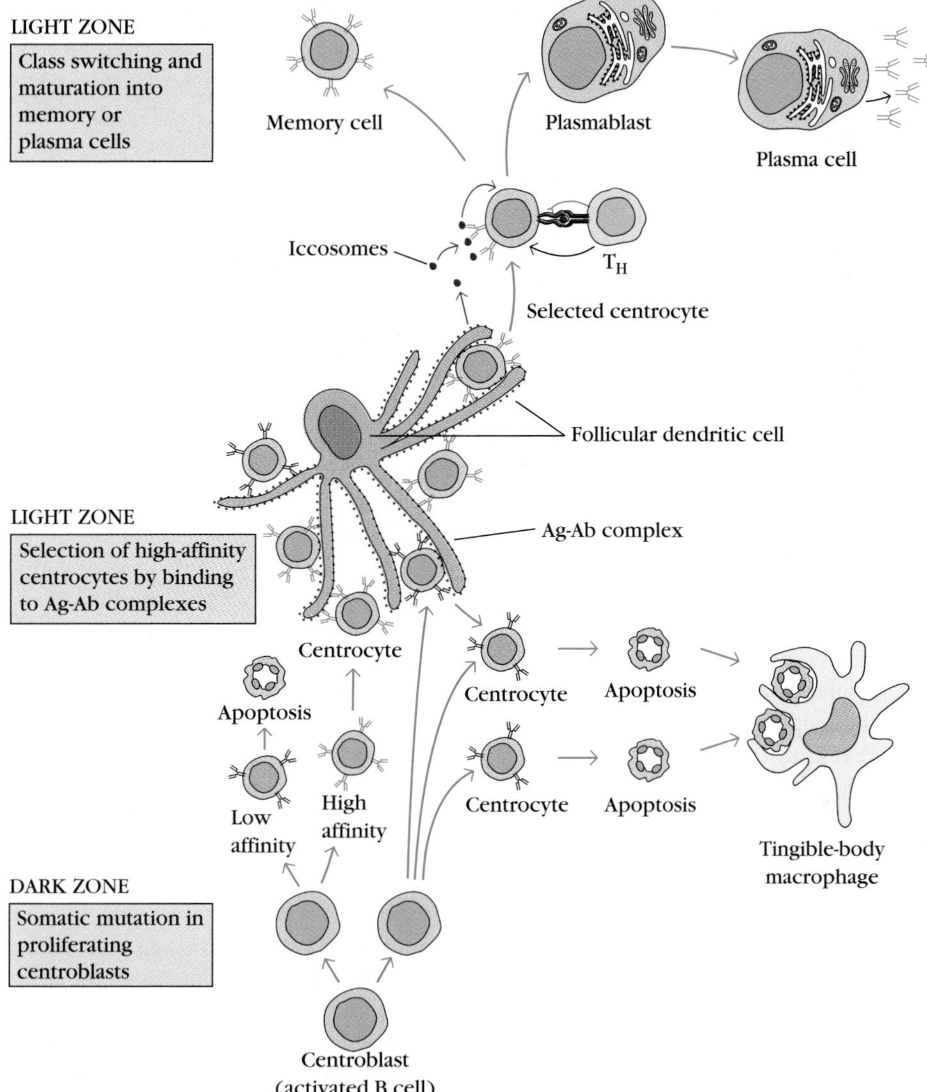

FIGURE 11-18 Overview of cellular events within secondary follicles of peripheral lymph nodes. Follicular dendritic cells bind antigen-antibody complexes along their long extensions. Small B cells (centrocytes) bearing high-affinity membrane immunoglobulin (antibodies shown in blue) are thought to interact with antigen presented as antigen-antibody complexes on the follicular dendritic cells; unselected centrocytes bearing low-affinity mIg (antibodies shown in black) die by apoptosis, and the debris is phagocytosed by tingible-body macrophages. Selected centrocytes, which may undergo class switching, then mature into memory B cells or plasmablasts; the latter develop into plasma cells.

depends upon the previous interaction of B cells in the foci with activated T_H cells and requires the CD40/CD40L interaction. If the CD40/CD40L interaction is blocked, then germinal centers fail to develop. Germinal centers characteristically arise within several (about 7–10) days after initial exposure to a thymus-dependent antigen.

During the first stage of formation of germinal centers, activated B cells undergo intense proliferation within the secondary follicle, filling the spaces between the network of follicular dendritic cells. The proliferating activated B cells, known as **centroblasts,** then move to one edge of the follicle. In humans, the densely packed centroblasts show up as a well-defined **dark zone** (Figure 11-18). Centroblasts are distinguished morphologically by their large size, expanded cytoplasm, diffuse chromatin, and lack of membrane Ig. The centroblasts become densely packed within the dark zone and divide to give rise to progeny called **centrocytes**, which are small, nondividing cells that now express membrane Ig. As the number of centrocytes increases, they move from the dark zone into a region containing numerous follicular dendritic cells called the **light zone**. Centrocytes make close contact with antigen displayed on the long extensions of follicular dendritic cells within this zone of the germinal center. As described later, contact with helper T cells is also an essential feature of the interactions of a centrocyte in the light zone.

Centrocytes bearing Ig that binds to antigen presented by the follicular dendritic cells in the light zone undergo differentiation within the light zone, forming two types of progeny: small memory B cells and large plasmablasts. The plasmablasts leave the germinal center and migrate to the medulla of the lymph node, where they develop into plasma cells and begin to secrete antibody molecules. Some memory B cells remain in the vicinity of the germinal center, while others leave the lymph node through the efferent lymphatic vessel and recirculate to other parts of the body.

The majority of centrocytes, however, cannot bind the antigen presented by the follicular dendritic cells. These cells die by apoptosis within the basal light zone of germinal centers and are phagocytosed by an unusual type of macrophage, the **tingible-body macrophage**, that specializes in phagocytosis of lymphoid cells (see Figure 11-18). The high rate of cell death by apoptosis provides a means of eliminating those B cells that bear mIg with low affinity for the antigen that is bound by the follicular dendritic cells or fail to recognize the antigen at all. As described in more detail below, this deletion of B cells that express mIg is believed to be one of the processes underlying the affinity maturation of the humoral response.

Germinal Centers and Antigen-Induced B-Cell Differentiation

As indicated in Figure 11-18, three important B-cell differentiation events take place in germinal centers: affinity maturation, class switching, and formation of plasma cells and memory B cells. In general, affinity maturation and memory cell formation require germinal centers. However some class switching and significant plasma-cell formation occur outside germinal centers.

Affinity Maturation

The average affinity of the antibodies produced during the course of the humoral response increases as much as 100-fold or more. These remarkable increases in antibody affinity were first noticed by H. N. Eisen and G. W. Siskind, who immunized two groups of rabbits with two different doses of the hapten-carrier complex DNP-BGG. Group I was immunized with 5 mg, and group II with 250 mg of DNP-BGG. The affinity of the serum anti-DNP antibodies produced in response to the antigen was then measured at 2 weeks, 5 weeks, and 8 weeks after immunization.

TABLE 11-6 EFFECT OF IMMUNIZING DOSE AND TIME ON AVERAGE AFFINITY OF INDUCED ANTI-DNP ANTIBODIES IN RABBITS

Group	DNP-BGG immunizing dose (mg per animal)	*K* of anti-DNP antibodies* (L/mol × 10^6)		
		2 weeks	5 weeks	8 weeks
I	5	0.86	14	120
II	250	0.18	0.13	0.15

*Values are averages for five animals per group and are based on binding of DNP-L-lysine with serum antibody samples obtained at indicated times after immunization.

SOURCE: Adapted from HN Eisen and GW Siskind, 1964, *Biochemistry* 3:966.

As the data in Table 11-6 show, the average affinity of the group I anti-DNP antibodies increased about 140-fold from 2 weeks to 8 weeks, whereas the affinity of the group II antibodies was initially lower and did not increase. The nearly fivefold lower average affinity of the group II antibodies at 2 weeks suggests that, at high immunizing doses, plasma cells arising from B cells expressing both high-affinity and low-affinity membrane antibody make significant contributions to the pool of serum antibody. In contrast, when the immunizing dose is low, plasma cells arising from B cells with high-affinity membrane antibody are the major source of antibody. Subsequent work has shown that affinity maturation is mainly the result of somatic hypermutation, although antigen-mediated selection of high-affinity B-cell clones may make a contribution in some immune responses.

The Role of Somatic Hypermutation

Monitoring of antibody genes during an immune response shows that extensive mutation of responding loci does not begin until the establishment of germinal centers, an event that occurs well into the primary response. Typically, significant numbers of germinal centers appear about a week after primary antigen challenge, reach peak activity during the next 4–10 days, and disappear by 4 weeks after immunization.

A direct demonstration that germinal centers are the sites of somatic hypermutation comes from the work of Kelsoe and his colleagues. These workers compared the mutation frequencies in B cells isolated from germinal centers with those from areas of intense B-cell activation outside the germinal centers. To do so, they prepared thin sections of spleen tissue from animals immunized with the hapten 4-hydroxy-3-nitrophenylacetyl (NP) conjugated with chicken gamma globulin as a carrier. This system is convenient because the initial response to this hapten is dominated by a particular heavy-chain gene rearrangement and the use of a λ light chain (in mice, >95% of antibodies bear κ light chains). Consequently, antibodies against the idiotype of this antibody can be used to readily distinguish responding B cells. Using antibodies to the idiotype and immunohistological staining techniques, these workers identified B cells bearing anti-NP antibody in germinal centers and nongerminal-center foci of B cell activation present in thin sections cut from the spleens of recently immunized mice. They isolated these B cells by microdissection, used PCR to amplify the immunoglobulin genes of each individual cell, and then cloned and sequenced the immunoglobulin genes. The sequences of immunoglobulin genes obtained from B cells in germinal centers had many mutations, but very few mutations were found in the genes obtained from activated B cells in nongerminal-center foci. When the mutated sequences of the collection of B cells from germinal centers was examined, it was apparent that many of the cells had sequences that were sufficiently similar that they were likely to be related by common descent from the same precursor cell. Detailed analysis of the sequences allowed these workers to build genealogic trees in which one could clearly see the descent of progeny from progenitors by progressive somatic hypermutation (Figure 11-19).

Somatic hypermutation of heavy- and light-chain variable-region genes probably occurs when centroblasts proliferate in the dark zone of the germinal center. The introduction of point mutations, deletions, and insertions into rearranged immunoglobulin genes is strikingly focused. Figure 11-20 shows that the overwhelming majority of these mutations occur in a region that extends from about 0.5 kb 5′ to about 1.5 kb 3′ of the V(D)J segments of rearranged immunoglobulin genes. Although the hypermutation process delivers mutations throughout the V region, antigen-driven selection results in the eventual emergence of immunoglobulin genes in which the majority of the mutations lie within the three complementarity-determining regions (CDRs).

It has been estimated that the mutation rate during somatic mutation is approximately 10^{-3}/base pair/division, which is a millionfold greater than the normal mutation rate for cells. Since the heavy- and light-chain V(D)J segments total about 700 base pairs, this rate of mutation means that, after two cell divisions, nearly every centroblast will acquire a mutation in either the heavy- or light-chain variable regions. On the basis of theoretical considerations, Perelson and his colleagues at Los Alamos have suggested that germinal-center B cells probably undergo several rounds of cell division in the dark zone and accumulate mutations, then leave and experience selection in the light zone. However, instead of departing the germinal center as memory B cells or plasma cells, some of the B cells return to the dark zone for additional rounds of division and mutation. Subsequent selection of these cells in the light zone allows the emergence of cells producing antibodies of higher affinity. The extremely high rates and precise targeting of somatic hypermutation are remarkable features that are unique to the immune

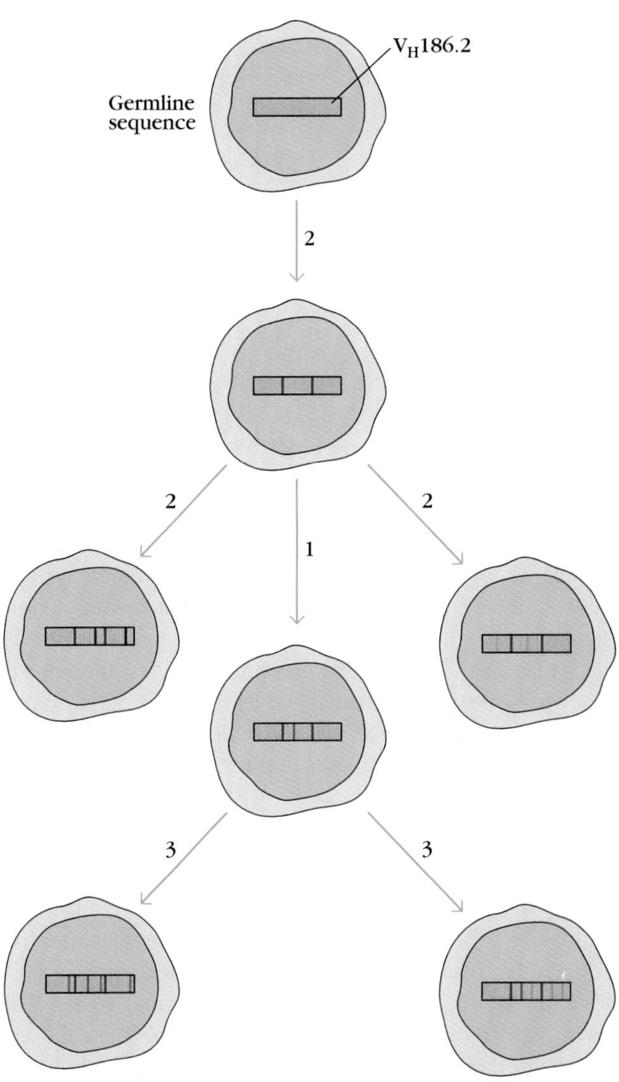

FIGURE 11-19 A B-cell family tree. By microdissection of B cells from the same area of a germinal center and using carefully executed PCR techniques on individual cells to determine the sequence of a V_H gene (mouse V_H 186.2) that dominates the NP response, it was possible to build a genealogic tree that showed the progenitor-progeny relationships among the cells. The numbers on the arrows indicate the numbers of mutations (colored lines) that occurred in the parent cell at each stage to produce its immediate descendents. The investigators thereby were able to show the in situ diversification of B cells within a germinal center by somatic point mutation. [As adapted by C Berek from Jacob et al, 1991, *Nature* **354:**389.]

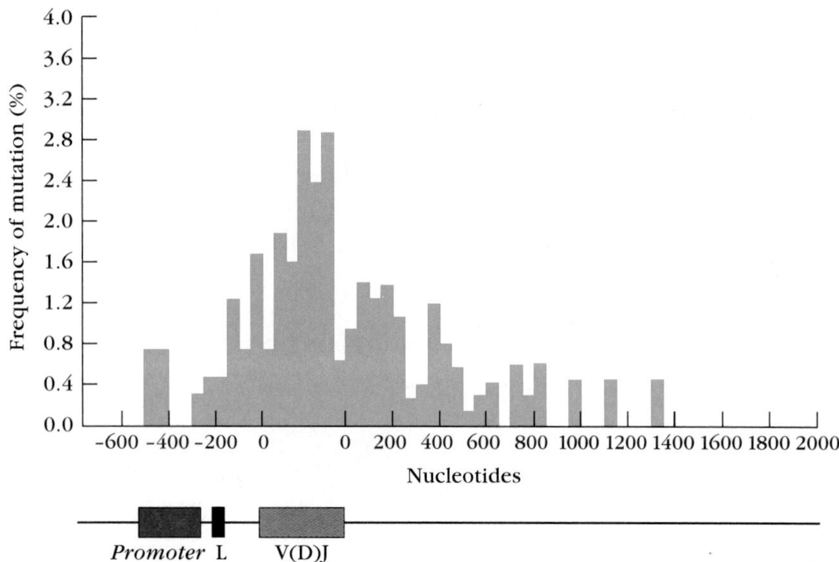

FIGURE 11-20 The frequency of somatic hypermutation decreases with the distance from the rearranged V(D)J gene. Experimental measurement of the mutation frequency shows that few if any mutations are seen beyond the promoter of the rearranged gene, and there are no mutations at positions more than about 1.5 kb 3′ of the rearranged gene. [Adapted from P Gearhart, in *Fundamental Immunology,* 3rd ed., 1993, p. 877.]

system. Determining the molecular basis of this extraordinary process remains a challenge in immunology.

Because somatic mutation occurs randomly, it will generate a few cells with receptors of higher affinity and many cells with receptors of unchanged, lower, or no affinity for a particular antigen. Therefore, selection is needed to derive a population of cells that has increased affinity. As mentioned above, the germinal center is not just a place where enormous diversity is generated, but also a site of selection. B cells that have high-affinity receptors for the antigen are likely to be positively selected and leave the germinal center, and those with low affinity are likely to undergo negative selection and die in the germinal center.

The Role of Selection

Selection in germinal centers takes place in the light zone, among the nondividing centrocyte population. A number of factors determine whether a centrocyte undergoes negative selection and dies in the germinal center or experiences positive selection and emerges from the germinal center. The most important factor influencing selection is the ability of the membrane Ig molecules on the centrocyte to recognize and bind antigen displayed by follicular dendritic cells (FDC). Because the surface of FDCs is richly endowed with both Fc receptors and complement receptors, antigen complexed with antibody or antigen that has been bound by C3 fragments generated during complement activation (see Chapter 13) can bind to FDCs by antibody or C3 bridges. A centrocyte whose membrane Ig binds and undergoes cross-linking by FDC-bound antigen receives a signal that is essential for its survival. Those that fail to receive such signals die. However, centrocytes must compete for the small amounts of antigen present on FDCs. Because the amount of antigen is limited, centrocytes with receptors of high affinity are more likely to be successful in binding antigen than those of lower affinity.

While antigen binding is necessary for centrocyte survival, it is not sufficient. A centrocyte must also receive signals generated by interaction with a $CD4^+$ T_H cell to survive. An indispensable feature of this interaction is the engagement of CD40 on the B cell (centrocyte) by CD40L on the helper T cell. It is also necessary that co-stimulatory molecules (B7) and processed antigen on class II MHC molecules of the B cell interact with CD28 and the TCR of the collaborating T_H-cell. Centrocytes that fail to receive either the T_H-cell or the antigen-membrane Ig signal undergo apoptosis in the germinal center. Indeed, one of the striking characteristics of the germinal center is the extensive cell death by apoptosis that takes place there. This is clearly evident in the presence of condensed chromatin fragments, indicative of apoptosis, in tingible-body macrophages.

Class Switching

Antibodies perform two important activities: the specific binding to an antigen, which is determined by the V_H and V_L domains; and participation in various biological effector functions, which is determined by the isotype of the heavy-chain constant domain. As described in Chapter 5, class switching allows any given V_H domain to associate with the constant region of any isotype. This enables antibody specificity to remain constant while the biological effector activities of the molecule vary. A number of cytokines affect the decision of what Ig class is chosen when an IgM-bearing cell undergoes the class switch (Figure 11-21). The role of cytokines in class switching is explored further in Chapter 12.

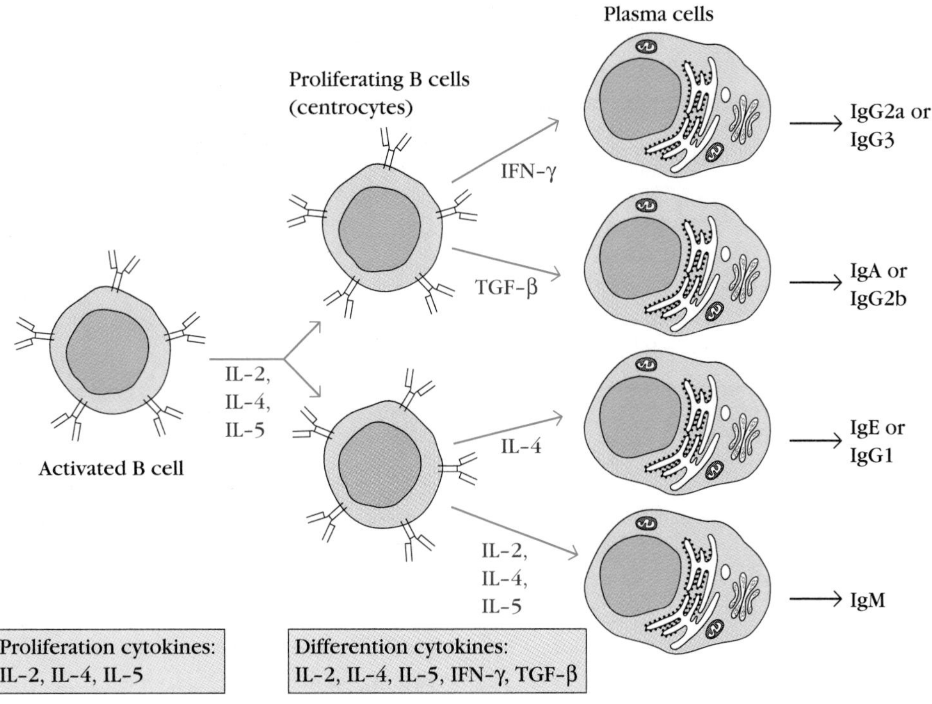

FIGURE 11-21 The interactions of numerous cytokines with B cells generate signals required for proliferation and class switching during the differentiation of B cells into plasma cells. Binding of the proliferation cytokines, which are released by activated T_H cells, provides the progression signal needed for proliferation of activated B cells. The effects of the indicated cytokines have been demonstrated; however, similar or identical effects may be mediated by other cytokines. Class switching in the response to thymus-dependent antigens also requires the CD40-CD40L interaction, which is not shown here.

As noted earlier, the humoral response to thymus-dependent antigens is marked by extensive class switching to isotypes other than IgM, whereas the antibody response to thymus-independent antigens is dominated by IgM. In the case of thymus-dependent antigens, membrane interaction between CD40 on the B cell and CD40L on the T_H cell is essential for the induction of class switching. The requirement for this interaction is highlighted by the **X-linked hyper-IgM syndrome,** an immunodeficiency disorder in which T_H cells fail to express CD40L. Patients with this disorder produce IgM but not other isotypes. Such patients also fail to generate memory-cell populations; they fail to form germinal centers, and their antibodies fail to undergo somatic hypermutation, which illustrates the importance of CD40/CD40 L interactions for the support of these processes.

Generation of Plasma Cells and Memory B Cells

After selection of centrocytes bearing high-affinity mIg for antigen displayed on follicular dendritic cells, the centrocytes differentiate into plasmablasts and memory B cells in the light zone (see Figure 11-18). Plasma cells generally lack detectable membrane-bound immunoglobulin and instead synthesize high levels of secreted antibody. Differentiation of mature B cells into plasma cells requires a change in RNA processing so that the secreted form of the heavy chain rather than the membrane form is synthesized. In addition, the rate of transcription of heavy- and light-chain genes is significantly greater in plasma cells than in less-differentiated B cells. Several authors have suggested that the increased transcription by plasma cells might be explained by their synthesis of higher levels of transcription factors that bind to immunoglobulin enhancers. Some mechanism also must coordinate the increase in transcription of heavy-chain and light-chain genes, even though these genes are on different chromosomes.

Memory cells also are generated from selected high-affinity centrocytes in the light zone of germinal centers. Some properties of naive and memory B cells are summarized in Table 11-7. Except for membrane-bound immunoglobulins, few membrane molecules have been identified that distinguish naive B cells from memory B cells. Naive B cells express only IgM and IgD; as a consequence of class switching, however, memory B cells express additional isotypes, including IgG, IgA, and IgE. In addition, the level of IgD often appears to be reduced on memory B cells.

TABLE 11-7 COMPARISON OF NAIVE AND MEMORY B CELLS

Properties	Naive B cell	Memory B cell
Membrane markers		
Immunoglobulin	IgM, IgD	IgM, IgD(?), IgG, IgA, IgE
Complement receptor	Low	High
Anatomic location	Spleen	Bone marrow, lymph node, spleen
Life span	Short-lived	May be long-lived
Recirculation	Yes	Yes
Receptor affinity	Lower average affinity	Higher average affinity due to affinity maturation*
Adhesion molecules	Low ICAM-1	High ICAM-1

*Affinity maturation results from somatic mutation during proliferation of centroblasts and subsequent antigen selection of centrocytes bearing high-affinity mIg.

Regulation of B-Cell Development

A number of transcription factors that regulate expression of various gene products at different stages of B-cell development have been identified. Among these are NF-κB, Ets-1, c-Jun, Ikaros, Oct-2, Pu.1, EBF, BCF, and E2A. Like all transcription factors, these DNA-binding proteins interact with promoter or enhancer sequences, thereby either stimulating or inhibiting transcription of the associated gene. Analyses of the effects of knocking out the gene that encodes a particular transcription factor have provided clues about the role of some factors in B-cell development. For example, in knockout mice that carry a disrupted *Ikaros* gene, there is a general failure of lymphocyte development, and pro-B cells fail to develop in the bone marrow.

One of the most critical B-cell transcription factors, *B-cell–specific activator protein (BSAP),* which has been previously mentioned (see Figure 11-3), appears to function as a master B-cell regulator. It is expressed only by B-lineage cells and influences all the cell stages during B-cell maturation. Moreover, recent evidence indicates that BSAP also influences the final differentiation events leading to the formation of memory B cells and plasma cells. The latter are the only B-lineage cells that do not express BSAP. BSAP binds to promoter or enhancer sequences of various B-cell–specific genes, including the λ5 and Vpre-B genes of the surrogate light chain, the J-chain gene of polymeric IgM, and the 3′α heavy-chain enhancer region, one of the two enhancers that lie 3′ of the α gene in heavy-chain germ-line DNA. In addition, BSAP binds to various immunoglobulin heavy-chain switch sites and to several genes involved in B-cell activation.

The heavy-chain 3′α enhancer ($E_{3'\alpha}$) contains binding sites for several transcription factors in addition to BSAP. Binding of BSAP to $E_{3'\alpha}$ appears to influence B-cell development by preventing the binding of other transcription factors. For example, when BSAP levels are high, this factor appears to block binding of NF-αP to the 3′α enhancer, thereby blocking transcription of the heavy-chain gene and promoting formation of memory B cells. When BSAP levels are low, NF-αP can bind to $E_{3'\alpha}$. As a result, transcription of the immunoglobulin heavy-chain gene is increased, leading to formation of plasma cells.

Regulation of the Immune Effector Response

Upon encountering an antigen, the immune system can either develop an immune response or enter a state of unresponsiveness called **tolerance**. The development of immunity or tolerance, both of which involve specific recognition of antigen by antigen-reactive T or B cells, needs to be carefully regulated since an inappropriate response—whether it be immunity to self-antigens or tolerance to a potential pathogen—can have serious and possibly life-threatening consequences.

Regulation of the immune response takes place in both the humoral and the cell-mediated branch. Every time an antigen is introduced, important regulatory decisions determine the branch of the immune system to be activated, the intensity of the response, and its duration. Chapter 12 describes the importance of the cytokines to the orchestration of appropriate immune responses. In addition to cytokines, other regulatory mechanisms may also play important immunoregulatory roles. Greater knowledge about these regulatory events, which are still not well understood, may produce two desirable outcomes. One is a better understanding of the humoral immune system. The other is the use of such an understanding to deliberately manipulate immune responses, selectively up-regulating desirable responses and down-regulating undesirable ones.

TABLE 11-8 ANTIGENIC COMPETITION BETWEEN SRBCS AND HRBCS

Immunizing antigen		Hemolytic plaque assay (day 8)*	
Agl (day 0)	Ag2 (day 3)	Test Ag	PFC/10^6 spleen cells
None	HRBC	HRBC	205
SRBC	HRBC	HRBC	13
None	SRBC	SRBC	626
HRBC	SRBC	SRBC	78

*See Figure 23-1 for a description of the plaque assay.

Antigen-Mediated Regulation

The immunologic history of an animal influences the quality and quantity of its immune response. A naive animal responds to antigen challenges very differently from a previously primed animal. Previous encounter with an antigen may have rendered the animal tolerant to the antigen or may have resulted in the formation of memory cells. In some cases, the presence of a competing antigen can regulate the immune response to an unrelated antigen. This **antigenic competition** is illustrated by injecting mice with a competing antigen a day or two before immunization with a test antigen. For example, the response to horse red blood cells (HRBCs) is severely reduced by prior immunization with sheep red blood cells (SRBCs) and vice versa (Table 11-8). Although antigenic competition is a well-established phenomenon, its molecular and cellular basis is not understood.

Antibody-Mediated Suppression

As in so many biochemical reactions subject to feedback inhibition by the end product, antibody exerts feedback inhibition on its own further production. If an animal is immunized with a specific antigen and is injected with preformed antibody to that same antigen just before or within 5 days after antigen priming, the immune response to the antigen is reduced as much as 100-fold.

One explanation for antibody-mediated suppression is that the passively administered antibody competes with antigen-reactive B cells for antigen, so that the B cells do not clonally expand. Evidence for such competition between passively administered antibody and antigen-reactive B cells comes from studies in which it took over 10 times more low-affinity anti-DNP antibody than high-affinity anti-DNP antibody to induce comparable suppression. Furthermore, the competition for antigen between passively administered antibody and antigen-reactive B cells drives the B-cell response toward higher-affinity antibody. Only the high-affinity antigen-reactive cells can compete successfully with the passively administered antibody for the available antigen.

Because of antibody-mediated suppression, certain vaccines (e.g., those for measles and mumps) are not administered to infants before the age of 1 year. The level of naturally acquired maternal IgG, which the fetus acquires by transplacental transfer, remains high for about 6 months after birth. If an infant is immunized with measles or mumps vaccine while this maternal antibody is still present, the humoral response is low and the production of memory cells is inadequate to confer long-lasting immunity.

Summary

1. Development of B cells involves antigen-independent maturation in the bone marrow and antigen-dependent activation and differentiation of mature B cells in the periphery, resulting in antibody-secreting plasma cells and memory B cells (see Figure 11-1).
2. During B-cell maturation, sequential Ig-gene rearrangement transforms the pro-B cell, the earliest distinctly B-lineage cell, into an immature B cell, which expresses mIgM with a single antigenic specificity (see Figure 11-3). Proliferation and development of pro-B cells into pre-B cells depends on the microenvironment provided by bone-marrow stromal cells (see Figure 11-2). Pre-B cells express the heavy chain and a surrogate light chain associated with the Ig-α/Ig-β heterodimer (see Figure 11-4). Although the function of this pre-B cell receptor is not entirely clear, it is required for maturation to continue to the immature B-cell stage. Further development, including changes in RNA processing, yields mature B cells, expressing both IgM and IgD.
3. The antigen-induced activation and differentiation of mature B cells occur in the periphery, generating the humoral response. The B-cell response to soluble protein antigens requires involvement of T_H cells; in contrast, the response to certain bacterial cell wall products (e.g., LPS) and highly polymeric molecules does not require T_H cells. The nature of the response to thymus-dependent and thymus-independent antigens differs considerably (see Table 11-2).
4. Activation of mature B cells involves signals generated by membrane events and, in some cases, cytokines. These signals are transduced by intracellular pathways, ultimately leading to changes in the expression of specific genes (see Figure 11-8).
5. B- and T-cell activation share many parallels, including: compartmentalization of function within receptor subunits; activation by membrane-associated protein tyrosine kinases; activating dephosphorylations by CD45; assembly of large signaling complexes with protein-tyrosine-kinase activity; and recruitment of several signal-transduction pathways. In both cell types, changes in

gene expression are a consequence of these signal transduction processes.

6. The B-cell coreceptor can intensify the activating signal resulting from crosslinkage of mIg (see Figure 11-9). This may be particularly important during the primary response to low concentrations of antigen, because many naive B cells express mIg with low affinity for antigen.
7. Activation induced by thymus-dependent antigens requires the delivery of contact-dependent help. The formation of T-B cell conjugates (see Figure 11-11) facilitates the interaction between CD40 on B cells and CD40L on activated T_H cells as well as the co-stimulation of T_H cells by interaction of B7 on the B cell with CD28 of its partnering T cell. The CD40/CD40L interaction is essential for B-cell survival, the formation of germinal centers, the generation of memory cell populations, and somatic mutation.
8. The kinetics of antibody formation and other properties of the primary and secondary humoral responses differ (see Figure 11-15 and Table 11-4). The primary response is marked by a long lag period, a logarithmic rise in antibody formation, a short plateau, and then a decline. During a primary response, IgM is the first antibody class produced. It is followed by a gradual switch to other classes, in particular, IgG subclasses. The secondary response has a shorter lag time, a more rapid logarithmic phase, a longer plateau phase and a slower decline than the primary response. Little IgM is produced in the secondary response, which is characterized by production of IgG or other isotypes and a higher average antibody affinity for antigen.
9. Generation of a humoral response to antigen in vivo occurs primarily in peripheral lymph nodes (see Figure 11-17). Within 1–2 weeks after exposure to a thymus-dependent antigen, secondary follicles form, composed of a few layers of cells surrounding a germinal center. Intense proliferation of activated B cells (centroblasts) occurs in the dark zone of germinal centers. About 90% of the resulting centrocytes undergo death by apoptosis in the light zone. The remaining centrocytes, which express high-affinity mIg, interact with antigen bound to follicular dendritic cells and undergo differentiation in the apical light zone, generating memory B cells and plasmablasts. The latter develop into antibody-secreting plasma cells.
10. Affinity maturation, class switching, and formation of plasma and memory B cells all take place during B-cell proliferation and differentiation within germinal centers. Somatic hypermutation during proliferation of centroblasts and antigen selection of high-affinity centrocytes lead to affinity maturation, so that the average affinity of the induced serum antibodies increases during the course of a T-dependent humoral response. Class switching depends on various cytokines (see Figure 11-21). The CD40/CD40L interaction is an essential additional signal that is required for the survival of centrocytes that bind antigen presented on FDCs. Such cells, many of which express mIg of higher affinity than the progenitor B cells that founded the germinal center, develop into memory B cells or plasma cells (see Figure 11-18).
11. Induction of immune responses by self-antigens can have serious, even fatal, consequences. When a self-antigen is expressed in the bone marrow, negative selection of self-reactive immature B cells occurs. The selected cells are deleted by apoptosis or undergo further light-chain gene rearrangement resulting in production of an edited mIg that is nonreactive with the self-antigen (see Figure 11-5). In contrast, when a self-antigen is expressed only in the periphery, negative selection of the self-reactive B cells occurs at the mature B-cell stage in the periphery; the selected cells are either deleted or rendered anergic. These processes assure that an individual does not mount autoimmune responses.

REFERENCES

Arulampalam, V, L Eckhardt, and S Pettersson. 1997. The enhancer shift: a model to explain the developmental control of IgH gene expression in B-lineage cells. *Immunology Today* **18:**549.

Benschop, RJ, and JC Cambier. 1999. B cell development: signal transduction by antigen receptors and their surrogates. *Curr. Opin. Immunol.* **11:**143.

Berek, C. 1999. Affinity Maturation. In *Fundamental Immunology,* 4th ed., edited by WE Paul. Lippincott-Raven, Philadelphia and New York.

Bruton, OC. 1952. Agammaglobulinemia. *Pediatrics* **9:**722.

Clevers, HC. 1996. Transcriptional control of lymphoid development: lessons from gene targeting. *Immunology Today* **17:**336.

Desiderio, S. 1997. Role of Btk in B cell development and signaling. *Curr. Opin. Immunol.* **9:**534.

Goodnow, CC, et al. 1988. Altered immunoglobulin expression and functional silencing of self-reactive B lymphocytes in transgenic mice. *Nature* **334:**676.

Hodgkin, PD, and A Basten. 1995. B cell activation, tolerance, and antigen-presenting function. *Curr. Opin. Immunol.* **7:**121.

Jacob, J, G Kelsoe, K Rajewsky, and U Weiss. 1991. Intraclonal generation of antibody mutants in germinal centres. *Nature* **354:**389.

Kurosaki, T. 1997. Molecular mechanisms in B cell antigen receptor signaling. *Curr. Opin. Immunol.* **9:**309.

Kelsoe, G. 1996. Life and death in germinal centers (redux). *Immunity* **4:**107.

Klinman, NR. 1994. Selection in the expression of functionally distinct B-cell subsets. *Curr. Opin. Immunol.* **6:**420.

Melchers, F, and A Rolink. 1999. B-lymphocyte development and biology. In *Fundamental Immunology,* 4th ed., edited by WE Paul. Lippincott-Raven, Philadelphia and New York.

Nemazee, DA, and K Burki. 1989. Clonal deletion of B lymphocytes in a transgenic mouse bearing anti-MHC class I antibody genes. *Nature* **337:**562.

Neuberger, MS, and C Milstein. 1995. Somatic hypermutation. *Curr. Opin. Immunol.* **7**:248.

O'Rourke, L, R Tooze R, and DT Fearon. 1997. Co-receptors of B lymphocytes. *Curr. Opin. Immunol.* **9**:324.

Reth, M. 1994. B cell antigen receptors. *Curr. Opin. Immunol.* **6**:3.

Rolink, A, and F Melchers. 1993. B lymphopoiesis in the mouse. *Adv. Immunol.* **53**:123.

Stavenezer, J. 1996. Immunoglobulin class switching. *Curr. Opin. Immunol.* **8**:199.

Storb, U. 1996. The molecular basis of somatic hypermutation of immunoglobulin genes. *Curr. Opin. Immunol.* **8**:206.

Tiegs, SL, DM Russell, and D Nemazee. 1993. Receptor editing in self-reactive bone marrow B cells. *Journal of Experimental Medicine* **177**:1009.

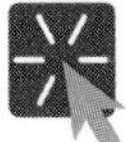

Useful Web Sites

http://www.ncbi.nlm.nih.gov/Omim/>
http://www.ncbi.nlm.nih.gov/htbinpost/Omim/getmim>
The Online Mendelian Inheritance in Man Web site contains a subsite that lists more than a dozen different inherited diseases that are associated with B cell defects. Any of those listed may be studied in detail by following the links in this database.

http://www.bioscience.org/knockout/knochome.htm>
Within the Frontiers in Bioscience Database of Gene Knockouts, one can find information on the effects of knockouts of many genes of significance to the development and function of cells of the B lineage.

STUDY QUESTIONS

1. Indicate whether each of the following statements concerning B-cell maturation is true or false. If you think a statement is false, explain why.

a. Heavy chain V_H-D_H-J_H rearrangement begins in the pre–B-cell stage.

b. Immature B cells express membrane IgM and IgD.

c. The enzyme terminal deoxyribonucleotidyl transferase (TdT) is active in the pre–B-cell stage.

d. The surrogate light chain is expressed by pre-B cells.

e. Self-reactive B cells can be rescued from negative selection by the expression of a different light chain.

f. In order to develop into immature B cells, pre-B cells must interact directly with bone-marrow stromal cells.

g. Most of the B cells generated every day never leave the bone marrow as mature B cells.

2. You have fluorescein (Fl)-labeled antibody to the μ heavy chain and a rhodamine (Rh)-labeled antibody to the δ heavy chain. Describe the fluorescent-antibody staining pattern of the following B-cell maturational stages assuming that you can visualize both membrane and cytoplasmic staining: (a) progenitor B cell (pro-B cell); (b) precursor B cell (pre-B cell); (c) immature B cell; (d) mature B cell; and (e) plasma cell before any class switching has occurred.

3. Describe the general structure and probable function of the B-cell–coreceptor complex.

4. In the Goodnow experiment demonstrating clonal anergy of B cells, two types of transgenic mice were compared: single transgenics carrying a transgene-encoded antibody against hen egg-white lysozyme (HEL) and double transgenics carrying the anti-HEL transgene and a HEL transgene linked to the zinc-activated metallothionine promoter.

a. In both the single and double transgenics, 60%–90% of the B cells expressed anti-HEL membrane-bound antibody. Explain why.

b. How could you show that the membrane antibody on these B cells is specific for HEL and how could you determine its isotype?

c. Why was the metallothionine promoter used in constructing the HEL transgene?

d. Design an experiment to prove that the B cells, not the T_H cells, from the double transgenics were anergic.

5. Discuss the origin of the competence and progression signals required for activation and proliferation of B cells induced by (a) soluble protein antigens and (b) bacterial lipopolysaccharide (LPS).

6. Fill in the blank(s) in each statement below (a–i) with the most appropriate term(s) from the following list. Terms may be used more than once or not at all.

dark zone	centroblasts	memory B cells
light zone	centrocytes	plasmablasts
paracortex	follicular dendritic cells	T_H cells
cortex	medulla	plasma cells

a. Most centrocytes die by apoptosis in the ________.

b. Initial activation of naive B cells induced by thymus-dependent antigens occurs within the ________ of lymph nodes.

c. ________ are rapidly dividing B cells located in the ________ of germinal centers.

d. ________ expressing high-affinity mIg interact with antigen captured by ________ in the light zone.

e. Class switching occurs in the ________ and requires direct contact between B cells and ________.

f. Centrocytes expressing mIg specific for a self-antigen present in the bone marrow are subjected to negative selection in the ________.

g. Within lymph nodes, plasma cells are found primarily in the ________ of secondary follicles.

h. Generation of ________ in the ________ of germinal centers is induced by interaction of centrocytes with IL-1 and CD3.

i. Somatic hypermutation, which occurs in proliferating ________, is critical to affinity maturation.

7. Activation and differentiation of B cells in response to thymus-dependent (TD) antigens requires T_H cells, whereas the B-cell response to thymus-independent (TI) antigens does not.

a. Discuss the differences in the structure of TD, TI-1, and TI-2 antigens and the characteristics of the humoral responses induced by them.

Go to www.whfreeman.com/immunology Self-Test
Review and quiz of key terms

b. Binding of which classes of antigen to mIg provides an effective competence signal for B-cell activation?

8. B-cell–activating signals must be transduced to the cell interior to influence developmental processes. Yet the cytoplasmic tails of all isotypes of mIg on B cells are too short to function in signal transduction.

a. How do naive B cells transduce the signal induced by crosslinkage of mIg by antigen?

b. Describe the general result of signal transduction in B cells during antigen-induced activation and differentiation.

9. In some of their experiments, Nemazee and Burki mated mice carrying a transgene encoding K^b, a class I MHC molecule, linked to a liver-specific promoter with mice carrying a transgene encoding antibody against K^b. In the resulting double transgenics, K^b-binding B cells were found in the bone marrow but not in lymph nodes. In contrast, the anti-K^b single transgenics had K^b-binding B cells in both the bone marrow and lymph nodes.

a. Was the haplotype of the mice that received the transgenes H-2^b or some other haplotype?

b. Why was the K^b transgene linked to a liver-specific promoter in these experiments?

c. What do these results suggest about the induction of B-cell tolerance to self-antigens?

10. Indicate whether each of the following statements is true or false. If you believe a statement is false, explain why.

a. Cytokines can regulate which branch of the immune system is activated.

b. Immunization with a hapten-carrier conjugate results in production of antibodies to both hapten and carrier epitopes.

c. All the antibodies secreted by a single plasma cell have the same idiotype and isotype.

d. If mice are immunized with HRBCs and then are immunized a day later with SRBCs, the antibody response to the SRBCs will be much higher than that achieved in control mice immunized only with SRBCs.

11. Four mice are immunized with antigen under the conditions listed below (a–d). In each case, indicate whether the induced serum antibodies will have high affinity or low affinity and whether they will be largely IgM or IgG.

a. A primary response to a low antigen dose

b. A secondary response to a low antigen dose

c. A primary response to a high antigen dose

d. A secondary response to a high antigen dose

12. DNA was isolated from three sources: liver cells, pre-B lymphoma cells, and IgM-secreting myeloma cells. Each DNA sample was digested separately with the restriction enzymes *Bam*HI and *Eco*RI, which cleave germ-line heavy-chain and κ light-chain DNA as indicated in part (a) of the accompanying figure. The digested samples were analyzed by Southern blotting using a radiolabeled $C_\mu 1$ probe with the *Bam*HI digests (blot #1) and a radiolabeled C_κ probe with the *Eco*RI digests (blot #2). The blot patterns are illustrated in part (b) of the figure. Based on this information, which DNA sample (designated A, B, or C) was isolated from the (a) liver cells, (b) pre-B lymphoma cells, and (c) IgM-secreting plasma cells? Explain your assignments.

For use with Question 12:

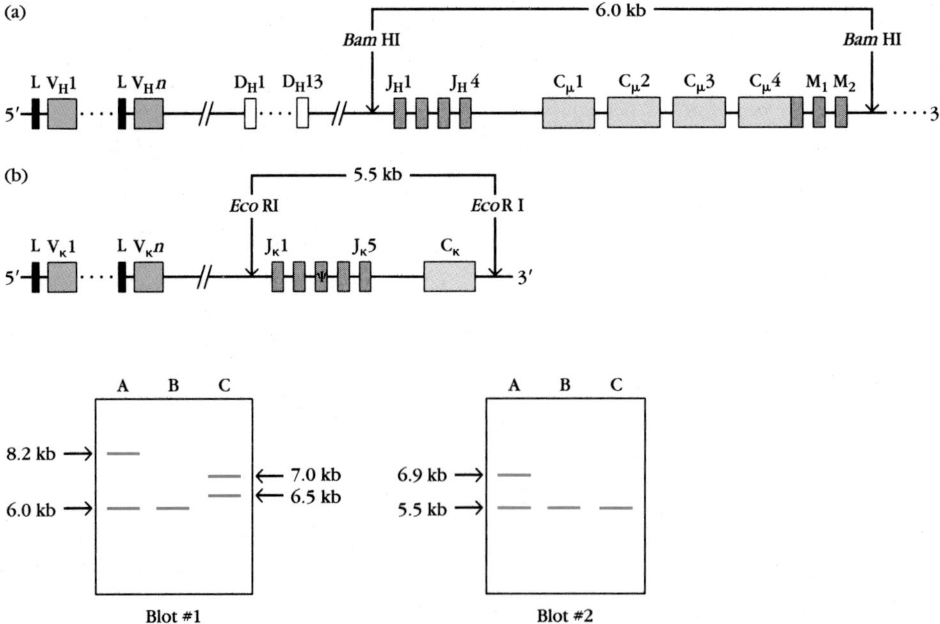

PART III | IMMUNE EFFECTOR MECHANISMS

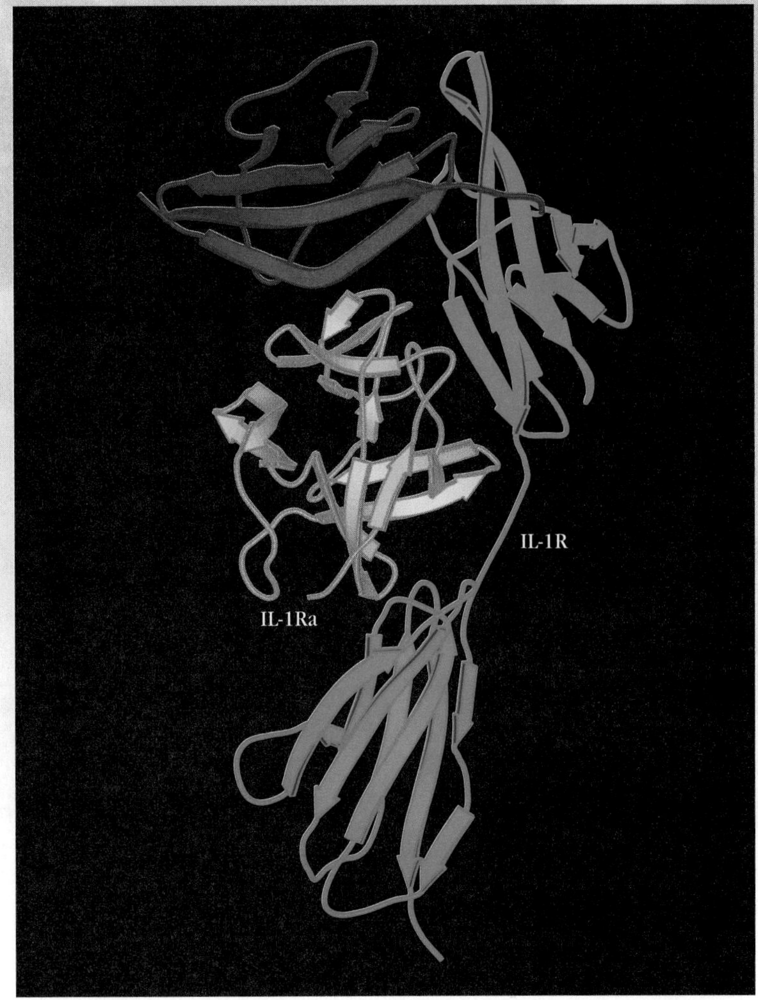

Interleukin-1 receptor (IL-1R) with IL-1R antagonist (IL-1Ra) bound.

Recognition of antigen by the immune system induces a variety of effector mechanisms associated with the humoral and cell-mediated responses. Part III concentrates on these effector mechanisms. Secreted antibodies and complement components are effectors of humoral immunity, whereas both specific and nonspecific cells are the key effectors of cell-mediated immunity. The humoral branch of the immune system functions primarily to eliminate extracellular bacteria and bacterial products, whereas the cell-mediated branch functions to eliminate altered self-cells (infected cells and tumor cells) and foreign grafts.

The cytokines described in Chapter 12 are small proteins that assist in regulating the development of immune effector cells and/or possess direct effector functions. Secreted by activated lymphocytes, macrophages, and certain other cells, cytokines are critical components of both humoral and cell-mediated immune responses. Many cytokines exert their biological effects by binding to specific receptors found on the membrane of target cells. These receptors can be grouped into five families of proteins. When a cytokine binds to its receptor, it triggers intracellular signals that lead to specific changes in gene expression. Some cytokines, called chemokines, chemotactically attract certain cell types, while others have direct cytotoxic or antiviral effects.

In vitro, the interaction of antibody and antigen leads to precipitation or agglutination of the antigen-antibody (immune) complexes. In vivo, however, activation of the complement system, consisting of nearly 30 serum and membrane proteins, is the primary effector mechanism of the humoral immune response. Chapter 13 will show how complement activation generates numerous products that function in clearance of immune complexes, lysis of invading microorganisms, and neutralization of viral infectivity. Some complement products also facilitate phagocytosis and play major roles in an inflammatory response.

Chapter 14 describes a major effector mechanism of cell-mediated immunity—direct cell-mediated cytotoxicity. Antigen-specific cytotoxic T lymphocytes (CTLs) and several nonspecific cell types, including natural killer (NK) cells, carry out the destruction of altered self-cells. Target-cell destruction results from the stimulation of intracellular pathways leading to apoptosis. This chapter describes common assays for measuring cell-mediated cytotoxicity and explores the mechanisms by which cell death is initiated by CTLs and NK cells.

Chapter 15 describes the movement of immune-system cells throughout the body and the chemokines and cell-adhesion molecules that direct their movement to specific sites. This trafficking delivers lymphocytes to lymphoid tissues, where they can encounter antigen and undergo proliferation and differentiation, as described in earlier chapters. Phagocytic cells directed to sites of tissue injury or local infection mediate inflammation, a localized nonspecific response that acts to contain infection or harmful substances within a confined site. Neutrophils, macrophages, and numerous mediators play critical roles in the inflammatory response. Under certain circumstances, the inflammatory response can be prolonged or excessive, with deleterious effects.

The four types of such hypersensitive reactions are covered in Chapter 16. Individuals who are allergic to pollens, mold spores, certain foods, or some drugs can blame type I hypersensitivity. A recipient who receives a blood transfusion that is not matched to their ABO blood group will develop a type II reaction, leading to destruction of the transfused blood cells. Some autoimmune diseases and infectious diseases are associated with type III reactions, which are triggered by antigen-antibody complexes. The manifestations of these three types of hypersensitivity occur within a few hours. Delayed type hypersensitivity (DTH), which is type IV hypersensitivity, is a response to intracellular pathogens and contact antigens (e.g., poison oak, poison ivy, certain organic compounds) that typically takes 2 to 3 days to develop.

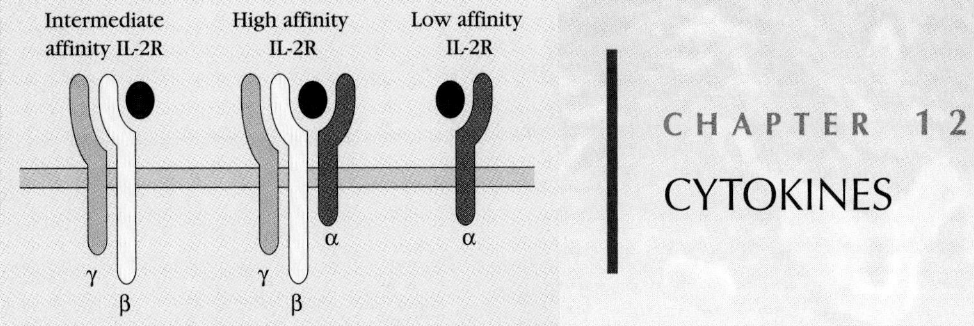

CHAPTER 12

CYTOKINES

The development of an effective immune response involves lymphoid cells, inflammatory cells, and hematopoietic cells. The complex interactions among these cells are mediated by a group of proteins that are collectively designated **cytokines** to denote their role in cell-to-cell communication. Cytokines are low-molecular-weight regulatory proteins or glycoproteins secreted by white blood cells and various other cells in the body in response to a number of stimuli. These proteins assist in regulating the development of immune effector cells, and some cytokines possess direct effector functions of their own. Just as hormones serve as messengers of the endocrine system, so cytokines serve as messengers of the immune system. Unlike endocrine hormones, though, which exert their effects over large distances, cytokines generally act locally.

This chapter focuses on the biological activity of cytokines, the structure of cytokines and their receptors, signal transduction by cytokine receptors, the role of cytokine abnormalities in the pathogenesis of certain diseases, and therapeutic uses of cytokines or their receptors. The important role of cytokines in the inflammatory response is described in Chapter 15.

Properties of Cytokines

Cytokines bind to specific receptors on the membrane of target cells, triggering signal-transduction pathways that ultimately alter gene expression in the target cells (Figure 12-1a). The susceptibility of the target cell to a particular cytokine is determined by the presence of specific membrane receptors. In general, the cytokines and their receptors exhibit very high affinity for each other, with dissociation constants ranging from 10^{-10} to 10^{-12} M. Because of this high affinity, picomolar concentrations of cytokines can mediate a biological effect.

A particular cytokine may bind to receptors on the membrane of the same cell that secreted it, exerting **autocrine** action; it may bind to receptors on a target cell in close proximity to the producer cell, exerting **paracrine** action; in a few cases, it may bind to target cells in distant parts of the body, exerting **endocrine** action (Figure 12-1b). Cytokines regulate the intensity and duration of the immune response by stimulating or inhibiting the activation, proliferation, and/or differentiation of various cells and by regulating the secretion of antibodies or other cytokines. As described later, binding of a given cytokine to responsive target cells generally stimulates increased expression of cytokine receptors as well as of other cytokines, which in turn affect other target cells. Thus, the cytokines secreted by even a small number of lymphocytes activated by antigen can influence the activity of various cells involved in the immune response. For example, cytokines produced by activated T_H cells can influence the activity of B cells, T_C cells, natural killer cells, macrophages, granulocytes, and hematopoietic stem cells, thereby activating an entire network of interacting cells.

Cytokines exhibit the attributes of pleiotropy, redundancy, synergy, antagonism, and cascade induction, which permit them to regulate cellular activity in a coordinated, interactive

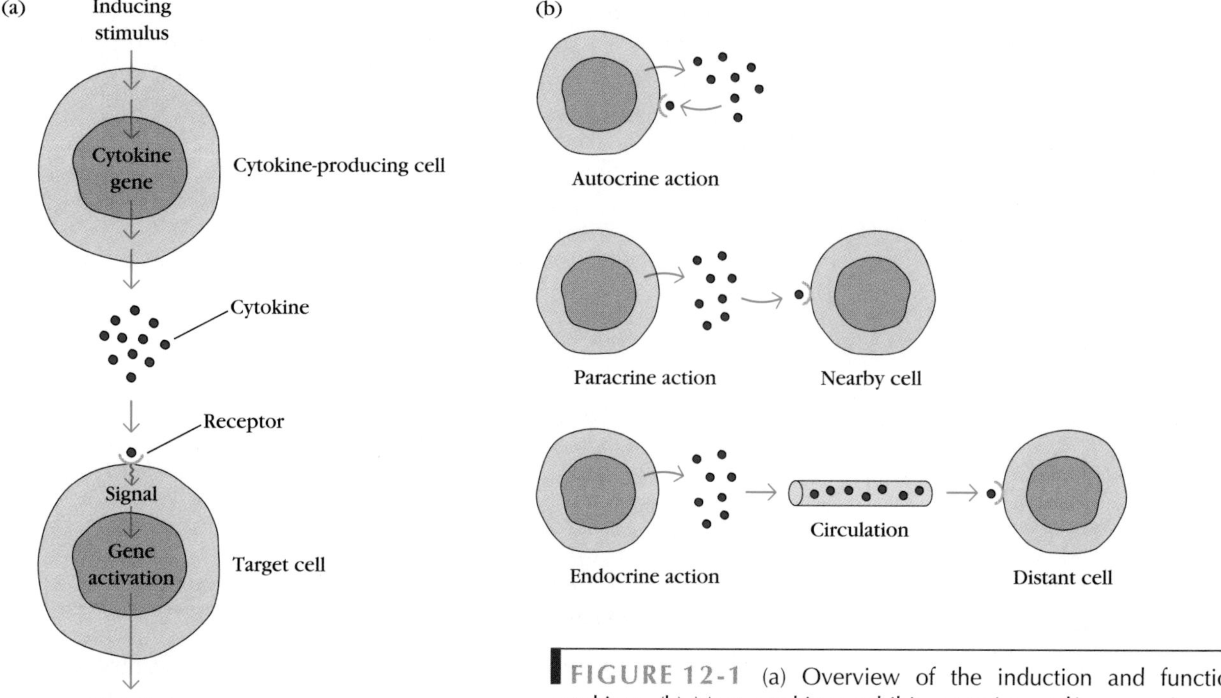

FIGURE 12-1 (a) Overview of the induction and function of cytokines. (b) Most cytokines exhibit autocrine and/or paracrine action; fewer exhibit endocrine action.

way (Figure 12-2). A given cytokine that has different biological effects on different target cells has a pleiotropic action. Two or more cytokines that mediate similar functions are said to be redundant; this property makes it difficult to ascribe a particular activity to a single cytokine. Cytokine synergism occurs when the combined effect of two cytokines on cellular activity is greater than the additive effects of the individual cytokines. In some cases, cytokines exhibit antagonism; that is, the effects of one cytokine inhibit or offset the effects of another cytokine. Cascade induction occurs when the action of one cytokine on a target cell induces that cell to produce one or more other cytokines, which in turn may induce other target cells to produce other cytokines.

The term *cytokine* encompasses those cytokines secreted by lymphocytes, substances formerly known as **lymphokines,** and those cytokines secreted by monocytes and macrophages, substances formerly known as **monokines.** Although these other two terms continue to be used, they are misleading because secretion of many lymphokines and monokines is not limited to lymphocytes and monocytes as these terms imply, but extends to a broad spectrum of cells and types. For this reason, the more inclusive term *cytokine* is preferred.

Many of the cytokines are referred to as **interleukins,** a name indicating that they are secreted by some leukocytes and act upon other leukocytes. Interleukins 1–18 have been identified. There is reason to suppose that still other cytokines will be discovered and that the interleukin group will likely expand further. Some cytokines are known by common names; these include the interferons and tumor necrosis factors. Yet another group of cytokines, **chemokines,** a group of low-molecular-weight cytokines including interleukin 8, that affect chemotaxis and other aspects of leukocyte behavior, have recently gained increased prominence. These molecules play an important role in the inflammatory response and are described in Chapter 15.

Because cytokines share many properties with hormones and growth factors, the distinction between these three classes of mediators is often blurred. All three classes of mediators are secreted soluble factors that elicit their biological effects at picomolar concentrations by binding to receptors on target cells. Growth factors tend to be produced constitutively, whereas cytokine production is carefully regulated. Cytokines generally are secreted after activation of a particular cell, and secretion is short-lived, generally ranging from a few hours to a few days. Unlike hormones, which generally act long range in an endocrine fashion, most cytokines act over a short distance in an autocrine or paracrine fashion. In addition, most hormones are produced by specialized glands and tend to have a unique action on one or a few types of target cell. In contrast, cytokines are often produced by a variety of cells and bind to receptors present on numerous types of cells.

The activity of cytokines was first recognized in the mid-1960s, when supernatants derived from in vitro cultures of lymphocytes were found to contain factors that could regulate proliferation, differentiation, and maturation of allogeneic immune-system cells. Soon after, it was discovered that production of these factors by cultured lymphocytes was induced by activation with antigen or with nonspecific mitogens. Biochemical isolation and purification of cytokines was hampered because of their low concentration in culture supernatants and the absence of well-defined assay systems for individual cytokines. The development of gene-cloning techniques during the 1970s and 1980s made it possible to produce pure cytokines by expressing the protein from cloned genes. The availability of such recombinant cytokines, made by recombinant-DNA technology, was a major advance. The discovery of cell lines whose growth depended on the presence of a particular cytokine provided researchers with the first simple assay systems. The derivation of monoclonal antibodies specific for each of the more important cytokines has made it possible to develop rapid quantitative immunoassays for each of them (Figure 12-3).

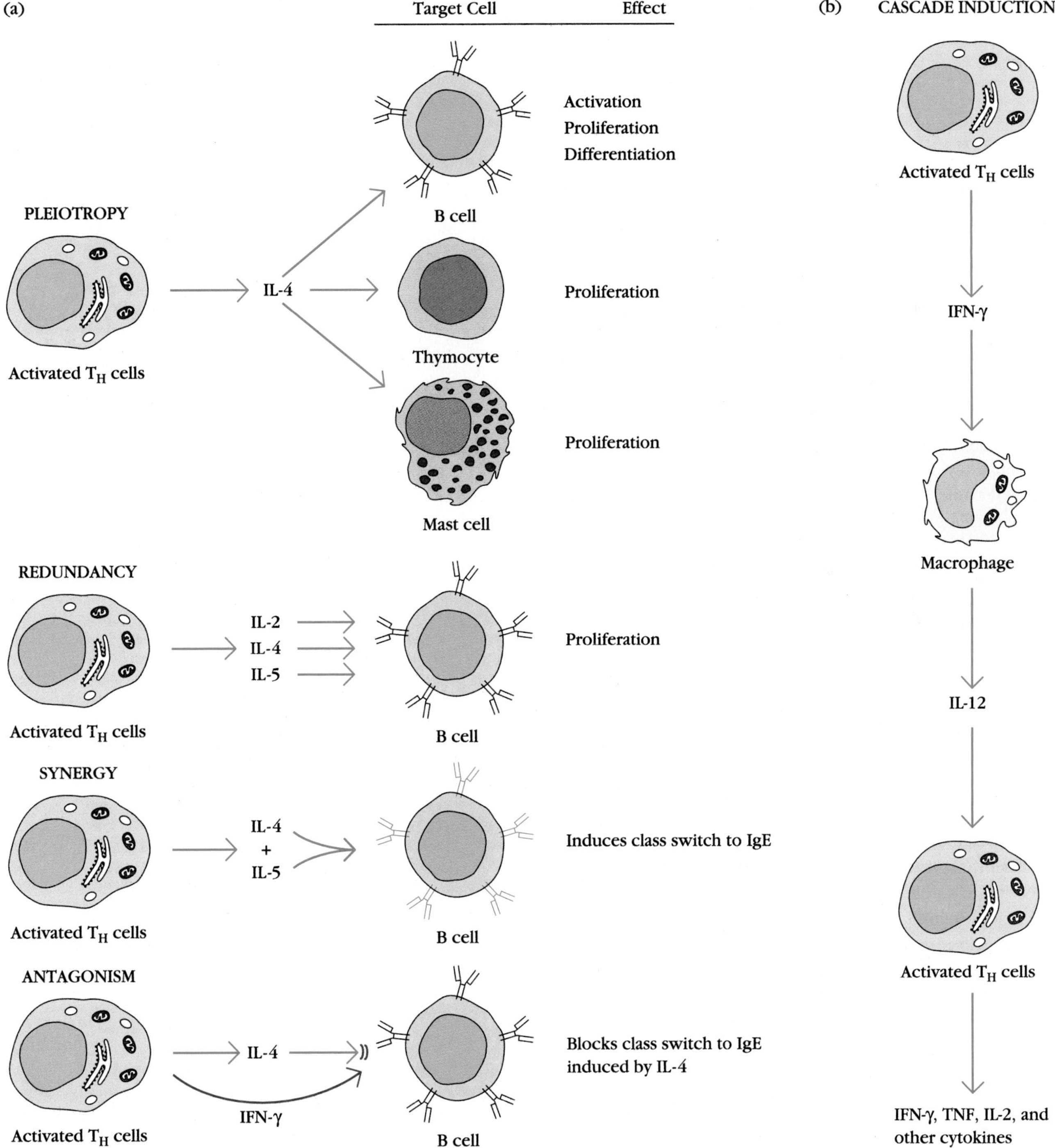

FIGURE 12-2 Cytokine attributes of (a) pleiotropy, redundancy, synergy (synergism), antagonism, and (b) cascade induction.

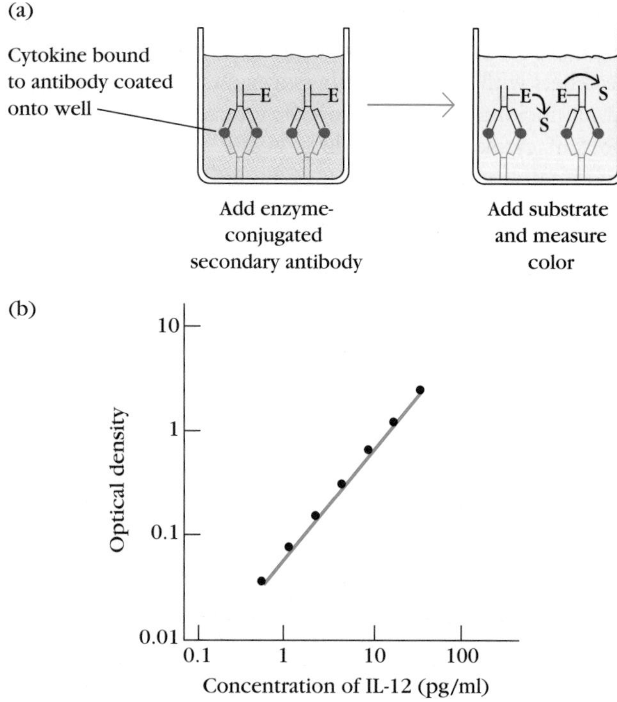

FIGURE 12-3 ELISA assay of a cytokine. (a) The sample containing the cytokine of interest is captured by specific antibody (blue) coated onto wells of a microtiter plate. A second specific antibody (blue), conjugated to an enzyme (E) such as horse radish peroxidase, forms a sandwich with the captured cytokine, immobilizing the enzyme in the microtiter well. A chromogenic substrate (S) is added, and the enzyme generates a color whose intensity is proportional to the amount of cytokine bound to the capture antibody. The optical density of this color produced by the unknown is compared with values on an appropriately determined standard curve. (b) The standard curve shown here is for human interleukin 12 (IL-12). It is clear that this assay is sufficiently sensitive to detect as little as 1 picogram of IL-12.

General Structure of Cytokines

Once the genes encoding various cytokines had been cloned, sufficient quantities of purified preparations became available for detailed studies on the structure and function of these important proteins. Cytokines generally have a molecular mass of less than 30 kDa. Structural studies have shown that the cytokines characterized so far belong to one of the following families: the hematopoietin family, the interferon family, the chemokine family, or the tumor necrosis factor (TNF) family. For example, many cytokines, GM-CSF, G-CSF, IL-2–7, IL-11–13, IL-15 and others, belong to the **hematopoietin family.**

The structures of two members of the hematopoietin family, IL-2 and IL-4, are depicted in Figure 12-4. Although the amino acid sequences of these family members differ considerably, all of them have a high degree of α-helical structure and little or no β-sheet structure. The molecules share a similar polypeptide fold, with four α-helical regions (A–D) in which the first and second helices and the third and fourth helices run roughly parallel to one another and are connected by loops.

Function of Cytokines

Cytokines generally function as intercellular messenger molecules that evoke particular biological activities after binding to a receptor on a responsive target cell. Although a variety of cells can secrete cytokines, the two principal producers are the T_H cell and the macrophage. Cytokines released from these two cell types activate an entire network of interacting cells (Figure 12-5). Among the numerous

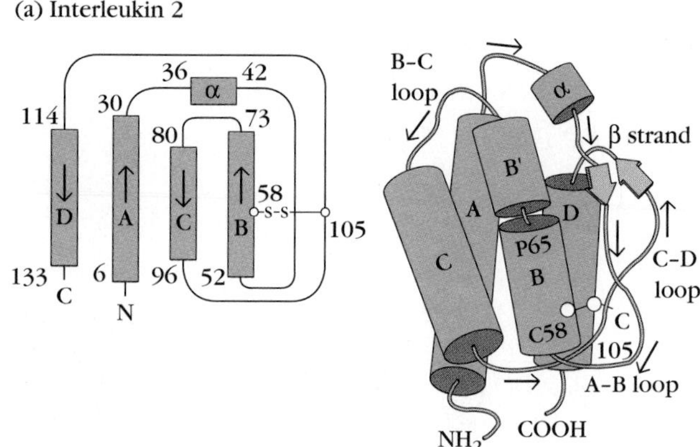

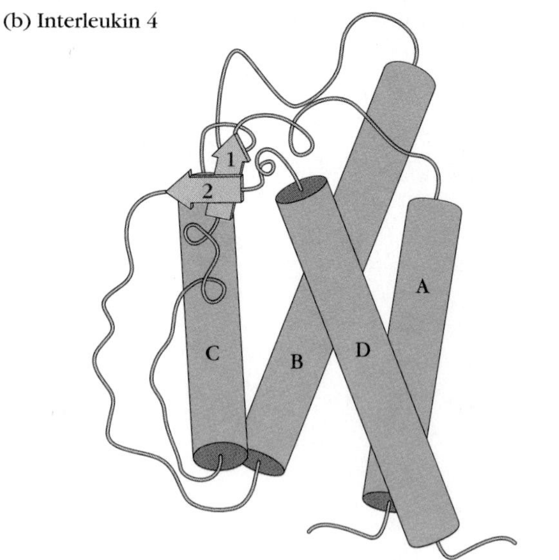

FIGURE 12-4 Several representations of structures in the hematopoietin family. (a) *Left:* Topographical representation of the primary structure of IL-2 showing α-helical regions (α and A–D) and connecting chains of the molecule. *Right:* Proposed three-dimensional model of IL-2. (b) Ribbon model of IL-4 deduced from x-ray crystallographic analysis of the molecule. In (a) and (b) the α helices are shown in red and the β sheets in blue. The structures of other cytokines belonging to the hematopoietin family are thought to be generally similar. [Part (b) from JL Boulay and WE Paul, 1993, *Curr. Biol.* **3**:573.]

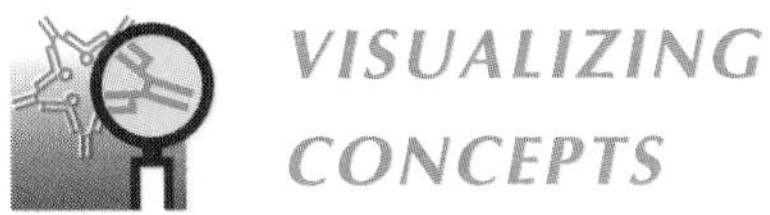

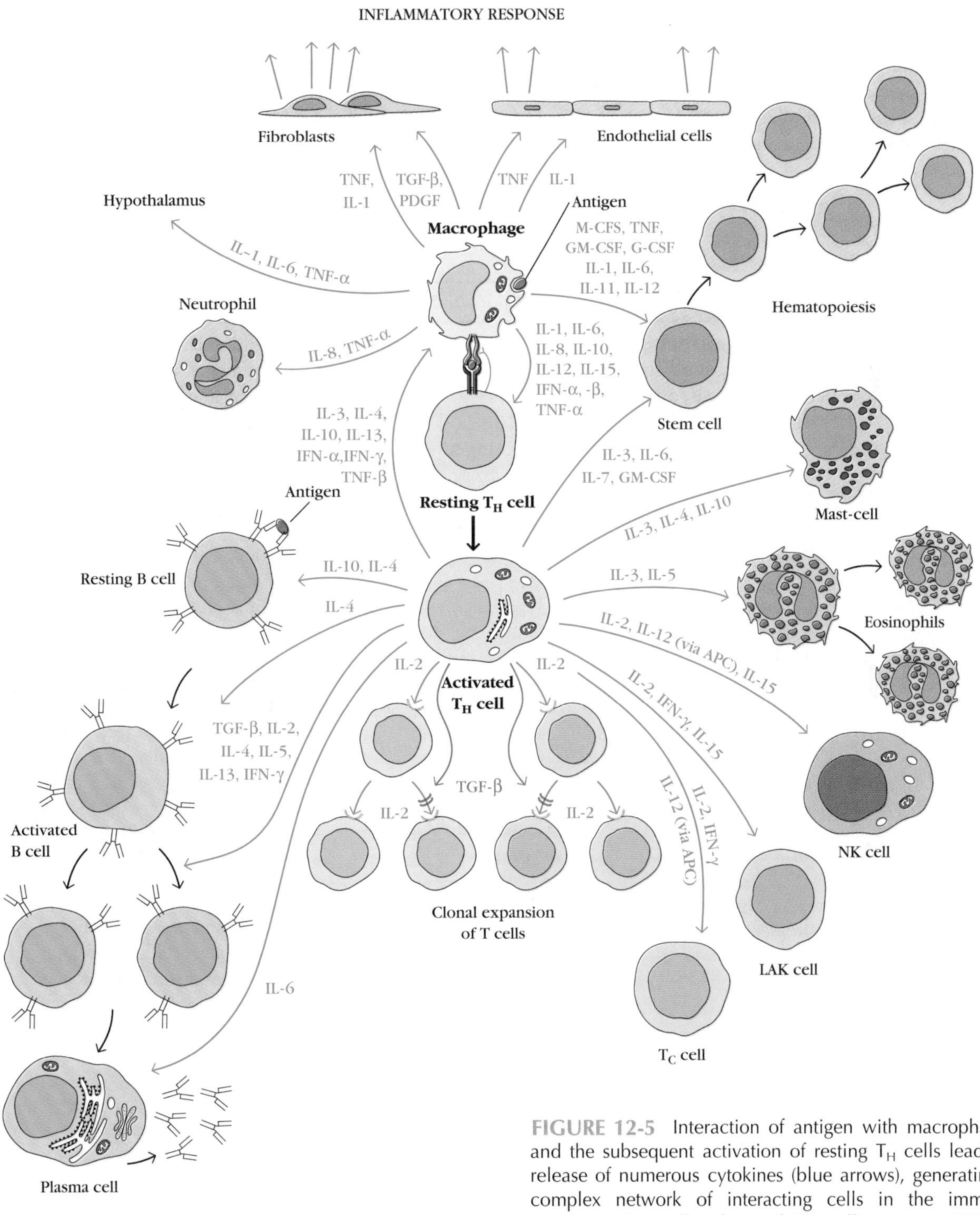

FIGURE 12-5 Interaction of antigen with macrophages and the subsequent activation of resting T_H cells leads to release of numerous cytokines (blue arrows), generating a complex network of interacting cells in the immune response. A small subset of T_H cells secretes TGF-β, a cytokine that can inhibit the proliferation of T cells (see red arrows).

physiologic responses that require cytokine involvement are development of cellular and humoral immune responses, induction of the inflammatory response, regulation of hematopoiesis, control of cellular proliferation and differentiation, and the healing of wounds. Although the immune response to a specific antigen may include the production of cytokines, it is important to remember that cytokines act in an antigen-nonspecific manner. That is, they affect whatever cells they encounter that bear appropriate receptors and are in a physiological state that allows them to respond.

Table 12-1 summarizes the main biological activities of a number of cytokines. It should be kept in mind that most of the listed functions have been identified from analysis of the effects of recombinant cytokines, often at nonphysiologic concentrations, added individually to in vitro systems. In vivo, however, cytokines rarely, if ever, act alone. Instead, a target cell is exposed to a milieu containing a mixture of cytokines, whose combined synergistic or antagonistic effects can have very different consequences. In addition, cytokines often induce the synthesis of other cytokines, resulting in cascades of activity in which cytokines produced at later steps in the cascade may influence the responses to cytokines released at earlier steps.

It is difficult to reconcile the nonspecificity of cytokines with the established specificity of the immune system. What keeps

TABLE 12-1 SELECTED FUNCTIONS OF SOME CYTOKINES

		Major biological functions	
Cytokine	Secreted by*	Target cells/tissues	Activity
Interleukin 1 (IL-1α, IL-1β)	Monocytes, macrophages, B cells, dendritic cells, endothelial cells, other cell types	T_H cells	Co-stimulates activation
		B cells	Promotes maturation and clonal expansion
		NK cells	Enhances activity
		Vascular endothelial cells	Increases expression of ICAMs†
		Macrophages and neutrophils	Chemotactically attracts
		Hepatocytes	Induces synthesis of acute-phase proteins
		Hypothalamus	Induces fever
Interleukin 2 (IL-2)	T_H1cells	Antigen-primed T_H and T_C cells	Induces proliferation
		Antigen-specific T-cell clones	Supports long-term growth
		NK cells (some) and T_C cells	Enhances activity
Interleukin 3 (IL-3)	T_H cells, NK cells, mast cells	Hematopoietic cells	Supports growth and differentiation
		Mast cells	Stimulates growth and histamine secretion
Interleukin 4 (IL-4)	T_H2 cells, mast cells, NK cells	Antigen-primed B cells	Co-stimulates activation
		Activated B cells	Stimulates proliferation and differentiation; induces class switch to IgG1 and IgE
		Resting B cells	Up-regulates class II MHC expression
		Thymocytes and T cells	Induces proliferation
		Macrophages	Up-regulates class II MHC expression; increases phagocytic activity
		Mast cells	Stimulates growth

*Activated cells generally secrete greater amounts of cytokine than unactivated cells do.

†ICAM = intercellular adhesion molecule.

the nonspecific cytokines from activating cells in a nonspecific fashion during the immune response? Clearly mechanisms must operate to ensure that the specificity of the immune response is maintained. One way in which specificity is maintained is by careful regulation of the expression of cytokine receptors on cells. Often cytokine receptors are expressed on a cell only after that cell has interacted with antigen. In this way cytokine activation is limited to antigen-activated lymphocytes. Another means of maintaining specificity may be a requirement for direct interaction between the cytokine-producing cell and the target cell to trigger cytokine secretion, thus ensuring that effective concentrations of the cytokine are released only in the vicinity of the intended target. In the case of the T_H cell, a major producer of cytokines, close cellular interaction occurs when the T-cell receptor recognizes an antigen-MHC complex on an appropriate antigen-presenting cell, such as a macrophage, dendritic cell, or B lymphocyte. Cytokines secreted at the junction of these interacting cells reach high enough local concentrations to affect the target APC but not more distant cells that are not complexed with the T_H cell. In addition, the half-life of cytokines in the bloodstream or other extracellular fluids into which they are secreted is usually very short, ensuring that they act for only a limited period of time and thus over a short distance.

Cytokine	Secreted by*	Major biological functions	
		Target cells/tissues	Activity
Interleukin 5 (IL-5)	T_H2 cells, mast cells	Activated B cells	Stimulates proliferation and differentation; induces class switch to IgA
		Eosinophils	Promotes growth and differentiation
Interleukin 6 (IL-6)	Monocytes, macrophages, T_H2 cells, bone-marrow stromal cells	Proliferating B cells	Promotes terminal differentiation into plasma cells
		Plasma cells	Stimulates antibody secretion
		Myeloid stem cells	Helps promote differentiation
		Hepatocytes	Induces synthesis of acute-phase proteins
Interleukin 7 (IL-7)	Bone-marrow, thymic stromal cells	Lymphoid stem cells	Induces differentiation into progenitor B and T cells
		Resting T cells	Increases expression of IL-2 and its receptor
Interleukin 8 (IL-8)	Macrophages, endothelial cells	Neutrophils	Chemokine; chemotactically attracts; induces adherence to vascular endothelium and extravasation into tissues
Interleukin 9 (IL-9)	T_H cells	Some T_H cells	Acts as mitogen, supporting proliferation in absence of antigen
Interleukin 10 (IL-10)	T_H2 cells	Macrophages	Suppresses cytokine production and thus indirectly reduces cytokine production by T_H1 cells
		Antigen-presenting cells	Down-regulates class II MHC expression

(continued)

TABLE 12-1 (CONTINUED) SELECTED FUNCTIONS OF SOME CYTOKINES

Cytokine	Secreted by*	Major biological functions	
		Target cells/tissues	Activity
Interleukin 11 (IL-11)	Bone-marrow stromal cells	Plasmacytomas	Supports growth
		Progenitor B cells	Promotes differentiation
		Megakaryocytes	Promotes differentiation
		Hepatocytes	Induces synthesis of acute-phase proteins
Interleukin 12 (IL-12)	Macrophages, B cells	Activated T_C cells	Acts synergistically with IL-2 to induce differentation into CTLs
		NK and LAK cells and activated T_H1 cells	Stimulates proliferation
Interleukin 13 (IL-13)	T_H cells	Macrophages	Inhibits activation and release of inflammatory cytokines; important regulator of inflammatory response
Interleukin 15 (IL-15)	T cells	T cells, intestinal epithelium	Stimulates growth of intestinal epithelium, T-cell proliferation
		NK	Supports proliferation
		Activated B cells	Co-mitogen for proliferation and differentiation
Interleukin 16 (IL-16)	T cells (primarily $CD8^+$) and eosinophils	$CD4^+$ T cells	Chemotaxis; induces expression of class II MHC; induces synthesis of cytokines; suppresses antigen-induced proliferation
		Monocytes	Chemotaxis; induces class II MHC
		Eosinophils	Chemotaxis; induces cell adhesion
Interleukin 17 (IL-17)	T cells	Macrophages	Initiates and maintains inflammation
Interleukin 18 (IL-18)	Activated macrophages	T cells	Induces IFN-γ production
		NK cells	Enhances NK cell cytotoxicity
Interferon alpha (IFN-α)	Leukocytes	Uninfected cells	Inhibits viral replication
Interferon beta (IFN-β)	Fibroblasts	Uninfected cells	Inhibits viral replication

Cytokine Receptors

As noted already, to exert their biological effects, cytokines must first bind to specific receptors expressed on the membrane of responsive target cells. Because these receptors are expressed by many types of cells, the cytokines can affect a diverse array of cells. Biochemical characterization of cytokine receptors initially progressed at a very slow pace because their levels on the membrane of responsive cells is quite low. As with the cytokines themselves, cloning of the genes encoding cytokine receptors has led to rapid advances in the identification and characterization of these receptors.

General Structure of Cytokine Receptors

Receptors for the various cytokines are quite diverse structurally, but almost all belong to one of five families of receptor proteins (Figure 12-6):

Cytokine	Secreted by*	Major biological functions: Target cells/tissues	Activity
Interferon gamma (IFN-γ)	T_H1, T_C, NK cells	Uninfected cells	Inhibits viral replication
		Macrophages	Enhances activity
		Many cell types	Increases expression of class I and class II MHC molecules
		Proliferating B cells	Induces class switch to IgG2a; blocks IL-4–induced class switch to IgE and IgG1
		T_H2 cells	Inhibits proliferation
		Inflammatory cells	Mediates various effects important in delayed-type hypersensitivity
Leukemia-inhibitory factor (LIF)	Thymic epithelial cells, bone-marrow stromal cells	Hepatocytes	Induces synthesis of acute-phase proteins
		Embryonic stem (ES) cells	Supports proliferation and differentiation
Oncostatin M (OSM)	Macrophages, T cells	Tumor cells	Inhibits growth
		Hepatocytes	Induces synthesis of acute-phase proteins
		Kaposi's sarcoma	Stimulates growth
Transforming growth factor β (TGF-β)	Platelets, macrophages, lymphocytes, mast cells	Monocytes and macrophages	Chemotactically attracts
		Activated macrophages	Induces increased IL-1 production
		Epithelial, endothelial, lymphoid, and hematopoietic cells	Inhibits proliferation, thus limiting inflammatory response and promoting wound healing
		Proliferating B cells	Induces class switch to IgA
Tumor necrosis factor α (TNF-α)	Macrophages, mast cells	Tumor cells	Has cytotoxic effect
		Inflammatory cells	Induces cytokine secretion and is responsible for extensive weight loss (cachexia) associated with chronic inflammation
Tumor necrosis factor β (TNF-β)	T_H1 and T_C cells	Tumor cells	Has cytotoxic and other effects similar to TNF-α
		Macrophages and neutrophils	Enhances phagocytic activity

- Immunoglobulin superfamily receptors
- Class I cytokine receptor family (also known as the hematopoietin receptor family)
- Class II cytokine receptor family (also known as the interferon receptor family)
- TNF receptor family
- Chemokine receptor family

Most of the cytokine-binding receptors that function in the immune and hematopoietic systems belong to the class I cytokine receptor family. The members of this receptor family have conserved amino acid sequence motifs in the extracellular domain consisting of four positionally conserved cysteine residues (CCCC) and a conserved sequence of tryptophan-serine-(any amino acid)-tryptophan-serine (WSXWS, where X is the nonconserved amino acid). The receptors for all the cytokines classified as hematopoietins belong to the class I cytokine receptor family, which also is called the hematopoietin receptor family. The class II cytokine receptors possess the conserved CCCC motifs, but lack the WSXWS motif present in class I cytokine receptors. Initially

RECEPTOR FAMILY	LIGANDS
(a) Immunoglobulin superfamily receptors	IL-1, M-CSF, C-Kit
(b) Class I cytokine receptors (hematopoietin)	IL-2, IL-3, IL-4, IL-5, IL-6, IL-7, IL-9, IL-11, IL-12, IL-13, IL-15, GM-CSF, G-CSF, OSM, LIF, CNTF, Growth hormone, Prolactin
(c) Class II cytokine receptors (interferon)	IFN-α, IFN-β, IFN-γ, IL-10
(d) TNF receptors	TNF-α, TNF-β, CD40, Nerve growth factor (NGF), FAS
(e) Chemokine receptors	IL-8, RANTES, MIP-1, PF4, MCAF, NAP-2

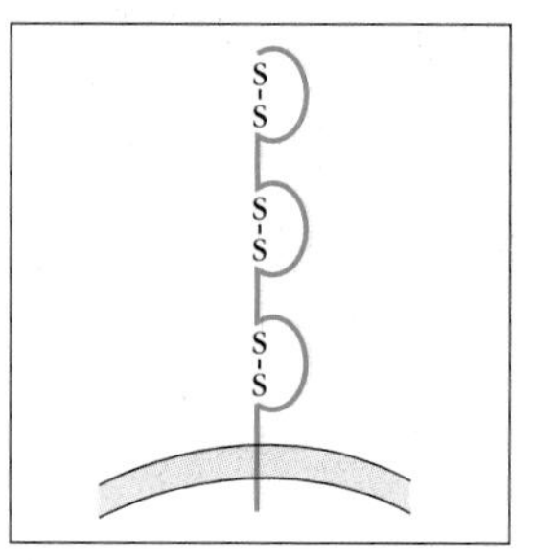

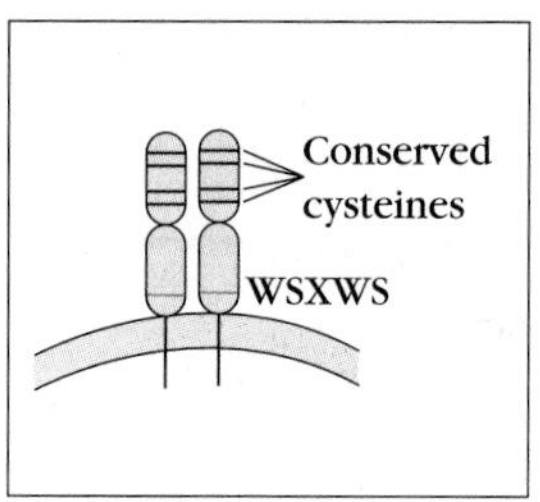

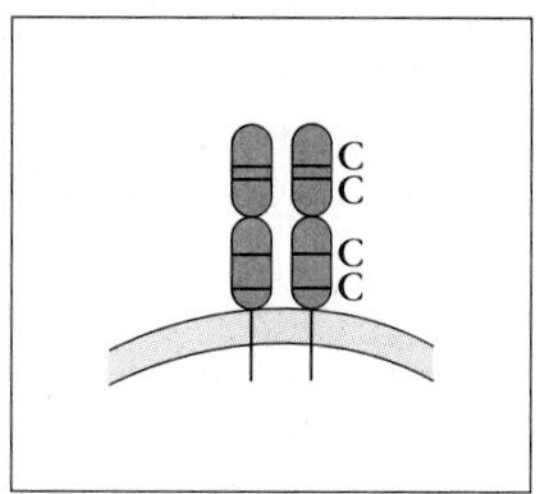

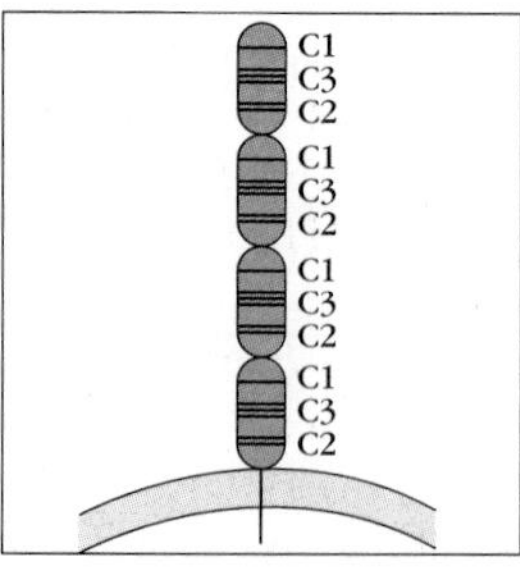

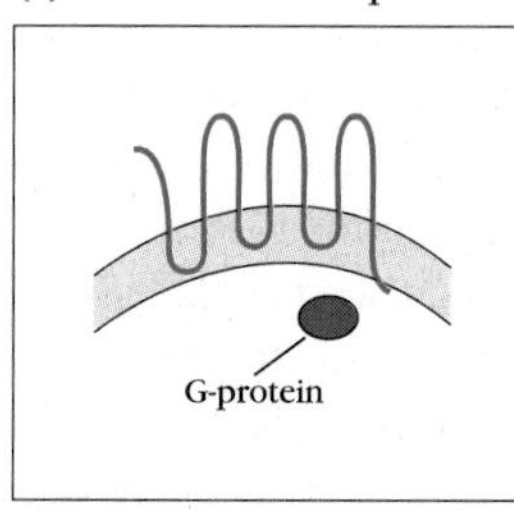

FIGURE 12-6 Schematic diagrams showing the structural features that define the five types of receptor proteins to which most cytokines bind. The receptors for most of the interleukins belong to the class I cytokine receptor family. C refers to conserved cysteine.

only the three interferons, α, β, and γ, were thought to be ligands for these receptors. However, recent work has shown that the IL-10 receptor is also a member of this group.

Another common feature of the hematopoietin (class I cytokine) and the class II cytokine receptor families is that most of these receptors are composed of more than one type of polypeptide chain and often include **cytokine-specific subunits** and a **signal-transducing subunit,** which often is not specific for the cytokine and plays only a minor role, if any, in ligand binding. Most of these receptors are dimers, consisting of one cytokine-specific subunit and one subunit whose major function is signal transduction, but a few are trimers. While there is a general pattern among cytokine receptors of assigning cytokine binding functions to one chain and signal transduction to another, this is not always the case. It is possible to find examples of receptor systems in which the cytokine-specific subunits also participate in signal transduction and signal-transducing subunits contribute to cytokine binding. Engagement of all of the class I and class II cytokine receptors studied to date has been shown to induce tyrosine phosphorylation of the receptor, although none of these receptors has tyrosine kinase activity in itself. This finding suggested that cytosolic domains of these receptors are closely associated with cytosolic protein tyrosine kinases. In fact, this has been found to be the case.

Subfamilies of Class I Cytokine Receptors

An important characteristic of many class I cytokine receptors is that they share common signal-transducing subunits with other members of the same family. Several subfamilies of class I cytokine receptors have been identified, with all the receptors in one subfamily having an identical signal-transducing subunit. Figure 12-7 schematically illustrates the members of three receptor subfamilies, named after GM-CSF, IL-2, and IL-6.

The sharing of signal-transducing subunits among receptors explains the redundancy and antagonism exhibited by some cytokines. Consider the GM-CSF receptor subfamily, which includes the receptors for IL-3, IL-5, and GM-CSF (see Figure 12-7a). Each of these cytokines binds to a unique low-affinity, cytokine-specific receptor consisting of an α subunit only. All three low-affinity subunits can associate noncovalently with a common signal-transducing β subunit. The resulting dimeric receptor not only exhibits increased affinity for the cytokine but also can transduce a signal across the membrane after binding the cytokine (Figure 12-8a). Interestingly, IL-3, IL-5, and GM-CSF exhibit considerable re-

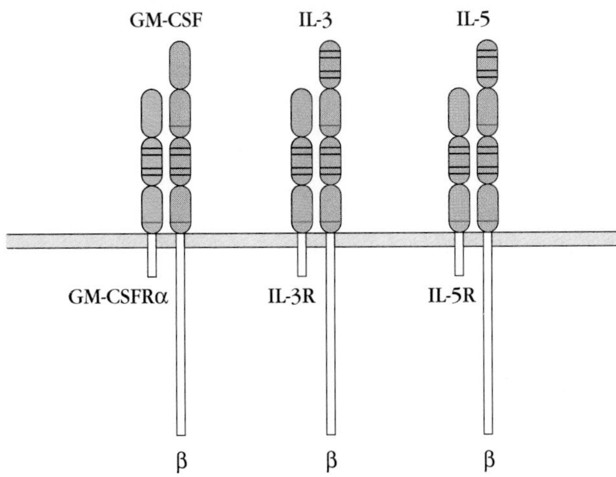

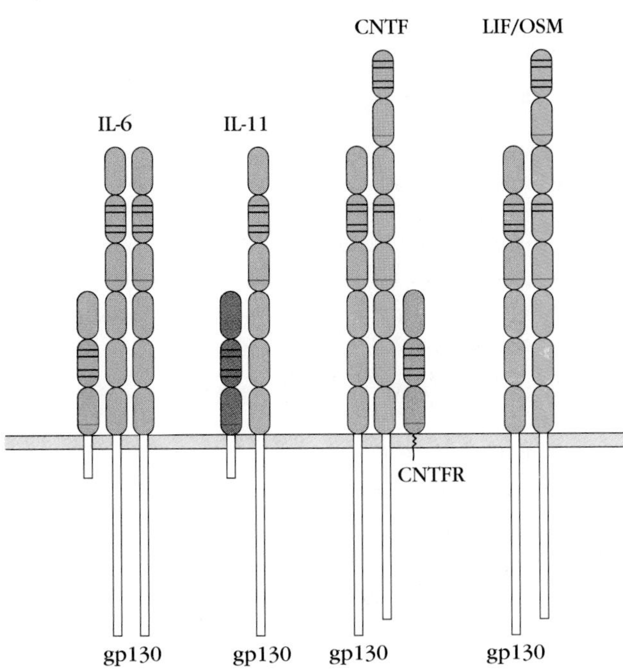

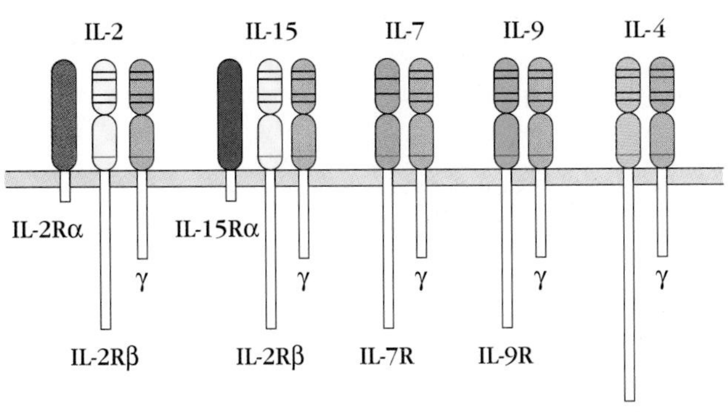

FIGURE 12-7 Schematic diagrams of the three subfamilies of class I cytokine receptors. All members of a subfamily have a common signal-transducing subunit (grayish-blue), but a unique cytokine-specific subunit. In addition to the conserved cysteines (double black lines) and WSXWS motifs (red lines) that characterize class I cytokine receptors, immunoglobulin-like domains are present in some of these receptors. CNTF = ciliary neurotrophic factor; LIF/OSM = leukemia-inhibitory factor/oncostatin. [Adapted from K Sugamura et al, 1996, *Annu. Rev. Immunol.* **14:**179.]

dundancy. Both IL-3 and GM-CSF act upon hematopoietic stem cells and progenitor cells, activate monocytes, and induce megakaryocyte differentiation. All three of these cytokines induce eosinophil proliferation and basophil degranulation with release of histamine.

Since the receptors for IL-3, IL-5, and GM-CSF share a common signal-transducing β subunit, each of these cytokines would be expected to transduce a similar activation signal, accounting for the redundancy among their biological effects (Figure 12-8b). In fact, all three cytokines induce the same patterns of protein phosphorylation. Furthermore, IL-3 and GM-CSF exhibit antagonism; IL-3 binding has been shown to be inhibited by GM-CSF, and conversely, the binding of GM-CSF has been shown to be inhibited by IL-3. Since the signal-transducing β subunit is shared between the receptors for these two cytokines, their antagonism is due to competition for a limited number of β subunits by the cytokine-specific α subunits of the receptors (Figure 12-8c).

A similar situation is found among the IL-6 receptor subfamily, which includes the receptors for IL-6, IL-11, IL-12, leukemia-inhibitory factor (LIF), oncostatin M (OSM), and ciliary neurotrophic factor (CNTF)(see Figure 12-7b). In this case, a common signal-transducing subunit, called gp130, associates with one or two different cytokine-specific subunits. LIF and OSM, which must share certain structural features, both bind to the same α subunit. As expected, the cytokines that bind to receptors in this subfamily display overlapping biological activities: IL-6, OSM, and LIF induce synthesis of acute-phase proteins by liver hepatocytes and differentiation of myeloid leukemia cells into macrophages; IL-6, LIF, and CNTF affect neuronal development, and IL-6, IL-11, and OSM stimulate megakaryocyte maturation and platelet production. The presence of gp130 in all receptors of the IL-6 subfamily explains their common signaling pathways as well as the binding competition for limited gp130 molecules that is observed among these cytokines.

A third signal-transducing subunit defines the IL-2 receptor subfamily, which includes receptors for IL-2, IL-4, IL-7, IL-9, and IL-15 (see Figure 12-7c). The IL-2 and the IL-15 receptors are heterotrimers, consisting of a cytokine-specific α chain and two chains—β and γ—responsible for signal transduction. The IL-2 receptor γ chain functions as the signal-transducing subunit in the other receptors in this subfamily, which are all dimers. Recently, it has been shown

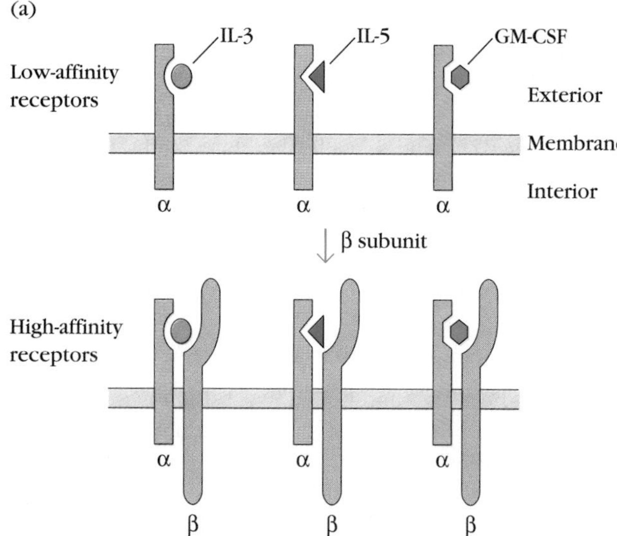

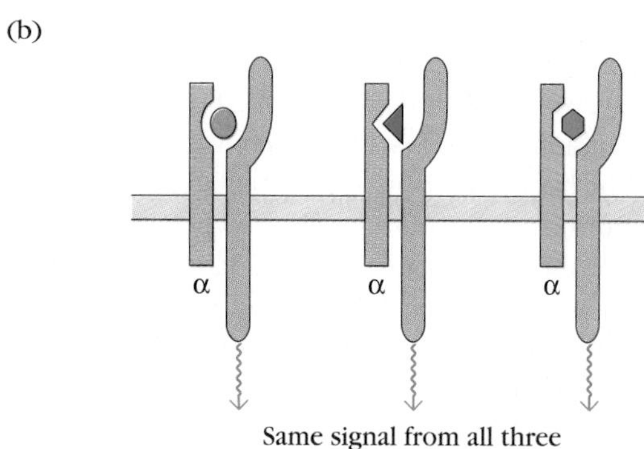

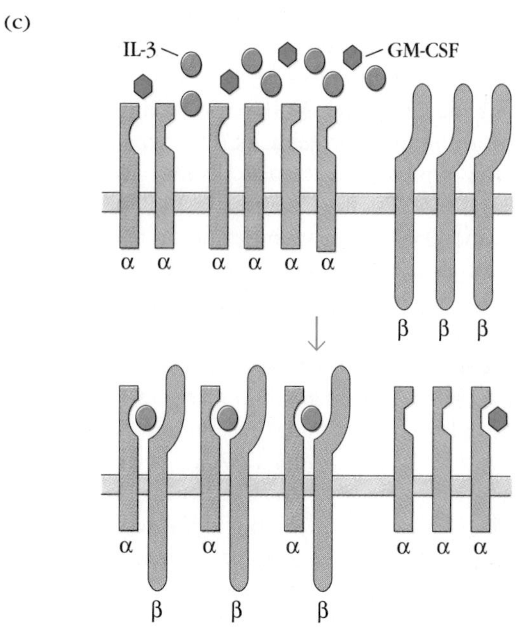

FIGURE 12-8 Interactions between cytokine-specific subunits and a common signal-transducing subunit of cytokine receptors. (a) Schematic diagram of the low-affinity and high-affinity receptors for IL-3, IL-5, and GM-CSF. The cytokine-specific subunits exhibit low-affinity binding and cannot transduce an activation signal. Noncovalent association of each subunit with a common β subunit yields a high-affinity dimeric receptor that can transduce a signal across the membrane. (b) Association of cytokine-specific subunits with a common signaling unit, the β subunit, allows the generation of cytokine-specific signals despite the generation of the same signal by the different cytokine receptors shown. (c) Competition of ligand-binding chains of different receptors for a common subunit can produce antagonistic effects between cytokines. Here binding of IL-3 by α subunits of the IL-3 receptor allows them to out-compete α chains of the GM-CSF receptor for β subunits. [Part (a) adapted from T Kishimoto et al, 1992, *Science* **258:**593.]

that the congenital **X-linked severe combined immunodeficiency (XSCID)** results from a defect in the γ-chain gene, which maps to the X chromosome. The immunodeficiencies observed in this disorder are due to the loss of all the cytokine functions mediated by the IL-2 subfamily receptors.

IL-2 Receptor

Because of the central role of IL-2 and its receptor in the clonal proliferation of T cells, the IL-2 receptor is one of the

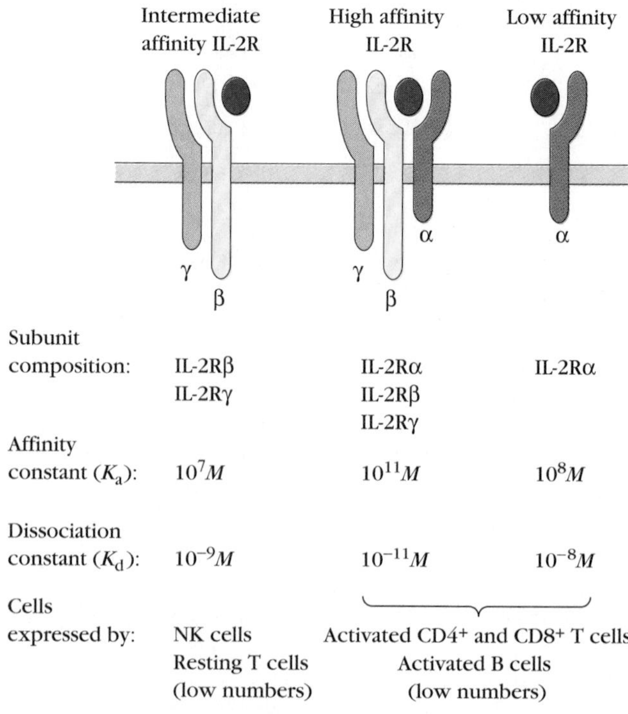

	Intermediate affinity IL-2R	High affinity IL-2R	Low affinity IL-2R
Subunit composition:	IL-2Rβ IL-2Rγ	IL-2Rα IL-2Rβ IL-2Rγ	IL-2Rα
Affinity constant (K_a):	$10^7 M$	$10^{11} M$	$10^8 M$
Dissociation constant (K_d):	$10^{-9} M$	$10^{-11} M$	$10^{-8} M$
Cells expressed by:	NK cells Resting T cells (low numbers)	Activated CD4+ and CD8+ T cells Activated B cells (low numbers)	

FIGURE 12-9 Comparison of the three forms of the IL-2 receptor. Signal transduction is mediated by the β and γ chains, but all three chains are required for high-affinity binding of IL-2.

most thoroughly studied of the cytokine receptors. As noted in the previous section, the complete trimeric receptor comprises three distinct subunits—the α, β, and γ chains. The β and γ chains belong to the class I cytokine receptor family, containing the characteristic CCCC and WSXWS motifs, whereas the α chain has a quite different structure and is not a member of this receptor family (see Figure 12-7c).

The IL-2 receptor occurs in three forms that exhibit different affinities for IL-2: the low-affinity monomeric IL-2Rα, the intermediate-affinity dimeric IL-2Rβγ, and the high-affinity trimeric IL-2Rαβγ (Figure 12-9). Because the α chain is expressed by activated but not resting T cells, it is often referred to as the TAC (T-cell activation) antigen. A monoclonal antibody, designated anti-TAC, which binds to the 55-kDa α chain, is often used to identify IL-2Rα on cells. Signal transduction by the IL-2 receptor requires both the β and γ chains, but only the trimeric receptor containing the α chain as well binds IL-2 with high affinity. Although the γ chain appears to be constitutively expressed on most lymphoid cells, expression of the α and β chains is more restricted and is markedly enhanced after antigen has activated resting lymphocytes. This phenomenon ensures that only antigen-activated $CD4^+$ and $CD8^+$ T cells will express the high-affinity IL-2 receptor and proliferate in response to physiologic levels of IL-2. Activated T cells express approximately 5×10^3 high-affinity receptors and ten times as many low-affinity receptors. NK cells express the β and γ subunits constitutively, accounting for their ability to bind IL-2 with an intermediate affinity and to be activated by IL-2.

Signal Transduction Mediated by Cytokine Receptors

While some important cytokine receptors lie outside the class I and class II families, the majority are included within these two families. As mentioned previously, class I and class II cytokine receptors lack signaling motifs (e.g., intrinsic tyrosine kinase domains). Yet, early observations demonstrated that one of the first events after the interaction of a cytokine with one of these receptors is a series of protein tyrosine phosphorylations. While these results were initially puzzling, they were explained when a unifying model emerged from studies of the molecular events triggered by binding of interferon gamma (INF-γ) to its receptor, a member of the class II family.

IFN-γ was originally discovered because of its ability to induce cells to block or inhibit the replication of a wide variety of viruses. Antiviral activity is a property it shares with IFN-α and IFN-β. However, unlike these other interferons, IFN-γ plays a central role in many immunoregulatory processes, including the regulation of mononuclear phagocytes, B-cell switching to certain IgG classes, and the support or inhibition of the development of T_H-cell subsets. The discovery of the major signaling pathway invoked by interaction of IFN-γ with its receptor led to the realization that signal transduction through most, if not all, class I and class II cytokine receptors begins with the cytokine-induced dimerization of receptors. This dimerization leads to a succession of reactions that ultimately generate an active transcription factor complex, which initiates the transcription of specific genes.

The following key features of the IFN-γ system are the basis of the unifying signaling model:

- *The cytokine receptor is composed of separate subunits.* As shown in Figure 12-10a, the IFN-γ receptor consists of two polypeptide chains, an α chain required for cytokine binding and for signal transduction, and a β chain necessary for signaling but with only a minor role in binding.
- *Different inactive protein tyrosine kinases are associated with different subunits of the receptor.* Studies of another cytokine receptor, the IL-6 receptor, showed that the subunit gp130 was associated with members of a novel family of protein tyrosine kinases known as Janus kinases (JAK).* Immunoprecipitation by subunit-specific antibodies showed that Janus kinases are associated with each of the subunits of the IFN-γ receptor. Treating cell lysates with antibody to the α subunit yielded an immunoprecipitate that contained JAK1 in addition to the expected α subunit. Alternatively, immunoprecipitation of the lysate with antibody to the β subunit gave a precipitate that contained a different Janus kinase, JAK2. Thus, the α chain of the IFN-γ receptor is associated with JAK1; the β chain is associated with JAK2 (Table 12-2). These JAKs were associated with chains of the IFN-γ receptor in cells that had not been treated with IFN-γ. Therefore the association of the JAK and the receptor subunit occurs spontaneously and does not require binding of cytokine. The protein tyrosine kinase of receptor-associated JAKs from cells that have not been treated with IFN-γ, were inactive, however.
- *Cytokine binding induces the association of the two separate cytokine receptor subunits and activation of the receptor-associated JAKs.* In particular, the binding of IFN-γ causes the association of the α and β subunits of the receptor. In addition, because IFN-γ is a dimer, it can bind to two receptors, forming a crosslinked oligomer. If cells are incubated with IFN-γ prior to lysis and immunoprecipitation with anti-α antibody, the precipitate contains not only α subunits and JAK1, but also β subunits and JAK2. Furthermore, JAK1 and JAK2 are no longer inactive; both have been phosphorylated and have full protein-kinase activity. Specifically, the JAK1 associated with the α subunit phosphorylates

*The Roman god Janus had two faces. Kinases of the Janus family have two sites, a binding site at which they link with the cytokine receptor subunit and a catalytic site that, when activated, has protein tyrosine kinase activity. Some biochemists, wearied by the multitude of different protein kinases that have been discovered, claim JAK means *J*ust *A*nother *K*inase.

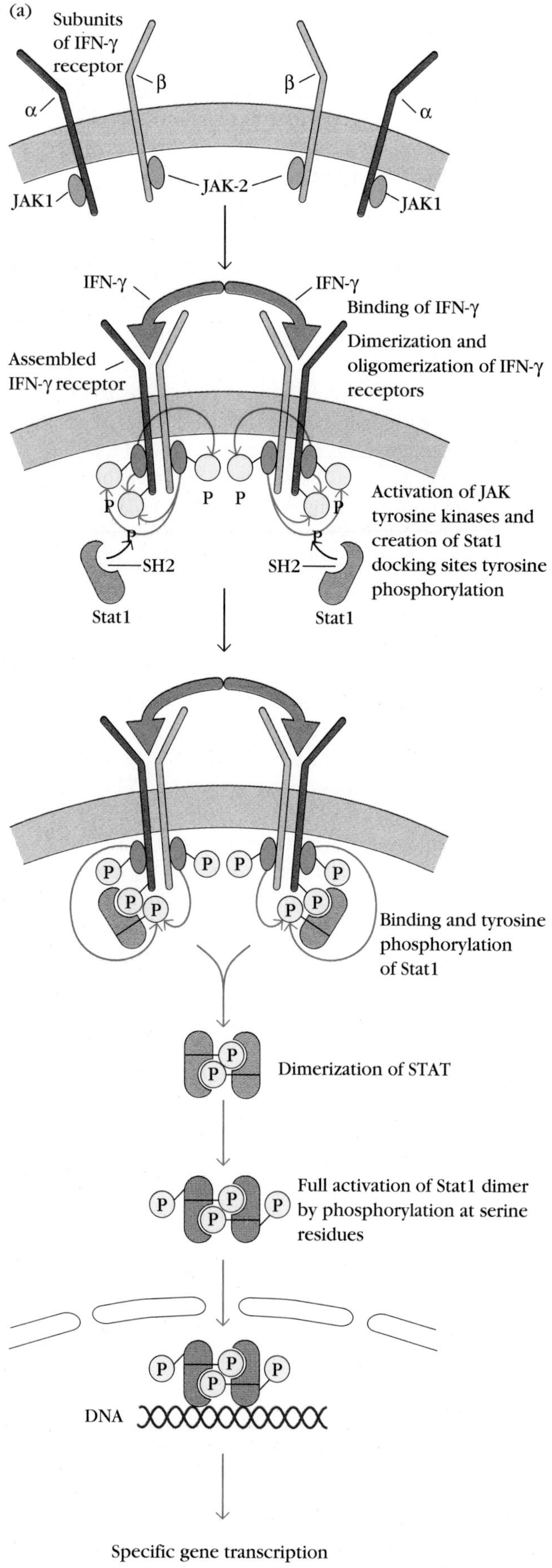

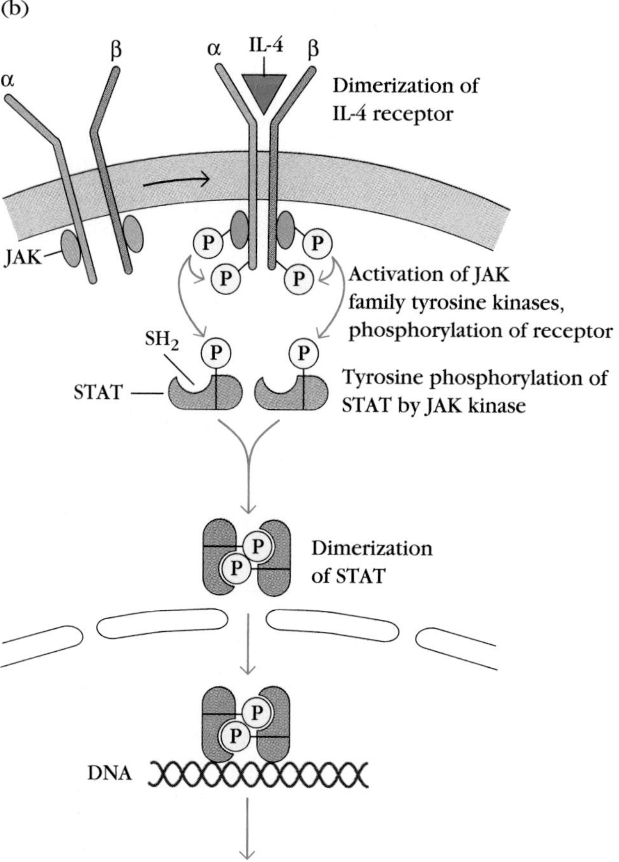

FIGURE 12-10 Signal transduction mediated by cytokine receptors. (a) The signal transduction pathway from the interferon-gamma receptor to the nucleus. The IFN-γ receptor consists of an α chain and a β chain, which are unassociated in the absence of ligand. The α subunit is associated with JAK1, an inactive protein tyrosine kinase, and the β subunit is associated with the inactive protein tyrosine kinase JAK2. Addition of ligand causes the association of the subunits, and the JAK kinases become active as a consequence of reciprocal phosphorylations. Because IFN-γ is a dimer, two assembled receptors are crosslinked. The α chain undergoes JAK-mediated tyrosine phosphorylation, thereby creating a docking site for Stat1, which binds via its SH2 domain. After JAK-mediated phosphorylation, Stat1 dissociates from the receptor and dimerizes with a second Stat1 molecule. Dimeric Stat1 then undergoes yet another phosphorylation at a serine residue and moves into the nucleus, where it initiates the transcription of a specific set of genes. (b) A general model of signal transduction mediated by most class I and class II cytokine receptors. Binding of a cytokine (in this view, IL-4) induces dimerization of the receptor subunits, which leads to the activation of receptor subunit-associated JAK tyrosine kinases by reciprocal phosphorylation. Subsequently, the activated JAKs phosphorylate various tyrosine residues, resulting in the creation of docking sites for STATs on the receptor and the activation of the one or more STAT transcription factors. The phosphorylated STATs dimerize and translocate to the nucleus, where they activate transcription of specific genes. [Part (a) adapted from Bach et al, 1997, *Annu. Rev. Immunol.* **15:**563.]

TABLE 12-2 STAT AND JAK INTERACTION WITH SELECTED CYTOKINE RECEPTORS DURING SIGNAL TRANSDUCTION

Cytokine receptor	JAK	STAT
IFN-γ	JAK1 and JAK2	Stat1
IFN-α/β	JAK1 and Tyk-2	Stat2
IL-2	JAK1 and JAK3	Stat5
IL-3	JAK2	Stat5
IL-4	JAK1 and JAK3	Stat6
IL-6	JAK1 (and sometimes others)	Stat3
IL-10	JAK1 and Tyk-2*	Stat3
IL-12	JAK2 and Tyk-2*	Stat4

*Despite its name, Tyk-2 is also a Janus kinase.
SOURCE: Adapted from Bach, Aguet, and Schreiber, 1997, *Annu. Rev. Immun.* **15:**563.

JAK2, and the JAK2 associated with the β subunit phosphorylates JAK1.

- *Activated JAKs create docking sites for the STAT transcription factors by phosphorylation of specific tyrosine residues on cytokine receptor subunits.* Once receptor-associated JAKs are activated, they phosphorylate specific tyrosines in the receptor subunits of the complex. Members of a family of transcription factors known as **STATs (signal transducers and activators of transcription)** bind to these phosphorylated tyrosine residues. Specific STATs (see Table 12-2) play essential roles in the signaling pathways of a wide variety of cytokines. The binding of STATs to receptor subunits is mediated by the joining of the SH2 domain on the STAT with the docking site created by the JAK-mediated phosphorylation of a particular tyrosine on receptor subunits. In the case of the IFN-γ receptor, Stat1 is the STAT family member used in signal transduction, and phosphorylation creates a docking site for it on the α subunit of the receptor. Mutation studies of the gene encoding the human α subunit show that, if the tyrosine at position 440 is changed to a phenylalanine, Stat1 is no longer able to dock with the α subunit of the IFN-γ receptor.
- *After undergoing JAK-mediated phosphorylation, STAT transcription factors translocate from receptor docking sites at the membrane to the nucleus, where they initiate the transcription of specific genes.* While docked to receptor subunits, STATs undergo JAK-catalyzed phosphorylation of a key tyrosine. This is followed by the dissociation of the STATs from the receptor subunits and their dimerization. Each of the STATs in the dimer then undergoes an additional phosphorylation, this time at a serine residue, which fully activates the dimer as a transcription factor. The STAT dimers then translocate into the nucleus and induce the expression of genes containing appropriate regulatory sequences in their promoter regions. Activated homodimers of the STAT family member that mediates the response induce transcription of a number of genes, including a group of genes called the interferon-stimulated genes (ISGs), which are rapidly induced within 15–30 minutes of ligand binding. These genes contain two types of conserved sequences in their promoter regions, the interferon-stimulated response element (ISRE) and the gamma-interferon activation site (GAS).

A summary of the signaling in the IFN-γ system appears in Figure 12-10a along with a general model for signaling by class I and class II receptors in Figure 12-10b. The ability of IFN-γ to bring about the association of the ligand-binding chains of its receptor has been directly demonstrated by x-ray crystallographic studies (Figure 12-11). In addition to IFN-γ a number of other class I and class II ligands have been shown to cause dimerization of their receptors. An important element of cytokine specificity derives from the exquisite specificity of the match between cytokines and their receptors. Another aspect of cytokine specificity is that each particular cytokine (or group of redundant cytokines) induces transcription of a specific subset of genes in a given

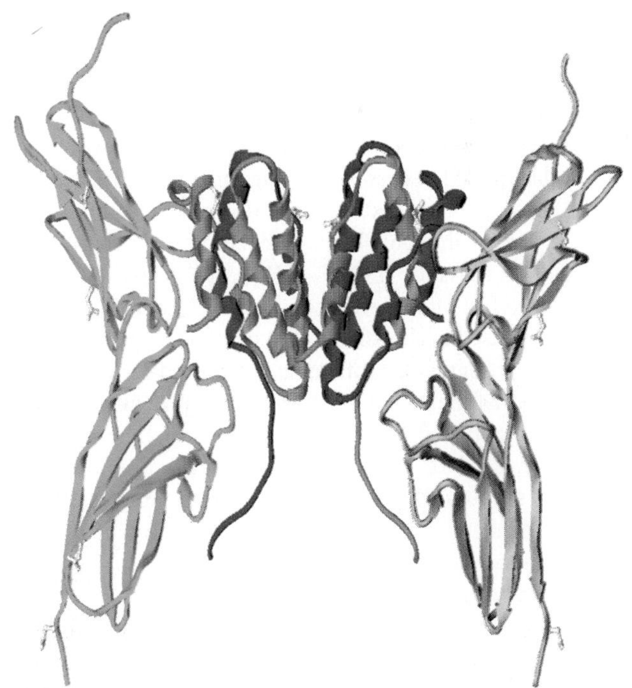

FIGURE 12-11 The complex between IFN-γ and the ligand-binding chains of its receptor. This model is based on the x-ray crystallographic analysis of a crystalline complex of interferon-γ (red and blue) bound to ligand-binding α chains of the receptor (green and yellow). Note that IFN-γ is shown in its native dimeric form. [From MR Walter et al, 1995, *Nature* **376:**230, courtesy M Walter, University of Alabama.]

cell type; the resulting gene products then mediate the various effects typical of that cytokine. The specificity of cytokine effects is then traceable to three factors. First, particular cytokine receptors start particular JAK-STAT pathways. Second, the transcriptional activity of activated STATs is specific because a particular STAT homodimer or heterodimer will only recognize certain sequence motifs and thus can interact only with the promoters of certain genes. Third, only those target genes whose expression is permitted by a particular cell type can be activated within that variety of cell. That is, in any given cell type only a subset of the potential target genes of a particular STAT may be permitted expression. For example, IL-4 induces one set of genes in T cells, another in B cells, and yet a third in eosinophils.

Cytokine Antagonists

A number of proteins that inhibit the biological activity of cytokines have been reported. These proteins act in one of two ways: either they bind directly to a cytokine receptor but fail to activate the cell, or they bind directly to a cytokine, inhibiting its activity. The best-characterized inhibitor is the IL-1 receptor antagonist (IL-1Ra), which binds to the IL-1 receptor but has no activity. Binding of IL-1Ra to the IL-1 receptor blocks binding of both IL-1α and IL-1β, thus accounting for its antagonistic properties. Production of IL-1Ra has been thought by some to play a role in regulating the intensity of the inflammatory response. It has been cloned and is currently being investigated as a potential treatment for chronic inflammatory diseases.

Cytokine inhibitors are found in the bloodstream and extracellular fluid. These soluble antagonists arise from enzymatic cleavage of the extracellular domain of cytokine receptors. Among the soluble cytokine receptors that have been detected are those for IL-2, IL-4, IL-6, IL-7, IFN-γ, TNF-α, TNF-β, and LIF. Of these, the soluble IL-2 receptor (sIL-2R), which is released in chronic T-cell activation, is the best characterized. A segment containing the amino-terminal 192 amino acids of the α subunit is released by proteolytic cleavage, forming a 45-kDa soluble IL-2 receptor. The shed receptor can bind IL-2 and prevent its interaction with the membrane-bound IL-2 receptor. The presence of sIL-2R has been used as a clinical marker of chronic T-cell activation and is observed in a number of diseases, including autoimmunity, transplant rejection, and AIDS.

Some viruses also produce cytokine-binding proteins or cytokine mimics. The evolution of such anti-cytokine strategies by microbial pathogens is good biological evidence of the importance of cytokines in organizing and promoting effective anti-microbial immune responses. The poxviruses, for example, have been shown to encode a soluble TNF-binding protein and a soluble IL-1–binding protein. Since both TNF and IL-1 exhibit a broad spectrum of activities in the inflammatory response, these soluble cytokine-binding proteins may prohibit or diminish the inflammatory effects of the cytokines, thereby conferring upon the virus a selective advantage. Epstein-Barr virus produces an IL-10–like molecule (viral IL-10 or vIL-10) that binds to the IL-10 receptor and, like cellular IL-10, suppresses T_H1-type cell-mediated responses (see the next section), which are effective against many intracellular parasites such as viruses. Molecules produced by viruses that mimic cytokines allow the virus to manipulate the immune response in ways that aid the survival of the pathogen. This is an interesting and powerful modification some viruses have undergone in their continuing struggle to overcome the formidable barrier of host immunity. Table 12-3 lists a number of viral products that mimic cytokines or their receptors.

TABLE 12-3 VIRAL MIMICS OF CYTOKINES AND CYTOKINE RECEPTORS

Virus	Product
Leporipoxvirus (a myxoma virus)	Soluble IFN-γ receptor
Several poxviruses	Soluble IFN-γ receptor
Vaccinia, smallpox virus	Soluble IL-1 β receptor
Epstein-Barr	IL-10 homolog
Human herpesvirus-8	IL-6 homolog; also homologs of the chemokines MIP-I and MIP II
Cytomegalovirus	Three different chemokine receptor homologs, one of which binds three different soluble chemokines (RANTES, MCP-1, and MIP-1α)

Cytokine Secretion by T_H1 and T_H2 Subsets

The immune response to a particular pathogen must induce an appropriate set of effector functions that can eliminate the disease agent or its toxic products from the host. For example, the neutralization of a soluble bacterial toxin requires antibodies, whereas the response to an intracellular virus or to a bacterial cell requires cell-mediated cytotoxicity or delayed-type hypersensitivity. A large body of evidence implicates differences in cytokine-secretion patterns among T_H-cell subsets as determinants of the type of immune response made to a particular antigenic challenge.

$CD4^+$ T_H cells exert most of their helper functions through secreted cytokines, which either act on the cells that produce them in an autocrine fashion or modulate the responses of other cells through paracrine pathways. Although $CD8^+$CTLs also secrete cytokines, their array of cytokines generally is more restricted than that of $CD4^+$ T_H cells. As briefly discussed in Chapter 10, two $CD4^+$ T_H-cell subpopulations can be distinguished in vitro by the cytokines they secrete. These two subsets of T cells, designated T_H1 and T_H2, both secrete IL-3 and GM-CSF but otherwise differ in the cytokines they secrete (Table 12-4). T_H1 and T_H2 cells are characterized by the following functional differences:

- The T_H1 subset is responsible for many cell-mediated functions (e.g., delayed-type hypersensitivity and activation of T_C cells) and for the production of opsonization-promoting IgG antibodies (i.e. antibodies that bind to the high-affinity Fc receptors of phagocytes and interact with the complement system). This subset is also associated with the promotion of excessive inflammation and tissue injury.
- The T_H2 subset stimulates eosinophil activation and differentiation; provides help to B cells, and promotes the production of relatively large amounts of IgM, IgE, and noncomplement-activating IgG isotypes. The T_H2 subset also supports allergic reactions.

TABLE 12-4 CYTOKINE SECRETION AND PRINCIPAL FUNCTIONS OF MOUSE T_H1 AND T_H2 SUBSETS

Cytokine/function	T_H1	T_H2
Cytokine secretion		
IL-2	+	−
IFN-γ	++	−
TNF-β	++	−
GM-CSF	++	+
IL-3	++	++
IL-4	−	++
IL-5	−	++
IL-10	−	++
IL-13	−	++
Functions		
Help for total antibody production	+	++
Help for IgE production	−	++
Help for IgG2a production	++	+
Eosinophil and mast-cell production	−	++
Macrophage activation	++	−
Delayed-type hypersensitivity	++	−
T_C-cell activation	++	−

SOURCE: Adapted from F Powrie and RL Coffman, 1993, *Immunol. Today* **14**:270.

The differences in the cytokines secreted by T_H1 and T_H2 cells determine the different biological functions of these two subsets. IFN-γ, a defining cytokine of the T_H1 subset, activates macrophages; it stimulates these cells to increase microbicidal activity, to up-regulate the level of class II MHC, and to secrete cytokines such as IL-12, which induces T_H cells to differentiate into the T_H1 subset. IFN-γ secretion by T_H1 cells also induces antibody-class switching to IgG classes (such as IgG2a in the mouse) that support phagocytosis and fixation of complement. TNF-β and IFN-γ are cytokines that mediate inflammation, and it is their secretion that accounts for the association of T_H1 cells with inflammatory phenomena such as delayed hypersensitivity (Chapter 16). T_H1 cells produce IL-2 and IFN-γ cytokines that promote the differentiation of fully cytotoxic T_C cells from CD8 precursors. This pattern of cytokine production makes the T_H1 subset particularly suited to respond to viral infections and intracellular pathogens. Finally, IFN-γ inhibits the expansion of the T_H2 population.

The secretion of IL-4 and IL-5 by cells of the T_H2 subset induces production of IgE and supports eosinophil-mediated attack on helminth (roundworm) infections. IL-4 promotes a pattern of class switching that produces IgG that does not fix complement (IgG1 in mice, for example). IL-4 also increases the extent to which B cells switch from IgM to IgE. This effect on IgE production meshes with eosinophil differentiation and activation by IL-5, because eosinophils are richly endowed with Fcε receptors, which bind IgE. Typically, roundworm infections induce T_H2 responses and evoke anti-roundworm IgE antibody. The antibody bound to the worm binds to the Fc receptors of eosinophils, thus forming an antigen-specific bridge between the worm and the eosinophils. The attack of the eosinophil on the worm is triggered by the crosslinking of the Fcε-bound IgE. Despite such beneficial actions of IgE, it is also the Ig class responsible for allergy. Finally, IL-4 and IL-10 suppress the expansions of T_H1 cell populations. This pattern suggests that the T_H2 subset may respond better to helminthic parasites and may mediate allergic reactions.

Because the T_H1 and T_H2 subsets were originally identified in long-term in vitro cultures of cloned T-cell lines, some researchers doubted that they represented true in vivo subpopulations. They suggested instead that these subsets might represent different maturational stages of a single lineage. Also, early observations in humans led some to believe that T_H1, T_H2, and other subsets of T helper cells did not occur in this species. However, further research corrected both these views. Experiments with transgenic mice demonstrated that T_H1 and T_H2 cells arise independently. Furthermore, T cells isolated from humans during chronic infectious diseases or chronic episodes of allergy consist of either T_H1 or T_H2 populations. Apparently, the full commitment of populations of T cells of either a T_H1 or a T_H2 phenotype often signals the endpoint of a chronic infection or allergy. Hence it was difficult to find clear T_H1 or T_H2 subsets in earlier studies, which often employed healthy human subjects, who would not be at this stage of a response. Finally, it is important to emphasize that many helper T cells are neither T_H1 nor T_H2. Sensitive assays of the profile of cytokines expressed by an individual cell have shown striking heterogeneity in the T_H-cell population. Many T cells do not show either a T_H1 or a T_H2 profile. Specifically, various cells produce IL-2, IL-4, IL-5, IFN-γ and IL-10, as well as other cytokines. One of the best described of these is the T_H0 subset, which secrete IL-2, IL-4, IL-5, IFN-γ, and IL-10, as well as IL-3 and GM-CSF. Some workers believe that the T_H1 and T_H2 subsets arise by differentiation from T_H0 cells, but this hypothesis has been difficult to prove and remains speculative.

Numerous reports of studies in both mice and humans now document that the in vivo outcome of the immune response can be critically influenced by the relative levels of T_H1-like or T_H2-like activity. The T_H1 profile of cytokines is higher in response to intracellular pathogens, and the T_H2 profile is higher in allergic diseases and helminthic infections.

Development of T_H1 and T_H2 Subsets

The cytokine environment in which antigen-primed T_H cells differentiate determines the subset that develops (Figure 12-12). In particular, IL-4 is essential for the development of a T_H2 response and IL-12 is important for T_H1 cells. Typically, macrophages activated by an encounter with intracellular bacteria, with bacterial products such as LPS, or with a number of other intracellular parasites are the source of IL-12. This cytokine then binds to those activated T cells that have functional IL-12 receptors and initiates differentiation to a T_H1 phenotype. T_H1 development also depends on IFN-γ because IFN-γ up-regulates IL-12 production by macrophages and dendritic cells and activates the IL-12 receptor on activated T cells by up-regulating expression of the β chain of the IL-12 receptor. At the beginning of an immune response, IFN-γ is generated by stimulation of T cells and can also come from activated NK cells. Yet another cytokine, IL-18 (IGIF, or interferon gamma inducing factor)

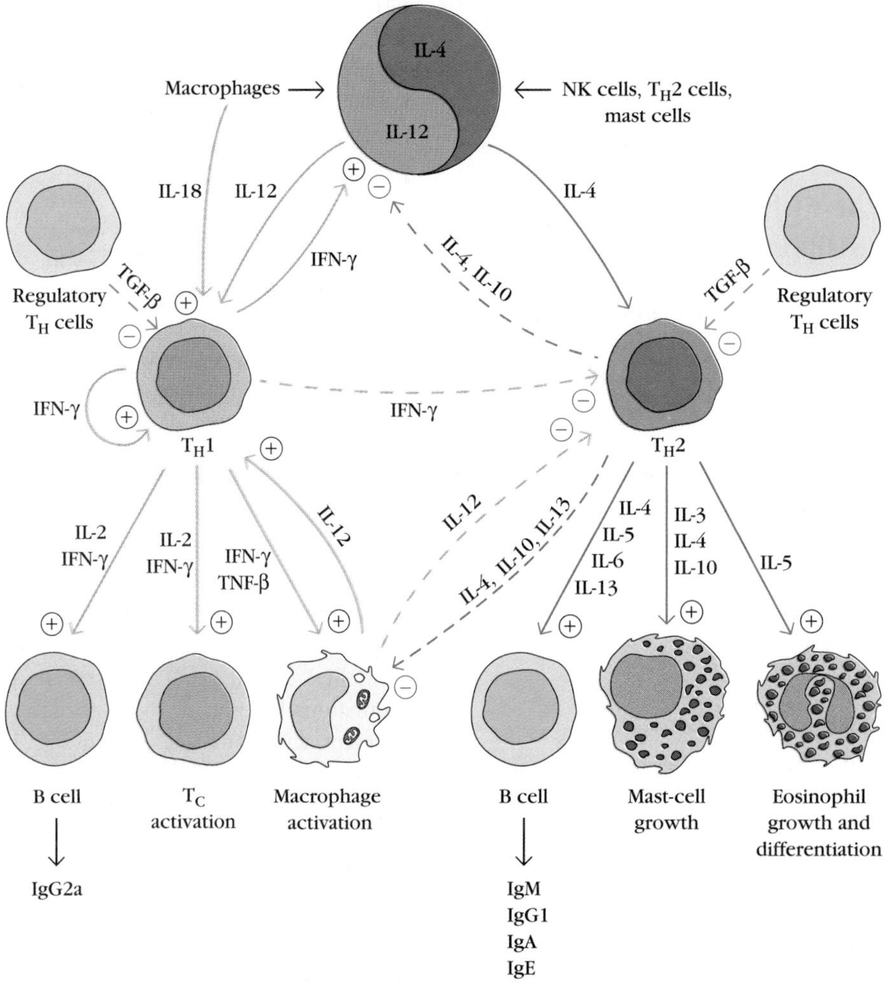

FIGURE 12-12 The regulation of T_H subsets by cytokines. Solid arrows indicate stimulatory effects (+); dashed arrows indicate inhibitory effects (−). Purple arrows indicate the cytokines of the T_H1 pathway; orange, the T_H2 pathway.

promotes proliferation and IFN-γ production by both developing and fully differentiated T_H1 cells and by NK cells. So a regulatory network of cytokines positively controls the generation of T_H1 cells. While IL-12 is central to the process, its level of expression is greatly increased by IFN-γ whose production is stimulated by IL-18. The whole process forms a sort of positive feedback loop, because increases in IFN-γ secretion by T_H1 cells result in more IL-12 secretion by macrophages, which results in more T_H1 cells, which produce more IFN-γ. The critical role played by each of these cytokines and their receptors has been demonstrated in a series of experiments in which either the cytokine or its receptor has been knocked out. Mice in which the genes for any of these critical components have been knocked out fail to generate populations of T_H1 cells.

Just as T_H1 cells require IL-12 and IFN-γ, the generation of T_H2 cells depends critically on IL-4. Exposing naive helper cells to IL-4 at the beginning of an immune response causes them to differentiate into T_H2 cells. In fact, this influence of IL-4 is predominant in directing T_H cells to the T_H1 route. Provided a threshold level of IL-4, T_H2 development is greatly favored over T_H1 even if IL-12 is present. The critical role of signals from IL-4 in T_H2 development is shown by the observation that knocking out the gene that encodes IL-4 prevents the development of this T-cell subset. Additional evidence supporting the central role of IL-4 comes from an experiment that interrupted the IL-4 signal-transduction pathway. Like so many other cytokines, IL-4 uses a pathway that involves JAK and STAT proteins. The Stat6 transcription factor is the one activated in signaling by IL-4. Consequently, in mice in which the gene for Stat6 has been disrupted (Stat6 knockouts), IL-4 mediated processes are severely inhibited or absent. The observation that Stat6 knockout mice have very few T_H2 cells confirms the importance of IL-4 for the differentiation of this subset.

Because T_H2 cells themselves are a major source of IL-4, what is the source of the IL-4 that initiates their differentiation? While final answers are not yet in, research has shown that, early in an immune response, the antigen-specific stimulation of both naive and memory $CD4^+$ T cells results in the secretion of some IL-4. Other cell types, such as mast cells, basophils, eosinophils, and $NK1^+$ T cells may also produce IL-4. Given the ability of threshold amounts of IL-4 to override signals for T_H1 differentiation, even small amounts of IL-4 early in the immune response may be sufficient to direct the development of T_H2 cells.

Cytokine Cross-Regulation

The critical cytokines produced by T_H1 and T_H2 subsets have three characteristic effects on subset development. First of all, they promote the growth of the subset that produces them, and second, they inhibit the development and activity of the opposite subset, an effect known as cross-regulation, (see Figure 12-12). For instance, IFN-γ (secreted by the T_H1 subset) preferentially inhibits proliferation of the T_H2 subset, and IL-4 and IL-10 (secreted by the T_H2 subset) down-regulate secretion of IL-12, the critical cytokine for T_H1 differentiation, by both macrophages and dendritic cells. Similarly, these cytokines have opposing effects on target cells other than T_H subsets. IFN-γ secreted by the T_H1 subset promotes IgG2a production by B cells but inhibits IgG1 and IgE production. On the other hand, IL-4 secreted by the T_H2 subset promotes production of IgG1 and IgE and suppresses production of IgG2a. The phenomenon of cross-regulation explains the observation that there is often an inverse relationship between antibody production and delayed-type hypersensitivity; that is, when antibody production is high, delayed-type hypersensitivity is low, and vice versa. Furthermore, recent research has shown that IL-4 and IFN-γ make members of the T-cell subset that releases them less responsive to the cytokine that directs differentiation of the other T-cell subset. Thus, IL-4 enhances T_H2 cell development by down-regulating the β subunit of the IL-12 receptor, thereby making T cells unresponsive to IL-12, which would direct T_H1 development. On the other hand, IFN-γ up-regulates the expression of this β subunit, making T cells more responsive to IL-12, thereby overriding the effects of IL-4 and favoring the differentiation and activity of T_H1 cells.

The cross-regulation of T_H1 cells by IL-10 secreted from T_H2 cells is not a direct inhibition of the T_H1 cells; instead, IL-10 acts on monocytes and macrophages, interfering with their ability to activate the T_H1 subset. This interference is thought to result from the demonstrated ability of IL-10 to down-regulate the expression of class II MHC molecules on these antigen-presenting cells. IL-10 has other potent immunosuppressant effects on the monocyte-macrophage lineage: it suppresses the production of nitric oxide and other bactericidal metabolites involved in the destruction of pathogens and also the production of various inflammatory mediators (e.g., IL-1, IL-6, IL-8, GM-CSF, G-CSF, and TNF-α). These suppressive effects on the macrophage serve to further diminish the biologic consequences of T_H1 activation.

In addition to cross-regulation of T_H1 and T_H2, recent research has revealed other regulatory phenomena that are mediated by subpopulations of $CD4^+$ T_H cells that are not as well characterized as are the T_H1 and T_H2 subsets. These regulatory T cells appear to use the cytokine TGF-β to inhibit a number of immune responses mediated by T_H1 and T_H2 cells. The production of TGF-β by these regulatory subsets is important because this cytokine is known to inhibit both T_H1 and T_H2 development. The action of such a regulatory T_H subset on the T_H1 cell-mediated responses is seen in oral tolerance to the induction of experimental allergic encephalitis (EAE). As described in Chapter 20, the injection of mice with myelin basic protein (MBP), a component of the myelin sheath, induces EAE. The pathology of EAE results from a T_H1-cell-mediated inflammatory attack on the myelinated cells of the central nervous system. Feeding the mice appropriate doses of MBP prior to the immunizing injections of MBP prevents the development of EAE. Thus, exposure of the animals to the antigen by the oral route induces tolerance. Investigation of the cellular basis of this phenomenon revealed that oral administration of EAE induced the appearance of antigen-specific T-cell populations. When these cells were cloned, lines of $CD4^+$ T cells that produced TGF-β were obtained. Surprisingly, these lines did not have a cytokine profile typical of either T_H1 or T_H2 cells and so belonged to a different subset. Additional studies of TGF-β-producing regulatory T-cell populations that are neither T_H1 nor T_H2 cells have shown that they play major roles in controlling T_H1-mediated inflammation, and studies of other immune responses in mice, rats, and in vitro human T-cell cultures have also implicated such cells in the inhibition of T_H1- and T_H2-mediated immune responses. The discovery of these new T_H subsets promises to significantly increase our understanding of the control of immune responses. However, much remains to be done to fully characterize these regulatory $CD4^+$ T-cell populations and to determine how they down-regulate T_H1 and T_H2 responses.

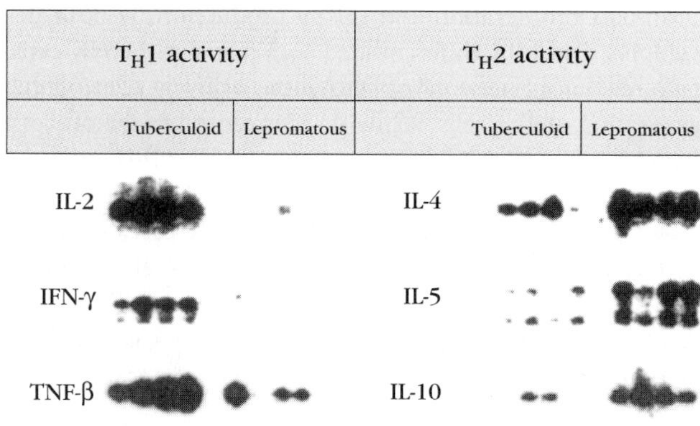

FIGURE 12-13 Correlation between type of leprosy and relative T_H1 or T_H2 activity. Messenger RNA isolated from lesions from tuberculoid and lepromatous leprosy patients was analyzed by Southern blotting using the cytokine probes indicated. Cytokines produced by T_H1 cells predominate in the tuberculoid patients, while cytokines produced by T_H2 cells predominate in the lepromatous patients. [From PA Sieling and RL Modlin, 1994, *Immunobiology* **191**:378.]

Role of T_H1/T_H2 Balance in Determining Disease Outcomes

The progression of some diseases may depend on the balance between the T_H1 and T_H2 subsets. In humans, a well-studied example of this phenomenon is leprosy, which is caused by *Mycobacterium leprae,* an intracellular pathogen that can survive within the phagosomes of macrophages. Leprosy is not a single clinical entity; rather, the disease presents as a spectrum of clinical responses, with two major forms of disease, tuberculoid and lepromatous, at each end of the spectrum. In **tuberculoid leprosy,** a cell-mediated immune response forms granulomas, resulting in the destruction of most of the mycobacteria, so that only a few organisms remain in the tissues. Although skin and peripheral nerves are damaged, tuberculoid leprosy progresses slowly and patients usually survive. In **lepromatous leprosy,** the cell-mediated response is depressed and, instead, humoral antibodies are formed, sometimes resulting in hypergammaglobulinemia. The mycobacteria are widely disseminated in macrophages, often reaching numbers as high as 10^{10} per gram of tissue. Lepromatous leprosy progresses into disseminated infection of the bone and cartilage with extensive nerve damage.

The development of lepromatous or tuberculoid leprosy depends on the balance of T_H1 and T_H2 cells (Figure 12-13). In tuberculoid leprosy, the immune response is characterized by a T_H1-type response with delayed-type hypersensitivity (T_{DTH}) and a cytokine profile consisting of high levels of IL-2, IFN-γ and TNF-β In lepromatous leprosy, there is a T_H2-type immune response, with high levels of IL-4, IL-5, and IL-10. This cytokine profile explains the diminished cell-mediated immunity and increased production of serum antibody in lepromatous leprosy.

There is also evidence for changes in T_H-subset activity in AIDS. Early in the disease, T_H1 activity is high, but as AIDS progresses, some workers have suggested, there may be a shift from a T_H1-like to a T_H2-like response. In addition, some pathogens may influence the activity of the T_H subsets. The Epstein-Barr virus, for instance, produces vIL-10, which has IL-10–like activity and, like cellular IL-10, tends to suppress T_H1 activity by cross-regulation. Some researchers have speculated that vIL-10 may reduce the cell-mediated response to the Epstein-Barr virus, thus conferring a survival advantage on the virus.

Cytokine-Related Diseases

Defects in the complex regulatory networks governing the expression of cytokines and cytokine receptors have been implicated in a number of diseases. This section describes several diseases resulting from overexpression or underexpression of cytokines or cytokine receptors.

Bacterial Septic Shock

The role of cytokine overproduction in pathogenesis can be illustrated by bacterial septic shock. This condition may develop a few hours after infection by certain gram-negative bacteria, including *E. coli, Klebsiella pneumoniae, Pseudomonas aeruginosa, Enterobacter aerogenes,* and *Neisseria meningitidis.* The symptoms of bacterial septic shock, which often is fatal, include a drop in blood pressure, fever, diarrhea, and widespread blood clotting in various organs. This condition afflicts about 500,000 Americans annually and causes more than 70,000 deaths. The annual cost for treating bacterial septic shock is estimated to be in excess of $5 billion.

Bacterial septic shock apparently develops because bacterial cell-wall **endotoxins** stimulate macrophages to overproduce IL-1 and TNF-α. It is the increased levels of IL-1 and

TNF-α that cause septic shock. In one study, for example, higher levels of TNF-α were found in patients who died of meningitis than in those who recovered. Furthermore, a condition resembling bacterial septic shock can be produced by injecting mice with recombinant TNF-α in the absence of gram-negative bacterial infection. Several studies offer some hope that neutralization of TNF-α or IL-1 activity with monoclonal antibodies or antagonists may prevent this fatal shock from developing in these bacterial infections. In one study, monoclonal antibody to TNF-α protected animals from endotoxin-induced shock. Another study has shown that injection of a recombinant IL-1 receptor antagonist (IL-1Ra), which prevents binding of IL-1 to the IL-1 receptor, reduced the mortality due to septic shock in humans from 45% to 16%. It is hoped that these experimental results will lead to clinically useful products for the treatment of bacterial septic shock in humans.

Bacterial Toxic Shock and Similar Diseases

A variety of microorganisms produce toxins that act as **superantigens.** As Chapter 10 described, superantigens bind simultaneously to a class II MHC molecule and to the V_β domain of the T-cell receptor, activating all T cells bearing a particular V_β domain. Unlike conventional antigens, superantigens are not internalized, processed, and presented by antigen-presenting cells. Instead, they bind directly to class II MHC molecules, apparently outside of the antigen-binding cleft. Likewise, superantigens are thought to bind to an exposed region of the β pleated sheet on the side of the T-cell receptor, well away from the sites that bind normal antigenic peptides. Because of their unique binding ability, superantigens can activate large numbers of T cells irrespective of their antigenic specificity.

Although less than 0.01% of T cells respond to a given conventional antigen, between 5% and 25% of T cells can respond to a given superantigen. The large proportion of T cells responsive to a particular superantigen results from the limited number of TCR V_β genes carried in the germ line. Mice, for example, have about 20 V_β genes. Assuming that each V_β gene is expressed with equal frequency, then each superantigen would be expected to interact with 1 in 20 T cells, or 5% of the total T-cell population.

A number of bacterial superantigens have been implicated as the causative agent of several diseases such as bacterial toxic shock and food poisoning. Included among these bacterial superantigens are several enterotoxins, exfoliating toxins, and toxic-shock syndrome toxin (TSST1) from *Staphylococcus aureus*; pyrogenic exotoxins from *Streptococcus pyrogenes*; and *Mycoplasma arthritidis* supernatant (MAS). The large number of T cells activated by these superantigens results in excessive production of cytokines. The toxic-shock syndrome toxin, for example, has been shown to induce extremely high levels of TNF and IL-1. As in bacterial septic shock, these elevated concentrations of cytokines can induce systemic reactions that include fever, widespread blood clotting, and shock.

Lymphoid and Myeloid Cancers

Abnormalities in the production of cytokines or their receptors have been associated with some types of cancer. For example, abnormally high levels of IL-6 are secreted by cardiac myxoma cells (a benign heart tumor), myeloma and plasmacytoma cells, and cervical and bladder cancer cells. In myeloma cells, IL-6 appears to operate in an autocrine manner to stimulate cell proliferation. When monoclonal antibodies to IL-6 are added to in vitro cultures of myeloma cells, their growth is inhibited. In addition, transgenic mice that express high levels of IL-6 have been found to exhibit a massive, fatal plasma-cell proliferation, called plasmacytosis. Although these plasma cells are not malignant, the high rate of plasma-cell proliferation possibly contributes to the development of cancer.

Chagas' Disease

The protozoan *Trypanosoma cruzi* is the causative agent of Chagas' disease, which is characterized by severe immune suppression. The ability of *T. cruzi* to mediate immune suppression can be observed by culturing peripheral-blood T cells in the presence and in the absence of *T. cruzi* and then evaluating their immune reactivity. Antigen, mitogen, or anti-CD3 monoclonal antibody normally can activate peripheral T cells, but in the presence of *T. cruzi,* T cells are not activated by any of these agents. The defect in these lymphocytes has been traced to a dramatic reduction in the expression of the 55-kDa α subunit of the IL-2 receptor. As noted earlier, the high-affinity IL-2 receptor contains the αβ and γ subunits, and the α subunit is specific for cytokine binding (see Figure 12-9). Co-culturing of T cells with *T. cruzi* and subsequent staining with fluorescein-labeled anti-TAC, which binds to the α subunit, revealed a 90% decrease in the level of the α subunit.

Although the mechanism by which *T. cruzi* suppresses expression of the α subunit is still unknown, the suppression can be induced across a filter that prevents contact between the lymphocytes and protozoa. This finding suggests that a diffusible factor mediates suppression. Such a factor, once isolated, might have numerous clinical applications for regulating the level of activated T cells in leukemias and autoimmune diseases.

Therapeutic Uses of Cytokines and Their Receptors

The availability of purified cloned cytokines and soluble cytokine receptors offers the prospect of specific clinical therapies to modulate the immune response. A few cytokines—notably, interferons (see Clinical Focus)—and colony-stimulating factors, such as GM-CSF, have proven to be therapeutically useful. However, despite the promise of cytokines as powerful mediators of immune and other

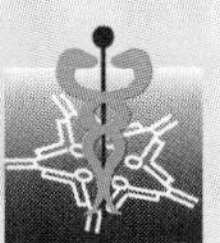

CLINICAL FOCUS

THERAPY WITH INTERFERONS

Interferons are an extraordinary group of proteins whose antiviral activity led to their discovery almost 50 years ago. Subsequent studies showed that interferons have other effects, including the capacity to induce cell differentiation, to inhibit proliferation by some cell types, to inhibit angiogenesis, and to function in various immunoregulatory roles. Their effects on the immune system are important and dramatic. Interferons induce increases in the expression of class I and class II MHC molecules, and augment NK-cell activity. Increased class I expression increases the display of antigen to $CD8^+$ cells, a class that includes most of the T_C population. This enhanced display of antigen not only makes the antigen-presenting cells more effective in inducing cytotoxic T-cell populations, it also makes them better targets for attack by T_C cells. In addition to up-regulating class I MHC expression of many cell types, IFN-γ increases the expression of class II MHC molecules on such antigen-presenting cells as macrophages and dendritic cells. This makes them better presenters of antigen to T_H cells. Gamma interferon is also a potent inducer of macrophage activation and general promoter of inflammatory responses. Cloning of the genes that encode all three types of interferon, IFN-α, IFN-β, and IFN-γ, has made it possible for the biotechnology industry to produce large amounts of all of these interferons at costs that make their clinical use practical. Some clinical uses of each type of interferon include:

- IFN-α (also known by its trade names Roferon and Intron-A) has been used for the treatment of hepatitis C and hepatitis B. It has also found a number of different applications in cancer therapy. A type of B-cell leukemia known as hairy-cell leukemia (because the cells are covered with fine, hairlike cytoplasmic projections) responds well to IFN-α Chronic myelogenous leukemia, a disease characterized by increased numbers of granulocytes, begins with a slowly developing chronic phase that changes to an accelerated phase and terminates in a blast phase, which is usually resistant to treatment. IFN-α is an effective treatment for this leukemia in the chronic phase (70% response rates have been reported) and some patients (as many as 20% in some studies) undergo complete remission. Kaposi's sarcoma, the cancer most often seen in American AIDS patients, also responds to treatment with IFN-α, and there are reports of a trend toward longer survival and fewer opportunistic infections in patients treated with this agent. IFN-α has also been used, with varying degrees of success, to treat a variety of malignancies that include non-Hodgkin's

biological responses, many have not yet made their way into clinical practice. A number of factors are likely to raise difficulties in adapting cytokines for safe and effective routine medical use. One of these is the need to provide effective dose levels and maintain them over a clinically significant period of time. During an immune response, interacting cells produce sufficiently high concentrations of cytokines in the vicinity of target cells, but achieving such local concentrations when cytokines must be administered systemically for clinical treatment is difficult. In addition, cytokines often have a very short half-life, so that continuous administration may be required. For example, recombinant human IL-2 has a half-life of only 7–10 min when administered intravenously. Finally, cytokines are extremely potent biological response modifiers and they can cause unpredictable and undesirable side effects. The side effects from administration of recombinant IL-2, for instance, range from mild ones (e.g., fever, chills, diarrhea, and weight gain) to more serious ones such as anemia, thrombocytopenia, shock, respiratory distress, and coma. Despite these difficulties, the promise of cytokines for clinical medicine is great and efforts to develop safe and effective cytokine-related strategies continue, particularly in areas such as inflammation, cancer therapy, and modification of the immune response during organ transplantation, infectious disease, and allergy.

Some specific examples of various approaches being explored include cytokine receptor blockade and the use of cytokine analogs and cytokine-toxin conjugates. For instance, proliferation of activated T_H cells and activation of T_C cells can be blocked by anti-TAC, a monoclonal antibody that binds to the α subunit of the high-affinity IL-2 receptor (Figure 12-14a, left panel). Administration of anti-TAC has prolonged the survival of heart transplants in rats. Similar results have been obtained with IL-2 analogs that retain their ability to bind the IL-2 receptor but have lost their biological activity (Figure 12-14a, right panel). Such analogs have been produced by site-directed mutagenesis of cloned IL-2 genes. Finally, cytokines conjugated to various toxins (e.g., the β chain of diphtheria toxin) have been shown to diminish rejection of kidney and heart transplants in animals. Such conjugates containing IL-2 selectively bind to and kill activated T_H cells (Figure 12-14b).

lymphoma, cutaneous T-cell lymphoma, and multiple myeloma. Most of the effects mentioned above have been obtained in clinical studies that used IFN-α alone. Future clinical trials in which IFN-α is used in combinations with other agents may improve the effectiveness of this interferon in cancer therapy.

- IFN-β has emerged as the first drug capable of producing clinical improvement in multiple sclerosis (MS). Young adults are the primary target of this autoimmune neurologic disease, in which nerves in the central nervous system (CNS) undergo demyelination. This results in progressive neurologic dysfunction, which leads to significant and, in many cases, severe disability. This disease is often characterized by periods of nonprogression and remission alternating with periods of relapse. Treatment with IFN-β provides longer periods of remission and reduces the severity of relapses. Furthermore, magnetic-resonance-imaging studies of CNS damage in treated and untreated patients revealed that MS-induced damage was less in a group of IFN-β–treated patients than in untreated ones.
- IFN-γ has found application in the clinic as an agent for the treatment of chronic granulomatous disease (CGD). This disease is hereditary and quite rare. Its central feature is a serious impairment of the ability of phagocytic cells to kill ingested microbes. Patients with CGD are beset with recurring infections by a number of bacteria (*Staphylococcus aureus, Klebsiella, Pseudomonas,* and others) and fungi such as *Aspergillus* and *Candida.* Before interferon therapy, standard treatment for the disease was attempts to avoid infection, aggressive administration of antibiotics, and surgical drainage of abscesses. A failure to generate microbicidal oxidants (H_2O_2, superoxide, and others) is the basis of CGD, and the administration of IFN-γ significantly reverses this defect. Therapy of CGD patients with IFN-γ significantly reduces the incidence of infections. Also, the infections that are contracted are less severe and the average number of days spent by patients in the hospital goes down.

The use of interferons in clinical practice is likely to expand, particularly as more is learned about their effects in combination with other therapeutic agents. Although, in common with other cytokines, interferons are powerful modifiers of biological responses, fortunately, the side effects accompanying their use are much milder. Typical side effects include flu-like symptoms, such as headache, fever, chills, and fatigue. These symptoms can largely be managed with acetaminophen (Tylenol) and diminish in intensity during continued treatment. Although interferon toxicity is usually not severe, serious manifestations such as anemia and depressed platelet and white-blood-cell counts have been seen. Experimental cytokine-related therapeutic agents offer the prospect of selectively modulating the immune response.

(a) Suppression of T_H-cell proliferation and T_C-cell activation

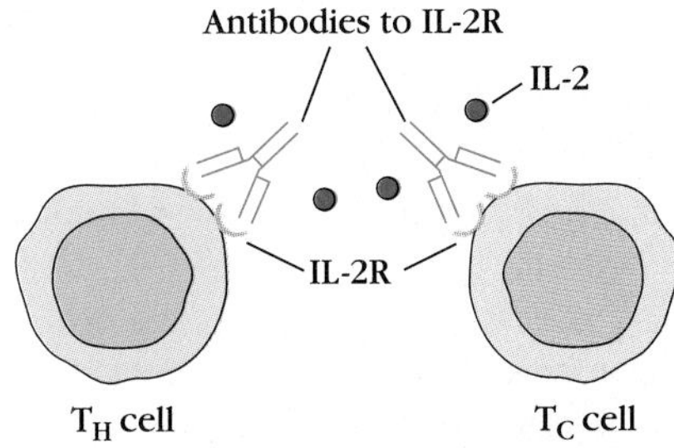

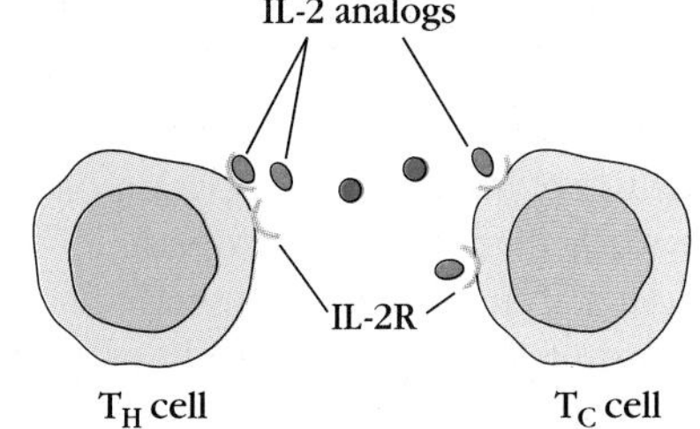

(b) Destruction of activated T_H cells

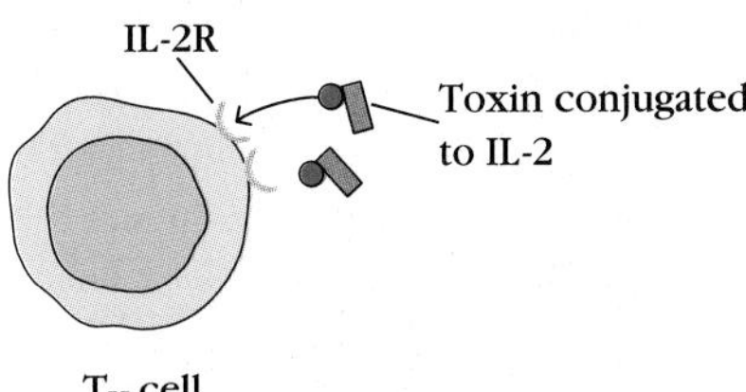

FIGURE 12-14 Experimental cytokine-related therapeutic agents offer the prospect of selectively modulating the immune response. (a) The anti-IL-2R monoclonal antibody binds to the cytokine receptor (IL-2R) on the cell surface, thereby preventing interaction of the cytokine with its receptor. (b) Conjugation of a toxin with a cytokine results in destruction of cells expressing the cytokine receptor.

Summary

1. The complex cellular interactions involving cells of the immune, inflammatory, and hematopoietic systems are mediated by a group of secreted, low-molecular-weight proteins, collectively called cytokines. Most cytokines act on nearby target cells, although in some cases a cytokine can act on the cell that secretes it or on a distant cell (see Figure 12-1). The biological activities of cytokines exhibit pleiotropy, redundancy, synergy, and antagonism, which contribute to the complexity of cytokine networks. Cytokines can also induce cascades (see Figure 12-2).
2. Studies on the structure and function of cytokines advanced greatly with cloning of cytokine genes. Cytokines are proteins or glycoproteins, usually with a molecular mass of less than 30 kDa. Most of the cytokines involved in immune responses share certain structural features that define the hematopoietin family of proteins (see Figure 12-4). The cytokines characterized to date include the interferons α, β, and γ; interleukins 1–18; tumor necrosis factors α and β; and transforming growth factor β.
3. A particular cytokine can act on any target cell that expresses receptors for that cytokine (see Figure 12-6). An important way in which the activity of cytokines is directed toward specific cells is by regulation of the expression of their receptors. For example, only activated T_H cells express the high-affinity IL-2 receptor.
4. The cell-surface proteins that bind cytokines can be classified into five types according to their structures (see Figure 12-6). Most of the cytokines critical in immune and inflammatory responses bind to class I or class II cytokine receptors, which possess certain conserved motifs in their extracellular domains. Most of these receptors are heterodimers, containing a cytokine-specific subunit and signal-transducing subunit (see Figure 12-8). Some class I cytokine receptors share a common signal-transducing subunit, accounting for the redundancy among the biological effects of these cytokines.
5. Cytokine-induced dimerization of the subunits of class I and class II cytokine receptors permits association of cytosolic JAK kinases with the receptor's cytoplasmic domain. This association activates the kinases; the activated JAKs create docking sites for STATs (a family of transcription factors) by phosphorylation of specific tyrosines on receptor subunits. JAKs also phosphorylate tyrosine residues on STAT proteins, and the phosphorylated STATs dimerize and move to the nucleus, where they activate transcription of specific genes (see Figure 12-10). The resulting gene products mediate the biological effects associated with various cytokines.
6. Antigen-stimulated T_H cells in the presence of certain cytokines develop preferentially into T_H1 and T_H2 subsets, with characteristic patterns of cytokine secretion (see Figure 12-12). The cytokines secreted by the T_H1 subset act primarily in cell-mediated responses, whereas those secreted by the T_H2 subset function mostly in B-cell activation and humoral response.
7. Abnormalities in the expression of either cytokines or their receptors may result in various diseases, including bacterial toxic shock, certain lymphoid and myeloid cancers, and Chagas' disease. Cytokine-related therapies that either increase or decrease the immune response offer promise of reducing graft rejection, treating certain cancers and immunodeficiency diseases, and reducing allergic reactions.
8. Therapeutic use of some cytokines of immunological interest, the interferons and colony-stimulating factors such as GM-CSF, has become standard medical practice. However, a number of barriers have prevented the use of many other cytokines for the treatment of disease. These include the need to maintain appropriate dose levels, to formulate effective combinations of cytokines with other drugs or cytokines, and, in some cases, to control cytokine toxicity.

REFERENCES

Abbas, A, KM Murphy, and A Sher. 1996. Functional diversity of helper T lymphocytes. *Nature* **383:**787.

Bach, EA, M Aguet, and RD Schreiber. 1998. The IFN-γ receptor: a paradigm for cytokine receptor signaling. *Ann. Rev. Immunol.* **15:**563.

Baron, S, et al. 1991. The interferons: mechanism of action and clinical applications. *JAMA* **266:**1375.

Bazan, JF. 1992. Unraveling the structure of IL-2. *Science* **257:**410.

Boulay, JL, and WE Paul. 1993. Hematopoietin sub-family classification based on size, gene organization and sequence homology. *Curr. Biol.* **3:**573.

Brennan, FM, and M Feldmann. 1996. Cytokines in autoimmunity. *Curr. Opin. Immunol.* **8:**872.

Dalton, DK, et al. 1993. Multiple defects of immune cell function in mice with disrupted interferon-γ genes. *Science* **259:**1739.

Herman, A, et al. 1991. Superantigens: mechanism of T-cell stimulation and role in immune responses. *Annu. Rev. Immunol.* **9:**745.

Hou, J, et al. 1994. An interleukin-4–induced transcription factor: IL-4 STAT. *Science* **265:**1701.

Huang, S, et al. 1993. Immune response in mice that lack the interferon-γ receptor. *Science* **259:**1742.

Ihle, JN, et al. 1995. Signaling through the hematopoietic cytokine receptors. *Annu. Rev. Immunol.* **13:**369.

Ivashkiv, LB, 1995. Cytokines and STATS: how can signals achieve specificity? *Immunity* **3:**1.

Mossman, TR, H Cherwinski, MW Bond, MA Gledlin, and RL Coffman. 1986. Two types of murine helper T cell clone. I. Definition according to profiles of lymphokine activities and secreted proteins. *J. Immunology* **136:**2348.

O'Garra, A. 1998. Cytokines induce the development of functionally heterogeneous T helper cell subsets. *Immunity* **8:**275.

Smith, K. 1990. Interleukin-2. *Sci. Am.* **262:**50.

Sugamura, K, et al. 1996. The interleukin-2 receptor γ chain: its role in the multiple cytokine receptor complexes and T cell development in XSCID. *Annu. Rev. Immunol.* **14:**179.

Szabo, SJ, LH Glimcher, and IC Ho 1997. Genes that regulate interleukin-4 expression in T cells. *Curr. Opin. Immunol.* **9:**776.

Takeda K, et al. 1998. Defective NK cell activity and T_H1 response in IL-18 deficient mice. *Immunity* **8:**383.

Trinchieri, G. 1995. Interleukin-12: a proinflammatory cytokine with immunoregulatory functions that bridge innate resistance and antigen-specific adaptive immunity. *Annu. Rev. Immunol.* **13:**251.

Waldmann, TA. 1993. The IL-2/IL-2 receptor system: a target for rational immune intervention. *Immunol. Today* **14:**264.

Walter, MR, et al. 1995. Crystal structure of a complex between interferon-γ and its soluble high-affinity receptor. *Nature* **376:**230.

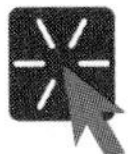

Useful Web Sites

http://www.psynix.co.uk/cytweb/index.html>
The Cytokines Web site provides information about cytokines and their receptors, including 3-D structural information. There are interesting notes on potential therapeutic uses for recently discovered human cytokines.

<http://www.copewithcytokines.de/>
Cytokines Online Pathfinder Encyclopaedia (COPE) created by H Ibelgauft has more than 6300 pages devoted to cytokine research and related subjects.

<http://www.rndsystems.com/>
The cytokine minireviews found at R&D Systems Web site provide extensive, detailed, well-referenced, and often strikingly illustrated reviews of many cytokines and their receptors.

STUDY QUESTIONS

1. Indicate whether each of the following statements is true or false. If you think a statement is false, explain why.

a. The high-affinity IL-2 receptor consists of two transmembrane proteins.

b. The anti-TAC monoclonal antibody recognizes the IL-1 receptor on T cells.

c. All cytokine-binding receptors contain two or three subunits.

d. Expression of the β subunit of the IL-2 receptor is indicative of T-cell activation.

e. Some cytokine receptors possess domains with tyrosine kinase activity that function in signal transduction.

f. All members of each subfamily of the class I cytokine (hematopoietin) receptors share a common signal-transducing subunit.

2. When IL-2 is secreted by one T cell in a peripheral lymphoid organ, do all the T cells in the vicinity proliferate in response to the IL-2 or only some of them? Explain.

3. Briefly describe the similarities and differences among cytokines, growth factors, and hormones.

4. Indicate which subunit(s) of the IL-2 receptor are expressed by the following types of cells:

a. _____ Resting T cells

b. _____ Activated T cells

c. _____ Activated T cells + cyclosporin A

d. _____ Resting T_C cells

e. _____ CTLs

f. _____ NK cells

5. Superantigens have been implicated in several diseases and have been useful as research tools.

a. What properties of superantigens distinguish them from conventional antigens?

b. By what mechanism are bacterial superantigens thought to cause symptoms associated with food poisoning and toxic-shock syndrome?

c. Does the activity of superantigens exhibit MHC restriction?

6. IL-3, IL-5, and GM-CSF exhibit considerable redundancy in their effects. What structural feature of the receptors for these cytokines might explain this redundancy?

7. Considerable evidence indicates the existence of two T_H-cell subsets, differing in the pattern of cytokines they secrete.

a. What type of immune response is mediated by the T_H1 subset? What type of antigen challenge is likely to induce a T_H1-mediated response?

b. What type of immune response is mediated by the T_H2 subset? What type of antigen challenge is likely to induce a T_H2-mediated response?

Go to www.whfreeman.com/immunology Self-Test
Review and quiz of key terms

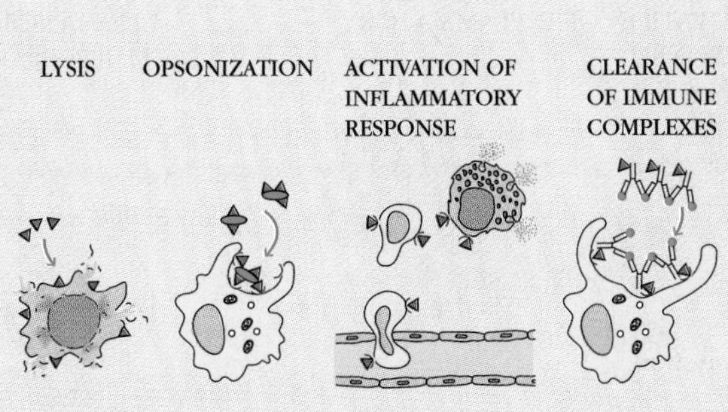

CHAPTER 13

THE COMPLEMENT SYSTEM

The Functions of Complement

The Complement Components

Complement Activation

Regulation of the Complement System

Biological Consequences of Complement Activation

Complement Deficiencies

The complement system is the major effector of the humoral branch of the immune system. Research on complement began in the 1890s, when Jules Bordet at the Institut Pasteur in Paris showed that sheep antiserum to the bacterium *Vibrio cholerae* caused lysis of the bacteria and that heating the antiserum destroyed its bacteriolytic activity. Surprisingly, the ability to lyse the bacteria was restored to the heated serum by adding fresh serum that contained no antibodies directed against the bacterium and by itself was unable to kill it. Bordet correctly reasoned that bacteriolytic activity requires two different substances: first, the specific antibacterial antibodies, which survive the heating process, and a second, heat-sensitive component responsible for the lytic activity. Bordet devised a simple test for the lytic activity, the easily detected lysis of antibody-coated red blood cells, called **hemolysis;** he designated the responsible substance *alexin* (from the Greek *alexein,* to ward off). Bordet's name for this activity did not survive long. Shortly afterward in Berlin, Paul Ehrlich independently carried out similar experiments and coined the term *complement,* defining it as "the activity of blood serum that completes the action of antibody." In ensuing years, researchers discovered that the action of complement was the result of interactions of a large and complex group of proteins. The reaction pathways, interactions, and activities of the components of the complement system were determined in a series of experiments with proteins that were isolated, purified, and then mixed in various combinations to reconstitute the ability to cause lysis. In this way, the activity of each component of the complement system was deduced.

This chapter describes the complement components and their activation pathways, the regulation of the complement system, the effector functions of various complement components, and the consequences of hereditary deficiencies in some of them.

The Functions of Complement

Research on complement now includes more than 30 soluble and cell-bound proteins. Biologic activities of this system impact both innate and acquired immunity and reach far beyond the original observations of antibody-mediated lysis of bacteria and red blood cells. After initial activation, the various complement components interact, in a highly regulated cascade, to carry out a number of basic functions (Figure 13-1) including:

- Lysis of cells, bacteria, and viruses
- Opsonization, which promotes phagocytosis of particulate antigens
- Binding to specific complement receptors on cells of the immune system, triggering activation of immune responses such as inflammation and secretion of immunoregulatory molecules that amplify or alter specific immune responses
- Immune clearance, which removes immune complexes from the circulation and deposits them in the spleen and liver

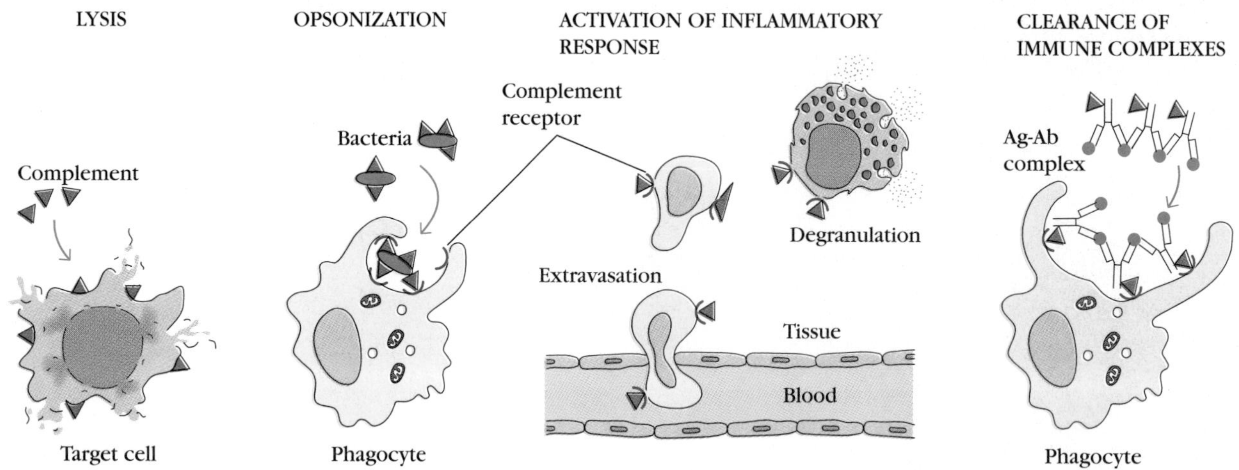

FIGURE 13-1 The multiple activities of the complement system. Serum complement proteins and membrane-bound complement receptors partake in a number of immune activities: lysis of foreign cells by antibody-dependent or antibody-independent pathways; opsonization or uptake of particulate antigens, including bacteria, by phagocytes; activation of inflammatory responses; and clearance of circulating immune complexes by cells in the liver and spleen. Soluble complement proteins are schematically indicated by a triangle and receptors by a semi-circle; no attempt is made to differentiate among individual components of the complement system here.

The Complement Components

The proteins and glycoproteins that compose the complement system are synthesized mainly by liver hepatocytes, although significant amounts of them are also produced by blood monocytes, tissue macrophages, and epithelial cells of the gastrointestinal and genitourinary tracts. These components constitute 5% (by weight) of the serum globulin fraction and most circulate in the serum in functionally inactive forms. Many components are proenzymes, or *zymogens,* which are inactive until proteolytic cleavage, which removes an inhibitory fragment and exposes the active site. The complement-reaction sequence starts with an enzyme cascade. Several of the activated components become inactivated shortly if they do not react with the next component in the sequence.

Complement components are designated by numerals (C1–C9), by letter symbols (e.g., factor D), or by trivial names (e.g., homologous restriction factor). The peptide fragments formed by activation of a component are denoted by small letters. In most cases, the smaller fragment resulting from cleavage of a component is designated "a" and the larger fragment designated "b" (e.g., C3a, C3b; note that C2 is an exception: C2a is the larger cleavage fragment). The larger fragments bind to the target near the site of activation, and the smaller fragments diffuse from the site and can initiate localized inflammatory responses by binding to specific receptors. The complement fragments interact with one another to form functional complexes. Those complexes that have enzymatic activity are designated by a bar over the number or symbol (e.g., $C\overline{4b2a}$, $C\overline{3bBb}$).

Complement Activation

Figure 13-2 outlines the pathways of complement activation. The early steps in complement activation, culminating in formation of C5b, can occur by the **classical pathway,** the **alternative pathway,** or the **lectin pathway.** The final steps that lead to a membrane attack are the same in all pathways.

Classical Pathway

Complement activation by the classical pathway commonly begins with the formation of soluble antigen-antibody complexes (immune complexes) or with the binding of antibody to antigen on a suitable target, such as a bacterial cell. IgM and certain subclasses of IgG (human IgG1, IgG2, and IgG3) can activate the classical complement pathway, as can certain nonimmunologic activators. The initial stage of activation involves C1, C2, C3, and C4, which are present in plasma in functionally inactive forms (Table 13-1). Because the components were named in order of their discovery and before their functional roles had been determined, the numbers in their names do not always reflect the order in which they react.

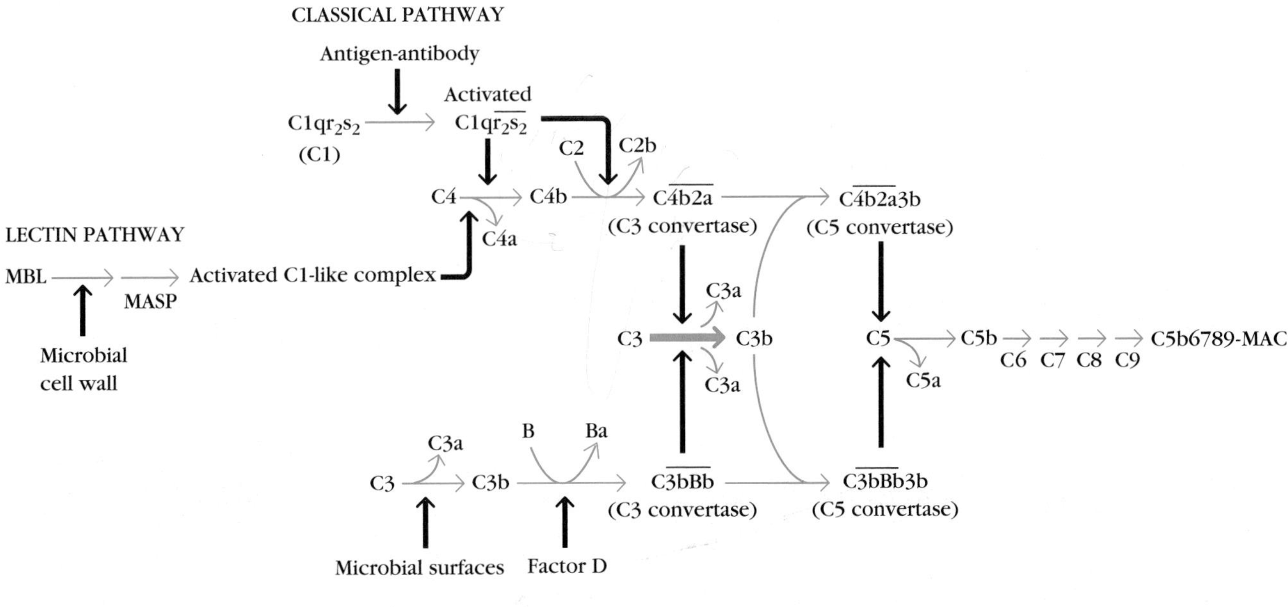

FIGURE 13-2 Overview of the complement activation pathways. The classical pathway is initiated by binding of C1 to antigen-antibody complexes. The alternative pathway is initiated by binding of C3b to activating surfaces such as microbial cell walls. The lectin pathway is initiated by binding of the serum protein MBL to the surface of a pathogen. The alternative pathway utilizes some components (or factors) that are unique, whereas the classical and the lectin pathways have all components in common after C1. All three pathways generate C3 and C5 convertases and bound C5b, which is converted into a membrane-attack complex (MAC) by a common sequence of terminal reactions. Hydrolysis of C3 is the major amplification step in all pathways, generating large amounts of C3b, which forms part of C5 convertase. C3b also can diffuse away from the activating surface and bind to immune complexes or foreign cell surfaces, where it functions as an opsonin. Blue arrows indicate reaction steps; black arrows indicate enzymatic or activating activity.

The complexing of antibody with antigen induces conformational changes in the Fc portion of the IgM molecule that expose a binding site for the C1 component of the complement system. C1 in serum is a macromolecular complex consisting of C1q and two molecules each of C1r and C1s, held together in a complex ($C1qr_2s_2$) stabilized by Ca^{2+} ions. The C1q molecule is composed of 18 polypeptide chains that associate to form six collagen-like triple helical arms, the tips of which bind to exposed C1q-binding sites in the C_H2 domain of the antibody molecule

TABLE 13-1 CLASSICAL COMPLEMENT PATHWAY: PROTEINS THAT PARTICIPATE IN FORMATION OF C5 CONVERTASE

Component	Active protein/split product	Immunologic function
C1	C1q	Binds to Fc region of IgM and IgG
	C1r	Serine protease: enzymatically activates C1s
	C1s	Serine protease: enzymatically activates C4 and C2
C4	C4a	Peptide mediator of inflammation (anaphylatoxin)
	C4b	Binds C2 forming complex that is cleaved by C1s to yield $\overline{C4b2a}$
C2	C2a	Serine protease: $\overline{C4b2a}$ acts as C3 convertase
	C2b	Unknown function
C3	C3a	Peptide mediator of inflammation (anaphylatoxin)
	C3b	Binds to $\overline{C4b2a}$ to form C5 convertase; major opsonin

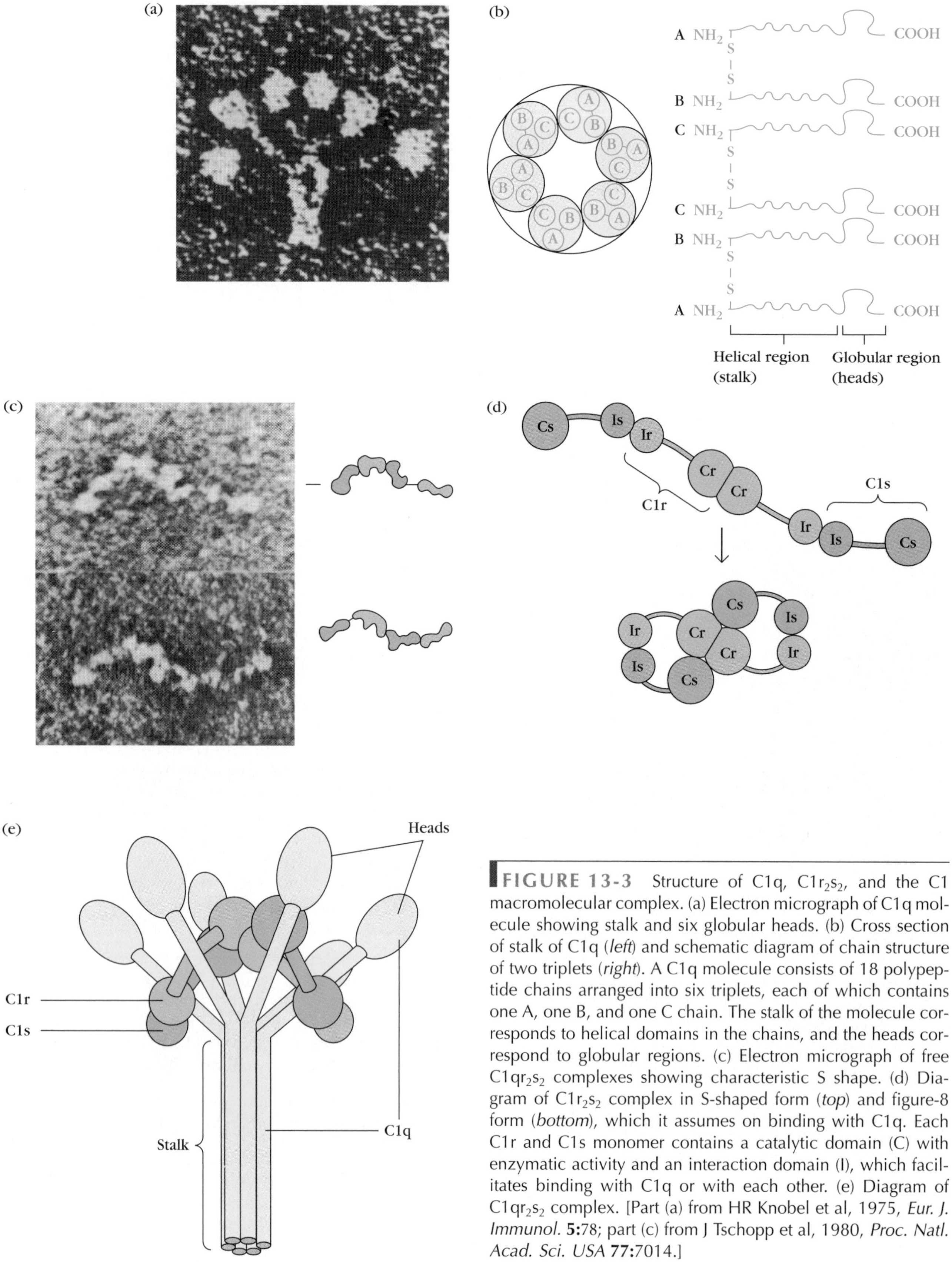

(a)

(b)

A NH_2 COOH
B NH_2 COOH
C NH_2 COOH
C NH_2 COOH
B NH_2 COOH
A NH_2 COOH
Helical region (stalk)
Globular region (heads)

(c)

(d)

Cs Is Ir Cr Cr Ir Is Cs
C1r
C1s

(e)

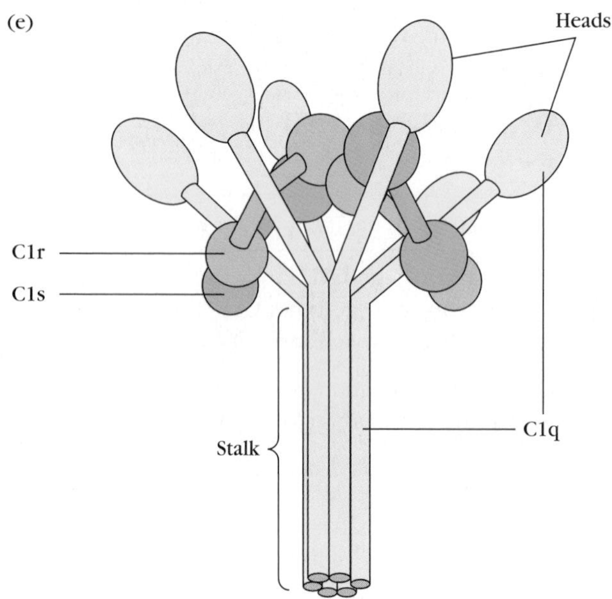

FIGURE 13-3 Structure of C1q, C1r$_2$s$_2$, and the C1 macromolecular complex. (a) Electron micrograph of C1q molecule showing stalk and six globular heads. (b) Cross section of stalk of C1q (*left*) and schematic diagram of chain structure of two triplets (*right*). A C1q molecule consists of 18 polypeptide chains arranged into six triplets, each of which contains one A, one B, and one C chain. The stalk of the molecule corresponds to helical domains in the chains, and the heads correspond to globular regions. (c) Electron micrograph of free C1qr$_2$s$_2$ complexes showing characteristic S shape. (d) Diagram of C1r$_2$s$_2$ complex in S-shaped form (*top*) and figure-8 form (*bottom*), which it assumes on binding with C1q. Each C1r and C1s monomer contains a catalytic domain (C) with enzymatic activity and an interaction domain (I), which facilitates binding with C1q or with each other. (e) Diagram of C1qr$_2$s$_2$ complex. [Part (a) from HR Knobel et al, 1975, *Eur. J. Immunol.* **5:**78; part (c) from J Tschopp et al, 1980, *Proc. Natl. Acad. Sci. USA* **77:**7014.]

(Figure 13-3a,b). The C1qr$_2$s$_2$ complex can exist in two configurations. When it is free and not bound to C1q, it assumes an S-shaped form; on binding to C1q, C1qr$_2$s$_2$ assumes a shape similar to a figure 8 (Figure 13-3c,d,e). Each C1r and C1s monomer contains a catalytic domain and an interaction domain; the latter facilitates interaction with C1q or with each other.

Each C1 molecule must bind, by its C1q globular heads, to at least two Fc sites for a stable C1–antibody interaction to occur. When pentameric IgM is bound to antigen on a target surface it assumes the so-called staple configuration, in which at least three binding sites for C1q are exposed. Circulating IgM, however, exists as a planar configuration in which the C1q-binding sites are not exposed (Figure 13-4). For this reason, circulating IgM cannot activate the complement cascade by itself. An IgG molecule, on the other hand, contains only a single C1q-binding site in the C_H2 domain of the Fc, so that firm C1q binding is achieved only when two IgG molecules are within 30–40 nm of each other on a target surface or in a complex, providing two attachment sites for C1q. This difference in the structure of IgM and IgG accounts for the observation that a single molecule of IgM bound to a red blood cell is enough to activate the classical complement pathway and lyse the red blood cell, whereas some 1000 molecules of IgG are required if two molecules, randomly distributed, are to end up close enough to each other to initiate C1q binding.

The intermediates in the classical activation pathway are depicted schematically in Figure 13-5. Binding of C1q to Fc binding sites induces a conformational change in C1r that converts C1r to an active serine protease enzyme, $\overline{\text{C1r}}$, which then cleaves C1s to a similar active enzyme, $\overline{\text{C1s}}$. $\overline{\text{C1s}}$ has two substrates, C4 and C2 (see Figure 13-2). The C4 component is a glycoprotein containing three polypeptide chains α, β, and γ. C4 is activated when $\overline{\text{C1s}}$ hydrolyzes a small fragment (C4a) from the amino terminus of the α chain, exposing a binding site on the larger fragment (C4b). The C4b fragment attaches to the target surface in the vicinity of C1, and the C2 proenzyme then attaches to the exposed binding site on C4b, where the C2 is then cleaved by the neighboring $\overline{\text{C1s}}$; the smaller fragment (C2b) diffuses away. The resulting $\overline{\text{C4b2a}}$ complex is called C3 convertase, referring to its role in converting the C3 proenzyme into an enzymatically active form. The smaller fragment from C4 cleavage, C4a, is an anaphylatoxin, or mediator of inflammation, which does not participate directly in the complement cascade; the anaphylatoxins, which include the smaller fragments of C4, C3, and C5 are discussed below.

The native C3 component consists of two polypeptide chains, α and β. Hydrolysis of a short fragment (C3a) from the amino terminus of the α chain by the C3 convertase generates C3b (Figure 13-6). A single C3 convertase molecule can generate over 200 molecules of C3b, resulting in tremendous amplification at this step of the sequence. Some of the C3b binds to $\overline{\text{C4b2a}}$ to form a trimolecular complex

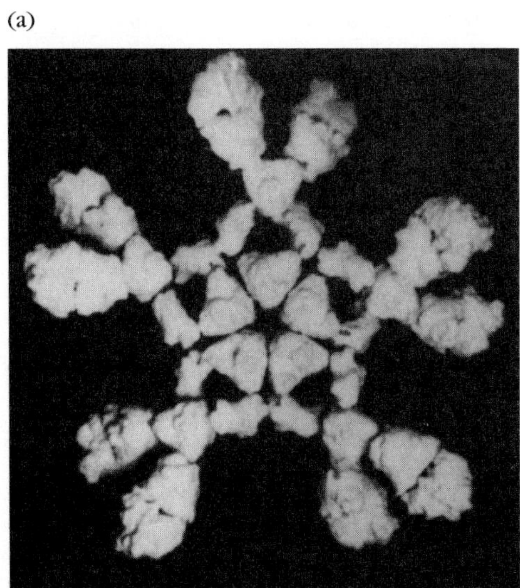

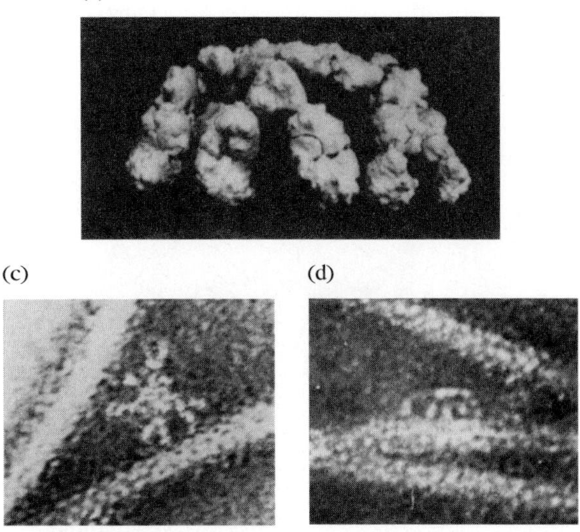

FIGURE 13-4 Models of pentameric IgM in planar form (a) and "staple" form (b). Several C1q-binding sites in the Fc region are accessible in the staple form, whereas none are exposed in the planar form. Electron micrographs of IgM antiflagellum antibody bound to flagella, showing the planar form (c) and staple form (d). [From A Feinstein et al, 1981, *Monogr. Allergy* **17:**28, and 1981, *Ann. N.Y. Acad. Sci.* **190:** 1104.]

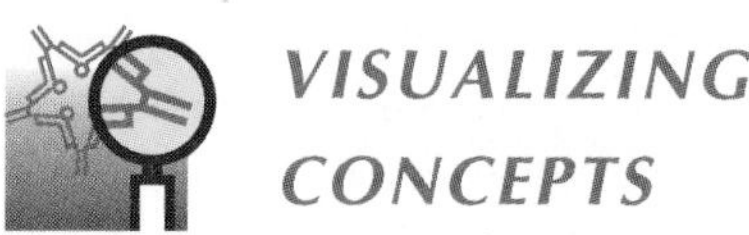

VISUALIZING CONCEPTS

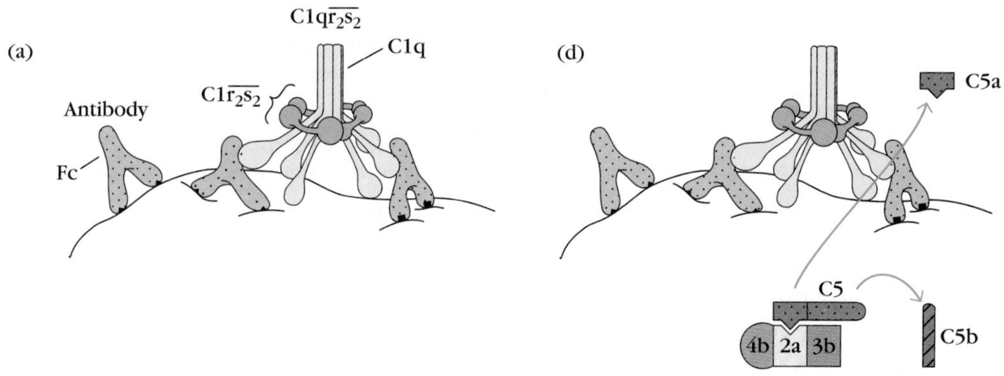

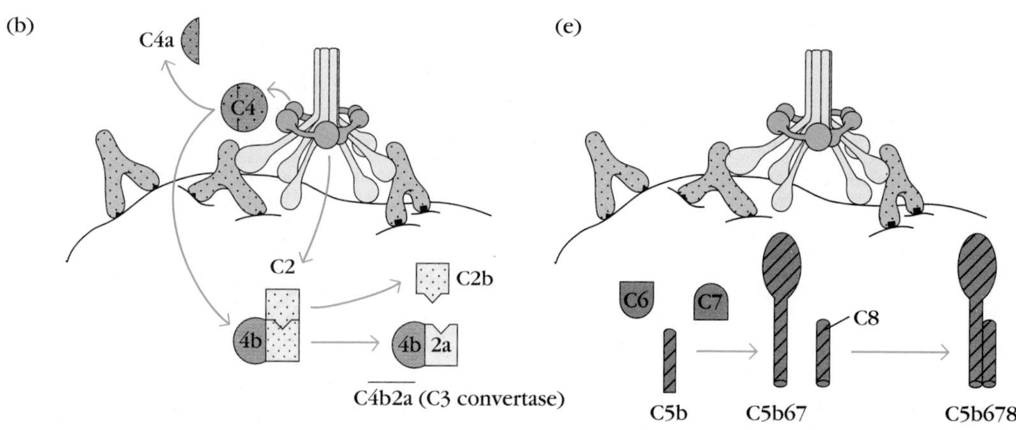

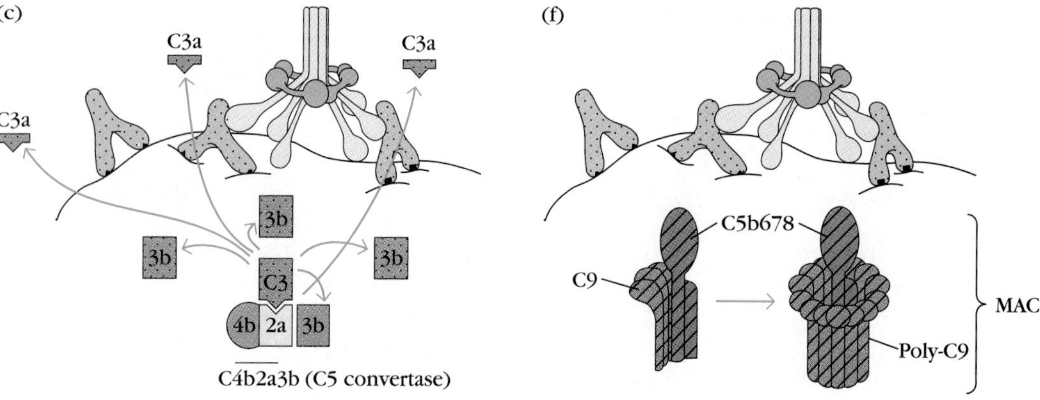

FIGURE 13-5 Schematic diagram of intermediates in the classical pathway of complement activation. Complement components, shown in solid colors, are bound to the antigenic surface but do not penetrate it; components that can insert into the cell membrane are marked with diagonal lines; and the freely diffusible components are stippled. The completed membrane-attack complex (MAC) forms a large pore in the membrane.

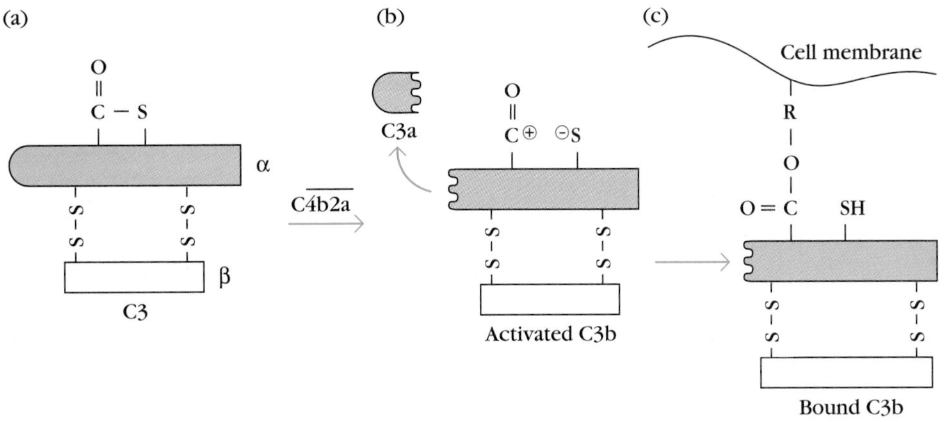

FIGURE 13-6 Hydrolysis of C3 by C3 convertase $\overline{C4b2a}$ (a) Native C3. (b) Activated C3 showing site of cleavage by $\overline{C4b2a}$ resulting in production of the C3a and C3b fragments. (c) A labile internal thioester bond in C3 is activated as C3b is formed, allowing the C3b fragment to bind to free hydroxyl or amino groups (R) on a cell membrane. Bound C3b exhibits various biological activities, including binding of C5 and binding to C3b receptors on phagocytic cells.

$\overline{C4b2a3b}$, called C5 convertase. The C3b component of this complex binds C5 and alters its conformation, so that the $\overline{C4b2a}$ component can cleave C5 into C5a, which diffuses away, and C5b, which attaches to C6 and initiates formation of the membrane-attack complex in a sequence described later. Some of the C3b generated by C3 convertase activity does not associate with $\overline{C4b2a}$; instead it diffuses away and then coats immune complexes and particulate antigens, functioning as an opsonin as discussed in a later section. C3b may also bind directly to cell membranes.

Alternative Pathway

The alternative pathway is an antibody-independent means to generate bound C5b, the same product as the classical pathway generates in a sequence of events requiring antigen-antibody complexes for initiation (see Figure 13-2). Because no antibody is required, the alternative pathway is a component of the innate immune system. This major pathway of complement activation involves four serum proteins: C3, factor B, factor D, and properdin (Table 13-2). Unlike the classical pathway, the alternative pathway is initiated without requiring antibody, in most cases by various cell-surface constituents that are foreign to the host (Table 13-3). For example, both gram-negative and gram-positive bacteria have cell-wall constituents that can activate the alternative pathway. The intermediates in the alternative pathway for generating C5b are depicted schematically in Figure 13-7.

In the classical pathway, C3 is cleaved to C3a and C3b rapidly by the enzymatic activity of the C3 convertase. In the alternative pathway, serum C3, which contains an unstable thioester bond, is subject to slow spontaneous hydrolysis to yield C3a and C3b. The C3b component can bind to foreign surface antigens (such as those on bacterial cells or viral

TABLE 13-2 ALTERNATIVE COMPLEMENT PATHWAY: PROTEINS THAT PARTICIPATE IN FORMATION OF C5 CONVERTASE

Component	Active protein/split product	Immunologic function
C3	C3a	Peptide mediator of inflammation (anaphylatoxin)
	C3b	Binds factor B, forming complex that is cleaved by factor D to yield $\overline{C3bBb}$
Factor B	Ba	Unknown function
	Bb	Serine protease: $\overline{C3bBb}$ acts as C3 convertase, which generates $\overline{C3bBb3b}$ (C5 convertase)
Factor D	D	Serine protease: cleaves factor B that is bound to C3b to form C3 convertase
Properdin		Binds to and stabilizes $\overline{C3bBb}$

VISUALIZING CONCEPTS

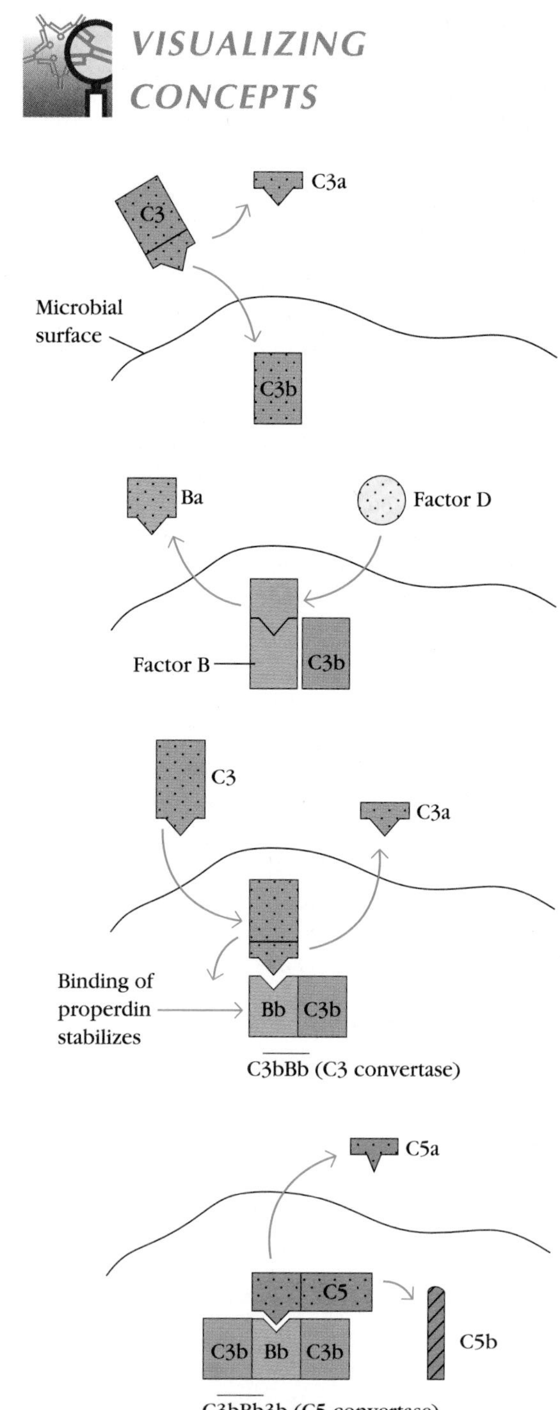

FIGURE 13-7 Schematic diagram of intermediates in formation of bound C5b by the alternative pathway of complement activation. The $\overline{C3bBb}$ complex is stabilized by binding of properdin. Membrane-bound intermediates are shown in solid colors; components that can penetrate the cell membrane are marked with diagonal lines; freely diffusible components are stippled. Conversion of bound C5b to the membrane-attack complex occurs by the same sequence of reactions as in the classical pathway (see Figure 13-5e and f).

particles) or even to the host's own cells (see Figure 13-6c). The membranes of most mammalian cells have high levels of sialic acid, which contributes to the rapid inactivation of bound C3b molecules on host cells; consequently this binding rarely leads to further reactions on the host cell membrane. Because many foreign antigenic surfaces (e.g., bacterial cell walls, yeast cell walls, and certain viral envelopes) have only low levels of sialic acid, C3b bound to these surfaces remains active for a longer time. The C3b present on the surface of the foreign cells can bind another serum protein called factor B by way of a Mg^{2+}-dependent bond. Binding to C3b exposes a site on factor B that serves as the substrate for an enzymatically active serum protein called factor D. Factor D cleaves the C3b-bound factor B, releasing a small fragment (Ba), which diffuses away, and generates $\overline{C3bBb}$. The $\overline{C3bBb}$ complex has C3 convertase activity and thus is analogous to the $\overline{C4b2a}$ complex in the classical pathway (Table 13-4). The C3 convertase activity of $\overline{C3bBb}$ has a half-life of only 5 minutes unless the serum protein properdin binds to it, stabilizing it and extending the half-life of this convertase activity to 30 minutes.

TABLE 13-3 INITIATORS OF THE ALTERNATIVE PATHWAY OF COMPLEMENT ACTIVATION

Pathogens and particles of microbial origin
Many strains of gram-negative bacteria
Lipopolysaccharides from gram-negative bacteria
Many strains of gram-positive bacteria
Teichoic acid from gram-positive cell walls
Fungal and yeast cell walls (zymosan)
Some viruses and virus-infected cells
Some tumor cells (Raji)
Parasites (trypanosomes)
Nonpathogens
Human IgG, IgA, and IgE in complexes
Rabbit and guinea pig IgG in complexes
Cobra venom factor
Heterologous erythrocytes (rabbit, mouse, chicken)
Anionic polymers (dextran sulfate)
Pure carbohydrates (agarose, inulin)

SOURCE: Adapted from MK Pangburn, 1986, in *Immunobiology of the Complement System*, Academic Press.

TABLE 13-4 COMPLEMENT COMPONENTS IN THE FORMATION OF C3 AND C5 CONVERTASES

	Classical pathway	Lectin pathway	Alternative pathway
Precursor proteins	C4 + C2	C4 + C2	C3 + factor B
Activating protease	C$\overline{1s}$	MASP	Factor D
C3 convertase	$\overline{C4b2a}$	$\overline{C4b2a}$	$\overline{C3bBb}$
C5 convertase	$\overline{C4b2a}$3b	$\overline{C4b2a}$3b	$\overline{C3bBb}$3b
C5-binding component	C3b	C3b	C3b

The $\overline{C3bBb}$ generated in the alternative pathway can activate unhydrolyzed C3 to generate more C3b autocatalytically. As a result, the initial steps are repeated and amplified, so that more than 2×10^6 molecules of C3b can be deposited on an antigenic surface in less than 5 minutes. The C3 convertase activity of $\overline{C3bBb}$ generates the $\overline{C3bBb}$3b complex, which exhibits C5 convertase activity, analogous to the $\overline{C4b2a}$3b complex in the classical pathway. The nonenzymatic C3b component binds C5, and the Bb component subsequently hydrolyzes the bound C5 to generate C5a and C5b; the latter binds to the antigenic surface (see Figure 13-7).

The Lectin Pathway

Recently, an additional means by which the complement cascade can be activated was described; this addition to the complement repertoire is called the lectin pathway. Lectins are proteins that bind to a carbohydrate. The lectin pathway, like the alternative pathway, does not depend on antibody for its activation. However, the mechanism is more like that of the classical pathway, because after initiation, it proceeds, through the action of C4 and C2, to produce a C5 convertase (see Figure 13-2). The pathway is activated by the binding of mannose-binding lectin (MBL) to mannose residues on glycoproteins or carbohydrates on the surface of microorganisms. MBL is an **acute phase protein** produced in inflammatory responses. Its function in the complement pathway is similar to that of C1q, which it resembles in structure. After MBL binds to the surface of a cell or pathogen, MBL-associated serine protease, or MASP, binds to it. The active complex formed by this association causes cleavage and activation of C4. MASP has structural similarity to C1r and C1s and mimics their activities. Details of the lectin pathway remain obscure, but this means of activating the C2–C4 components to form a C5 convertase without need for specific antibody binding certainly represents an important innate defense mechanism comparable to the alternative pathway.

Terminal Sequence: Formation of Membrane-Attack Complex

The terminal sequence of complement activation involves C5b, C6, C7, C8, and C9, which interact sequentially to form a macromolecular structure called the **membrane-attack complex (MAC).** This complex displaces the membrane phospholipids, forming a large transmembrane channel that disrupts the membrane of the target cell and enables ions and small molecules to diffuse through it freely.

As noted previously, in the classical, lectin, and alternative pathways, a C5 convertase cleaves C5, which contains two protein chains (α and β). After binding of C5 to the nonenzymatic C3b component of the convertase, the amino terminus of the α chain is cleaved. This generates the small C5a fragment, which diffuses away, and the large C5b fragment, which binds to the surface of the target cell and provides a binding site for the subsequent components of the membrane-attack complex (see Figure 13-5d). The C5b component is extremely labile and is inactivated within 2 minutes unless C6 binds to it and stabilizes its activity.

Up to this point, all the complement reactions take place on the hydrophilic surface of membranes or on immune complexes in the fluid phase. As C5b6 binds to C7, the resulting complex undergoes a hydrophilic-amphiphilic structural transition that exposes hydrophobic regions, which serve as binding sites for membrane phospholipids. If the reaction occurs on a target-cell membrane, the hydrophobic binding sites enable the C5b67 complex to insert into the phospholipid bilayer (see Figure 13-5e). If, however, the reaction occurs on an immune complex or other noncellular activating surface, then the hydrophobic binding sites cannot anchor the complex and it is released. Released C5b67 complexes can insert into the membrane of nearby cells and mediate "innocent-bystander" lysis, although this rarely occurs. In a number of diseases in which immune complexes are produced, tissue damage may result from such innocent-bystander lysis. This autoimmune process will be discussed in Chapter 20.

Binding of C8 to membrane-bound C5b67 induces a conformational change in C8, so that it too undergoes a hydrophilic-amphiphilic structural transition, exposing a hydrophobic region, which interacts with the plasma membrane. The C5b678 complex creates a small pore 10 Å in diameter; formation of this pore can lead to lysis of red blood cells but not of nucleated cells. The final step in formation of the MAC is the binding and polymerization of C9, a perforin-like molecule, to the C5b678 complex.

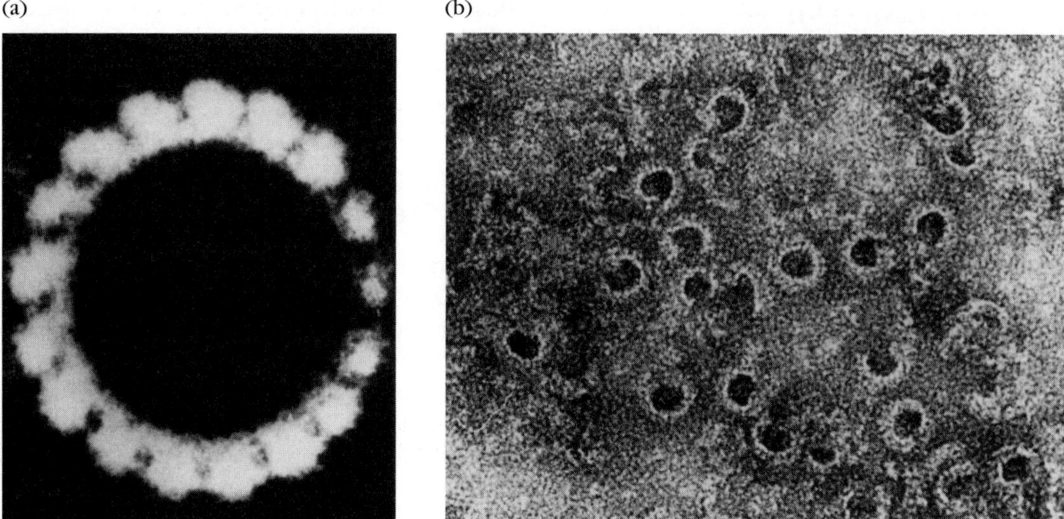

FIGURE 13-8 (a) Photomicrograph of poly-C9 complex formed by in vitro polymerization of C9. (b) Photomicrograph of complement-induced lesions on the membrane of a red blood cell. These lesions result from formation of membrane-attack complexes. [Part (a) from ER Podack, 1986, in *Immunobiology of the Complement System*, Academic Press; part (b) from J Humphrey and R Dourmashkin, 1969, *Adv. Immunol.* **11**:75.]

As many as 10–17 molecules of C9 can be bound and polymerized by a single C5b678 complex. During polymerization, the C9 molecules undergo a hydrophilic-amphophilic transition, so that they also can insert into the membrane (see Figure 13-5f). The completed MAC, which has a tubular form and functional pore size of 70–100 Å, consists of a C5b678 complex surrounded by a poly-C9 complex (Figure 13-8). Since ions and small molecules can diffuse freely through the central channel of the MAC, the cell cannot maintain its osmotic stability and is killed by an influx of water and loss of electrolytes. The components of the terminal sequence of the complement pathways are summarized in Table 13-5.

Regulation of the Complement System

Because the complement system is nonspecific and thus capable of attacking host cells as well as microorganisms, elaborate regulatory mechanisms have evolved to restrict its activity to designated targets. A general mechanism of regulation in all complement pathways is the inclusion of a number of extremely labile components, which undergo spontaneous inactivation as they diffuse away from target cells. In addition, the complement system includes a series of regulatory proteins that inactivate various complement

TABLE 13-5 TERMINAL COMPLEMENT PATHWAY: PROTEINS INVOLVED IN THE FORMATION OF THE MEMBRANE-ATTACK COMPLEX (MAC)

Component	Active protein/split product	Immunologic function
C5	C5a	Peptide mediator of chemotaxis and inflammation (anaphylatoxin)
	C5b	Binds C6 to initiate formation of MAC
C6	C6	C5b6 binds C7
C7	C7	After an amphophilic transition of C5b67, the resulting complex inserts into the lipid bilayer
C8	C8	C5b678 binds multiple C9 molecules, initiating their polymerization
C9	C9	Polymerizes to complete formation of MAC pore

components (Table 13-6). For example, the glycoprotein C1 inhibitor (C1Inh) can form a complex with $C1r_2s_2$, causing it to dissociate from C1q and preventing further activation of C4 or C2 (Figure 13-9a).

The reaction catalyzed by the C3 convertase enzymes of the classical, lectin, and alternative pathways is the major amplification step in complement activation, generating hundreds of molecules of C3b. The C3b generated by these enzymes has the potential to bind to nearby cells, mediating damage to the healthy cells through opsonization by phagocytic cells bearing C3b receptors or by induction of the membrane-attack complex. Damage to normal host cells is prevented because C3b undergoes spontaneous hydrolysis by the time it has diffused 40 nm away from the $\overline{C4b2a}$ or $\overline{C3bBb}$ convertase enzymes, so that it can no longer bind to its target site. The potential destruction of healthy host cells by C3b is limited not only by its rapid spontaneous inactivation but also by a family of related proteins that regulate C3 convertase activity in the classical and alternative pathways. These C3 convertase regulatory proteins all contain repeating amino acid sequences (or motifs) of about 60 residues, termed short consensus repeats (SCRs). All these proteins are encoded at a single location on chromosome 1 in humans, known as the regulators of complement activation (RCA) gene cluster.

TABLE 13-6 PROTEINS THAT REGULATE COMPLEMENT SYSTEM

Protein	Type of protein	Pathway affected	Immunologic function
C1 inhibitor (C1Inh)	Soluble	Classical	Serine protease inhibitor: causes $C1r_2s_2$ to dissociate from C1q
C4b-binding protein (C4bBP)*	Soluble	Classical and lectin	Blocks formation of C3 convertase by binding C4b; cofactor for cleavage of C4b by factor I
Factor H*	Soluble	Alternative	Blocks formation of C3 convertase by binding C3b; cofactor for cleavage of C3b by factor I
Complement-receptor type 1 (CR1)* Membrane-cofactor protein (MCP)*	Membrane bound	Classical, alternative, and lectin	Block formation of C3 convertase by binding C4b or C3b; cofactor for factor I-catalyzed cleavage of C4b or C3b
Decay-accelerating factor (DAF)*	Membrane bound	Classical, alternative, and lectin	Accelerates dissociation of $\overline{C4b2a}$ and $\overline{C3bBb}$ (classical and alternative C3 convertases)
Factor I	Soluble	Classical, alternative, and lectin	Serine protease: cleaves C4b or C3b using C4bBP, CR1, factor H, DAF, or MCP as cofactor
S protein	Soluble	Terminal	Binds soluble C5b67 and prevents its insertion into cell membrane
Homologous restriction factor (HRF) Membrane inhibitor of reactive lysis (MIRL)	Membrane bound	Terminal	Bind to C5b678 on autologous cells, blocking binding of C9
Anaphylatoxin inactivator	Soluble	Effector	Inactivates anaphylatoxin activity of C3a, C4a, and C5a by carboxypeptidase N removal of C-terminal Arg

*An RCA (regulator of complement activation) protein. In humans, all RCA proteins are encoded on chromosome 1 and contain short consensus repeats.

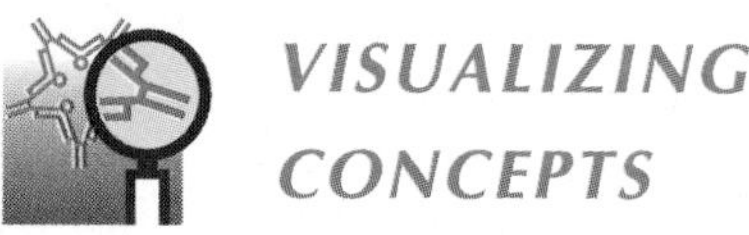

(a)
$C\overline{1r_2s_2}$
$C1q\overline{r_2s_2}$
C1Inh
Antibody

(d)
C2a
C4c
Decay-
accelerating
factor
$C\overline{4b2a}$
C4b
Factor I
C4d

(b)
C2a
C4c
Factor I
C4b
C4bBP
C4d

(e)
Free
C5b67
S protein
Cannot attack
nearby cells
Bound
C5b67

(c)
Factor B
C3f
C3c
Factor I
Factor I
Factor H
C3b
iC3b
C3dg

(f)
Bound
C5b678
C9
HRF
Cannot
polymerize

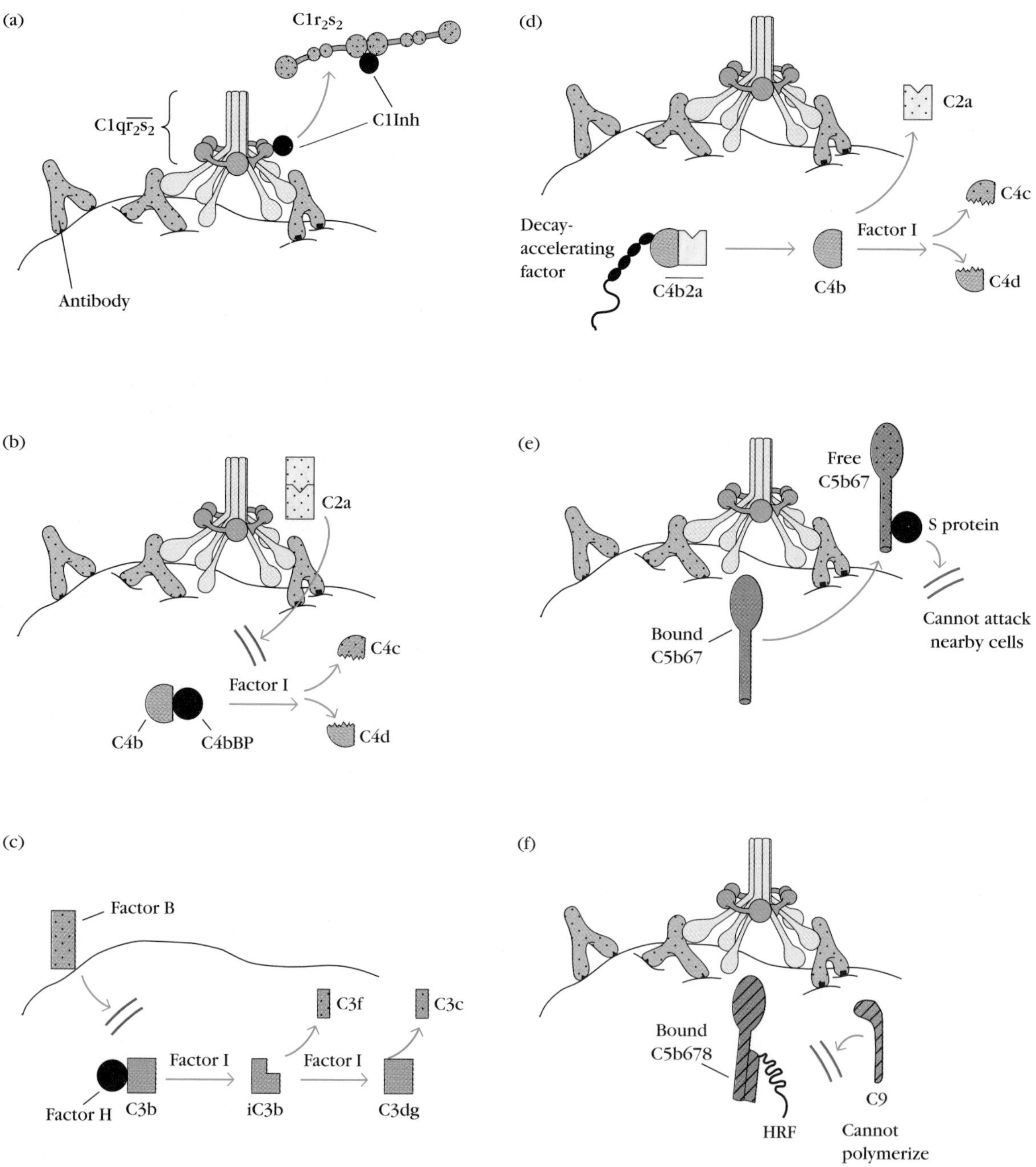

FIGURE 13-9 Schematic diagram of regulation of complement system by regulatory proteins (black), which either cause dissociation of various intermediates or block their formation. Membrane-bound intermediates are shown in solid colors; components that can penetrate the cell membrane are marked with diagonal lines; freely diffusible components are stippled. C1Inh = C1 inhibitor; C4bBP = C4b-binding protein; HRF = homologous restriction factor. See Table 13-6.

In the classical and lectin pathways, three structurally different RCA proteins act similarly to prevent assembly of C3 convertase (Figure 13-9b). These regulatory proteins include soluble C4b-binding protein (C4bBP) and two membrane-bound proteins, complement receptor type 1 (CR1) and membrane cofactor protein (MCP). Each of these regulatory proteins binds to C4b and prevents its association with C2a. Once C4bBP, CR1, or MCP is bound to C4b, another regulatory protein, factor I, cleaves the C4b into bound C4d and soluble C4c (Figure 13-10a). A similar regulatory sequence operates to prevent assembly of the C3 convertase $\overline{C3bBb}$ in the alternative pathway. In this case CR1, MCP, or a regulatory component called factor H binds to C3b and prevents its association with factor B (Figure 13-9c). Once CR1, MCP, or factor H is bound to C3b, factor I cleaves the C3b into a bound iC3b fragment and a soluble C3f fragment. Further cleavage of iC3b by factor I releases C3c and leaves C3dg bound to the membrane (Figure 13-10b).

Several RCA proteins also act on the assembled C3 convertase, causing it to dissociate; these include the previously mentioned C4bBP, CR1, and factor H. In addition, decay-accelerating factor (DAF), which is a glycoprotein anchored covalently to a glycophospholipid membrane protein, has the ability to dissociate C3 convertase. Each of these RCA proteins accelerates decay (dissociation) of C3 convertase, by releasing the component with enzymatic activity (C2a or Bb) from the cell-bound component (C4b or C3b). Once dissociation of the C3 convertase occurs, factor I cleaves the remaining membrane-bound C4b or C3b component to irreversibly inactivate the convertase (Figure 13-9d).

Regulatory proteins also operate at the level of the membrane-attack complex. The ability of the C5b67 complex to be released and then bind to nearby cells poses a threat of innocent-bystander lysis of healthy cells. A number of serum proteins can counter this threat by binding to released C5b67 and preventing its insertion into the membrane of nearby cells. A serum protein called S protein can bind to C5b67, inducing a hydrophilic transition and thereby preventing insertion of C5b67 into the membrane of nearby cells (Figure 13-9e).

Complement-mediated lysis of cells is more effective if the complement is from a species different from that of the cells being lysed. This phenomenon depends on two membrane proteins that block MAC formation. These two proteins, present on the membrane of many cell types, are homologous restriction factor (HRF) and membrane inhibitor

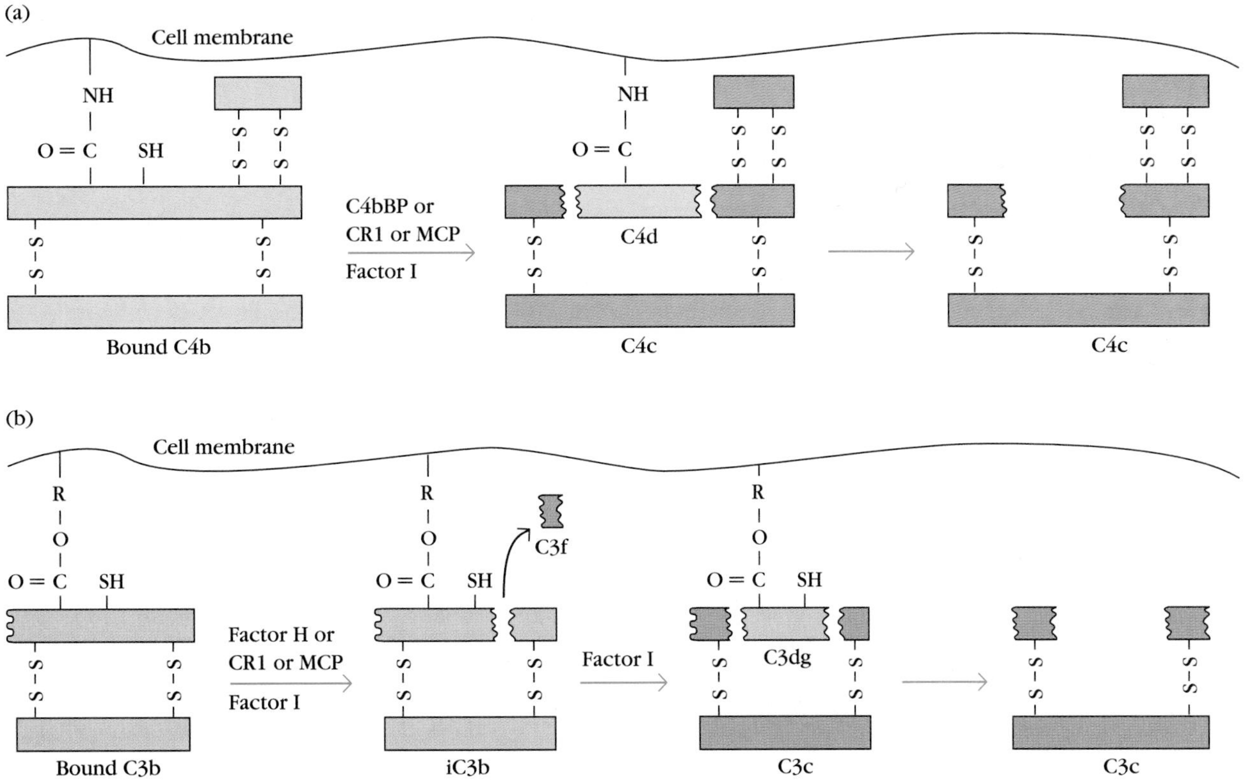

FIGURE 13-10 Inactivation of bound C4b and C3b by regulatory proteins of the complement system. (a) In the classical pathway, C4bBP (C4b-binding protein), CR1 (complement receptor type 1), or MCP (membrane cofactor protein) bind to C4b and act as cofactors for factor I–mediated cleavage of C4b. (b) In the alternative pathway, factor H, CR1, or MCP bind to C3b and act as cofactors for factor I–mediated cleavage of C3b. Free diffusible fragments are shown in dark shades; membrane bound components in light shades.

of reactive lysis (MIRL, now called CD59). Both HRF and CD59 protect cells from nonspecific complement-mediated lysis by binding to C8, preventing assembly of poly-C9 and its insertion into the plasma membrane (Figure 13-9f). However, this inhibition occurs only if the complement components are from the same species as the target cells. For this reason, CD59 and HRF are said to display homologous restriction, for which the latter was named.

Biological Consequences of Complement Activation

Complement serves as an important mediator of the humoral response by amplifying the response and converting it into an effective defense mechanism to destroy invading microorganisms and viruses. The MAC mediates cell lysis, while other complement components or split products participate in the inflammatory response, opsonization of antigen, viral neutralization, and clearance of immune complexes (Table 13-7).

Many of the biological activities of the complement system depend on the binding of complement fragments to complement receptors, which are expressed by various cells. In addition, some complement receptors play an important role in regulating complement activity by binding biologically active complement components and degrading them into inactive products. The complement receptors and their primary ligands, which include various complement components and their proteolytic breakdown products, are listed in Table 13-8.

Cell Lysis

The membrane-attack complex formed by complement activation is capable of lysing a broad spectrum of microorganisms, viruses, erythrocytes, and nucleated cells. Because the alternative and lectin pathways of activation generally occur without an initial antigen-antibody interaction, these pathways serve as important innate systems of nonspecific defense against infectious microorganisms. The requirement for an initial antigen-antibody reaction in the classical pathway supplements these nonspecific innate defenses with a more specific defense mechanism.

The importance of cell-mediated immunity in host defense against viral infections has been emphasized in previous chapters. Nevertheless, antibody and complement do play a role in host defense against viruses and are often crucial in containing viral spread during acute infection and in protecting against reinfection. Most—perhaps all—enveloped viruses are susceptible to complement-mediated lysis. The viral envelope is largely derived from the plasma membrane of the infected host cell and is therefore susceptible to pore

TABLE 13-7 SUMMARY OF BIOLOGICAL EFFECTS MEDIATED BY COMPLEMENT PRODUCTS

Effect	Complement product mediating*
Cell lysis	C5b–9, the membrane-attack complex (MAC)
Inflammatory response	
Degranulation of mast cells and basophils†	C3a, C4a, and C5a (anaphylatoxins)
Degranulation of eosinophils	C3a, C5a
Extravasation and chemotaxis of leukocytes at inflammatory site	C3a, **C5a,** C5b67
Aggregation of platelets	C3a, C5a
Inhibition of monocyte/macrophage migration and induction of their spreading	Bb
Release of neutrophils from bone marrow	C3c
Release of hydrolytic enzymes from neutrophils	C5a
Increased expression of complement receptors type 1 and 3 (CR1 and CR3) on neutrophils	C5a
Opsonization of particulate antigens, increasing their phagocytosis	**C3b,** C4b, iC3b
Viral neutralization	C3b, C5b–9 (MAC)
Solubilization and clearance of immune complexes	C3b

*Boldfaced component is most important in mediating indicated effect.

†Degranulation leads to release of histamine and other mediators that induce contraction of smooth muscle and increased permeability of vessels.

TABLE 13-8 COMPLEMENT-BINDING RECEPTORS

Receptor	Major ligands	Activity	Cellular distribution
CR1 (CD35)	C3b, C4b	Blocks formation of C3 convertase; binds immune complexes to cells	Erthrocytes, neutrophils, monocytes, macrophages, eosinophils, follicular dendritic cells, B cells, some T cells
CR2 (CD21)	C3d, C3dg,* iC3b	Part of B-cell coreceptor; binds Epstein-Barr virus	B cells, some T cells
CR3 (CD11b/18) CR4 (CD11c/18)	iC3b	Bind cell-adhesion molecules on neutrophils, facilitating their extravasation; blind immune complexes, enhancing their phagocytosis	Monocytes, macrophages, neutrophils, natural killer cells, some T cells
C3a/C4a receptor	C3a, C4a	Induces degranulation of mast cells and basophils	Mast cells, basophils, granulocytes
C5a receptor	C5a	Induces degranulation of mast cells and basophils	Mast cells, basophils, granulocytes, monocytes, macrophages, platelets, endothelial cells

*Cleavage of C3dg by serum proteases generates C3d and C3g.

formation by the membrane-attack complex. Among the pathogenic viruses shown to be lysed by complement-mediated lysis are herpesviruses, orthomyxoviruses, paramyxoviruses, and retroviruses.

The complement system is generally quite effective in lysing gram-negative bacteria (Figure 13-11). However, some gram-negative bacteria and most gram-positive bacteria have mechanisms for evading complement-mediated damage (Table 13-9). For example, a few gram-negative bacteria can develop resistance to complement-mediated lysis that correlates with the virulence of the organism. In *Escherichia coli* and *Salmonella,* resistance to complement is associated with the smooth bacterial phenotype, which is characterized by the presence of long polysaccharide side chains in the cell-wall lipopolysaccharide (LPS) component. It has been proposed that the increased LPS in the wall of resistant strains may prevent insertion of the MAC into the bacterial membrane, so that the complex is released from the bacterial cell rather than forming a pore. Strains of *Neisseria gonorrheae* resistant to complement-mediated killing have been associated with disseminated gonococcal infections in humans. Some evidence suggests that the membrane proteins of resistant *Neisseria* strains undergo noncovalent interactions with the MAC that prevent its insertion into the outer membrane of the bacterial cells. These examples of resistant gram-negative bacteria are the exception; most gram-negative bacteria are susceptible to complement-mediated lysis.

In contrast, gram-positive bacteria are generally resistant to complement-mediated lysis because the thick peptidoglycan layer in their cell wall prevents insertion of the MAC into the inner membrane. Although complement activation can occur on the cell membrane of encapsulated bacteria such as *Streptococcus pneumoniae,* the capsule prevents interaction between C3b deposited on the membrane and the CR1 on phagocytic cells. Some bacteria possess an elastase that inactivates C3a and C5a, preventing these split products from inducing an inflammatory response. In addition to these mechanisms of evasion, various bacteria, viruses, fungi, and protozoans contain proteins that can interrupt the complement cascade on their surfaces, thus mimicking the effects of the normal complement regulatory proteins C4bBP, CR1, and DAF.

Nucleated cells tend to be more resistant to complement-mediated lysis than red blood cells are. Lysis of nucleated cells requires formation of multiple membrane attack complexes, whereas a single MAC can lyse a red blood cell. Many nucleated cells, including the majority of cancer cells, can endocytose the MAC. If the complex is removed soon enough, the cell can repair any membrane damage and restore its osmotic stability. This is the reason why complement-mediated lysis by antibody specific for tumor-cell antigens is often not effective. Experimental studies indicate that tumor-specific monoclonal

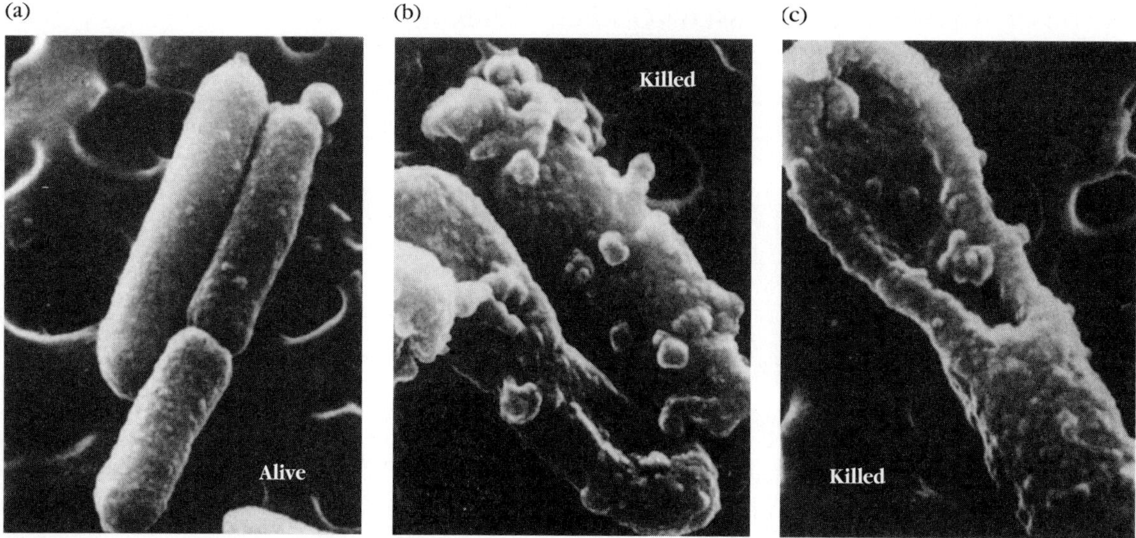

FIGURE 13-11 Scanning electron micrographs of *E. coli* showing (a) intact cells and (b, c) cells killed by complement-mediated lysis. Note membrane blebbing on lysed cells. [From RD Schreiber et al, 1979, *J. Exp. Med.* **149:**870.]

TABLE 13-9 MICROBIAL EVASION OF COMPLEMENT-MEDIATED DAMAGE

Microbial component	Mechanism of evasion	Examples
	Gram-negative bacteria	
Long polysaccharide chains in cell-wall LPS	Side chains prevent insertion of MAC into bacterial membrane	Resistant strains of *E. coli* and *Salmonella*
Outer membrane protein	MAC interacts with membrane protein and fails to insert into bacterial membrane	Resistant strains of *Neisseria gonorrhoeae*
Elastase	Anaphylatoxins C3a and C5a are inactivated by microbial elastase	*Pseudomonas aeruginosa*
	Gram-positive bacteria	
Peptidoglycan layer of cell wall	Insertion of MAC into bacterial membrane is prevented by thick layer of peptidoglycan	*Streptococcus*
Bacterial capsule	Capsule provides physical barrier between C3b deposited on bacterial membrane and CR1 on phagocytic cells	*Streptococcus pneumoniae*
	Other microbes	
Proteins that mimic complement regulatory proteins	Proteins present in various bacteria, viruses, fungi, and protozoans inhibit the complement cascade	Vaccinia virus, herpes simplex, Epstein-Barr virus, *Trypanosoma cruzi, Candida albicans*

KEY: CR1 = type 1 complement receptor; LPS = lipopolysaccharide; MAC = membrane-attack complex (C5b–9).

antibodies must be conjugated with toxins or radioactive isotopes to be effective tumor-killing agents.

Inflammatory Response

The complement cascade is often viewed in terms of the final outcome of cell lysis, but various peptides generated during formation of the MAC play a decisive role in the development of an effective inflammatory response (see Table 13-7). The smaller fragments resulting from complement cleavage, C3a, C4a, and C5a, called **anaphylatoxins,** bind to receptors on mast cells and blood basophils and induce degranulation with release of histamine and other pharmacologically active mediators. The anaphylatoxins induce smooth-muscle contraction and increased vascular permeability. Activation of the complement system thus results in influxes of fluid that carries antibody and phagocytic cells to the site of antigen entry. The activities of these highly reactive anaphylatoxins are regulated by a serum protease called carboxypeptidase N, which cleaves an Arg residue from the C terminus of the molecules, resulting in what are termed the des-Arg forms (see Table 13-6). The des-Arg forms of C3a and C4a are completely inactive while that of C5a retains about 10% of its chemotactic activity and 1% of its ability to cause smooth muscle contraction.

Each of C3a, C5a, and C5b67 can induce monocytes and neutrophils to adhere to vascular endothelial cells, extravasate through the endothelial lining of the capillary, and migrate toward the site of complement activation in the tissues. C5a is most potent in mediating these processes, with picomolar quantities being effective. The role of complement in leukocyte chemotaxis is discussed more fully in Chapter 15.

Opsonization of Antigen

C3b is the major **opsonin** of the complement system, although C4b and iC3b also have opsonizing activity. The amplification that occurs with C3 activation results in a coating of C3b on immune complexes and particulate antigens. Phagocytic cells, as well as some other cells, express complement receptors (CR1, CR3, and CR4) that bind C3b, C4b, or iC3b (see Table 13-8). When antigen has been coated with C3b during complement activation, the coated antigen binds to cells bearing CR1. If the cell is a phagocyte (e.g., a neutrophil, monocyte, or macrophage), phagocytosis will be enhanced (Figure 13-12). Activation of phagocytic cells by various agents, including C5a anaphylatoxin, has been shown to increase the number of CR1s from 5000 on resting phagocytes to 50,000 on activated cells, greatly facilitating their phagocytosis of C3b-coated antigen.

Viral Neutralization

The complement system plays an important role in host defense by neutralizing viral infectivity. Some viruses (e.g., retroviruses, Epstein-Barr virus, Newcastle disease virus, and rubella virus) can activate the alternative, lectin, or even the classical pathway in the absence of antibody. For most viruses, the binding of serum antibody to the repeating subunits of the viral structural proteins creates particulate immune complexes ideally suited for complement activation by the classical pathway.

The complement system mediates viral neutralization by a number of mechanisms. Some degree of neutralization is

(a)

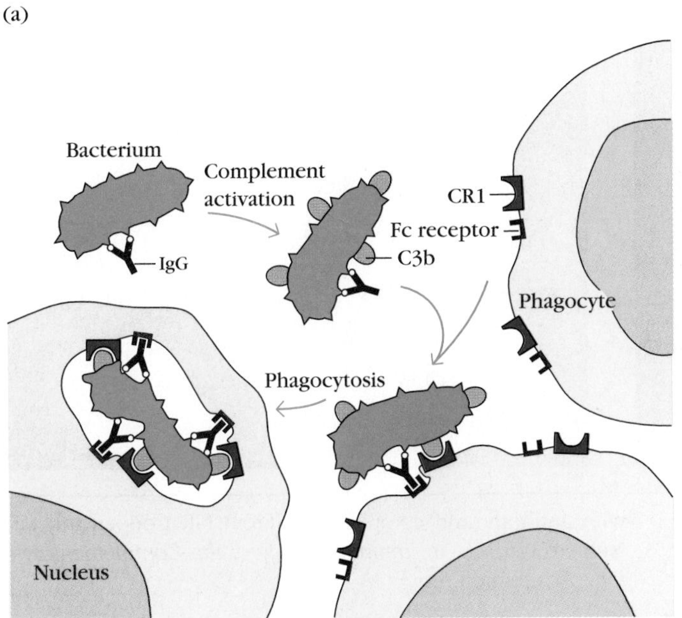

(b)

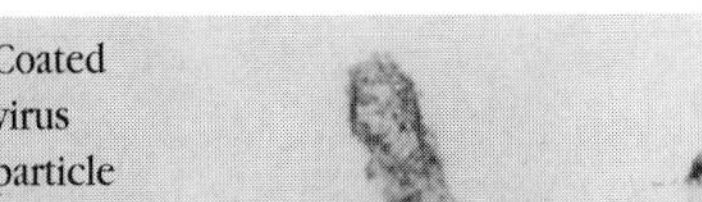

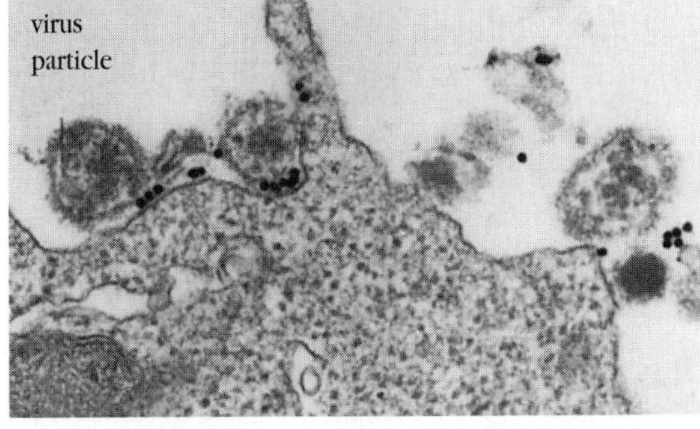

FIGURE 13-12 (a) Schematic representation of the role of C3b and antibody in opsonization. (b) Electron micrograph of Epstein-Barr virus coated with antibody and C3b and bound to the Fc and C3b receptor (CR1) on a B lymphocyte. [From NR Cooper and GR Nemerow, 1986, in *Immunobiology of the Complement System*, Academic Press.]

achieved through the formation of larger viral aggregates, simply because these aggregates reduce the net number of infectious viral particles. Although antibody does play a role in the formation of viral aggregates, in vitro studies show that the C3b component facilitates aggregate formation in the presence of as little as two molecules of antibody per virion. For example, polyoma virus coated with antibody is neutralized when serum containing activated C3 is added.

The binding of antibody and/or complement to the surface of a viral particle creates a thick protein coating that can be visualized by electron microscopy (Figure 13-13). This coating neutralizes viral infectivity by blocking attachment to susceptible host cells. The deposits of antibody and complement on viral particles also facilitate binding of the viral particle to cells possessing Fc or type 1 complement receptors (CR1). In the case of phagocytic cells, such binding can be followed by phagocytosis and intracellular destruction of the ingested viral particle. Finally, complement is effective in lysing most, if not all, enveloped viruses, resulting in fragmentation of the envelope and disintegration of the nucleocapsid.

Solubilization of Immune Complexes

The role of the complement system in clearing immune complexes can be seen in patients with the autoimmune disease systemic lupus erythematosus (SLE). These individuals produce large quantities of immune complexes and suffer tissue damage as a result of complement-mediated lysis and the induction of type II or type III hypersensitivity (see Chapter 16). Although complement plays a significant role in the development of tissue damage in SLE, the paradoxical finding is that deficiencies in C1, C2, C4, and CR1 predispose an individual to SLE; indeed, 90% of individuals who completely lack C4 develop SLE. The complement deficiencies are thought to interfere with effective solubilization and clearance of immune complexes; the result is the persistence of these complexes and subsequent tissue damage by the very system whose deficiency was to blame.

The coating of soluble immune complexes with C3b is thought to facilitate their binding to CR1 on erythrocytes. Although red blood cells express lower levels of CR1 ($\sim 5 \times 10^2$ per cell) than granulocytes do ($\sim 5 \times 10^4$ per cell), there are about 10^3 red blood cells for every white blood cell; therefore, erythrocytes account for about 90% of the CR1 in the blood. For this reason, erythrocytes play an important role in binding C3b-coated immune complexes and carrying these complexes to the liver and spleen. In these organs, immune complexes are stripped from the red blood cells and are phagocytosed, thereby preventing their deposition in tissues (Figure 13-14). In SLE patients, deficiencies in C1, C2, and C4 each contribute to reduced levels of C3b on immune complexes and hence inhibit their clearance. The lower levels of CR1 expressed on the erythrocytes of SLE patients also may interfere with the proper binding and clearance of immune complexes.

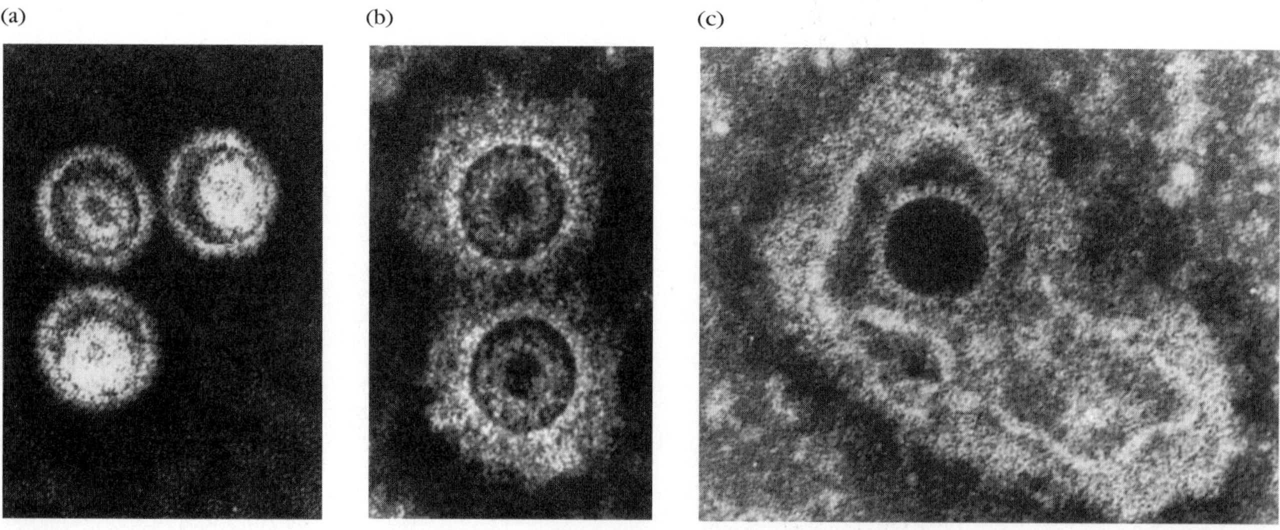

FIGURE 13-13 Electron micrographs of negatively stained preparations of Epstein-Barr virus. (a) Control without antibody. (b) Antibody-coated particles. (c) Particles coated with antibody and complement. [From NR Cooper and GR Nemerow, 1986, in *Immunobiology of the Complement System*, Academic Press.]

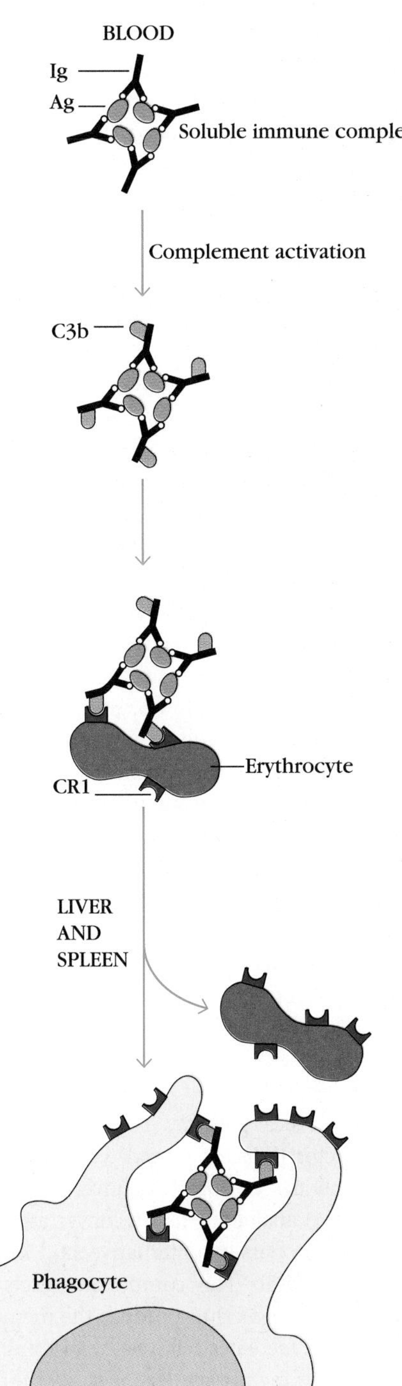

FIGURE 13-14 Clearance of circulating immune complexes by reaction with receptors for complement products on erythrocytes and removal of these complexes by receptors on macrophages in the liver and spleen. Because the erythrocytes have fewer receptors than the macrophages do, the latter can strip the complexes from the erythrocytes as they pass through the liver or spleen. Deficiency in this process can lead to renal damage due to accumulation of immune complexes.

Complement Deficiencies

Clinical Observations

Genetic deficiencies have been described for each of the complement components. Homozygous deficiencies in any of the early components of the classical pathway (C1q, C1r, C1s, C4, and C2) exhibit similar symptoms, notably a marked increase in immune-complex diseases such as systemic lupus erythematosus, glomerulonephritis, and vasculitis. These deficiencies highlight the important role of the early complement reactions in generating C3b and the critical importance of C3b for solubilization and clearance of immune complexes. In addition to immune-complex diseases, individuals with such complement deficiencies may suffer from recurrent infections by pyogenic bacteria such as streptococci and staphylococci. These organisms are gram-positive and therefore resistant in any case to the lytic effects of the MAC. Nonetheless, the early complement components ordinarily prevent recurrent infection by mediating a localized inflammatory response and opsonizing the bacteria. Deficiencies in factor D and properdin—early components of the alternative pathway—appear to be associated with *Neisseria* infections but with immune-complex disease.

Patients with C3 deficiencies have the most severe clinical manifestations, reflecting the central role of C3 in activation of C5 and formation of the MAC. The first patient identified with a C3 deficiency was a child who suffered from frequent severe bacterial infections and was erroneously thought to have agammaglobulinemia. When tests revealed normal immunoglobulin levels, a deficiency in C3 was discovered. This case highlights the critical function of the complement system in converting a humoral antibody response into an effective defense mechanism. The majority of patients with C3 deficiency have recurrent bacterial infections and may have immune-complex diseases.

Individuals with homozygous deficiencies in the components involved in the MAC develop recurrent meningococcal and gonococcal infections caused by *Neisseria* species. In normal individuals, these gram-negative bacteria are generally susceptible to complement-mediated lysis or are cleared by the opsonizing activity of C3b. MAC-deficient individuals rarely have immune-complex disease, which suggests that they produce enough C3b to clear immune complexes. Interestingly, a deficiency in C9 results in no clinical symptoms, suggesting that in some cases the entire MAC is not necessary for complement-mediated lysis.

Congenital deficiencies of complement regulatory proteins have also been reported. The C1 inhibitor (C1Inh) regulates activation of the classical pathway by preventing excessive C4 and C2 activation by C1. Deficiency of C1Inh is an autosomal dominant condition with a frequency of 1 in 1000. The deficiency gives rise to a disease called hereditary angioedema, which manifests clinically as localized edema of the tissue, often following trauma, but sometimes with no known cause. The edema can be in subcutaneous tissues or within the bowel or upper respiratory tract, where it causes abdominal pain or obstruction of the airway.

A number of the membrane-bound regulatory components, including decay-accelerating factor (DAF) and homologous restriction factor (HRF) are anchored to the plasma membrane by glycosyl phosphatidylinositol membrane anchors. In individuals with paroxysmal nocturnal hemoglobinuria the glycosyl phosphatidylinositol membrane anchor is defective, resulting in an absence of DAF and HRF on the cell membrane. As a consequence of this defect, red blood cells can be lysed by levels of complement that are much lower than normally required. The lack of these inhibitors gives rise to increased lysis of host red blood cells, causing chronic hemolytic anemia. The hemoglobin released by the broken red blood cells appears in the patient's urine (hemoglobinuria).

Experimental Studies

Clinical case studies in individuals with homozygous deficiencies in complement components have provided the major source of information concerning the role of individual complement components in immunity. Use of experimental animals that are deficient in complement either by virtue of genetic background or because of depletion with a chemical or biologic agent have supplemented this information and allow tests of immune function by inoculating the deficient animals with pathogens. Use of mice genetically engineered to lack expression of specific complement components by knockout of the corresponding genes provides a means to study the deficiencies in a controlled manner that is not always possible in human patients or more traditional animal models in which only partial depletion of a given component is sometimes possible. Investigations of in vivo complement activity in genetically engineered knockout mice are in their infancy but promise to allow dissection of the complex system of complement proteins in a manner that will allow the assignment of precise biologic roles to each.

The type of information that may result from use of knockout mice is exemplified by studies of factor B in this system. No well-documented reports of homozygous deficiency in human factor B exist, and this deficiency was presumed to be a lethal trait because of extraordinary susceptibility to infection. However, studies of mice with a disrupted factor B gene showed no gross differences from normal littermates, although the alternative pathway was not functional in these animals. However, mice deficient in factor B were at a reproductive disadvantage compared to heterozygous littermates, providing a possible explanation for the scarcity of this trait in human populations. As with humans, mice with disrupted C3 and C4 genes survive and can mount normal immune responses to most pathogens. By contrast, loss of complement receptors 1 and 2 in mice causes serious impairment of immune function.

Summary

1. The complement system, which plays a central role in immune function (see Figure 13-1), comprises a group of serum proteins, many of which exist in inactive and active forms. Complement activation involves an enzymatic cascade that generates various complement proteins, which play an important role in antigen clearance. The three pathways of complement activation, the classical pathway, the alternative pathway, and the lectin pathway, involve different complement proteins and are initiated differently (see Figure 13-2). All pathways converge in a common terminal reaction sequence that generates a membrane-attack complex (MAC) responsible for cell lysis.
2. The classical pathway, which involves in order the C1, C4, C2, and C3 components, is initiated by binding of IgM and certain subclasses of IgG to soluble antigen or cell-surface antigens. The reaction sequence generates the enzymatically active C$\overline{4a2b}$ complex (C3 convertase), which can split C3 into C3a and C3b, and the C$\overline{4a2b}$3b complex (C5 convertase), which can split C5 into C5a and C5b. The alternative and lectin pathways are most commonly initiated by surface constituents of a variety of microorganisms (bacteria, fungi, some viruses, and some parasites); however, the alternative pathway also can be initiated by IgG-, IgA-, and IgE-antigen complexes (see Table 13-3). The lectin pathway is initiated by binding of a serum protein, MBL (mannose binding lectin), to carbohydrate residues on microbial cell surfaces and its reaction with MASP (MBL-associated serine protease). MBL and MASP have structural similarities to the C1 components and form a complex with activity analogous to the active C1qr_2s_2. After initiation, the lectin pathway proceeds through C4 and C2 in a manner identical with the classical pathway. The alternative pathway involves C3, factor B, factor D, and properdin. The reaction sequence generates C$\overline{3bBb}$ (C3 convertase) and C$\overline{3bBb}$3b (C5 convertase) analogous to the convertases in the classical pathway. The classical, alternative, and lectin pathways generate bound C5b. This component reacts sequentially with C6, C7, C8, and C9 to produce the membrane-attack complex, which mediates cell lysis by forming a large pore in the target cell membrane (see Figures 13–5 and 13–7).
3. Because of its nonspecific nature, the complement system requires elaborate regulatory mechanisms to prevent damage to normal tissues. A number of passive and active regulatory mechanisms have evolved. Passive control is exerted by the extreme lability of many of the active components, which lose activity quickly unless they react with a subsequent component. Active control is exerted by a number of regulatory components that function to inactivate complement products and prevent excessive buildup of enzymatically active components (see Figure 13-9 and Table 13-6).
4. The complement system serves as an important effector of the humoral immune response with various components mediating specific effects (see Figure 13-1 and Table 13-7).

It destroys foreign cells through the process of MAC-mediated lysis and acts to neutralize viral infectivity by several mechanisms. The complement system also induces a localized inflammatory response with a buildup of fluid and inflammatory cells, and it facilitates phagocytosis of antigen through its effect as an opsonin (see Figure 13-12). Complement also plays an essential function in clearance of circulating immune complexes (see Figure 13-14).

5. Inherited deficiencies of most of the complement components have been described. The consequences of these conditions depend on which complement component is deficient. Deficiencies in the components of the classical pathway, of which C3 deficiencies are clinically the most severe, are often associated with immune-complex disease and susceptibility to recurrent bacterial infections. The severity of C3 deficiency reflects the central role of C3 in the classical, alternative, and lectin pathways of complement activation. Deficiency of the regulatory protein C1 inhibitor (C1Inh) is fairly common and is associated with a localized edema called hereditary angioedema.

REFERENCES

Adinolfi, M. 1997. Ontogeny of human natural and acquired immunity. *Curr. Top. Microbiol. Immunol.* **222:**67.

Ahearn, JM, and DT Fearon. 1989. Structure and function of the complement receptors CR1 (CD35) and CR2 (CD21). *Adv. Immunol.* **46:**183.

Brekke, OH, TE Michaelsen, and I Sandlie. 1995. The structural requirements for complement activation by IgG: does it hinge on the hinge? *Immunol. Today* **16:**85.

Carroll MC. 1998. The role of complement and complement receptors in induction and regulation of immunity. *Ann. Rev. Immunol.* **16:**545.

Davies, A. 1996. Policing the membrane: cell surface proteins which regulate complement. *Res. Immunol.* **147:**82.

Frank, MM. 1995. Animal models for complement deficiencies. *J. Clin. Immunol.* **6 (Suppl):**113S–121S

Frank, MM, and LF Fries. 1991. The role of complement in inflammation and phagocytosis. *Immunol. Today* **12:**322.

Hostetter, MK. 1993. The third component of complement: new functions for an old friend. *J. Lab. Clin. Med.* **122:**491.

Johnston, RB, Jr. 1993. The complement system in host defense and inflammation: the cutting edges of a double-edged sword. *Pediatr. Infect. Dis. J.* **12:**933.

Kinoshita, T. 1991. Biology of complement: the overture. *Immunol. Today* **12:**291.

Kolble, K, and KB Reid. 1993. Genetic deficiencies of the complement system and association with disease—early components. *Int. Rev. Immunol.* **10:**17.

Law, SK, and AW Dodds. 1997. The internal thioester and the covalent binding properties of the complement proteins C3 and C4. *Protein Sci.* **2:**263.

Liszewski, MK, et al. 1996. Control of the complement system. *Adv. Immunol.* **61:**201.

Lokki, ML, and HR Colten. 1995. Genetic deficiencies of complement. *Ann. Med.* **27:**451.

Matsushita, M. 1996. The lectin pathway of the complement system. *Microbiol. Immunol.* **12:**887.

Matsumoto, M, et al. 1997. Abrogation of the the alternative complement pathway by targeted deletion of murine factor B. *Proc. Natl. Acad. Sci. USA* **94:**8720.

Molina, H, and VM Holers. 1996. Markedly impaired humoral immune response in mice deficient in complement receptors 1 and 2. *Proc. Natl. Acad. Sci. USA* **93:**3357.

Morgan, BP, and P Gasque. 1997. Extrahepatic complement biosynthesis: where, when and why? *Clin. Exp. Immunol.* **107:**1.

Morgan, BP, and MJ Walport. 1991. Complement deficiency and disease. *Immunol. Today* **12:**301.

Muller-Eberhard, HJ. 1988. Molecular organization and function of the complement system. *Annu. Rev. Biochem.* **57:**321.

Pascual, M, and LE French. 1995. Complement in human disease: looking toward the 21st century. *Immunol. Today* **16:**58.

Stoiber, H, MD Dierich, and A Clivio. 1997. Role of complement in HIV infection. *Ann. Rev. Immunol.* **15:**649.

Sultan, AA, et al. 1997. Sporozoites of *Plasmodium yoelii* infect mice with targeted deletions in ICAM-1 and ICAM-2 or complement components C3 and C4. *Mol. Biochem. Parasitol.* **88:**263.

Sylvestre, D, et al. 1996. Immunoglobulin G-mediated inflammatory responses develop normally in complement deficient mice. *J. Exp. Med.* **184:**2385.

Turner, MW. 1996. The lectin pathway of complement activation. *Res. Immunol.* **147:**110.

Walport, MJ, et al. 1997. Complement deficiency and autoimmunity. *Ann. NY Acad. Sci.* **815:**267.

Wilson JG, et al. 1987. Deficiency of the C3b/C4b receptor (CR1) of erythrocytes in systemic lupus erythematosus. *J. Immunol.* **138:**2706.

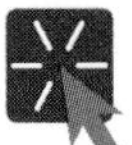

Useful Web Sites

http://www.cehs.siu.edu/fix/medmicro/cfix.htm
A clever graphic representation of the basic assay for complement activity using red blood cell lysis, from D Fix at University of Southern Illinois, Carbondale.

http://athena.bioc.uvic.ca/AJC/Tutorials/Complement/Comp1b.html
Tutorial describing complement pathways with multiple choice questions and graphic illustrations; from the University of Victoria, Canada.

http://www.gla.ac.uk/Acad/Immunology/compsyst.htm.
Notes from DF Lappin at University of Glasgow, UK, on complement system. The site includes a listing of all complement proteins and their properties.

STUDY QUESTIONS

1. Indicate whether each of the following statements is true or false. If you think a statement is false, explain why.

Go to www.whfreeman.com/immunology 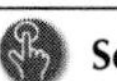 **Self-Test**
Review and quiz of key terms

a. A single molecule of bound IgM can activate the C1q component of the classical complement pathway.

b. C3a and C3b are fragments of C3.

c. The C4 and C2 complement components are present in the serum in a functionally inactive proenzyme form.

d. Nucleated cells tend to be more resistant to complement-mediated lysis than red blood cells.

e. Enveloped viruses cannot be lysed by complement because their outer envelope is resistant to pore formation by the membrane-attack complex.

f. C4-deficient individuals have difficulty eliminating immune complexes.

2. Explain why serum IgM cannot activate complement by itself.

3. Would you expect a C1 or C3 complement deficiency to be more serious clinically? Why?

4. Some microorganisms produce enzymes that can degrade the Fc portion of antibody molecules. Why would such enzymes be advantageous for the survival of microorganisms that possess them?

5. Complement activation can occur via the classical, alternative, or lectin pathway.

a. How do the three pathways differ in the substances that can initiate activation?

b. Which portion of the overall activation sequence differs in the three pathways? Which portion is similar?

c. How do the biological consequences of complement activation via these pathways differ?

6. Enucleated cells, such as red blood cells, are more susceptible to complement-mediated lysis than nucleated cells.

a. Explain why the red blood cells of an individual are not normally destroyed as the result of innocent-bystander lysis by complement.

b. Under what conditions might complement cause lysis of an individual's own red blood cells?

7. Briefly explain the mechanism of action of the following complement regulatory proteins. Indicate which pathway(s) each protein regulates.

a. C1 inhibitor (C1Inh)

b. C4b-binding protein (C4bBP)

c. Homologous restriction factor (HRF)

d. Decay-accelerating factor (DAF)

e. Factor H

f. Membrane cofactor protein (MCP)

8. For each complement component(s) or reaction (a–l), select the most appropriate description listed below (1–13). Each description may be used once, more than once, or not at all.

Complement Component(s)/Reactions

a. C3b
b. C1, C4, C2, and C3
c. C9
d. C3, factor B, and factor D
e. C1q
f. $\overline{C4b2a3b}$
g. C5b, C6, C7, C8, and C9
h. C3 → C3a + C3b
i. C3a, C5a, and C5b67
j. C3a, C4a, and C5a
k. $\overline{C4b2a}$
l. C3b + B → $\overline{C3bBb}$ + Ba

Descriptions

(1) Reaction that produces major amplification during activation
(2) Are early components of alternative pathway
(3) Compose the membrane-attack complex
(4) Mediates opsonization
(5) Are early components of classical pathway
(6) Has perforin-like activity
(7) Binds to Fc region of antibodies
(8) Have chemotactic activity
(9) Has C3 convertase activity
(10) Induce degranulation of mast cells (are anaphylatoxins)
(11) Has C5 convertase activity
(12) Reaction catalyzed by factor D
(13) Reaction catalyzed by $C1qr_2s_2$

9. You have prepared knockout mice with mutations in the genes that encode various complement components. Each knockout strain cannot express one of the complement components listed across the top of the table below. Predict the effect of each mutation on the steps in complement activation and on the complement effector functions indicated in the table below using the following symbols: NE = no effect; D = process/function decreased but not abolished; A = process/function abolished.

	Component knocked out						
	C1q	C4	C3	C5	C6	C9	Factor B
Complement activation							
Formation of C3 convertase in classical pathway							
Formation of C3 convertase in alternative pathway							
Formation of C5 convertase in classical pathway							
Formation of C5 convertase in alternative pathway							
Effector functions							
C3b-mediated opsonization							
Neutrophil chemotaxis							
Cell lysis							

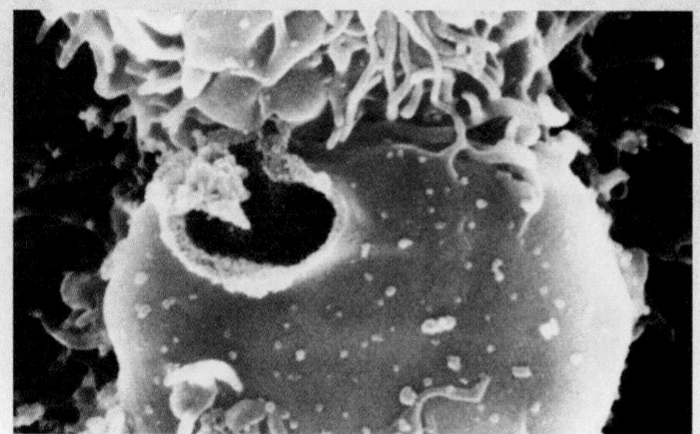

CHAPTER 14
CELL-MEDIATED EFFECTOR RESPONSES

The cell-mediated and humoral branches of the immune system assume different roles in protecting the host. The effectors of the humoral branch are secreted antibodies, highly specific molecules that can bind and neutralize antigens on the surface of cells and in the extracellular spaces. The primary domain of antibody protection lies outside the cell. If antibodies were the only agents of immunity, pathogens that managed to evade them and colonize the intracellular environment would escape the immune system. This is not the case. The principal role of cell-mediated immunity is to detect and eliminate cells that harbor intracellular pathogens. Cell-mediated immunity also can recognize and eliminate cells, such as tumor cells, that have undergone genetic modifications so that they express antigens not typical of normal cells.

Both antigen-specific and nonspecific cells can contribute to the cell-mediated immune response. Specific cells include cytokine-secreting $CD4^+$ T_H cells and $CD8^+$ cytotoxic T lymphocytes (T_C or CTL); nonspecific cells include NK cells and nonlymphoid cell types such as macrophages, neutrophils, and eosinophils. The activity of both specific and nonspecific components depends usually on effective local concentrations of various cytokines. T cells, NK cells, and macrophages are the most important sources of the cytokines that organize and support cell-mediated immunity. Finally, although humoral and cell-mediated immunity have many distinctive features, they are not completely independent. Cells such as macrophages, NK cells, neutrophils, and eosinophils can use antibodies as receptors to recognize and target cells for killing. Also, chemotactic peptides generated by the activation of complement by antigen-antibody complexes can contribute to assembling the cell types required for a cell-mediated response.

In the preceding chapters, various aspects of the humoral and cell-mediated effector responses have been described. This chapter addresses cytotoxic effector mechanisms mediated by T_C cells, NK cells, antibody-dependent cell-mediated cytotoxicity (ADCC); the experimental assay of cytotoxicity; and the delayed-type hypersensitivity (DTH) response mediated by effector T_H cells.

Effector Responses

The importance of cell-mediated immunity becomes evident when the system is defective. Children with DiGeorge syndrome, who are born without a thymus and therefore lack the T-cell component of the cell-mediated immune system, generally are able to cope with infections of extracellular bacteria, but they cannot effectively eliminate intracellular pathogens. Their lack of functional cell-mediated immunity results in repeated infections with viruses, intracellular bacteria, and fungi. The severity of the cell-mediated immunodeficiency in these children is such that even the attenuated virus present in a vaccine, capable of only limited growth in normal individuals, can produce life-threatening infections.

Cell-mediated immune responses can be divided into two major categories according to different effector populations. One group contains effector cells that have direct cytotoxic activity. These effectors eliminate foreign cells and altered self-cells by mounting a cytotoxic reaction that lyses their target. The various cytotoxic effector cells can be grouped into two general categories: antigen-specific cytotoxic T lymphocytes (CTLs) and nonspecific cells, such as natural killer (NK) cells and macrophages. The target cells to which these effectors are directed include allogeneic cells, malignant cells, virus-infected cells, and chemically conjugated cells. The other group is a subpopulation of effector $CD4^+$ T cells that mediates delayed-type hypersensitivity reactions. The next section reviews the general properties of effector T cells and their differences from naive T cells.

General Properties of Effector T Cells

The three types of effector T cells—$CD4^+$ T_H1 and T_H2 cells and $CD8^+$ CTLs—exhibit several properties that set them apart from naive helper and cytotoxic T cells (Table 14-1). In particular, effector cells are characterized by their less stringent activation requirements, increased expression of cell-adhesion molecules, and production of both membrane-bound and soluble effector molecules.

Activation Requirements

T cells at different stages of differentiation may respond with different efficiencies to signals mediated by the T-cell receptor and may consequently require different levels of a second set of co-stimulatory signals. As described in Chapter 10, activation of naive T cells and their subsequent proliferation and differentiation into effector T cells require both a primary signal, delivered when the TCR complex and CD4 or CD8 coreceptor interact with a foreign peptide–MHC molecule complex, and a co-stimulatory signal, delivered by interaction between particular membrane molecules on the T cell and the antigen-presenting cell. In contrast, antigen-experienced effector cells (as well as memory cells) are able to respond to TCR-mediated signals with little, if any co-stimulation.

The reason for the different activation requirements of naive and activated T cells is an area of continuing research. However, some clues to these differences have been found. One is that many populations of naive and effector T cells express different isoforms of CD45, designated CD45RA and CD45RO, which are produced by alternative splicing of the RNA transcript of the CD45 gene. This membrane molecule has phosphatase activity and mediates TCR signal transduction by catalyzing dephosphorylation of a tyrosine residue on the protein tyrosine kinases Lck and Fyn; this change activates these kinases and triggers the subsequent steps in T-cell activation (see Figures 10-11 and 10-12). The CD45RO isoform, which is expressed on effector T cells, associates with the TCR complex and its coreceptors CD4 and CD8 much better than does the CD45RA isoform, which is expressed by naive T cells. Memory T cells have both isoforms, but the CD45RO is predominant. As a result, effector and memory T cells are more sensitive to TCR-mediated activation by a peptide-MHC complex. They also have less stringent requirements for the co-stimulatory signals and therefore are able to respond to peptide-MHC complexes displayed on target cells or antigen-presenting cells that lack the co-stimulatory B7 molecules.

Cell-Adhesion Molecules

Compared with naive T cells, effector T cells also express higher densities of several cell-adhesion molecules, including CD2 and the integrin LFA-1, which bind, respectively, to LFA-3 and ICAMs on antigen-presenting cells and various target cells (see Figure 9-13). The level of LFA-1 and CD2 is twofold to fourfold higher on effector T cells than on naive T cells, enabling the effector T cells to bind more effectively to antigen-presenting cells and to various target cells that express low levels of ICAMs or LFA-3.

As Chapter 9 showed, the initial interaction of an effector T cell with an antigen-presenting cell or target cell is weak, allowing the TCR to scan the membrane for specific peptides presented by self-MHC molecules. If no peptide-MHC complex is recognized by the effector cell, then it will disengage from the APC or target cell. Recognition of a peptide-MHC complex by the TCR, however, produces a signal that increases the affinity of LFA-1 for ICAMs on the APC or target-cell membrane, prolonging the interaction between the cells. For example, T_H1 effector cells remain bound to macrophages that

TABLE 14-1 COMPARISON OF NAIVE AND EFFECTOR T CELLS

Property	Naive T cells	Effector T cells
Co-stimulatory signal (CD28-B7 interaction)	Required for activation	Not required for activation
CD45 isoform	CD45RA	CD45RO
Cell-adhesion molecules (CD2 and LFA-1)	Low	High
Trafficking patterns	HEVs* in secondary lymphoid tissue	Tertiary lymphoid tissues; inflammatory sites

*HEV = high endothelial venules, sites in blood vessel used by lymphocytes for extravasation.

display peptide–class II MHC complexes; T_H2 effector cells remain bound to B cells that display peptide–class II MHC complexes; and CTL effector cells bind tightly to virus-infected target cells that display peptide–class I MHC complexes.

As Chapter 15 will show, effector T cells and naive T cells circulate to different lymphoid tissues. While naive T cells are limited to secondary lymphoid tissues, effector T cells can enter tertiary lymphoid tissue (such as skin and mucosal epithelia) and sites of inflammation, as well as secondary lymphoid tissue.

Effector Molecules

Unlike naive T cells, effector T cells express certain effector molecules, which may be membrane bound or soluble (Table 14-2). The membrane-bound molecules belong to the tumor necrosis factor (TNF) family of membrane proteins and include the Fas ligand (FAS) on $CD8^+$ CTLs, TNF-β on T_H1 cells, and the CD40 ligand on T_H2 cells. Each of the effector T-cell populations also secretes distinct panels of soluble effector molecules. CTLs secrete cytotoxins (perforins and granzymes) as well as two cytokines, IFN-γ and TNF-β. As described in Chapter 12, the T_H1 and T_H2 subsets secrete largely nonoverlapping sets of cytokines.

Each of these membrane-bound and secreted molecules plays an important role in various T-cell effector functions. The Fas ligand, perforins, and granzymes, for example, mediate target-cell destruction by the CTL; membrane-bound TNF-β and soluble IFN-γ and GM-CSF promote macrophage activation by the T_H1 cell; and the membrane-bound CD40 ligand and soluble IL-4, IL-5, and IL-6 all play a role in B-cell activation by the T_H2 cell.

Cytotoxic T Cells

Cytotoxic T lymphocytes, or CTLs, are generated by immune activation of T cytotoxic (T_C) cells. These effector cells have lytic capability and are critical in the recognition and elimination of altered self-cells (e.g., virus-infected cells and tumor cells) and in graft-rejection reactions. In general, CTLs are $CD8^+$ and are therefore class I MHC restricted, although in rare instances $CD4^+$ class II–restricted T cells have been shown to function as CTLs. Since virtually all nucleated cells in the body express class I MHC molecules, CTLs can recognize and eliminate almost any altered body cell.

The CTL-mediated immune response can be divided into two phases, reflecting different aspects of the response. The first phase activates and differentiates naive T_C cells into functional effector CTLs. In the second phase, effector CTLs recognize antigen–class I MHC complexes on specific target cells, which leads them to destroy the target cells.

Generation of CTLs

Naive T_C cells are incapable of killing target cells and are therefore referred to as CTL precursors (CTL-Ps) to denote their functionally immature state. Only after a CTL-P has been activated will the cell differentiate into a functional CTL with cytotoxic activity. Generation of CTLs from CTL-Ps appears to require at least three sequential signals (Figure 14-1):

- An antigen-specific signal 1 transmitted by the TCR complex upon recognition of a peptide–class I MHC molecule complex
- A co-stimulatory signal transmitted by the CD28-B7 interaction of the CTL-P and the antigen-presenting cell
- A signal induced by the interaction of IL-2 with the high-affinity IL-2 receptor, resulting in proliferation and differentiation of the antigen-activated CTL-P into an effector CTL

Unactivated CTL-Ps do not express IL-2 or IL-2 receptors, do not proliferate, and do not display cytotoxic activity. Antigen activation induces a CTL-P to begin expressing the IL-2 receptor and to a lesser extent IL-2, the principal cytokine required for proliferation and differentiation of activated CTL-Ps into effector CTLs. In some cases, the amount of IL-2 secreted by an antigen-activated CTL-P may be sufficient to induce its own proliferation and differentiation; this is particularly true of memory CTL-Ps, which have lower activation requirements than naive cells do (Figure 14-2a). In general, though, most activated CTL-Ps require additional IL-2 produced by proliferating T_H1 cells to proliferate and differentiate into effector CTLs. The fact that the IL-2 receptor is not expressed until after a CTL-P has been activated by antigen plus a class I MHC molecule favors the clonal expansion and acquisition of cytotoxicity by only the antigen-specific CTL-Ps.

TABLE 14-2 EFFECTOR MOLECULES PRODUCED BY EFFECTOR T CELLS

Cell type	Soluble effectors	Membrane-bound effectors
CTL	Cytotoxins (perforins and granzymes), IFN-γ, TNF-β,	Fas ligand (FAS)
T_H1	IL-2, IL-3, TNF-β, IFN-γ, GM-CSF (high)	Tumor necrosis factor β (TNF-β)
T_H2	IL-3, IL-4, IL-5, IL-6, IL-10, IL-13, GM-CSF (low)	CD40 ligand

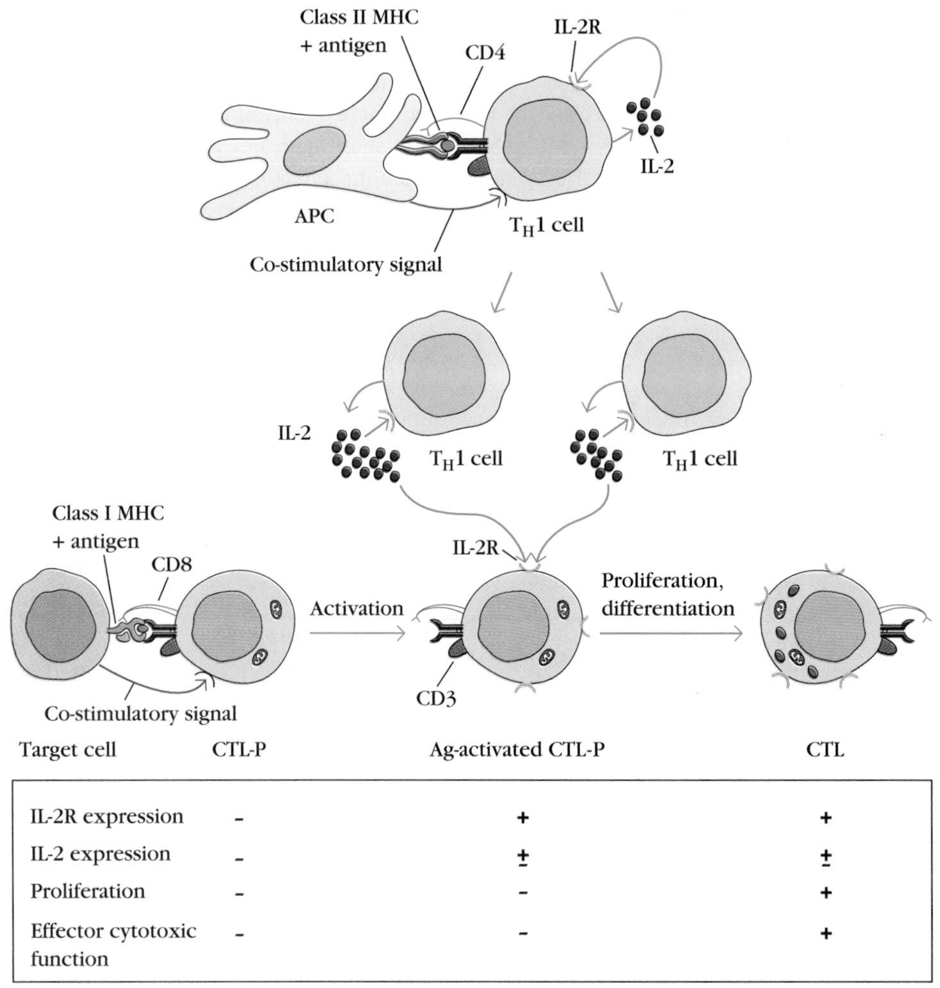

	CTL-P	Ag-activated CTL-P	CTL
IL-2R expression	-	+	+
IL-2 expression	-	±	±
Proliferation	-	-	+
Effector cytotoxic function	-	-	+

FIGURE 14-1 Generation of effector CTLs. Upon interaction with antigen–class I MHC complexes on appropriate target cells, CTL-Ps begin to express IL-2 receptors (IL-2R) and lesser amounts of IL-2. Proliferation and differentiation of antigen-activated CTL-Ps generally require additional IL-2 secreted by T_H1 cells resulting from antigen activation and proliferation of $CD4^+$ T cells. In the subsequent effector phase, CTLs destroy specific target cells.

The proliferation and differentiation of both antigen-activated T_H1 cells and CTL-Ps depend on IL-2. In IL-2 knockout mice, the absence of IL-2 has been shown to abolish CTL-mediated cytotoxicity. After clearance of antigen, the level of IL-2 declines. This decline in IL-2 induces T_H1 cells and CTLs to undergo programmed cell death by apoptosis. In this way, the immune response is rapidly terminated, lessening the likelihood of nonspecific tissue damage from the inflammatory response.

The role of T_H1 cells in the generation of CTLs from naive CTL-Ps is not completely understood, and it is unlikely that a T_H1 cell and CTL-P interact directly. However, IL-2 and co-stimulation are important in the transformation of naive CTL-Ps into effector cells, and T_H1 cells can be mediators in the provision of these essential requirements. As shown in Figure 14-2b, the interaction of helper cells with antigen-presenting cells can result in production of IL-2 by the T_H1 cell. The paracrine action of this cytokine on nearby naive CTL-Ps whose TCRs are engaged can cause them to proliferate and differentiate into active CTLs. Additionally, T_H1 can induce the up-regulation of co-stimulatory molecules on the surface of antigen-presenting cells. In this manner, T_H1 cells help CTL-P division and differentiation by causing the generation of adequate levels of co-stimulation.

Destruction of Target Cells by CTLs

The effector phase of a CTL-mediated response involves a carefully orchestrated sequence of events culminating in the destruction of the target cells (Figure 14-3). Long-term cultures of CTL clones have been used to identify many of the membrane molecules and membrane events involved in this process. As described below, studies with mouse strains carrying mutations that affect the ability of CTLs to induce death have led to the identification of the necessary molecules.

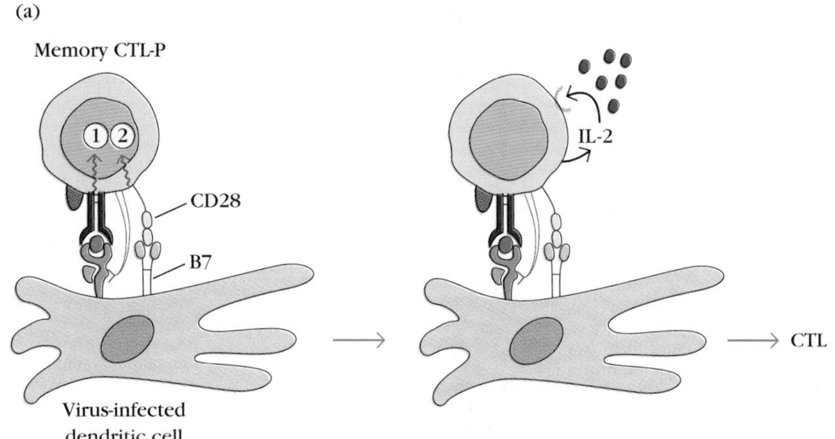

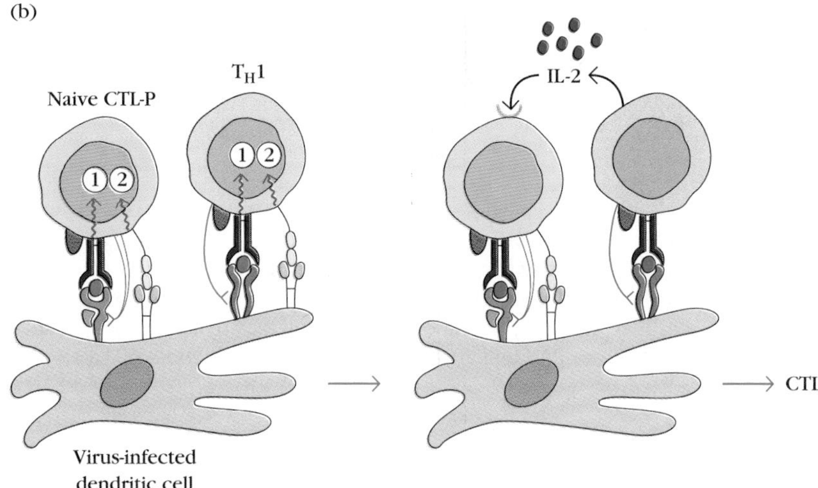

FIGURE 14-2 Proliferation of memory CTL-Ps may not require help from T_H cells. (a) Antigen-activated memory CTL-Ps appear to secrete sufficient IL-2 to stimulate their own proliferation and differentiation into effector CTLs. They also may not require the CD28-B7 co-stimulatory signal for activation. (b) A T_H cell may provide the IL-2 necessary for proliferation of an antigen-activated naive CTL-P when it binds to the same APC as the CTL-P. Also, T_H cells may alter the behavior of APCs in a number of ways, such as increasing the display of co-stimulatory molecules by the APC.

The primary events in CTL-mediated death are conjugate formation, membrane attack, CTL dissociation, and target-cell destruction (Figure 14-4). When antigen-specific CTLs are incubated with appropriate target cells, the two cell types interact and undergo conjugate formation. Formation of a CTL–target cell conjugate is followed within several minutes by a Ca^{2+}-dependent, energy-requiring step in which the CTL programs the target cell for death. The CTL then dissociates from the target cell and goes on to bind to another target cell. Within a variable period of time (up to a few hours) after CTL dissociation, the target cell dies by apoptosis. Each of the steps in this process has been studied in more detail with cloned CTLs.

The TCR-CD3 membrane complex on a CTL recognizes antigen in association with class I MHC molecules on a target cell. After this antigen-specific recognition, the integrin receptor LFA-1 on the CTL membrane binds to intercellular cell-adhesion molecules (ICAMs) on the target-cell membrane, resulting in the formation of a conjugate.

(a)

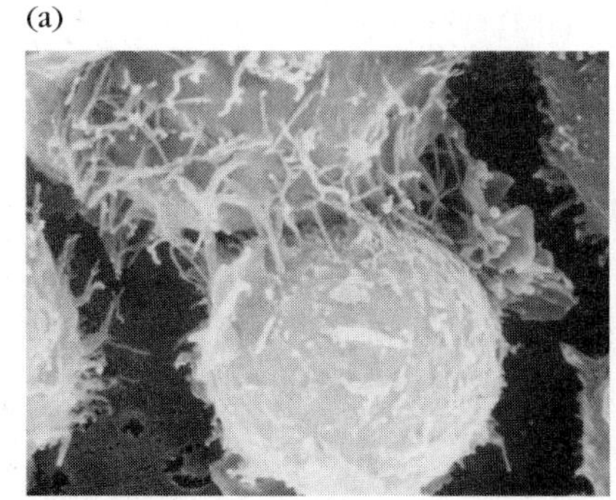

(b)

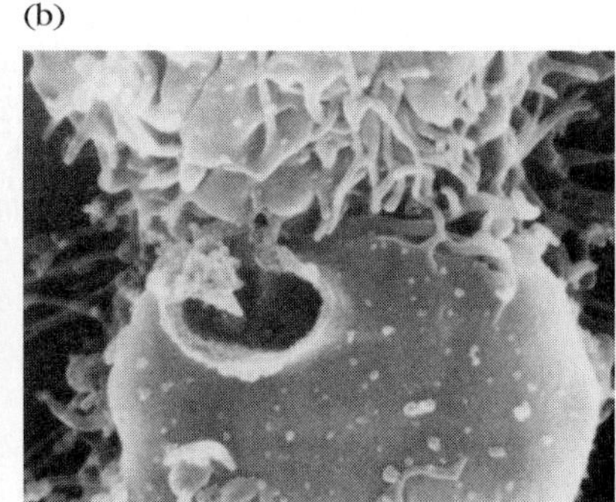

FIGURE 14-3 Scanning electron micrographs of tumor-cell destruction by a CTL. (a) A CTL (*top left*) makes contact with a smaller tumor cell. (b) Membrane damage to the tumor cell. [From JDE Young and ZA Cohn, 1988, *Sci. Am.* **258**(1):38.]

Go to www.whfreeman.com/immunology Animation
Cell Death

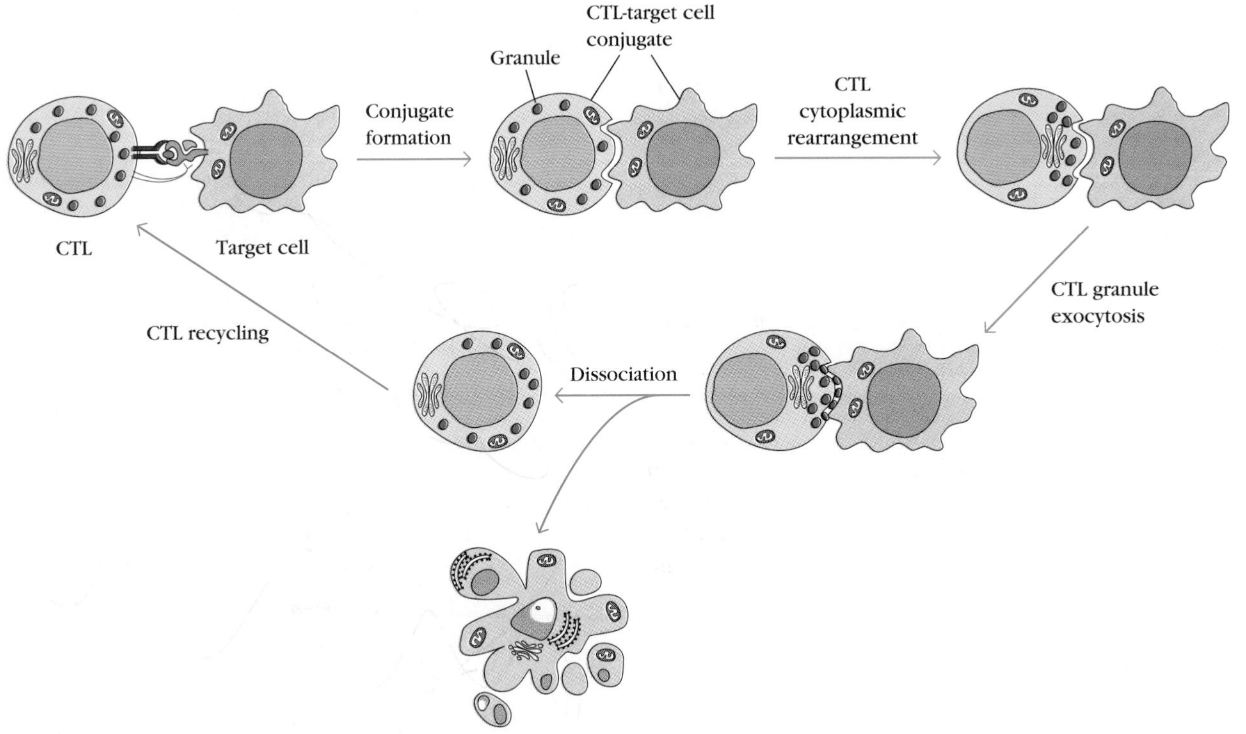

FIGURE 14-4 Stages in CTL-mediated killing of target cells. T-cell receptors on a CTL interact with processed antigen–class I MHC complexes on an appropriate target cell, leading to formation of a CTL/target-cell conjugate. The Golgi stacks and granules in the CTL reorient towards the point of contact with the target cell, and the granules' contents are released by exocytosis. After dissociation of the conjugate, the CTL is recycled and the target cell dies by apoptosis. [Adapted from PA Henkart, 1985, *Annu. Rev. Immunol.* **3**:31.]

Antigen-mediated CTL activation converts LFA-1 from a low-avidity state to a high-avidity state (Figure 14-5). Because of this phenomenon, CTLs adhere to and form conjugates only with appropriate target cells that display antigenic peptides associated with class I MHC molecules. LFA-1 persists in the high-avidity state for only 5–10 min after antigen-mediated activation, and then it returns to the low-avidity state. This downshift in LFA-1 avidity is thought to facilitate dissociation of the CTL from the target cell.

Electron microscopy of cultured CTL clones reveals the presence of intracellular electron-dense storage granules. These granules have been isolated by fractionation and shown to mediate target-cell damage by themselves. Analysis of isolated CTL storage granules has shown that they contain 65-kDA monomers of a pore-forming protein called **perforin** and several serine proteases called **granzymes** (or **fragmentins**). Although CTL-Ps lack cytoplasmic granules and perforin, their activation results in the appearance of these cytoplasmic granules and expression of perforin monomers within them.

Immediately after formation of a CTL–target cell conjugate, the Golgi stacks and storage granules reorient within the cytoplasm of the CTL to concentrate near the junction with the target cell (Figure 14-6). Evidence suggests that perforin monomers and the granzyme proteases then are released from the granules by exocytosis into the junctional space between the two cells. As the perforin monomers contact the

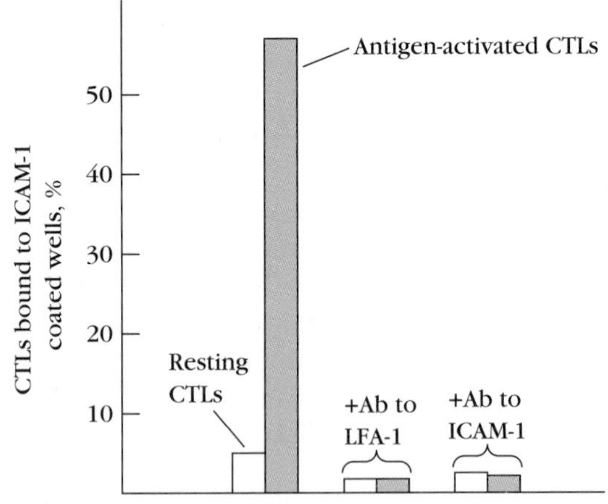

FIGURE 14-5 Effect of antigen activation on the ability of CTLs to bind to the intercellular cell-adhesion molecule ICAM-1. Resting mouse CTLs were first incubated with anti-CD3 antibodies. Crosslinkage of CD3 molecules on the CTL membrane by anti-CD3 has the same activating effect as interaction with antigen–class I MHC complexes on a target cell. Adhesion was assayed by binding radiolabeled CTLs to microwells coated with ICAM-1. Antigen activation increased CTL binding to ICAM-1 more than 10-fold. The presence of excess monoclonal antibody to LFA-1 or ICAM-1 in the microwell abolished binding, demonstrating that both molecules are necessary for adhesion. [Based on ML Dustin and TA Springer, 1989, *Nature* **341:**619.]

FIGURE 14-6 Formation of a conjugate between a CTL and target cell and reorientation of CTL cytoplasmic granules as recorded by time-lapse cinematography. (a) A motile mouse CTL (thin arrow) approaches an appropriate target cell (TC). The thick arrow indicates direction of movement. (b) Initial contact of the CTL and target cell has occurred. (c) Within 2 min of initial contact, the membrane-contact region has broadened and the rearrangement of dark cytoplasmic granules within the CTL (thin arrow) is under way. (d) Further movement of dark granules toward the target cell is evident 10 min after initial contact. [From JR Yanelli et al, 1986, *J. Immunol.* **136:**377].

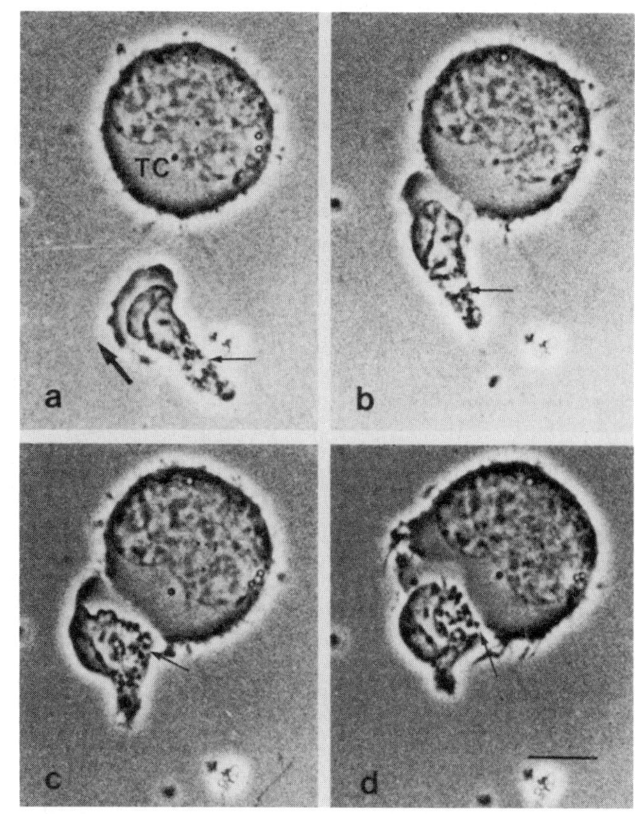

target-cell membrane, they undergo a conformational change, exposing an amphipathic domain that inserts into the target-cell membrane; the monomers then polymerize (in the presence of Ca^{2+}) to form cylindrical pores with an internal diameter of 5–20 nm (Figure 14-7a). A large number of perforin pores are visible on the target-cell membrane in the region of conjugate formation (Figure 14-7b). Interestingly, perforin exhibits some sequence homology with the terminal C9 component of the complement system, and the membrane pores formed by perforin are similar to those observed in complement-mediated lysis. The importance of perforin to CTL-mediated killing is demonstrated by perforin-deficient knockout mice, which are unable to eliminate lymphocytic choriomeningitis virus (LCMV) even though they mount a significant $CD8^+$ immune response to the virus.

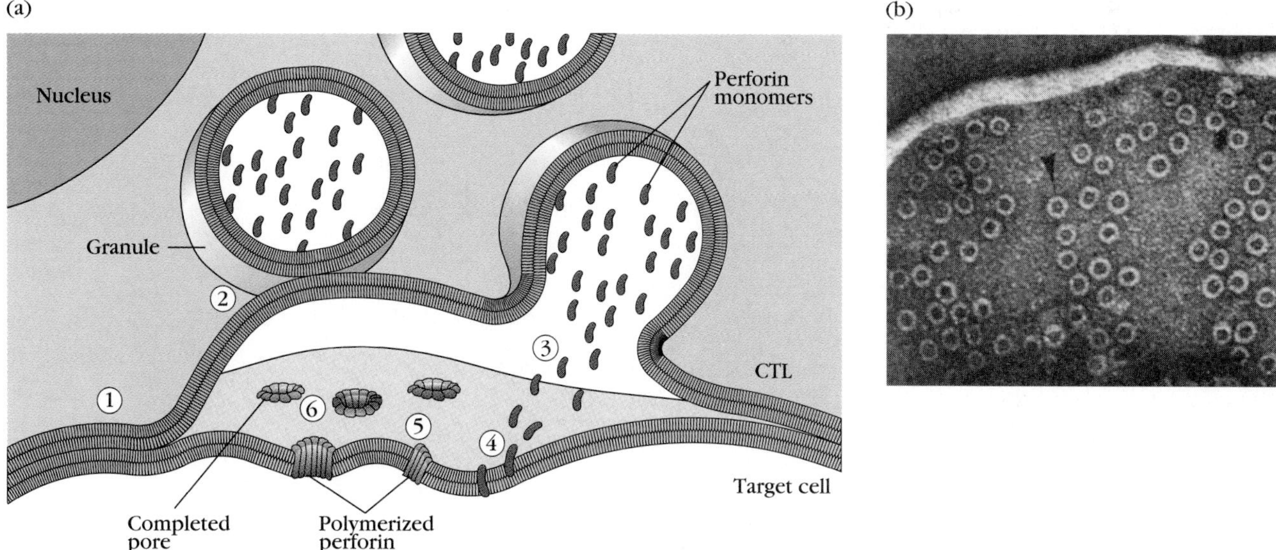

FIGURE 14-7 CTL-mediated pore formation in target-cell membrane. (a) In this model, a rise in intracellular Ca^{2+} triggered by CTL-target cell interaction (1) induces exocytosis, in which the granules fuse with the CTL cell membrane (2) and release monomeric perforin into the small space between the two cells (3). The released perforin monomers undergo a Ca^{2+}-induced conformational change that allows them to insert into the target-cell membrane (4). In the presence of Ca^{2+}, the monomers polymerize within the membrane (5), forming cylindrical pores (6). (b) Electron micrograph of perforin pores on the surface of a rabbit erythrocyte target cell. [Part (a) adapted from JDE Young and ZA Cohn, 1988, *Sci. Am.* **258**(1):38; part (b) from ER Podack and G Dennert, 1983, *Nature* **301:**442.1

The pores facilitate entry of granzyme proteases into the target cell. One result of the introduction of granzymes is the fragmentation of the target-cell DNA into oligomers of 200 bp; this type of DNA fragmentation is typical of apoptosis. Since granzymes are proteases, they cannot directly mediate DNA fragmentation. Rather, they activate an apoptotic pathway within the target cell. This apoptotic process does not require mRNA or protein synthesis in either the CTL or the target cell. Within 5 min of CTL contact, target cells begin to exhibit DNA fragmentation. Interestingly, viral DNA within infected target cells has also been shown to be fragmented during this process. This observation shows that CTL-mediated killing not only kills virus-infected cells but can also destroy the viral DNA in those cells. It has been suggested that the rapid onset of DNA fragmentation after CTL contact may prevent continued viral replication and assembly during the time before destruction of the target cell.

While perforin and granzymes play important roles in the induction of cell death, other observations demonstrate that they are not the sole inducers. Some potent CTL lines have been shown to lack perforin and granzymes. In these cases, cytotoxicity is mediated by Fas. As Chapter 10 showed, this transmembrane protein, which is a member of the TNF-receptor family, can deliver a death signal when crosslinked by its natural ligand, a member of the tumor necrosis family called Fas ligand (see Figure 10-20). Fas ligand (FasL) is found on the membrane of CTLs, and the interaction of FasL with Fas on a target cell triggers apoptosis.

Key insight into the role of perforin and the Fas-FasL system in CTL-mediated cytolysis came from experiments with mutant mice. These experiments used two types of mutant mice, the perforin knockout mice mentioned above and a strain of mice known as lpr (Figure 14-8). Mice that are homozygous for the lpr mutation express little or no Fas and, consequently, cells from these mice cannot be killed by inter-

(a) Generation of CTLs

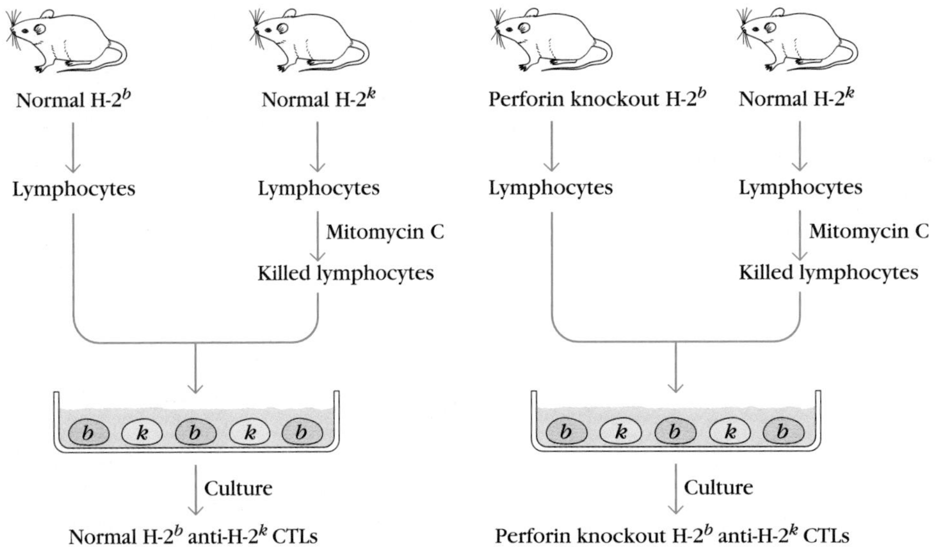

Normal H-2^b → Lymphocytes

Normal H-2^k → Lymphocytes → (Mitomycin C) → Killed lymphocytes

b k b k b → Culture → Normal H-2^b anti-H-2^k CTLs

Perforin knockout H-2^b → Lymphocytes

Normal H-2^k → Lymphocytes → (Mitomycin C) → Killed lymphocytes

b k b k b → Culture → Perforin knockout H-2^b anti-H-2^k CTLs

(b) Interaction of CTLs with Fas^+ and Fas^- targets

CTLs	Target cells: Normal H-2^k	lpr mutant H-2^k (no Fas)
Normal H-2^b anti-H-2^k	Killed	Killed
Perforin knockout H-2^b anti-H-2^k	Killed	Survive

FIGURE 14-8 Experimental demonstration that CTLs use Fas and perforin pathways. (a) Generation of CTLs. Lymphocytes were harvested from mice of H-2^b and H-2^k MHC haplotypes. H-2^k haplotype cells were killed by treatment with mitomycin C and co-cultured with H-2^b haplotype cells to stimulate the generation of anti-H-2^k CTLs. If the H-2^b lymphocytes were derived from normal mice, they gave rise to CTLs that had both perforin and Fas ligand. If the CTLs were raised by stimulation of lymphocytes from perforin knockout (KO) mice, they expressed Fas ligand but not perforin. (b) Interaction of CTLs with Fas^+ and Fas^- targets. Normal H-2^b anti-H-2^k CTLs that express both Fas ligand and perforin kill normal H-2^k target cells and H-2^k lpr mutant cells, which do not express Fas. In contrast, H-2^b anti-H-2^k CTLs from perforin KO mice kill Fas^+ normal cells by engagement of Fas with Fas ligand but are unable to kill the lpr cells, which lack Fas.

action with Fas ligand. If lymphocytes from normal H-2^b mice are incubated with killed cells from H-2^k mice, anti-H-2^k CTLs are generated. These H-2^b CTLs will kill target cells from normal H-2^k mice or from H-2^k animals that are homozygous for the lpr mutation. Incubation of H-2^b cells of perforin knockout mice with killed cells from H-2^k mice resulted in CTLs that killed wild-type target cells but failed to induce lysis in target cells from H-2^k mice homozygous for the lpr mutation.

The results of these experiments taken together with other studies allowed the investigators to make the following interpretation. CTLs raised from normal mice can kill target cells by a perforin-mediated mechanism, by a mechanism involving engagement of target cell Fas with Fas ligand displayed on the CTL membrane, or, in some cases, perhaps by a combination of both mechanisms. Such CTLs can kill target cells that lack membrane Fas by using the perforin mechanism alone. On the other hand, CTLs from perforin-knockout mice can kill only by the Fas-FasL mechanism. Consequently, CTLs from perforin-knockout mice can kill Fas-bearing normal target cells but not lpr cells, which lack Fas. These workers also concluded that all of the CTL-mediated killing they observed could be traced to the action of perforin-dependent killing, Fas-mediated killing, or a combination of the two. No other mechanism was detected.

This experiment taken together with a number of other studies shows that two mechanisms are responsible for initiating all CTL-mediated apoptotic death of target cells:

- Directional delivery of cytotoxic proteins (perforin and granzymes) that are released from CTLs and enter target cells
- Interaction of the membrane-bound Fas ligand on CTLs with the Fas receptor on the surface of target cells

Either of these initiating events results in the activation of a signaling pathway that culminates in the death of the target cell by apoptosis (Figure 14-9). A feature of cell death by apoptosis is the involvement of the caspase family of cysteine proteases, which cleave after an aspartic acid residue. The name **caspase** incorporates all of these elements (*c*ysteine, *asp*artate prote*ase*). Normally, caspases are present in the cell as inactive proenzymes, procaspases, that require proteolytic cleavage for conversion to the active forms. There are many different caspases, each with its own specificity, and more than a dozen different ones have been found. Cleavage of a procaspase produces an active initiator caspase, which cleaves other procaspases, thereby activating their proteolytic activity. The end result is the systematic and orderly disassembly of the cell that is the hallmark of apoptosis.

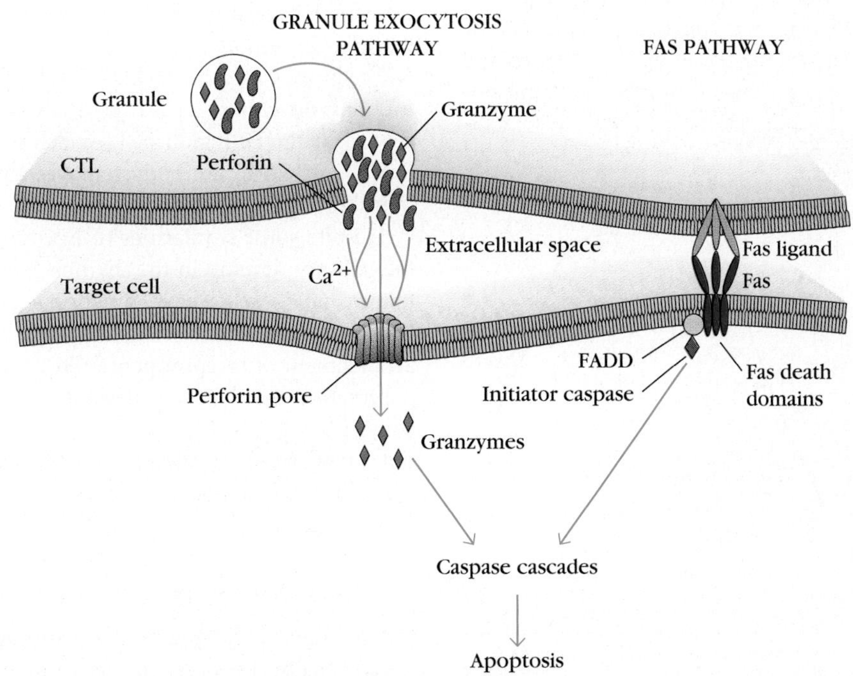

FIGURE 14-9 Proposed model of target-cell apoptosis stimulated by CTLs. The introduction of granzymes by the granule exocytosis pathway or the engagement of Fas by CTL-borne Fas ligand activates a caspase cascade, a chain of proteolytic reactions mediated by cysteine proteases, that culminates in the death of the target cell. In the granule-exocytosis pathway (*left*), granule contents are released into the space between the CTL and the target cell. In this space, the released perforin undergoes a Ca^{2+}-dependent polymerization and forms pores in the target cell membrane, which permit the entry of granzymes. Granzymes enter these pores and initiate a caspase cascade that results in the apoptotic death of the target. CTLs can also use the Fas pathway (*right*), which begins with ligation of trimeric Fas units by CTL-borne Fas ligand. This results in association of the death domains of Fas with FADD, which in turn results in activation of caspases, initiating a caspase cascade, which finally causes apoptosis of the target cell. [Adapted from Shresta et al, 1998, *Curr. Opin. Immunol.* **10:**581.]

CTLs use granzymes and Fas ligand to initiate caspase cascades in their targets. The granzymes introduced into the target cell from the CTL mediate proteolytic events that activate an initiator caspase. Similarly, the engagement of Fas on a target cell by Fas ligand on the CTL causes the activation of an initiator caspase in the target cell. Fas is associated with a protein known as FADD (*F*as-*a*ssociated protein with *d*eath *d*omain), which in turn associates with a procaspase form of caspase 8. Upon Fas crosslinking, procaspase 8 is converted to caspase 8 and initiates an apoptotic caspase cascade. As one immunologist has so aptly put it, CTLs don't so much kill target cells as persuade them to commit suicide.

Natural Killer Cells

Natural killer cells were discovered quite by accident when immunologists were measuring in vitro activity of tumor-specific cells taken from mice with tumors. Normal unimmunized mice and mice with unrelated tumors served as negative controls. Much to the consternation of the investigators, the controls showed significant lysis of the tumor cells, too. Characterization of this nonspecific tumor-cell killing revealed that a population of large granular lymphocytes was responsible. The cells, which were named natural killer (NK) cells for their nonspecific cytotoxicity, make up 5%–10% of the recirculating lymphocyte population. These cells are involved in immune defenses against viruses and tumors. Because NK cells produce a number of immunologically important cytokines (IFN-γ, for example), they also can play important roles in immune regulation.

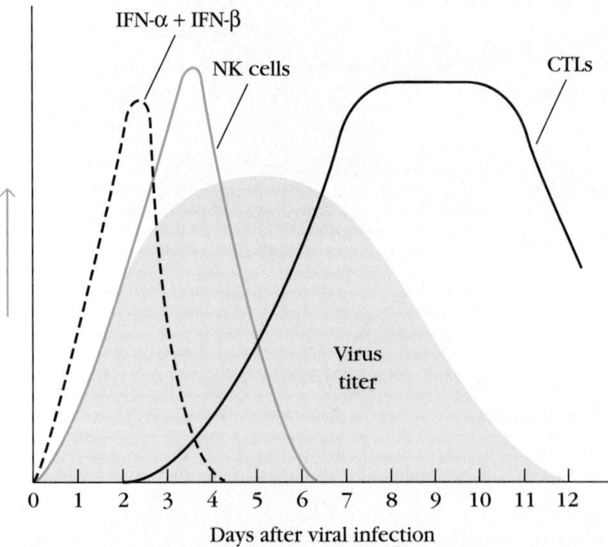

FIGURE 14-10 Time course of viral infection. IFN-α and IFN-β (dashed curve) are released from virus-infected cells soon after infection. These cytokines stimulate the NK cells, quickly leading to a rise in the NK-cell population (blue curve). NK cells help contain the infection during the period required for generation of CTLs (black curve). Once the CTL population reaches a peak, the virus titer (blue area) rapidly decreases.

NK cells are involved in the early response to infection with certain viruses and intracellular bacteria. NK activity is stimulated by IFN-α, IFN-β, and IL-12. In the course of a viral infection, the level of these cytokines rapidly rises, followed closely by a wave of NK cells that peaks in about 3 days (Figure 14-10). NK cells are the first line of defense against virus infection, controlling viral replication during the time required for activation, proliferation, and differentiation of CTL-P cells into functional CTLs at about day 7. The importance of NK cells in defense against viral infections is illustrated by the case of a young woman who completely lacked these cells. Even though this patient had normal T- and B-cell counts, she suffered severe varicella virus infections and a life-threatening cytomegalovirus infection.

NK-Cell Lineage

NK cells are lymphoid cells derived from bone marrow that share a common early progenitor with T cells, but their detailed lineage remains to be worked out. They express some membrane markers that are found on monocytes and granulocytes as well as some that are typical of T cells. Different NK cells express different sets of membrane molecules. It is not known whether this heterogeneity reflects subpopulations of NK cells or different stages in their activation or maturation. Among the membrane molecules expressed by NK cells are CD2, the 75-kDa β subunit of the IL-2 receptor, and, on almost all NK cells, CD16 (or FcγRIII), a receptor for the Fc region of IgG. Cell depletion with monoclonal anti-CD16 antibody removes almost all NK-cell activity from peripheral blood.

Despite some similarities of NK cells to T lymphocytes, they do not develop in the thymus. Nude mice, which have few or no T cells, have functional NK-cell populations. Unlike T cells and B cells, NK cells do not undergo rearrangement of receptor genes. This is demonstrated by the observation that NK cells develop in mice in which the recombinase genes *RAG-1* or *RAG-2* have been knocked out. Furthermore, while no T or B cells are found in SCID mice, functional populations of NK cells can be readily demonstrated.

Mechanism of NK-Cell Killing

Natural killer cells appear to kill tumor cells and virus-infected cells by a process similar to that employed by CTLs. The cytoplasm of NK cells contains numerous granules containing perforin and granzymes. Unlike CTLs, which need to be activated before granules appear, NK cells are constitutively cytotoxic, always having large granules in their cytoplasm. After an NK cell adheres to a target cell, degranulation occurs with release of perforin and granzymes at the junction of the interacting cells. The roles of perforin and granzymes in NK-mediated killing of target cells by apoptosis are thought to be similar to their roles in the CTL-mediated process.

Despite these similarities, NK cells differ from CTLs in several significant ways. First, NK cells do not express antigen-specific T-cell receptors or CD3. In addition, recognition of target cells by NK cells is not MHC restricted; that is, in many cases the same levels of NK-cell activity are observed with syngeneic and allogeneic tumor cells. Moreover, although prior priming enhances CTL activity, NK-cell activity does not increase after a second injection with the same tumor cells. In other words, the NK-cell response generates no immunologic memory.

NK-Cell Receptors

Given that NK cells do not express antigen-specific receptors, the mechanism by which NK cells recognize altered self-cells and distinguish them from normal body cells baffled immunologists for years. The solution to the problem emerged with the realization that NK cells employ two different categories of receptors, one that delivers inhibition signals to NK cells, and another that delivers activation signals. Initially, it was thought that there were two receptors, one that activated and another that inhibited NK cells—the so-called two-receptor model. It is now clear that there are many different cell-surface receptors for activation signals and a number of different kinds for inhibitory ones. Consequently, it is more appropriate to think in terms of an "opposing-signals model" rather than a "two-receptor model." It is the balance between activating signals and inhibitory signals that is believed to enable NK cells to distinguish healthy cells from infected or cancerous ones. It is important to be aware that additional NK-activating signals can be delivered by soluble factors. These include cytokines such as α and β interferons, TNF-α, IL-12, and IL-15.

The exact nature of the membrane-bound receptors on NK cells that produce activation is not completely clear. Antibody crosslinking of many molecules found on the surface of NK cells can activate these cells artificially, but the natural ligands for many of these putative activation receptors (ARs) are not known. Some of the candidate ARs are members of a class of carbohydrate-binding proteins known as C-type lectins, so named because they have calcium-dependent carbohydrate-recognition domains. NKR-P1 is an example of a C-type lectin with activation properties found on NK cells. In addition to lectins, other molecules on NK cells might be involved in activation, including CD28 (receptor for B-7 family of co-stimulatory molecules), CD2 (receptor for the adhesion molecule LFA-3), and the FcγIII receptor, CD16. Although CD16 is responsible for antibody-mediated recognition and killing of target cells by NK cells, it is probably not involved in killing that does not involve such recognition.

Clues to the sources of inhibitory signals came from studies of the killing of tumor cells and virus-infected cells by NK cells. In murine systems, it was noticed that the preferential killing of mouse tumor cells compared with normal cells correlated with a lack of expression of MHC molecules by the tumor cells. Experiments with human cells showed that NK cells lysed a B-cell line that was MHC deficient because it had been transformed by Epstein-Barr virus. However, when this cell line was transformed with human HLA genes so that it expressed high levels of MHC molecules, NK cells failed to lyse it. These observations led to the idea that NK cells target cells for killing that have aberrant MHC expression. Since many virus-infected and tumor cells have reduced MHC expression, this model made good physiological sense. Vindication of this proposal has come from the discovery of receptors on NK cells that produce inhibitory signals when they recognize MHC molecules on potential target cells. These inhibitory receptors on the NK cell then prevent NK-cell killing, proliferation, and cytokine release.

Two major groups of inhibitory receptors have been found on NK cells. One of these is a family of C-type-lectin–inhibitory receptors (CLIR), and the other is a group of Ig-superfamily–inhibitory receptors (ISIR) known as the killer-cell–inhibitory (KIR) receptors. Even though these groups are chemically quite different, they are together referred to as the inhibitory-receptor superfamily (IRS). In humans, the C-type-lectin–inhibitory receptor is CD94/NKG2, a disulfide-bonded heterodimer made up of two glycoproteins, one of which is CD94 and the other a member of the NKG2 family. The CD94/NKG2 receptors recognize HLA-E on potential target cells. Because HLA-E is not transported to the surface of a cell unless it has bound a peptide derived from HLA-A, HLA-B, or HLA-C, the amount of HLA-E on the surface serves as indicator of the overall level of class I MHC biosynthesis in the cells. These inhibitory CD94/NKG2 receptors are thus not specific for a particular HLA allele and will send inhibitory signals to the NK cell with the net result that killing of potential target cells is inhibited if they are expressing adequate levels of class I. In contrast, KIR receptors, of which more than 50 family members have been found, are specific for one or a limited number of polymorphic products of particular HLA loci. Unlike B and T cells, NK cells are not limited to expressing a single MHC receptor, but may express several, each specific for a different MHC molecule or for a set of closely related MHC molecules. For example, individual clones of human NK cells expressing a CD94/NKG2 receptor and as many as six different KIR receptors have been found. Because signals from inhibitory receptors have veto power over signals from activating receptors, a negative signal from any inhibitory receptor, whether of the CD94/NKG2 or KIR type, can block the lysis of target cells by NK cells. Thus, cells expressing normal levels of unaltered MHC class I molecules tend to escape all forms of NK-cell–mediated killing.

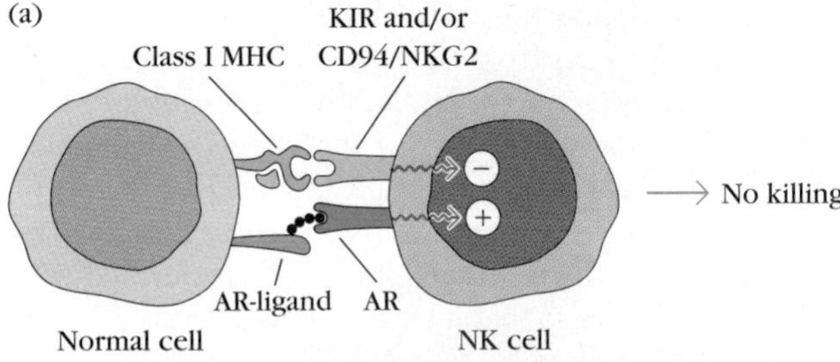

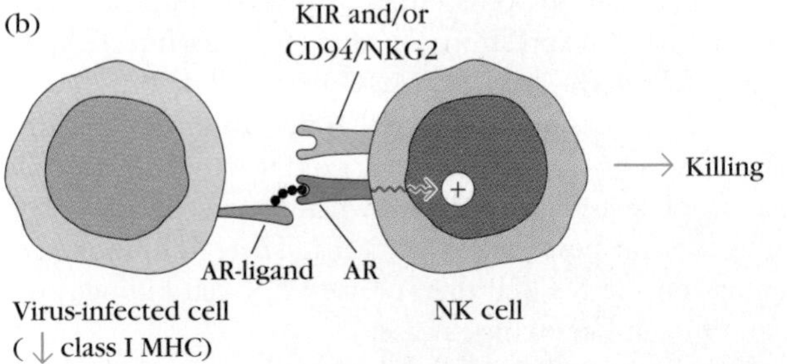

FIGURE 14-11 Opposing-signals model of how cytotoxic activity of NK cells is restricted to altered self-cells. An activation receptor (AR) on NK cells interacts with its ligand on normal and altered self-cells, inducing an activation signal that results in killing. However, engagement of inhibitory NK cell receptors such as KIR and CD94/NKG2 by class I MHC molecules delivers an inhibitory signal that counteracts the activation signal. Expression of class I molecules on normal cells thus prevents their destruction by NK cells. Because class I expression is often decreased on altered self-cells, the killing signal predominates, leading to their destruction.

In the opposing-signals model of NK-cell regulation that is emerging from studies of NK cells (Figure 14-11), activating receptors engage ligands on the target cell. These ligands may be abnormal forms or patterns of glycosylation on the surface of tumor or virus-infected cells. Recognition of these determinants by ARs on NK cells would signal NK cells to kill the target cells. Ligand engagement by NKR-P1-type lectin receptors, or a number of other ARs, such as CD16, in some cases CD2, and perhaps CD28, generates signals that direct the NK cell to kill the target cell. Any of these killing signals can be overridden by a signal from inhibitory receptors. As we have already seen, members of the inhibitory superfamily of receptors (ISRs) provide a signal that decisively overrides activation signals when these inhibitory receptors detect normal levels of MHC class I expression on potential target cells. This prevents the death of the target cell. It also prevents NK-cell proliferation and the induction of secretion of cytokines such as IFN-γ and TNF-α. The overall consequence of the opposing-signals model is to spare cells that express critical indicators of normal self, the MHC class I molecules, and to kill cells that lack indicators of self (absence of normal levels of class I MHC).

Antibody-Dependent Cell-Mediated Cytotoxicity

A number of cells that have cytotoxic potential express membrane receptors for the Fc region of the antibody molecule. When antibody is specifically bound to a target cell, these receptor-bearing cells can bind to the antibody Fc region, and thus to the target cells and subsequently cause lysis of the target cell. Although these cytotoxic cells are nonspecific for antigen, the specificity of the antibody directs them to specific target cells. This type of cytotoxicity is referred to as **antibody-dependent cell-mediated cytotoxicity (ADCC).**

Among the cells that can mediate ADCC are NK cells, macrophages, monocytes, neutrophils, and eosinophils. Antibody-dependent cell-mediated killing of cells infected with the measles virus can be observed in vitro by adding anti-measles antibody together with macrophages to a culture of measles-infected cells. Similarly, cell-mediated killing of helminths, such as schistosomes or blood flukes, can be observed in vitro by incubating larvae (schistosomules) with antibody to the schistosomules together with eosinophils.

Target-cell killing by ADCC does not involve complement-mediated lysis, but appears to involve a number of different cytotoxic mechanisms (Figure 14-12). When macrophages, neutrophils, or eosinophils bind to a target cell by way of the Fc receptor, they become more active metabolically; as a result, the lytic enzymes in their cytoplasmic lysosomes or granules increase. Release of these lytic enzymes at

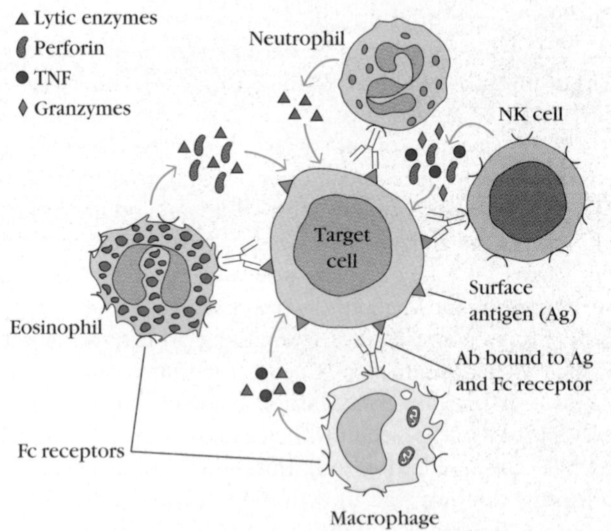

FIGURE 14-12 Antibody-dependent cell-mediated cytotoxicity (ADCC). Nonspecific cytotoxic cells are directed to specific target cells by binding to the Fc region of antibody bound to surface antigens on the target cells. Various substances (e.g., lytic enzymes, TNF, perforin, granzymes) secreted by the nonspecific cytotoxic cells then mediate target-cell destruction.

the site of the Fc-mediated contact may result in damage to the target cell. In addition, activated monocytes, macrophages, and NK cells have been shown to secrete tumor necrosis factor (TNF), which may have a cytotoxic effect on the bound target cell. Since both NK cells and eosinophils contain perforin in cytoplasmic granules, their target-cell killing also may involve perforin-mediated membrane damage similar to the mechanism described for CTL-mediated cytotoxicity.

Experimental Assessment of Cell-Mediated Cytotoxicity

Three experimental systems have been particularly useful for measuring the activation and effector phases of cell-mediated cytotoxic responses. The mixed-lymphocyte reaction (MLR) is an in vitro system for assaying T_H-cell proliferation in a cell-mediated response; cell-mediated lympholysis (CML) is an in vitro assay of effector cytotoxic function; and the graft-versus-host reaction (GVH) in experimental animals provides an in vivo system for studying cell-mediated cytotoxicity.

Mixed-Lymphocyte Reaction (MLR)

During the 1960s, early in the history of modern cellular immunology, it was observed that when rat lymphocytes were cultured on a monolayer of mouse fibroblast cells, the rat lymphocytes proliferated and destroyed the mouse fibroblasts. In 1970 it was discovered that functional CTLs could also be generated by co-culturing allogeneic spleen cells in a system termed the mixed-lymphocyte reaction (MLR). The T lymphocytes in an MLR undergo extensive blast transformation and cell proliferation. The degree of proliferation can be assessed by adding [^{3}H]thymidine to the culture medium and monitoring uptake of label into DNA in the course of repeated cell divisions.

Both populations of allogeneic T lymphocytes proliferate in an MLR unless one population is rendered unresponsive by treatment with mitomycin C or lethal x-irradiation (Figure 14-13). In the latter system, called a one-way MLR, the unresponsive population provides stimulator cells that express alloantigens foreign to the responder T cells. Within 24–48 h the responder T cells begin dividing in response to the alloantigens of the stimulator cells, and by 72–96 h an expanding population of functional CTLs is generated. With

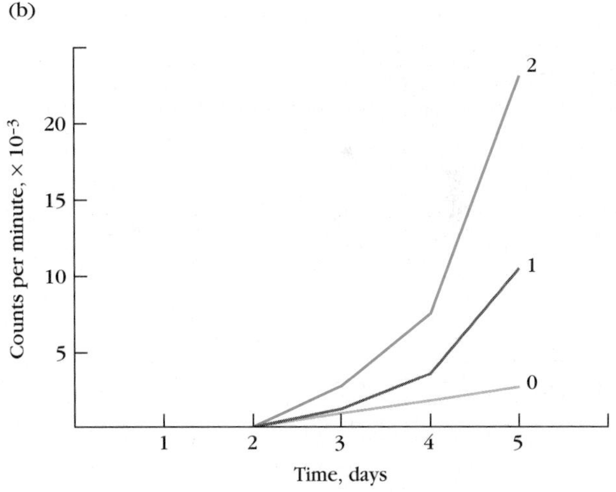

FIGURE 14-13 One-way mixed-lymphocyte reaction (MLR). (a) This assay measures the proliferation of lymphocytes from one strain (responder cells) in response to allogeneic cells that have been x-irradiated or treated with mitomycin C to prevent proliferation (stimulator cells). The amount of [^{3}H]-thymidine incorporated into the DNA is directly proportional to the extent of responder-cell proliferation. (b) The amount of [^{3}H]-thymidine uptake in a one-way MLR depends on the degree of differences in class II MHC molecules between the stimulator and responder cells. Curve 0 = no class II MHC differences; curve 1 = one class II MHC difference; curve 2 = two class II MHC differences. These results demonstrate that the greater the class II MHC differences, the greater the proliferation of responder cells.

this experimental system, functional CTLs can be generated entirely in vitro, after which their activity can be assessed with various effector assays.

The significant role of T_H cells in the one-way MLR can be demonstrated by use of antibodies to the T_H-cell membrane marker CD4. In a one-way MLR, responder T_H cells recognize allogeneic class II MHC molecules on the stimulator cells and proliferate in response to these differences. Removal of the $CD4^+$ T_H cells from the responder population with anti-CD4 plus complement abolishes the MLR and prevents generation of CTLs. In addition to T_H cells, accessory cells such as macrophages also are necessary for the MLR to proceed. When adherent cells (mostly macrophages) are removed from the stimulator population, the proliferative response in the MLR is abolished and functional CTLs are no longer generated. It is now known that the function of these macrophages is to activate the class II MHC–restricted T_H cells whose proliferation is measured in the MLR. In the absence of T_H-cell activation, there is no proliferation.

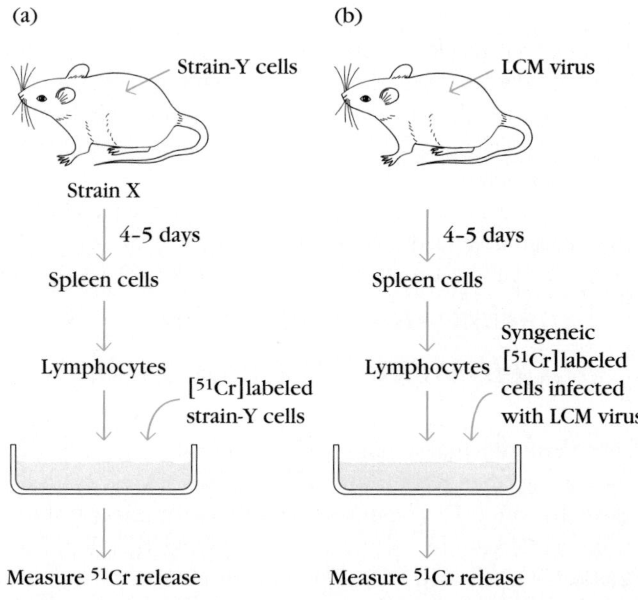

FIGURE 14-14 In vitro cell-mediated lympholysis (CML) assay. This assay can measure the activity of cytotoxic T lymphocytes (CTLs) against allogeneic cells (a) or virus-infected cells (b). In both cases the release of ^{51}Cr into the supernatant indicates the presence of CTLs that can lyse the target cells.

Cell-Mediated Lympholysis (CML)

Development of the cell-mediated lympholysis (CML) assay was a major experimental advance that contributed to understanding of the mechanism of target-cell killing by CTLs. In this assay, suitable target cells are labeled intracellularly with chromium-51 (^{51}Cr) by incubating the target cells with $Na_2^{51}CrO_4$. After the ^{51}Cr diffuses into a cell, it binds to cytoplasmic proteins, reducing passive diffusion of the label out of the cell. When specifically activated CTLs are incubated for 1–4 h with such labeled target cells, the cells lyse and the ^{51}Cr is released. The amount of ^{51}Cr released is directly related to the number of target cells lysed by the CTLs. By means of this assay, the specificity of CTLs for allogeneic cells, tumor cells, virus-infected cells, and chemically modified cells has been demonstrated (Figure 14-14).

The T cells responsible for CML were identified by selectively depleting different T-cell subpopulations by means of antibody-plus-complement lysis. In general, the activity of CTLs exhibits class I MHC restriction. That is, they can kill only target cells that present antigen associated with syngeneic class I MHC molecules. Occasionally, however, $CD4^+$, class II–restricted T cells have been shown to function as CTLs.

Graft-Versus-Host Reaction

The graft-versus-host (GVH) reaction is an in vivo indication of cell-mediated cytotoxicity. The reaction develops when immunocomponent lymphocytes are injected into an allogeneic recipient whose immune system is compromised. Because the donor and recipient are not genetically identical, the grafted lymphocytes begin to attack the host, and the host's compromised state prevents an immune response against the graft. In humans, GVH reactions often develop after transplantation of bone marrow into patients who have had radiation exposure or who have leukemia, immunodeficiency diseases, or autoimmune anemias. The clinical manifestations of the GVH reaction include diarrhea, skin lesions, jaundice, spleen enlargement, and death. Epithelial cells of the skin and gastrointestinal tract often become necrotic, causing the skin and intestinal lining to be sloughed.

Experimentally, GVH reactions develop when immunocompetent lymphocytes are transferred into an allogeneic neonatal or x-irradiated animal. The recipients, especially neonatal ones, often exhibit weight loss. The grafted lymphocytes generally are carried to a number of organs, including the spleen, where they begin to proliferate in response to the allogeneic MHC antigens of the host. This proliferation induces an influx of host cells and results in visible spleen enlargement, or splenomegaly. The intensity of a GVH reaction can be assessed by calculating the spleen index as follows:

$$\text{Spleen index} = \frac{\text{weight of experimental spleen/total body weight}}{\text{weight of control spleen/total body weight}}$$

A spleen index of 1.3 or greater is considered to be indicative of a positive GVH reaction. Spleen enlargement results from proliferation of both $CD4^+$ and $CD8^+$ T-cell populations. NK cells also have been shown to play a role in the GVH reaction, and these cells may contribute to some of the skin lesions and intestinal wall damage observed.

Delayed-Type Hypersensitivity

When some subpopulations of activated T_H cells encounter certain types of antigens, they secrete cytokines that induce a localized inflammatory reaction called **delayed-type hypersensitivity (DTH).** The reaction is characterized by large influxes of nonspecific inflammatory cells, in which the macrophage is a major participant. This type of reaction was first described in 1890 by Robert Koch, who observed that individuals infected with *Mycobacterium tuberculosis* developed a localized inflammatory response when injected intradermally with a filtrate derived from a mycobacterial culture. He called this localized skin reaction a "tuberculin reaction."

Later, as it became apparent that a variety of other antigens could induce this response, its name was changed to delayed-type hypersensitivity in reference to the delayed onset of the reaction and to the extensive tissue damage (hypersensitivity) that is often associated with it. The term *hypersensitivity* is somewhat misleading, for it suggests that a DTH response is always detrimental. Although in some cases a DTH response does cause extensive tissue damage and is in itself pathologic, in many cases tissue damage is limited, and the response plays an important role in defense against intracellular pathogens and contact antigens. (Contact antigens are synthetic or naturally occuring substances, such as poison ivy, that induce DTH reactions when brought into contact with skin or mucous membranes.)

Phases of the DTH Response

The development of the DTH response requires an initial sensitization phase of 1–2 weeks after primary contact with the antigen. During this period, T_H cells are activated and clonally expanded by antigen presented together with the requisite class II MHC molecule on an appropriate antigen-presenting cell (Figure 14-15a). A variety of antigen-presenting cells have been shown to be involved in the activation of a DTH response, including Langerhans cells and macrophages. Langerhans cells are dendritic cells found in the epidermis. These cells are thought to pick up antigen that enters through the skin and transport it to regional lymph nodes, where T cells are activated by the antigen. In some species, including humans, the vascular endothelial cells express class II MHC molecules and also function as antigen-presenting cells in the development of the DTH response. Generally, the T cells activated during the sensitization phase are $CD4^+$, primarily of the T_H1 subtype, but in a few cases $CD8^+$ cells have also been shown to induce a DTH response. The activated T cells are often designated as T_{DTH} cells to denote their function in the DTH response, although in reality they are simply a subset of T_H cells (or, in some cases, T_C cells).

A subsequent exposure to the antigen induces the effector phase of the DTH response (see Figure 14-15). In the effector phase, T_{DTH} cells secrete a variety of cytokines that are responsible for the recruitment and activation of macrophages and other nonspecific inflammatory cells. A DTH response normally does not become apparent until an average of 24 h after secondary contact with the antigen; the response generally peaks 48–72 h after secondary contact. The delayed onset of this response reflects the time required for the cytokines to induce localized influxes of macrophages and their activation. Once a DTH response begins, a complex interplay of nonspecific cells and mediators is set in motion that can result in tremendous amplification. By the time the DTH response is fully developed, only about 5% of the participating cells are antigen-specific T_{DTH} cells; the remainder are macrophages and other nonspecific cells.

Macrophages function as the principal effector cells of the DTH response. Cytokines elaborated by T_{DTH} cells induce blood monocytes to adhere to vascular endothelial cells and migrate from the blood into the surrounding tissues. During this process the monocytes differentiate into activated macrophages. As Chapter 2 described, activated macrophages exhibit increased levels of phagocytosis and an increased ability to kill microorganisms through various cytotoxic mediators. In addition, activated macrophages express increased levels of class II MHC molecules and cell-adhesion molecules and therefore function as more effective antigen-presenting cells.

The influx and activation of macrophages in the DTH response are an effective host defense against intracellular pathogens. Generally, the pathogen is cleared rapidly with little tissue damage. However, in some cases, especially if the antigen is not easily cleared, a prolonged DTH response can itself become destructive to the host as the intense inflammatory response develops into a visible granulomatous reaction. A granuloma develops when continuous activation of macrophages induces the macrophages to adhere closely to one another, assuming an epithelioid shape and sometimes fusing to form multinucleated giant cells (Figure 14-16). These giant cells displace the normal tissue cells, forming palpable nodules, and release high concentrations of lytic enzymes, which destroy the surrounding tissue. In these cases the response can damage blood vessels and lead to extensive tissue necrosis.

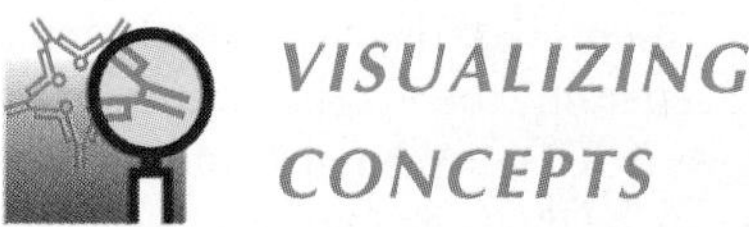

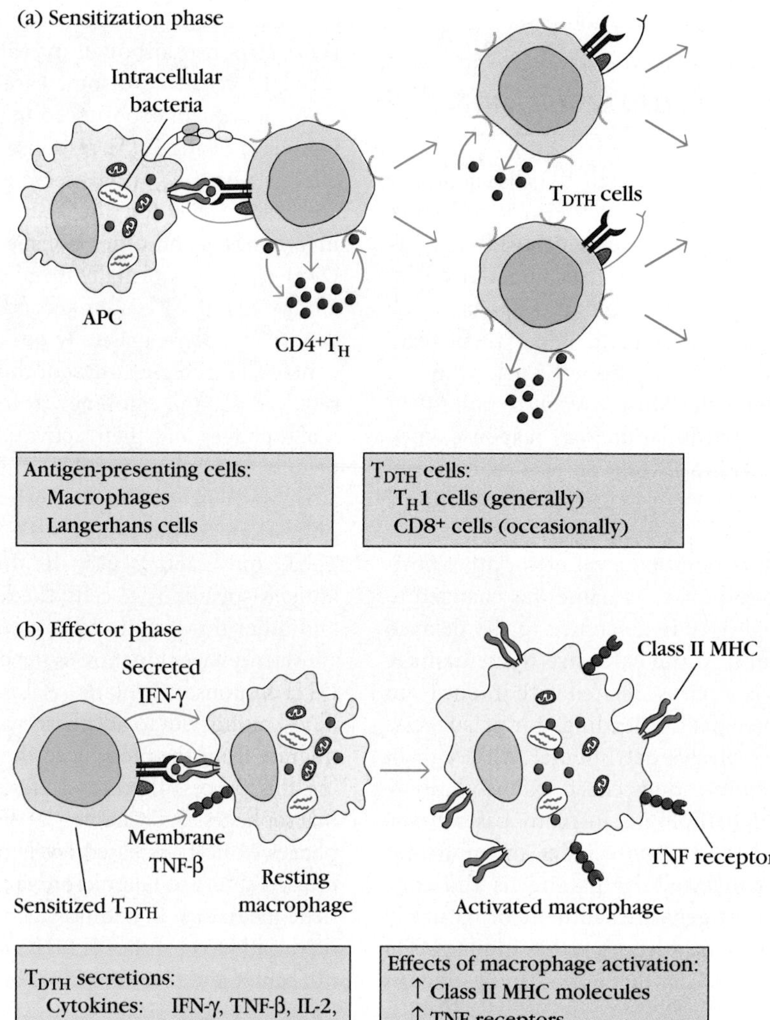

FIGURE 14-15 Overview of the DTH response. (a) In the sensitization phase after initial contact with antigen (e.g., peptides derived from intracellular bacteria), T_H cells proliferate and differentiate into T_{DTH} cells. Cytokines secreted by these T cells are indicated by the dark blue balls. (b) In the effector phase after subsequent exposure of sensitized T_{DTH} cells to antigen, the T_{DTH} cells secrete a variety of cytokines and chemokines. These factors attract and activate macrophages and other nonspecific inflammatory cells. Activated macrophages are more effective in presenting antigen, thus perpetuating the DTH response, and function as the primary effector cells in this reaction. MCAF = macrophage chemotactic and activating factor; MIF = macrophage-inhibition factor.

Cytokines Involved in the DTH Reaction

Numerous cytokines play a role in generating a DTH reaction. The pattern of cytokines implicated in a DTH response suggest that T_{DTH} cells may be primarily of the T_H1 subset (see Table 14-2). IL-2 functions in an autocrine manner to amplify the population of cytokine-producing T cells. Among the cytokines produced by T_{DTH} cells are a number that serve to activate and attract macrophages to the site of activation. IL-3 and GM-CSF induce localized hematopoiesis of the granulocyte-monocyte lineage. IFN-γ

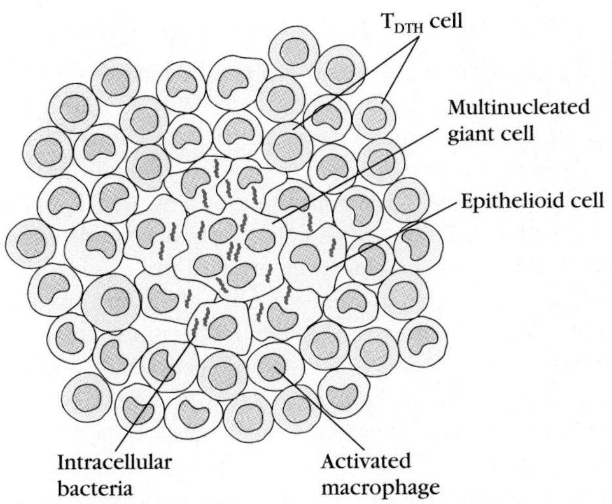

FIGURE 14-16 A prolonged DTH response can lead to formation of a granuloma, a nodule-like mass. Lytic enzymes released from activated macrophages in a granuloma can cause extensive tissue damage.

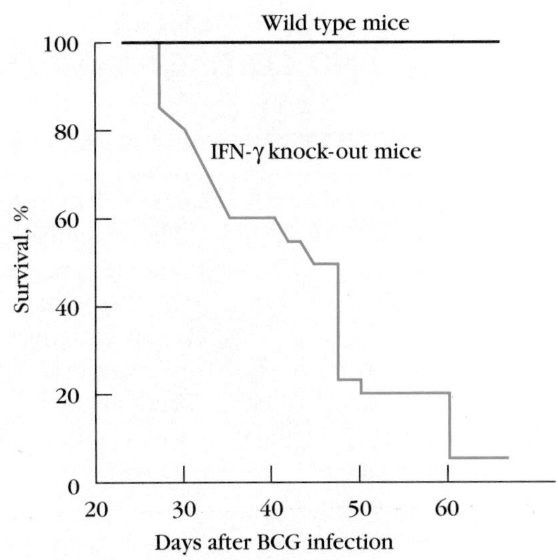

FIGURE 14-17 Experimental demonstration of role of IFN-γ in host defense against intracellular pathogens. Knock-out mice were produced by introducing a targeted mutation in the gene encoding IFN-γ. The mice were then infected with 10^7 colony-forming units of attenuated *Mycobacterium bovis* (BCG) and their survival monitored. [Adapted from DK Dalton et al, 1993, *Science* **259:**1739.]

and TNF-β (together with macrophage-derived TNF-α and IL-1) act on nearby endothelial cells, inducing a number of changes that facilitate extravasation of monocytes and other nonspecific inflammatory cells. Circulating neutrophils and monocytes adhere to the adhesion molecules displayed on the vascular endothelial cells and extravasate into the tissue spaces. Neutrophils appear early in the reaction, peaking by about 6 h and then declining in numbers. The monocyte infiltration occurs between 24 and 48 h after antigen exposure.

As the monocytes enter the tissues to become macrophages, they are chemotactically drawn to the site of the DTH response by chemokines such as monocyte chemotactic and activating factor (MCAF). Another chemokine, called migration-inhibition factor (MIF), inhibits further macrophage migration and thus prevents the macrophages from migrating beyond the site of a DTH reaction. As macrophages accumulate at the site of a DTH reaction, they are activated by cytokines, particularly IFN-γ and membrane-bound TNF-β produced by T_{DTH} cells. As noted earlier, activated macrophages are more effective antigen-presenting cells than unactivated macrophages are. Thus, the activated macrophages can efficiently mediate activation of more T cells, which in turn secrete more cytokines that recruit and activate even more macrophages. This self-perpetuating response, however, is a double-edged sword, with a fine line existing between a beneficial, protective response and a detrimental response characterized by extensive tissue damage.

A report of experiments with knockout mice that could not produce IFN-γ demonstrated the importance of this cytokine in the DTH response. When these knockout mice were infected with an attenuated strain of *Mycobacterium bovis* known as BCG (Bacille Calmette Guérin), nearly all the animals died within 60 days, whereas wild-type mice survived (Figure 14-17). Macrophages from the IFN-γ knockout mice were shown to have reduced levels of class II MHC molecules and of bactericidal metabolites such as nitric oxide and superoxide anion.

Protective Role of the DTH Response

A variety of intracellular pathogens and contact antigens can induce a DTH response (Table 14-3). Cells harboring intracellular pathogens are rapidly destroyed by lytic enzymes released by activated macrophages that accumulate at the site of a DTH reaction (Figure 14-18). The initial response, however, is nonspecific and often results in significant damage to healthy tissue. Generally, this is the price the body pays for successful elimination of cells harboring intracellular and fungal pathogens. The response to *Mycobacterium tuberculosis* illustrates the double-edged nature of the DTH response. Immunity to this intracellular bacterium involves a DTH response in which activated macrophages wall off the organism in the lung and contain it within a granuloma-type lesion called a tubercle.

TABLE 14-3 INTRACELLULAR PATHOGENS AND CONTACT ANTIGENS THAT INDUCE DELAYED-TYPE HYPERSENSITIVITY

Intracellular bacteria	Intracellular viruses
Mycobacterium tuberculosis	Herpes simplex virus
Mycobacterium leprae	Variola (smallpox)
Listeria monocytogenes	Measles virus
Brucella abortus	Contact antigens
Intracellular fungi	Picrylchloride
Pneumocystis carinii	Hair dyes
Candida albicans	Nickel salts
Histoplasma capsulatum	Poison ivy
Cryptococcus neoformans	Poison oak
Intracellular parasites	
Leishmania sp.	

Often, however, the concentrated release of lytic enzymes from the activated macrophages within tubercles damages lung tissue.

The vitally important role of the DTH response in protecting the host against various intracellular pathogens is illustrated by AIDS. In this disease, $CD4^+$ T cells are severely depleted, resulting in a loss of the DTH response. Often patients suffering with AIDS develop life-threatening infections from intracellular bacteria, fungi, or protozoans that would not be able to establish a serious infection in individuals whose DTH response was intact. AIDS is described in greater depth in Chapter 19.

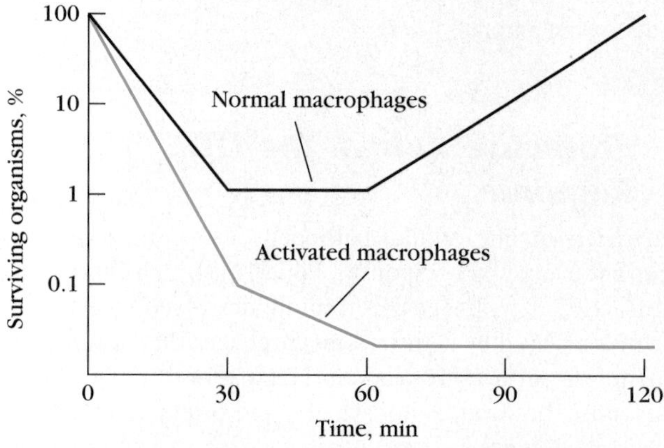

FIGURE 14-18 Survival of the intracellular pathogen *Listeria monocytogenes* when mixed with normal macrophages (not activated by IFN-γ) or activated macrophages in vitro. Note the logarithmic scale. The much greater ability of activated macrophages to destroy intracellular pathogens is evident.

Detection of the DTH Reaction

The presence of a DTH reaction can be measured experimentally by injecting antigen intradermally into an animal and observing whether a characteristic skin lesion develops at the injection site. A positive skin-test reaction indicates that the individual has a population of sensitized T_{DTH} cells specific for the test antigen. For example, to determine whether an individual has been exposed to *M. tuberculosis*, PPD, a protein derived from the cell wall of this mycobacterium, is injected intradermally. Development of a red, slightly swollen, firm lesion at the site between 48 and 72 h later indicates that the individual has been exposed to *M. tuberculosis* antigens. However, a positive test does not allow one to conclude whether the exposure was to a pathogenic form of *M. tuberculosis* or to a vaccine form received through immunization, which is performed in some parts of the world. Development of a skin lesion in a previously sensitized individual results from the intense infiltration of cells to the site of injection during a DTH reaction; 80%–90% of these cells are macrophages.

Pathologic DTH Responses

In some cases, the DTH response to an intracellular pathogen can cause such extensive tissue damage that the response itself is pathologic and constitutes a truly hypersensitive condition. Much of the tissue damage in tuberculosis results from the accumulation of activated macrophages whose lysosomal enzymes destroy healthy lung tissue. Delayed-type hypersensitive reactions can also develop to poison oak and to other contact antigens. Some examples of truly hypersensitive conditions, in which tissue damage far outweighs any beneficial effects, are described in Chapter 17.

Summary

1. The cell-mediated branch of the immune system involves three types of antigen-specific effector cells: $CD4^+$ T_H1 and T_H2 cells and cytotoxic T lymphocytes (CTLs). Compared with naive T_H and T_C cells, the effector cells are more easily activated, express higher levels of cell-adhesion molecules, exhibit different trafficking patterns, and produce both soluble and membrane effector molecules (see Tables 14-1 and 14-2).
2. The first phase of the CTL-mediated immune response involves the activation and differentiation of T_C cells, called CTL precursors (CTL-Ps). Interaction of a CTL-P with an antigen–class I MHC complex leads to expression of IL-2 receptors and of IL-2 on the activated CTL-P. IL-2 produced by the CTL-P itself and/or by proliferating T_H cells then binds to the IL-2 receptors, in-

ducing proliferation and differentiation of the CTL-P into an effector CTL (see Figure 14-1).

3. The second phase of the CTL-mediated response involves several steps: recognition of specific target cells bearing antigen and class I MHC molecules, formation of CTL/target-cell conjugates, reorientation of cytoplasmic granules within the CTL towards the region of contact with the target cell, release of the granular contents within the zone of cellular adhesion, formation of pores in the target-cell membrane, dissociation of the CTL from the target cell, and the subsequent destruction of the target cell (see Figure 14-4). Perforin monomers released from the CTL granules insert into target-cell membrane and polymerize, forming pores through which granzyme proteases released from the CTL can enter the target cell (see Figure 14-7). Target-cell killing by CTLs appears to occur through apoptosis induced by the soluble granzymes released from the CTL or induced by the membrane-bound Fas ligand (see Figure 14-9).
4. Various nonspecific cytotoxic cells also can kill target cells without having to interact with antigen-MHC complexes. NK cells, for example, mediate lysis of tumor cells and virus-infected cells by perforin-induced pore formation, by a mechanism similar to that employed by CTLs. The expression of relatively high levels of class I MHC molecules on normal cells appears to protect them against NK cell–mediated killing. NK cell killing is regulated by the balance between positive signals generated by the engagement of activating receptors (NKR-P1 and others) and negative signals from inhibitory receptors (CD94/NKG2 and the KIR family) (see Figure 14-11).
5. NK cells and several other types of nonspecific cytotoxic cells can bind to the Fc region of antibody on target cells and subsequently release lytic enzymes, perforin, or TNF, which damage the target-cell membrane. This process, called antibody-dependent cell-mediated cytotoxicity (ADCC), thus directs nonspecific cytotoxic cells to specific target cells.
6. Cell-mediated immunity involving delayed-type hypersensitivity plays an important role in host defense against intracellular pathogens. DTH-associated T cells, or T_{DTH} cells, which differentiate from activated T_H cells, secrete a number of T_H1-like cytokines that cause macrophages to accumulate and to become activated. The activated macrophages, which are more effective killers of intracellular pathogens, are the primary effector cells in the DTH response (see Figure 14-15 and Table 14-3).

REFERENCES

Atkinson, EA, and RC Bleackley. 1995. Mechanisms of lysis by cytotoxic T cells. *Crit. Rev. Immunol.* **15**:359.

Berke, G. 1995. Unlocking the secrets of CTL and NK cells. *Immunol. Today* **16**:343.

Braud, VM, et al. 1998. HLA-E binds to natural killer cell receptors CD94/NKG2A, B, and C. *Nature* **391**:795–799.

Croft, M. 1994. Activation of naive, memory and effector T cells. *Curr. Opin. Immunol.* **6**:431.

Gray, D. 1994. Regulation of immunological memory. *Curr. Opin. Immunol.* **6**:425.

Griffiths, GM. 1995. The cell biology of CTL killing. *Curr. Opin. Immunol.* **7**:343.

Henkart, PA, and MV Sitkovsky. 1994. Two ways to kill target cells. *Curr. Biol.* **4**:923.

Kagi, D, et al. 1994. Fas and perforin as major mechanisms of T cell-mediated cytotoxicity. *Science* **265**:528.

Lanier, LL. 1998. NK cell receptors. *Annu. Rev. of Immunol.* **16**:359.

Long, EO. 1999. Regulation of immune responses through inhibitory receptors. *Annu. Rev. Immunol.* **17**:875–904.

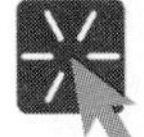

Useful Web Sites

http://www.cellsalive.com/ctl.htm
This Cells Alive subsite has a motion picture of cytotoxic T lymphocytes (CTLs) recognizing, attacking, and killing a much larger influenza virus-infected target. The sequence recorded by MT Esser and V Lam Braciale, of the University of Virginia Beirne B. Carter Center for Immunology Research represents 30 minutes elapsed time.

http://www.antibodyassay.com/nkcell.htm
The AAL Reference Laboratories Web site provides the rationale for clinical tests of NK cell function and tells how such tests are performed.

STUDY QUESTIONS

1. Indicate whether each of the following statements is true or false. If you believe a statement is false, explain why.

a. Cytokines can regulate which branch of the immune system is activated.

b. Both CTLs and NK cells release perforin after interacting with target cells.

c. Antigen activation of naive CTL-Ps requires a co-stimulatory signal delivered by interaction of CD28 and B7.

d. CTLs use a single mechanism to kill target cells.

e. The secretion of certain critical cytokines is the basis of the role played by T cells in DTH reactions.

2. You have a monoclonal antibody specific for LFA-1. You perform CML assays of a CTL clone, using target cells for which the clone is specific, in the presence and absence of this antibody. Predict the relative amounts of ^{51}Cr released in the two assays. Explain your answer.

Go to www.whfreeman.com/immunology Self-Test
Review and quiz of key terms

3. You decide to co-culture lymphocytes from the strains listed in the table below in order to observe the mixed-lymphocyte reaction (MLR). In each case, indicate which lymphocyte population(s) you would expect to proliferate.

Population 1	Population 2	Proliferation
C57BL/6 (H-2^b)	CBA (H-2^k)	
C57BL/6 (H-2^b)	CBA (H-2^k) mitomycin C-treated	
C57BL/6 (H-2^b)	(CBA × C57BL/6) F_1 (H-$2^{k/b}$)	
C57BL/6 (H-2^b)	C57L (H-2^b)	

4. In the mixed-lymphocyte reaction (MLR), the uptake of [^{3}H]thymidine often is used to assess cell proliferation.

a. Which cell type proliferates in the MLR?

b. How could you prove the identity of the proliferating cell?

c. Explain why production of IL-2 also can be used to assess cell proliferation in the MLR.

5. Indicate whether each of the properties listed below is exhibited by T_H cells, CTLs, both T_H cells and CTLs, or neither cell type.

a. ______ Can make IL-1

b. ______ Can make IL-2

c. ______ Is class I MHC restricted

d. ______ Expresses CD8

e. ______ Is required for B-cell activation

f. ______ Is cytotoxic for target cells

g. ______ Is the main proliferating cell in an MLR

h. ______ Is the effector cell in a CML assay

i. ______ Is class II MHC restricted

j. ______ Expresses CD4

k. ______ Is the primary effector cell in a DTH response

l. ______ Expresses CD3

m. ______ Adheres to target cells by LFA-1

n. ______ Can express the IL-2 receptor

o. ______ Expresses the αβ T-cell receptor

p. ______ Is the principal target of HIV

q. ______ Responds to soluble antigens alone

r. ______ Produces perforin

s. ______ Expresses the CD40 ligand on its surface

6. Mice from several different inbred strains were infected with LCM virus, and several days later their spleen cells were isolated. The ability of the primed spleen cells to lyse LCM-infected, ^{51}Cr-labeled target cells from various strains was determined. In the accompanying table, indicate with a (+) or (−) whether the spleen cells listed in the left column would cause ^{51}Cr release from the target cells listed in the headings across the top of the table.

7. A mouse is infected with influenza virus. How could you assess whether the mouse has T_H and T_C cells specific for influenza?

8. Explain why NK cells from a given host will kill many types of virus-infected cells but do not kill normal cells from that host.

9. Consider the following genetically altered mice and predict the outcome of the indicated procedures. H-2^d mice in which both perforin and Fas ligand have been knocked out are immunized with LCM virus. One week after immunization, T cells from these mice are harvested and tested for cytotoxicity on the following:

a. Target cells from normal LCM-infected H-2^b mice

b. Target cells from normal H-2^d mice

c. Target cells from H-2^d mice in which both perforin and Fas have been knocked out

d. Target cells from LCM infected normal H-2^d mice

e. Target cells from H-2^d mice in which both perforin and FasL have been knocked out

For use with Question 6:

Source of primed spleen cells	^{51}Cr release from LCM-infected target cells			
	B10.D2 (H-2^d)	B10 (H-2^b)	B10.BR (H-2^k)	(BALB/c × B10) F_1 (H-$2^{b/d}$)
B10.D2 (H-2^d)				
B10 (H-2^b)				
BALB/c (H-2^d)				
BALB/c × B10) (H-$2^{b/d}$)				

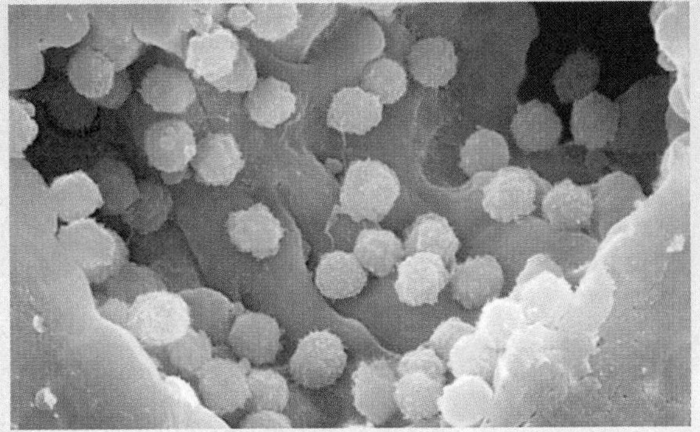

CHAPTER 15

LEUKOCYTE MIGRATION AND INFLAMMATION

Lymphocyte Recirculation

Cell-Adhesion Molecules

Neutrophil Extravasation

Lymphocyte Extravasation

Mediators of Inflammation

The Inflammatory Process

Anti-Inflammatory Agents

Many types of leukocytes move from one part of the body to another. This is especially true of lymphocytes, which circulate continually in the blood and lymph and, in common with other types of leukocytes, migrate into the tissues at sites of infection or tissue injury. This recirculation not only increases the chance that lymphocytes specific for a particular antigen will encounter that antigen but also is critical to development of an **inflammatory response.** Inflammation is a complex response to local injury or other trauma; it is characterized by redness, heat, swelling, and pain. Inflammation involves various immune-system cells and numerous mediators. Assembling and regulating inflammatory responses would be impossible without the controlled migration of leukocyte populations. This chapter covers the molecules and processes that play a role in leukocyte migration, various molecules that mediate inflammation, and the characteristic physiologic changes that accompany inflammatory responses.

Lymphocyte Recirculation

Lymphocytes are capable of a remarkable level of recirculation, continually moving through the blood and lymph to the various lymphoid organs (Figure 15-1). After a brief transit time of approximately 30 min in the bloodstream, nearly 45% of all lymphocytes are carried from the blood directly to the spleen, where they reside for approximately 5 h. Almost equal numbers (42%) of lymphocytes exit from the blood into various peripheral lymph nodes, where they reside for about 12 h. A smaller number of lymphocytes (10%) migrate to tertiary extralymphoid tissues by crossing between endothelial cells that line the capillaries. These tissues normally have few, if any, lymphoid cells but can import them during an inflammatory response. The most immunologically active tertiary extralymphoid tissues are those that interface with the external environment, such as the skin and various mucosal epithelia of the gastrointestinal, pulmonary, and genitourinary tracts.

The process of continual lymphocyte recirculation allows maximal numbers of antigenically committed lymphocytes to encounter and interact with antigen. An individual lymphocyte may make a complete circuit from the blood to the tissues and lymph and back again as often as 1–2 times per day. Since only about one in 10^5 lymphocytes recognizes a particular antigen, it would appear that a large number of antigen-committed T or B cells must contact antigen on a given antigen-presenting cell within a short time in order to generate a specific immune response. The odds of the small percentage of lymphocytes committed to a given antigen actually making contact with that antigen when it is present are elevated by the extensive recirculation of lymphocytes. The likelihood of such contacts is profoundly increased also by factors that regulate, organize, and direct the circulation of lymphocytes and antigen-presenting cells.

Cell-Adhesion Molecules

The vascular endothelium serves as an important "gatekeeper," regulating the movement of blood-borne molecules and leukocytes into the tissues. In order for circulating

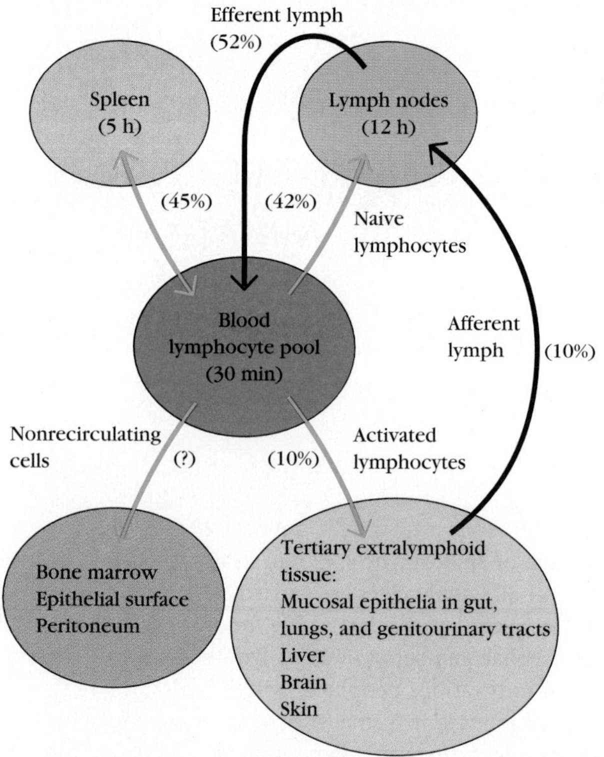

FIGURE 15-1 Lymphocyte recirculation routes. The percentage of the lymphocyte pool that circulates to various sites and the average transit times in the major sites are indicated. Lymphocytes migrate from the blood into lymph nodes through specialized areas in postcapillary venules called high-endothelial venules (HEVs). Although most lymphocytes circulate, some sites appear to contain lymphocytes that do not. [Adapted from A Ager, 1994, *Trends Cell Biol.* **4**:326.]

leukocytes to enter inflamed tissue or peripheral lymphoid organs, the cells must adhere to and pass between the endothelial cells lining the walls of blood vessels, a process called **extravasation.** Endothelial cells express leukocyte-specific **cell-adhesion molecules (CAMs).** Some of these membrane proteins are expressed constitutively; others are expressed only in response to local concentrations of cytokines produced during an inflammatory response. Recirculating lymphocytes, monocytes, and granulocytes bear receptors that bind to CAMs on the vascular endothelium, enabling these cells to extravasate into the tissues.

In addition to their role in leukocyte adhesion to vascular endothelial cells, CAMs on leukocytes also serve to increase the strength of the functional interactions between cells of the immune system. Various adhesion molecules have been shown to contribute to the interactions between T_H cells and APCs, T_H and B cells, and CTLs and target cells.

A number of endothelial and leukocyte CAMs have been cloned and characterized, providing new details about the extravasation process. Most of these CAMs belong to four families of proteins: the selectin family, the mucin-like family, the integrin family, and the immunoglobulin (Ig) superfamily (Figure 15-2).

Selectin Family

The **selectin** family of membrane glycoproteins has a distal lectin-like domain that enables these molecules to bind to specific carbohydrate groups. Selectins interact primarily with sialylated carbohydrate moieties, which are often linked to mucin-like molecules. The selectin family includes three molecules, designated L, E, and P. Most circulating leukocytes express L-selectin, whereas E-selectin and P-selectin are expressed on vascular endothelial cells. Selectin molecules are responsible for the initial stickiness of leukocytes to vascular endothelium.

Mucin-Like Family

Mucins are a group of serine- and threonine-rich proteins that are heavily glycosylated. Their extended structure allows them to present sialylated carbohydrate ligands to selectins. For example, L-selectin on leukocytes recognizes sialylated carbohydrates on two mucin-like molecules (CD34 and GlyCAM-1) expressed on certain endothelial cells of lymph nodes. Another mucin-like molecule (PSGL-1) found on neutrophils interacts with E- and P-selectin expressed on inflamed endothelium.

Integrin Family

The **integrins** are heterodimeric proteins (consisting of an α and a β chain) that are expressed by leukocytes and facilitate both adherence to the vascular endothelium and other cell-to-cell interactions. The integrins are grouped into categories according to which β subunit they contain. Different integrins are expressed by different populations of leukocytes, allowing these cells to bind to different CAMs that belong to the immunoglobulin superfamily expressed along the vascular endothelium. As described later, some integrins must be activated before they can bind with high affinity to their ligands. The importance of integrin molecules in leukocyte extravasation is demonstrated by **leukocyte-adhesion deficiency (LAD)**, an autosomal recessive disease described later in this chapter (see the Clinical Focus). It is characterized by recurrent bacterial infections and impaired healing of wounds.

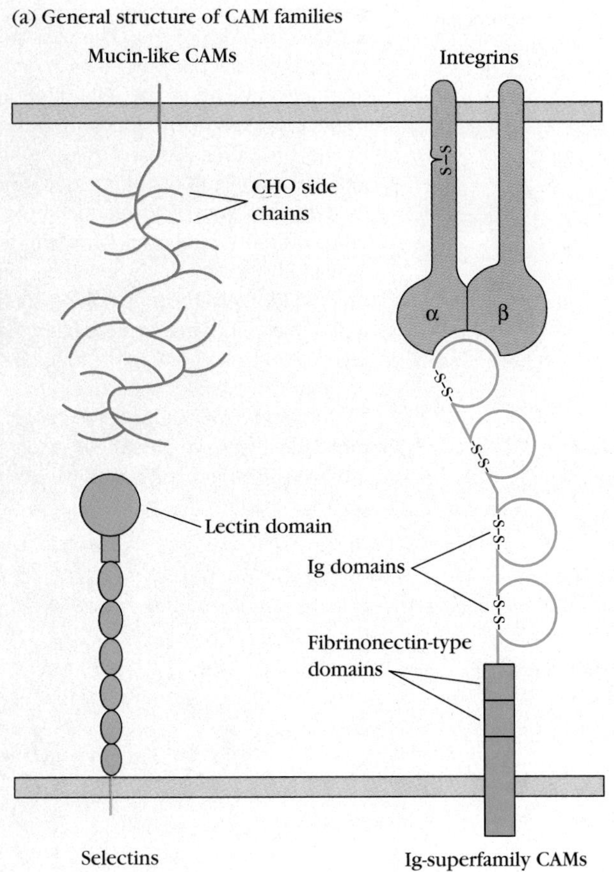

(b) Selected CAMs belonging to each family

Mucin-like CAMs:	Selectins:
GlyCAM-1	L-selectin
CD34	P-selectin
PSGL-1	E-selectin
MAdCAM-1	
Ig-superfamily CAMs:	**Integrins:**
ICAM-1, -2, -3	α4β1 (VLA-4, LPAM-2)
VCAM-1	α4β7 (LPAM-1)
LFA-2 (CD2)	α6β1 (VLA-6)
LFA-3 (CD58)	αLβ2 (LFA-1)
MAdCAM-1	αMβ2 (Mac-1)
	αXβ2 (CR4, p150/95)

FIGURE 15-2 Schematic diagrams depicting the general structures of the four families of cell-adhesion molecules (a) and a list of representative molecules in each family (b). The lectin domain in selectins interacts primarily with carbohydrate (CHO) moieties on mucin-like molecules. Both component chains in integrin molecules contribute to the binding site, which interacts with an Ig domain in CAMs belonging to the Ig superfamily. MAdCAM-1 contains both mucin-like and Ig-like domains and can bind to both selectins and integrins.

Immunoglobulin Superfamily

Several adhesion molecules contain a variable number of immunoglobulin-like domains and thus are classified in the **immunoglobulin superfamily.** Included in this group are ICAM-1, ICAM-2, ICAM-3, and VCAM, which are expressed on vascular endothelial cells and bind to various integrin molecules. An important cell-adhesion molecule called MAdCAM-1 has both Ig-like domains and mucin-like domains. This molecule is expressed on mucosal endothelium and directs lymphocyte entry into mucosa. It binds to integrins by its immunoglobulin-like domain and to selectins by its mucin-like domain.

Neutrophil Extravasation

As an inflammatory response develops, various cytokines and other inflammatory mediators act upon the local blood vessels, inducing increased expression of endothelial CAMs. The vascular endothelium is then said to be **activated,** or **inflamed.** Neutrophils are generally the first cell type to bind to inflamed endothelium and extravasate into the tissues. To accomplish this, neutrophils must recognize the inflamed endothelium and adhere strongly enough so that they are not swept away by the flowing blood. The bound neutrophils must then penetrate the endothelial layer and migrate into the underlying tissue. Monocytes and eosinophils extravasate by a similar process, but the steps have been best established for the neutrophil, so this description will focus on this cell.

The process of neutrophil extravasation can be divided into four sequential steps: (1) rolling, (2) activation by chemoattractant stimulus, (3) arrest and adhesion, and (4) transendothelial migration (Figure 15-3a). In the first step, neutrophils attach loosely to the endothelium by a low-affinity selectin-carbohydrate interaction. During an inflammatory response, cytokines and other mediators act upon the local endothelium, inducing expression of adhesion molecules of the selectin family. These E- and P-selectin molecules bind to mucin-like cell-adhesion molecules on the neutrophil membrane or with a sialylated lactosaminoglycan called sialyl Lewis^{x} (Figure 15-3b). This interaction tethers the neutrophil briefly to the endothelial cell, but the shear force of the circulating blood soon detaches the neutrophil.

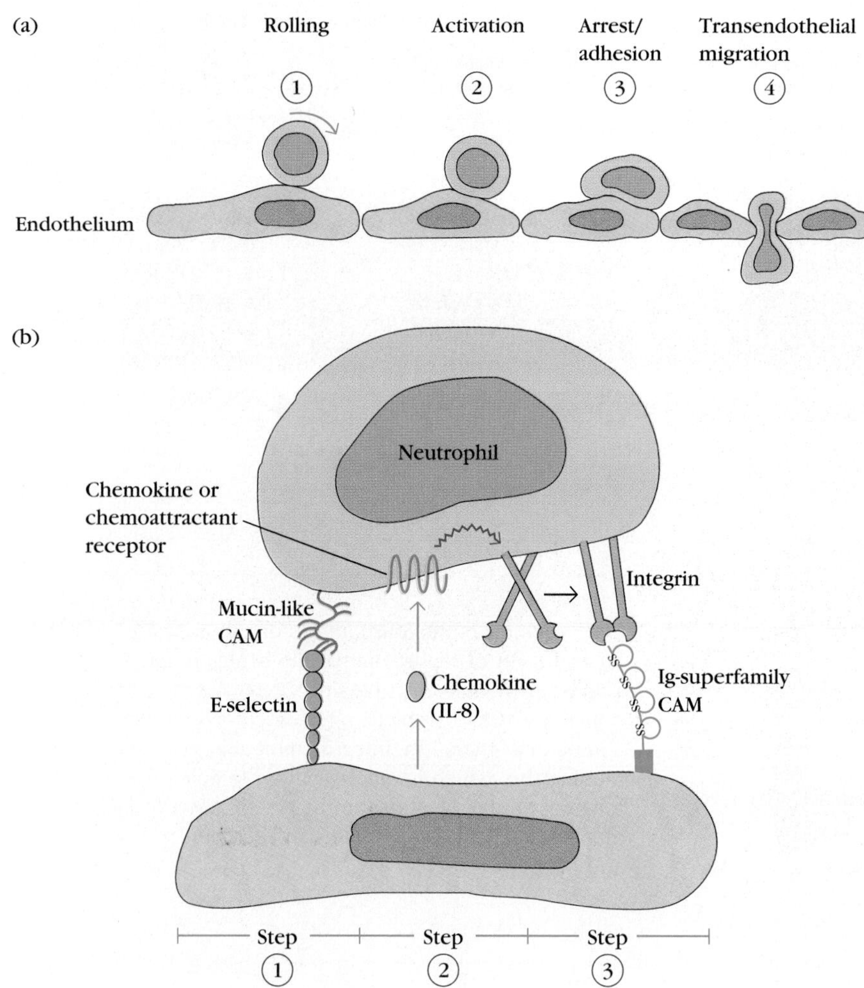

FIGURE 15-3 (a) The four sequential but overlapping steps in neutrophil extravasation. (b) Cell-adhesion molecules and chemokines involved in the first three steps of neutrophil extravasation. Initial rolling is mediated by binding of E-selectin molecules on the vascular endothelium to sialylated carbohydrate moieties on mucin-like CAMs. A chemokine such as IL-8 then binds to a G-protein–linked receptor on the neutrophil, triggering an activating signal. This signal induces a conformational change in the integrin molecules, enabling them to adhere firmly to Ig-superfamily molecules on the endothelium.

Selectin molecules on another endothelial cell again tether the neutrophil; this process is repeated so that the neutrophil tumbles end-over-end along the endothelium, a type of binding called rolling.

As the neutrophil rolls, it is activated by various **chemoattractants;** these are either permanent features of the endothelial cell surface or secreted locally by cells involved in the inflammatory response. Among the chemoattractants are members of a large family of chemoattractive cytokines called **chemokines.** Two chemokines involved in the activation process are interleukin 8 (IL-8) and macrophage inflammatory protein (MIP-1β). However, not all chemoattractants belong to the chemokine group. Other chemoattractants are platelet-activating factor (PAF), the complement split products C5a, C3a, and C5b67 and various *N*-formyl peptides produced by the breakdown of bacterial proteins during an infection. Binding of these chemoattractants to receptors on the neutrophil membrane triggers an activating signal mediated by **G proteins** associated with the receptor. This signal induces a conformational change in the integrin molecules in the neutrophil membrane, increasing their affinity for the Ig-superfamily adhesion molecules on the endothelium. Subsequent interaction between integrins and Ig-superfamily CAMs stabilizes adhesion of the neutrophil to the endothelial cell, enabling the cell to adhere firmly to the endothelial cell.

Subsequently, the neutrophil migrates through the vessel wall into the tissues. The steps in transendothelial migration and how it is directed are still largely unknown; they are thought to be mediated by further activation by chemoattractants and subsequent integrin-Ig superfamily interactions or by a separate migration stimulus.

Lymphocyte Extravasation

Various subsets of lymphocytes exhibit directed extravasation at inflammatory sites and secondary lymphoid organs. The recirculation of lymphocytes thus is carefully controlled to ensure that appropriate populations of B and T cells are recruited into different tissues. As with neutrophils, extravasation of lymphocytes involves interactions among a number of cell-adhesion molecules (Table 15-1). The overall

Go to www.whfreeman.com/immunology **Animation**
Leukocyte Extravasation

TABLE 15-1 SOME INTERACTIONS BETWEEN CELL-ADHESION MOLECULES IMPLICATED IN LEUKOCYTE EXTRAVASATION*

Receptor on cells	Expression	Ligands on endothelium	Step involving interaction†	Main function
CLA or ESL-1	Effector T cells	E-selectin	Tethering/rolling	Homing to skin and migration into inflamed tissue
L-selectin	All leukocytes	GlyCAM-1, CD34, MAdCAM-1	Tethering/rolling	Lymphocyte recirculation via HEVs to peripheral lymph nodes and migration into inflamed tertiary sites
LFA-1 (αLβ2)	Leukocyte subsets	ICAM-1, 2, 3	Adhesion/arrest	General role in lymphocyte extravasation via HEVs and leukocyte migration into inflamed tissue
LPAM-1 (α4β7)	Effector T cells, monocytes	MAdCAM-1, VCAM-1	Rolling/adhesion	Homing of T cells to gut via mucosal HEV; migration into inflamed tissue
Mac-1 (αMβ2)	Monocytes	VCAM-1	—	Monocyte migration into inflamed tissue
PSGL-1	Neutrophils	E- and P-selectin	Tethering/rolling	Neutrophil migration into inflamed tissue
VLA-4 (α4β1)	Neutrophils, T cells, monocytes	VCAM-1, MAdCAM-1, fibronectin	Rolling/adhesion	General role in leukocyte migration into inflamed tissue
VLA-6 (α6β1)	T cells,	Laminin	—	Homing of progenitor T cells to thymus; possible role in T-cell homing to nonmucosal sites

*Most endothelial and leukocyte CAMs belong to four groups of proteins as shown in Figure 15-2. In general, molecules in the integrin family bind to Ig-superfamily CAMs, and molecules in the selectin family bind to mucin-like CAMs. Members of the selectin and mucin-like families can be expressed on both leukocytes and endothelial cells, whereas integrins are expressed only on leukocytes, and Ig-superfamily CAMs are expressed only on endothelium.

†See Figures 15-3a and 15-7 for an illustration of steps in the extravasation process.

process is similar to what happens during neutrophil extravasation and comprises the same four stages of contact and rolling, activation, arrest and adhesion, and, finally, transendothelial migration.

High-Endothelial Venules

Some regions of vascular endothelium in postcapillary venules of various lymphoid organs are composed of specialized cells with a plump, cuboidal ("high") shape; such regions are called **high-endothelial venules**, or **HEVs** (Figure 15-4a, b). Their cells contrast sharply in appearance with the flattened endothelial cells that line the rest of the capillary. Each of the secondary lymphoid organs, with the exception of the spleen, contains HEVs. When frozen sections of lymph nodes, Peyer's patches, or tonsils are incubated with lymphocytes and washed to remove unbound cells, over 85% of the bound cells are found adhering to HEVs, even though HEVs account for only 1%–2% of the total area of the frozen section (Figure 15-4c).

It has been estimated that as many as 1.4×10^4 lymphocytes extravasate every second through HEVs into a single lymph node. The development and maintenance of HEVs in lymphoid organs is influenced by cytokines produced in response to antigen capture. For example, HEVs fail to develop in animals raised in a germ-free environment. The role of antigenic activation of lymphocytes in the maintenance of HEVs has been demonstrated by surgically blocking the afferent lymphatic vasculature to a node, so that antigen entry to the node is blocked. Within a short period of time, the HEVs show impaired function and eventually revert to a more flattened morphology.

(a)

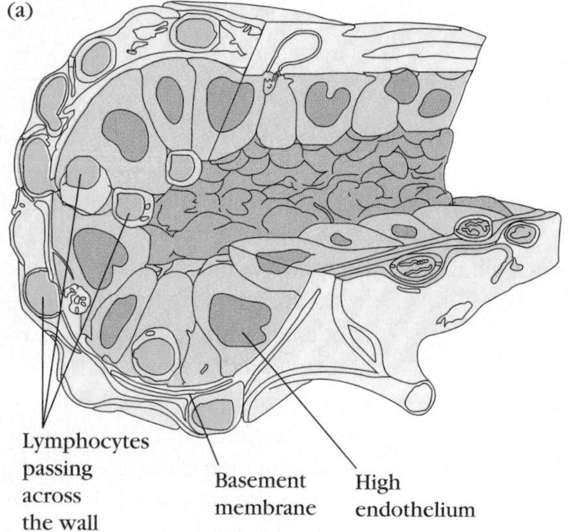

(b)

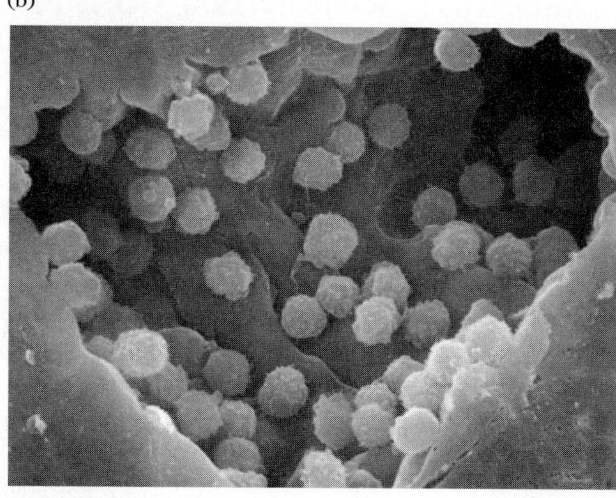

(c)

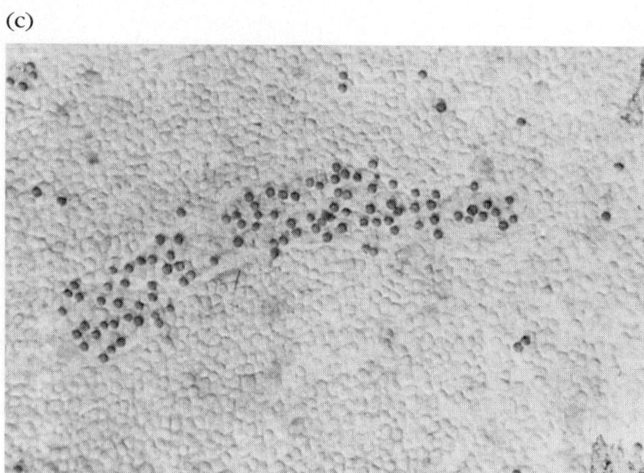

FIGURE 15-4 (a) Schematic cross-sectional diagram of a lymph-node postcapillary venule with high endothelium. Lymphocytes are shown in various stages of attachment to the HEV and in migration across the wall into the cortex of the node. (b) Scanning electron micrograph showing numerous lymphocytes bound to the surface of a high-endothelial venule. (c) Micrograph of frozen sections of lymphoid tissue. Some 85% of the lymphocytes (darkly stained) are bound to HEVs (in cross section), which comprise only 1%–2% of the total area of the tissue section. [Part (a) adapted from AO Anderson and ND Anderson, 1981, in *Cellular Functions in Immunity and Inflammation*, JJ Oppenheim et al (eds.), Elsevier, North-Holland; part (b) from SD Rosen and LM Stoolman, 1987, *Vertebrate Lectins*, Van Nostrand Reinhold; part (c) from SD Rosen, 1989, *Curr. Opin. Cell Biol.* **1**:913.]

High-endothelial venules express a variety of cell-adhesion molecules. Like other vascular endothelial cells, HEVs express CAMs of the selectin family (E- and P-selectin), the mucin-like family (GlyCAM-1 and CD34), and the immunoglobulin superfamily (ICAM-1, ICAM-2, ICAM-3, VCAM-1, and MAdCAM-1). Some of these adhesion molecules are distributed in a tissue-specific manner. These tissue-specific adhesion molecules have been called **vascular addressins (VAs)** because they serve to direct the extravasation of different populations of recirculating lymphocytes to particular lymphoid organs.

Homing of Lymphocytes

The general process of lymphocyte extravasation is similar to neutrophil extravasation. An important feature distinguishing the two processes is that different subsets of lymphocytes migrate differentially into different tissues. This process is called **trafficking,** or **homing.** The different trafficking patterns of lymphocyte subsets are mediated by receptors on the surface of recirculating lymphocytes that recognize particular vascular addressins on the HEVs of different secondary lymphoid tissues and endothelium at sites of inflammation. Because these receptors direct the circulation of various populations of lymphocytes to particular lymphoid and inflammatory tissues, they have been called **homing receptors.** Researchers have identified a number of lymphocyte and endothelial cell-adhesion molecules that participate in the interaction of lymphocytes with HEVs and with endothelium at tertiary sites or sites of inflammation (see Table 15-1). It has become apparent that a variety of factors, including differences in vascular addressins and homing receptors, contribute to trafficking differences among lymphocyte subsets. As is described later, in the section on chemokines, these molecules play a major role in determining the heterogeneity of lymphocyte circulation patterns.

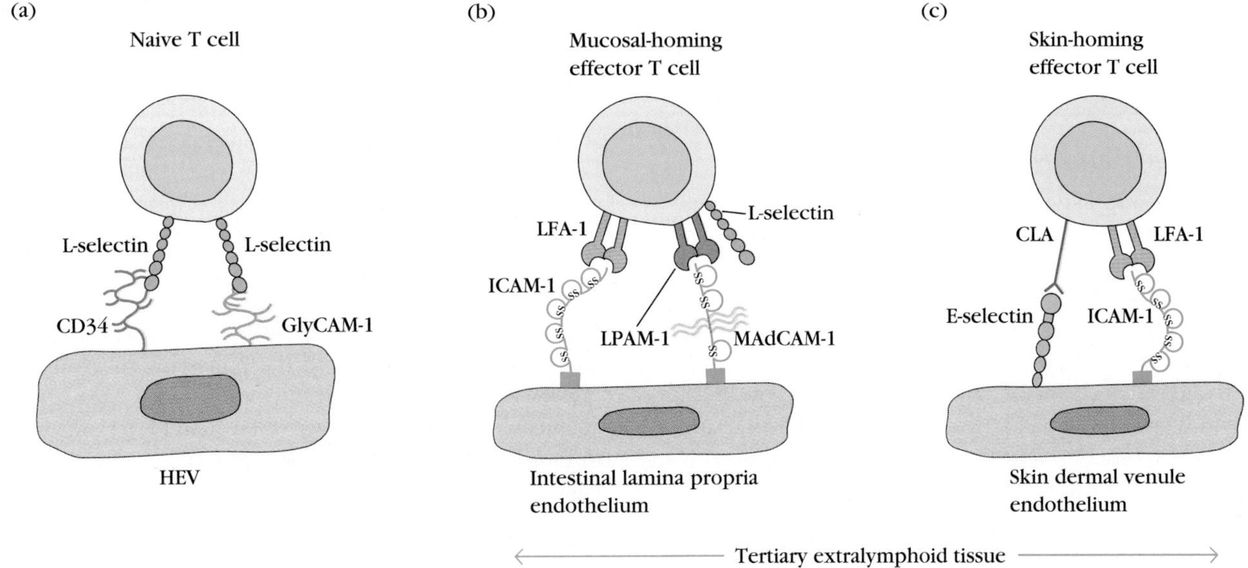

FIGURE 15-5 Examples of homing receptors and vascular addressins involved in selective trafficking of naive and effector T cells. (a) Naive T cells tend to home to secondary lymphoid tissues through their HEV regions. The initial interaction involves the homing receptor L-selectin and mucin-like cell-adhesion molecules such as CD34 or GlyCAM-1 expressed on HEV cells. (b, c) Various subsets of effector T cells express high levels of particular homing receptors that allow them to home to endothelium in particular tertiary extralymphoid tissues. The initial interactions in homing of effector T cells to mucosal and skin sites are illustrated.

Naive Lymphocytes

A naive lymphocyte is not able to mount an immune response until it has been activated to become an effector cell. Activation of a naive cell occurs in specialized microenvironments within secondary lymphoid tissue (e.g., peripheral lymph nodes, Peyer's patches, tonsils, and spleen). Within these specialized microenvironments, dendritic cells capture antigen and present it to the naive lymphocyte, resulting in its activation. Naive cells do not exhibit a preference for a particular type of secondary lymphoid tissue but instead circulate indiscriminately to secondary lymphoid tissue throughout the body by recognizing adhesion molecules on HEVs.

The initial attachment of naive lymphocytes to HEVs is generally mediated by the binding of the homing receptor L-selectin to adhesion molecules such as GlyCAM-1 and CD34 on HEVs (Figure 15-5a). The trafficking pattern of naive cells is designed to keep these cells constantly recirculating through secondary lymphoid tissue, whose primary function is to trap blood-borne or tissue-borne antigen. Since only about 1 in 10^5 lymphocytes is specific for a particular antigen, this type of trafficking helps to maximize the probability that the antigen will be encountered by a lymphocyte that recognizes it.

Once naive lymphocytes encounter antigen trapped in a secondary lymphoid tissue, they become activated and enlarge into lymphoblasts. Activation takes about 48 h, and during this time the blast cells are retained in the paracortical region of the secondary lymphoid tissue. During this phase, called the shut-down phase, the antigen-specific lymphocytes cannot be detected in the circulation (Figure 15-6). Rapid proliferation and differentiation of naive cells occurs

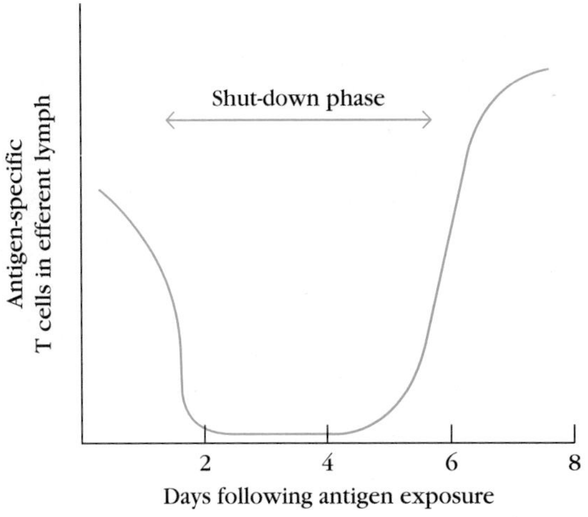

FIGURE 15-6 T-cell activation in the paracortical region of a lymph node results in the brief loss of lymphocyte recirculation. During this shut-down phase, antigen-specific T cells cannot be detected leaving the node in the efferent lymph.

during the shut-down phase. The effector and memory cells that are generated by this process then leave the lymphoid tissue and begin to recirculate.

Effector and Memory Lymphocytes

The trafficking patterns of effector and memory lymphocytes differ from those of naive lymphocytes. Effector cells tend to home to regions of infection by recognizing inflamed vascular endothelium and chemoattractant molecules that are generated during the inflammatory response. Memory lymphocytes, on the other hand, home selectively to the type of tissue in which they first encountered antigen. Presumably this ensures that a particular memory cell will return to the tissue where it is most likely to reencounter a subsequent threat by the antigen it recognizes.

Effector and memory cells express increased levels of certain cell-adhesion molecules, such as LFA-1, that are capable of interacting with ligands present on tertiary extralymphoid tissue (such as skin and mucosal epithelia) and at sites of inflammation, in addition to the ligands in secondary lymphoid organs. Such interactions allow effector and memory cells to enter these sites, while naive cells, which express a high level of L-selectin and low levels of molecules interacting with these sites, do not home to these sites. Inflamed endothelium expresses a number of adhesion molecules, including E- and P-selectin and the Ig-superfamily molecules VCAM-1 and ICAM-1, that bind to the receptors expressed at high levels on memory and effector cells.

Unlike naive lymphocytes, which do not exhibit a preference for a particular type of secondary lymphoid tissue, subsets of the memory and effector populations exhibit tissue-selective homing behavior. Such tissue specificity is imparted not by a single adhesion receptor but by different combinations of adhesion molecules. For example, a mucosal homing subset of memory/effector cells has high levels of the integrins LPAM-1 ($\alpha4\beta7$) and LFA-1 ($\alpha L\beta2$), which bind to MAdCAM and various ICAMs on intestinal lamina propria venules (see Figure 15-5b). However, these cells avoid direction to secondary lymphoid tissues because they have low levels of the L-selectin that would facilitate their entry into secondary lymphoid tissue. A second subset of memory/effector cells displays preferential homing to the skin. This subset also expresses low levels of L-selectin but displays high levels of cutaneous lymphocyte antigen (CLA) and LFA-1, which bind to E-selectin and ICAMs on dermal venules of the skin (see Figure 15-5c). Although effector and memory cells that express reduced levels of L-selectin do not tend to home through HEVs into peripheral lymph nodes, they can enter peripheral lymph nodes through the afferent lymphatic vessels.

Adhesion-Molecule Interactions

The extravasation of lymphocytes into secondary lymphoid tissue or regions of inflammation is a multistep process involving a cascade of adhesion-molecule interactions similar to those involved in neutrophil emigration from the bloodstream. Figure 15-7 depicts the typical interactions in extravasation of naive T cells across HEVs into lymph nodes. The first step is usually a selectin-carbohydrate interaction similar to that seen with neutrophil adhesion. Naive lymphocytes initially bind to HEVs by L-selectin, which serves

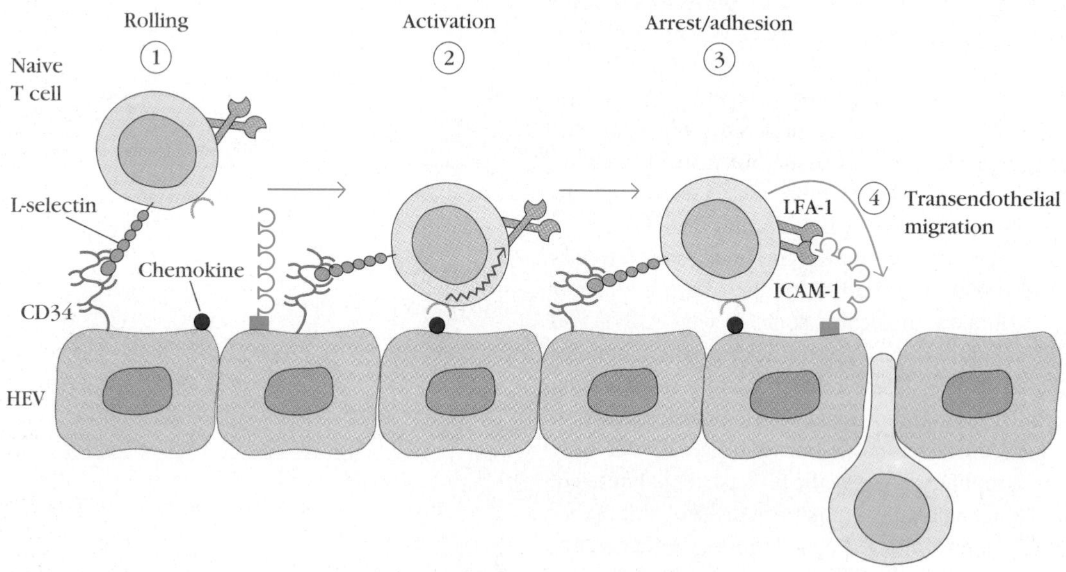

FIGURE 15-7 Steps in extravasation of a naive T cell through a high-endothelial venule into a lymph node. Extravasation of lymphocytes includes the same basic steps as neutrophil extravasation but some of the cell-adhesion molecules differ. Activation of the integrin LFA-1, induced by chemokine binding to the lymphocyte, leads to firm adhesion followed by migration between the endothelial cells into the tissue.

as a homing receptor that directs the lymphocytes to particular tissues expressing a corresponding mucin-like vascular addressin such as CD34 or GlyCAM-1. Lymphocyte rolling is less pronounced than that of neutrophils. Although the initial selectin-carbohydrate interaction is quite weak, the slow rate of blood flow in postcapillary venules, particularly in regions of HEVs, reduces the likelihood that the shear force of the flowing blood will dislodge the tethered lymphocyte.

In the second step, an integrin-activating stimulus is mediated by chemokines that are either localized on the endothelial surface or secreted locally. The thick glycocalyx covering of the HEVs may function to retain these soluble chemoattractant factors on the HEVs. If, as some have proposed, HEVs secrete lymphocyte-specific chemoattractants, it would explain why neutrophils do not extravasate into lymph nodes at the HEVs even though they express L-selectin. Chemokine binding to G protein–coupled receptors on the lymphocyte leads to activation of integrin molecules on the membrane, as occurs in neutrophil extravasation. Once activated, the integrin molecules interact with Ig-superfamily adhesion molecules (e.g., ICAM-1), so the lymphocyte adheres firmly to the endothelium. The molecular mechanisms involved in the final step, transendothelial migration, are poorly understood.

Mediators of Inflammation

During an inflammatory response, a variety of mediators are released by cells of the innate and acquired immune systems. These mediators serve to trigger or enhance specific aspects of the inflammatory response. They are released by tissue mast cells, blood platelets, and a variety of leukocytes, including neutrophils, monocytes/macrophages, eosinophils, basophils, and lymphocytes.

Chemokines

Chemokines are a superfamily of small polypeptides, most of which contain 90–130 amino acid residues. They selectively, and often specifically, control the adhesion, chemotaxis, and activation of many types of leukocyte populations and subpopulations. Consequently, they are major regulators of leukocyte traffic. A variety of lymphoid and nonlymphoid tissues can produce chemokines, often in connection with the initiation or progress of inflammation. However, members of this group are also involved in the regulation of normal leukocyte traffic into, out of, and within lymphoid tissues and organs. Chemokines cause leukocytes to move into various tissue sites by inducing the adherence of these cells to the vascular endothelium. After migrating into tissues, leukocytes are attracted toward high localized concentrations of chemokines. Recent work has also shown that some chemokines are involved in the development of nonlymphoid tissues, such as the heart.

The chemokines possess four conserved cysteine residues and can be separated into two distinctive subgroups based on the position of two of the four invariant cysteine residues.

- **C-C subgroup** chemokines, in which the conserved cysteines are contiguous
- **C-X-C subgroup** chemokines, in which the conserved cysteines are separated by some other amino acid (X)

Chemokine action is mediated by receptors whose polypeptide chain traverses the membrane seven times. Because of their snakelike pattern of repeated penetration and emergence from the membrane, they are called serpentine receptors. When they bind the appropriate chemokine, these receptors activate large GTP-binding proteins, which are heterotrimeric G proteins. This initiates signal transduction processes that generate such potent second messengers as cAMP, IP_3, Ca^2, and activated small G proteins (Figure 15-8).

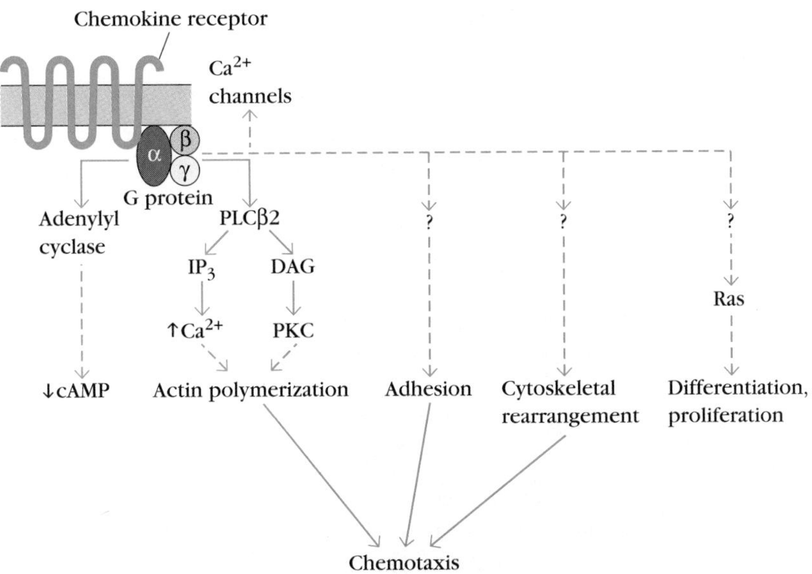

FIGURE 15-8 Chemokines signal through receptors coupled with large heterotrimeric G proteins. Binding of a chemokine to its receptor activates many signal-transduction pathways, resulting in a variety of modifications in the physiology of the target cell. If the signal-transduction pathway is not known or incompletely worked out, dashed lines and question marks are used here to represent probable pathways. [Adapted from Premack et al, 1996, *Nature Medicine* **2:**1174.]

Dramatic changes are effected by the chemokine-initiated activation of these signal transduction pathways. Within seconds, the addition of an appropriate chemokine to leukocytes causes abrupt and extensive changes in shape, the promotion of greater adhesiveness to endothelial walls by activation of leukocyte integrins, and the generation of microbicidal oxygen radicals in phagocytes. These signal-transduction pathways promote other changes such as the release of granular contents, proteases in neutrophils and macrophages, histamine from basophils, and cytotoxic proteins from eosinophils. As might be expected, processes that depend on chemokine signaling are inhibited by *Bordetella pertussis* toxin, a protein that blocks the action of the Gα subunit of large G proteins.

A large number (more than 50) of chemokines and multiple (14) chemokine receptors have been described (Table 15-2). There are two subgroups of receptors, CXC receptors (CXCRs), which recognize CXC chemokines, and CC receptors (CCRs), which recognize CC chemokines. As with cytokines, the interaction between chemokines and their receptors is of high affinity ($K_a > 10^9$) and high specificity. However, as Table 15-2 shows, most receptors bind more than one chemokine. For example, CXCR2 recognizes at least six different chemokines, and many chemokines can bind to more than one receptor. For example, RANTES can be bound by CCR1, CCR3, CCR4, CCR5, and CCR10. Different cells display different profiles of chemokine receptors (Figure 15-9). Among major populations of human leukocytes, neutrophils express CXCR1, CXCR2, and CXCR4; eosinophils have CCR1 and CCR3. While resting naive T cells display few types of chemokine receptors, some activated T cells have CCR1, CCR2, CCR3, CCR5, CXCR3, CXCR4, and possibly others. Clearly, a cell can respond to a chemokine only if it possesses a receptor that recognizes it. Consequently, differences in the expression of chemokine receptors by leukocytes coupled with the production of distinctive profiles of chemokines by destination tissues and sites provide rich opportunities for the differential regulation of activities of different leukocyte populations. Indeed, differences in patterns of chemokine receptor expression occur within leukocyte populations as well as between different ones. Recall that T_H1 and T_H2 subsets of T_H cells can be distinguished by their different patterns of cytokine production. These subsets also display different profiles of chemokine receptors. T_H2 cells express CCR3, CCR4, and a number of other receptors not expressed by T_H1 cells. On the other hand, T_H1 cells express CCR5 and CXCR3, but most T_H2 cells do not.

TABLE 15-2 HUMAN CHEMOKINES AND THEIR RECEPTORS*

Chemokine receptors	Chemokines bound by receptor
CXC subgroup	
CXCR1	IL-8, GCP-2
CXCR2	IL-8, Gro-α, Gro-β, Gro-γ, NAP-2, ENA-78
CXCR3	IP-10, Mig, I-TAC
CXCR4	SDF-1, PBSF
CXCR5	BCA-1
CC subgroup	
CCR1	MIP-1, RANTES, MCP-2, MIP-5
CCR2	MCP-1, MCP-2, MCP-3
CCR3	Eotaxin, RANTES, MCP-2, MCP-3, MCP-4, Eotaxin-2, MIP-5
CCR4	TARC, RANTES
CCR5	MIP-1α RANTES, MIP-1β
CCR6	Exodus-1
CCR7	ELC
CCR8	1-309
CCR10	MCP-1, MCP-2, MCP-3, RANTES
Both CC and CXC subgroups	
DARC (the Duffy antigen of RBCs)	Binds to a number of CC and CXC chemokines

*This table lists most known chemokine receptors but not all chemokines. The full names for a number of the chemokines abbreviated in the table are as follows: ELC (Ebl1 ligand chemokine); ENA-78 (epithelial-cell-derived neutrophil-activating protein); GCP-2 (granulocyte chemotactic protein 2); Gro-α, β, γ (growth-related oncogene α, β, γ); MCP-1, 2, 3, or 4 (monocyte chemoattractant protein 1, 2, 3, or 4); Mig (monokine induced by interferon γ); MIP-1α, 1β, or 5 (macrophage inflammatory protein 1α, 1β, or 5); NAP-2 (neutrophil-activating protein 2); RANTES (*r*egulated upon *a*ctivation, *n*ormal *T*-cell *e*xpressed and *s*ecreted); TARC (thymus- and activation-regulated chemokine).

SOURCE: Adapted from Nelson and Krensky, 1998, *Curr. Opin. Immunol.* **10:**265, and Baggiolini, 1998, *Nature* **392:**565.

Plasma Enzyme Mediators

Plasma contains four interconnected mediator-producing systems: the kinin system, the clotting system, the fibrinolytic system, and the complement system. With the exception of the complement system, these systems share a common intermediate, as illustrated in Figure 15-10. When tissue damage occurs, these four systems are activated to form a web of interacting systems that generate a number of mediators of inflammation.

Kinin System

The kinin system is an enzymatic cascade that begins when a plasma clotting factor, called Hageman factor, is activated following tissue injury. The activated Hageman factor then activates prekallikrein to form kallikrein, which cleaves

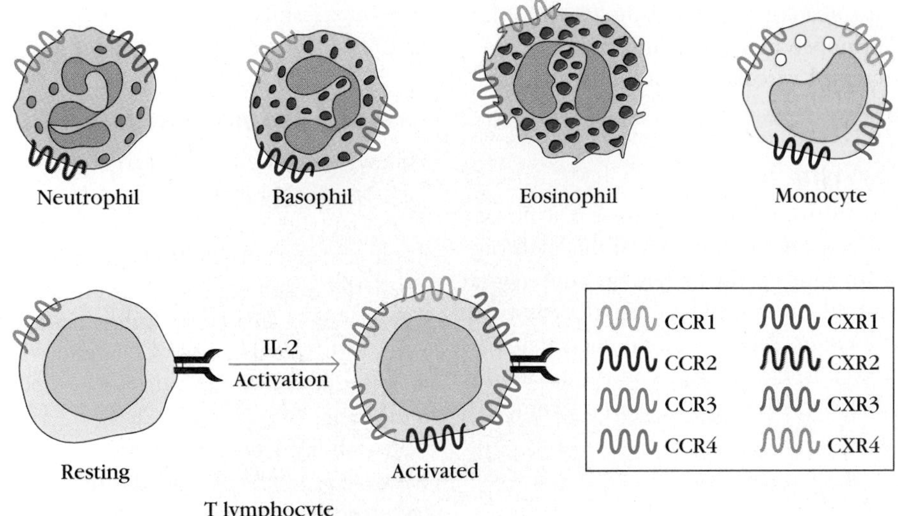

FIGURE 15-9 Patterns of expression of some principal chemokine receptors on different classes of human leukocytes. So far the greatest variety of chemokine receptors has been observed on activated T lymphocytes. (Adapted from M Baggiolini, 1998, *Nature* **392:**565.)

kininogen to produce **bradykinin** (see Figure 15-10). This inflammatory mediator is a potent vasoactive basic peptide that increases vascular permeability, causes vasodilation, induces pain, and induces contraction of smooth muscle. Kallikrein also acts directly on the complement system by cleaving C5 into C5a and C5b. The C5a complement component is an anaphylatoxin that induces mast cell degranulation, resulting in the release of a number of inflammatory mediators from the mast cell.

Clotting System

Another enzymatic cascade that is triggered by damage to blood vessels yields large quantities of thrombin. Thrombin acts on soluble fibrinogen in tissue fluid or plasma to produce insoluble strands of **fibrin** and **fibrinopeptides.** The insoluble fibrin strands crisscross one another to form a **clot,** which serves as a barrier to the spread of infection. The clotting system is triggered very rapidly after tissue injury to prevent

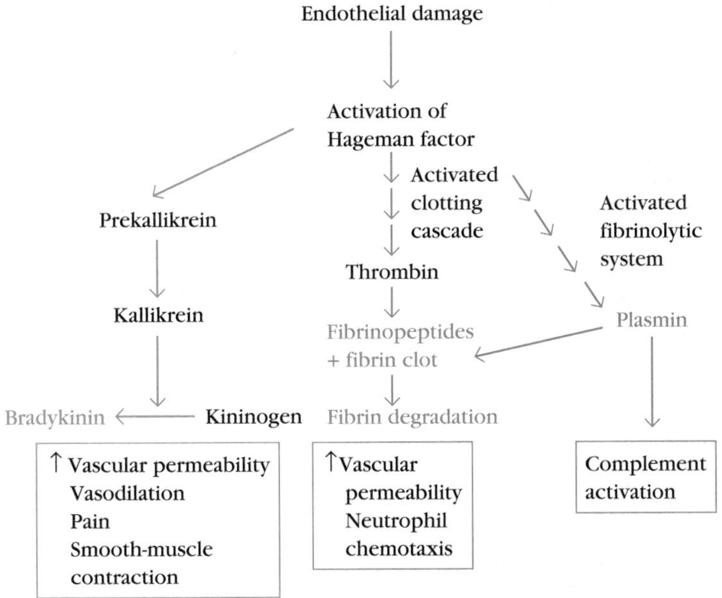

FIGURE 15-10 Tissue damage induces formation of plasma enzyme mediators by the kinin system, the clotting system, and the fibrinolytic system. These mediators cause vascular changes, among the earliest signs of inflammation, and various other effects. Plasmin not only degrades fibrin clots but also activates the classical complement pathway.

bleeding and limit the spread of invading pathogens into the bloodstream. The fibrinopeptides act as inflammatory mediators, inducing increased vascular permeability and neutrophil chemotaxis.

Fibrinolytic System

Removal of the fibrin clot from the injured tissue is achieved by the fibrinolytic system. The end product of this pathway is the enzyme **plasmin,** which is formed by the conversion of plasminogen. Plasmin, a potent proteolytic enzyme, breaks down fibrin clots into degradation products that are chemotactic for neutrophils. Plasmin also contributes to the inflammatory response by activating the classical complement pathway.

Complement System

Activation of the complement system by both classical and alternative pathways results in the formation of a number of complement split products that serve as important mediators of inflammation. Binding of the **anaphylatoxins** (C3a, C4a, and C5a) to receptors on the membrane of tissue mast cells induces degranulation with release of histamine and other pharmacologically active mediators. These mediators induce smooth-muscle contraction and increases in vascular permeability. C3a, C5a, and C5b67 act together to induce monocytes and neutrophils to adhere to vascular endothelial cells, extravasate through the endothelial lining of the capillary, and migrate toward the site of complement activation in the tissues. Activation of the complement system thus results in influxes of fluid that carries antibody and phagocytic cells to the site of antigen entry.

Lipid Inflammatory Mediators

Following membrane perturbations, phospholipids in the membrane of several cell types (e.g., macrophages, monocytes, neutrophils, and mast cells) are degraded into arachidonic acid and lyso–platelet-activating factor (Figure 15-11). The latter is subsequently converted into platelet-activating factor (PAF). This factor causes platelet activation and has many inflammatory effects, including eosinophil chemotaxis and the activation and degranulation of neutrophils and eosinophils.

Metabolism of arachidonic acid by the cyclooxygenase pathway produces **prostaglandins** and **thromboxanes.** Different prostaglandins are produced by different cells: monocytes and macrophages produce large quantities of PGE2 and PGF2; neutrophils produce moderate amounts of PGE2; mast cells produce PGD2. Prostaglandins have diverse physiological effects, including increased vascular permeability, increased vascular dilation, and induction of neutrophil chemotaxis. The thromboxanes cause platelet aggregation and constriction of blood vessels.

Arachidonic acid is also metabolized by the lipoxygenase pathway to yield **leukotrienes.** There are four leukotrienes: LTB4, LTC4, LTD4, and LTE4. Three of these (LTC4, LTD4, and LTE4) together make up what was formerly called **slow-reacting substance of anaphylaxis (SRS-A)**; these mediators induce smooth muscle contraction. LTB4 is a potent chemoat-

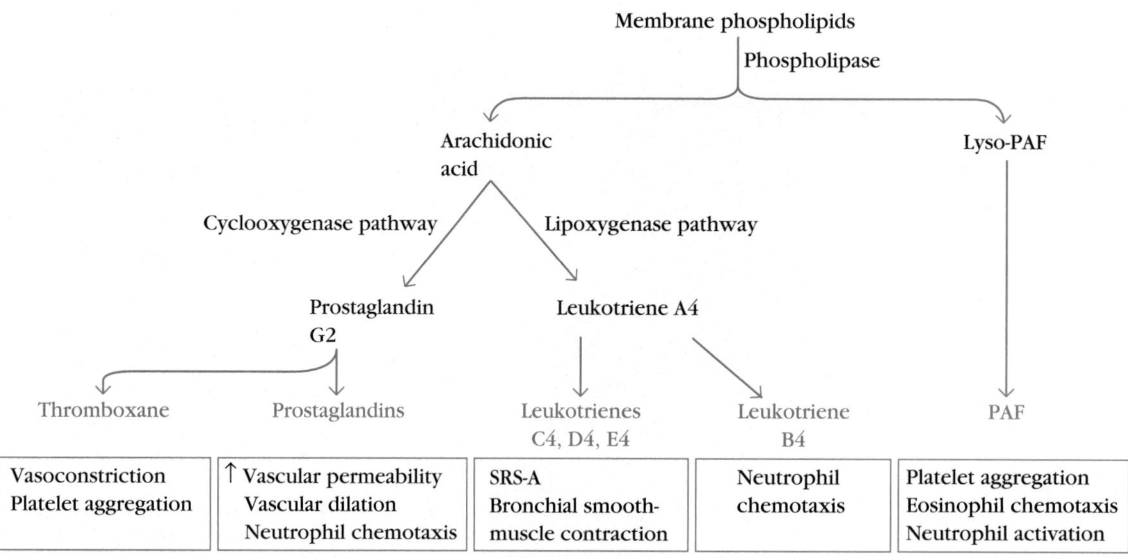

FIGURE 15-11 The breakdown of membrane phospholipids generates important mediators of inflammation, including thromboxane, prostaglandins, leukotrienes, and platelet-activating factor (PAF).

tractant of neutrophils. The leukotrienes are produced by a variety of cells, including monocytes, macrophages, and mast cells.

Cytokine Inflammatory Mediators

A number of cytokines play a significant role in the development of an acute or chronic inflammatory response. IL-1, IL-6, TNF-α, IL-12, and many chemokines exhibit redundant and pleiotropic effects that together contribute to the inflammatory response. Some of the effects mediated by IL-1, IL-6, and TNF-α are listed in Table 15-3. In addition, IFN-γ contributes to the inflammatory response, acting later in the acute response and contributing in a major way to chronic inflammation by attracting and activating macrophages. IL-12 induces the differentiation of the proinflammatory T_H1 subset. The role of several of these inflammatory cytokines in the development of acute and chronic inflammation will be described more fully in the next section.

TABLE 15-3 REDUNDANT AND PLEIOTROPIC EFFECTS OF IL-1, TNF-α, AND IL-6

Effect	IL-1	TNF-α	IL-6
Endogenous pyrogen fever	+	+	+
Synthesis of acute-phase proteins by liver	+	+	+
Increased vascular permeability	+	+	+
Increased adhesion molecules on vascular endothelium	+	+	−
Fibroblast proliferation	+	+	−
Platelet production	+	−	+
Chemokine induction (e.g., IL-8)	+	+	−
Induction of IL-6	+	+	−
T-cell activation	+	+	+
B-cell activation	+	+	+
Increased immunoglobulin synthesis	−	−	+

The Inflammatory Process

Inflammation is a physiologic response to a variety of stimuli such as infections and tissue injury. In general, an acute inflammatory response has a rapid onset and lasts a short while. Acute inflammation is generally accompanied by a systemic response, known as the acute-phase response, which is characterized by a rapid alteration in the levels of several plasma proteins. In some diseases persistent immune activation can result in chronic inflammation, which often has pathologic consequences.

Central Role of Neutrophils in Inflammation

In the early stages of an inflammatory response, the predominant cell type infiltrating the tissue is the neutrophil. Neutrophil infiltration into the tissue peaks within the first 6 h of an inflammatory response. Neutrophil production in the bone marrow increases to meet this need. A normal adult produces more than 10^{10} neutrophils per day, but during a period of acute inflammation, neutrophil production may increase as much as tenfold.

The neutrophils leave the bone marrow and circulate within the blood. In response to mediators of acute inflammation, vascular endothelial cells increase their expression of E- and P-selectin. Thrombin and histamine induce increased expression of P-selectin; cytokines such as IL-1 or TNF-α induce increased expression of E-selectin. The circulating neutrophils express mucins such as PSGL-1 or the tetrasaccharides sialyl Lewis^a and sialyl Lewis^x, which bind to E- and P-selectin.

As described earlier, this binding mediates the attachment or tethering of neutrophils to the vascular endothelium, allowing the cells to roll in the direction of the blood flow. During this time, chemokines such as IL-8 or other chemoattractants act upon the neutrophils, triggering a G-protein–mediated activating signal that leads to a conformational change in the integrin adhesion molecules, resulting in neutrophil adhesion and subsequent transendothelial migration (see Figure 15-3).

Once in tissues, the activated neutrophils also express increased levels of receptors for chemoattractants and therefore exhibit **chemotaxis,** migrating up a gradient of the chemoattractant. Among the inflammatory mediators that are chemotactic for neutrophils are several chemokines, complement split products (C3a, C5a, and C5b67), fibrinopeptides, prostaglandins, and leukotrienes. In addition, molecules released by microorganisms, such as formyl methionyl peptides, are also chemotactic for neutrophils. Activated neutrophils express increased levels of Fc receptors for antibody and receptors for complement, enabling these cells to bind more effectively to antibody- or complement-coated pathogens, thus increasing phagocytosis.

The activating signal also stimulates metabolic pathways to a respiratory burst, which produces **reactive oxygen intermediates** and **reactive nitrogen intermediates**. Release of some of these reactive intermediates and the release of mediators from neutrophil primary and secondary granules (proteases, phospholipases, elastases, and collagenases) play an important role in killing various pathogens. These substances also contribute to the tissue damage that can result from an inflammatory response. The accumulation of dead cells and microorganisms, together with accumulated fluid and various proteins, makes up what is known as pus.

Acute Inflammatory Response

Infection or tissue injury induces a complex cascade of nonspecific events, known as the inflammatory response, that provides early protection by restricting the tissue damage to the site of infection or tissue injury. The acute inflammatory response involves both localized and systemic responses.

Localized Response

The hallmarks of a localized acute inflammatory response, first described almost 2000 years ago, are swelling (*tumor*), redness (*rubor*), heat (*calor*), pain (*dolor*), and loss of function. Within minutes after tissue injury, there is an increase in vascular diameter (vasodilation), resulting in an increase in the volume of blood in the area and a reduction in the flow of blood. The increased blood volume heats the tissue and causes it to redden. Vascular permeability also increases, leading to leakage of fluid from the blood vessels, particularly at postcapillary venules. This results in an accumulation of fluid (**edema**) in the tissue and, in some instances, extravasation of leukocytes, contributing to the swelling and redness in the area. When fluid exudes from the bloodstream, the kinin, clotting, and fibrinolytic systems are activated (see Figure 15-10). Many of the vascular changes that occur early in a local response are due to the direct effects of plasma enzyme mediators such as bradykinin and fibrinopeptides, which induce vasodilation and increased vascular permeability. Some of the vascular changes are due to the indirect effects of the complement anaphylatoxins (C3a, C4a, and C5a), which induce local mast-cell degranulation with release of histamine. Histamine is a potent mediator of inflammation, causing vasodilation and smooth-muscle contraction. The prostaglandins can also contribute to the vasodilation and increased vascular permeability associated with the acute inflammatory response.

Within a few hours of the onset of these vascular changes, neutrophils adhere to the endothelial cells, and migrate out of the blood into the tissue spaces (Figure 15-12). These neutrophils phagocytose invading pathogens and release mediators that contribute to the inflammatory response. Among the mediators are the macrophage inflammatory proteins (MIP-1α and MIP-1β), chemokines that attract macrophages to the site of inflammation. Macrophages arrive about 5–6 hours after an inflammatory response begins. These macrophages are activated cells that exhibit increased phagocytosis and increased release of mediators and cytokines that contribute to the inflammatory response.

Activated tissue macrophages secrete three cytokines (IL-1, IL-6, and TNF-α) that induce many of the localized and systemic changes observed in the acute inflammatory response (see Table 15-3). All three cytokines act locally, inducing coagulation and an increase in vascular permeability. Both TNF-α and IL-1 induce increased expression of adhesion molecules on vascular endothelial cells. For instance, TNF-α stimulates expression of E-selectin, an endothelial adhesion molecule that selectively binds adhesion molecules on neutrophils. IL-1 induces increased expression of ICAM-1 and VCAM-1, which bind to integrins on lymphocytes and monocytes. Circulating neutrophils, monocytes, and lymphocytes adhere to the wall of a blood vessel by recognizing these adhesion molecules and then move through the vessel wall into the tissue spaces. IL-1 and TNF-α also act on macrophages and endothelial cells to induce production of the chemokines that contribute to the influx of neutrophils by increasing their adhesion to vascular endothelial cells and by acting as potent chemotactic factors. In addition, IFN-γ and TNF-α activate macrophages and neutrophils, promoting increased phagocytic activity and increased release of lytic enzymes into the tissue spaces.

A local acute inflammatory response can occur without the overt involvement of the immune system. Often, however, cytokines released at the site of inflammation facilitate both the adherence of immune-system cells to vascular endothelial cells and their migration through the vessel wall into the tissue spaces. The result is an influx of lymphocytes, neutrophils, monocytes, eosinophils, basophils, and mast cells to the site of tissue damage, where these cells participate in clearance of the antigen and healing of the tissue.

The duration and intensity of the local acute inflammatory response must be carefully regulated to control tissue damage and facilitate the tissue-repair mechanisms that are necessary for healing. TGF-β has been shown to play an important role in limiting the inflammatory response. It also promotes accumulation and proliferation of fibroblasts and the deposition of an extracellular matrix that is required for proper tissue repair.

Clearly, the processes of leukocyte adhesion are of great importance in the inflammatory response. A failure of proper leukocyte adhesion can result in disease as exemplified by leukocyte-adhesion deficiency (see Clinical Focus).

Systemic Acute-Phase Response

The local inflammatory response is accompanied by a systemic response known as the **acute-phase response** (Figure 15-13). This response is marked by the induction of fever, increased synthesis of hormones such as ACTH and hydrocortisone, increased production of white blood cells (leukocytosis), and production of a large number of **acute-phase proteins** in the liver. The increase in body temperature inhibits the growth of a number of pathogens and appears to enhance the immune response to the pathogen.

C-reactive protein is a prototype acute-phase protein whose serum level increases 1000-fold during an acute-phase

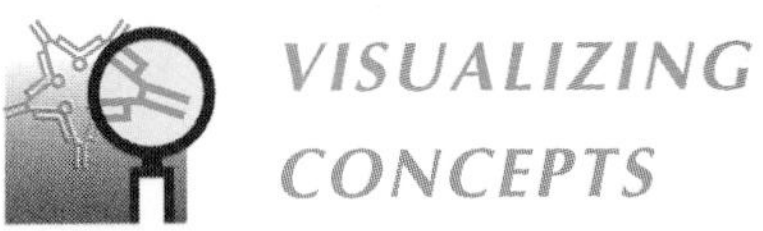

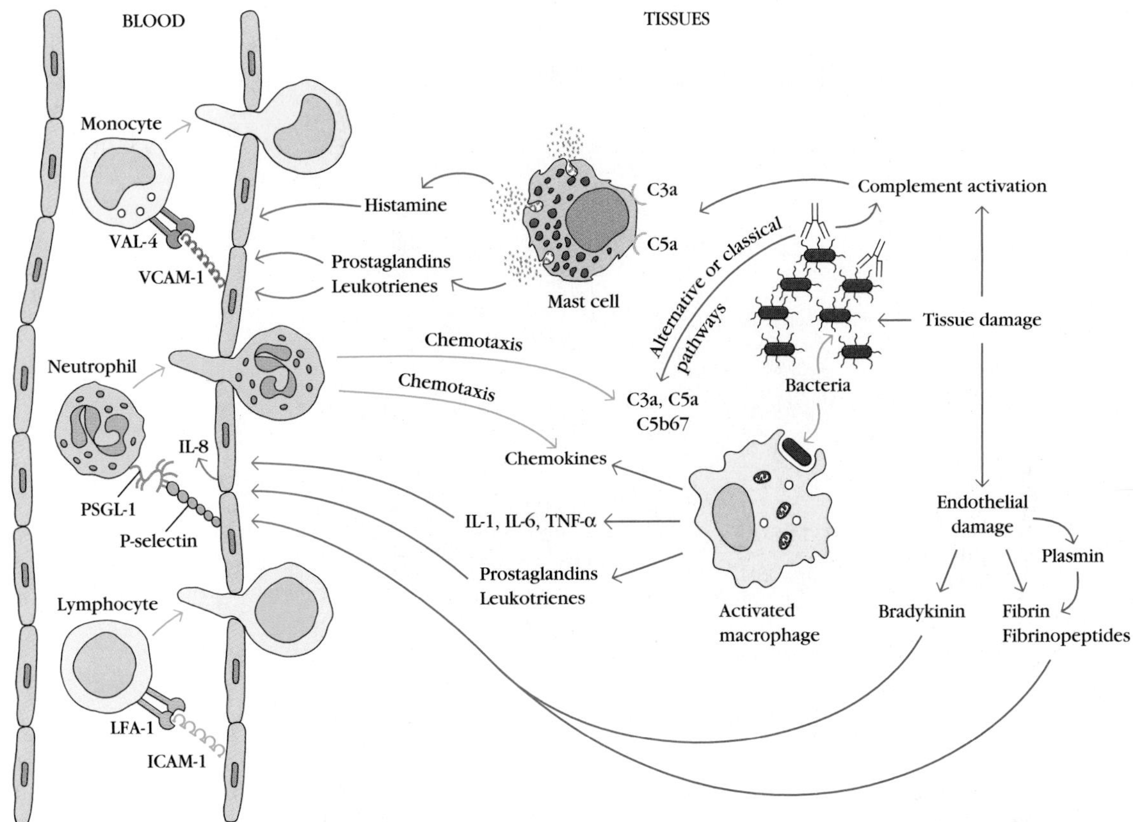

FIGURE 15-12 Overview of the cells and mediators involved in a local acute inflammatory response. Tissue damage leads to the formation of complement products that act as opsonins, anaphylatoxins, and chemotactic agents. Bradykinin and fibrinopeptides induced by endothelial damage mediate vascular changes. Neutrophils generally are the first leukocytes to migrate into the tissue, followed by monocytes and lymphocytes. Only some of the interactions involved in the extravasation of leukocytes are depicted.

response. It is composed of five identical polypeptides held together by noncovalent interactions. C-reactive protein binds to a wide variety of microorganisms and activates complement, resulting in deposition of the opsonin C3b on the surface of microorganisms. Phagocytic cells, which express C3b receptors, can then readily phagocytose the C3b-coated microorganisms.

Many systemic acute-phase effects are due to the combined action of IL-1, TNF-α and IL-6 (see Figure 15-13). Each of these cytokines acts on the hypothalamus to induce a fever response. Within 12–24 h of the onset of an acute-phase inflammatory response, increased levels of IL-1, TNF-α and IL-6 (as well as LIF and OSM) induce production of acute-phase proteins by hepatocytes. TNF-α also acts on vascular endothelial cells and macrophages to induce secretion of colony-stimulating factors (M-CSF, G-CSF, and GM-CSF). These CSFs stimulate hematopoiesis, resulting in transient increases in the number of white blood cells needed to fight the infection.

The redundancy in the ability of at least five cytokines (TNF-α, IL-1, IL-6, LIF, and OSM) to induce production of acute-phase proteins by the liver results from the induction of a common transcription factor, NF-IL6, after each of these cytokines interacts with its receptor. Amino acid sequencing of cloned NF-IL6 revealed that it has a high degree of sequence homology with C/EBP, a liver-specific transcription faction (Figure 15-14a). Both NF-IL6 and C/EBP contain a leucine-zipper domain and a basic DNA-binding domain, and both proteins bind to the same nucleotide sequence in the promoter or enhancer of the genes encoding various liver proteins. C/EBP, which stimulates production of albumin and transthyretin, is expressed constitutively by hepatocytes.

VISUALIZING CONCEPTS

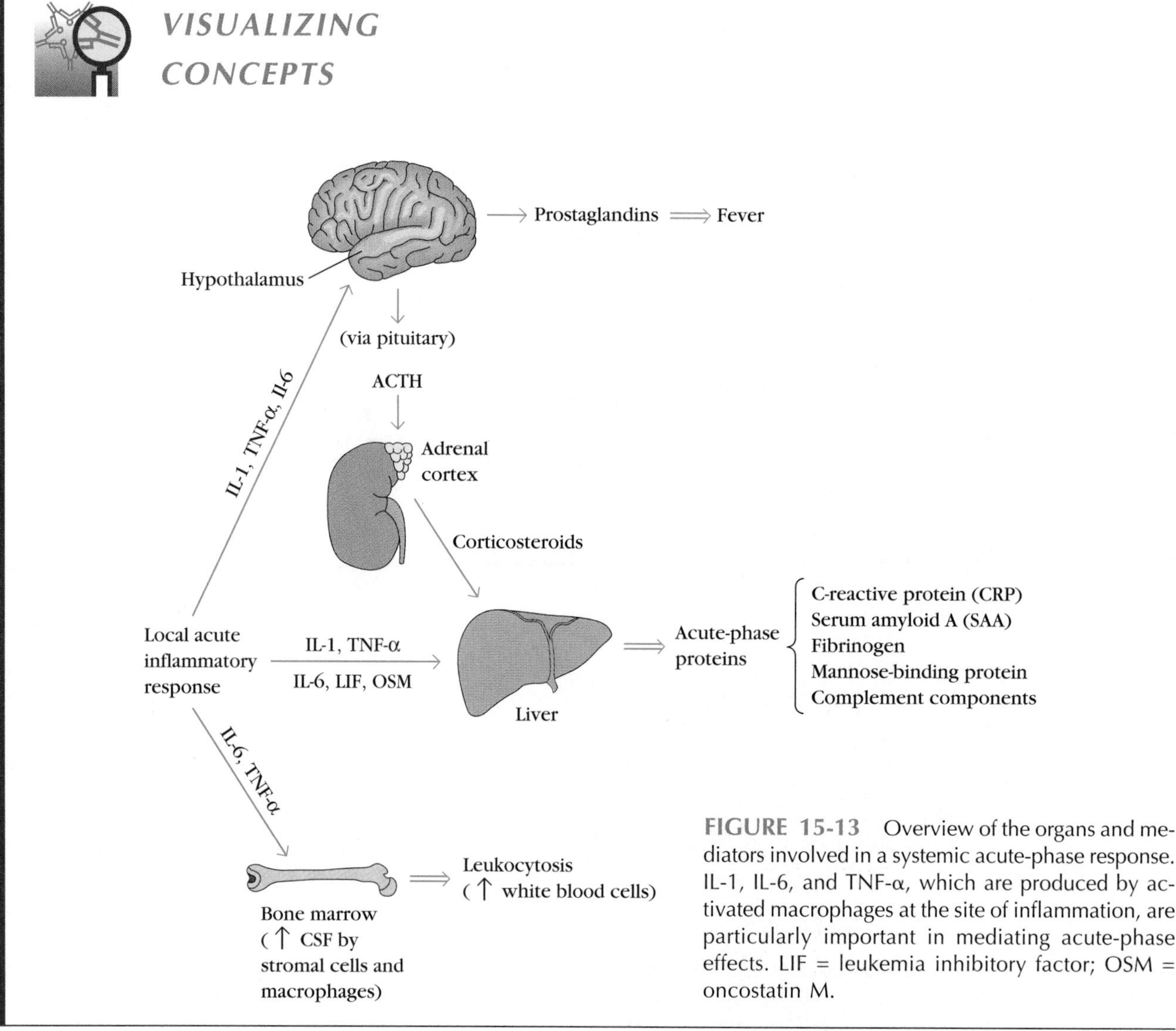

FIGURE 15-13 Overview of the organs and mediators involved in a systemic acute-phase response. IL-1, IL-6, and TNF-α, which are produced by activated macrophages at the site of inflammation, are particularly important in mediating acute-phase effects. LIF = leukemia inhibitory factor; OSM = oncostatin M.

As an inflammatory response develops and the cytokines interact with their respective receptors on liver hepatocytes, expression of NF-IL6 increases and that of C/EBP decreases (Figure 15-14b). The inverse relationship between these two transcription factors accounts for the observation that serum levels of proteins such as albumin and transthyretin decline while those of acute-phase proteins increase during an inflammatory response.

Chronic Inflammatory Response

Chronic inflammation develops because of the persistence of an antigen. Some microorganisms, for example, have cell-wall components that enable them to resist phagocytosis. Such organisms often induce a chronic inflammatory response, resulting in significant tissue damage. Chronic inflammation also occurs in a number of autoimmune diseases in which self-antigens continually activate T cells. Finally, chronic inflammation also contributes to the tissue damage and wasting associated with many types of cancer.

The accumulation and activation of macrophages is the hallmark of chronic inflammation. Cytokines released by the chronically activated macrophages also stimulate fibroblast proliferation and collagen production. A type of scar tissue develops at sites of chronic inflammation by a process called **fibrosis.** Although fibrosis is a wound-healing reaction, it can interfere with normal tissue function. Chronic inflammation often leads to formation of a **granuloma.** This is a tumor-like mass consisting of a central area of activated macrophages surrounded by activated lymphocytes. The center of the granuloma often contains multinucleated giant cells formed by the fusion of activated macrophages. These giant cells typically are surrounded by large modified macrophages that resemble epithelial cells and therefore are called epithelioid cells.

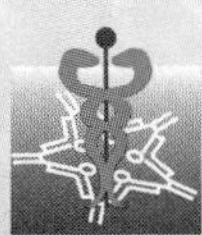

CLINICAL FOCUS

LEUKOCYTE-ADHESION DEFICIENCY (LAD) IN HUMANS AND CATTLE

The immune system uses inflammation to assemble the components of an effective response and focus these resources at the site of infection. Inflammation is complex and involves many processes (vasodilation, increased vascular permeability, exudation of plasma proteins, and a gathering of inflammatory cells). Chemoattractants are key elements in calling leukocytes to sites of inflamation. These include chemokines such as IL-8, monocyte chemoattractant protein 1 (MCP-1), macrophage inflammatory protein 1 (MIP-1) and peptide fragments, such as C5a, generated during complement fixation. Chemoattractants signal passing leukocytes to adhere tightly to the vascular surface, and, using adhesive interactions for traction, these cells push their way between lining endothelial cells and gain entry into the surrounding tissue. Once in, they are guided by gradients of chemoattractants to the sites of the inflammatory responses and become participants in the process. The key players in the adhesive interactions that are central to adhesion and extravasation are heterodimeric integrin molecules on the surface of the migrating leukocytes. There are a number of integrins, among which are LFA-1 (comprised of CD11a and CD18); Mac-1, also called CR3 (components: CD11b and CD18); and p150/95 or CR4 (components: CD11c and CD18). When leukocytes encounter the appropriate chemokine or other chemoattractant, their complement of membrane integrin molecules undergoes a conformational change that transforms them from a slightly adhesive to a highly adhesive state.

In 1979, a paper entitled "Delayed separation of the umbilical cord, widespread infections, and defective neutrophil mobility" appeared in *Lancet*, a British medical journal. This turned out to be the first in a series of reports that have appeared over the years describing patients afflicted with a rare autosomal recessive disease in which the first indication is quite often omphalitis, a swelling and reddening around the stalk of the umbilical cord. Although no more susceptible to virus infections than normal controls, those afflicted with this disorder suffer recurrent and often chronic bacterial infections, and sites where one would expect to find pus are instead pus-free. This observation is particularly striking because the patients are not deficient in granulocytes; in fact, they typically have greatly elevated numbers of granulocytes in the circulation. Detailed immunological workups of these patients showed that Ig levels were in the normal range and that they had nearly normal B-, T-, and NK-cell function. However, examination of leukocyte migration in response to tissue damage revealed the root cause of the disease in these patients.

One method of evaluating leukocyte migration involves gently scraping the skin from a small area of the arm; the cell populations that move into the abraded area are then sampled by capturing some of those cells on a glass coverslip placed onto the wounded skin. A series of glass coverslips is sequentially placed, incubated, and removed over a period of several hours. Typically, each coverslip is left in place for two hours, and the procedure is repeated four times over an eight-hour period. Examination of the coverslips under a microscope reveals whether leukocytes have adhered to the coverslips. In normal individuals, the response of the immune system to tissue injury is to deliver leukocytes to the damaged area, and one finds these cells on the coverslips. However, in the patients described here, the coverslips were largely negative for leukocytes. Examination of white blood cells in these patients revealed an absence of CD18, an essential component of a number of integrins. A key element in the migration of leukocytes is integrin-mediated cell adhesion, and these patients suffer from an inability of their leukocytes to undergo adhesion-dependent migration into sites of inflammation. Hence, this syndrome has been named leukocyte-adhesion deficiency (LAD).

Bacterial infections in these patients can be treated with antibiotics, but they recur. Furthermore, there are antibiotic-resistant strains of many pathogenic bacteria, and LAD patients must live under this microbial Sword of Damocles, never knowing when the life-saving thread of antibiotics will fail. If a suitable bone-marrow donor can be found (almost always a close relative), though, there is a curative strategy. The LAD patient's hematopoietic system is destroyed, perhaps by treatment with cytotoxic chemicals, and then bone-marrow transplantation is performed. If successful, this procedure provides the patient with leukocytes that have normal levels of functional integrin and display the full range of migratory capacities.

This disease is not limited to humans. A strikingly similar version known as bovine leukocyte adhesion disease (BLAD) occurs in cattle. The cause of BLAD in

(continued)

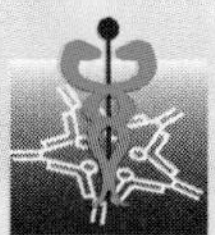

CLINICAL FOCUS (continued)

these animals is identical to the cause of LAD in human patients—the lack of a functional integrin subunit. What is different in some dairy herds is the incidence of the disease; though rare in humans, it can occur at economically important frequencies in cattle. This is a consequence of the high degree of inbreeding that exists in populations of dairy cattle. Typically, dairy herds are sired by the artificial insemination of semen from very few bulls. As a consequence of this practice, by the 1980s, almost 1 in 20 dairy bulls could be traced back to a single Holstein bull who happened to be heterozygous for BLAD. Such a high frequency of this recessive trait in the sire population dramatically raised the frequency of this disease in dairy herds. During the early 1990s, in some countries, the incidence of the BLAD gene was as high as 10% in a number of dairy herds. The gene for bovine CD18 has been cloned; this has allowed the design of a PCR-based assay for the aberrant forms of this gene. It is now possible to routinely screen sires and recipients for the BLAD allele. As a result, bulls that are carriers of the BLAD gene have been identified and eliminated from the breeding pool. This has led to a dramatic reduction in the frequency of new BLAD cases and in the overall frequency of the BLAD allele in dairy herd populations.

Role of IFN-γ and TNF-α

Two cytokines in particular, IFN-γ and TNF-α, play a central role in the development of chronic inflammation. T_H1 cells, NK cells, and T_C cells release IFN-γ, while activated macrophages secrete TNF-α.

All three members of the interferon family of glycoproteins (IFN-α, IFN-β, and IFN-γ) are released from virus-infected cells and confer antiviral protection on neighboring cells. Exactly which interferon is produced depends on the type of cell infected. IFN-α is produced by leukocytes, IFN-β, often called fibroblast interferon, is made largely by fibroblasts, and IFN-γ is produced exclusively by T cells and NK cells. However, IFN-γ has a number of pleiotropic activities that distinguish it from IFN-α and IFN-β and contribute to the inflammatory response (Figure 15-15). One of the most striking effects of IFN-γ is its ability to activate macrophages. Activated macrophages exhibit increased expression of class II MHC molecules, increased cytokine production, and increased microbicidal activity compared with nonactivated macrophages; thus, they are more effective in antigen pres-

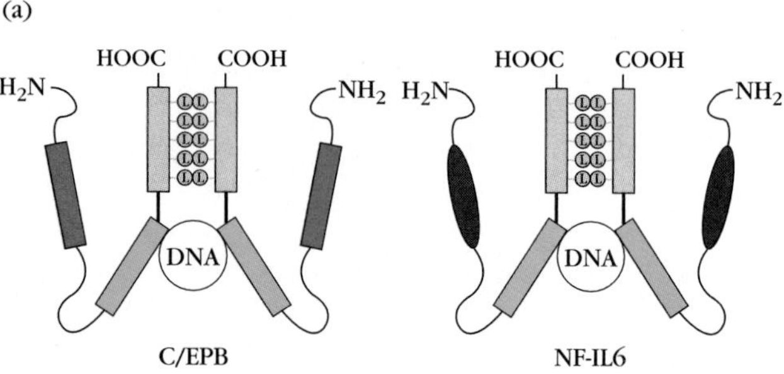

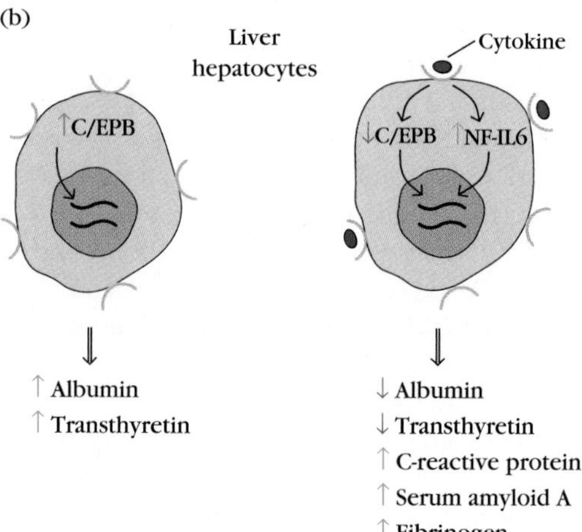

FIGURE 15-14 Comparison of the structure and function of C/EBP and NF-IL6. (a) Both transcription factors are dimeric proteins containing a leucine-zipper domain (light orange) and a basic DNA-binding domain (blue). (b) C/EBP is expressed constitutively in liver hepatocytes and promotes transcription of albumin and transthyretin genes. During an inflammatory response, binding of IL-1, IL-6, TNF-α, LIF, or OSM to receptors on liver hepatocytes induces production of NF-IL6, which promotes transcription of the genes encoding various acute-phase proteins. Concurrently, C/EBP levels decrease and the levels of albumin and transthyretin consequently decrease.

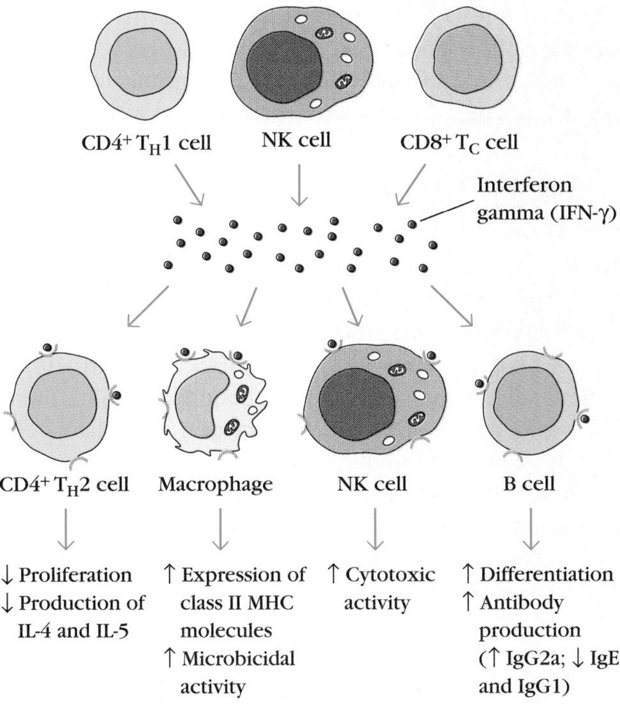

FIGURE 15-15 Summary of pleiotropic activity of interferon gamma (IFN-γ). The activation of macrophages induced by IFN-γ plays a critical role in chronic inflammation. This cytokine is secreted by T_H1 cells, NK cells, and T_C cells and acts on numerous cell types. [Adapted from Research News, 1993, *Science* **259:**1693.]

entation and killing of intracellular microbial pathogens. In a chronic inflammatory response, the accumulation of large numbers of activated macrophages is responsible for much of the tissue damage. These cells release various hydrolytic enzymes and reactive oxygen and nitrogen intermediates, which damage the surrounding tissue.

One of the principal cytokines secreted by activated macrophages is TNF-α. The activity of this cytokine was first observed around the turn of the century by a surgeon, William Coley. He noted that when cancer patients developed certain bacterial infections, the tumors would become necrotic. In the hope of providing a cure for cancer, Coley began to inject cancer patients with supernatants derived from various bacterial cultures. These culture supernatants, called "Coley's toxins," did induce hemorrhagic necrosis in the tumors but had numerous undesirable side effects, making them unsuitable for cancer therapy. Decades later, the active component of Coley's toxin was shown to be a lipopolysaccharide (endotoxin) component of the bacterial cell wall. This endotoxin does not itself induce tumor necrosis but instead induces macrophages to produce TNF-α. This cytokine has a direct cytotoxic effect on tumor cells but not on normal cells (Figure 15-16a). Potential immunotherapeutic approaches using TNF-α for the treatment of cancer are examined in Chapter 22.

Several lines of evidence indicate that TNF-α also contributes to much of the tissue wasting that characterizes chronic inflammation. For example, mice carrying a TNF-α transgene become severely wasted (Figure 15-16b). In studies by A. Cerami and coworkers, rabbits were found to lose nearly half of their body mass within 2 months of being infected with trypanosomes. These workers subsequently discovered that a macrophage-derived factor was responsible for the profound wasting; they called the factor cachetin.

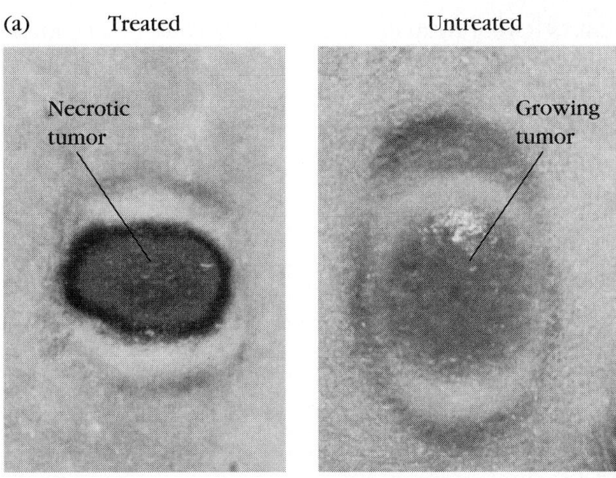

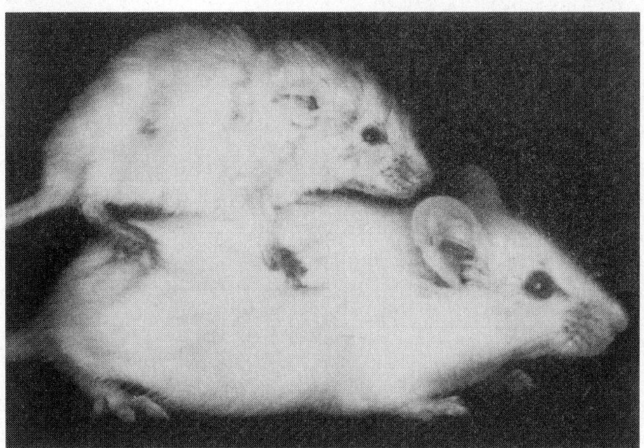

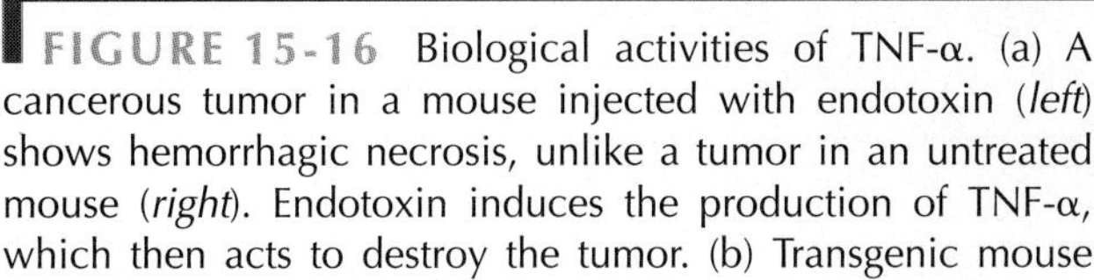
FIGURE 15-16 Biological activities of TNF-α. (a) A cancerous tumor in a mouse injected with endotoxin (*left*) shows hemorrhagic necrosis, unlike a tumor in an untreated mouse (*right*). Endotoxin induces the production of TNF-α, which then acts to destroy the tumor. (b) Transgenic mouse (*top*) bearing a TNF-α transgene becomes anorectic and severely wasted. Normal mouse is shown on the bottom. [Part (a) from LJ Old, 1988, *Sci. Am.* **258:**59; part (b) from B Beutler, 1993, *Hosp. Prac.* (April 15):45.]

Cloning of the genes for TNF-α and cachetin revealed that they were the same protein.

Activation of macrophages by IFN-γ promotes increased transcription of the TNF-α gene and increases the stability of TNF-α mRNA. Both effects result in increased TNF-α production. TNF-α acts synergistically with IFN-γ to initiate a chronic inflammatory response. Both cytokines together induce much greater increases in ICAM-1, E-selectin, and class I MHC molecules than either cytokine alone. The increase in intercellular adhesion molecules facilitates the recruitment of large numbers of cells in a chronic inflammatory response.

Chronic Inflammatory Diseases

Recent studies suggest that regions of plump endothelial cells resembling HEVs appear along the vasculature in tertiary extralymphoid sites of chronic infection. These HEV-like regions, which appear to be sites of lymphocyte extravasation into the inflamed tissue, express several mucins (e.g., GlyCAM-1, MAdCAM-1, and CD34) that are often displayed on normal HEVs. Several cytokines, notably IFN-γ and TNF-α, that are associated with chronic inflammation may play a role in the induction of HEV-like regions along the vasculature.

These HEV-like regions have been observed in a number of chronic inflammatory diseases in humans, including rheumatoid arthritis, Crohn's disease, ulcerative colitis, Graves' disease, Hashimoto's thyroiditis, and diabetes mellitus (Table 15-4). Development of this HEV-like vasculature is likely to facilitate a large-scale influx of leukocytes, contributing to chronic inflammation. These observations suggest that an effective approach for treating chronic inflammatory diseases may be to try to control the development of these HEV-like regions.

Anti-Inflammatory Agents

Although development of an effective inflammatory response can play an important role in the body's defense, the response can sometimes be detrimental. Allergies, autoimmune diseases, microbial infections, transplants, and burns may initiate a chronic inflammatory response. Various therapeutic approaches are available for reducing long-term inflammatory responses and thus the complications associated with them.

Agents That Reduce Leukocyte Extravasation

Because leukocyte extravasation is an integral part of the inflammatory response, one approach for reducing inflammation is to impede this process. Theoretically, one way to reduce leukocyte extravasation is to block the activity of various adhesion molecules with antibodies. In animal models, for example, antibodies to the integrin LFA-1 have been used to reduce neutrophil buildup in inflammatory tissue. Antibodies to ICAM-1 have also been used, with some success, in preventing the tissue necrosis associated with burns and in reducing the likelihood of kidney-graft rejection in animal models. The results with antibodies specific for these adhesins have been so encouraging that a combination of antibodies (anti-ICAM-1 and anti-LFA-1) was used in clinical trials on human kidney-transplant patients. A combination of two anti-adhesins had to be used because failure to block both LFA-1 and ICAM-1 results in rejection.

Corticosteroids

The corticosteroids, which are cholesterol derivatives, include prednisone, prednisolone, and methylprednisolone. These potent anti-inflammatory agents exert various effects that result in a reduction in the numbers and activity of immune-system cells. They are regularly used in anti-inflammatory therapy.

Corticosteroid treatment causes a decrease in the number of circulating lymphocytes as the result either of steroid-induced lysis of lymphocytes (lympholysis) or of alterations in lymphocyte-circulation patterns. Some species (e.g., hamster, mouse, rat, and rabbit) are particularly sensitive to cor-

TABLE 15-4 CHRONIC INFLAMMATORY DISEASES ASSOCIATED WITH HEV-LIKE VASCULATURE

Disease	Affected organ	Plump endothelium	Mucin-like CAMs on endothelium*
Crohn's disease	Gut	+	+
Diabetes mellitus	Pancreas	+	+
Graves' disease	Thyroid	+	+
Hashimoto's thyroiditis	Thyroid	+	+
Rheumatoid arthritis	Synovium	+	+
Ulcerative colitis	Gut	+	+

*Includes GlyCAM-1, MAdCAM-1, and CD34.

SOURCE: Adapted from JP Girard and TA Springer, 1995, *Immunol. Today* **16**:449.

ticosteroid-induced lympholysis. In these animals, corticosteroid treatment at dosages as low as 10^{-7} M causes such widespread lympholysis that the weight of the thymus is reduced by 90%; the spleen and lymph nodes also shrink visibly. Immature thymocytes in these species appear to be particularly sensitive to corticosteroid-mediated killing. In rodents, corticosteroids induce programmed cell death of immature thymocytes, whereas mature thymocytes are resistant to this activity. Within 2 h following in vitro incubation with corticosteroids, immature thymocytes begin to show the characteristic morphology of apoptosis, and 90% of the chromatin is degraded into the characteristic nucleosome ladder by 24 h after treatment. The steps involved in the induction of apoptosis by corticosteroids remain to be determined. In humans, guinea pigs, and monkeys, corticosteroids do not induce apoptosis but instead affect lymphocyte-circulation patterns, causing a decrease in thymic weight and a marked decrease in the number of circulating lymphocytes.

Like other steroid hormones, the corticosteroids are lipophilic and thus can cross the plasma membrane and bind to receptors in the cytosol. The resulting receptor-hormone complexes are subsequently transported to the nucleus, where they bind to specific regulatory DNA sequences, either up-regulating or down-regulating transcription. The corticosteroids have been shown to induce increased transcription of the NF-κB inhibitor (I-κB). Binding of this inhibitor to NF-κB in the cytosol prevents the translocation of NF-κB into the nucleus and consequently prevents NF-κB activation of a number of genes, including genes involved in T-cell activation and cytokine production.

Corticosteroids also reduce both the phagocytic and killing ability of macrophages and neutrophils, and this effect may contribute to their anti-inflammatory action. In addition, they reduce chemotaxis, so that fewer inflammatory cells are attracted to the site of T_H-cell activation. In the presence of corticosteroids, expression of class II MHC molecules and IL-1 production by macrophages is dramatically reduced; such reductions would be expected to lead to corresponding reductions in T_H-cell activation. Corticosteroids also stabilize the lysosomal membrane, so that decreased levels of lysosomal enzymes are released at the site of inflammation.

Nonsteroidal Anti-Inflammatory Drugs

Since the time of Hippocrates, extracts of willow bark have been used for relief of pain. The active ingredient, salicylate, which is found in aspirin, is just one of many nonsteroidal anti-inflammatory drugs (NSAIDs). NSAIDs are the most frequently used medication for treating pain and inflammation. One mechanism by which these drugs exert anti-inflammatory effects is by inhibiting the cyclooxygenase pathway by which prostaglandins and thromboxanes are produced from arachidonic acid (see Figure 15-11). The reduction in prostaglandin production limits the increase in vascular permeability and neutrophil chemotaxis in the inflammatory response. Clinically, NSAIDs have been shown to be effective for treatment of many acute and chronic inflammatory reactions.

Summary

1. Lymphocytes undergo constant recirculation between the blood, lymph, lymphoid organs, and tertiary extralymphoid tissues (see Figure 15-1). This extensive recirculation greatly increases the chances that the small number of lymphocytes specific for a given antigen (about 1 in 10^5 cells) will actually encounter that antigen when it is present in the body. Although the tertiary extralymphoid tissues normally contain few lymphoid cells, migration of lymphoid cells into these sites occurs during the inflammatory response.
2. Migration of leukocytes into inflamed tissue or into lymphoid organs requires interaction between cell-adhesion molecules (CAMs) on the vascular endothelium and those on the circulating cells. Most of these CAMs fall into one of four protein families: the selectins, the mucin-like family, integrins, or the Ig superfamily (see Figure 15-2). Selectins and mucin-like CAMs interact with each other, and members of each family are expressed on both leukocytes and endothelial cells. Integrins, expressed on leukocytes, interact with Ig-superfamily CAMs, expressed on endothelial cells.
3. Neutrophils are generally the first cell type to move from the bloodstream into inflammatory sites. Extravasation of both neutrophils and lymphocytes involves four steps: rolling, chemoattractant-activating signal, arrest and adhesion, and transendothelial migration (see Figures 15-3 and 15-7). Unlike neutrophils, various lymphocyte populations exhibit differential extravasation into various tissues. Homing receptors on lymphocytes interact with tissue-specific adhesion molecules, called vascular addressins, on high-endothelial venules (HEVs) in lymphoid organs and on the endothelium in tertiary extralymphoid tissues (see Table 15-1). Naive lymphocytes home to secondary lymphoid organs, extravasating across HEVs, whereas effector lymphocytes selectively home to inflamed vascular endothelium (see Figure 15-5).
4. Several types of mediators play a role in the inflammatory response. Chemokines are a group of small polypeptides that act as chemoattractants and activating molecules during leukocyte extravasation (see Table 15-2 and Figures 15-8 and 15-9). Plasma enzyme mediators include bradykinin and fibrinopeptides, which increase vascular permeability; plasmin, a proteolytic enzyme that degrades fibrin clots into chemotactic products and activates complement; and various complement products that act as

anaphylatoxins, opsonins, and chemotactic molecules for neutrophils and monocytes (see Figure 15-10). Lipid inflammatory mediators, derived from membrane phospholipids, include thromboxanes, prostaglandins, leukotrienes, and platelet-activating factor (see Figure 15-11). Three cytokines, IL-1, IL-6, and TNF-α, mediate many of the local and systemic features of the acute inflammatory response (see Table 15-3).

5. Inflammation is a physiologic response to a variety of stimuli such as tissue injury and infection. An acute inflammatory response involves both localized and systemic effects. The localized response begins when tissue and endothelial damage induces formation of plasma enzyme mediators that lead to vasodilation and increased vascular permeability (see Figure 15-12). Neutrophils and then monocytes extravasate into the site. Activation of tissue macrophages and degranulation of mast cells lead to release of numerous inflammatory mediators, some of which induce systemic acute-phase effects. The systemic response includes induction of fever, leukocytosis, and production of corticosteroids and acute-phase proteins, including C-reactive protein (see Figure 15-13).
6. Chronic inflammation results from persistence of antigen due to infection with certain resistant microorganisms or to various pathologic conditions. Two cytokines, IFN-γ and TNF-α are central to the chronic inflammatory response, which often involves granuloma formation and tissue wasting. Several human chronic inflammatory diseases are marked by the presence of an HEV-like vasculature in the affected organs (see Table 15-4).
7. A chronic inflammatory response may accompany allergies, autoimmune diseases, microbial infections, transplants, and burns. Antibodies to cell-adhesion molecules involved in leukocyte extravasation have shown promise in reducing chronic inflammation associated with burns and graft rejection. Corticosteroids have numerous effects that contribute to their anti-inflammatory action. A variety of nonsteroidal anti-inflammatory drugs (NSAIDs) are available and are the most commonly used medications for pain and inflammation.

REFERENCES

Ager, A. 1994. Lymphocyte recirculation and homing: roles of adhesion molecules and chemoattractants. *Trends Cell Biol.* **4:**326.

Baggiolini, M. 1998. Chemokines and leukocyte traffic. *Nature* **392:**565.

Bargatze, RF, MA Jutila, and EC Butcher. 1995. Distinct roles of L-selectin and integrins $\alpha 4\beta 7$ and LFA-1 in lymphocyte homing to Peyer's patch-HEV in situ: the multistep model confirmed and refined. *Immunity* **3:**99.

Baumann, H, and J Gauldie. 1994. The acute response. *Immunol. Today* **15:**74.

Bradley, LM, and SR Watson. 1996. Lymphocyte migration into tissue: the paradigm derived from CD4 subsets. *Curr. Opin. Immunol.* **8:**312.

Butcher, E, and LJ Picker. 1996. Lymphocyte homing and homeostasis. *Science* **272:**60.

Dianzani, U, and F Malavasi. 1995. Lymphocyte adhesion to endothelium. *Crit. Rev. Immunol.* **15:**167.

Dinarello, CA. 1996. Biological basis for interleukin-1 in disease. *Blood* **87:**2095.

Girard, JP, and TA Springer. 1995. High endothelial venules (HEVs): specialized endothelium for lymphocyte migration. *Immunol. Today* **16:**449.

Hayward, AR, et al. 1979. Delayed separation of the umbilical cord, widespread infections, and defective neutrophil mobility. *Lancet* **1:**1099.

Hogg, N, and C Berlin. 1995. Structure and function of adhesion receptors in leukocyte trafficking. *Immunol. Today* **16:**327.

Hynes, RO. 1994. The impact of molecular biology on models for cell adhesion. *Bioessays* **16:**663.

Hynes, RO, and AD Lander. 1992. Contact and adhesive specificities in the associations, migrations, and targeting of cells and axons. *Cell* **68:**303.

Kuijpers, TW, et al. 1997. Leukocyte adhesion deficiency type 1 (LAD-1)/variant. A novel immunodeficiency syndrome characterized by dysfunctional beta2 integrins. *Journal of Clinical Investigation* **100:**1725.

Marx, J. 1995. How the glucocorticoids suppress immunity. *Science* **270:**232.

Nelson, PJ, and AM Krensky. 1998. Chemokines, lymphocytes and viruses: what goes around, comes around. *Curr. Opin. Immunol.* **10:**265.

Shuster, DE, et al. 1992. Identification and prevalence of a genetic defect that causes leukocyte adhesion deficiency in Holstein cattle. *Proceedings of the National Academy of Sciences (USA)* **89:**9225.

Springer, TA. 1994. Traffic signals for lymphocyte recirculation and leukocyte emigration: the multistep paradigm. *Cell* **76:**301.

Steel, DM, and AS Whitehead. 1994. The major acute phase reactants: C-reactive protein, serum amyloid P component and serum amyloid A protein. *Immunol. Today* **15:**81.

Trincheri, G. 1996. Interleukin 12: a proinflammatory cytokine with immunoregulatory functions that bridge innate resistance and antigen-specific adaptive immunity. *Annu. Rev. Immunol.* **13:**251.

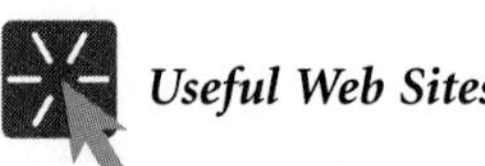

Useful Web Sites

http://www.mdsystems.com

The Cytokine Mini-Reviews Section (Site Map/Reviews & Technical Notes) of the R&D Systems site contains extensive, detailed, and well-illustrated reviews of many chemokines and chemokine receptors.

http://www.ncbi.nlm.nih.gov/Omim/

OMIM: Online Mendelian Inheritance in Man is a catalog of human genes and genetic disorders authored and edited by Dr. V. A. McKusick and his colleagues at Johns Hopkins and elsewhere, and developed for the World Wide Web by the National Center for Biotechnology Information (NCBI). It contains, pictures, and references on many diseases, including LAD.

STUDY QUESTIONS

1. Indicate whether each of the following statements is true or false. If you think a statement is false, explain why.

a. Chemokines are chemoattractants for lymphocytes but not other leukocytes.

b. Integrins are expressed on both leukocytes and endothelial cells.

c. Leukocyte extravasation involves multiple interactions between cell-adhesion molecules.

d. Most secondary lymphoid organs contain high-endothelial venules (HEVs).

e. Mucin-like CAMs interact with selectins.

f. An acute inflammatory response involves only localized effects in the region of tissue injury or infection.

g. MAdCAM-1 is an endothelial adhesion molecule that binds to L-selectin and to several integrins.

h. Granuloma formation is a common symptom of local inflammation.

2. Various inflammatory mediators induce expression of ICAMs on a wide variety of tissues. What effect might this induction have on the localization of immune cells?

3. Extravasation of neutrophils and of lymphocytes occurs by generally similar mechanisms, although some differences distinguish the two processes.

a. List in order the four basic steps in leukocyte extravasation.

b. At which sites are neutrophils most likely to extravasate? Why?

c. Different lymphocyte subpopulations migrate preferentially into different tissues, a process called homing (or trafficking). Discuss the roles of the three types of molecules that permit homing of lymphocytes.

4. Which three cytokines secreted by activated macrophages play a major role in mediating the localized and systemic effects associated with an acute inflammatory response?

5. An effective inflammatory response requires differentiation and proliferation of various nonlymphoid white blood cells. Explain how hematopoiesis in the bone marrow is induced by tissue injury or local infection.

6. For each pair of molecules listed below, indicate whether the molecules interact during the 1st, 2nd, 3rd, or 4th step in neutrophil extravasation at an inflammatory site. Use N to indicate any molecules that do not interact.

a. ______Chemokine and L-selectin

b. ______E-selectin and mucin-like CAM

c. ______IL-8 and E-selectin

d. ______Ig-superfamily CAM and integrin

e. ______ICAM and chemokine

f. ______Chemokine and G-protein–coupled receptor

g. ______ICAM and integrin

7. Discuss the main effects of IFN-γ and TNF-α during a chronic inflammatory response.

8. Five cytokines (IL-1, IL-6, TNF-α, LIF, and OSM) induce production of C-reactive protein and other acute-phase proteins by hepatocytes. Briefly explain how these different cytokines can exert the same effect on hepatocytes.

9. For each inflammation-related term (a–h), select the descriptions listed below (1–11) that apply. Each description may be used once, more than once, or not at all; more than one description may apply to some terms.

Terms

a. ______Tertiary extralymphoid tissue

b. ______P- and E-selectin

c. ______Prostaglandins

d. ______Nonsteroidal anti-inflammatory drugs

e. ______ICAM-1, -2, -3

f. ______MAdCAM

g. ______Bradykinin

h ______Inflamed endothelium

Descriptions

(1) Bind to sialylated carbohydrate moieties

(2) Inhibit cyclooxygenase pathway

(3) Induce expression of NF-κB inhibitor

(4) Has both Ig domains and mucin-like domains

(5) Region of vascular endothelium found in postcapillary venules

(6) Expressed by inflamed endothelium

(7) Exhibits HEV-like vasculature in chronic inflammation

(8) Belong to Ig-superfamily of CAMs

(9) Exhibits increased expression of CAMs

(10) Increase vascular permeability and induce fever

(11) Induce fever

Go to www.whfreeman.com/immunology Self-Test
Review and quiz of key terms

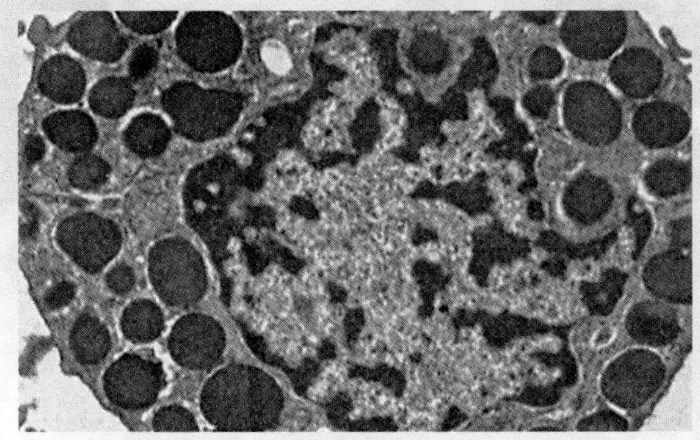

CHAPTER 16
HYPERSENSITIVE REACTIONS

Gell and Coombs Classification

IgE-Mediated (Type I) Hypersensitivity

Antibody-Mediated Cytotoxic (Type II) Hypersensitivity

Immune Complex–Mediated (Type III) Hypersensitivity

T_{DTH}-Mediated (Type IV) Hypersensitivity

An immune response evokes a battery of effector molecules that act to remove antigen by various mechanisms described in previous chapters. Generally, these effector molecules induce a subclinical, localized inflammatory response that eliminates antigen without extensively damaging the host's tissue. Under certain circumstances, however, this inflammatory response can have deleterious effects, resulting in significant tissue damage or even death. This inappropriate immune response is termed **hypersensitivity** or **allergy.** Although the word *hypersensitivity* implies an increased response, the response is not always heightened but may, instead, be an inappropriate immune response to an antigen. Hypersensitive reactions may develop in the course of either humoral or cell-mediated responses.

The ability of the immune system to respond inappropriately to antigenic challenge was recognized early in this century, when the Prince of Monaco became aware that bathers in the Mediterranean were plagued by the stings of the Portuguese Man-of-War jellyfish. To alleviate this problem, the Prince engaged the help of two French scientists, Paul Portier and Charles Richet. After investigating the situation, Portier and Richet concluded that the localized reaction of the bathers to the stings of the jellyfish was the result of toxins. To counteract this reaction, the scientists isolated toxins from the jellyfish and planned to use them as an immunogen to vaccinate the susceptible bathers. This would protect them, the scientists reasoned, from future encounters with the annoying jellyfish. However, their first attempts met with disastrous results. To test their vaccine, Portier and Richet injected dogs with the purified toxins. This initial injection was followed with a boost of toxins. Instead of reacting to the boost by producing antibodies against the toxins, the dogs immediately reacted with vomiting, diarrhea, asphyxia, and, in some instances, death. Clearly this was an instance where the animals "overreacted" to the antigen. Portier and Richet coined the term *anaphylaxis,* loosely translated from Greek to mean the opposite of *prophylaxis,* to describe this overreaction. Richet was subsequently awarded the Nobel Prize in Medicine in 1913 for his work on anaphylaxis.

We currently refer to anaphylactic reactions within the humoral branch initiated by antibody or antigen-antibody complexes as **immediate hypersensitivity,** because the symptoms are manifest within minutes or hours after a sensitized recipient encounters antigen. Three types of such hypersensitive reactions are commonly recognized: IgE-mediated (type I), antibody-mediated (type II), and immune complex–mediated (type III) hypersensitivity. A fourth type of hypersensitivity depends on reactions within the cell-mediated branch. These are initiated by T_{DTH} cells and are referred to as **delayed-type hypersensitivity (DTH),** in recognition of the delay of symptoms until days after exposure. Although DTH reactions, as described in Chapter 14, provide an important line of defense against intracellular pathogens, they sometimes cause extensive tissue damage that is pathologic and truly hypersensitive. This chapter examines the mechanisms and consequences of the four primary types of hypersensitive reactions.

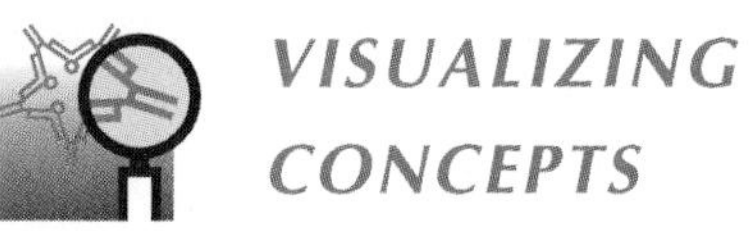

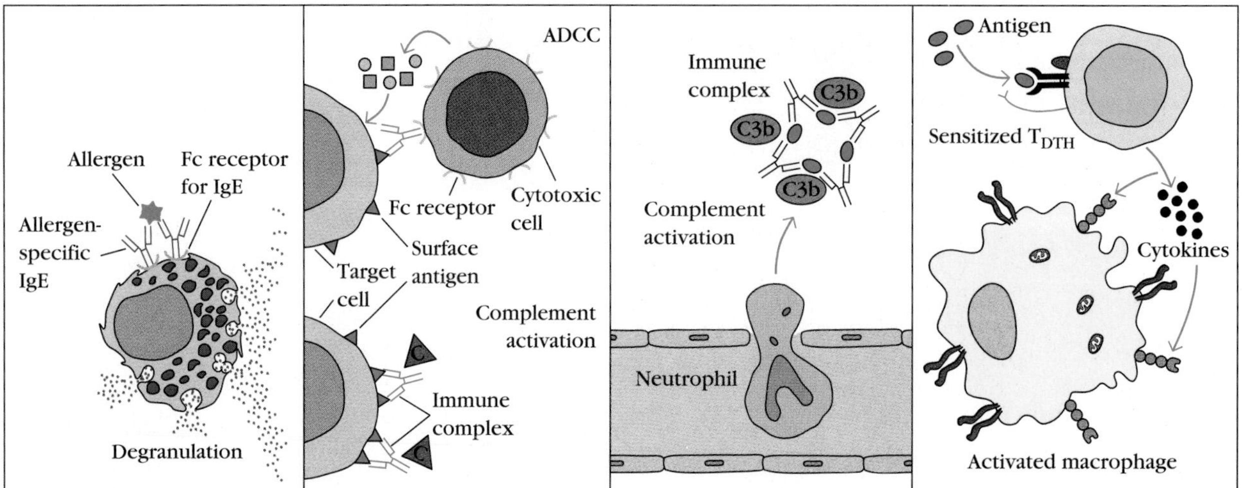

Type I	Type II	Type III	Type IV
IgE-Mediated Hypersensitivity	IgG-Mediated Cytotoxic Hypersensitivity	Immune Complex-Mediated Hypersensitivity	Cell-Mediated Hypersensitivity
Ag induces crosslinking of IgE bound to mast cells and basophils with release of vasoactive mediators	Ab directed against cell surface antigens meditates cell destruction via complement activation or ADCC	Ag-Ab complexes deposited in various tissues induce complement activation and an ensuing inflammatory response mediated by massive infiltration of neutrophils	Sensitized T_{DTH} cells release cytokines that activate macrophages or T_C cells which mediate direct cellular damage
Typical manifestations include systemic anaphylaxis and localized anaphylaxis such as hay fever, asthma, hives, food allergies, and eczema	Typical manifestations include blood transfusion reactions, erythroblastosis fetalis, and autoimmune hemolytic anemia	Typical manifestations include localized Arthus reaction and generalized reactions such as serum sickness, necrotizing vasculitis, glomerulnephritis, rheumatoid arthritis, and systemic lupus erythematosus	Typical manifestations include contact dermatitis, tubercular lesions and graft rejection

FIGURE 16-1 The four types of hypersensitive responses.

Gell and Coombs Classification

Several forms of hypersensitive reaction can be distinguished, reflecting differences in the effector molecules generated in the course of the reaction. In immediate hypersensitive reactions, different antibody isotypes induce different immune effector molecules. IgE antibodies, for example, induce mast-cell degranulation with release of histamine and other biologically active molecules. IgG and IgM antibodies, on the other hand, induce hypersensitive reactions by activating complement. The effector molecules in these reactions are the membrane-attack complex and such complement split products as C3a, C4a, and C5a. In delayed-type hypersensitivity reactions, the effector molecules are various cytokines secreted by T_{DTH} cells.

As it became clear that different immune mechanisms can give rise to hypersensitive reactions, P. G. H. Gell and R. R. A. Coombs proposed a classification scheme in which hypersensitive reactions are divided into four types, I, II, III, and IV, each involving distinct mechanisms, cells, and mediator molecules (Figure 16-1). This classification scheme has served an important function in identifying the mechanistic differences among various hypersensitive reactions, but it is important to point out that a great deal more complexity exists in a vast array of secondary effects that blur the boundaries between the four categories.

IgE-Mediated (Type I) Hypersensitivity

A type I hypersensitive reaction is induced by certain types of antigens, referred to as **allergens,** and has all the hallmarks of a normal humoral response. That is, an allergen induces a humoral antibody response by the same mechanisms as described in Chapter 11 for other soluble antigens, resulting in the generation of antibody-secreting plasma cells and memory cells. What distinguishes a type I hypersensitive response from a normal humoral response is that the plasma cells secrete IgE. This class of antibody binds with high affinity to **Fc receptors** on the surface of tissue mast cells and blood basophils. Such IgE-coated mast cells and basophils are said to be sensitized. A later exposure to the same allergen cross-links the membrane-bound IgE on sensitized mast cells and basophils, causing **degranulation** of these cells (Figure 16-2). The pharmacologically active mediators released from the granules act on the surrounding tissues. The principal effects—vasodilation and smooth-muscle contraction—may be either systemic or localized, depending on the extent of mediator release.

Components of Type I Reactions

As depicted in Figure 16-2, several components are critical to development of type I hypersensitive reactions. This section will consider these components first and then describe the mechanism of degranulation.

Allergens

The majority of humans mount significant IgE responses only as a defense against parasitic infections. After an individual has been exposed to a parasite, serum IgE levels increase and remain high until the parasite is successfully cleared from the body. Some persons, however, may have an abnormality called **atopy,** a hereditary predisposition to the development of immediate hypersensitivity reactions against common environmental antigens. The IgE regulatory defects

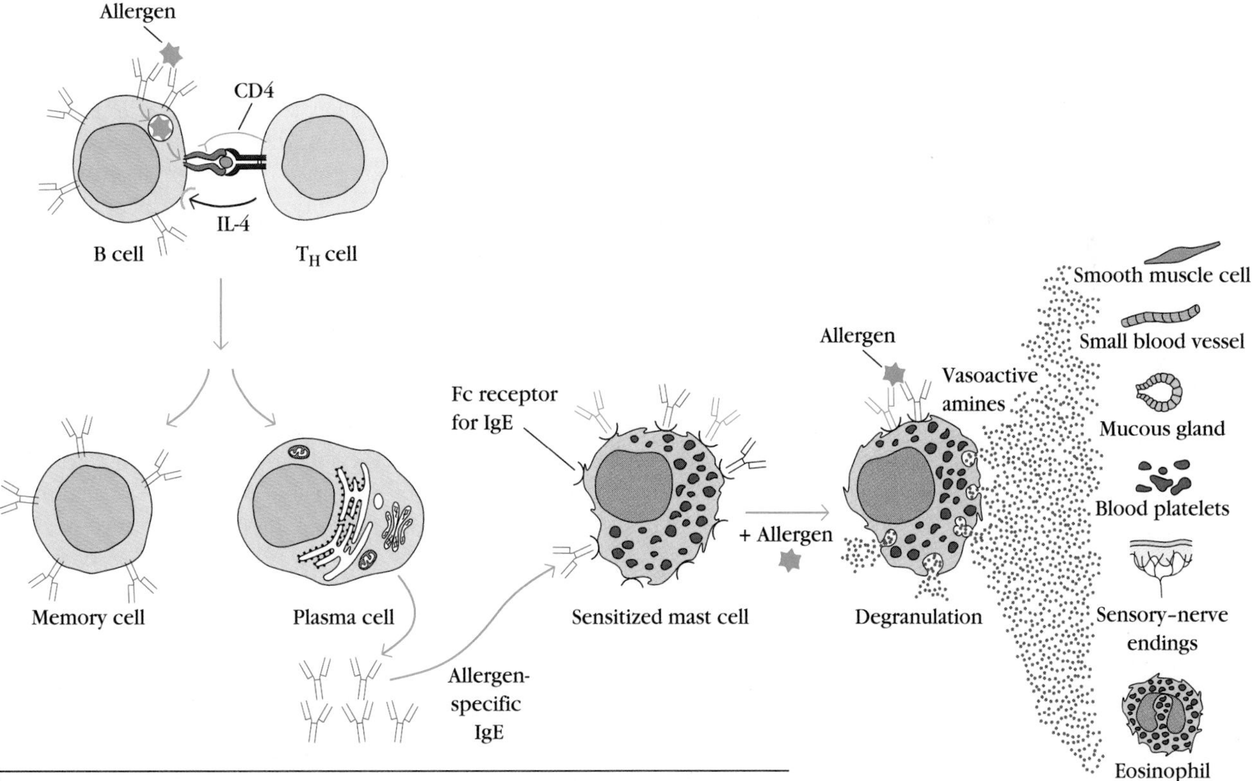

FIGURE 16-2 General mechanism underlying a type I hypersensitive reaction. Exposure to an allergen activates B cells to form IgE-secreting plasma cells. The secreted IgE molecules bind to IgE-specific Fc receptors on mast cells and blood basophils. (Many molecules of IgE with various specificities can bind to the IgE-Fc receptor.) Second exposure to the allergen leads to crosslinking of the bound IgE, triggering the release of pharmacologically active mediators, vasoactive amines, from mast cells and basophils. The mediators cause smooth-muscle contraction, increased vascular permeability, and vasodilation.

suffered by atopic individuals allow nonparasitic antigens to stimulate inappropriate IgE production, leading to tissue-damaging type I hypersensitivity. The term *allergen* refers specifically to nonparasitic antigens capable of stimulating type I hypersensitive responses in allergic individuals.

The abnormal IgE response of atopic individuals is at least part genetic—it often runs in families. Atopic individuals have abnormally high levels of circulating IgE and also more than normal numbers of circulating eosinophils. These individuals are more susceptible to allergies such as hay fever, eczema, and asthma. The genetic propensity to atopic responses has been mapped to several candidate loci. One locus, on chromosome 5q, is linked to a region that encodes a variety of cytokines, including IL-3, IL-4, IL-5, IL-9, IL-13, and GM-CSF. A second locus, on chromosome 11q, is linked to a region that encodes the β chain of the high-affinity IgE receptor. It is known that inherited atopy is multigenic and that other loci probably also are involved. Indeed, as the sequencing of the human genome progresses, these other candidate genes may be revealed.

Most allergic IgE responses occur on mucous membrane surfaces in response to allergens that enter the body by either inhalation or ingestion. Of the common allergens listed in Table 16-1, few have been purified and characterized. Those that have include the allergens from rye grass pollen, ragweed pollen, codfish, birch pollen, timothy grass pollen, and bee venom. Each of these allergens has been shown to be a multiantigenic system that contains a number of allergenic components. Ragweed pollen, a major allergen in the United States, is a case in point. It has been reported that a square mile of ragweed yields 16 tons of pollen in a single season. The pollen particles are inhaled, and their tough outer wall is dissolved by enzymes in the mucous secretions, releasing the allergenic substances. Chemical fractionation of ragweed has revealed a variety of substances, most of which are not allergenic but are capable of eliciting an IgM or IgG response. Of the five fractions that are allergenic (i.e., able to induce an IgE response), two evoke allergenic reactions in about 95% of ragweed-sensitive individuals and are called major allergens; these are designated the E and K fractions. The other three, called Ra3, Ra4, and Ra5, are minor allergens that induce an allergic response in only 20%–30% of sensitive subjects.

What makes these agents allergens? Why are some pollens (e.g., ragweed) highly allergenic, whereas other equally abundant pollens (e.g., nettle) are rarely allergenic? No single physicochemical property seems to distinguish the highly allergenic E and K fractions of ragweed from the less allergenic Ra3, Ra4, and Ra5 fractions and from the nonallergenic fractions. Rather, allergens as a group appear to possess diverse properties. Some allergens, including foreign serum and egg albumin, are potent antigens; others, such as plant pollens, are weak antigens. Although most allergens are small proteins or protein-bound substances having a molecular weight between 15,000 and 40,000, attempts to identify some common chemical property of these antigens, one that would render them all allergenic, have failed. It appears that allergenicity is a consequence of a complex series of interactions involving not only the allergen but also the dose, the sensitizing route, sometimes an adjuvant, and—most important, as noted above—the genetic constitution of the recipient.

TABLE 16-1 COMMON ALLERGENS ASSOCIATED WITH TYPE I HYPERSENSITIVITY

Proteins	*Foods*
Foreign serum	Nuts
Vaccines	Seafood
	Eggs
Plant pollens	Peas, beans
Rye grass	Milk
Ragweed	
Timothy grass	*Insect products*
Birch trees	Bee venom
	Wasp venom
Drugs	Ant venom
Penicillin	Cockroach calyx
Sulfonamides	Dust mites
Local anesthetics	
Salicylates	*Mold spores*
	Animal hair and dander

Reaginic Antibody (IgE)

As described in Chapter 4, the existence of a human serum factor that reacted with allergens was first demonstrated by K. Prausnitz and H. Kustner in 1921. The local wheal and flare response that occurs when an allergen is injected into a sensitized individual is called the P-K reaction. Because the serum components responsible for the P-K reaction displayed specificity for allergen, they were assumed to be antibodies, but the nature of these P-K antibodies, or **reagins,** was not demonstrated for many years.

Experiments conducted by K. and T. Ishizaka in the mid-1960s showed that the biological activity of reaginic antibody in a P-K test could be neutralized by rabbit antiserum against whole atopic human sera but not by rabbit antiserum specific for the four human immunoglobulin classes known at that time (IgA, IgG, IgM, and IgD) (Table 16-2). In addition, when rabbits were immunized with sera from ragweed-sensitive individuals, the rabbit antiserum could inhibit (neutralize) a positive ragweed P-K test even after precipitation of the rabbit antibodies specific for the human IgG, IgA, IgM, and IgD isotypes. The Ishizakas called this new isotype IgE in reference to the E antigen of ragweed that they used to characterize it.

TABLE 16-2 IDENTIFICATION OF IgE BASED ON REACTIVITY OF ATOPIC SERUM IN P-K TEST

Serum	Treatment	Allergen added	P-K reaction at skin site
Atopic	None	−	−
Atopic	None	+	+
Nonatopic	None	+	−
Atopic	Rabbit antiserum to human atopic serum*	+	−
Atopic	Rabbit antiserum to human IgM, IgG, IgA, and IgD†	+	+

*Serum from an atopic individual was injected into rabbits to produce antiserum against human atopic serum. When this antiserum was reacted with human atopic serum, it neutralized the P-K reaction.

†Serum from an atopic individual was reacted with rabbit antiserum to the known classes of human antibody (IgM, IgA, IgG, and IgD) to remove these isotypes from the atopic serum. The treated atopic serum continued to give a positive P-K reaction, indicating that a new immunoglobulin isotype was responsible for this reactivity.

SOURCE: Based on K Ishizaka and T Ishizaka, 1967, *J. Immunol.* **99:**1187.

Serum IgE levels in normal individuals fall within the range of 0.1–0.4 μg/ml; even the most severely allergic individuals rarely have IgE levels greater than 1 μg/ml. These low levels made physiochemical studies of IgE difficult; it was not until the discovery of an IgE myeloma by S. G. O. Johansson and H. Bennich, in 1967, that extensive chemical analysis of IgE could be undertaken. IgE was found to be composed of two heavy (ε) and two light chains with a combined molecular weight of 190,000. The higher molecular weight compared with IgG (150,000) is due to the presence of an additional constant-region domain (see Figure 4-13). This additional domain (C_H4) contributes to an altered conformation of the Fc portion of the molecule that enables it to bind to glycoprotein receptors on the surface of basophils and mast cells. Although the half-life of IgE in the serum is only 2–3 days, once IgE has been bound to its receptor on mast cells and basophils, it is stable in that state for a number of weeks.

Mast Cells and Basophils

The cells that bind IgE were identified by incubating human leukocytes and tissue cells with either ^{125}I-labeled IgE myeloma protein or ^{125}I-labeled anti-IgE. In both cases, autoradiography revealed that the labeled probe bound with high affinity to blood basophils and tissue mast cells. Basophils are granulocytes that circulate in the blood of most vertebrates; in humans, they account for 0.5%–1.0% of the circulating white blood cells. Their granulated cytoplasm stains with basic dyes, hence the name basophil. Electron microscopy reveals a multilobed nucleus, few mitochondria, numerous glycogen granules, and electron-dense membrane-bound granules, which contain pharmacologically active mediators, scattered throughout the cytoplasm (see Figure 2-10c).

Mast-cell precursors are formed in the bone marrow during hematopoiesis and are carried to virtually all vascularized peripheral tissues, where they differentiate into mature cells. Mast cells are found throughout connective tissue, particularly near blood and lymphatic vessels. Some tissues, including the skin and mucous membrane surfaces of the respiratory and gastrointestinal tracts, contain high concentrations of mast cells; skin, for example, contains 10,000 mast cells per mm^3. Electron micrographs of mast cells reveal numerous membrane-bounded granules, which, like basophils, contain pharmacologically active mediators, distributed throughout the cytoplasm (Figure 16-3). After activation, these mediators are released from the granules, resulting in the clinical manifestations of the type I hypersensitive reaction.

Mast cell populations in different anatomic sites differ significantly in the types and amounts of allergic mediators they contain and in their sensitivity to activating stimuli and cytokines. Mast cells also secrete a variety of cytokines, including IL-1, IL-3, IL-4, IL-5, IL-6, GM-CSF, TGF-β, and TNF-α. Because these cytokines exert diverse biological effects (see Table 12-1), mast cells contribute to a broad spectrum of physiologic, immunologic, and pathologic processes.

IgE-Binding Fc Receptors

The reaginic activity of IgE depends on its ability to bind to a receptor specific for the Fc region of the ε heavy chain. Two classes of FcεR have been identified, designated FcεRI and FcεRII, which are expressed by different cell types and differ by 1000-fold in their affinity for IgE.

High-Affinity Receptor (FcεRI) Mast cells and basophils express FcεRI, which binds IgE with a high affinity (K_D = 1–2 × 10^{-9} M). The high affinity of this receptor enables

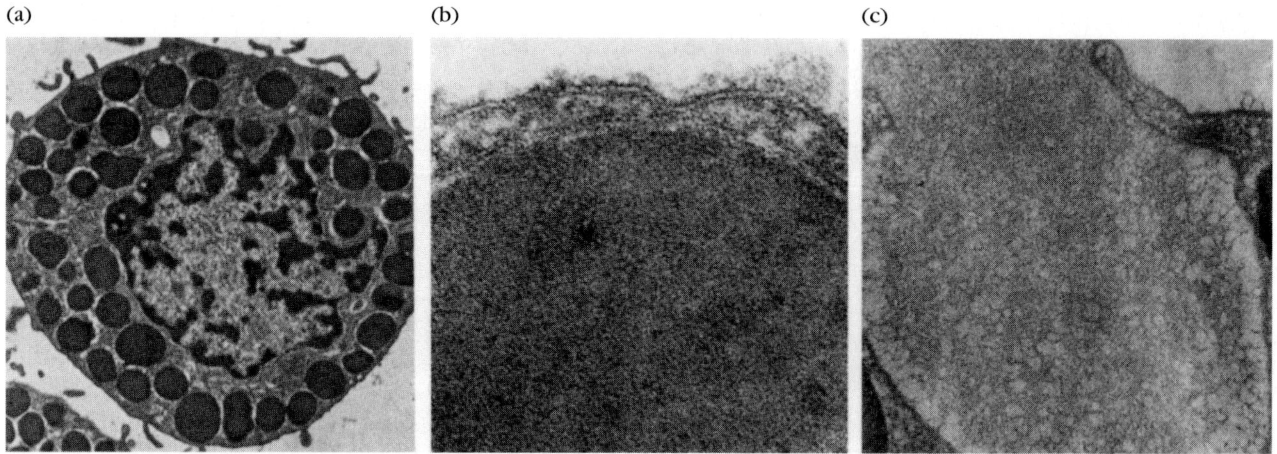

FIGURE 16-3 (a) Electron micrograph of a typical mast cell reveals numerous electron-dense membrane-bounded granules prior to degranulation. (b) Close-up of intact granule underlying the plasma membrane of a mast cell. (c) Granule releasing its contents (towards top left) during degranulation. [From S Burwen and B Satir, 1977, *J. Cell Biol.* **73:**662.]

it to bind IgE despite the low serum concentration of IgE (1×10^{-7} M). Between 40,000 and 90,000 FcεRI molecules have been shown to be present on a human basophil.

The FcεRI receptor contains four polypeptide chains: an α and a β chain and two identical disulfide-linked γ chains (Figure 16-4a). The external region of the α chain contains two 90-aa domains that exhibit homology with the immunoglobulin-fold structure, placing the molecule in the immunoglobulin superfamily (see Figure 4-19). FcεRI interacts with the C_H3/C_H3 and C_H4/C_H4 domains of the IgE molecule via the two Ig-like domains of the α chain. The β chain spans the plasma membrane four times and is thought

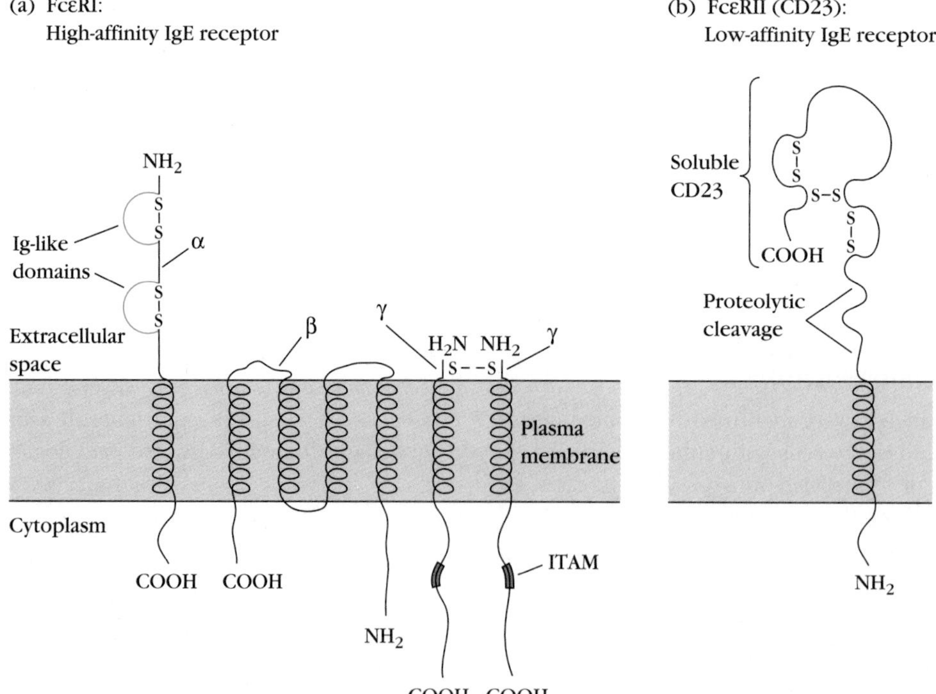

FIGURE 16-4 Schematic diagrams of the high-affinity (FcεRI) and low-affinity (FcεRII) receptors that bind the Fc region of IgE. (a) Each γ chain of the high-affinity receptor contains an ITAM, a motif also present in the Ig-α/Ig-β heterodimer of the B-cell receptor and in the CD3 complex of the T-cell receptor. (b) The low-affinity receptor is unusual because it is oriented in the membrane with its NH_2-terminus directed toward the cell interior and its COOH-terminus directed toward the extracellular space.

to link the α chain to the γ homodimer. The two γ chains are disulfide-linked and extend a considerable distance into the cytoplasm. Each γ chain has a conserved sequence in its cytosolic domain known as an immunoreceptor tyrosine-based activation motif (ITAM). As described earlier, two other membrane receptors that have this motif are CD3 and the associated ζ chains of the T-cell receptor complex (see Figure 10-11) and the Ig-α/Ig-β chains associated with membrane immunoglobulin on B cells (see Figure 11-7). The ITAM motif on these three receptors is thought to interact with protein tyrosine kinases to transduce an activating signal to the cell. Allergen-mediated crosslinkage of the bound IgE results in aggregation of the FcεRI receptors and rapid tyrosine phosphorylation, which initiates the process of mast-cell degranulation. The role of FcεRI in anaphylaxis is confirmed by experiments conducted in mice that lack FcεRI. These mice have normal levels of mast cells but are resistant to localized and systemic anaphylaxis.

Low-Affinity Receptor (FcεRII) The other IgE receptor, designated FcεRII (or CD23), is specific for the C_H3/C_H3 domain of IgE and has a lower affinity for IgE $1K_D = 1 \times 10^{-6}$ M2 than does FcεRI (Figure 16-4b). The FcεRII receptor appears to play a variety of roles in regulating the intensity of the IgE response. Allergen crosslinkage of IgE bound to FcεRII has been shown to activate B cells, alveolar macrophages, and eosinophils. When this receptor is blocked with monoclonal antibodies, IgE secretion by B cells is diminished. A soluble form of FcεRII (or sCD23), which is generated by autoproteolysis of the membrane receptor, has been shown to enhance IgE production by B cells. Interestingly, atopic individuals have higher levels of CD23 on their lymphocytes and macrophages and higher levels of sCD23 in their serum than do nonatopic individuals.

Mechanism of IgE-Mediated Degranulation

The biochemical events that mediate degranulation of mast cells and blood basophils have many features in common. For simplicity, this section presents a general overview of mast-cell degranulation mechanisms without calling attention to the slight differences between mast cells and basophils. Although mast-cell degranulation generally is initiated by allergen crosslinkage of bound IgE, a number of other stimuli can also initiate the process, including the anaphylatoxins (C3a, C4a, and C5a); various drugs, such as synthetic ACTH (adrenocorticotropic hormone), codeine, and morphine; and compounds such as the calcium ionophore. This section focuses on the biochemical events that follow allergen crosslinkage of bound IgE.

Receptor Crosslinkage

IgE-mediated degranulation begins when an allergen crosslinks IgE that is bound (fixed) to the Fc receptor on the surface of a mast cell or basophil. In itself, the binding of IgE to FcεRI apparently has no effect on a target cell. It is only after allergen crosslinks the fixed IgE-receptor complex that degranulation proceeds. The importance of crosslinkage is indicated by the inability of monovalent allergens, which cannot crosslink the fixed IgE, to trigger degranulation. Experimental studies with preformed IgE-allergen complexes, in which the ratio of IgE to allergen was carefully monitored, revealed that only complexes having IgE:allergen ratios of 2:1 or greater could induce degranulation. Complexes in antigen excess (having an IgE:allergen ratio of 1:2) failed to induce degranulation because the requisite crosslinkage of receptors did not occur.

Other experiments have revealed that it is actually the crosslinkage of two or more FcεRI molecules—with or without bound IgE—that is essential for degranulation. Although crosslinkage is normally effected by the interaction of fixed IgE with divalent or multivalent allergen, it also can be effected by a variety of experimental means that bypass the need for allergen and in some cases even for IgE (Figure 16-5).

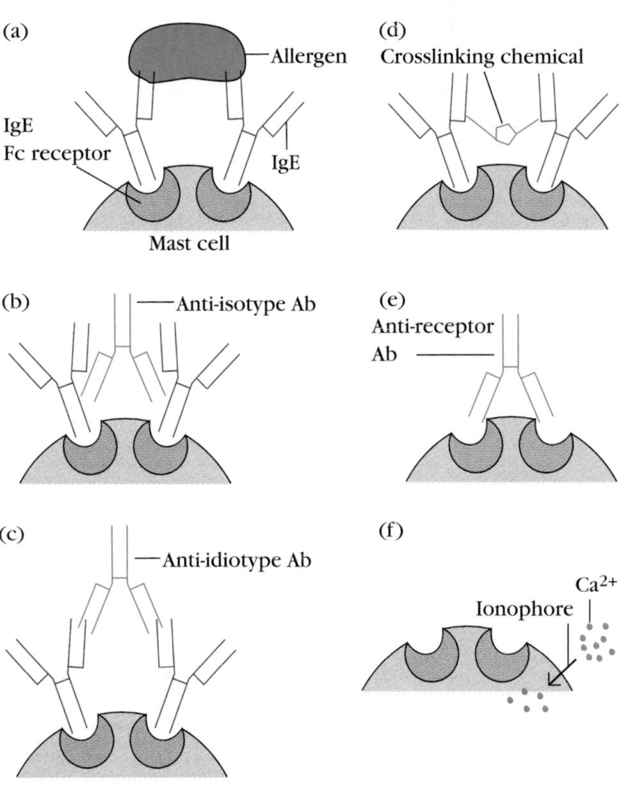

FIGURE 16-5 Schematic diagrams of mechanisms that can trigger degranulation of mast cells. (a) Allergen crosslinkage of cell-bound IgE molecules. (b, c) Antibody crosslinkage of IgE. (d) Chemical crosslinkage of IgE. (e) Crosslinkage of IgE Fc receptors by anti-receptor antibody. (f) Enhanced Ca^{2+} influx stimulated by an ionophore that increases membrane permeability to Ca^{2+} ions. Note that mechanisms (b), (c), and (d) do not require allergen; mechanisms (e) and (f) require neither allergen nor IgE; and mechanism (f) does not even require receptor crosslinkage.

Intracellular Events Leading to Mast-Cell Degranulation

The cytoplasmic domains of the β and γ chains of FcεRI are associated with protein tyrosine kinases (PTKs). Crosslinkage of the FcεRI receptors activates the associated PTKs, resulting in the phosphorylation of tyrosines within the ITAMs of the γ subunit as well as phosphorylation of residues on the β subunit and on phospholipase C. These phosphorylation events induce the production of a number of second messengers that mediate the process of degranulation (Figure 16-6).

Within 15 s after crosslinkage of FcεRI, methylation of various membrane phospholipids is observed, resulting in an increase in membrane fluidity and the formation of Ca^{2+} channels. An increase of Ca^{2+} reaches a peak within 2 min of FcεRI crosslinkage (Figure 16-7). This increase is due both to the uptake of extracellular Ca^{2+} and to a release of Ca^{2+} from intracellular stores in the endoplasmic reticulum (see Figure 16-6). The Ca^{2+} increase eventually leads to the formation of arachidonic acid, which is converted into two classes of potent mediators: the **prostaglandins** and the **leukotrienes** (see Figure 16-6). The increase of Ca^{2+} also

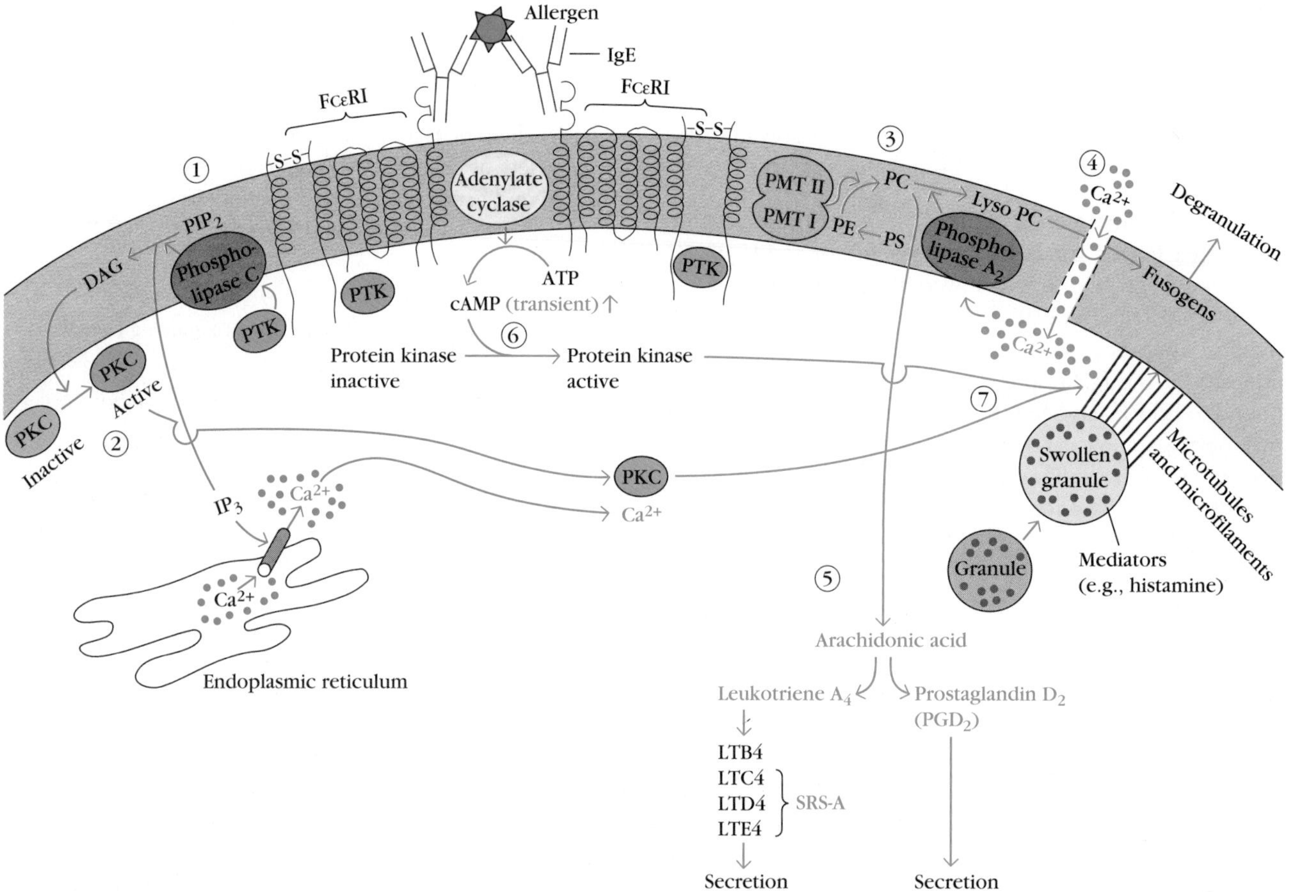

FIGURE 16-6 Diagrammatic overview of biochemical events in mast-cell activation and degranulation. Allergen crosslinkage of bound IgE results in FcεRI aggregation and activation of protein tyrosine kinase (PTK). (1) PTK then phosphorylates phospholipase C, which converts phosphatidylinositol-4,5 bisphosphate (PIP_2) into diacylglycerol (DAG) and inositol triphosphate (IP_3). (2) DAG activates protein kinase C (PKC), which with Ca^{2+} is necessary for microtubular assembly and the fusion of the granules with the plasma membrane. IP_3 is a potent mobilizer of intracellular Ca^{2+} stores. (3) Crosslinkage of FcεRI also activates an enzyme that converts phosphatidylserine (PS) into phosphatidylethanolamine (PE). Eventually, PE is methylated to form phosphatidylcholine (PC) by the phospholipid methyl transferase enzymes I and II (PMT I and II). (4) The accumulation of PC on the exterior surface of the plasma membrane causes an increase in membrane fluidity and facilitates the formation of Ca^{2+} channels. The resulting influx of Ca^{2+} activates phospholipase A_2, which promotes the breakdown of PC into lysophosphatidylcholine (lyso PC) and arachidonic acid. (5) Arachidonic acid is converted into potent mediators: the leukotrienes and prostaglandin D_2. (6) FcεRI crosslinkage also activates the membrane adenylate cyclase, leading to a transient increase of cAMP within 15 s. A later drop in cAMP levels is mediated by protein kinase and is required for degranulation to proceed. (7) cAMP-dependent protein kinases are thought to phosphorylate the granule-membrane proteins, thereby changing the permeability of the granules to water and Ca^{2+}. The consequent swelling of the granules facilitates fusion with the plasma membrane and release of the mediators.

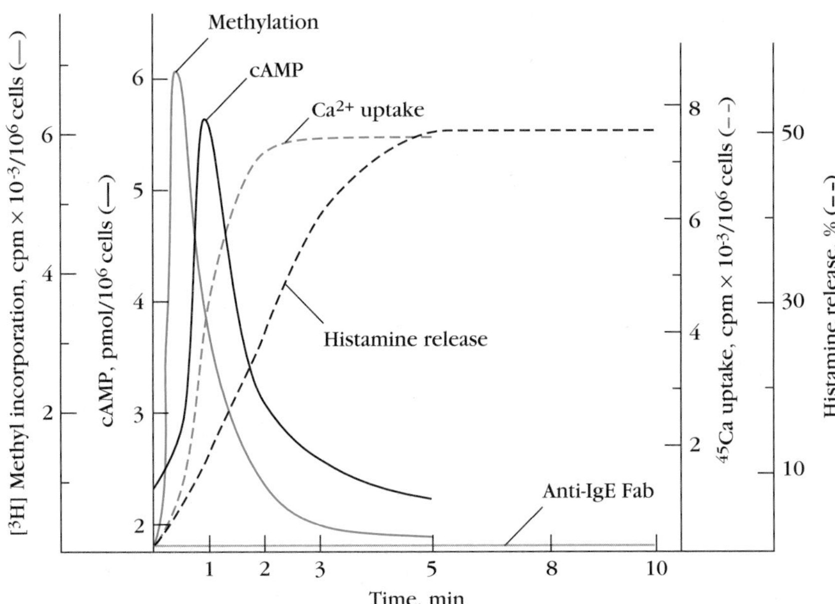

FIGURE 16-7 Kinetics of major biochemical events that follow crosslinkage of bound IgE on cultured human basophils with $F(ab')_2$ fragments of anti-IgE. Curves are shown for phospholipid methylation (solid blue), cAMP production (solid black), Ca^{2+} influx (dashed blue), and histamine release (dashed black). In control experiments with anti–IgE Fab fragments, no significant changes were observed. [Adapted from T Ishizaka et al, 1985, *Int. Arch. Allergy Appl. Immunol.* **77**:137.]

promotes the assembly of microtubules and the contraction of microfilaments, both of which are necessary for the movement of granules to the plasma membrane. The importance of the Ca^{2+} increase in mast-cell degranulation is highlighted by the use of drugs, such as cromolyn sodium, that block this influx as a treatment for allergies.

Concomitant with phospholipid methylation and Ca^{2+} increase, there is a transient increase in membrane-bound adenylate cyclase activity, with a rapid peak of cAMP reached about 1 min after crosslinkage of FcεRI (see Figure 16-7). The effects of cAMP are exerted through the activation of cAMP-dependent protein kinases, which phosphorylate the granule-membrane proteins, thereby changing the permeability of the granules to water and Ca^{2+} (see Figure 16-6). The consequent swelling of the granules facilitates their fusion with the plasma membrane, releasing their contents. The increase in cAMP is transient and is followed by a drop in cAMP to levels below baseline (see Figure 16-7). This drop in cAMP appears to be necessary for degranulation to proceed; when cAMP levels are increased by certain drugs, the degranulation process is blocked. Several of these drugs are given to treat allergic disorders and are considered later in this section.

Mediators of Type I Reactions

The clinical manifestations of type I hypersensitive reactions are related to the biological effects of the mediators released during mast cell or basophil degranulation. These mediators are pharmacologically active agents that act on local tissues as well as on populations of secondary effector cells, including eosinophils, neutrophils, T lymphocytes, monocytes, and platelets. The mediators thus serve as an amplifying terminal effector mechanism, much as the complement system serves as an amplifier and effector of an antigen-antibody interaction. When generated in response to parasitic infection, these mediators initiate a beneficial defense process. Vasodilation and increased vascular permeability result from the release of mediators and bring an influx of plasma and inflammatory cells to attack the pathogen. On the other hand, mediator release induced by inappropriate antigens, such as allergens, results in unnecessary increases in vascular permeability and inflammation whose detrimental effects far outweigh any beneficial effect.

The mediators can be classified as either primary or secondary (Table 16-3). The primary mediators are produced before degranulation and are stored in the granules. The most significant primary mediators are histamine, proteases, eosinophil chemotactic factor, neutrophil chemotactic factor, and heparin. The secondary mediators either are synthesized after target-cell activation or are released by the breakdown of membrane phospholipids during the degranulation process. The secondary mediators include platelet-activating factor, leukotrienes, prostaglandins, bradykinin, and various cytokines. The differing manifestations of type I hypersensitivity in different species or different tissues partly reflect variations in the primary and secondary mediators present. The main biological effects of several of these mediators are described briefly in the next sections.

Histamine

Histamine, which is formed by decarboxylation of the amino acid histidine, is a major component of mast cell granules, accounting for about 10% of granule weight. Because it is stored—preformed—in the granules, its biological effects are observed within minutes of mast-cell activation. Once released from mast cells, histamine initially binds to specific receptors on various target cells. Three types of histamine

TABLE 16-3 PRINCIPAL MEDIATORS INVOLVED IN TYPE I HYPERSENSITIVITY

Mediator	Effects
Primary	
Histamine	Increased vascular permeability; smooth-muscle contraction
Serotonin	Increased vascular permeability; smooth-muscle contraction
Eosinophil chemotactic factor (ECF-A)	Eosinophil chemotaxis
Neutrophil chemotactic factor (NCF-A)	Neutrophil chemotaxis
Proteases	Bronchial mucus secretion; degradation of blood-vessel basement membrane; generation of complement split products
Secondary	
Platelet-activating factor	Platelet aggregation and degranulation; contraction of pulmonary smooth muscles
Leukotrienes (slow reactive substance of anaphylaxis, SRS-A)	Increased vascular permeability; contraction of pulmonary smooth muscles
Prostaglandins	Vasodilation; contraction of pulmonary smooth muscles; platelet aggregation
Bradykinin	Increased vascular permeability; smooth-muscle contraction
Cytokines	
IL-1 and TNF-α	Systemic anaphylaxis; increased expression of CAMs on venular endothelial cells
IL-2, IL-3, IL-4, IL-5, IL-6, TGF-β, and GM-CSF	Various effects (see Table 12-1)

receptors—designated H_1, H_2, and H_3—have been identified; these receptors have different tissue distributions and mediate different effects when they bind histamine.

Most of the biologic effects of histamine in allergic reactions are mediated by the binding of histamine to H_1 receptors. This binding induces contraction of intestinal and bronchial smooth muscles, increased permeability of venules, and increased mucus secretion by goblet cells. Interaction of histamine with H_2 receptors increases vasopermeability and dilation and stimulates exocrine glands. Binding of histamine to H_2 receptors on mast cells and basophils suppresses degranulation; thus, histamine exerts negative feedback on the release of mediators.

Leukotrienes and Prostaglandins

As secondary mediators, the leukotrienes and prostaglandins are not formed until the mast cell undergoes degranulation and the enzymatic breakdown of phospholipids in the plasma membrane. An ensuing enzymatic cascade generates the prostaglandins and the leukotrienes (see Figure 16-6). It therefore takes a longer time for the biological effects of these mediators to become apparent. Their effects are more pronounced and longer lasting, however, than those of histamine. The leukotrienes mediate bronchoconstriction, increased vascular permeability, and mucus production. Prostaglandin D_2 causes bronchoconstriction.

The contraction of human bronchial and tracheal smooth muscles appears at first to be mediated by histamine, but, within 30–60 s, further contraction is mediated by the leukotrienes and prostaglandins. Being active at nanomole levels, the leukotrienes are as much as 1000 times more potent as bronchoconstrictors than histamine is, and they are also more potent stimulators of vascular permeability and mucus secretion. In humans, the leukotrienes are thought to contribute to the prolonged bronchospasm and buildup of mucus seen in asthmatics.

Cytokines

Adding to the complexity of the type I reaction is the variety of cytokines released from mast cells and eosinophils. Some of these may contribute to the clinical manifestations of type I hypersensitivity. Human mast cells secrete IL-4, IL-5, IL-6, and TNF-α. These cytokines alter the local microenvironment, eventually leading to the recruitment of inflammatory cells such as neutrophils and eosinophils. IL-4 increases IgE production by B cells. IL-5 is especially important in the recruitment and activation of eosinophils. The high concentrations of TNF-α secreted by mast cells may contribute to shock in systemic anaphylaxis. (This effect may parallel the role of TNF-α in bacterial septic shock and toxic-shock syndrome described in Chapter 12.)

Consequences of Type I Reactions

The clinical manifestations of type I reactions can range from serious life-threatening conditions, such as systemic anaphylaxis and asthma, to hay fever and eczema, which are merely annoying.

Systemic Anaphylaxis

Systemic anaphylaxis is a shock-like and often fatal state whose onset occurs within minutes of a type I hypersensitive reaction. This was the response observed by Portier and Richet in dogs after antigenic challenge. Systemic anaphylaxis can be induced in a variety of experimental animals and is seen occasionally in humans. Each species exhibits characteristic symptoms, which reflect differences in the distribution of mast cells and in the biologically active contents of their granules. The animal model of choice for studying systemic anaphylaxis has been the guinea pig. Anaphylaxis can be induced in guinea pigs with ease, and its symptoms closely parallel those observed in humans.

Active sensitization in guinea pigs is induced by a single injection of a foreign protein such as egg albumin. After an incubation period of about 2 weeks, the animal is usually challenged with an intravenous injection of the same protein. Within 1 min, the animal becomes restless, its respiration becomes labored, and its blood pressure drops. As the smooth muscles of the gastrointestinal tract and bladder contract, the guinea pig defecates and urinates. Finally bronchiole constriction results in death by asphyxiation within 2–4 min of the injection. These events all stem from the systemic vasodilation and smooth-muscle contraction brought on by mediators released in the course of the reaction. Postmortem examination reveals that massive edema, shock, and bronchiole constriction are the major causes of death.

Systemic anaphylaxis in humans is characterized by a similar sequence of events. A wide range of antigens have been shown to trigger this reaction in susceptible humans, including the venom from bee, wasp, hornet, and ant stings; drugs, such as penicillin, insulin, and antitoxins; and seafood and nuts. If not treated quickly, these reactions can be fatal. Epinephrine is the drug of choice for systemic anaphylactic reactions. Epinephrine counteracts the effects of mediators such as histamine and the leukotrienes by relaxing the smooth muscles and reducing vascular permeability. Epinephrine also improves cardiac output, which is necessary to prevent vascular collapse during an anaphylactic reaction. In addition, epinephrine increases cAMP levels in the mast cell, thereby blocking further degranulation.

Localized Anaphylaxis (Atopy)

In localized anaphylaxis, the reaction is limited to a specific target tissue or organ, often involving epithelial surfaces at the site of allergen entry. The tendency to manifest localized anaphylactic reactions is inherited and is called atopy. Atopic allergies, which afflict at least 20% of the population in developed countries, include a wide range of IgE-mediated disorders, including allergic rhinitis (hay fever), asthma, atopic dermatitis (eczema), and food allergies.

Allergic Rhinitis The most common atopic disorder, affecting 10% of the U. S. population, is allergic rhinitis, commonly known as hay fever. This results from the reaction of airborne allergens with sensitized mast cells in the conjunctivae and nasal mucosa to induce the release of pharmacologically active mediators from mast cells; these mediators then cause localized vasodilation and increased capillary permeability. The symptoms include watery exudation of the conjunctivae, nasal mucosa, and upper respiratory tract, as well as sneezing and coughing.

Asthma Another common manifestation of localized anaphylaxis is asthma. In some cases, airborne or blood-borne allergens, such as pollens, dust, fumes, insect products, or viral antigens, trigger an asthmatic attack (allergic asthma); in other cases, an asthmatic attack can be induced by exercise or cold, apparently independently of allergen stimulation (intrinsic asthma). Like hay fever, asthma is triggered by degranulation of mast cells with release of mediators, but instead of occurring in the nasal mucosa, the reaction develops in the lower respiratory tract. The resulting contraction of the bronchial smooth muscles leads to bronchoconstriction. Airway edema, mucus secretion, and inflammation contribute to the bronchial constriction and to airway obstruction. Asthmatic patients may have abnormal levels of receptors for neuropeptides. For example, asthmatic patients have been reported to have increased expression of receptors for substance P, a peptide that contracts smooth muscles, and decreased expression of receptors for vasoactive intestinal peptide, which relaxes smooth muscles.

Most clinicians view asthma as primarily an inflammatory disease. The asthmatic response can be divided into early and late responses (Figure 16-8). The early response occurs within minutes of allergen exposure and primarily involves histamine, leukotrienes (LTC_4), and prostaglandin D_2 (PGD_2). The effects of these mediators lead to bronchoconstriction, vasodilation, and some buildup of mucus. The late response occurs hours later and involves additional mediators, including IL-4, IL-5, IL-16, TNF-α, eosinophil chemotactic factor (ECF), and platelet-activating factor (PAF). The overall effects of these mediators is to increase endothelial cell adhesion as well as to recruit inflammatory cells, including eosinophils and neutrophils, into the bronchial tissue.

The neutrophils and eosinophils are capable of causing significant tissue injury by releasing toxic enzymes, oxygen radicals, and cytokines. These events lead to occlusion of the bronchial lumen with mucus, proteins, and cellular debris;

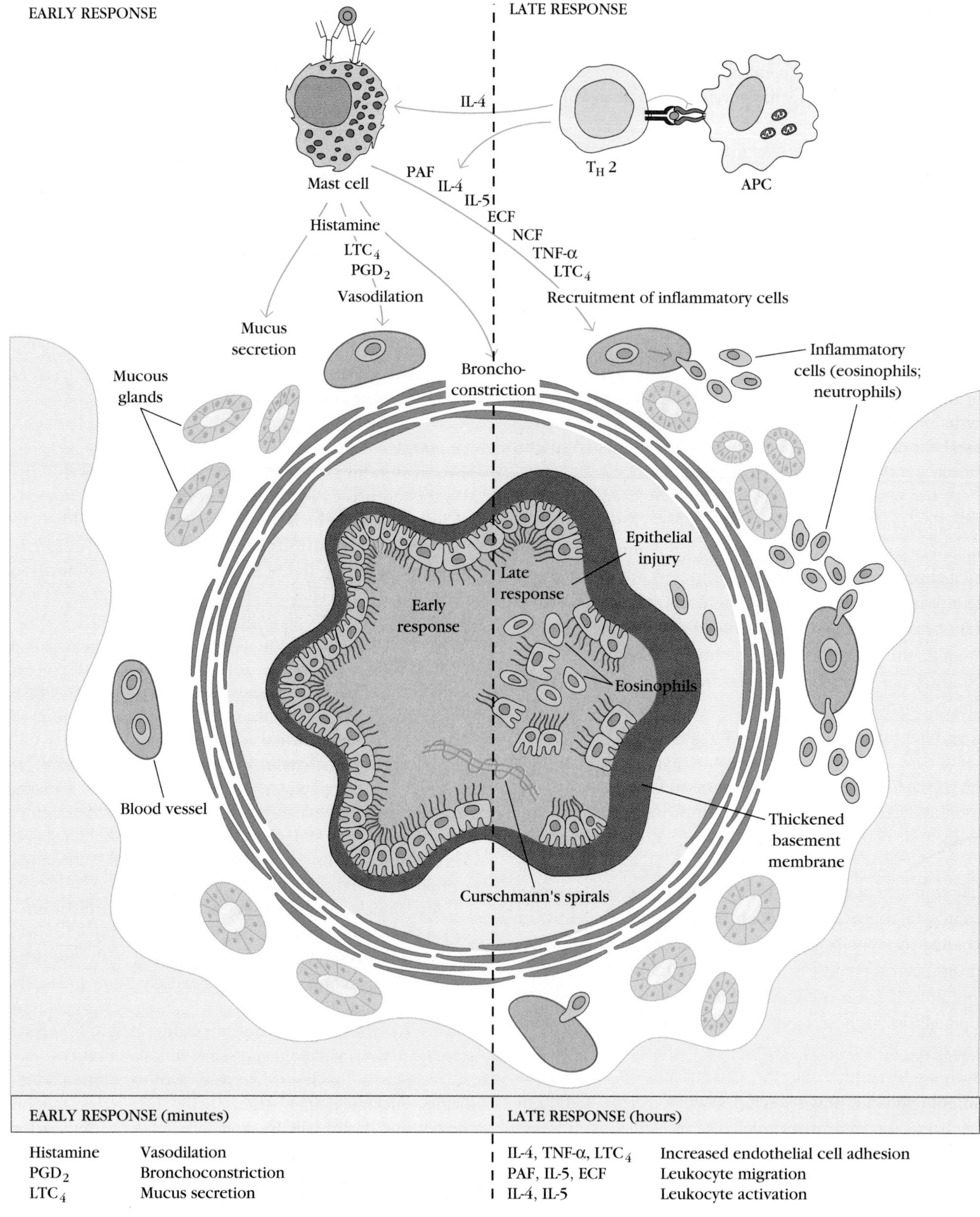

FIGURE 16-8 The early and late inflammatory response in asthma. The immune cells involved in the early and late responses are represented at the top. The effects of various mediators on an airway, represented in cross section, are illustrated in the center.

sloughing of the epithelium; thickening of the basement membrane; fluid buildup (edema); and hypertrophy of the bronchial smooth muscles. A mucus plug often forms and adheres to the bronchial wall. The mucus plug contains clusters of detached epithelial-cell fragments, eosinophils, some neutrophils, and spirals of bronchial tissue known as Curschmann's spirals. Asthma is increasing in prevalence in the United States, particularly among children in inner-city environments (see Clinical Focus).

Food Allergies Various foods also can induce localized anaphylaxis in allergic individuals. Allergen crosslinking of IgE on mast cells along the upper or lower gastrointestinal tract can induce localized smooth-muscle contraction and vasodilation and thus such symptoms as vomiting or diarrhea. Mast-cell degranulation along the gut can increase the permeability of mucous membranes, so that the allergen enters the bloodstream. Various symptoms can ensue, depending on where the allergen is deposited. For example, some individuals develop asthmatic attacks after ingesting certain foods. Others develop atopic urticaria, commonly known as hives, when a food allergen is carried to sensitized mast cells in the skin, causing swollen (edematous) red (erythematous) eruptions; this response is called a **wheal and flare reaction.**

Atopic Dermatitis Atopic dermatitis (allergic eczema) is an inflammatory disease of skin that is frequently associated with a family history of atopy. The disease is observed most frequently in young children, often developing during infancy. Serum IgE levels are often elevated. The allergic individual develops skin eruptions that are erythematous and filled with pus. Unlike a delayed-type hypersensitive reaction, which involves T_H1 cells, the skin lesions in atopic dermatitis have T_H2 cells and an increased number of eosinophils.

Late-Phase Reaction

As a type I hypersensitive reaction begins to subside, mediators released during the course of the reaction often induce a localized inflammatory reaction, called the late-phase reaction. The late-phase reaction, distinct from the late response seen in asthma, begins to develop 4–6 h after the initial type I reaction and persists for 1–2 days. The reaction is characterized by infiltration of neutrophils, eosinophils, macrophages, lymphocytes, and basophils. The localized late-phase response also may be mediated partly by cytokines released from mast cells. Both TNF-α and IL-1 increase the expression of cell-adhesion molecules on venular endothelial cells, thus facilitating the buildup of neutrophils, eosinophils, and monocytes that characterizes the late-phase response.

Eosinophils play a principal role in the late-phase reaction, accounting for some 30% of the cells that accumulate. Eosinophil chemotactic factor, released by mast cells during the initial reaction, attracts large numbers of eosinophils to the affected site. Various cytokines released at the site, including IL-3, IL-5, and GM-CSF, contribute to the growth and differentiation of the eosinophils. Eosinophils express Fc receptors for IgG and IgE isotypes and bind directly to antibody-coated allergen. Much as in mast-cell degranulation, binding of antibody-coated antigen activates eosinophils, leading to their degranulation and release of inflammatory mediators, including leukotrienes, major basic protein, platelet-activation factor, cationic protein, and eosinophil-derived neurotoxin. The release of these eosinophil-derived mediators may play a protective role in parasitic infections. However, in response to allergens, these mediators contribute to extensive tissue damage in the late-phase reaction. The influx of eosinophils in the late-phase response has been shown to contribute to the chronic inflammation of the bronchial mucosa that characterizes persistent asthma.

Neutrophils are another major participant in late-phase reactions, also accounting for 30% of the inflammatory cells. Neutrophils are attracted to the area of a type I reaction by neutrophil chemotactic factor, released from degranulating mast cells. In addition, a variety of cytokines released at the site, including IL-8, have been shown to activate neutrophils, resulting in release of their granule contents, including lytic enzymes, platelet-activating factor, and leukotrienes.

Regulation of the Type I Response

As noted earlier, the genetic constitution of an animal, the antigen dose, and the mode of antigen presentation influence the level of the IgE response induced by an antigen (i.e., its allergenicity). For example, inbred strains of mice have been shown to differ in their tendency to mount an IgE response. Some strains (e.g., SJL) fail to produce an IgE response to allergens, whereas other strains (e.g., BDF1) have an increased propensity for IgE production. Breeding experiments have shown that this genetic variation is not linked to the MHC. A genetic component also has been shown to influence susceptibility to type I hypersensitive reactions in humans. If both parents are allergic, there is a 50% chance that a child will also be allergic; when only one parent is allergic, there is a 30% chance that a child will manifest some kind of type I reaction.

The effect of antigen dosage on the IgE response is illustrated by immunization of BDF1 mice. Repeated low doses of an appropriate antigen induce a persistent IgE response in these mice, but higher antigen doses result in transient IgE production and a shift toward IgG. The mode of antigen presentation also influences the development of the IgE response. For example, immunization of Lewis-strain rats with keyhole limpet hemocyanin (KLH) plus aluminum hydroxide gel or *Bordetella pertussis* as an adjuvant induces a strong IgE response, whereas injection of KLH with complete Freund's adjuvant produces a largely IgG response. Similar experimental findings have been reported in mice.

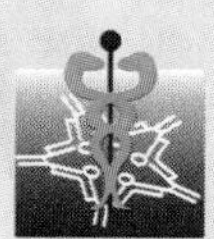

CLINICAL FOCUS

THE GENETICS OF ASTHMA

Asthma is a common disease that affects almost 5% of the population of the United States. For reasons that are still unclear, the incidence of asthma recently has increased dramatically in developed countries. Even more alarming is that the severity of the disease also appears to be increasing. The increase in asthma mortality is highest among children, and in the United States the mortality is highest among African-American children of the inner city. In 1995, 4.8 million children had asthma and more than 2000 of them died of the disease. These statistics are increasing each year. In addition to its human costs, asthma imposes high financial costs on society. During 1994, the cost for the treatment of asthma in the United States was more than $12 billion.

Asthma is commonly defined as an inflammatory disease of the airway, and it is characterized by bronchial hyperresponsiveness. Atopic individuals, those with a predisposition to the type I hypersensitive response, are most susceptible to the development of bronchial hyperresponsiveness and asthma, but only 10%–30% of atopic individuals actually develop asthma. The evidence that asthma has a genetic component originally was derived from family studies, which estimated that the relative contribution of genetic factors to atopy and asthma is 40%–60%. While genetic factors are important, further studies have indicated that environmental factors also play a large role. Additionally, asthma is a complex genetic disease, controlled by several genes, so that susceptibility to it is likely to involve the interaction of multiple genetic and environmental factors.

How do we determine which genes contribute to a complex multigenic disease such as this? One approach is the candidate-gene approach, in which a hypothesis suggests that a particular gene or set of genes may have some relation to the disease. After such a gene has been identified, families with apparent predisposition to the disease are examined for polymorphic alleles of the gene in question. Comparison of individuals within these families that have the disease and those that do not allows correlation between a particular allele and the presence of the disease. The problem with this approach is its bias toward identification of genes already suspected to play a role in the disease, which precludes identification of new genes. A good example of the use of the candidate-gene approach is the identification of a region on chromosome 5, region 5q31–33, that appears to be linked to the development of asthma. Using a candidate gene approach, this region was investigated because it includes a cluster of cytokine genes, among them the genes that encode interleukins 3, 4, 5, 9, and 13, as well as the gene that encodes granulocyte-macrophage colony-stimulating factor. *Interleukin-4* is thought to be a good candidate gene, since IL-4 induces the Ig class-switch to IgE. Several groups of investigators have examined this region in different populations and concluded that there is a polymorphism associated with predisposition to asthma that maps to the promotor region of *IL-4*. Addi-

Infection with the nematode *Nippostrongylus brasiliensis* (Nb), like certain adjuvants, preferentially induces an IgE response. For example, Nb-infected mice develop higher levels of IgE specific for an unrelated antigen than do uninfected control mice.

The relative levels of the T_H1 and T_H2 subsets also are key to the regulation of type I hypersensitive responses. T_H1 cells reduce the response, whereas T_H2 cells enhance it. Cytokines secreted by T_H2 cells—namely, IL-3, IL-4, IL-5, and IL-10—stimulate the type I response in several ways. IL-4 enhances class switching to IgE and regulates the clonal expansion of IgE-committed B cells; IL-3, IL-4, and IL-10 enhance mast-cell production; and IL-3 and IL-5 enhance eosinophil maturation, activation, and accumulation. In contrast, T_H1 cells produce IFN-γ, which inhibits the type I response.

The pivotal role of IL-4 in regulation of the type I response was demonstrated in experiments by W. E. Paul and coworkers. When these researchers activated normal, unprimed B cells in vitro with LPS, only 2% of the cells expressed membrane IgG1 and only 0.05% expressed membrane IgE. However, when unprimed B cells were incubated with LPS plus IL-4, the percentage of cells expressing IgG1 increased to 40%–50% and the percentage expressing IgE increased to 15%–25%. In an attempt to determine whether IL-4 plays a role in regulating IgE production in vivo, Paul primed Nb-infected mice with TNP-KLH in the presence or in the absence of monoclonal antibody to IL-4. The antibody to IL-4 reduced the production of IgE specific for TNP-KLH in these Nb-infected mice to 1% of the level in control animals.

Further support for the role of IL-4 in the IgE response comes from the experiments of K. Rajewsky and coworkers with IL-4 knockout mice. These IL-4–deficient mice were unable to mount an IgE response to helminthic antigens.

tionally, two alleles of *IL-9* associated with atopy have been identified.

Another approach to identifying genes associated with a particular disease is a random genomic search. In this method, the entire genome is scanned for polymorphisms associated with the disease in question. Using the random genomic approach, a British study (Lympany et al, 1992) identified a linkage between a polymorphism on chromosome 11—more specifically, region 11q13—associated with atopy in British families. This region maps to the vicinity of the β subunit of the high-affinity IgE receptor (FcεRIB). This association is exciting, since we know how important IgE is in mediating type I reactions. However, some caution in interpreting these results is necessary. This study looked at associations between polymorphisms and atopy, but most individuals who are atopic do not develop asthma. Therefore this association, while important in identifying factors in developing atopy, may not be relevant to the development of asthma.

More recently, a large genome-wide screen for loci linked to asthma susceptibility was conducted in ethnically diverse populations that included Caucasians, Hispanics, and African-Americans. This study, published by a large collaborative group from medical centers throughout the United States identified many candidate loci associated with asthma. One locus on chromosome 5 coincided with the already identified region at 5q. Interestingly, however, this locus was associated with asthma in Caucasians but not in Hispanics or African-Americans. This discrepancy was seen with several other genes identified in this screen as well. Some loci appeared to have a high correlation with asthma in Hispanics but not in African-Americans or Caucasians, and other loci were identified as unique to African-Americans. Another interesting conclusion was that the association between chromosome 11q and atopy did not appear to be correlated with asthma. This could indicate that asthma and atopy have different molecular bases. More important, it suggests that genetic linkage to atopy should not be confused with genetic linkage to asthma. Overall, this study identified several genes linked to asthma and found that the number and relative importance of these genes may differ among ethnic groups. This suggests that genetic differences as well as differences in environment may be the underlying basis of the differences observed in the prevalence as well as the severity of the disease among ethnic groups in the United States.

It is well documented that a higher than average percentage of African-American inner city children have serious complications with asthma. This has raised the question whether there is a genetic predisposition for asthma in African-Americans. Recently, however, a report from Rosenstreich and colleagues has indicated an important environmental linkage to asthma in the inner city. This group assessed the role of allergies to the cockroach in the development of asthma; they found that a combination of cockroach allergy and exposure to high levels of cockroach allergen can help explain the high frequency of asthma-related health problems in inner-city children. These data also point to defects in the public-health systems in large cities. Clearly, a concerted effort by public agencies to eradicate insect infestations would benefit the health of those who live in inner-city communities.

Thus environmental factors, coupled with genetic predispositions unique among ethnic groups, may predispose some groups to disease at a higher frequency than other groups. It is only when both the environmental factors and the genes have been identified that the most effective and rational approach to disease prevention can be designed.

Furthermore, increased levels of $CD4^+$ T_H2 cells and increased levels of IL-4 have been detected in atopic individuals. When allergen-specific $CD4^+$ T cells from atopic individuals are cloned and added to an autologous B-cell culture, the B cells synthesize IgE, whereas allergen-specific $CD4^+$ T cells from nonatopic individuals do not support IgE production.

In contrast to IL-4, IFN-γ decreases IgE production, suggesting that the balance of IL-4 and IFN-γ may determine the amount of IgE produced (Figure 16-9). Since IFN-γ is secreted by the T_H1 subset and IL-4 by the T_H2 subset, the relative activity of these subsets may influence an individual's response to allergens. According to this proposal, atopic and nonatopic individuals would exhibit qualitatively different type I responses to an allergen: the response in atopic individuals would involve the T_H2 subset and result in production of IgE; the response in nonatopic individuals would involve the T_H1 subset and result in production of IgM or IgG. To test this hypothesis, allergen-specific T cells were cloned from atopic and nonatopic individuals. The cloned T cells from the atopic individuals were predominantly of the T_H2 phenotype (secreting IL-4), whereas the cloned T cells from nonatopic individuals were predominantly of the T_H1 phenotype (secreting IFN-γ2 Needless to say, there is keen interest in down-regulating IL-4 as a possible treatment for allergic individuals.

Detection of Type I Hypersensitivity

Type I hypersensitivity is commonly identified and assessed by skin testing. Small amounts of potential allergens are introduced at specific skin sites either by intradermal injection or by superficial scratching. A number of tests can be applied to sites on the forearm or back of an individual at one

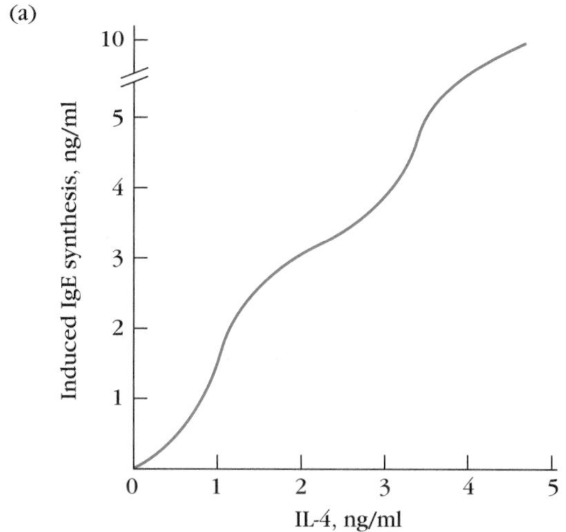

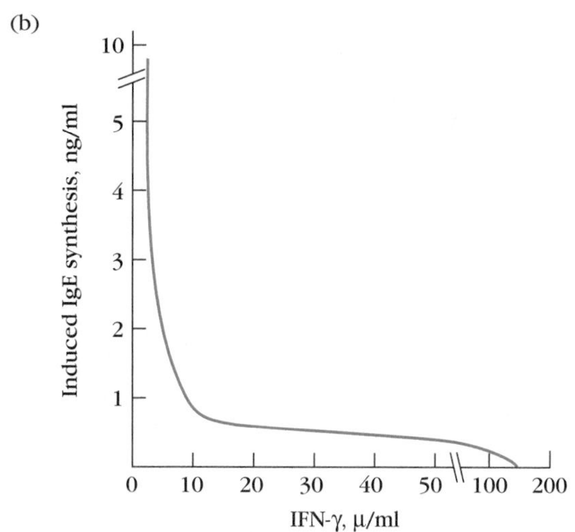

FIGURE 16-9 Effect of IL-4 and IFN-γ on in vitro production of IgE. These plots show the amount of IgE produced by plasma cells cultured in the presence of various concentrations of IL-4 (a) or IFN-γ (b). [Adapted from G Del Prete, 1988, *J. Immunol.* **140:**4193.]

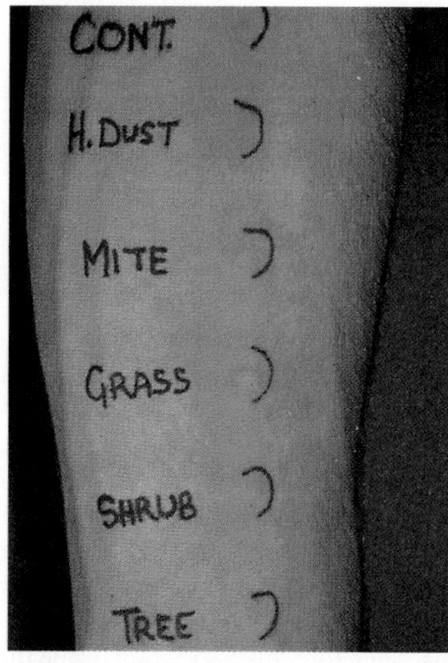

FIGURE 16-10 Skin testing by intradermal injection of allergens into the forearm. In this individual, a wheal and flare response developed within a few minutes at the site where grass was injected, indicating that the individual is allergic to grass. [From LM Lichtenstein, 1993, *Sci. Am.* **269**(2):117. Used with permission.]

time. If a person is allergic to the allergen, local mast cells degranulate and the release of histamine and other mediators produces a wheal and flare within 30 min (Figure 16-10). The advantage of skin testing is that it is relatively inexpensive and allows screening of a large number of allergens in a single sitting. The disadvantage of skin testing is that it sometimes sensitizes the allergic individual to new allergens and in some rare cases may induce systemic anaphylactic shock. A few individuals also manifest a late-phase reaction, which comes 4–6 h after testing and sometimes lasts for up to 24 h. As noted already, eosinophils accumulate during a late-phase reaction, and release of eosinophil-granule contents contributes to the tissue damage in a late-phase reaction site.

Another method of assessing type I hypersensitivity is to determine the serum level of total IgE antibody by the radioimmunosorbent test (RIST). This highly sensitive technique, based on the radioimmunoassay, can detect nanogram levels of total IgE. The patient's serum is reacted with agarose beads or paper disks coated with rabbit anti-IgE. After the beads or disks are washed, ^{125}I-labeled rabbit anti-IgE is added. The radioactivity of the beads or disks is measured with a gamma counter; it is proportional to the level of IgE in the patient's serum (Figure 16-11a).

The similar radioallergosorbent test (RAST) detects the serum level of IgE specific for a given allergen. The allergen is coupled to beads or disks, the patient's serum is added, and unbound antibody is washed away. The amount of specific IgE bound to the solid-phase allergen is then measured by adding ^{125}I-labeled rabbit anti-IgE, washing the beads, and counting the bound radioactivity (Figure 16-11b).

Therapy for Type I Hypersensitivities

The obvious first step in controlling type I hypersensitivities is to identify the offending allergen and avoid contact if possible. Often the removal of house pets, dust-control measures, or avoidance of offending foods can eliminate a type I response. Elimination of inhalant allergens (such as pollens) is a physical impossibility, however, and other means of intervention must be pursued.

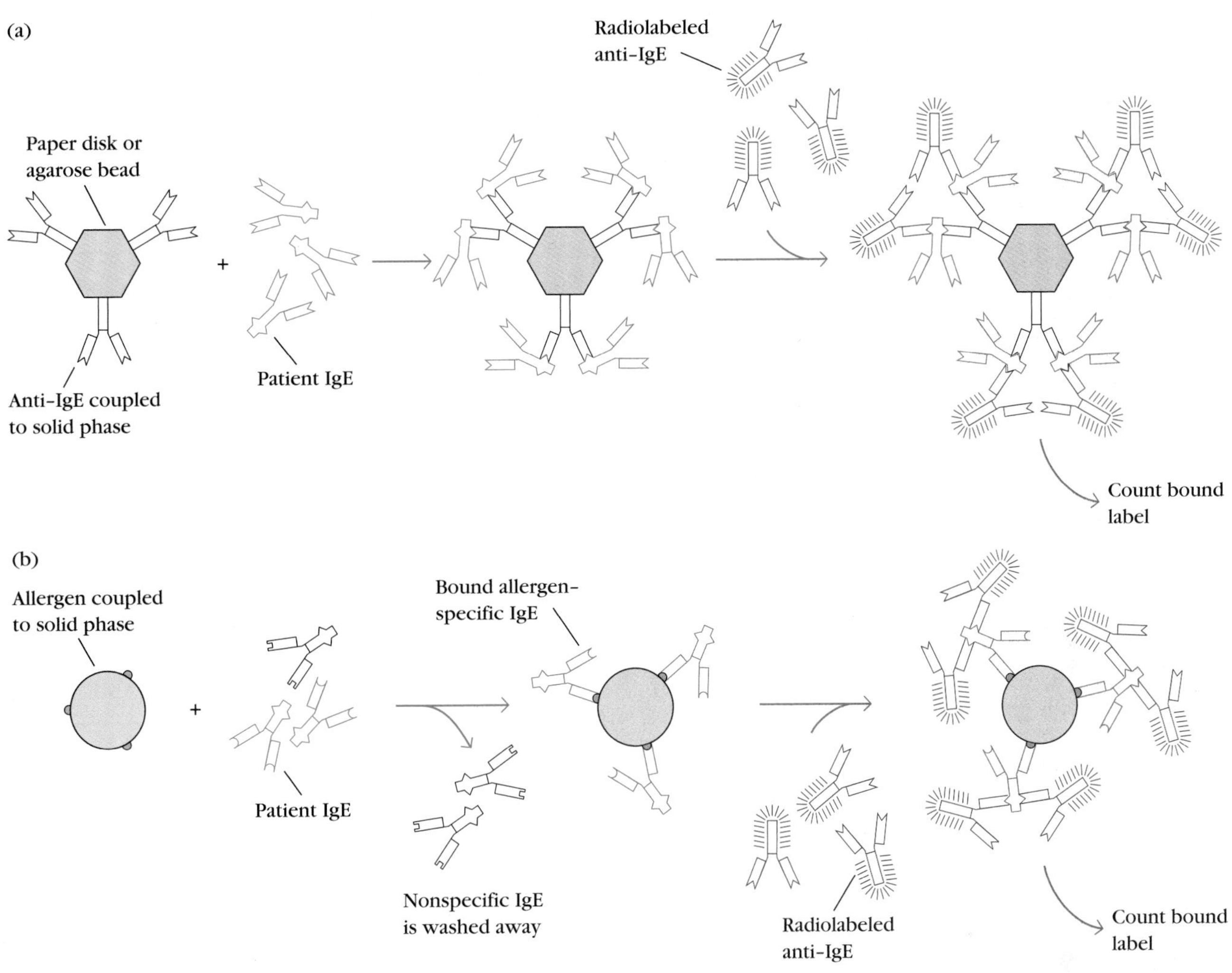

FIGURE 16-11 Procedures for assessing type I hypersensitivity. (a) Radioimmunosorbent test (RIST) can quantify nanogram amounts of total serum IgE. (b) Radioallergosorbent test (RAST) can quantify nanogram amounts of serum IgE specific for a particular allergen.

Immunotherapy with repeated injections of increasing doses of allergens (hyposensitization) has been known for some time to reduce the severity of type I reactions, or even eliminate them completely, in a significant number of individuals suffering from allergic rhinitis. Such repeated introduction of allergen by subcutaneous injections appears to cause a shift toward IgG production or to induce T-cell–mediated suppression (possibly by a shift to the T_H1 subset and IFN-γ production) that turns off the IgE response (Figure 16-12). In this situation, the IgG antibody is referred to as blocking antibody because it competes for the allergen, binds to it, and forms a complex that can be removed by phagocytosis; as a result, the allergen is not available to crosslink the fixed IgE on the mast cell membranes, so that allergic symptoms decrease.

Another approach for treating allergies stems from the finding that soluble antigens tend to induce a state of anergy by activating T cells in the absence of the necessary co-stimulatory signal (see Figure 10-15). Presumably, a soluble antigen is internalized by endocytosis, processed, and presented with class II MHC molecules, but fails to induce expression of the requisite co-stimulatory ligand (B7) on antigen-presenting cells.

Knowledge of the mechanism of mast-cell degranulation and the mediators involved in type I reactions opened the way to drug therapy for allergies. Antihistamines have been the most useful drugs for symptoms of allergic rhinitis. These drugs act by binding to the histamine receptors on target cells and blocking the binding of histamine. The H_1 receptors are blocked by the classical antihistamines, and the H_2 receptors by a newer class of antihistamines.

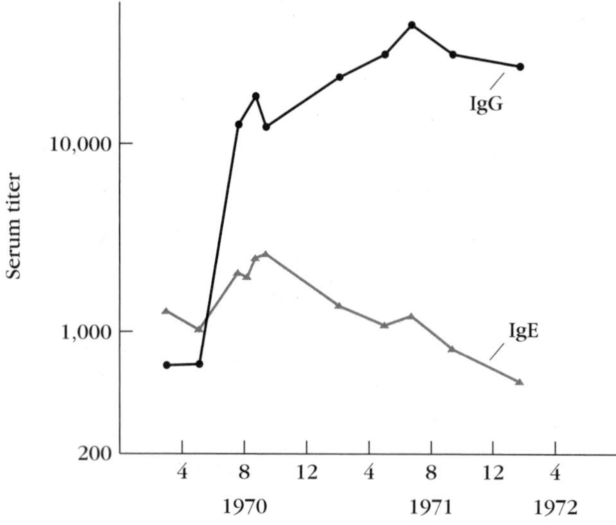

FIGURE 16-12 Hyposensitization treatment of type I allergy. Injection of ragweed antigen periodically for 2 years into a ragweed-sensitive individual induced a gradual decrease in IgE levels and a dramatic increase in IgG. Both antibodies were measured by a radioimmunoassay. [Adapted from K Ishizaka and T Ishizaka, 1973, in *Asthma Physiology, Immunopharmacology and Treatment,* KF Austen and LM Lichtenstein (eds.), Academic Press.]

TABLE 16-4 MECHANISM OF ACTION OF SOME DRUGS USED TO TREAT TYPE I HYPERSENSITIVITY

Drug	Action
Antihistamines	Block H_1 and H_2 receptors on target cells
Cromolyn sodium	Blocks Ca^{2+} influx into mast cells
Theophylline	Prolongs high cAMP levels in mast cells by inhibiting phosphodiesterase, which cleaves cAMP to 5′-AMP*
Epinephrine (adrenalin)	Stimulates cAMP production by binding to β-adrenergic receptors on mast cells*
Cortisone	Reduces histamine levels by blocking conversion of histidine to histamine and stimulates mast-cell production of cAMP*

*Although cAMP rises transiently during mast cell activation, degranulation is prevented if cAMP levels remain high.

Several drugs block release of allergic mediators by interfering with various biochemical steps in mast-cell activation and degranulation (Table 16-4). Disodium cromoglycate (cromolyn sodium) prevents Ca^{2+} influx into mast cells. Theophylline, which is commonly administered to asthmatics orally or through inhalers, blocks phosphodiesterase, which catalyzes conversion of cAMP to 5 -AMP. The resulting prolonged increase in cAMP levels blocks degranulation. A number of drugs stimulate the β-adrenergic system by stimulating β receptors. As mentioned earlier, epinephrine (also known as adrenaline) is commonly administered during anaphylactic shock. It acts by binding to β receptors on bronchial smooth muscles and mast cells, elevating the cAMP levels within these cells. The increased levels of cAMP lead to relaxation of the bronchial muscles and decreased mast-cell degranulation. A number of epinephrine analogs have been developed that bind to selected β receptors and induce cAMP increases with fewer side effects than seen with epinephrine. Cortisone and various other anti-inflammatory drugs also have been used to reduce type I reactions.

Antibody-Mediated Cytotoxic (Type II) Hypersensitivity

Type II hypersensitive reactions involve antibody-mediated destruction of cells. This type of reaction is best exemplified by blood-transfusion reactions, in which host antibodies react with foreign antigens on the incompatible transfused blood cells and mediate destruction of these cells. Antibody can mediate cell destruction by activating the complement system to create pores in the membrane of the foreign cell (see Figure 13-5). Antibody can also mediate cell destruction by antibody-dependent cell-mediated cytotoxicity (ADCC). In this process, cytotoxic cells with Fc receptors bind to the Fc region of antibodies on target cells and promote killing of the cells (see Figure 14-12). Antibody bound to a foreign cell also can serve as an opsonin, enabling phagocytic cells with Fc or C3b receptors to bind and phagocytose the antibody-coated cell (see Figure 13-12).

This section examines three examples of type II hypersensitive reactions. Certain autoimmune diseases involve auto-antibody-mediated cellular destruction by type II mechanisms. These diseases are described in Chapter 20.

Transfusion Reactions

A large number of proteins and glycoproteins on the membrane of red blood cells are encoded by different genes, each of which has a number of alternative alleles. An individual possessing one allelic form of a blood-group antigen can recognize other allelic forms on transfused blood as foreign and mount an antibody response. In some cases, the antibodies have already been induced by natural exposure to similar antigenic determinants on a variety of microorganisms thought to be normal flora of the gut. This is the case with the ABO blood-group antigens (Figure 16-13a).

(a)

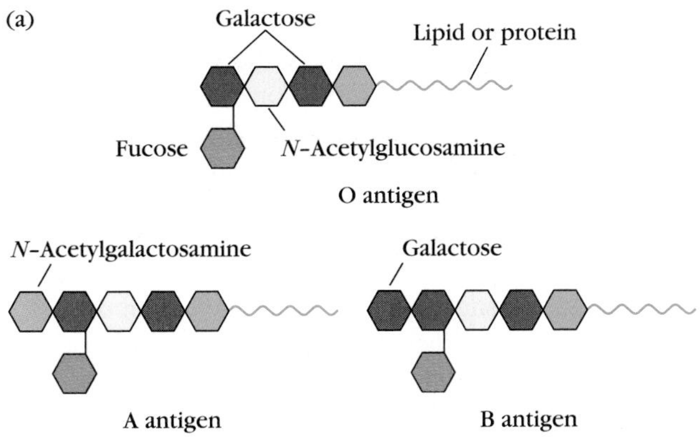

(b)

Genotype	Blood-group phenotype	Antigens on erythrocytes (*agglutinins*)	Serum antibodies (*isohemagglutinins*)
AA or AO	A	A	Anti-B
BB or BO	B	B	Anti-A
AB	AB	A and B	None
OO	O	None	Anti-A and anti-B

FIGURE 16-13 ABO blood group. (a) Structure of terminal sugars, which constitute the distinguishing epitopes, in the A, B, and O blood antigens. (b) ABO genotypes and corresponding phenotypes, agglutinins, and isohemagglutinins.

Antibodies to the A, B, and O antigens, called isohemagglutinins, are usually of the IgM class. An individual with blood type A, for example, recognizes B-like epitopes on intestinal microorganisms and produces isohemagglutinins to the B-like epitopes. This same individual does not respond to A-like epitopes on the same intestinal microorganisms because these A-like epitopes are too similar to self and a state of self-tolerance to these epitopes should exist (Figure 16-13b). If a type A individual is accidentally transfused with blood containing type B cells, the anti-B isohemagglutinins will bind to the B blood cells and mediate their destruction by means of complement-mediated lysis. Antibodies to other blood-group antigens may result from repeated blood transfusions because minor allelic differences in these antigens can stimulate antibody production. These antibodies are usually of the IgG class.

Transfusion of blood into a recipient possessing antibodies to one of the blood-group antigens can result in a transfusion reaction. The clinical manifestations of transfusion reactions result from massive intravascular hemolysis of the transfused red blood cells by antibody plus complement. These manifestations may be either immediate or delayed. Reactions that begin immediately are most commonly associated with ABO blood-group incompatibilities, which lead to complement-mediated lysis triggered by the IgM isohemagglutinins. Within hours, free hemoglobin can be detected in the plasma; it is filtered through the kidneys, resulting in hemoglobinuria. Some of the hemoglobin gets converted to bilirubin, which at high levels is toxic. Typical symptoms include fever, chills, nausea, clotting within blood vessels, pain in the lower back, and hemoglobin in the urine. Treatment involves prompt termination of the transfusion and maintenance of urine flow with a diuretic, because the accumulation of hemoglobin in the kidney can cause acute tubular necrosis.

Delayed hemolytic transfusion reactions generally occur in individuals who have received repeated transfusions of ABO-compatible blood that is incompatible for other blood-group antigens. The reactions develop between 2 and 6 days after transfusion and reflect the secondary nature of these reactions. The transfused blood induces clonal selection and production of IgG against a variety of blood-group membrane antigens. The most common blood-group antigens that induce delayed transfusion reactions are Rh, Kidd, Kell, and Duffy. The predominant isotype involved in these reactions is IgG, which is less effective than IgM in activating complement. For this reason, complement-mediated lysis of the transfused red blood cells is incomplete, and many of the transfused cells are destroyed at extravascular sites by agglutination, opsonization, and subsequent phagocytosis by macrophages. Symptoms include fever, low hemoglobin, increased bilirubin, mild jaundice, and anemia. Free hemoglobin is usually not detected in the plasma or urine in these reactions because RBC destruction occurs in extravascular sites.

Transfusion reactions can be prevented by proper cross-matching between the donor's and the recipient's blood. Cross-matching can reveal the presence of the antibodies in donor or recipient sera that can cause these reactions.

Hemolytic Disease of the Newborn

Hemolytic disease of the newborn develops when maternal IgG antibodies specific for fetal blood-group antigens cross the placenta and destroy fetal red blood cells. The consequences of such transfer can be minor, serious, or lethal. Severe hemolytic disease of the newborn, called **erythroblastosis fetalis,** most commonly develops when an Rh^+ fetus expresses an **Rh antigen** on its blood cells that the Rh^- mother does not express.

During pregnancy, fetal red blood cells are separated from the mother's circulation by a layer of cells in the placenta called the trophoblast. During her first pregnancy with an Rh^+ fetus, an Rh^- woman is usually not exposed to enough fetal red blood cells to activate her Rh-specific B cells. At the time of delivery, however, separation of the placenta from the uterine wall allows larger amounts of fetal umbilical-cord blood to enter the mother's circulation. These fetal red blood cells activate Rh-specific B cells, resulting in production of Rh-specific plasma cells and memory B cells in the mother. The secreted IgM antibody clears the Rh^+ fetal red cells from the mother's circulation, but the memory cells remain, a threat to any subsequent pregnancy with an Rh^+ fetus. Activation of these memory cells in a subsequent pregnancy results in the formation of IgG anti-Rh antibodies, which cross the placenta and damage the fetal red blood cells (Figure 16-14). Mild to severe anemia can develop in the fetus, sometimes with fatal consequences. In addition, conversion of hemoglobin to bilirubin can present an additional threat to the newborn because the lipid-soluble bilirubin may accumulate in the brain and cause brain damage.

Hemolytic disease of the newborn caused by Rh incompatibility in a subsequent pregnancy can be almost entirely prevented by administering antibodies against the Rh antigen to the mother within 24–48 h after the first delivery. These antibodies, called **Rhogam,** bind to any fetal red blood cells that enter the mother's circulation at the time of delivery and facilitate their clearance before B-cell activation and ensuing memory-cell production can take place. In a subsequent pregnancy with an Rh^+ fetus, a mother who has been treated with Rhogam is unlikely to produce IgG anti-Rh antibodies; thus, the fetus is protected from the damage that occurs when these antibodies cross the placenta.

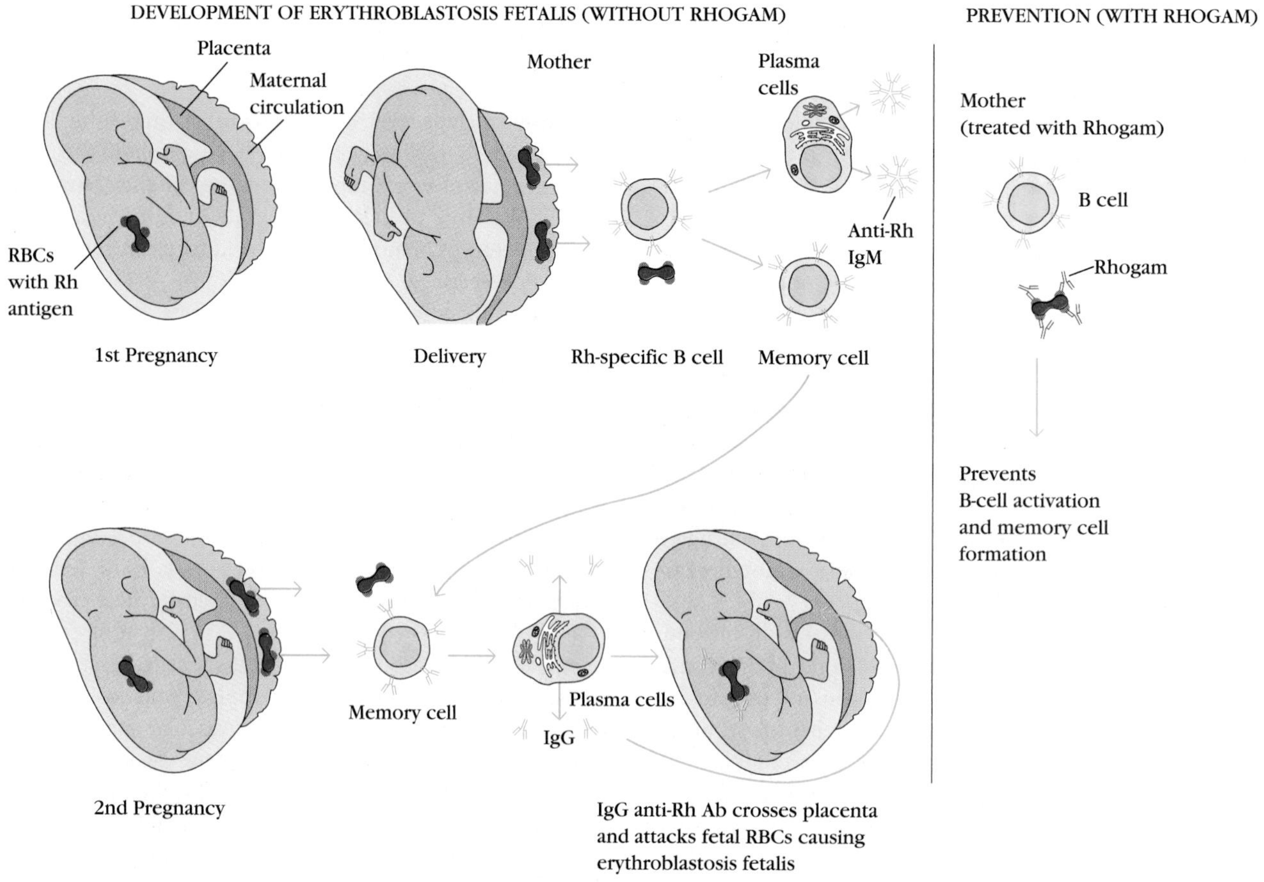

FIGURE 16-14 Development of erythroblastosis fetalis (hemolytic disease of the newborn) caused when an Rh^- mother carries an Rh^+ fetus (*left*), and effect of treatment with anti-Rh antibody, or Rhogam (*right*).

The development of hemolytic disease of the newborn caused by Rh incompatibility can be detected by testing maternal serum at intervals during pregnancy for antibodies to the Rh antigen. A rise in the titer of these antibodies as pregnancy progresses indicates that the mother has been exposed to Rh antigens and is producing increasing amounts of antibody. The presence of maternal IgG on the surface of fetal red blood cells can be detected by a Coombs test. Isolated fetal red blood cells are incubated with the Coombs reagent, goat antibody to human IgG antibody. If maternal IgG is bound to the fetal red blood cells, the cells agglutinate with the Coombs reagent.

If hemolytic disease caused by Rh incompatibility is detected during pregnancy, the treatment depends on the severity of the reaction. For a severe reaction, the fetus can be given an intrauterine blood-exchange transfusion to replace fetal Rh^+ red blood cells with Rh^- cells. These transfusions are given every 10–21 days until delivery. In less severe cases, a blood-exchange transfusion is not given until after birth, primarily to remove bilirubin; the infant is also exposed to low levels of UV light to break down the bilirubin and prevent any cerebral damage. The mother can also be treated during the pregnancy by **plasmapheresis.** In this procedure, a cell-separation machine is used to separate the mother's blood into two fractions, cells and plasma. The plasma containing the anti-Rh antibody is discarded, and the cells are reinfused into the mother in an albumin or fresh plasma solution.

The majority of cases (65%) of hemolytic disease of the newborn have minor consequences and are caused by ABO blood-group incompatibility between the mother and fetus. Type A or B fetuses carried by type O mothers most commonly develop these reactions. A type O mother is most likely to develop IgG antibody to the A or B blood-group antigens either through natural exposure or through exposure to fetal blood-group A or B antigens in successive pregnancies. Usually the fetal anemia resulting from this incompatibility is mild; the major clinical manifestation is a slight elevation of bilirubin, with jaundice. Depending on the severity of the anemia and jaundice, a blood-exchange transfusion may be required in these infants. In general the reaction is mild, however, and exposure of the infant to low levels of UV light is enough to break down the bilirubin and avoid any cerebral damage.

Drug-Induced Hemolytic Anemia

Certain antibiotics (e.g., penicillin, cephalosporin, and streptomycin) can adsorb nonspecifically to proteins on RBC membranes, forming a complex similar to a hapten-carrier complex. In some patients, such drug-protein complexes induce formation of antibodies, which then bind to the adsorbed drug on red blood cells, inducing complement-mediated lysis and thus progressive anemia. When the drug is withdrawn, the hemolytic anemia disappears. Penicillin is notable in that it can induce all four types of hypersensitivity with various clinical manifestations (Table 16-5).

TABLE 16-5 PENICILLIN-INDUCED HYPERSENSITIVE REACTIONS

Type of reaction	Antibody or lymphocytes induced	Clinical manifestations
I	IgE	Urticaria, systemic anaphylaxis
II	IgM, IgG	Hemolytic anemia
III	IgG	Serum sickness, glomerulonephritis
IV	T_{DTH} cells	Contact dermatitis

Immune Complex–Mediated (Type III) Hypersensitivity

The reaction of antibody with antigen generates immune complexes. Generally this complexing of antigen with antibody facilitates the clearance of antigen by phagocytic cells. In some cases, however, large amounts of immune complexes can lead to tissue-damaging type III hypersensitive reactions. The magnitude of the reaction depends on the quantity of immune complexes as well as their distribution within the body. Depending on where these complexes are carried, different tissue-damaging reactions can be observed. When the complexes are deposited in tissue very near the site of antigen entry, a localized reaction develops. When the complexes are formed in the blood, a reaction can develop wherever the complexes are deposited. In particular, complex deposition is frequently observed on blood-vessel walls, in the synovial membrane of joints, on the glomerular basement membrane of the kidney, and on the choroid plexus of the brain. The deposition of these complexes initiates a reaction that results in the recruitment of neutrophils to the site. The tissue there is injured as a consequence of granular release from the neutrophil.

Type III hypersensitive reactions develop when immune complexes activate the complement system's array of immune effector molecules (see Figure 13-2). As explained in Chapter 13, the C3a, C4a, and C5a complement split products are anaphylatoxins that cause localized mast-cell degranulation and consequent increase in local vascular permeability. C3a, C5a, and C5b67 are also chemotactic factors for neutrophils, which can accumulate in large numbers at the site of immune-complex deposition. Larger immune complexes are deposited on the basement membrane of blood-vessel walls or kidney glomeruli, whereas smaller complexes may pass through the basement membrane and be deposited in the subepithelium. The type of lesion that results depends on the site of deposition of the complexes.

Much of the tissue damage in type III reactions stems from release of lytic enzymes by neutrophils as they attempt to phagocytose immune complexes. The C3b complement component acts as an opsonin, coating immune complexes. A neutrophil binds to a C3b-coated immune complex by means of the type I complement receptor, which is specific for C3b. Because the complex is deposited on the basement-membrane surface, phagocytosis is impeded, so that lytic enzymes are released during the unsuccessful attempts of the neutrophil to ingest the adhering immune complex. Further activation of the membrane-attack mechanism of the complement system can also contribute to the destruction of tissue. In addition, the activation of complement can induce aggregation of platelets, and the resulting release of clotting factors can lead to formation of microthrombi.

Localized Type III Reactions

Injection of an antigen intradermally or subcutaneously into an animal that has high levels of circulating antibody specific for that antigen leads to formation of localized immune complexes, which mediate an acute Arthus reaction within 4–8 h (Figure 16-15). Microscopic examination of the tissue reveals neutrophils adhering to the vascular endothelium and then migrating into the tissues at the site of immune-complex deposition. As the reaction develops, localized tissue and vascular damage results in an accumulation of fluid (edema) and red blood cells (erythema) at the site. The severity of the reaction can vary from mild swelling and redness to tissue necrosis.

After an insect bite, a sensitive individual may have a rapid, localized type I reaction at the site. Often, some 4–8 h later, a typical Arthus reaction also develops at the site,

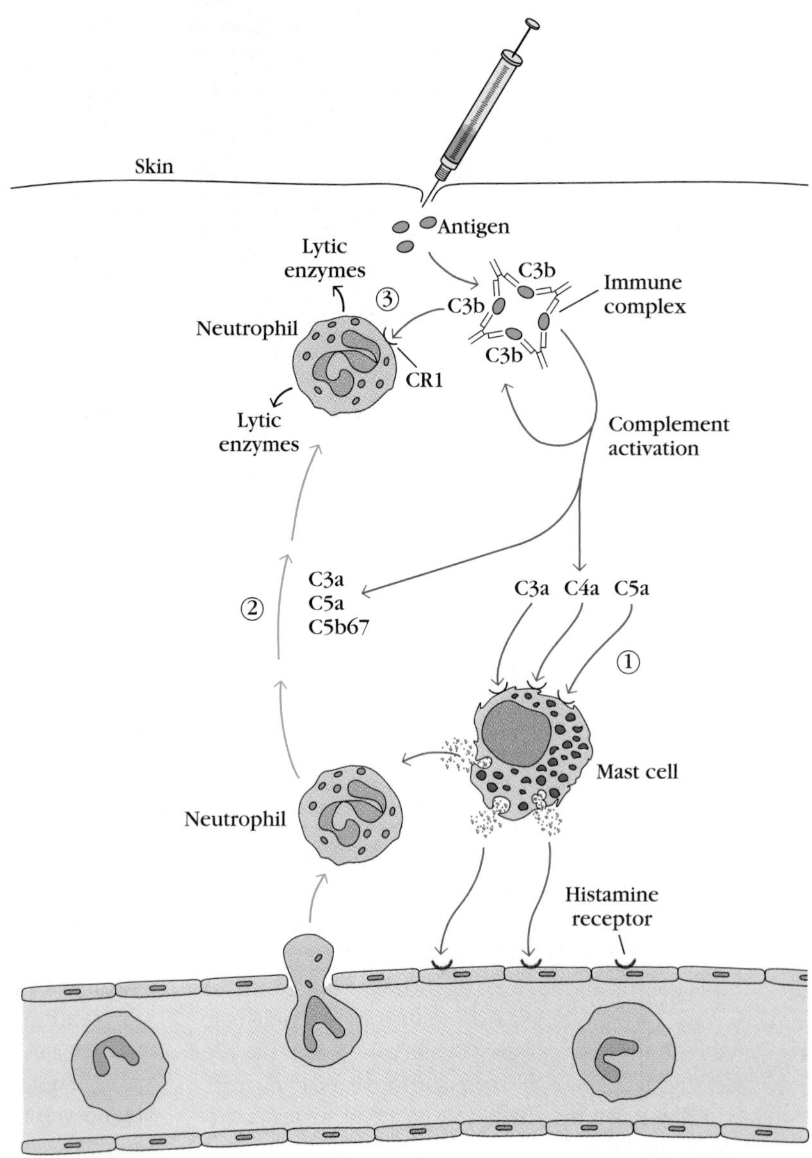

FIGURE 16-15 Development of a localized Arthus reaction (type III hypersensitive reaction). Complement activation initiated by immune complexes (classical pathway) produces complement intermediates that (1) mediate mast-cell degranulation, (2) chemotactically attract neutrophils, and (3) stimulate release of lytic enzymes from neutrophils trying to phagocytose C3b-coated immune complexes.

with pronounced erythema and edema. Intrapulmonary Arthus-type reactions induced by bacterial spores, fungi, or dried fecal proteins can also cause pneumonitis or alveolitis. These reactions are known by a variety of common names reflecting the source of the antigen. For example, "farmer's lung" develops after inhalation of thermophilic actinomycetes from moldy hay, and "pigeon fancier's disease" results from inhalation of a serum protein in dust derived from dried pigeon feces.

Generalized Type III Reactions

When large amounts of antigen enter the bloodstream and bind to antibody, circulating immune complexes can form. If antigen is in excess, small complexes form; because these are not easily cleared by the phagocytic cells, they can cause tissue-damaging type III reactions at various sites. Historically, generalized type III reactions were often observed after the administration of antitoxins containing foreign serum, such as horse antitetanus or antidiphtheria serum. In such cases, the recipient of a foreign antiserum develops antibodies specific for the foreign serum proteins; these antibodies then form circulating immune complexes with the foreign serum antigens. Typically, within days or weeks after exposure to foreign serum antigens, an individual begins to manifest a combination of symptoms that are called **serum sickness** (Figure 16-16). These symptoms include fever, weakness, generalized vasculitis (rashes) with edema and erythema, lymphadenopathy, arthritis, and sometimes glomerulonephritis. The precise manifestations of serum sickness depend on the quantity of immune complexes formed as well as the overall size of the complexes, which determine the site of their deposition. As mentioned above, the sites of deposition vary but, in general, complexes accumulate in tissues where filtration of plasma occurs. This explains the high incidence of glomerulonephritis (complex deposition in the kidney) and vasculitis (deposition in the arteries) and arthritis (deposition in the synovial joints) caused by serum sickness.

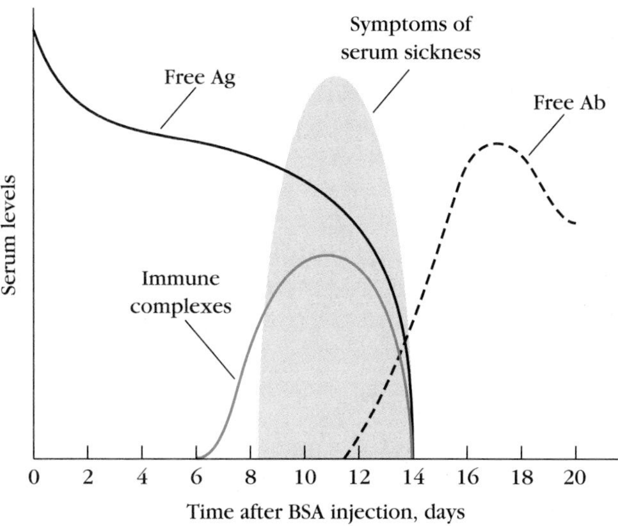

FIGURE 16-16 Correlation between formation of immune complexes and development of symptoms of serum sickness. A large dose of antigen (BSA) was injected into a rabbit at day 0. As antibody formed, it complexed with the antigen and was deposited in the kidneys, joints, and capillaries. The symptoms of serum sickness (light blue area) corresponded to the peak in immune-complex formation. As the immune complexes were cleared, free circulating antibody (dashed black curve) was detected and the symptoms of serum sickness subsided. [Based on FG Germuth, Jr, 1953, *J. Exp. Med.* **97**:257.]

Formation of circulating immune complexes contributes to the pathogenesis of a number of conditions other than serum sickness. These include the following:

- *Autoimmune Diseases*
  Systemic lupus erythematosus
  Rheumatoid arthritis
  Goodpasture's syndrome
- *Drug Reactions*
  Allergies to penicillin and sulfonamides
- *Infectious Diseases*
  Poststreptococcal glomerulonephritis
  Meningitis
  Hepatitis
  Mononucleosis
  Malaria
  Trypanosomiasis

Complexes of antibody with various bacterial, viral, and parasitic antigens have been shown to induce a variety of type III hypersensitive reactions, including skin rashes, arthritic symptoms, and glomerulonephritis. Poststreptococcal glomerulonephritis, for example, develops when circulating complexes of antibody and streptococcal antigens are deposited in the kidney and damage the glomeruli. A number of autoimmune diseases stem from circulating complexes of antibody with self-proteins, with glycoproteins, or even with DNA. In systemic lupus erythematosus, complexes of DNA and anti-DNA antibodies accumulate in synovial membranes, causing arthritic symptoms, or accumulate on the basement membrane of the kidney, causing progressive kidney damage.

T_{DTH}-Mediated (Type IV) Hypersensitivity

Type IV hypersensitive reactions develop when antigen activates sensitized T_{DTH} cells; these cells generally appear to be a T_H1 subpopulation, although sometimes T_C cells are involved. Activation of T_{DTH} cells by antigen on appropriate antigen-presenting cells results in the secretion of various cytokines, including interleukin 2 (IL-2), interferon gamma

(IFN-γ), macrophage-inhibition factor (MIF), and tumor necrosis factor β (TNF-β) (see Figure 14-15). The overall effect of these cytokines is to draw macrophages into the area and activate them, promoting increased phagocytic activity and increased concentrations of lytic enzymes for more effective killing. As lytic enzymes leak out of the activated macrophages into the surrounding tissue, localized tissue destruction can ensue. These reactions typically take 48–72 h to develop, the time required for initial T_{DTH}-cell activation and cytokine secretion to mediate accumulation of macrophages and the subsequent release of their lytic enzymes. The hallmarks of a type IV reaction are the delay in time required for the reaction to develop and the recruitment of macrophages as opposed to neutrophils, as found in a type III reaction. Macrophages are the major component of the infiltrate that surrounds the site of inflammation.

As explained in Chapter 14, several lines of evidence suggest that the type IV (or DTH) reaction is important in host defense against parasites and bacteria that can live within cells. Once these organisms are inside the host's cells, circulating antibodies cannot reach them. However, the heightened phagocytic activity and the buildup of lytic enzymes from macrophages in the area of infection lead to nonspecific destruction of cells, and thus of the intracellular pathogen. When this defense process is not entirely effective, the continued presence of the pathogen's antigens can provoke a chronic DTH reaction, which is characterized by excessive numbers of macrophages, continual release of lytic enzymes, and consequent tissue destruction. The granulomatous skin lesions seen with *Mycobacterium leprae* and the lung cavitation seen with *Mycobacterium tuberculosis* are examples of the tissue damage that can result when chronic delayed-type hypersensitive reactions develop (see Figures 14-16 and 17-9).

The reaction to an intradermal injection of an antigen can serve as a test for the presence of T_{DTH} cells previously sensitized by that antigen. The use of the PPD antigen to detect previous exposure to *M. tuberculosis* was described in Chapter 14. Similar skin tests to detect previous exposure to the bacterium that causes leprosy and the fungus that causes coccidiomycosis use lepromin and coccidiodin, respectively, as test antigens. In these tests, the appearance of swelling and redness at the injection site within 48–72 h is a positive reaction. The depletion in $CD4^+$ T cells associated with AIDS can be monitored by repeated skin testing with any of the various antigens, such as haptens (e.g., nickle or chromate) or antigens (e.g., tuberculin), that induce a type IV DTH response in most normal individuals. As AIDS progresses, the decline in T_{DTH} cells is reflected in decreased skin reactivity to such antigens.

Many contact-dermatitis reactions, including the responses to formaldehyde, trinitrophenol, nickel, turpentine, various cosmetics and hair dyes, poison oak, and poison ivy, are mediated by T_{DTH} cells. Most of these substances are small molecules that can complex with skin proteins. This complex is internalized by antigen-presenting cells in the skin (e.g., Langerhans cells), then processed and presented together with class II MHC molecules, causing activation of sensitized T_{DTH} cells. In the reaction to poison oak, for example, a pentadecacatechol compound from the leaves of the plant complexes with skin proteins. When T_H cells react with this compound appropriately displayed by local antigen-presenting cells, they differentiate into sensitized T_{DTH} cells. A subsequent exposure to pentadecacatechol will elicit activation of T_{DTH} cells and induce cytokine production (Figure 16-17). Approximately 48–72 h after this secondary exposure, the secreted cytokines cause macrophages to accumulate at the site. Activation of these macrophages and release of their lytic enzymes result in the redness and pustules that characterize a reaction to poison oak.

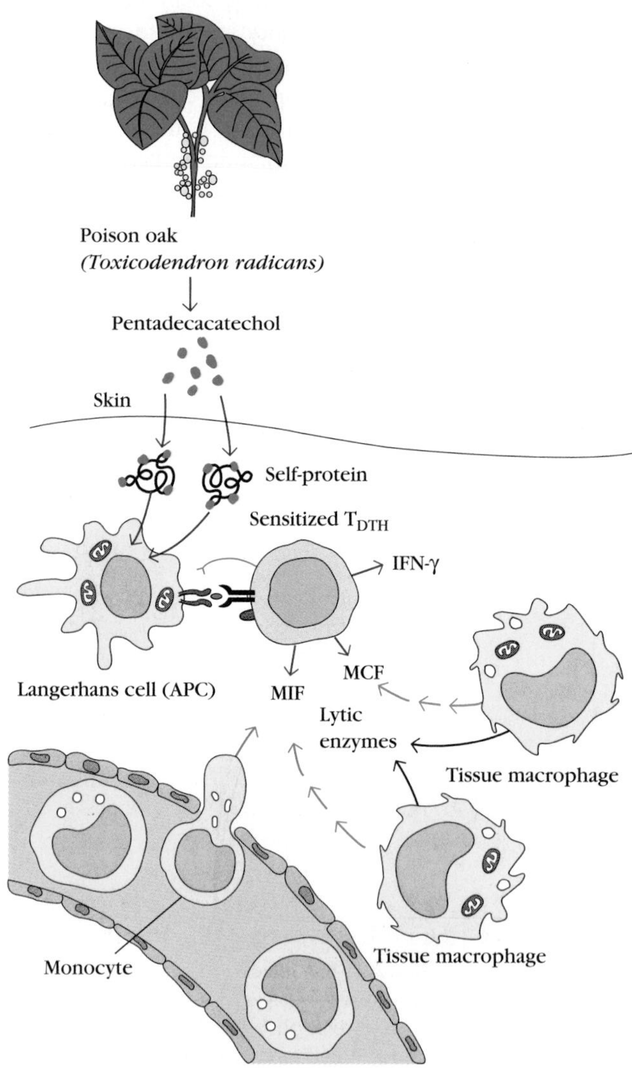

FIGURE 16-17 Development of delayed-type hypersensitivity reaction after a second exposure to poison oak. Cytokines such as IFN-γ, MCF, and MIF released from sensitized T_{DTH} cells mediate this reaction. Tissue damage results from lytic enzymes released from activated macrophages. MCF = macrophage-chemotactic factor; MIF = migration-inhibition factor. See also Figure 14-15.

Summary

1. Hypersensitive reactions are inflammatory reactions within the humoral or cell-mediated branches of the immune system that lead to extensive tissue damage or even death. These reactions are classified into four main types according to the mechanism that induces them (see Figure 16-1). Each type generates characteristic effector molecules and clinical manifestations.
2. A type I hypersensitive reaction is mediated by IgE antibodies, whose Fc region binds to receptors on mast cells or blood basophils (see Figure 16-2). Crosslinkage of the fixed IgE by allergen initiates a sequence of intracellular events leading to mast cell or basophil degranulation with release of pharmacologically active mediators (see Table 16-3). The mediators are the immune effector molecules in this reaction. The principal effects of these mediators are smooth-muscle contraction and vasodilation. Clinical manifestations of type I reactions include potentially life-threatening systemic anaphylaxis and localized responses such as hay fever and asthma (see Figure 16-8).
3. A type II hypersensitive reaction occurs when antibody reacts with antigenic determinants present on the surface of cells, leading to cell damage or death through complement-mediated lysis or antibody-dependent cell-mediated cytotoxicity (ADCC). Transfusion reactions, resulting from mismatching of donor and recipient blood, and hemolytic disease of the newborn are two clinical conditions caused by type II reactions. The latter is most likely when an Rh^- mother carries an Rh^+ fetus (see Figure 16-14).
4. A type III hypersensitive reaction is mediated by the formation of immune complexes and the ensuing activation of complement. Complement split products serve as immune effector molecules that elicit localized vasodilation and chemotactically attract neutrophils. Deposition of immune complexes near the site of antigen entry can induce an Arthus reaction, in which lytic enzymes released by the accumulated neutrophils and the complement membrane-attack complex cause localized tissue damage (see Figure 16-15). Generalized type III reactions occur when circulating immune complexes are deposited at various sites; the manifestations of these reactions vary depending on the site of tissue deposition.
5. A type IV hypersensitive reaction involves the cell-mediated branch of the immune system. Antigen activation of sensitized T_{DTH} cells induces release of various cytokines, which serve as the immune effector molecules in this reaction (see Figure 16-17). The net effect of these cytokines is to cause an accumulation and activation of macrophages, which release lytic enzymes that cause localized tissue damage.

REFERENCES

Ansari, AA, et al. 1989. Human immune responsiveness to *Lolium perenne* pollen allergen Lol p III (rye III) is associated with HLA-DR3 and DR5. *Hum. Immunol.* **25:**59.

Aubry, JP, et al. 1992. CD21 is a ligand for CD23 and regulates IgE production. *Nature* **358:**505.

Barnes, KC, and DG Marsh. 1998. The genetics and complexity of allergy and asthma. *Immunol. Today* **19:**325.

Bonnefoy, JY, et al. 1993. A new pair of surface molecules involved in human IgE regulation. *Immunol. Today* **14:**1.

Borish, L. 1999. Genetics of allergy and asthma. *Ann. Allergy Asthma Immunol.* **82:**413.

The Collaborative Study on the Genetics of Asthma (CSGA). 1997. A genome-wide search for asthma susceptibility loci in ethnically diverse populations. *Nat. Genet.* **15:**389.

Daser, A, et al. 1995. Role and modulation of T-cell cytokines in allergy. *Curr. Opin. Immunol.* **7:**762.

Finkelman, FD, et al. 1988. IL-4 is required to generate and sustain in vivo IgE response. *J. Immunol.* **141:**2335.

Gordon, JR, PR Burd, and SJ Gali. 1990. Mast cells as a source of multifunctional cytokines. *Immunol. Today* **11:**457.

Holt, PG. 1994. Immunoprophylaxis of atopy: light at the end of the tunnel? *Immunol. Today* **15:**484.

Hoyne, GF, et al. 1995. Peptide modulation of allergen-specific immune responses. *Curr. Opin. Immunol.* **7:**757.

Kawakami, T, et al. 1992. Tyrosine phosphorylation is required for mast cell activation by FcεRI crosslinking. *J. Immunol.* **148:**3513.

Kuhn, R, K Rajewsky, and W Muller. 1991. Generation and analysis of interleukin-4 deficient mice. *Science* **254:**707.

Lympany, P, et al. 1992. Genetic analysis of the linkage between chromosome 11q and atopy. *Clin. Exp. Allergy* **22:**1085.

Marsh, DG, et al. 1994. Linkage analysis of IL-4 and other chromosome 5q31.1 markers and total serum immunoglobulin E concentrations. *Science* **264:**1152.

Metzger, H. 1999. It's spring, and thoughts turn to . . . allergies. *Cell* **97:**287.

Paul-Eugène, N, et al. 1993. Functional interaction between β_2-adrenoceptor agonists and interleukin-4 in the regulation of CD23 expression and release and IgE production in humans. *Molec. Immunol.* **30:**157.

Razin, E, I Pecht, and J Rivera. 1995. Signal transduction in the activation of mast cells and basophils. *Immunol. Today* **16:**370.

Rosenstreich, DL, et al. 1997. The role of cockroach allergy and exposure to cockroach allergen in causing morbidity among inner-city children with asthma. *N. Engl. J. Med.* **336:**1356.

Teixeira, MM, TJ Williams, and PG Hellewell. 1995. Mechanisms and pharmacological manipulation of eosinophil accumulation. *Trends Pharmacol. Sci.* **16:**418.

Thomas, P, et al. 1992. Glycosylation-inhibiting factor from human T cell hybridomas constructed from peripheral blood lymphocytes of a bee venom–sensitive allergic patient. *J. Immunol.* **148:**729.

Williams, J, et al. 1992. Regulation of low-affinity IgE receptor (CD23) expression on mononuclear phagocytes in normal and asthmatic subjects. *J. Immunol.* **149**:2823.

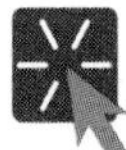

Useful Web Sites

http://www.niaid.nih.gov/
National Institute of Allergy and Infectious Diseases homepage. NIAID is the NIH Institute that sponsors research in infectious diseases. Their Web site provides a number of links to other relevant sites.

http://allergy.mcg.edu/home.html
A site maintained by the American College of Allergy, Asthma & Immunology. An excellent source of patient information about many allergies. This site contains many valuable links.

http//:www.glaxowellcome.co.uk/health/actiontb/
Action TB—A review of tuberculosis for a general audience that appears on the Glaxo-Wellcome company's Web site.

http//:www.aaaai.org/
The American Association of Allergy, Asthma and Immunology Web site. A good site for exploring the many aspects of asthma.

STUDY QUESTIONS

1. Indicate whether each of the following statements is true or false. If you think a statement is false, explain why.

a. Mice infected with *Nippostrongylus brasiliensis* exhibit decreased production of IgE.

b. IL-4 decreases IgE production by B cells.

c. The initial step in the process of mast-cell degranulation is crosslinking of Fc receptors.

d. Antihistamines are effective for the treatment of type III hypersensitivity.

e. Most pollen allergens contain a single allergenic component.

f. Babies can acquire IgE-mediated allergies by passive transfer of maternal antibody.

g. Transfusion reactions are a manifestation of type II hypersensitivity.

h. Most T_{DTH} cells belong to the T_H1 subset.

2. In an immunology laboratory exercise, you are studying the response of mice injected intradermally with complete antibodies to the IgE Fc receptor (FcεRI) or with Fab fragments of such antibodies.

a. Predict the response expected with each type of antibody.

b. Would the responses observed depend on whether the mice were allergic? Explain.

1. Serum sickness can result when an individual is given a large dose of antiserum such as a mouse antitoxin to snake venom. How could you take advantage of recent technological advances to produce an antitoxin that would not produce serum sickness in patients who receive it?

4. What immunologic mechanisms most likely account for a person's developing each of the following reactions after an insect bite?

a. Within 1–2 min after being bitten, swelling and redness appear at the site and then disappear by 1 h.

b. 6–8 h later, swelling and redness again appear and persist for 24 h.

c. 72 h later, the tissue becomes inflamed, and tissue necrosis follows.

5. Indicate which type(s) of hypersensitive reaction (I–IV) apply to the following characteristics. Each characteristic can apply to one, or more than one, type.

a. Is an important defense against intracellular pathogens.

b. Can be induced by penicillin.

c. Involves histamine as an important mediator.

d. Can be induced by poison oak in sensitive individuals.

e. Can lead to symptoms of asthma.

f. Occurs as result of mismatched blood transfusion.

g. Systemic form of reaction is treated with epinephrine.

h. Can be induced by pollens and certain foods in sensitive individuals.

i. May involve cell destruction by antibody-dependent cell-mediated cytotoxicity.

j. One form of clinical manifestation is prevented by Rhogam.

k. Localized form characterized by wheal and flare reaction.

6. In the table on the facing page, indicate whether each immunologic event listed does (+) or does not (−) occur in each type of hypersensitive response.

Go to www.whfreeman.com/immunology Self-Test
Review and quiz of key terms

For Question 6:

Immunologic event	Hypersensitivity			
	Type I	Type II	Type III	Type IV
IgE-mediated degranulation of mast cells				
Lysis of antibody-coated blood cells by complement				
Tissue destruction in response to poison oak				
C3a- and C5a-mediated mast-cell degranulation				
Chemotaxis of neutrophils				
Chemotaxis of eosinophils				
Activation of macrophages by IFN-γ				
Deposition of antigen-antibody complexes on basement membranes of capillaries				
Sudden death due to vascular collapse (shock) shortly after injection or ingestion of antigen				

PART IV | THE IMMUNE SYSTEM IN HEALTH AND DISEASE

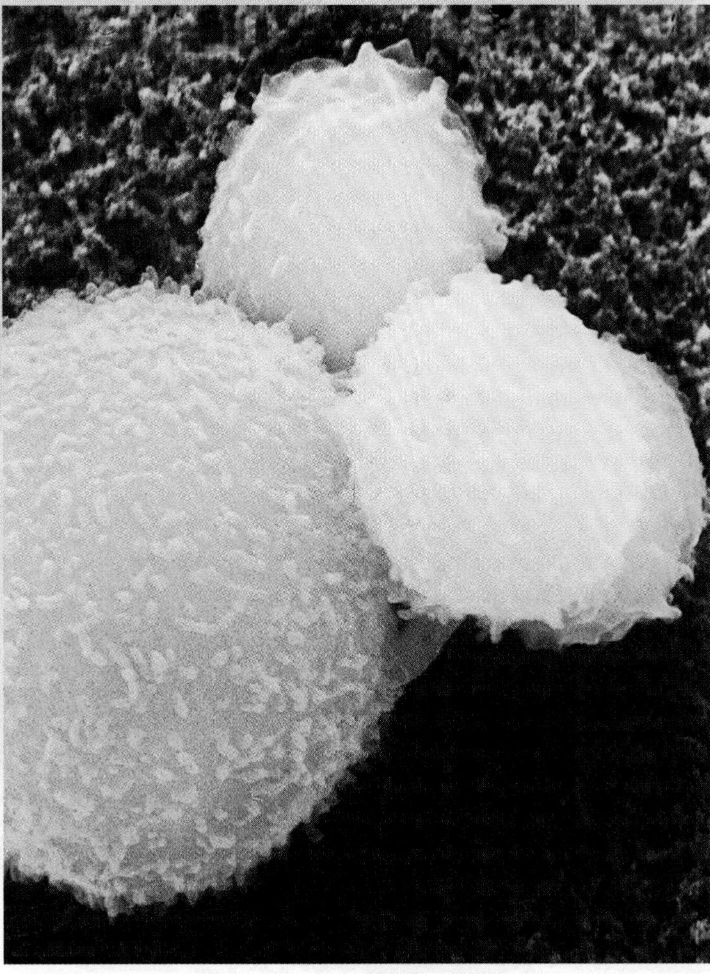

T lymphocytes destroying a tumor cell.

Immunology provides many clues for understanding the pathogenesis of numerous diseases and for developing various measures to either prevent or treat disease. The chapters in Part IV deal with these direct medical applications.

If the human immune system were 100% effective, we would never suffer serious infectious diseases. However, each year millions of people become infected with pathogens, and, especially in less-developed countries, many die from such infections. Chapter 17 reviews the response of the immune system to the four major types of pathogens—viruses, bacteria, protozoans, and parasitic worms—focusing on specific diseases as examples. It also describes the strategies used by various pathogens to evade immune destruction so that they can become established within a host. A section on emerging diseases introduces new emerging infectious diseases that pose potential health risks. By knowing in detail how the immune system responds to a particular pathogen and how that pathogen evades the response, researchers are better able to devise preventive and therapeutic measures.

Since Pasteur's public demonstration of the technique of vaccination a little more than 100 years ago, immunologists have developed vaccines against many of the most devastating infectious diseases. The routine immunization of children in many countries has dramatically reduced the toll taken by common childhood illnesses during the past 50 years. Chapter 18 first describes the common types of vaccines; then it shows how modern advances in immunology are being applied to design new vaccines that pose less risk to recipients.

Chapter 19 examines the causes and devastating consequences of immunodeficiency diseases. Those afflicted with such disorders suffer from frequent, prolonged, severe infections, often caused by pathogens that a normal immune system can combat effectively. A wide array of congenital defects give rise to various primary immunodeficiency diseases. Some disorders are marked by defects in phagocytic cells; others lead to abnormalities in antibody production or in the complement system. Those afflicted with combined immunodeficiencies, the most serious of these disorders, are unable to mount effective humoral or cell-mediated immune responses. Many of these patients die in infancy, although bone-marrow transplants and gene therapy offer therapeutic possibilities.

In addition to congenital defects, secondary causes (e.g., infection, malnutrition, and certain drugs) can compromise the immune system. The most significant of these acquired immunodeficiencies—AIDS—renders its victims susceptible to numerous opportunistic infections and rare forms of cancer, which usually are the immediate causes of death. The rapid worldwide spread of AIDS that began in the early 1980s led to an explosion of research about its cause, its effects on the immune system, and approaches for treating or preventing it. This vast body of research is summarized in Chapter 19. The causative agent is human immunodeficiency virus (HIV), a retrovirus that infects $CD4^+$ T cells as well as certain other cell types. HIV infection in most individuals remains asymptomatic throughout a chronic phase, during which there is a dynamic equilibrium between the amount of virus produced (viral load) and the number of $CD4^+$ T cells. After the chronic phase, which may last up to 10 years, the viral load increases and the $CD4^+$ T-cell count falls; at this point, the host becomes susceptible to a variety of infections and eventually succumbs to them.

Lymphocytes that recognize self-antigen normally either are eliminated during B-cell and T-cell maturation or are rendered nonfunctional by various processes. The sometimes devastating consequences of a breakdown in the mechanisms for generating this self-tolerance are described in Chapter 20. Autoimmune reactions are the cause of several fairly common chronic disorders, including insulin-dependent diabetes mellitus, myasthenia gravis, multiple sclerosis, and rheumatoid arthritis. Most current therapies for autoimmune disease reduce the immune response nonspecifically; although these may alleviate the autoimmune symptoms, they compromise the patient's ability to ward off infections. Researchers are devising more specific therapies based on knowledge about the molecular mechanisms involved in the immune response.

In the past several decades, great strides have been made in transplantation of tissues and organs. The main obstacle to successful transplantation is rejection of the graft by the recipient's immune system. Chapter 21 analyzes the immunologic basis for graft rejection and describes the methods for promoting acceptance. Graft rejection results primarily from a cell-mediated response to histocompatibility antigens (primarily but not exclusively MHC molecules) on the graft cells that differ from those on the recipient's cells. Tissue typing to minimize the differences in histocompatibility antigens between donor and recipient greatly increases the chances of graft acceptance. Drugs that suppress the immune system are helpful, but they increase the recipient's risk of infection. Efforts now under way promise to develop more specific techniques, including the use of monoclonal antibodies, for promoting graft acceptance.

Under certain conditions, normal cells undergo transformation into tumor (cancer) cells, which are characterized by unregulated cell growth. Chapter 22 shows that tumor cells can be viewed as altered self-cells, which express cell-membrane antigens that may induce a cell-mediated immune response. Although the immune response to tumor cells is often ineffective, promotion or supplementation of these natural defense mechanisms is the basis for some cancer treatments. This chapter concludes with a discussion of various cancer immunotherapies.

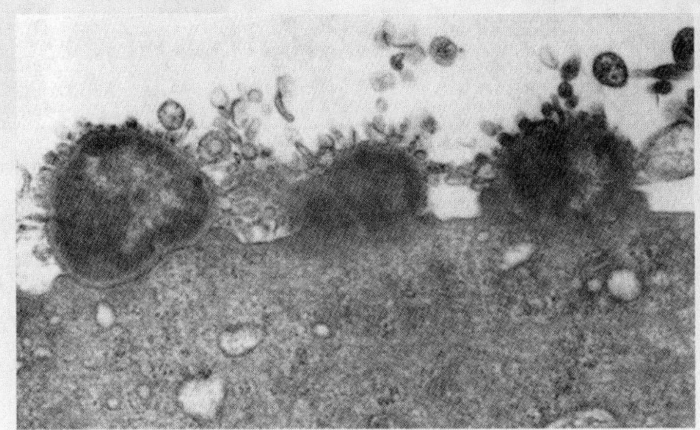

CHAPTER 17

IMMUNE RESPONSE TO INFECTIOUS DISEASES

Viral Infections

Bacterial Infections

Protozoan Diseases

Diseases Caused by Parasitic Worms (Helminths)

Emerging Infectious Diseases

If a pathogen is to establish an infection in a susceptible host, a series of coordinated events must circumvent the nonspecific (innate) and specific (adaptive) host defenses. One of the first and most important features of host innate immunity is the barrier provided by the epithelial surfaces of the skin and the lining of the gut. The difficulty of penetrating this epithelial barrier ensures that most pathogens never gain productive entry into the host and instead pass through it without establishing a productive infection. In addition to providing a physical barrier to infection, the epithelia also produce chemicals that are useful in preventing infection. The secretion of gastric enzymes by specialized epithelial cells lowers the pH of the stomach and upper gastrointestinal tract. Other specialized cells produce antibacterial peptides in the gut.

A major feature of innate immunity is the presence of the normal gut flora, which can competitively inhibit the binding of pathogens to gut epithelial cells. Innate responses also can block the establishment of infection. For example, the cell walls of some Gram-positive bacteria contain a peptidoglycan that activates the alternate complement pathway, resulting in the generation of C3b, which opsonizes bacteria and enhances phagocytosis (see Chapter 13). Some bacteria produce endotoxins such as LPS, which stimulate the production of cytokines such as TNF, IL-1, and IL-6 by macrophages or endothelial cells. These cytokines can activate macrophages. Phagocytosis of bacteria by macrophages and other phagocytic cells is another highly effective line of innate defense. However, some types of bacteria that commonly grow intracellularly have developed mechanisms that allow them to resist degradation within the phagocyte.

Viruses are well known for the stimulation of innate responses. In particular, many viruses induce the production of interferons, which can inhibit viral production by inducing an anti-viral response. Viruses are controlled also by NK cells. As described in Chapter 14, NK cells frequently form the first line of defense against viral infections.

Generally, pathogens use a variety of strategies to escape destruction by the adaptive immune system. Many pathogens reduce their own antigenicity either by growing within host cells, where they are sequestered from immune attack, or by shedding their membrane antigens. Other pathogens camouflage themselves by mimicking the surfaces of host cells, either by expressing molecules with amino acid sequences similar to those of host cell-membrane molecules or by acquiring a covering of host membrane molecules. Some pathogens are able to suppress the immune response selectively or to regulate it so that a branch of the immune system is activated that is ineffective against the pathogen. Continual variation in surface antigens is another strategy that enables a pathogen to elude the immune system. This antigenic variation may be due to the gradual accumulation of mutations, or it may involve an abrupt change in surface antigens.

Both innate and adaptive immune responses to pathogens provide critical defense, but infectious diseases, which have plagued human populations throughout history, still cause the death of millions each year. Although widespread use of vaccines and drug therapy has drastically reduced mortality from infectious diseases in developed countries, such diseases continue to be the leading cause of death in the Third World. It is estimated that nearly 1 billion people are infected worldwide, resulting in close to 20 million deaths every year

(Table 17-1). Despite these alarming numbers, estimated expenditures for research on infectious diseases prevalent in the Third World are less than 5% of total health-research expenditures worldwide. Not only is this a tragedy for these countries, but some of these diseases are beginning to emerge or re-emerge in developed countries. For example, some United States troops returned from the Persian Gulf with leishmaniasis; cholera cases have recently increased worldwide, with more than 47 cases reported in the United States in 1994; and a new drug-resistant strain of *Mycobacterium tuberculosis* is spreading at an alarming rate in the United States.

In this chapter, the concepts described in earlier chapters, antigenicity (Chapter 3) and immune effector mechanisms (Chapters 12–16), as well as vaccine development (which will be considered in Chapter 18) are applied to selected infectious diseases caused by viruses, bacteria, protozoa, and helminths—the four main types of pathogens.

Viral Infections

A number of specific immune effector mechanisms, together with nonspecific defense mechanisms, are called into play to eliminate an infecting virus (Table 17-2). At the same time, the virus acts to subvert one or more of these mechanisms to prolong its own survival. The outcome of the infection depends on how effectively the host's defensive mechanisms resist the offensive tactics of the virus.

TABLE 17-1 INFECTIOUS DISEASES: THE LEADING KILLERS IN 1996

Cause of death	Estimated number of deaths worldwide
Acute respiratory infections	4,000,000
Diarrheal diseases	4,200,000
Tuberculosis	3,300,000
Malaria	1,000,000–2,000,000
Hepatitis	1,000,000–2,000,000
Measles	1,200,000
Meningitis, bacterial	200,000
Pertussis (whooping cough)	250,000
African trypanosomiasis (sleeping sickness)	150,000 or more
Leishmaniasis	80,000
Rabies	40,000–70,000
Amoebiasis	40,000–70,000
Hookworm	65,000
Roundworm	60,000
Yellow fever (epidemic)	30,000
Schistosomiasis (parasitic tropical disease)	20,000

SOURCE: World Health Organization, U.S. Agency for International Development, and National Institute of Allergy and Infectious Diseases.

TABLE 17-2 MECHANISMS OF HUMORAL AND CELL-MEDIATED IMMUNE RESPONSES TO VIRUSES

Response type	Effector molecule or cell	Activity
Humoral	Antibody (especially, secretory IgA)	Blocks binding of virus to host cells, thus preventing infection or reinfection
	IgG, IgM, and IgA antibody	Blocks fusion of viral envelope with host-cell plasma membrane
	IgG and IgM antibody	Enhances phagocytosis of viral particles (opsonization)
	IgM antibody	Agglutinates viral particles
	Complement activated by IgG or IgM antibody	Mediates opsonization by C3b and lysis of enveloped viral particles by membrane-attack complex
Cell-mediated	IFN-γ secreted by T_H or T_C cells	Has direct antiviral activity
	Cytotoxic T lymphocytes (CTLs)	Kill virus-infected self-cells
	NK cells and macrophages	Kill virus-infected cells by antibody-dependent cell-mediated cytotoxicity (ADCC)

The innate immune response to viral infection is primarily through the induction of type I interferons (IFN-α and IFN-β) and the activation of NK cells. Double stranded RNA (dsRNA) produced during the viral life cycle can induce the expression of IFN-α and IFN-β by the infected cell. Macrophages, monocytes, and fibroblasts also are capable of synthesizing these cytokines, but the mechanisms that induce the production of type I interferons in these cells are not completely understood. IFN-α and IFN-β can induce an antiviral response or resistance to viral replication by binding to the IFN α/β receptor. Once bound, IFN-α and IFN-β activate the JAK-STAT pathway, which in turn induces the synthesis of several genes. One of these genes encodes an enzyme known as 2′-5′-oligo-adenylate synthetase [2-5(A) synthetase], which activates a ribonuclease (RNAse L) that degrades viral RNA. Other genes activated by IFN-α/β binding to its receptor also contribute to the inhibition of viral replication. For example, IFN-α/β binding induces a specific protein kinase called dsRNA-dependent protein kinase (PKR), which inactivates protein synthesis, thus blocking viral replication in infected cells (Figure 17-1).

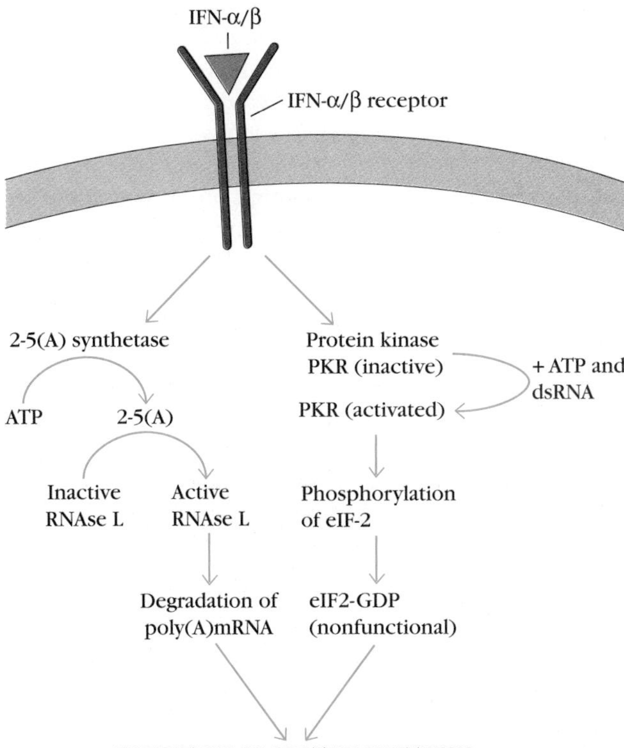

FIGURE 17-1 Induction of antiviral activity by IFN-α and -β. These interferons bind to the IFN receptor, which in turn induces the synthesis of both 2-5(A) synthetase and protein kinase (PKR). The action of of 2-5(A) synthetase results in the activation of RNAse L, which can degrade mRNA. PKR inactivates the translation initiation factor e1F-2 by phosphorylating it. Both pathways thus result in the inhibition of protein synthesis and thereby effectively block viral replication.

The binding of IFN-α and IFN-β to NK cells induces lytic activity, making them very effective in killing virally infected cells. The activity of NK cells is also greatly enhanced by IL-12, a cytokine that is produced very early in a response to viral infection.

Viral Neutralization by Humoral Antibody

Antibodies specific for viral surface antigens are often crucial in containing the spread of a virus during acute infection and in protecting against reinfection. Antibodies are particularly effective in protecting against infection if they are localized at the site of viral entry into the body. Most viruses express surface receptor molecules that enable them to initiate infection by binding to specific host-cell membrane molecules. For example, influenza virus binds to sialic acid residues in cell-membrane glycoproteins and glycolipids; rhinovirus binds to intercellular adhesion molecules (ICAMs); and Epstein-Barr virus binds to type 2 complement receptors on B cells. If antibody to the viral receptor is produced, it can block infection altogether by preventing the binding of viral particles to host cells. Secretory IgA in mucous secretions plays an important role in host defense against viruses by blocking viral attachment to mucosal epithelial cells. The advantage of the attenuated oral polio vaccine, considered in Chapter 18, is that it induces production of secretory IgA, which effectively blocks attachment of poliovirus along the gastrointestinal tract.

Viral neutralization by antibody sometimes involves mechanisms that operate after viral attachment to host cells. In some cases, antibodies may block viral penetration by binding to epitopes that are necessary to mediate fusion of the viral envelope with the plasma membrane. If the induced antibody is of a complement-activating isotype, lysis of enveloped virions can ensue. Antibody or complement can also agglutinate viral particles and function as an opsonizing agent to facilitate Fc- or C3b-receptor–mediated phagocytosis of the viral particles.

Cell-Mediated Antiviral Mechanisms

Although antibodies have an important role in containing the spread of a virus in the acute phases of infection, they are not usually able to eliminate the virus once infection has occurred—particularly if the virus is capable of entering a latent state in which its DNA is integrated into host chromosomal DNA. Once an infection is established, cell-mediated immune mechanisms are most important in host defense. In general, $CD8^+$ T_C cells and $CD4^+$ T_H1 cells are the main components of cell-mediated antiviral defense, although in some cases $CD4^+$ T_C cells have also been implicated. Activated T_H1 cells produce a number of cytokines, including IL-2, IFN-γ, and TNF, that defend against viruses either directly or indirectly. IFN-γ acts directly by inducing an antiviral state in cells. IL-2 acts indirectly by assisting in the recruitment of CTL precursors into an effector population. Both IL-2 and IFN-γ activate NK cells, which play an important role in host defense during the first days of many viral infections until a specific CTL response develops.

In most viral infections, specific CTL activity arises within 3–4 days after infection, peaks by 7–10 days, and then declines. Within 7–10 days of primary infection, most virions have been eliminated, paralleling the development of CTLs. CTLs specific for the virus eliminate virus-infected self-cells and thus eliminate potential sources of new virus. The role of CTLs in defense against viruses is demonstrated by the ability of virus-specific CTLs to confer protection for the specific virus on nonimmune recipients by adoptive transfer. The viral specificity of the CTL as well can be demonstrated with adoptive transfer: adoptive transfer of a CTL clone specific for influenza virus strain X protects mice against influenza virus X but not against influenza virus strain Y.

Viral Evasion of Host-Defense Mechanisms

Despite their restricted genome size, a number of viruses have been found to encode proteins that interfere at various levels with specific or nonspecific host defenses. Presumably, the advantage of such proteins is that they enable viruses to replicate more effectively amidst host antiviral defenses. As described above, the induction of IFN-α and IFN-β is a major innate defense against viral infection, but some viruses have developed strategies to evade the action of IFN-α/β. These include hepatitis C virus, which has been shown to overcome the antiviral effect of the interferons by blocking or inhibiting the action of PKR (see Figure 17-1).

Another mechanism for evading host responses, utilized in particular by herpes simplex viruses (HSV) is inhibition of antigen presentation by infected host cells. HSV-1 and HSV-2 both express an immediate-early protein (a protein synthesized shortly after viral replication) called ICP47, which very effectively inhibits the human transporter molecule needed for antigen processing (TAP; see Figure 8-8). Inhibition of TAP blocks antigen delivery to class I MHC receptors on HSV-infected cells, thus preventing presentation of viral antigen to $CD8^+$ T cells. This results in the trapping of empty class I MHC molecules in the ER and effectively shuts down a $CD8^+$ T-cell response to HSV-infected cells.

The targeting of MHC molecules is not unique to HSV. Other viruses have been shown to down-regulate class I MHC expression shortly after infection. In two of the best-characterized examples, the adenoviruses and cytomegalovirus (CMV) use distinct molecular mechanisms to reduce the surface expression of class I MHC molecules, again inhibiting antigen presentation to $CD8^+$ T cells. Some viruses—CMV, measles virus, and HIV—have been shown to reduce levels of class II MHC molecules on the cell surface, thus blocking the function of antigen-specific anti-viral helper T cells.

Antibody-mediated destruction of viruses requires complement activation, resulting either in direct lysis of the viral particle or opsonization and elimination of the virus by phagocytic cells. A number of viruses have strategies for evading complement-mediated destruction. Vaccinia virus, for example, secretes a protein that binds to the C4b complement component, inhibiting the classical complement pathway; and herpes simplex viruses have a glycoprotein component that binds to the C3b complement component, inhibiting both the classical and alternative pathways.

A number of viruses escape immune attack by constantly changing their antigens. In the influenza virus, continual antigenic variation results in the frequent emergence of new infectious strains. The absence of protective immunity to these newly emerging strains leads to repeated epidemics of influenza. Antigenic variation among rhinoviruses, the causative agent of the common cold, is responsible for our inability to produce an effective vaccine for colds. Nowhere is antigenic variation greater than in the human immunodeficiency virus (HIV), the causative agent of AIDS. Estimates suggest that HIV accumulates mutations at a rate 65 times faster than does influenza virus. Because of the importance of AIDS, a section of Chapter 19 addresses this disease.

A large number of viruses evade the immune response by causing generalized immunosuppression. Among these are the paramyxoviruses that cause mumps, the measles virus, Epstein-Barr virus (EBV), cytomegalovirus, and HIV. In some cases, immunosuppression is caused by direct viral infection of lymphocytes or macrophages. The virus can then either directly destroy the immune cells by cytolytic mechanisms or alter their function. In other cases, immunosuppression is the result of a cytokine imbalance. For example, EBV produces a protein, called BCRF1, that is homologous to IL-10; like IL-10, BCRF1 suppresses cytokine production by the T_H1 subset, resulting in decreased levels of IL-2, TNF, and IFN-γ.

Influenza

The influenza virus infects the upper respiratory tract and major central airways in humans, horses, birds, pigs, and even seals. It has been responsible for some of the worst pandemics (worldwide epidemics) in human history, one of which killed more than 20 million people in 1918–1919, a toll surpassing the number of casualties in World War I. Some areas, such as Alaska and the Pacific Islands, lost more than half of their population during that pandemic.

Properties of the Influenza Virus

Influenza viral particles, or virions, are roughly spherical or ovoid in shape, with an average diameter of 90–100 nm. The virions are surrounded by an outer envelope—a lipid bilayer

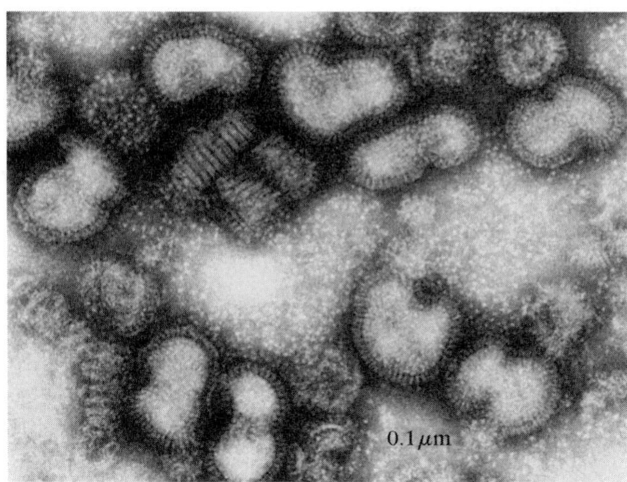

FIGURE 17-2 Electron micrograph of influenza virus reveals roughly spherical viral particles enclosed in a lipid bilayer with protruding hemagglutinin and neuraminidase glycoprotein spikes. [Courtesy of G Murti, Department of Virology, St. Jude Children's Research Hospital, Memphis, Tenn.]

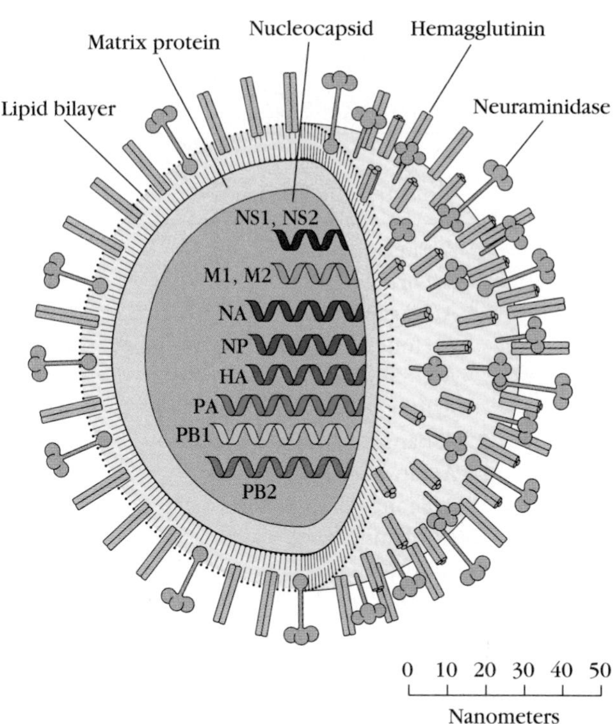

FIGURE 17-3 Schematic representation of influenza structure. The envelope is covered with neuraminidase and hemagglutinin spikes. Inside is an inner layer of matrix protein surrounding the nucleocapsid, which consists of eight ssRNA molecules associated with nucleoprotein. The eight RNA strands encode ten proteins: PB1, PB2, PA, HA (hemagglutinin), NP (nucleoprotein), NA (neuraminidase), M1, M2, NS1, and NS2.

acquired from the plasma membrane of the infected host cell during the process of budding. Inserted into the envelope are two glycoproteins, **hemagglutinin (HA)** and neuraminidase (NA), which form radiating projections that are visible in electron micrographs (Figure 17-2). The hemagglutinin projections, in the form of trimers, are responsible for the attachment of the virus to host cells. There are approximately 1000 hemagglutinin projections per influenza virion. The hemagglutinin trimer binds to sialic acid groups on host-cell glycoproteins and glycolipids by way of a conserved amino acid sequence that forms a small groove in the hemagglutinin molecule. Neuraminidase, as its name indicates, cleaves *N*-acetylneuraminic (sialic) acid from nascent viral glycoproteins and host-cell membrane glycoproteins, an activity that presumably facilitates viral budding from the infected host cell. Within the envelope, an inner layer of matrix protein surrounds the nucleocapsid, which consists of eight different strands of single-stranded RNA (ssRNA) associated with protein and RNA polymerase (Figure 17-3). Each RNA strand encodes one or more different influenza proteins.

Three basic types of influenza (A, B, and C), can be distinguished by differences in their nucleoprotein and matrix proteins. Type A, which is the most common, is responsible for the major human pandemics. Antigenic variation in hemagglutinin and neuraminidase distinguishes subtypes of type A influenza virus. According to the nomenclature of the World Health Organization, each virus strain is defined by its animal host of origin (specified, if other than human), geographical origin, strain number, year of isolation, and antigenic description of HA and NA (Table 17-3). For example, A/Sw/Iowa/15/30 (H1N1) designates strain-A isolate 15 that arose in swine in Iowa in 1930 and has antigenic subtypes 1 of HA and NA, and A/Hong Kong/1/68 (H3N2) denotes strain-A isolate 1 that arose in humans in Hong Kong in 1968 and has antigenic subtypes 3 of HA and 2 of NA, respectively. Notice that the H and N spikes are antigenically distinct in these two strains. There are 13 different hemagglutinins and 9 neuraminidases among the type A influenza viruses.

The distinguishing feature of influenza virus is its variability. The virus can change its surface antigens so completely that the immune response to infection with the virus that caused a previous epidemic gives little or no protection against the virus causing a subsequent epidemic. The antigenic variation results primarily from changes in the hemagglutinin and neuraminidase spikes protruding from the viral envelope (Figure 17-4). Two different mechanisms generate antigenic variation in HA and NA: antigenic drift and antigenic shift. **Antigenic drift** involves a series of spontaneous point mutations that occur gradually, resulting in minor changes in HA and NA. **Antigenic shift** results in the sudden emergence of a new subtype of influenza whose HA and possibly also NA are considerably different from that of the virus present in a preceding epidemic.

TABLE 17-3 SOME INFLUENZA A STRAINS AND THEIR HEMAGGLUTININ (H) AND NEURAMINIDASE (N) SUBTYPE

Species	Virus strain designation	Antigenic subtype
Human	A/Puerto Rico/8/34	H0N1
	A/Fort Monmouth/1/47	H1N1
	A/Singapore/1/57	H2N2
	A/Hong Kong/1/68	H3N2
	A/USSR/80/77	H1N1
	A/Brazil/11/78	H1N1
	A/Bangkok/1/79	H3N2
	A/Taiwan/1/86	H1N1
	A/Shanghai/16/89	H3N2
	A/Johannesburg/33/95	H3N2
	A/Wuhan/359/95	H3N2
	A/Texas/36/95	H1N1
	A/Hong Kong/156/97	H5N1
Swine	A/Sw/Iowa/15/30	H1N1
	A/Sw/Taiwan/70	H3N2
Horse (equine)	A/Eq/Prague/1/56	H7N7
	A/Eq/Miami/1/63	H3N8
Birds	A/Fowl/Dutch/27	H7N7
	A/Tern/South America/61	H5N3
	A/Turkey/Ontario/68	H8N4
	A/Chicken/Hong Kong/258/97	H5N1

The first time a human influenza virus was isolated was in 1934; this virus was given the subtype designation H0N1. The H0N1 subtype persisted until 1947, when a major antigenic shift generated a new subtype, H1N1, which supplanted the previous subtype and became prevalent worldwide until 1957, when H2N2 emerged. The H2N2 subtype prevailed for the next decade and was replaced in 1968 by H3N2. Antigenic shift in 1977 saw the re-emergence of H1N1. The most recent antigenic shift, in 1989, brought the re-emergence of H3N2, which remained dominant throughout the next several years. However, an H1N1 strain re-emerged in Texas in 1995, and current influenza vaccines contain both H3N2 and H1N1 strains. With each antigenic shift, hemagglutinin and neuraminidase undergo major sequence changes, resulting in major antigenic variations for which the immune system lacks memory. Thus, each antigenic shift finds the population immunologically unprepared, resulting in major outbreaks of influenza, which sometimes reach pandemic proportions.

Between pandemic-causing antigenic shifts, the influenza virus undergoes antigenic drift, generating minor antigenic variations, which account for strain differences within a subtype. The immune response contributes to the emergence of these different influenza strains. As individuals infected with a given influenza strain mount an effective immune response, the strain is eliminated. However, the accumulation of point mutations sufficiently alters the antigenicity of some variants so that they are able to escape immune elimination (Figure 17-5a). These variants become a new strain of influenza, causing another local epidemic cycle. The role of antibody in such immunologic selection can be demonstrated in the laboratory by mixing an influenza strain with a monoclonal antibody specific for that strain and then culturing the virus in cells. The antibody has neutralized all unaltered viral particles and only those viral particles with mutations resulting in altered antigenicity escape neutralization and are able to continue the infection. Within a short time in culture, a new influenza strain can be shown to emerge.

Antigenic shift is thought to occur through genetic reassortment between influenza virions from humans and from various animals, including horses, pigs, and ducks (Figure 17-5b). The fact that influenza contains eight separate strands of ssRNA makes possible the reassortment of the

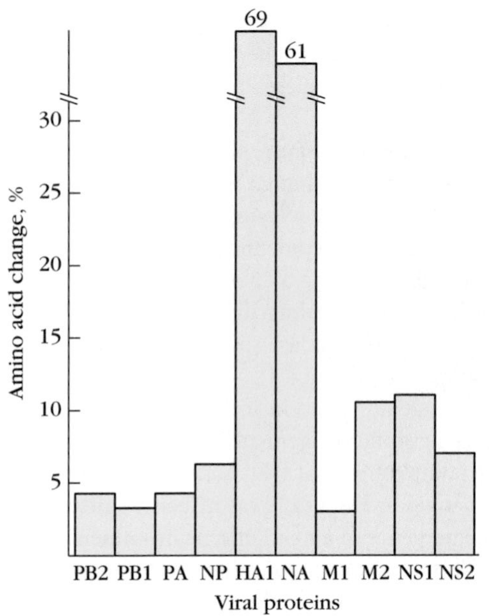

FIGURE 17-4 Amino acid sequence variation in 10 influenza viral proteins from two H3N2 strains and one H1N1 strain. The surface glycoproteins hemagglutinin (HA1) and neuraminidase (NA) show significant sequence variation; in contrast, the sequences of internal viral proteins, such as matrix proteins (M1 and M2) and nucleoprotein (NP), are largely conserved. [Adapted from GG Brownlee, 1986, in *Options for the Control of Influenza,* Alan R. Liss.]

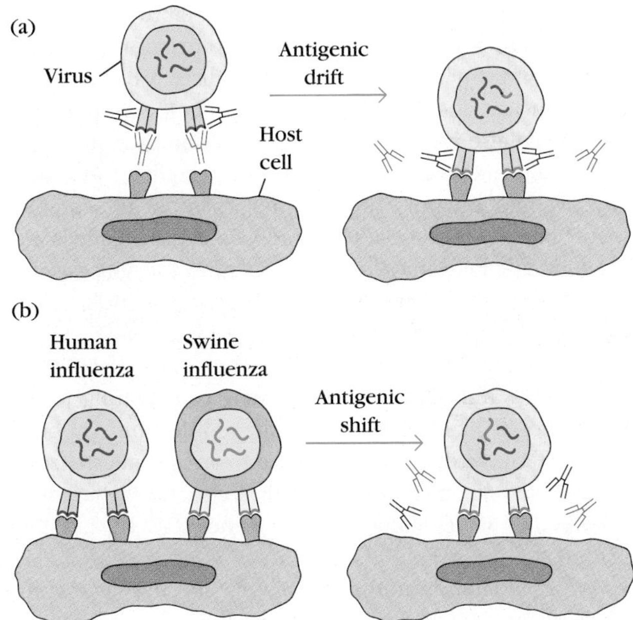

FIGURE 17-5 Two mechanisms generate variations in influenza surface antigens. (a) In antigenic drift, the accumulation of point mutations eventually yields a variant protein that is no longer recognized by antibody to the original antigen. (b) Antigenic shift may occur by reassortment of an entire ssRNA between human and animal virions infecting the same cell. Only four of the eight RNA strands are depicted.

RNA strands of human and animal virions within a single cell infected with both viruses. Evidence for in vivo genetic reassortment between influenza A viruses from humans and domestic pigs was obtained in 1971. After infecting a pig simultaneously with human Hong Kong influenza (H3N2) and with swine influenza (H1N1), investigators were able to recover virions expressing H3N1. In some cases, an apparent antigenic shift may represent the re-emergence of a previous strain that has remained hidden for several decades. In May of 1977, a strain of influenza, A/USSR/77 (H′1N1), appeared that proved to be identical to a strain that had caused an epidemic 27 years earlier. The virus could have been preserved over the years in a frozen state or in an animal reservoir. When such a re-emergence occurs, the HA and NA antigens expressed are not really new; however, they will be seen by the immune system of anyone not previously exposed to that strain (people under the age of twenty-seven in the 1977 epidemic, for example) as if they were new because no memory cells specific for these antigenic subtypes will exist in the susceptible population. Thus, from an immunologic point of view, the re-emergence of an old influenza A strain can have the same effect as an antigenic shift that generates a new subtype.

Host Response to Influenza Infection

Humoral antibody specific for the HA molecule is produced during an influenza infection. This antibody protects against influenza infection, but its specificity is strain-specific and is readily bypassed by antigenic drift. Antigenic drift in the HA molecule results in amino acid substitutions in several antigenic domains at the molecule's distal end (Figure 17-6). Two of these domains are on either side of the conserved sialic-acid–binding cleft, which is necessary for binding of virions to target cells. Serum antibodies specific for these two regions are important in blocking initial viral infectivity. These antibody titers peak within a few days of infection and then decrease over the next 6 months; the titers then plateau and

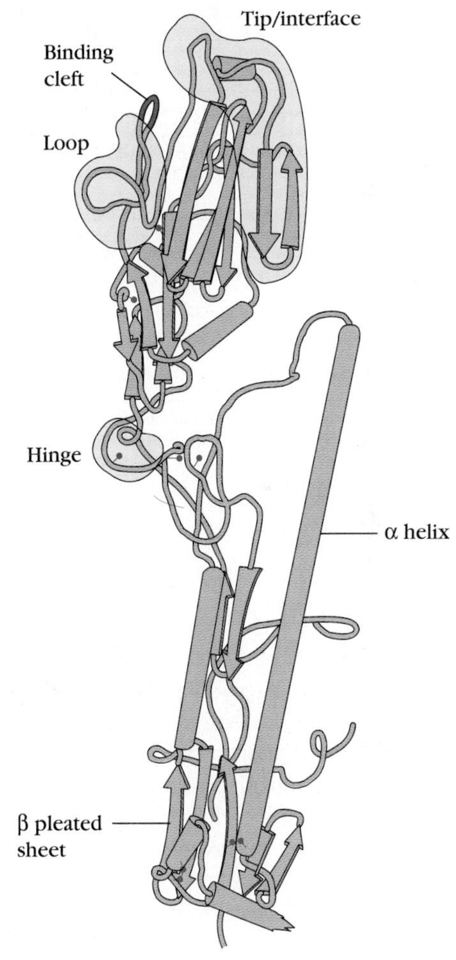

FIGURE 17-6 Structure of hemagglutinin molecule. Sialic acid on host cells interacts with the binding cleft, which is bounded by regions—designated the loop and tip/interface—where antigenic drift is prevalent (blue areas). Antibodies to these regions are important in blocking viral infections. Continual changes in amino acid residues in these regions allow the influenza virus to evade the antibody response. Small red dots represent residues that exhibit a high degree of variation among virus strains. [Adapted from DC Wiley et al, 1981, *Nature* **289**:373.]

Go to www.whfreeman.com/immunology **Molecular Visualization**
Viral Antigens *See Introduction and Flu Virus Hemagglutinin.*

remain fairly stable for the next several years. This antibody does not appear to be required for recovery from influenza, as patients with agammaglobulinemia recover from the disease. Instead, the serum antibody appears to play a significant role in resistance to reinfection by the same strain. When serum-antibody levels are high for a particular HA molecule, both mice and humans are resistant to infection by virions expressing that HA molecule. If mice are infected with influenza virus and antibody production is experimentally suppressed, the mice recover from the infection but can be reinfected with the same viral strain. In addition to humoral responses, CTLs can play a role in immune responses to influenza.

Bacterial Infections

Immunity to bacterial infections is achieved by means of antibody unless the bacterium is capable of intracellular growth, in which case delayed-type hypersensitivity has an important role. Bacteria enter the body either through a number of natural routes (e.g., the respiratory tract, the gastrointestinal tract, and the genitourinary tract) or through unnatural routes opened up by breaks in mucous membranes or skin. Depending on the number of organisms entering and their virulence, different levels of host defense are enlisted. If the inoculum size and the virulence are both low, then localized tissue phagocytes may be able to eliminate the bacteria with an innate, nonspecific defense. Larger inoculums or organisms with greater virulence tend to induce an adaptive, specific immune response.

Immune Response to Extracellular and Intracellular Bacteria

Infection by extracellular bacteria induces production of humoral antibodies, which are ordinarily secreted by plasma cells in regional lymph nodes and the submucosa of the respiratory and gastrointestinal tracts. The humoral immune response is the main protective response against extracellular bacteria. The antibodies act in several ways, including removal of the bacteria and inactivation of bacterial toxins, to protect the host from the invading organisms (Figure 17-7). Extracellular bacteria can be pathogenic because they induce a localized inflammatory response or because they produce toxins. The toxins, endotoxin or exotoxin, can be cytotoxic but also may cause pathogenesis in other ways. An excellent example of this is the toxin produced by diphtheria, which exerts a toxic effect on the cell by blocking protein synthesis. Endotoxins, such as lipopolysaccharides (LPS), are generally components of bacterial cell walls, while exotoxins, such as diphtheria toxin, are secreted by the bacteria.

Antibody that binds to accessible antigens on the surface of a bacterium can, together with the C3b component of complement, act as an opsonin that increases phagocytosis and thus clearance of the bacterium (see Figure 17-7). In the case of some bacteria—notably, the gram-negative organisms—complement activation can lead directly to lysis of the organism. Antibody-mediated activation of the complement system can also induce localized production of immune effector molecules that help to develop an amplified and more effective inflammatory response. For example, the complement split products C3a, C4a, and C5a act as anaphylatoxins, inducing local mast-cell degranulation and thus vasodilation and the extravasation of lymphocytes and neutrophils from the blood into tissue space (see Figure 17-7). Other complement split products serve as chemotactic factors for neutrophils and macrophages, thereby contributing to the buildup of phagocytic cells at the site of infection. Antibody to a bacteria toxin may bind to the toxin and neutralize it; the antibody-toxin complexes are then cleared by phagocytic cells in the same manner as any other antigen-antibody complex.

While innate immunity is not very effective against intracellular bacterial pathogens, intracellular bacteria can activate NK cells which, in turn, provide an early defense against these bacteria. Intracellular bacterial infections tend to induce a cell-mediated immune response, specifically, delayed-type hypersensitivity. In this response, cytokines secreted by $CD4^+$ T cells are important—notably IFN-γ, which activates macrophages to kill ingested pathogens more effectively (see Figure 14-15).

Bacterial Evasion of Host Defense Mechanisms

There are four primary steps in bacterial infection:

- Attachment to host cells
- Proliferation
- Invasion of host tissue
- Toxin-induced damage to host cells

Host-defense mechanisms act at each of these steps, and many bacteria have evolved ways to circumvent some of these host defenses (Table 17-4).

Some bacteria have surface structures or molecules that enhance their ability to attach to host cells. A number of gram-negative bacteria, for instance, have pili (long hairlike projections), which enable them to attach to the membrane of the intestinal or genitourinary tract (Figure 17-8). Other bacteria, such as *Bordetella pertussis*, secrete adhesion molecules that attach to both the bacterium and the ciliated epithelial cells of the upper respiratory tract.

Secretory IgA antibodies specific for such bacterial structures can block bacterial attachment to mucosal epithelial cells and are the main host defense against bacterial attachment. However, some bacteria (e.g., *Neisseria gonorrhoeae*, *Haemophilus influenzae*, and *Neisseria meningitidis*) evade the IgA response by secreting proteases that cleave secretory

Go to www.whfreeman.com/immunology Animation
Vaccine Strategies *See pathogenenisis sections.*

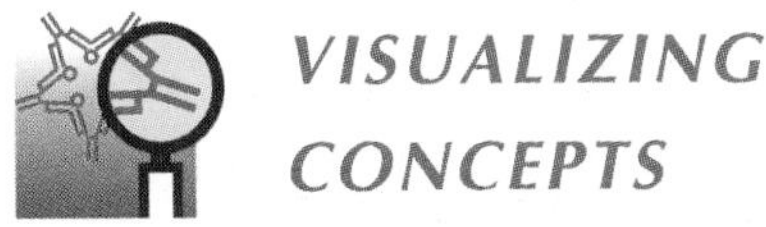

VISUALIZING CONCEPTS

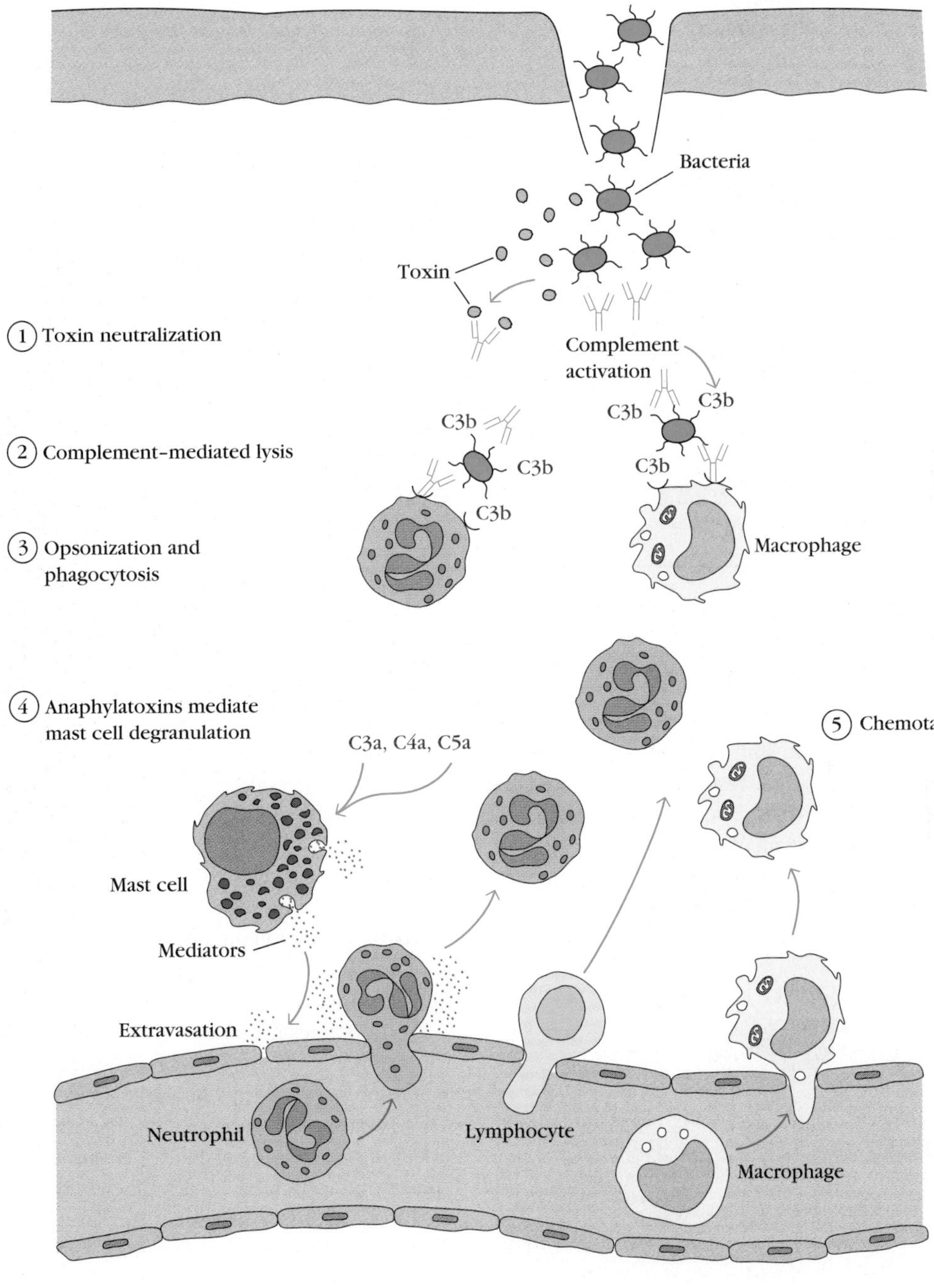

FIGURE 17-7 Antibody-mediated mechanisms for combating infection by extracellular bacteria. (1) Antibody neutralizes bacterial toxins. (2) Complement activation on bacterial surfaces leads to complement-mediated lysis of bacteria. (3) Antibody and the complement split product C3b bind to bacteria, serving as opsonins to increase phagocytosis. (4) C3a and C5a, generated by antibody-initiated complement activation, induce local mast cell degranulation, releasing substances that mediate vasodilation and extravasation of lymphocytes and neutrophils. (5) Other complement split products are chemotactic for neutrophils and macrophages.

TABLE 17-4 HOST IMMUNE RESPONSES TO BACTERIAL INFECTION AND BACTERIAL EVASION MECHANISMS

Infection process	Host defense	Bacterial evasion mechanisms
Attachment to host cells	Blockage of attachment by secretory IgA antibodies	Secretion of proteases that cleave secretory IgA dimers (*Neisseria meningitidis, N. gonorrhoeae, Haemophilus influenzae*) Antigenic variation in attachment structures (pili of *N. gonorrhoeae*)
Proliferation	Phagocytosis (Ab- and C3b-mediated opsonization)	Production of surface structures (polysaccharide capsule, M protein, fibrin coat) that inhibit phagocytic cells Mechanisms for surviving within phagocytic cells Induction of apoptosis in macrophages (*Shigella flexneri*)
	Complement-mediated lysis and localized inflammatory response	Generalized resistance of gram-positive bacteria to complement-mediated lysis Insertion of membrane-attack complex prevented by long side chain in cell-wall LPS (some gram-negative bacteria)
Invasion of host tissues	Ab-mediated agglutination	Secretion of elastase that inactivates C3a and C5a (*Pseudomonas*)
Toxin-induced damage to host cells	Neutralization of toxin by antibody	Secretion of hyaluronidase, which enhances bacterial invasiveness

IgA at the hinge region; the resulting Fab and Fc fragments have a shortened half-life in mucous secretions and are not able to agglutinate microorganisms.

Some bacteria evade the IgA response of the host by changing these surface antigens. In *N. gonorrhoeae*, for example, pilin, the protein component of the pili, has a highly variable structure. Variation in the pilin amino acid sequence is generated by gene rearrangements of its coding sequence.

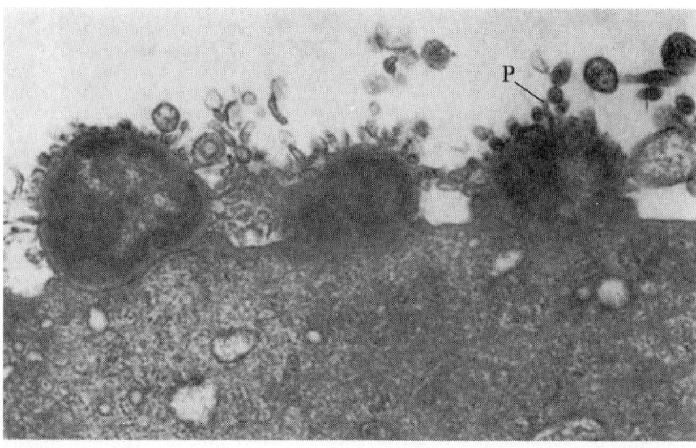

FIGURE 17-8 Electron micrograph of *Neisseria gonorrhoeae* attaching to urethral epithelial cells. Pili (P) extend from the gonococcal surface and mediate the attachment. [From ME Ward and PJ Watt, 1972, *J. Inf. Dis.* **126**:601.]

The pilin locus consists of one or two expressed genes and 10–20 silent genes. Each gene is arranged into six regions called "minicassettes." Pilin variation is generated by a process of gene conversion, in which one or more minicassettes from the silent genes replace a minicassette of the expression gene. This process generates enormous antigenic variation, which may contribute to the pathogenicity of *N. gonorrhoeae* by increasing the likelihood that expressed pili will bind firmly to epithelial cells. In addition, the continual changes in the pilin sequence allow the organism to evade neutralization by IgA.

Some bacteria possess surface structures that serve to inhibit phagocytosis. A classic example is *Streptococcus pneumoniae*, whose polysaccharide capsule prevents phagocytosis very effectively. There are 84 serotypes of *S. pneumoniae* that differ from one another by distinct capsular polysaccharides. During infection, the host produces antibody against the infecting serotype. This antibody protects against reinfection with the same serotype but will not protect against infection by a different serotype. In this way, *S. pneumoniae* can cause disease many times in the same individual. On other bacteria, such as *Streptococcus pyogenes*, a surface protein projection called the M protein inhibits phagocytosis. Some pathogenic staphylococci are able to assemble a protective coat from host proteins. These bacteria secrete a coagulase enzyme that precipitates a fibrin coat around them, shielding them from phagocytic cells.

Mechanisms for interfering with the complement system help other bacteria survive. In some gram-negative bacteria, for example, long side chains on the lipid A moiety of the cell-wall core polysaccharide help to resist complement-mediated lysis. *Pseudomonas* secretes an enzyme, elastase, that inactivates both the C3a and C5a anaphylatoxins, thereby diminishing the localized inflammatory reaction.

A number of bacteria escape host defense mechanisms by their ability to survive within phagocytic cells. Some, such as *Listeria monocytogenes*, do this by escaping from the phagolysosome to the cytoplasm, which is a more favorable environment for their growth. Other bacteria, such as *Mycobacterium avium*, block lysosomal fusion with the phagolysosome; and some mycobacteria are resistant to the oxidative attack that takes place within the phagolysosome.

Contribution of the Immune Response to Bacterial Pathogenesis

In some cases, disease is caused not by the bacterial pathogen itself but by the immune response to the pathogen. As described in Chapter 12, pathogen-stimulated overproduction of cytokines leads to the symptoms of bacterial septic shock, food poisoning, and toxic-shock syndrome. For instance, cell-wall endotoxins of some gram-negative bacteria activate macrophages, resulting in release of high levels of IL-1 and TNF-α, which can cause septic shock. In staphylococcal food poisoning and toxic-shock syndrome, exotoxins produced by the pathogens function as superantigens, which can activate all T cells that express T-cell receptors with a particular V_β domain (see Table 10-4). The resulting overproduction of cytokines by activated T_H cells causes many of the symptoms of these diseases.

The ability of some bacteria to survive intracellularly within infected cells can result in chronic antigenic activation of $CD4^+$ T cells, leading to tissue destruction by a cell-mediated response with the characteristics of a delayed-type hypersensitivity reaction (see Chapter 14). Cytokines secreted by these activated $CD4^+$ T cells can lead to extensive accumulation and activation of macrophages, resulting in formation of a **granuloma**. The localized concentrations of lysosomal enzymes in these granulomas can cause extensive tissue necrosis. Much of the tissue damage seen with *M. tuberculosis* is due to a cell-mediated immune response.

Diphtheria (Corynebacterium diphtheriae)

Diphtheria is the classic example of a bacterial disease caused by a secreted exotoxin to which immunity can be induced by immunization with an inactivated **toxoid**. The causative agent, a gram-positive, rodlike organism called *Corynebacterium diphtheriae*, was first described by Klebs in 1883 and was shown a year later by Loeffler to cause diphtheria in guinea pigs and rabbits. Autopsies on the infected animals revealed that, while bacterial growth was limited to the site of inoculation, there was widespread damage to a variety of organs, including the heart, liver, and kidneys. This finding led Loeffler to speculate that the neurologic and cardiologic manifestations of the disease were caused by a toxic substance elaborated by the organism.

Loeffler's hypothesis was validated in 1888, when Roux and Yersin produced the disease in animals by injecting them with a sterile filtrate from a culture of *C. diphtheriae.* Two years later, von Behring showed that an antiserum to the toxin was able to prevent death in infected animals. He prepared a toxoid by treating the toxin with iodine trichloride and demonstrated that it could induce protective antibodies in animals. However, the toxoid was still quite toxic and therefore unsuitable for use in humans. In 1923, Ramon found that exposing the toxin to heat and formalin rendered it nontoxic but did not destroy its antigenicity. Clinical trials showed that formaldehyde-treated toxoid conferred a high level of protection against diphtheria.

As immunizations with the toxoid increased, the number of cases of diphtheria decreased rapidly. In the 1920s, there were approximately 200 cases of diphtheria per 100,000 population in the United States. In 1989, the Centers for Disease Control reported only three cases of diphtheria in the entire United States. Recently in the former Soviet Union, there has been an alarming epidemic of diphtheria due to a reduction in vaccinations.

Natural infection with *C. diphtheriae* occurs only in humans. The disease is spread from one individual to another by airborne respiratory droplets. The organism colonizes the nasopharyngeal tract, remaining in the superficial layers of the respiratory mucosa. Growth of the organism itself causes little tissue damage, and only a mild inflammatory reaction develops. The virulence of the organism is due completely to its potent exotoxin. The toxin causes destruction of the underlying tissue, resulting in the formation of a tough fibrinous membrane ("pseudomembrane") composed of fibrin, white blood cells, and dead respiratory epithelial cells. The membrane itself can cause suffocation. The exotoxin also is responsible for widespread systemic manifestations. Pronounced myocardial damage (often leading to congestive heart failure) and neurologic damage (ranging from mild weakness to complete paralysis) are common.

The exotoxin that causes diphtheria symptoms is encoded by the *tox* gene carried by phage β. Within some strains of *C. diphtheriae,* phage β can exist in a state of **lysogeny,** in which the β-prophage DNA persists within the bacterial cell. Only strains that carry lysogenic phage β are able to produce the exotoxin. The diphtheria exotoxin contains two disulfide-linked chains, a binding chain and toxin chain. The binding chain interacts with ganglioside receptors on susceptible cells, facilitating internalization of the exotoxin. Toxicity results from the inhibitory effect of the toxin chain on protein synthesis. The diphtheria exotoxin is extremely potent; a single molecule has been shown to kill a cell. Removal of the binding chain prevents the exotoxin from entering the cell, thus rendering the exotoxin nontoxic. As described in Chapter 4, an immunotoxin can be prepared by replacing the binding chain with a monoclonal antibody specific for a tumor-cell surface antigen; in this way the toxin chain can be targeted to tumor cells (see Figure 4-23).

Today, diphtheria toxoid is prepared by treating diphtheria toxin with formaldehyde. The reaction with formaldehyde cross-links the toxin, resulting in an irreversible loss in its toxicity while enhancing its antigenicity. The toxoid is administered together with tetanus toxoid and inactivated *Bordetella pertussis* in a combined vaccine that is given to children beginning at 6–8 weeks of age. Immunization with the toxoid induces the production of antibodies (antitoxin), which can bind to the toxin and neutralize its activity. Because antitoxin levels decline slowly over time, booster doses are recommended at 10-year intervals to maintain antitoxin levels within the protective range. Interestingly, antibodies specific for epitopes on the binding chain of the diphtheria exotoxin are critical for toxin neutralization because these antibodies block internalization of the active toxin chain.

Tuberculosis (*Mycobacterium tuberculosis*)

Tuberculosis is the leading cause of death in the world from a single infectious agent, killing about 3 million individuals every year and accounting for 18.5% of all deaths in adults between the ages of 15 and 59. About 1.79 billion people, roughly one-third of the world's population, are infected with the causative agent *M. tuberculosis* and are at risk of developing the disease. Long thought to have been eliminated as a public health problem in the United States, tuberculosis re-emerged in the early 1990s, particularly in the inner cities and in areas where HIV-infection levels are high (See the last section of this chapter). In 1995, approximately 23,000 individuals were diagnosed with tuberculosis in the United States.

Although several *Mycobacterium* species can cause tuberculosis, *M. tuberculosis* is the principal causative agent. This organism is spread easily, and pulmonary infection usually results from inhalation of small droplets of respiratory secretions containing a few bacilli. The inhaled bacilli are ingested by alveolar macrophages and are able to survive and multiply intracellularly by inhibiting formation of phagolysosomes. When the infected macrophages lyse, as they eventually do, large numbers of bacilli are released. A cell-mediated response involving $CD4^+$ T cells, which is required for immunity to tuberculosis, may be responsible for much of the tissue damage in the disease. $CD4^+$ T-cell activity is the basis for the tuberculin skin test to the purified protein derivative (PPD) from *M. tuberculosis* (see Chapter 14).

Upon infection with *M. tuberculosis*, the most common clinical pattern, termed pulmonary tuberculosis, appears in about 90% of those infected. In this pattern, $CD4^+$ T cells are activated within 2–6 weeks after infection, inducing the infiltration of large numbers of activated macrophages. These cells wall off the organism inside a granulomatous lesion called a tubercle (Figure 17-9). A tubercle consists of a few small lymphocytes and a compact collection of activated macrophages, which sometimes differentiate into epithelioid cells or multinucleated giant cells. The massive activation of macrophages that occurs within tubercles often results in the concentrated release of lytic enzymes. These enzymes destroy nearby healthy cells, resulting in circular regions of necrotic tissue, which eventually form a lesion with a caseous (cheese-like) consistency (see Figure 17-9). As these caseous lesions heal, they become calcified and are readily visible on x-rays, where they are called Ghon complexes.

Because the activated macrophages suppress proliferation of the phagocytosed bacilli, infection is contained. Cytokines produced by $CD4^+$ T cells (T_H1 subset) play an important role in the response by activating macrophages, so that they are able to kill the bacilli or inhibit their growth. The role of IFN-γ in the immune response to mycobacteria has been demonstrated with knockout mice lacking IFN-γ. These mice died when they were infected with an attenuated strain of mycobacteria (BCG), whereas IFN-γ^+ normal mice survive.

Recent studies have revealed high levels of IL-12 in the pleural effusions of tuberculosis patients. The high levels of IL-12, produced by activated macrophages, are not surpris-

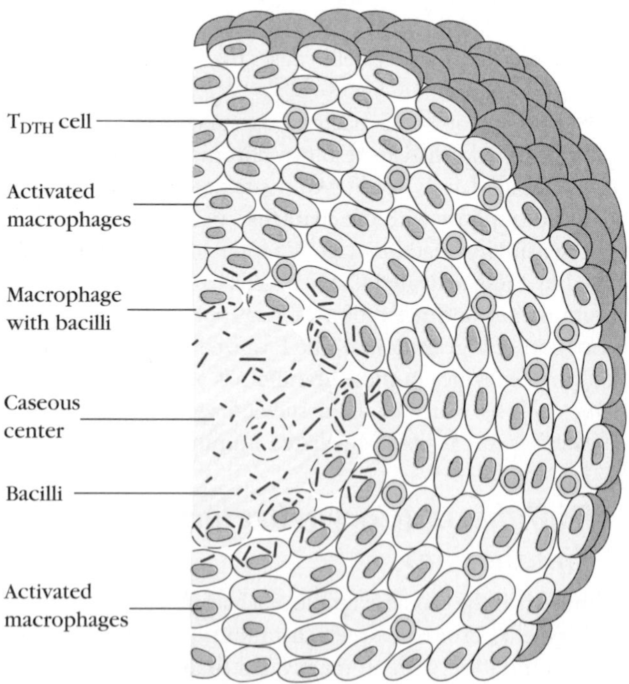

FIGURE 17-9 A tubercle formed in pulmonary tuberculosis. [Modified from AM Dannenberg, 1993, *Hosp. Prac.* (Jan. 15):51.]

ing, given the decisive role of IL-12 in stimulating T_H1-mediated responses (see Figure 12-12). In mouse models of tuberculosis, IL-12 has been shown to increase resistance to the disease. Not only does IL-12 stimulate development of T_H1 cells, but it also may contribute to resistance by inducing the production of chemokines that attract macrophages to the site of infection. When IL-12 is neutralized by antibody to IL-12, granuloma formation in tuberculous mice is blocked.

The $CD4^+$ T-cell–mediated immune response mounted by the majority of people exposed to *M. tuberculosis* thus controls the infection and later protects against reinfection. However, about 10% of individuals infected with *M. tuberculosis* follow a different clinical pattern: the disease progresses to chronic pulmonary tuberculosis or extrapulmonary tuberculosis. This progression may occur years after the primary infection. In this clinical pattern, accumulation of large concentrations of mycobacterial antigens within tubercles leads to extensive and continual chronic $CD4^+$ T-cell activation and ensuing macrophage activation. The resulting high concentrations of lytic enzymes cause the necrotic caseous lesions to liquefy, creating a rich medium that allows the tubercle bacilli to proliferate extracellularly. Eventually the lesions rupture, and the bacilli disseminate in the lung and/or are spread through the blood and lymphatic vessels to the pleural cavity, bone, urogenital system, meninges, peritoneum, or skin.

Tuberculosis is treated with several drugs, used in combination, including isoniazid, rifampin, streptomycin, pyrazinamide, and ethambutol. The combination therapy of isoniazid and rifampin has been particularly effective. The intracellular growth of *M. tuberculosis* makes it difficult for drugs to reach the bacilli. For this reason, drug therapy must be continued for at least 9 months to eradicate the bacteria. Some patients with tuberculosis do not exhibit any clinical symptoms, and some patients with symptoms begin to feel better within 2–4 weeks after treatment begins. The side effects associated with the usual antibiotic therapy, in addition to the fact that they feel better, lead many patients to stop taking the medications long before the recommended treatment period is completed. Because briefer treatment may not eradicate organisms that are somewhat resistant to the antibiotics, a multidrug-resistant strain can emerge. Noncompliance with required treatment regimes, one of the most troubling aspects of the large number of current tuberculosis cases, clearly compromises efforts to contain the spread of the disease.

Presently, the only vaccine for *M. tuberculosis* is an attenuated strain of *M. bovis* called BCG (Bacillus Calmette-Guerin). The vaccine appears to provide fairly effective protection against extrapulmonary tuberculosis but has been inconsistent against pulmonary tuberculosis. In different studies, BCG has provided protection in anywhere from 0% to 80% of vaccinated individuals; in some cases, BCG vaccination has even increased the risk of infection. Moreover, after BCG vaccination, the tuberculin skin test cannot be used as an effective monitor of exposure to *M. tuberculosis*. Because of the variable effectiveness of the BCG vaccine and the inability to monitor for exposure with the skin test after vaccination, this vaccine is not used in the United States. However, the alarming increase in multidrug-resistant strains has stimulated renewed efforts to develop a more effective tuberculosis vaccine.

Lyme Disease (Borrelia burgdorferi)

In 1975, about 60 cases of a newly observed disease were reported in Lyme, Connecticut. The disease symptoms included unexplained "bull's-eye" rashes, headaches, and arthritis; in some cases, severe neurologic complications developed, including excruciating headaches, meningitis, loss of memory, and mood swings. An epidemiologic study was initiated in the hope of identifying the causative agent. The disease was shown to have a higher incidence in heavily wooded areas, and a close geographic clustering of infected individuals was found. In addition, the disease was shown to be contracted during the summer months between June and September. In 1977, nine patients with the disease remembered having been bitten by a tick at the site of the characteristic rash. Fortuitously, the tick had been saved by one patient and was examined by Willy Burgdorfer, a noted authority on tick-borne diseases. He found the tick (an *Ixodes* species) to be teeming with a new species of gram-negative spirochete, which was subsequently named *Borrelia burgdorferi.*

As an infected tick takes a blood meal, *B. burgdorferi* enters the bloodstream. Staining with fluorescent antibodies to *B. burgdorferi* revealed the presence of low numbers of the spirochete at the site of the bite and in various organs, including the kidneys, spleen, liver, cerebrospinal fluid, and brain. The clinical symptoms of Lyme disease generally begin with a characteristic rash, which first appears as a red papule and spreads to form what appears as a bull's-eye 10–50 cm in diameter (Figure 17-10). After the rash, arthritic and neurologic symptoms often develop. Roughly 80% of individuals with Lyme disease develop some arthritic symptoms, ranging from joint pain to chronic joint destruction. Neurologic symptoms develop in about 60% of patients. Most report headaches, and about 15% develop meningitis and encephalitis. The disease can be successfully treated with broad-spectrum antibiotics such as penicillin and tetracycline.

Antibodies to a protein associated with the flagella of *B. burgdorferi* can often be detected after infection. However, these antibodies do not appear to confer protection against the spirochete and may even contribute to the pathogenesis of Lyme disease. Immune complexes consisting of spirochete antigens and antibody are thought to result in a type III hypersensitive reaction. Deposition of complexes near the original bite results in the characteristic rash; deposition of com-

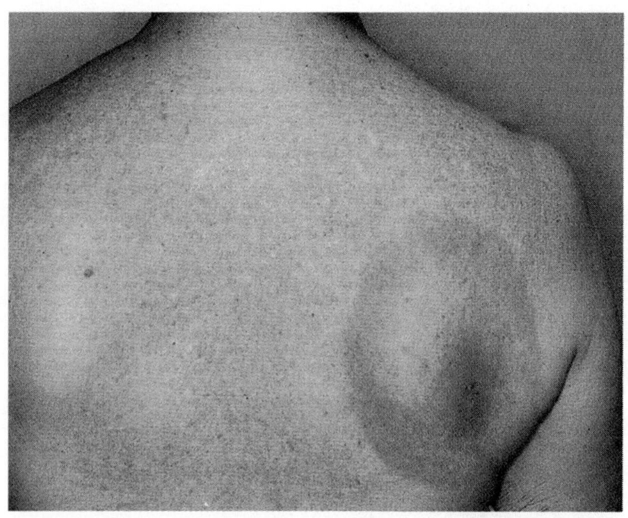

FIGURE 17-10 Bull's-eye rash is an early symptom of Lyme disease. [Courtesy MS Klempner, New England Medical Center.]

plexes in the joints is thought to induce an inflammatory response resulting in arthritic symptoms; deposition of the complexes in the vasculature and along the meninges leads to neurologic symptoms. These antigen-antibody complexes can activate the complement system, resulting in direct lytic damage to the joints or vasculature. Alternatively, complement split products, such as C3a and C5a, will induce neutrophil chemotaxis and activation. Some of the tissue damage may then result from lytic enzymes released by the activated neutrophils.

Some investigators have suggested that interleukin 1 (IL-1) is involved in the pathogenesis of Lyme disease. Like other Gram-negative bacteria, *Borrelia* has a cell wall containing lipopolysaccharide (LPS), and LPS is a well-known inducer of IL-1 in macrophages. When macrophages are cultured together with *B. burgdorferi,* the macrophages secrete high levels of IL-1, which may be responsible for many of the symptoms of the disease. For example, when IL-1 is injected into rabbit skin, a characteristic rash appears. Furthermore, when IL-1 is added to cultured synovial cells, the cells begin to secrete collagenase and prostaglandins. The release of collagenase in a joint could lead to the degradation of collagen and destruction of the joint. This mechanism would explain the mysterious observation that there is a temporary exacerbation of symptoms (called the Jarish-Herxheimer reaction) soon after antibiotic is administered. It suggests that the exacerbation may result from massive killing of *B. burgdorferi,* releasing large quantities of LPS from the Gram-negative cell wall. The LPS in turn is hypothesized to induce excessive release of IL-1, resulting in increased severity of symptoms until the LPS levels subside.

Although mice are a major reservoir of *B. burgdorferi,* mice infected with *B. burgdorferi* do not develop Lyme disease, suggesting that they can mount a protective immune response. Comparison of the immune responses to *B. burgdorferi* in mice and humans has shown that mice produce high levels of antibodies to two proteins on the outer surface of the bacterial envelope, whereas humans fail to do so; instead, most infected humans produce antibodies to a flagellar antigen. The ability of mouse antibodies to protect against Lyme disease was studied in SCID mice, which, unlike normal mice, are susceptible to the disease. Monoclonal antibodies, made in normal mice, to the outer-surface proteins protected SCID mice from disease, whereas monoclonal antibodies to the flagellar antigen did not. Recent human clinical trials with a vaccine based on outer-surface protein A (OspA) strongly suggest that it offers significant protection. This vaccine was approved for release in January 1999.

Protozoan Diseases

Protozoans are unicellular eukaryotic organisms. They are responsible for several serious diseases in humans, including amoebiasis, Chagas' disease, African sleeping sickness, malaria, leishmaniasis, and toxoplasmosis. The type of immune response that develops to protozoan infection and the effectiveness of the response depend in part on the location of the parasite within the host. Many protozoans have life-cycle stages in which they are free within the bloodstream, and it is during these stages that humoral antibody is most effective. Many of these same pathogens are also capable of intracellular growth; during these stages, cell-mediated immune reactions are effective in host defense. In the development of vaccines for protozoan diseases, the branch of the immune system that is most likely to confer protection must be carefully considered.

Malaria (Plasmodium Species)

Malaria, one of the most devastating diseases in the world today, is estimated to infect 600 million people worldwide and to cause 1–2 million deaths every year. Malaria is caused by various species of the genus *Plasmodium,* of which *P. falciparum* is the most virulent and prevalent. The alarming development of multiple-drug resistance in *Plasmodium* and the increased resistance of its vector, the *Anopheles* mosquito, to DDT underscore the importance of developing new strategies to hinder the spread of malaria.

Plasmodium Life Cycle and Pathogenesis of Malaria

Plasmodium progresses through a remarkable series of developmental and maturational stages in its extremely complex life cycle. Female *Anopheles* mosquitoes, which feed on blood meals, serve as the vector for *Plasmodium,* and part of the parasite's life cycle takes place within the mosquito. (Because male *Anopheles* mosquitoes feed on plant juices, they do not transmit *Plasmodium.*)

Human infection begins when sporozoites, one of the *Plasmodium* stages, are introduced into an individual's bloodstream as an infected mosquito takes a blood meal (Figure 17-11). Within 30 min, the sporozoites disappear from the blood as they migrate to the liver, where they infect hepatocytes. Sporozoites are long, slender cells that are covered by a 45-kDa protein called circumsporozoite (CS) antigen, which probably mediates their adhesion to hepatocytes. Such adhesion has been demonstrated in vitro, and recombinant CS antigens have been shown to bind to hepatocytes in vitro. The binding site on the CS antigen is a conserved region in the carboxyl-terminal end (called region II) that has a high degree of sequence homology with known cell-adhesion molecules.

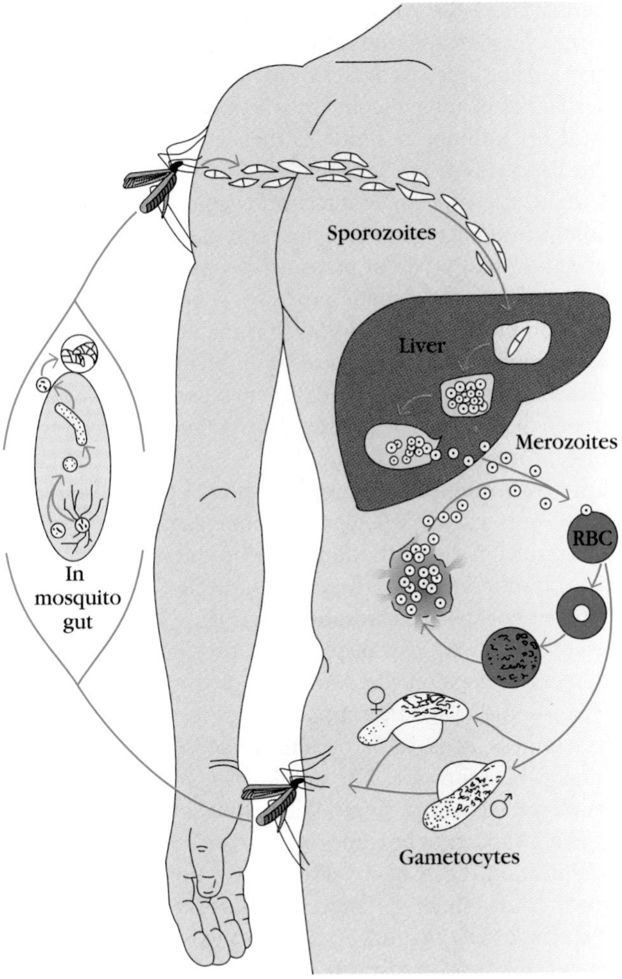

FIGURE 17-11 The life cycle of *Plasmodium*. Sporozoites enter the bloodstream when an infected mosquito takes a blood meal. The sporozoites migrate to the liver, where they multiply, transforming liver hepatocytes into giant multinucleate schizonts, which release thousands of merozoites into the bloodstream. The merozoites infect red blood cells, which eventually rupture, releasing more merozoites. Eventually some of the merozoites differentiate into male and female gametocytes, which are ingested by a mosquito and differentiate into gametes. The gametes fuse to form a zygote that differentiates to the sporozoite stage within the salivary gland of the mosquito.

Within the liver, the sporozoites multiply extensively and undergo a complex series of transformations that culminate in the formation and release of merozoites in about a week. It has been estimated that a liver hepatocyte infected with a single sporozoite can release 5,000–10,000 merozoites. The released merozoites infect red blood cells, initiating the symptoms and pathology of malaria. Within a red blood cell, merozoites replicate and undergo successive differentiations; eventually the cell ruptures and releases new merozoites, which go on to infect more red blood cells. Eventually some of the merozoites differentiate into male and female gametocytes, which may be ingested by a female *Anopheles* mosquito during a blood meal. Within the mosquito's gut, the male and female gametocytes differentiate into gametes that fuse to form a zygote, which multiplies and differentiates into sporozoites within the salivary gland. The infected mosquito is now set to initiate the cycle once again.

The symptoms of malaria are recurrent chills, fever, and sweating. The symptoms peak roughly every 48 h, when successive generations of merozoites are released from infected red blood cells. An infected individual eventually becomes weak and anemic and shows splenomegaly. The large numbers of merozoites formed can block capillaries, causing intense headaches, renal failure, heart failure, or cerebral damage—often with fatal consequences. There is speculation that some of the symptoms of malaria may be caused not by *Plasmodium* itself but instead by excessive production of cytokines. This hypothesis stemmed from the observation that cancer patients treated in clinical trials with recombinant tumor necrosis factor (TNF) developed symptoms that mimicked malaria. The relation between TNF and malaria symptoms was studied by infecting mice with a mouse-specific strain of *Plasmodium*, which causes rapid death by cerebral malaria. Injection of these mice with antibodies to TNF was shown to prevent the rapid death.

Host Response to Plasmodium Infection

In regions where malaria is endemic, the immune response to *Plasmodium* infection is poor. Children less than 14 years old mount the lowest immune response and consequently are most likely to develop malaria. In some regions, the childhood mortality rate for malaria reaches 50%, and worldwide the disease kills about a million children a year. The low immune response to *Plasmodium* among children can be demonstrated by measuring serum antibody levels to the sporozoite stage. Only 22% of the children living in endemic areas have detectable antibodies to the sporozoite stage, whereas 84% of the adults have such antibodies. Even in adults, the degree of immunity is far from complete, however, and most people living in endemic regions have lifelong low-level *Plasmodium* infections.

A number of factors may contribute to the low levels of immune responsiveness to *Plasmodium*. The maturational changes from sporozoite to merozoite to gametocyte allow the organism to keep changing its surface molecules, resulting in continual changes in the antigens seen by the immune system. The intracellular phases of the life cycle in liver cells and erythrocytes also reduce the degree of immune activation generated by the pathogen and allow the organism to multiply while it is shielded from attack. Furthermore, the most accessible stage, the sporozoite, circulates in the blood for only about 30 min before it infects liver hepatocytes; it is unlikely that much immune activation can occur in such a short period of time. And even when an antibody response does develop to sporozoites, *Plasmodium* has evolved a way of overcoming that response by sloughing off the surface CS-antigen coat, thus rendering the antibodies ineffective.

Design of Malaria Vaccines

An effective vaccine for malaria should maximize the most effective immune defense mechanisms. Unfortunately, little is known of the roles that humoral and cell-mediated responses play in the development of protective immunity to this disease. Current approaches to design of malaria vaccines focus largely on the sporozoite stage. One experimental vaccine, for example, consists of *Plasmodium* sporozoites attenuated by x-irradiation. In one study, nine volunteers were repeatedly immunized by the bite of *P. falciparum*–infected, irradiated mosquitoes. Later challenge by the bites of mosquitoes infected with virulent *P. falciparum* revealed that six of the nine recipients were completely protected. As encouraging as these results are, the need to breed mosquitoes to obtain *Plasmodium* sporozoites makes this approach impracticable for immunizing the millions of people living in endemic malaria regions. Sporozoites do not grow well in cultured cells, so large numbers of mosquitoes are needed, making this an unreasonable approach. For example, an enormous insectory would be required to breed mosquitoes in which to prepare enough irradiated sporozoites to vaccinate just one small village in such regions.

Current vaccine strategies are aimed at producing synthetic subunit vaccines consisting of epitopes that can be recognized by T cells and B cells. While no effective vaccine has been developed, this is an active area of investigation.

African Sleeping Sickness (*Trypanosoma* Species)

Two species of African trypanosomes, which are flagellated protozoans, can cause sleeping sickness, a chronic, debilitating disease transmitted to humans and cattle by the bite of the tsetse fly. In the bloodstream, a trypanosome differentiates into a long, slender form that continues to divide every 4–6 h. The disease progresses through several stages, beginning with an early (systemic) stage in which trypanosomes multiply in the blood and progressing to a neurologic stage in which the parasite infects the central nervous system, causing meningoencephalitis and eventually the loss of consciousness.

As parasite numbers increase after infection, an effective humoral antibody response develops to the glycoprotein coat, called variant surface glycoprotein (VSG), that covers the trypanosomal surface. These antibodies eliminate most of the parasites from the bloodstream, both by complement-mediated lysis and by opsonization and subsequent phagocytosis. However, about 1% of the organisms, which bear an antigenically different VSG, escape the initial antibody response. These surviving organisms now begin to proliferate in the bloodstream, and a new wave of parasitemia is observed. The successive waves of parasitemia reflect a unique mechanism of antigenic shift by which the trypanosomes can evade the immune response to their glycoprotein antigens. This process is so effective that each new variant that arises in the course of a single infection is able to escape the humoral antibodies generated in response to the preceding variant, so that waves of parasitemia recur (Figure 17-12a).

Several unusual genetic processes generate the extensive variation in trypanosomal VSG that enables the organism to escape immunologic clearance. An individual trypanosome carries a large repertoire of VSG genes, each encoding a different VSG primary sequence. *Trypanosoma brucei*, for example, contains more than 1000 VSG genes in its genome, clustered at multiple chromosomal sites. A trypanosome expresses only a single VSG gene at a time. Activation of a VSG gene results in duplication of the gene and its transposition to a transcriptionally active expression site (ES) at the telomeric end of specific chromosomes (Figure 17-12b). Activation of a new VSG gene displaces the previous gene from the telomeric expression site. A number of chromosomes in the trypanosome have transcriptionally active expression sites at the telomeric ends, so that a number of VSG genes can potentially be expressed, but unknown control mechanisms limit expression to a single VSG expression site at a time.

There appears to be some order in the VSG variation during infection. Each new variant arises not by clonal outgrowth from a single variant cell but instead from the growth of multiple cells that have activated the same VSG gene in the current wave of parasite growth. It is not known how this process is regulated among individual trypanosomes. The continual shifts in epitopes displayed by the VSG make the development of a vaccine for African sleeping sickness extremely difficult.

Leishmaniasis

The protozoan parasite *Leishmania major* provides a powerful and illustrative example of how host responses can differ between individuals. These differences can lead to either

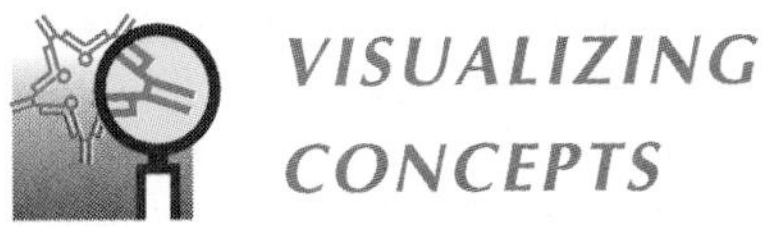

VISUALIZING CONCEPTS

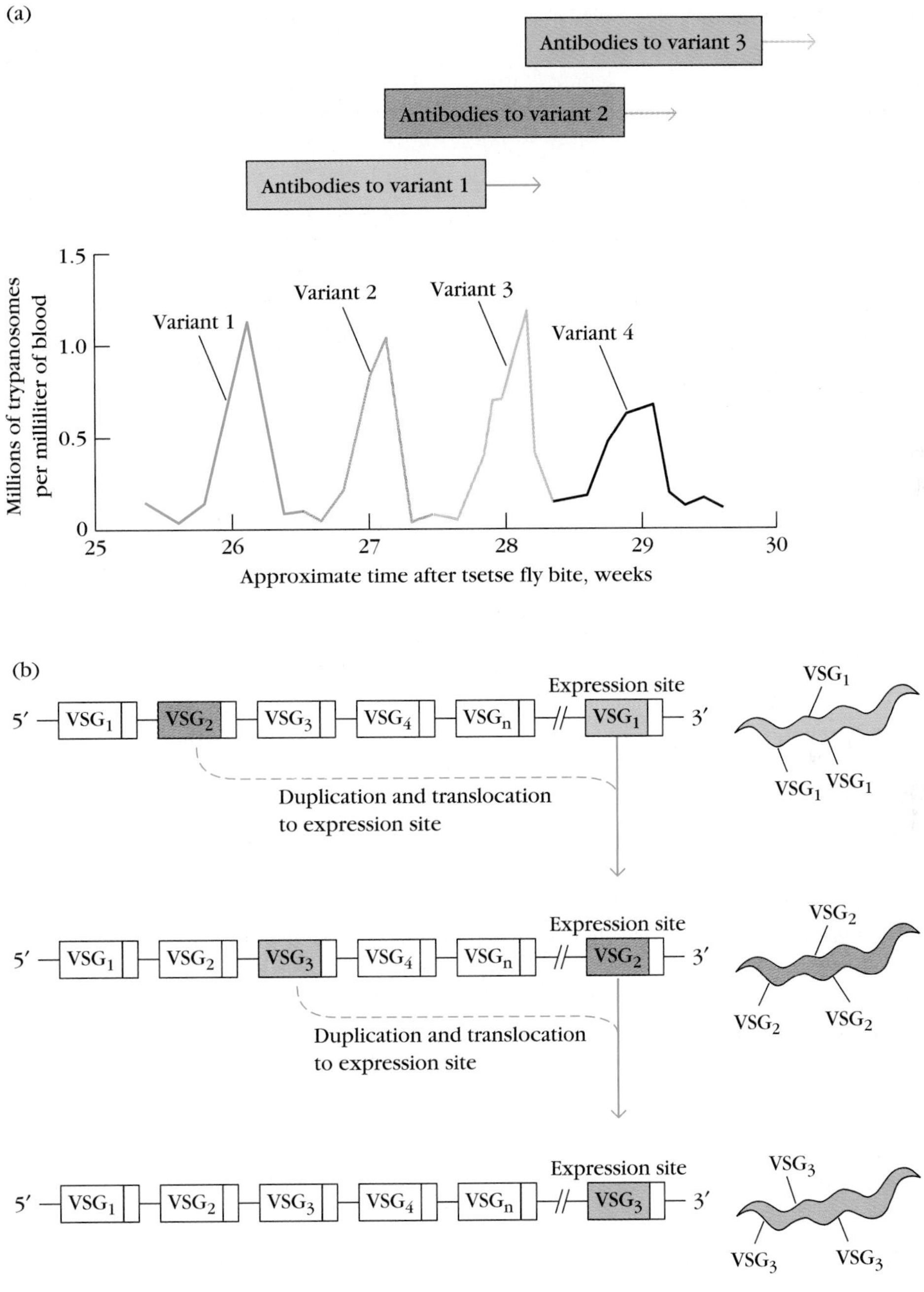

(a)

Antibodies to variant 3
Antibodies to variant 2
Antibodies to variant 1

Variant 1
Variant 2
Variant 3
Variant 4

Millions of trypanosomes per milliliter of blood
1.5
1.0
0.5
0
25 26 27 28 29 30
Approximate time after tsetse fly bite, weeks

(b)

5′ — VSG$_1$ — VSG$_2$ — VSG$_3$ — VSG$_4$ — VSG$_n$ // Expression site VSG$_1$ — 3′
VSG$_1$ VSG$_1$ VSG$_1$
Duplication and translocation to expression site

5′ — VSG$_1$ — VSG$_2$ — VSG$_3$ — VSG$_4$ — VSG$_n$ // Expression site VSG$_2$ — 3′
VSG$_2$ VSG$_2$ VSG$_2$
Duplication and translocation to expression site

5′ — VSG$_1$ — VSG$_2$ — VSG$_3$ — VSG$_4$ — VSG$_n$ // Expression site VSG$_3$ — 3′
VSG$_3$ VSG$_3$ VSG$_3$

FIGURE 17-12 (a) Successive waves of parasitemia after infection with *Trypanosoma* result from antigenic shifts in the parasite's variant surface glycoprotein (VSG). Each variant that arises is unaffected by the humoral antibodies induced by the previous variant. (b) Antigenic shifts in trypanosomes occur by the duplication of gene segments encoding variant VSG molecules and their translocation to an expression site located close to the telomere.[Part (a) adapted from J Donelson, 1988, *The Biology of Parasitism,* Alan R. Liss.]

clearance of the parasite or fatality from the infection. *Leishmania* is a protozoan the lives in the phagosomes of macrophages. Resistance to the infection correlates well with the production of IFN-γ and the development of a T_H1 response. Elegant studies in mice have demonstrated that strains that are resistant to *Leishmania* develop a T_H1 response and produce IFN-γ upon infection. Such strains of mice become highly susceptible to *Leishmania*-induced fatality if they lose either IFN-γ or the IFN-γ receptor, further underscoring the importance of IFN-γ in containing the infection. A few strains of mice, such as BALB/c, are highly susceptible to *Leishmania*, and these animals frequently succumb to infection. These mice mount a T_H2-type response to *Leishmania* infection; they produce high levels of IL-4 and essentially no IFN-γ. Thus, one difference between an effective and an ineffective defense against the parasite is the development of a T_H1 response or a T_H2 response. Recent studies demonstrate that one difference between the resistant strains of mice and BALB/c is that a small restricted subset of BALB/c $CD4^+$ T cells are capable of recognizing a particular epitope on *L. major*, and this subset produces high levels of IL-4 early in the response to the parasite. This skews the response toward a predominantly T_H2 type. Understanding how these different T-helper responses affect the outcome of infection could provide a more rational approach to the design of effective treatments and successful vaccines for other pathogens.

Diseases Caused by Parasitic Worms (Helminths)

Unlike protozoans, which are unicellular and often grow within human cells, helminths are large, multicellular organisms that reside in humans but do not ordinarily multiply there and are not intracellular pathogens. Although helminths are more accessible to the immune system than protozoans are, most infected individuals carry few of these parasites; for this reason, the immune system is not strongly engaged and the level of immunity generated to helminths is often very poor.

Parasitic worms are responsible for a wide variety of diseases in both humans and animals. More than a billion people are infected with *Ascaris*, a parasitic roundworm that infects the small intestine, and more than 300 million people are infected with *Schistosoma*, a trematode worm that causes a chronic debilitating infection. Several helminths are important pathogens of domestic animals and invade humans who ingest contaminated food. These helminths include *Taenia*, a tapeworm of cattle and pigs, and *Trichinella*, the roundworm of pigs that causes trichinosis.

Several *Schistosoma* species are responsible for the chronic, debilitating, and sometimes fatal disease **schistosomiasis** (formerly known as *bilharzia*). Three species, *S. mansoni*, *S. japonicum*, and *S. haematobium*, are the major pathogens in humans, infecting individuals in Africa, the Middle East, South America, the Caribbean, China, Southeast Asia, and the Philippines. A rise in the incidence of schistosomiasis in recent years has paralleled the increasing worldwide use of irrigation, which has expanded the habitat of the freshwater snail that serves as the intermediate host for schistosomes.

Infection occurs through contact with free-swimming infectious larvae, called cercariae, which are released from an infected snail at the rate of 300–3000 per day. When cercariae contact human skin, they secrete digestive enzymes that help them to bore into the skin, where they shed their tails and are transformed into schistosomules. The schistosomules enter the capillaries and migrate to the lungs, then to the liver, and finally to the primary site of infection, which varies with the species. *S. mansoni* and *S. japonicum* infect the intestinal mesenteric veins; *S. haematobium* infects the veins of the urinary bladder. Once established in their final tissue site, schistosomules mature into male and female adult worms. The worms mate and the females produce at least 300 spiny eggs a day. Unlike protozoan parasites, schistosomes and other helminths do not multiply within their hosts. The eggs produced by the female worm do not mature into adult worms in humans; instead, some of them pass into the feces or urine and are excreted to infect more snails. The number of worms in an infected individual increases only through repeated exposure to the free-swimming cercariae, and so most infected individuals carry rather low numbers of worms.

Most of the symptoms of schistosomiasis are initiated by the eggs. As many as half of the eggs produced remain in the host, where they invade the intestinal wall, liver, or bladder and cause hemorrhage. A chronic state can then develop in which the adult worms persist and the unexcreted eggs induce cell-mediated delayed-type hypersensitive reactions, resulting in large granulomas that are gradually walled off by fibrous tissue. Although the eggs are contained by the formation of the granuloma, often the granuloma itself obstructs the venous blood flow to the liver or bladder.

Although an immune response does develop to the schistosomes, in most individuals it is not sufficient to eliminate the adult worms, even though the intravascular sites of schistosome infestation should make the worm an easy target for immune attack. Instead, the worms survive for up to 20 years. The schistosomules would appear to be the forms most susceptible to attack, but because they are motile, they can evade the localized cellular buildup of immune and inflammatory cells. Adult schistosome worms also have several unique mechanisms that protect them from immune defenses. The adult worm has been shown to decrease the expression of antigens on its outer membrane and also to enclose itself in a glycolipid and glycoprotein coat derived from the host, masking the presence of its own antigens. Among the antigens observed on the adult worm are the host's own ABO blood-group antigens and histocompatibility antigens! The

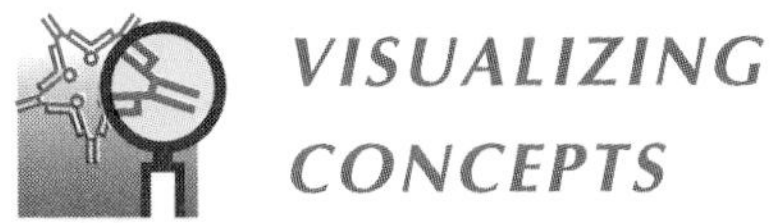

VISUALIZING CONCEPTS

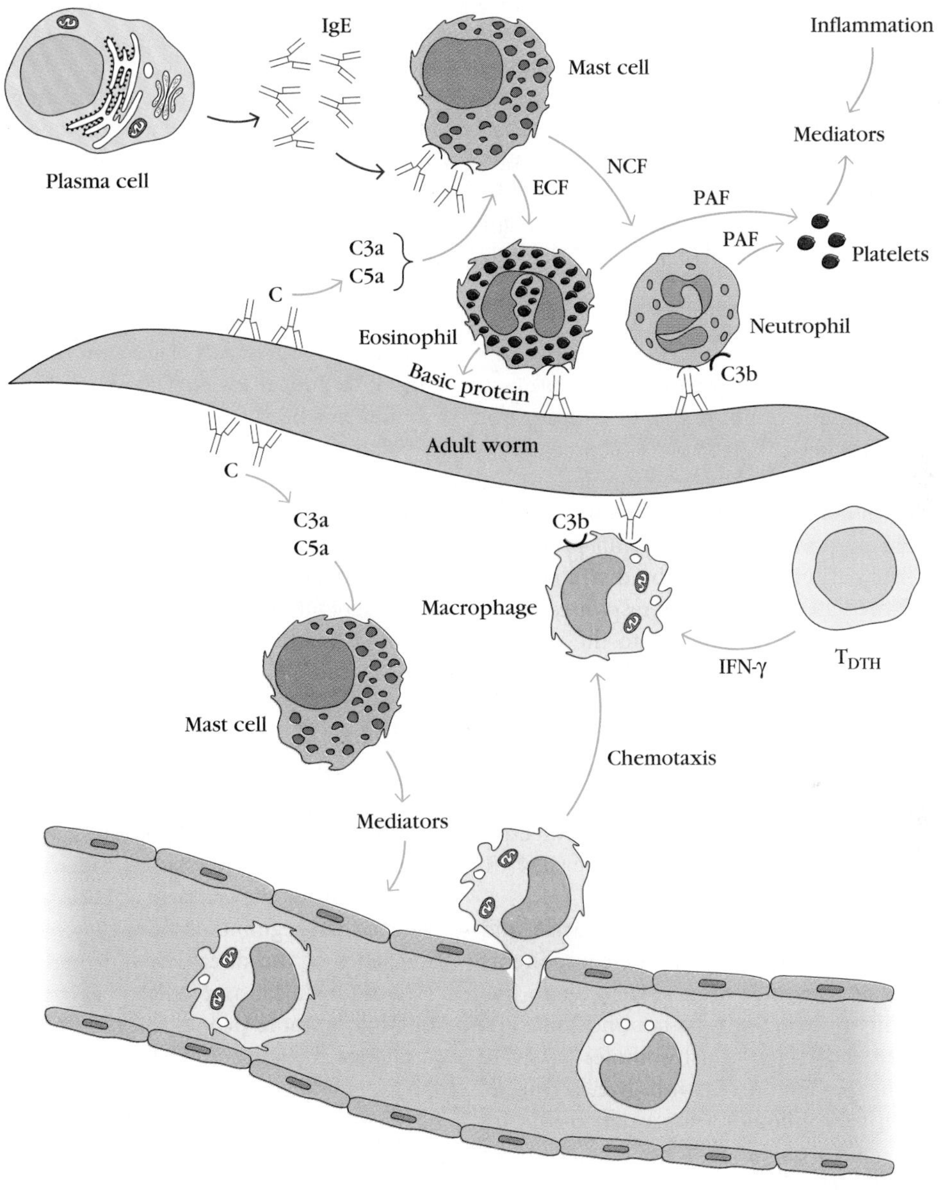

FIGURE 17-13 Overview of the immune response generated against *Schistosoma mansoni*. The response includes an IgE humoral component (*top*) and a cell-mediated component involving $CD4^+$ T cells (*bottom*). C = complement; ECF = eosinophil chemotactic factor; NCF = neutrophil chemotactic factor; PAF = platelet-activating factor.

immune response is, of course, diminished by this covering made of the host's self-antigens, which must contribute to the lifelong persistence of these organisms.

The relative importance of the humoral and cell-mediated responses in protective immunity to schistosomiasis is controversial. The humoral response to infection with *S. mansoni* is characterized by high titers of antischistosome IgE antibodies, localized increases in mast cells and their subsequent degranulation, and increased numbers of eosinophils (Figure 17-13, *top*). These manifestations suggest that cytokines produced by a T_H2-like subset are important for the immune response: IL-4, which induces B cells to class-switch to IgE production; IL-5, which induces bone-marrow precursors to differentiate into eosinophils; and IL-3, which (along with IL-4) stimulates growth of mast cells. Degranulation of mast cells releases mediators that increase the infiltration of such inflammatory cells as macrophages and eosinophils. The eosinophils express Fc receptors for IgE and IgG and bind to the antibody-coated parasite. Once bound to the parasite, an eosinophil can participate in antibody-dependent cell-mediated cytotoxicity (ADCC), releasing mediators from its granules that damage the parasite (see Figure 14-12). One eosinophil mediator, called basic protein, is particularly toxic to helminths.

Immunization studies with mice, however, suggest that this humoral IgE response may not provide protective immunity. When mice are immunized with *S. mansoni* vaccine, the protective immune response that develops is not an IgE response, but rather a T_H1 response characterized by IFN-γ production and macrophage accumulation (see Figure 17-13, *bottom*). Furthermore, inbred strains of mice with deficiencies in mast cells or IgE develop protective immunity from vaccination, whereas inbred strains with deficiencies in cell-mediated $CD4^+$ T-cell responses fail to develop protective immunity in response to the vaccine. These studies suggest that the $CD4^+$ T-cell response may be the most important in immunity to schistosomiasis. It has been suggested that the ability to induce an ineffective T_H2-like response may have evolved in schistosomes as a clever defense mechanism to ensure that T_H2 cells produced sufficient levels of IL-10 to inhibit protective immunity mediated by the T_H1-like subset in the $CD4^+$ T response.

Antigens present on the membrane of cercariae and young schistosomules are promising vaccine components because these stages appear to be most susceptible to immune attack. Injecting mice and rats with monoclonal antibodies to cercariae and young schistosomules passively transferred resistance to infection with live cercariae. When these protective antibodies were used in affinity columns to purify schistosome membrane antigens from crude membrane extracts, it was found that mice immunized and boosted with these purified antigens exhibited increased resistance to a later challenge with live cercariae. Schistosome cDNA libraries were then established and screened with the protective monoclonal antibodies to identify those cDNAs encoding surface antigens. Experiments using cloned cercariae or schistosomule antigens are presently under way to assess their ability to induce protective immunity in animal models. However, in developing an effective vaccine for schistosomiasis, a fine line separates a beneficial immune response, which at best limits the parasite load, from a detrimental response, which in itself may become pathologic.

Emerging Infectious Diseases

A cursory glance at the current offerings in your local bookstore or video rental store brings into focus the preoccupation of the public and the press with new infectious agents. Several times a year, it seems, we hear about a new virus or bacterium that arises in a particular location and causes severe illness or death in a population. Newly described pathogens are referred to as emerging pathogens. Some of the emerging pathogens that have been described since the early 1970s appear in Table 17-5. These new pathogens are thought to have emerged within the recent past. HIV is an example of a newly emerged pathogen.

In other instances, diseases that were no longer causing widespread infection suddenly began to infect an ever-larger number of individuals. These are referred to as "re-emerging" infectious diseases. The re-emergence of these diseases should not be surprising if we consider that bacteria can adapt to living in almost any environment. If they can adapt to living at the high temperatures of the thermal vents deep within the oceans, it is not difficult to accept that they can evolve to evade antimicrobial drugs.

Tuberculosis is a well-known re-emerging disease. Ten years ago, public health officials were convinced that tuberculosis would soon disappear as a major health consideration in the United States. Then, because of a number of events, including the AIDS epidemic, thousands of infected individuals developed strains of *M. tuberculosis* resistant to the conventional battery of antibiotics. These individuals then passed on the newly emerged, antibiotic-resistant strains of *M. tuberculosis* to others. While the rate of infection with *M. tuberculosis* in the United States increased sharply during the early part of this decade, by 1995 the incidence had begun to decline again. However, the worldwide incidence of the disease is still increasing, and the World Health Organization predicts that, between 1998 and 2020, one billion more people will become infected and over 70 million will die from this disease if preventive measures are not adopted.

Another a re-emerging disease is diphtheria. This disease was almost non-existent throughout Europe in recent years because of vaccination; in 1994, however, scattered cases were reported in some of the republics of the former Soviet Union. By 1995, there were over 50,000 cases reported in the same region, and thousands died from diphtheria infection. The social upheaval and instability that came with the breakup of the Soviet Union was almost certainly a major factor in the re-emergence of this disease, because of the resultant lapses in public health measures—perhaps most important was the loss of immunization programs. Since 1995, immunization programs have been re-established and the trend has reversed, with only 13,687 cases of diphtheria reported in Russian republics in 1996 and 6,932 in 1998.

TABLE 17-5 EMERGING PATHOGENS RECOGNIZED SINCE 1973

Year	Pathogen	Disease
1973	Rotavirus	Major cause of infantile diarrhea globally
1974	Hepatitis C	Non-A, non-B hepatitis commonly transmitted via transfusions
1976	*Cryptosporidium parvum*	Acute chronic diarrhea
1977	Ebola virus	Ebola haemorrhagic fever
	Legionella pneumophilia	Legionnaires' disease
	Hantavirus	Haemorrhagic fever with renal syndrome
	Campylobacter jejuni	Enteric diseases distributed globally
1980	Human T-lymphotrophic virus I (HTLV-1)	T-cell lymphoma
1981	Toxin-producing strains of *Staphylococcus aureus*	Toxic shock syndrome
1982	*Escherichia coli* 0157:H7	Haemorrhagic colitis
	HTLV-II	Hairy cell leukemia
	Borrelia burgdorferi	Lyme disease
1983	HIV	AIDS
	Helicobacter pylori	Peptic ulcers
1988	Hepatitis E	Enteric non-A, non-B hepatitis
1990	Guanarito virus	Venezuelan haemorrhagic fever
1991	*Encephalitozzon hellem*	Conjunctivitis, disseminated disease
1992	*Vibrio cholerae* 0139	New strain of epidemic cholera
	Bartonella henselae	Cat scratch disease
1994	Sabia virus	Brazilian haemorrhagic fever
1995	Human herpes virus-8	Associated with Kaposi sarcoma in AIDS patients
1996	TSE causing agent	New variant of Creutzfeldt-Jakob disease (mad cow disease)
1997	Influenza A subtype H5N1	Avian influenza
1999	Influenza A subtype H9N2	New strain of human influenza
	Nipah virus	Encephalitis

Other diseases have appeared seemingly from nowhere and, as far as we know, are new pathogens. These include such pathogens as the widely publicized Ebola virus and *Legionella pneumophilia*, the bacterial causative agent for Legionnaires' disease. Ebola was first recognized after an outbreak in Africa, in 1976. By 1977, the virus that causes this disease had been isolated and classified as a filovirus, a type of RNA virus that includes Marburg virus, a close relative of Ebola. Ebola causes a particularly severe haemorrhagic fever that kills more than 50% of those infected. Because of the severity of disease and the rapid progression to death after the initial appearance of symptoms, this virus has received a great deal of attention. However, while the risk of death is very high if you are infected with Ebola, it is fairly easy to control the spread of the virus. Through isolation of infected individuals, hospital workers and medical personnel can be protected. In such ways, the spread of Ebola virus has been contained during the two most recent outbreaks.

Another emerging disease recently described is Legionnaires' disease, a virulent pneumonia first reported in 221 individuals who had attended an American Legion convention in Philadelphia in 1976. Of the 221 afflicted, 34 died from the infection. The organism causing the disease was not known, but further investigation led to the identification of a bacterium that was named *Legionella pneumophilia*. This bacterium proliferates in cool, damp areas and can be found in the condensing units of large commercial air-conditioning systems. The air-conditioning system can produce an aerosol that contains the bacteria, thus spreading the infection throughout the area served by the unit. This was determined to be the source of the bacteria at the 1976 convention in Philadelphia. Because the hazard of such aerosols is now recognized, improved design of air-conditioning and plumbing systems has greatly reduced the incidence of the disease.

Why are these new diseases emerging and others re-emerging? One possible reason suggested by public-health officials is the crowding of the world's poorest populations into very small places within huge cities. Another factor is the great increase in international travel. Additionally, it is now easy to traverse the globe in a very short time, making it possible for an individual to become infected on one continent and then spread the disease to another continent tens of thousands of miles distant. Other features of modern life that may contribute include mass distribution of food, which exposes large populations to potentially contaminated food, and unhygienic food preparation. The World Health Organization and the U. S. Center for Disease Control both actively monitor new infections and work together closely to detect and identify new infectious agents and to provide up-to-date information for travelers to parts of the world where such agents may pose a risk.

Summary

1. Innate immune responses form the primary defense against pathogens. These include physical barriers, such as skin, as well as the nonspecific production of complement components and certain cytokines in response to infection by various pathogens.
2. The immune response to viral infections involves both humoral and cell-mediated components (see Table 17-2). Antibody to a viral receptor can block viral infections of host cells. However, a number of viruses, including influenza, are able to mutate their receptor molecules and thus evade the humoral antibody response (see Figure 17-5). Once a viral infection has been established, cell-mediated immunity appears to be more important than humoral, and it acts to eliminate infected cells.
3. The immune response to extracellular bacterial infections is generally mediated by antibody (see Figure 17-7). Antibody can induce localized production of immune effector molecules of the complement system, thus facilitating development of an inflammatory response. Antibody can also activate complement-mediated lysis of the bacterium, neutralize toxins, and serve as an opsonin to increase phagocytosis. Bacteria can evade the humoral antibody response by several mechanisms (see Table 17-4). Some bacteria secrete protease enzymes that cleave IgA dimers, thus reducing the effectiveness of IgA in the mucous secretions. Other bacteria escape phagocytosis by producing surface capsules or proteins that inhibit adherence to phagocytes, by secreting toxins that kill phagocytes, or by their ability to survive within phagocytes. Host defense against intracellular bacteria depends largely on $CD4^+$ T-cell mediated responses.
4. Both humoral and cell-mediated immune responses have been implicated in immunity to protozoan infections. The effectiveness of the response depends in part on the location of the parasite, which typically changes with stages of its life cycle. In general, humoral antibody is effective against blood-borne stages, but once protozoans have infected host cells, cell-mediated immunity is necessary. Protozoans escape the immune response through several mechanisms. Some—notably *Trypanosoma brucei*—are covered by a glycoprotein coat that is constantly changed by a genetic-switch mechanism (see Figure 17-12). Others (including *Plasmodium*, the causative agent of malaria) slough off their glycoprotein coat after antibody has bound to it.
5. Helminths are large parasites, which normally do not multiply within cells. Because few of these organisms are carried by an affected individual and because they do not multiply within the host, immune-system exposure to helminths is limited; consequently, only a low level of immunity is induced. Although helminths generally are attacked by antibody-mediated defenses, these may be ineffective. A cell-mediated response by $CD4^+$ T cells plays a critical role in the response to *Schistosoma* (see Figure 17-13).
6. Emerging and re-emerging pathogens have become increasingly prominent in recent years (see Table 17-5). These pathogens include some that are newly described and others that had been thought to be controlled by public-health practices. Among the factors leading to the emergence of such pathogens are our increased ability to travel long distances in a short time and the intense crowding of some populations into small urban environments.

REFERENCES

Biron, CA. 1998. Role of early cytokines, including α and β interferons (IFN-α/β), in innate and adaptive immune responses to viral infections. *Semin. Immunol.* **10:**383.

Bloom, BR, and CJL Murray. 1992. Tuberculosis: commentary on a reemergent killer. *Science* **257:**1055.

Borst, P, et al. 1998. Control of VSG gene expression sites in *Trypanosoma brucei. Mol. Biochem. Parasitol.* **91:**67.

Bretscher, PA. 1992. A strategy to improve the efficacy of vaccination against tuberculosis and leprosy. *Immunol. Today* **13:**342.

Cooper, AM, and JL Flynn. 1995. The protective immune response to *Mycobacterium tuberculosis. Curr. Opin. Immunol.* **7:**512.

Cox, FE. 1997. Designer vaccines for parasitic diseases. *Int. J. Parasitol.* **27:**1147.

Doherty, PC. 1997. Effector $CD4^+$ and $CD8^+$ T-cell mechanisms in the control of respiratory virus infections. *Immunol. Rev.* **159:**105.

Evans, J. 1998. Lyme disease. *Curr. Opin. Rheumatol.* **10:**339.

Finkelman, FD, et al. 1997. Cytokine regulation of host defense against parasitic gastrointestinal nematodes: lessons from studies with rodent models. *Annu. Rev. Immunol.* **15:**505.

Good, MF, et al. 1998. Pathways and strategies for developing a malaria blood-stage vaccine. *Annu. Rev. Immunol.* **16:**57.

Gooding, LR. 1992. Virus proteins that counteract host immune defenses. *Cell* **71:**5.

Hollingdale, MR, et al. 1998. Biology of malarial liver stages: implications for vaccine design. *Ann. Trop. Med. Parasitol.* **92:**411.

Huebner, RE, and KG Castro. 1995. The changing face of tuberculosis. *Annu. Rev. Med.* **46:**47.

Kaufmann, SHE. 1993. Immunity to intracellular bacteria. *Annu. Rev. Immunol.* **11:**129.

Krause, RM, et al. 1997. Summary of antibody workshop: The role of humoral immunity in the treatment and prevention of emerging and extant infectious diseases. *J. Infect. Dis.* **176:**549.

Lachmann, PJ, and A Davies. 1997. Complement and immunity to viruses. *Immunol. Rev.* **159:**69.

Lamm, ME. 1997. Interaction of antigens and antibodies at mucosal surfaces. *Annu. Rev. Microbiol.* **51:**311.

Louis, J., et al. 1998. Regulation of protective immunity against *Leishmania major* in mice. *Curr. Opin. Immunol.* **10**:459.

Mims, CA. 1987. *Pathogenesis of Infectious Disease,* 2nd ed. New York: Academic Press.

Nardin, EH, and RS Nussenzweig. 1993. T cell responses to pre-erythrocyte stages of malaria: role in protection and vaccine development against pre-erythrocyte stages. *Annu. Rev. Immunol.* **11**:687.

Ramshaw, IA, et al. 1997. Cytokines and immunity to viral infections. *Immunol. Rev.* **159**:119.

Robertson, BD, and TF Meyer. 1992. Genetic variation in pathogenic bacteria. *Trends Genet.* **8**:422.

Scott, P. 1998. Differentiation, regulation, and death of T helper cell subsets during infection with *Leishmania major. Immunol. Res.* **17**:229.

Sher, A, and RL Coffman. 1992. Regulation of immunity to parasites by T cells and T-cell derived cytokines. *Annu. Rev. Immunol.* **10**:385.

Weiss, R. 1992. On the track of "killer" TB. *Science* **255**:148.

Welsh, RM. 1997. Alpha beta and gamma delta T-cell networks and their roles in natural resistance to viral infections. *Immunol. Rev.* **159**:79.

Useful Web Sites

http://www.cdc.gov/ncidod/

National Center for Infectious Diseases home page—a superb site for monitoring emerging diseases. This is a subdivision of the Centers for Disease Control (CDC), and links to CDC are found at this site.

http://www.niaid.nih.gov/

National Institute of Allergy and Infectious Diseases home page—NIAID is the NIH institute that sponsors research in infectious diseases, and its Web site provides a number of links to other relevant sites.

http://www.who.int/

World Health Organization home page—the international organization that monitors infectious diseases worldwide.

STUDY QUESTIONS

1. The effect of the MHC on the immune response to peptides of the influenza virus nucleoprotein was studied in H-2^b mice that had been previously immunized with live influenza virions. The CTL activity of primed lymphocytes was determined by in vitro CML assays using H-2^k fibroblasts as target cells. The target cells had been transfected with different H-2^b class I MHC genes and were infected either with live influenza or incubated with nucleoprotein synthetic peptides. The results of these assays are shown in the table.

a. Why was there no killing of the target cells in system A even though the target cells were infected with live influenza?

b. Why was a CTL response generated to the nucleoprotein in system C, even though it is an internal viral protein?

c. Why was there a good CTL response in system C to peptide 365–380, whereas there was no response in system D to peptide 50–63?

d. If you were going to develop a synthetic peptide vaccine for influenza in humans, how would these results obtained in mice influence your design of a vaccine?

Target cell (H-2^k fibroblast)	Test antigen	CTL activity of influenza-primed H-2^b lymphocytes (% lysis)
(A) Untransfected	Live influenza	0
(B) Transfected with class I D^b	Live influenza	60
(C) Transfected with class I D^b	Nucleoprotein peptide 365–380	50
(D) Transfected with class I D^b	Nucleoprotein peptide 50–63	2
(E) Transfected with class I K^b	Nucleoprotein peptide 365–380	0.5
(F) Transfected with class I K^b	Nucleoprotein peptide 50–63	1

2. Describe the nonspecific defenses that operate when a disease-producing microorganism first enters the body.

3. Describe the various specific defense mechanisms that the immune system employs to combat various pathogens.

4. What is the role of the humoral response in immunity to influenza?

5. Describe the unique mechanisms each of the following pathogens has for escaping the immune response: (a) African trypanosomes, (b) *Plasmodium* species, and (c) influenza virus.

6. M. F. Good and coworkers analyzed the effect of MHC haplotype on the antibody response to a malarial circumsporozoite (CS) peptide antigen in several recombinant congenic mouse strains. Their results are shown in the table below.

a. Based on the results of this study, which MHC molecule(s) serve(s) as restriction element(s) for this peptide antigen?

b. Since antigen recognition by B cells is not MHC restricted, why is the humoral antibody response influenced by the MHC haplotype?

Strain	H-2 alleles					Antibody response to CS peptide
	K	IA	IE	S	D	
B10.BR	*k*	*k*	*k*	*k*	*k*	6 1
B10.A (4R)	*k*	*k*	*b*	*b*	*b*	6 1
B10.HTT	*s*	*s*	*k*	*k*	*d*	6 1
B10.A (5R)	*b*	*b*	*k*	*d*	*d*	67
B10	*b*	*b*	*b*	*b*	*b*	73
B10.MBR	*b*	*k*	*k*	*k*	*q*	6 1

SOURCE: Adapted from MF Good et al, 1988, *Annu. Rev. Immunol.* **6**:633.

Go to www.whfreeman.com/immunology Self-Test
Review and quiz of key terms

7. Fill in the blanks in the following statements.

a. The current vaccine for tuberculosis consists of an attenuated strain of *M. bovis* called ________________.

b. Variation in influenza surface proteins is generated by ________________ and ________________.

c. Variation in pilin, which is expressed by many gram-negative bacteria, is generated by the process of ________________.

d. The mycobacteria causing tuberculosis are walled off in granulomatous lesions called ________________, which contain a small number of ________________ and many ________________.

e. The diphtheria vaccine is a formaldehyde-treated preparation of the exotoxin, called a ________________.

f. A major contribution to nonspecific host defense against viruses is provided by ________________ and ________________.

g. The primary host defense against viral and bacterial attachment to epithelial surfaces is ________________.

h. Two cytokines of particular importance in the response to infection with *M. tuberculosis* are ________________, which stimulates development of T_H1 cells, and ________________, which promotes activation of macrophages.

8. Discuss the factors that contribute to the emergence of new pathogens or the re-emergence of pathogens previously thought to be controlled in human populations.

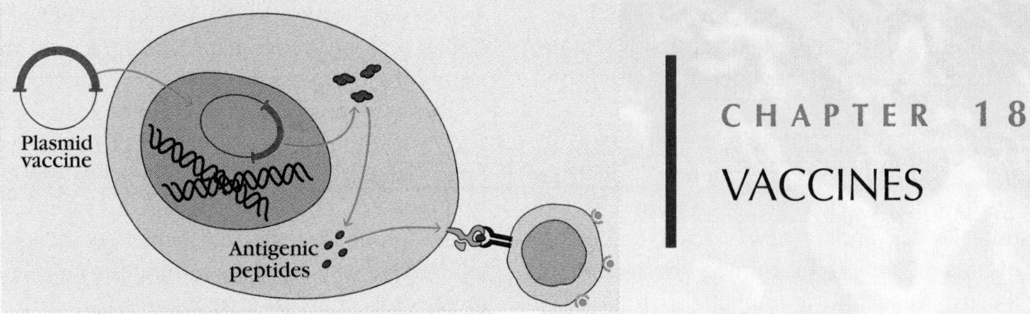

CHAPTER 18
VACCINES

Active and Passive Immunization

Designing Vaccines for Active Immunization

Whole-Organism Vaccines

Purified Macromolecules as Vaccines

Recombinant-Vector Vaccines

DNA Vaccines

Synthetic-Peptide Vaccines

Multivalent Subunit Vaccines

The discipline of immunology has its roots in the early vaccination trials of Edward Jenner and Louis Pasteur. Since these pioneering efforts, vaccines have been developed for many diseases that were once major afflictions of mankind. The incidence of diseases such as diphtheria, measles, mumps, pertussis (whooping cough), rubella (German measles), poliomyelitis, and tetanus has declined dramatically as vaccination has become more common. Clearly, vaccination is a cost-effective weapon for disease prevention. Perhaps in no other case have the benefits of vaccination been as dramatically evident as in the eradication of smallpox, one of mankind's long-standing and most terrible scourges. Since October 1977, not a single naturally acquired smallpox case has been reported anywhere in the world. Equally encouraging is the predicted eradication of polio. There were no cases of polio in the United States last year and the World Health Organization (WHO) predicts that paralytic polio will be eradicated throughout the world by the year 2003. A new addition to the weapons against childhood disease is a vaccine against rotavirus, the major cause of infant diarrhea. Use of this vaccine can save the lives of millions of infants worldwide and prevent a majority of the almost 250,000 episodes of infant diarrhea in the United States that require hospitalization.

The control of a number of the diseases that cause significant mortality and morbidity has made outstanding progress, but there remains a crying need for vaccines against others. Every year, millions of deaths throughout the world are caused by malaria, tuberculosis, and AIDS, diseases for which there are no effective vaccines. It is estimated by the World Health Organization that 16,000 individuals a day, or 5.8 million a year, become infected with HIV-1, the virus that causes AIDS. Forty million deaths from AIDS are projected by the end of the 1990s, leaving more than 9 million orphans. An effective vaccine could have an immense impact on the control of this tragic spread of death and disaster. In addition to the challenges presented by diseases for which no vaccines exist, there remains the need to improve the safety and efficacy of present vaccines and to find ways to lower their cost and deliver them efficiently to all who need them, especially in developing countries of the world. The WHO estimates that 20%–35% of infant deaths in the world are due to diseases that could be prevented by existing vaccines.

The road to successful development of a vaccine that can be approved for human use, manufactured at reasonable cost, and efficiently delivered to at-risk populations is costly, long, and tedious. Methods for producing materials that can be tested in humans and the ways they are tested in clinical trials are regulated closely. Even those candidate vaccines that survive initial scrutiny and are approved for use in human trials are not guaranteed to find their way into common usage. Experience has shown that not every vaccine candidate that was successful in laboratory or animal studies prevents disease in humans. Some potential vaccines cause unacceptable side effects, and others worsen the disease they were meant to prevent. Live virus vaccines pose a special threat to those with primary or acquired immunodeficiency (see Chapter 19). Stringent testing is an absolute necessity, because vaccines will be given to large numbers of well persons. Adverse side effects, even those that occur very seldom, must be balanced against the potential benefit of protection by the vaccine.

The beginnings of any vaccine development pathway are in basic research. Recent advances in immunology and molecular biology have led to effective new vaccines and to promising strategies for finding new vaccine candidates. Knowledge of the differences in epitopes recognized by T cells and B cells has enabled immunologists to begin to design vaccine candidates to maximize activation of either the humoral or the cell-mediated branch of the immune system. As differences in antigen-processing pathways became evident, scientists began to design vaccines and to use adjuvants that maximize antigen presentation with class I or class II MHC molecules. Genetic engineering techniques can be used to develop vaccines to maximize the immune response to selected epitopes and to simplify delivery of the vaccines. This chapter describes the vaccines now in use and describes vaccine strategies, including experimental designs that may lead to the vaccines of the future.

Active and Passive Immunization

Immunity to infectious microorganisms can be achieved by active or passive **immunization**. In each case, immunity can be acquired either by natural processes (usually by transfer from mother to fetus or by previous infection by the organism) or by artificial means such as injection of antibodies or vaccines (Table 18-1). The agents used for inducing passive immunity include antibodies from humans or animals, whereas active immunization is achieved by inoculation with microbial pathogens that induce immunity but do not cause disease or with antigenic components from the pathogens. This section describes current usage of passive and active immunization techniques.

Passive Immunization

Jenner and Pasteur are recognized as the immunologists who pioneered vaccination, or induction of active immunity, but just as much recognition is due to Emil von Behring and Hidesaburo Kitasato for their contributions to passive immunity. These investigators were the first to show that immunity elicited in one animal can be transferred to another by injecting it with serum from the first (see Clinical Focus, Chapter 4).

Passive immunization, in which preformed antibodies are transferred to a recipient, occurs naturally by transfer of maternal antibodies across the placenta to the developing fetus. Maternal antibodies to diphtheria, tetanus, streptococci, rubeola, rubella, mumps, and poliovirus all afford passively acquired protection to the developing fetus. Maternal antibodies present in colostrum and milk also provide passive immunity to the infant.

Passive immunization can also be achieved by injecting a recipient with preformed antibodies. In the past, before vaccines and antibiotics became available, passive immunization provided a major defense against various infectious diseases. Despite the risks (see Chapter 16) incurred by injecting animal sera, usually horse serum, this was the only effective therapy for otherwise fatal diseases. Currently, there are several conditions that warrant the use of passive immunization. These include:

- Deficiency in synthesis of antibody as a result of congenital or acquired B-cell defects, alone or together with other immunodeficiencies.
- When a susceptible person is exposed or likely to be exposed to a disease that will cause complications (e.g., a child with leukemia exposed to varicella or measles), or when time does not permit adequate protection by active immunization.
- When a disease is already present and the antibody may ameliorate or help suppress the effects of toxin (tetanus, diphtheria, or botulism).

TABLE 18-1 ACQUISITION OF PASSIVE AND ACTIVE IMMUNITY

Type	Acquired through
Passive immunity	Natural maternal antibody
	Immune globulin*
	Antitoxin†
Active immunity	Natural infection
	Vaccines‡
	Attenuated organisms
	Inactivated organisms
	Purified microbial macromolecules
	Cloned microbial antigens (alone or in vectors)
	Multivalent complexes
	Toxoid§

*An antibody-containing solution derived from human blood, obtained by cold ethanol fractionation of large pools of plasma; available in intramuscular and intravenous preparations.

†An antibody derived from the serum of animals that have been stimulated with specific antigens.

‡A suspension of attenuated live or killed microorganisms, or antigenic portions of them, presented to a potential host to induce immunity and prevent disease.

§A bacterial toxin that has been modified to be nontoxic but retains the capacity to stimulate the formation of antitoxin.

For example, if individuals who have not received up-to-date active immunization against tetanus suffer a puncture wound, they are given an injection of horse antiserum to tetanus toxin. The preformed horse antibody neutralizes any tetanus toxin produced by *Clostridium tetani* in the wound.

Passive immunization is routinely administered to individuals exposed to botulism, tetanus, diphtheria, hepatitis, measles, and rabies (Table 18-2). Passively administered antiserum is also used to provide protection from snake bites and black widow spider bites. Passive immunization can provide immediate protection to travelers or health care workers who will soon be exposed to an infectious organism and lack active immunity to it. Because passive immunization does not activate the immune system, it generates no memory response and the protection provided is transient.

For certain diseases such as the acute respiratory failure in children caused by respiratory syncytial virus (RSV), passive immunization is the best treatment currently available. Modern immunologic techniques have improved the methods used. Currently, a monoclonal antibody or a combination of two monoclonal antibodies may be administered to children suffering from RSV disease. These monoclonal antibodies are prepared in mice but have been "humanized" by splicing the constant regions of human IgG to the mouse variable regions (see Chapter 5). This modification prevents many of the complications that may follow a second injection of the complete mouse antibody, which is a highly immunogenic foreign protein.

Although passive immunization may be the treatment of choice, it should be used only when necessary because certain risks are associated with the injection of preformed antibody. If the antibody was produced in another species, such as a horse, the recipient can mount a strong response to the isotypic determinants of the foreign antibody. This anti-isotype response can have serious complications. Some individuals, for example, produce IgE antibody specific for a passive antibody. Immune complexes of this IgE bound to the passively administered antibody can mediate systemic mast cell degranulation, leading to systemic anaphylaxis. Other individuals produce IgG or IgM antibodies specific for the foreign antibody, which form complement-activating immune complexes. The deposition of these complexes in the tissues can lead to type III hypersensitive reactions. Even when human gamma globulin is administered passively, the recipient can generate an anti-allotype response to the human immunoglobulin, although its intensity is usually much less than that of an anti-isotype response.

TABLE 18-2 COMMON AGENTS USED FOR PASSIVE IMMUNIZATION

Disease	Agent
Black widow spider bite	Horse antivenin
Botulism	Horse antitoxin
Diphtheria	Horse antitoxin
Hepatitis A and B	Pooled human immune gamma globulin
Measles	Pooled human immune gamma globulin
Rabies	Pooled human immune gamma globulin
Snake bite	Horse antivenin
Tetanus	Pooled human immune gamma globulin or horse antitoxin

Active Immunization

Whereas the aim of passive immunization is transient protection or alleviation of an existing condition, the goal of active immunization is to elicit protective immunity and immunologic memory. When active immunization is successful, a subsequent exposure to the pathogenic agent elicits a heightened immune response that successfully eliminates the pathogen or at least prevents disease mediated by its products. Active immunization can be achieved by natural infection with a microorganism, or it can be acquired artificially by administration of a **vaccine** (see Table 18-1). In active immunization, as the name implies, the immune system plays an active role—proliferation of antigen-reactive T and B cells results in the formation of memory cells. Active immunization with various types of vaccines has played an important role in the reduction of deaths from infectious diseases, especially among children.

Vaccination of children is begun at about 2 months of age. The recommended program of childhood immunizations in this country, updated in 1999 by the American Academy of Pediatrics, is outlined in Table 18-3. The program includes the following vaccines:

- Hepatitis B vaccine
- Diphtheria-pertussis-tetanus (DPT) combined vaccine (a recently developed acellular pertussis vaccine is recommended to replace the whole pertussis vaccine; the combined vaccine is now called DTaP)
- Trivalent (Sabin) oral polio vaccine (OPV) and inactivated (Salk) polio vaccine (IPV)
- Measles-mumps-rubella (MMR) combined vaccine
- *Haemophilus influenzae* (Hib) vaccine
- Varicella zoster (Var) vaccine for chickenpox
- Rotavirus (Rv) vaccine for infant diarrhea (new)

The introduction and spreading use of various vaccines for childhood immunization has led to a dramatic decrease in the incidence of common childhood diseases in the United

States (Figure 18-1). The comparisons of disease incidence in 1996 to that reported in the peak years show dramatic drops and, in one case, complete elimination of the disease in the United States. As long as widespread, effective immunization programs are maintained, the incidence of these childhood diseases should remain low. However, the occurrence of side reactions to a vaccine may cause a drop in its use, which can lead to re-emergence of that disease. For example, the side effects from the pertussis attenuated bacterial vaccine include seizures, encephalitis, brain damage, and even death. Although these consequences are rare and much less frequent than similar episodes caused by natural infection, their occurrence has led to decreased usage of the vaccine. This has led to an increase in the incidence of whooping cough. Hopefully, the recent development of an acellular pertussis vaccine that is as effective as the older vaccine but that carries none of the side effects will reverse this trend.

As indicated in Table 18-3, children typically require multiple boosters (repeated inoculations) at appropriately timed intervals to achieve effective immunity. In the first months of life, the reason for this may be persistence of circulating maternal antibodies in the young infant. For example, passively acquired maternal antibodies bind to epitopes on the DPT vaccine and block adequate activation of the immune system; therefore, this vaccine must be given several times after the maternal antibody has been cleared from an infant's circulation in order to achieve adequate immunity. Passively acquired maternal antibody also interferes with the effectiveness of the measles vaccine; for this reason, the MMR vaccine is not given before 12–15 months of age. In Third World

TABLE 18-3 RECOMMENDED CHILDHOOD IMMUNIZATION SCHEDULE IN THE UNITED STATES, JANUARY–DECEMBER 2000

	Age								
Vaccine*	Birth	1 mo	2 mos	4 mos	6 mos	12 mos	15 mos	18 mos	4–6 yrs
Hepatitis B†		+							
			+			+			
Diphtheria, tetanus, pertussis‡			+	+	+		+		+
H. influenzae, type b			+	+	+	+			
Poliovirus§			+	+		+			+
Measles, mumps, rubella						+			+
Varicella#							+		
Hepatitis A¶									

*This schedule indicates the recommended ages for routine administration of currently licensed childhood vaccines. Bars indicate ranges of recommended ages. Any dose not given at the recommended age should be given as a "catch-up" immunization at any subsequent visit when indicated and feasible.

†Different schedules exist depending upon the HBsAg status of the mother.

‡DTaP (diphtheria and tetanus toxoids and acellular pertussis vaccine) is the preferred vaccine for all doses in the immunization series. Td (tetanus and diphtheria toxoids) is recommended at 11–12 years of age if at least 5 years have elapsed since the last dose.

§Two poliovirus vaccines currently are licensed in the United States: inactivated poliovirus (IPV) vaccine and oral poliovirus (OPV) vaccine. To eliminate the risk of vaccine-associated paralytic polio (VAPP), an all-IPV schedule is now recommended for routine childhood polio vaccination in the United States. All children should receive four doses of IPV at 2 months, 4 months, 6–18 months, and 4–6 years. However, OPV remains the vaccine of choice for mass immunization campaigns to control outbreaks due to wild poliovirus.

#Varicella (Var) vaccine is recommended at any visit on or after the first birthday for susceptible children, i.e., those who lack a reliable history of chickenpox (as judged by a health care provider) and who have not been immunized. Susceptible persons 13 years of age or older should receive 2 doses, given at least 4 weeks apart.

¶Hepatitis A vaccine is recommended for use in selected states and/or regions; local public health authorities should be consulted. (Also see *Morb. Mortal. Wkly. Rep.*, Oct. 01, 1999;**48**(RR-12): 1–37).

SOURCE: Adapted from the ECBT Web site (see references); approved by the American Academy of Pediatrics.

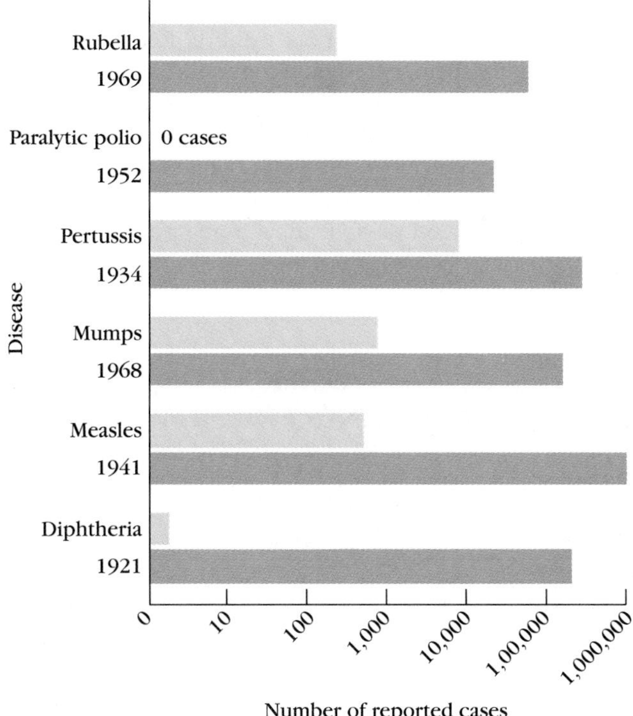

FIGURE 18-1 Reported annual number of cases of rubella (German measles), polio, pertussis (whooping cough), mumps, measles, and diphtheria in the United States in the peak year for which data are available (orange) compared with the number of cases of each disease in 1996 (green). Currently, vaccines are available for each of these diseases, and vaccination is recommended for all children in the United States. [Data from Centers for Disease Control.]

countries, however, the measles vaccine is administered at 9 months, even though maternal antibodies are still present, because 30%–50% of young children in these countries contract the disease before 15 months of age. Multiple immunizations with the oral polio vaccine are required to ensure that an adequate immune response is generated to each of the three strains of poliovirus that make up the vaccine.

Recommendations for vaccination of adults depend on the risk group. Vaccines for meningitis, pneumonia, and influenza are often given to groups living in close quarters (e.g., military recruits) or to individuals with reduced immunity (e.g., the elderly). Depending on their destination, international travelers are also routinely immunized against such endemic diseases as cholera, yellow fever, plague, typhoid, hepatitis, typhus, and polio. Immunization against the deadly disease anthrax had been reserved for workers coming into close contact with infected animals or products from them. Recently, however, suspected use of anthrax spores by terrorists or in biological warfare has widened use of the vaccine to military personnel and civilians in areas at risk of attack with this deadly agent.

Vaccination is not 100% effective. Instead, with any vaccine a small percentage of recipients will respond poorly and therefore will not be adequately protected. This is not a serious problem if the majority of the population is immune to an infectious agent. In this case, the chance of a susceptible individual contacting an infected individual is so low that the susceptible one is not likely to become infected. This phenomenon is known as herd immunity. The appearance of measles epidemics among college students and unvaccinated preschool-age children in the United States during the mid- to late-1980s resulted partly from an overall decrease in vaccinations, which had lowered the herd immunity of the population (Figure 18–2).

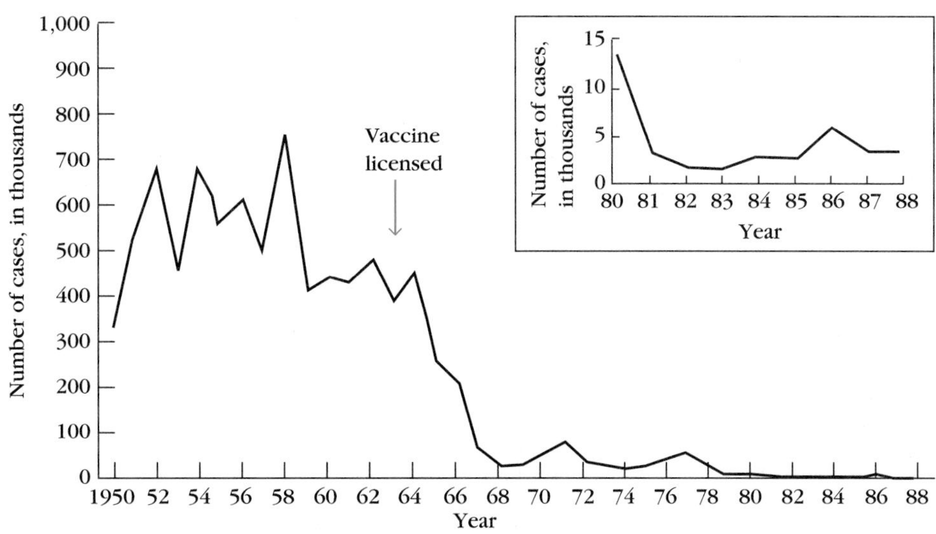

FIGURE 18-2 Introduction of the measles vaccine in 1962 led to a dramatic decrease in the annual incidence of this disease in the United States. Occasional outbreaks of measles in the 1980s (*inset*) occurred mainly among unvaccinated young children and among college students; most of the latter had been vaccinated, but only once, when they were young. [Data from Centers for Disease Control.]

Among preschool-age children, 88% of those who developed measles were unvaccinated. Most of the college students who contracted measles had been vaccinated as children, but only once; the failure of the single vaccination to protect them may have resulted from the presence of passively acquired maternal antibodies that reduced their overall response to the vaccine. This increase in the incidence of measles prompted the Immunization Practices Advisory Committee of the Centers for Disease Control to recommend that children receive two immunizations with the combined measles-mumps-rubella vaccine, one at 12–15 months of age and one at entry to kindergarten.

The CDC has called attention to the decline in vaccination rates and herd immunity among American children. For example, a 1995 publication reports that in California nearly one-third of all infants are unvaccinated and that about half of all children under the age of 2 are behind schedule on their vaccinations. Such a decrease in herd immunity portends serious consequences, as illustrated by recent events in the newly independent states of the former Soviet Union. By the mid-1990s, a diphtheria epidemic was raging in many regions of these new countries, linked to a decrease in herd immunity resulting from decreased vaccination rates after the breakup of the Soviet Union.

Designing Vaccines for Active Immunization

Several factors must be kept in mind in developing a successful vaccine. First and foremost, the development of an immune response does not necessarily mean that a state of protective immunity has been achieved. What is often critical is which branch of the immune system is activated, and therefore vaccine designers must recognize the important differences between activation of the humoral and the cell-mediated branches. A second factor is the development of immunologic memory. For example, a vaccine that induces a protective primary response may fail to induce the formation of memory cells, leaving the host unprotected after the primary response to the vaccine subsides.

The role of memory cells in immunity depends, in part, on the incubation period of the pathogen. In the case of influenza virus, which has a very short incubation period (1 or 2 days), disease symptoms are already under way by the time memory cells are activated. Effective protection against influenza therefore depends on maintaining high levels of neutralizing antibody by repeated reimmunizations. For pathogens with a longer incubation period, demonstrable neutralizing antibody at the time of infection is not necessary. The poliovirus, for example, requires more than 3 days to begin to infect the central nervous system. An incubation period of this length gives the memory B cells time to respond by producing high levels of serum antibody. Thus, the vaccine for polio is designed to induce high levels of immunologic memory. After immunization with the Salk vaccine, serum antibody levels peak within 2 weeks and then decline, but the memory response continues to climb, reaching maximal levels at 6 months and persisting for years (Figure 18-3). If an immunized individual is later exposed to the poliovirus, these memory cells will respond by differentiating into plasma cells that produce high levels of serum antibody, which protect the individual from infection.

Go to www.whfreeman.com/immunology Animation
Vaccine Strategies

TABLE 18-4 CLASSIFICATION OF COMMON VACCINES FOR HUMANS

Disease or pathogen	Type of vaccine
Whole organisms	
Bacterial cells	
Anthrax	Inactivated
Cholera	Inactivated
Pertussis*	Inactivated
Plague	Inactivated
Tuberculosis	Live attenuated BCG†
Typhoid	Live attenuated
Viral particles	
Hepatitis A	Inactivated
Influenza	Inactivated
Measles	Live attenuated
Mumps	Live attenuated
Polio (Sabin)	Live attenuated
Polio (Salk)	Inactivated
Rabies	Inactivated
Rubella	Live attenuated
Varicella zoster (chickenpox)	Live attenuated
Yellow fever	Live attenuated
Purified macromolecules	
Toxoids	
Diphtheria	Inactivated exotoxin
Tetanus	Inactivated exotoxin
Capsular polysaccharides	
Haemophilus influenzae type b	Polysaccharide + protein carrier
Neissera meningitidis	Polysaccharide
Streptococcus pneumoniae	23 distinct capsular polysaccharides
Surface antigen	
Hepatitis B	Recombinant surface antigen (HbsAg)

*There is an now also an acellular pertussis vaccine consisting of toxoids and inactivated bacteria components.

†Bacillus Calmette-Guerin (BCG) is an avirulent strain of *Mycobacterium bovis*.

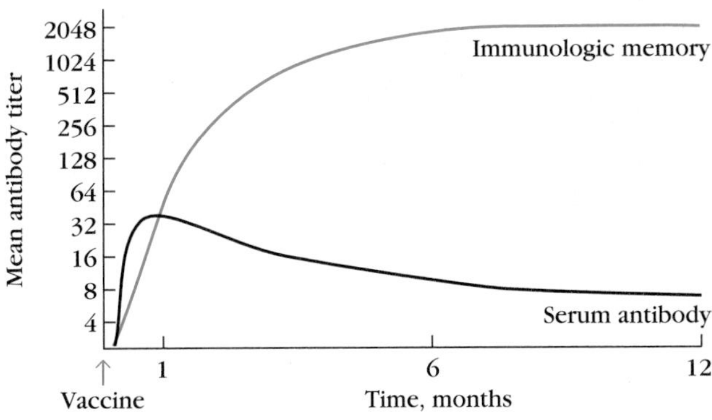

FIGURE 18-3 Immunization with a single dose of the Salk polio vaccine induces a rapid increase in serum antibody levels, which peak by 2 weeks and then decline. Induction of immunologic memory follows a slower time course, reaching maximal levels 6 months after vaccination. The persistence of the memory response for years after primary vaccination is responsible for immunity to poliomyelitis. [From M Zanetti et al, 1987, *Immunol. Today* **8:**18.]

In the remainder of this chapter, various approaches to the design of vaccines—both currently used vaccines and experimental ones—are described and examined in terms of their ability to induce humoral and cell-mediated immunity and the production of memory cells.

Whole-Organism Vaccines

As Table 18-4 indicates, many of the common vaccines currently in use consist of inactivated (killed) or live but attenuated (avirulent) bacterial cells or viral particles. The primary characteristics of these two types of vaccines are compared in Table 18-5.

Attenuated Viral or Bacterial Vaccines

In some cases, microorganisms can be attenuated so that they lose their ability to cause significant disease (pathogenicity) but retain their capacity for transient growth within an inoculated host. Attenuation often can be achieved by growing a pathogenic bacterium or virus for prolonged periods under abnormal culture conditions. This procedure selects mutants that are better suited to growth in the abnormal culture conditions and are therefore less capable of growth in the natural host. For example, an attenuated strain of *Mycobacterium bovis* called **Bacillus Calmette-Guerin (BCG)** was developed by growing *M. bovis* on a medium containing increasing concentrations of bile. After 13 years, this strain had adapted to growth with increased bile and had become sufficiently attenuated that it was suitable as a vaccine for tuberculosis. The Sabin polio vaccine and the rubella vaccine consist of viral strains that have been successfully attenuated and now serve as successful vaccines. The poliovirus used in the Sabin vaccine was attenuated by growth in monkey kidney epithelial cells. The rubella vaccine contains a strain of rubella virus that was grown in duck embryo cells and later in human cell lines.

Attenuated vaccines have some advantages and some disadvantages. Because of their capacity for transient growth, such vaccines provide prolonged immune-system exposure to the individual epitopes on the attenuated organisms, resulting in increased immunogenicity and production of memory cells. As a consequence, these vaccines often require only a single immunization, eliminating the need for repeated boosters. This property is a major advantage in Third World countries, where epidemiologic studies have shown that roughly 20% of individuals fail to return for each subsequent booster. The ability of many attenuated vaccines to replicate within host cells makes them particularly suitable for inducing a cell-mediated response.

TABLE 18-5 COMPARISON OF ATTENUATED (LIVE) AND INACTIVATED (KILLED) VACCINES

Characteristic	Attenuated vaccine	Inactivated vaccine
Production	Selection for avirulent organisms: virulent pathogen is grown under adverse culture conditions or prolonged passage of a virulent human pathogen through different hosts	Virulent pathogen is inactivated by chemicals or irradiation with γ-rays
Booster requirement	Generally requires only a single booster	Requires multiple boosters
Relative stability	Less stable	More stable (advantageous for Third World countries where refrigeration is limited)
Type of immunity induced	Produces humoral and cell-mediated immunity	Produces mainly humoral immunity
Reversion tendency	May revert to virulent form	Cannot revert to virulent form

The Sabin polio vaccine, consisting of three attenuated strains of poliovirus, is administered orally to children on a sugar cube or in sugar liquid. The attenuated viruses colonize the intestine and induce protective immunity to all three strains of virulent poliovirus. The ability of the attenuated Sabin vaccine to colonize the intestines enables it to induce production of secretory IgA, which serves as an important defense against naturally acquired poliovirus. The vaccine also induces IgM and IgG classes of antibody. Unlike most other attenuated vaccines, which require a single immunizing dose, the Sabin polio vaccine requires boosters, because the three strains of attenuated poliovirus in the vaccine interfere with each other's replication in the intestine. With the first immunization, one strain will predominate in its growth, inducing immunity to that strain. With the second immunization, the immunity generated by the previous immunization will limit the growth of the previously predominant strain in the vaccine, enabling one of the two remaining strains to predominate and induce immunity. Finally, with the third immunization, immunity to all three strains is achieved.

A major disadvantage of attenuated vaccines is the possibility of their reversion to a virulent form. The rate of reversion of the Sabin polio vaccine (OPV) leading to subsequent paralytic disease is about one case in four million doses of vaccine. This reversion implies that pathogenic forms of the virus are being passed by a few immunized individuals and can find their way into the water supply, especially in areas where sanitation standards are not rigorous or where waste water must be recycled. This possibility has led some to argue that the projected eradication of polio (Figure 18-4) will be impossible as long as OPV is used and that the alternative inactivated Salk vaccine should be substituted as the number of cases decreases.

Another concern with attenuated vaccines is the presence of other viruses as contaminants. In 1960 it was discovered that the oncogenic virus SV40 had contaminated some monkey kidney cultures used in the production of the Sabin vaccine. Although no adverse reactions caused by this contaminant have been recorded, more stringent vaccine testing was required to eliminate SV40 from the oral polio vaccine. Attenuated vaccines also may be associated with complications similar to those seen in the natural disease. A small percentage of recipients of the measles vaccine, for example, develop postvaccine encephalitis. Although these complications are undesirable, the risk of such complications is far less than that observed in a naturally acquired measles infection.

In some cases, however, postvaccine complications may render a potential vaccine unacceptable. This situation is illustrated by trials conducted several years ago with an experimental measles vaccine. This vaccine—an attenuated strain of the virus called the Edmonston-Zagreb strain—is immunogenic in infants as young as 4–6 months old. Maternal antibodies render the standard measles vaccine ineffective when it is given before 9 months of age. The new vaccine was developed for use in Third World countries, where many infants are infected with the measles virus at a very early age. Unfortunately, trials of the Edmonston-Zagreb vaccine in Guinea-Bissau, Senegal, and Haiti had to be halted when many vaccinated children began dying from common endemic disorders such as diarrhea, pneumonia, and parasitic diseases. Mortality rates were higher in girls than boys, an unexplained finding. The high rate of postvaccine complications with the Edmonston-Zagreb strain may result from vaccine-mediated immunosuppression, since the measles virus is known to cause

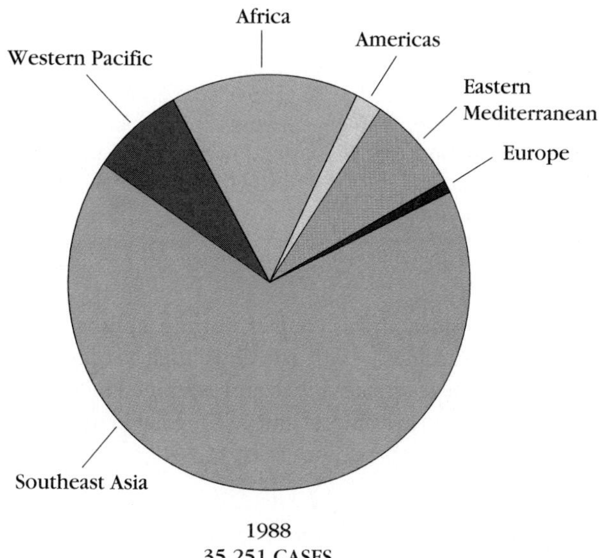

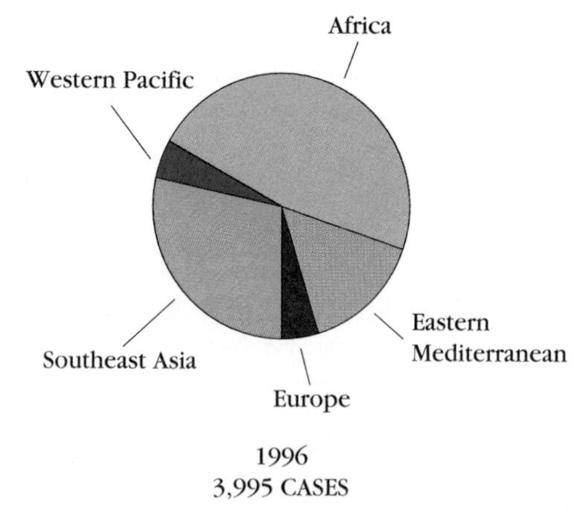

FIGURE 18-4 Progress toward the worldwide eradication of polio. Considerable progress has been made in most parts of the world. Some experts questions whether the use of live attentuated oral polio vaccine will cause reversion to pathogenic forms at a rate sufficiently high to prevent total eradication of this once prevalent crippling disease. [Adapted from *Polio: The Beginning of the End,* 1997, World Health Organization, Geneva; document available from the WHO Web site on vaccines and vaccination.]

transient immunosuppression. Some have speculated that the potent immunogenicity of the Edmonston-Zagreb strain, even in the presence of maternal antibodies, may be associated with potent immunosuppressive effects, placing vaccinated infants at risk for infection by other endemic pathogens that unvaccinated infants can resist.

Genetic engineering techniques provide a way to attenuate a virus irreversibly by selectively removing genes that are necessary for virulence. This has been done with a herpes virus vaccine for pigs, in which the thymidine kinase gene was removed. Because thymidine kinase is required for the virus to grow in certain types of cells (e.g., neurons), removal of this gene rendered the virus incapable of causing disease. It is possible that similar genetic engineering techniques could eliminate the risk of reversion of the attenuated polio vaccine. More recently, a vaccine against rotavirus, a major cause of infant diarrhea, was developed using genetic engineering techniques to modify an animal rotavirus to contain antigens present on the human viruses (see Clinical Focus).

Inactivated Viral or Bacterial Vaccines

Another common approach in vaccine production is to inactivate the pathogen by heat or by chemical means so that it is no longer capable of replication in the host. It is critically important to maintain the structure of epitopes on surface antigens during inactivation. Heat inactivation is generally unsatisfactory because it causes extensive denaturation of proteins; thus, any epitopes that depend on higher orders of protein structure are likely to be altered significantly. Chemical inactivation with formaldehyde or various alkylating agents has been successful. The Salk polio vaccine and the pertussis (whooping cough) vaccine are produced by formaldehyde inactivation.

Unlike immunization with attenuated vaccines, which generally requires only one dose to induce long-lasting immunity, repeated boosters of killed vaccines are often needed to maintain the immune status of the host. In addition, killed vaccines induce a predominantly humoral antibody response; they are less effective than attenuated vaccines in inducing cell-mediated immunity and in eliciting a secretory IgA response.

Even though they contain killed pathogens, inactivated whole-organism vaccines are still associated with certain risks. A serious complication with the first Salk vaccines arose when formaldehyde failed to kill all the virus in two vaccine lots, which caused paralytic polio in a high percentage of recipients. As mentioned above, the pertussis vaccine highlights another problem that can arise with a complex whole-organism vaccine. The encephalitis-type reactions that occurred in a small percentage of infants receiving this vaccine have led to development of a new acellular vaccine for pertussis.

Purified Macromolecules as Vaccines

Some of the risks associated with attenuated or killed whole-organism vaccines can be avoided with vaccines that consist of specific, purified macromolecules derived from pathogens. Three general forms of such vaccines are in current use: inactivated exotoxins, capsular polysaccharides, and recombinant surface antigens (see Table 18-4).

Polysaccharide Vaccines

The virulence of some pathogenic bacteria depends primarily on the antiphagocytic properties of their hydrophilic polysaccharide capsule. Coating of the capsule with antibodies and/or complement greatly increases the ability of macrophages and neutrophils to phagocytose such pathogens. These findings provide the rationale for vaccines consisting of purified capsular polysaccharides.

The current vaccine for *Streptococcus pneumoniae*, which causes pneumococcal pneumonia, consists of 23 antigenically different capsular polysaccharides. It is marketed as Pneumovax 23 by Merck and as Pnu-Immune 23 by Lederle Laboratories. The vaccine induces formation of opsonizing antibodies and is administered to high-risk groups such as infants, splenectomized patients, other immune-suppressed individuals, and the elderly. The vaccine for *Neisseria meningitidis*, a common cause of bacterial meningitis, also consists of purified capsular polysaccharides.

One limitation of polysaccharide vaccines is their inability to activate T_H cells. They activate B cells in a thymus-independent type 2 (TI-2) manner, resulting in IgM production but little class switching, no affinity maturation, and little, if any, development of memory cells. Several investigators have reported the induction of IgA-secreting plasma cells in humans receiving subcutaneous immunization with the pneumococcal polysaccharide vaccine. In this case, since T_H cells are not involved in the response, the vaccine may activate IgA-specific memory B cells previously generated by naturally occurring bacterial antigens at mucosal surfaces. Because these bacteria have both polysaccharide and protein epitopes, they would activate T_H cells, which in turn could mediate class switching and memory-cell formation.

One way to involve T_H cells directly in the response to a polysaccharide antigen is to conjugate the antigen to some sort of protein carrier. For example, the vaccine for *Haemophilus influenzae* type b (Hib), the major cause of bacterial meningitis in children under 5 years of age, consists of type b capsular polysaccharide covalently linked to a protein carrier, tetanus toxoid. The polysaccharide-protein conjugate is considerably more immunogenic than the polysaccharide alone, and because it activates T_H cells, it

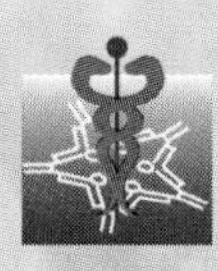

CLINICAL FOCUS

ENGINEERING A LIVE VIRUS VACCINE FOR INFANT DIARRHEA

A recent development in vaccine research combined use of an attenuated animal virus with techniques in modern immunology and molecular biology to construct a vaccine that has the potential to save millions of lives and prevent severe diarrheal disease throughout the world. In developing countries, infant diarrhea is a serious cause of mortality accounting for about 2 million deaths per year. Approximately half of these fatalities are caused by infection with rotavirus. This intestinal pathogen also causes severe diarrhea in infants in developed countries and, while mortality is rare, almost fifty thousand infants in the United States are hospitalized and another five hundred thousand visit a physician every year to combat the effects of rotavirus. It has been evident since the discovery of rotavirus in the 1970s and its linkage to infant diarrhea that a vaccine against this agent is necessary.

In a painstaking series of experiments that began by identifying the diarrhea-causing rotavirus particles in infant stool samples by electron microscopy, the major antigens that give rise to protective antibodies were characterized. These investigations revealed the major antigens to be the outer capsid proteins VP4 and VP7. Correlation between presence of antibodies to the VP7 antigen and resistance to diarrheal disease was shown in newborn nurseries where certain rotavirus-infected infants escaped disease. The presence of maternally-acquired antibodies to the rotavirus protein or of those acquired by natural infection did not prevent subsequent infection by rotavirus, but it was highly effective in preventing disease. Further investigation of immunity to rotavirus revealed several different serotypes, which reflect variation in the VP7 antigen. This variation mandates that any widely effective protection must include immunity to all the major serotypes, of which there are four. Because there are bovine and simian viruses similar in structure to human rotavirus, a "Jennerian" approach to vaccination could be considered; that is, live animal viruses might be tested as vaccines against human disease. Initial trials showed that the viruses from calves or rhesus monkeys were attenuated in infant humans and could be administered without causing disease or other side effects. The immunity shown in early trials of the bovine virus was not significantly protective for use as a vaccine, but the rhesus rotavirus was somewhat more effective. However, this monkey rotavirus was not highly protective—it prevented disease caused by virus of only one of the four prevalent serotypes; by itself, it could not provide universal protection.

The problem of conferring immunity to all of the major rotavirus serotypes was solved by Dr. Albert Kapikian and his coworkers at the National Institute for Allergy and Infectious Diseases, NIH, who gave a modern twist to the Jennerian approach. In a strategy that may be applicable to other diseases for which vaccine development has proven difficult, these investigators modified the monkey rotavirus, using genetic engineering techniques, to produce chimeric viruses that include genes for the VP7 antigens of the four major human serotypes. This product, which is called a quadrivalent (containing antigens of the four major serotypes) live rotavirus vaccine, was tested

enables class switching from IgM to IgG. Although this type of vaccine can induce memory B cells, it cannot induce memory T cells specific for the pathogen. In the case of the Hib vaccine, it appears that the memory B cells can be activated to some degree in the absence of a population of memory T_H cells, thus accounting for the efficacy of this vaccine.

Toxoid Vaccines

Some bacterial pathogens, including those that cause diphtheria and tetanus, produce exotoxins. These exotoxins produce many of the disease symptoms that result from infection. Diphtheria and tetanus vaccines, for example, can be made by purifying the bacterial exotoxin and then inactivating the toxin with formaldehyde to form a **toxoid.** Vaccination with the toxoid induces antitoxoid antibodies, which are also capable of binding to the toxin and neutralizing its effects. In production of toxoid vaccines the conditions must be closely controlled to achieve detoxification without excessive modification of the epitope structure.

One of the problems with vaccines consisting of purified macromolecules is the difficulty of obtaining sufficient quantities of the purified starting materials. In the case of the diphtheria and tetanus toxoid vaccines, this limitation has been overcome by cloning the exotoxin

in large-scale clinical trials in the United States, Finland, and Venezuela. The outcome of these trials was highly encouraging: this oral vaccine prevented diarrhea in the majority of vaccinated infants and no vaccinated infant had diarrhea sufficiently severe to require hospitalization. The efficacy of the vaccine and the absence of significant side effects led to approval by the Food and Drug Administration in December of 1997. The quadrivalent rhesus rotavirus vaccine was placed on the list of vaccinations recommended by the American Academy of Pediatrics and on the international list published by the World Health Organization. Widespread use of this vaccine began, and millions of vaccinated infants were followed closely to confirm that it prevents severe diarrhea and to look for side effects.*

*In 1999, data collected by the program for monitoring vaccine side effects in the United States suggested there was an increased incidence of intussusception (a condition where one segment of the intestine enfolds within another, causing an obstruction that may require surgery) in vaccinated infants during the first two weeks after immunization with rotavirus vaccine. Pending a more complete and statistically valid evaluation of the data, the U.S. Advisory Committee on Immunization Practices (ACIP) temporarily suspended its recommendation for administration of this vaccine in the United States. Although this decision may be appropriate for areas, such as the United States, where the death rate from rotavirus diarrhea is low, it is not accepted universally as the proper course of action (N Gay et al, 1999, *Lancet* **354:**956). Evaluation of the balance between a low increased risk of intussusception and the protective benefit of the vaccine may indicate that the vaccine should be used in areas where there is a high infant death rate from rotavirus diarrhea (see *J. Am. Med. Assoc.* **282:**2113, 1999).

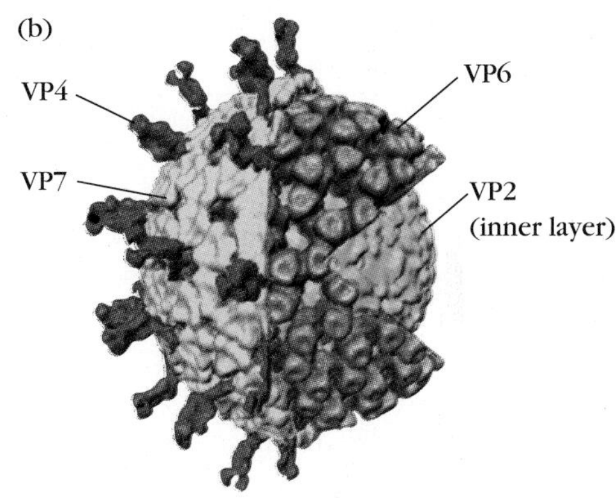

(a) Electron micrograph of rotavirus from filtrate of stool sample from a child with acute diarrhea. (b) Schematic of rotavirus showing surface proteins; VP7 is the protein to which protective immunity is raised. Mutant forms of human VP7 representing all four major serotypes of rotavirus are contained in the vaccine, which is based upon a rhesus monkey rotavirus that causes infection but no disease in infants. [Part (a) from A Kapikian et al, 1976, *New England Journal of Medicine* **294:**965–972, courtesy of AZ Kapikian, NIAID, NIH; part (b) courtesy BVV Prasad, Baylor College of Medicine.]

genes and then expressing them in easily grown host cells. In this way, large quantities of the exotoxin can be produced, purified, and subsequently inactivated.

Recombinant Antigen Vaccines

Theoretically, the gene encoding any immunogenic protein can be cloned and expressed in bacterial, yeast, or mammalian cells using recombinant DNA technology. A number of genes encoding surface antigens from viral, bacterial, and protozoan pathogens have been successfully cloned into bacterial, yeast, insect, or mammalian expression systems, and the expressed antigens used for vaccine development. The first such recombinant antigen vaccine approved for human use is the hepatitis B vaccine. This vaccine was developed by cloning the gene for the major surface antigen of hepatitis B virus (HBsAg) in yeast cells. The recombinant yeast cells are grown in large fermenters, and HBsAg accumulates intracellularly in the cells. The yeast cells are harvested and disrupted by high pressure, releasing the recombinant HBsAg, which is then purified by conventional biochemical techniques. This recombinant hepatitis B vaccine has been shown to induce the production of protective antibodies. This vaccine holds much promise for the 250 million carriers of chronic hepatitis B worldwide!

Recombinant-Vector Vaccines

It is possible to introduce genes that encode major antigens of especially virulent pathogens into attenuated viruses or bacteria. The attenuated organism serves as a vector, replicating within the host and expressing the gene product of the pathogen. A number of organisms have been used for vector vaccines, including vaccinia virus, the canarypox virus, attenuated poliovirus, adenoviruses, attenuated strains of *Salmonella*, and the BCG strain of *Mycobacterium bovis*.

Vaccinia virus, the attenuated vaccine used to eradicate smallpox, has been widely employed as a vector vaccine. This large, complex virus, with a genome of about 200 genes, can be engineered to carry several dozen foreign genes without impairing its capacity to infect host cells and replicate. The procedure for producing a vaccinia vector that carries a foreign gene from a pathogen is outlined in Figure 18-5. The genetically engineered vaccinia expresses high levels of the inserted gene product, which can then serve as a potent immunogen in an inoculated host. Like the smallpox vaccine, genetically engineered vaccinia vector vaccines can be administered simply by scratching the skin, causing a localized infection in host cells. If the foreign gene product expressed by the vaccinia is a viral envelope protein, it is inserted into the membrane of the infected host cell, inducing development of cell-mediated immunity as well as antibody-mediated immunity.

Other attenuated vector vaccines may prove to be safer than the vaccinia vaccine. The canarypox virus has recently been tried as a vector vaccine. Like its relative vaccinia, the canarypox virus is a large virus that can easily be engineered to carry multiple genes. Unlike vaccinia, the canarypox virus does not appear to be virulent even in individuals with severe immune suppression. Another possible vector is an attenuated strain of *Salmonella typhimurium*, which has been engineered with genes from the bacterium that causes cholera. The advantage of this vector vaccine is that *Salmonella* infects cells of the mucosal lining of the gut and therefore will induce secretory IgA production. Effective immunity against a number of diseases, including cholera and gonorrhea, depends on increased production of secretory IgA at mucous membrane surfaces. One of the poliovirus strains used in the Sabin vaccine is another candidate for a safe and effective vector vaccine. In this case, the poliovirus vector is engineered so that a portion of the gene that encodes the outer capsid protein of poliovirus is replaced by DNA that encodes the epitope of choice. The resulting poliovirus chimera will express the desired epitope in a highly accessible presentation that protrudes from the nucleocapsid.

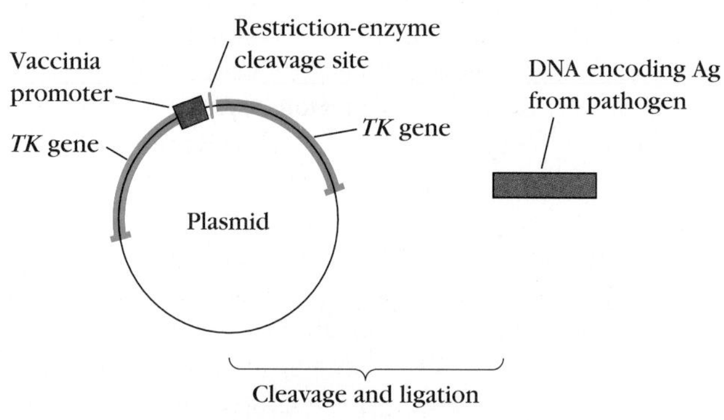

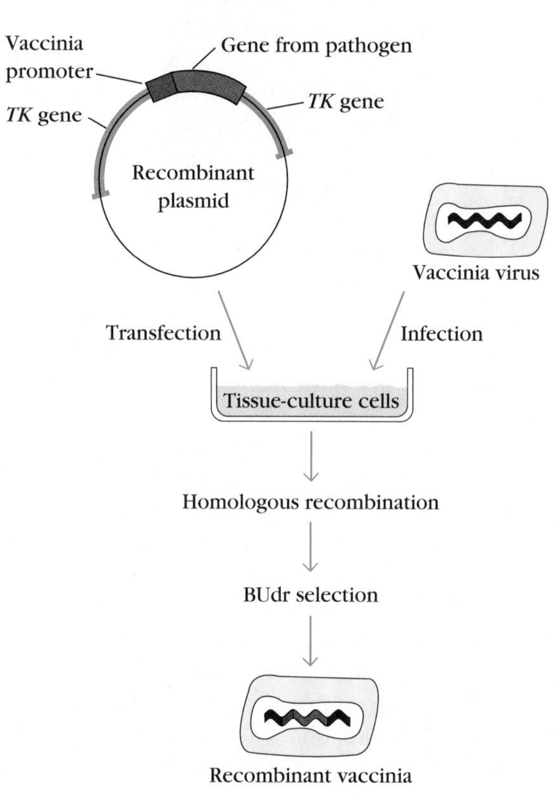

FIGURE 18-5 Production of vaccinia vector vaccine. The gene that encodes the desired antigen (orange) is inserted into a plasmid vector adjacent to a vaccinia promoter (magenta) and flanked on either side by the vaccinia thymidine kinase (*TK*) gene (green). When tissue-culture cells are incubated simultaneously with vaccinia virus and the recombinant plasmid, the antigen gene and promoter are inserted into the vaccinia virus genome by homologous recombination at the site of the nonessential *TK* gene, resulting in a TK^- recombinant virus. Cells containing the recombinant vaccinia virus are selected by addition of bromodeoxyuridine (BUdr), which kills TK^+ cells. [Adapted from B Moss, 1985, *Immunol. Today* **6**:243.]

DNA Vaccines

In a recently developed vaccination strategy, plasmid DNA encoding antigenic proteins is injected directly into the muscle of the recipient. The DNA is taken up by muscle cells and the encoded protein antigen is expressed, leading to both a humoral antibody response and a cell-mediated response. What is most surprising about this finding is that the injected DNA is taken up and expressed by the muscle cells with much greater efficiency than in tissue culture. The DNA appears either to integrate into the chromosomal DNA or to be maintained for long periods in an episomal form. The viral antigen is expressed not only by the muscle cells but also by dendritic cells in the area that take up the plasmid DNA and express the viral antigen. The fact that muscle cells express rather low levels of class I MHC molecules and do not express co-stimulatory molecules suggests that dendritic cells in the area may be crucial to the development of antigenic responses to DNA vaccines (Figure 18-6).

DNA vaccines offer advantages over many of the existing vaccines. The encoded protein is expressed in the host in its natural form—there is no denaturation or modification. The immune response will be directed to the antigen exactly as it is expressed by the pathogen. DNA vaccines induce both humoral and cell-mediated immunity. This stimulation of both arms of the immune response normally requires immunization with a live attenuated vaccine. DNA vaccines cause prolonged expression of the antigen, which generates significant immunological memory.

The practical aspects of DNA vaccines are also very promising. Refrigeration is not required for the handling and storage of the plasmid DNA, a feature that greatly lowers the cost and complexity of delivery. The same plasmid vector can be custom tailored to make a variety of proteins, so that the same manufacturing techniques can be used for different DNA vaccines, each encoding an antigen from a different pathogen. An improved method for administering these vaccines is to coat microscopic gold beads with the plasmid DNA and then deliver the coated particles through the skin into the underlying muscle with an air gun (called a *gene gun*). This will allow rapid delivery of a vaccine to large populations without the requirement for massive quantities of needles and syringes.

Tests of DNA vaccines in animal models have shown that these vaccines are able to induce protective immunity against a number of pathogens, including the influenza virus. At present, there are human trials underway with several different DNA vaccines, including those for malaria, AIDS, influenza, and herpesvirus. Future experimental trials of DNA vaccines will mix genes for antigenic proteins with those for cytokines or chemokines that direct the immune response to the optimum pathway. For example, the IL-12 gene may be included in a DNA vaccine. The expression of IL-12 at the site of immunization will stimulate TH_1 type immunity induced by the vaccine.

Results to date with DNA vaccines are very promising, and they will likely be used for human immunization within the next few years. Some drawbacks might preclude their universal application; for example, only protein antigens can be encoded—certain vaccines, such as those for pneumococcal and meningococcal infections, use protective polysaccharide antigens. Another shortcoming is the present inability to use DNA immunization with vaccines, such as the oral vaccines or those given as a nasal spray, that are applied to mucosal surfaces.

Synthetic Peptide Vaccines

Although considered very promising, the use of synthetic peptides as vaccines has not progressed as quickly as originally projected. Peptides are not as immunogenic as proteins, and it is difficult to elicit both humoral and cellular immunity to them. The use of conjugates and adjuvants can assist in raising protective immunity to peptides, but barriers to the widespread use of peptide vaccines remain and pose an interesting problem for immunologists. Construction of synthetic peptides for use as vaccines to induce either humoral or cell-mediated immunity requires an understanding of the nature of T-cell and B-cell epitopes.

Although the amino acid sequence of many important antigens from pathogens is known, few have been subjected to x-ray crystallographic analysis, so their three-dimensional structure is unknown. However, because B-cell epitopes must constitute accessible surface regions, vaccine designers commonly analyze the primary structure of an antigen to identify strongly hydrophilic sequences, which most likely correspond to such surface regions. Synthetic peptides corresponding to these potential B-cell epitopes are then prepared. Ideally, vaccines for inducing humoral immunity should include peptides that compose immunodominant B-cell epitopes. Such epitopes can be identified by determining the dominant antibody in the sera of individuals who are recovering from a disease and then testing various synthetic peptides for their ability to react with that antibody with a high affinity. In one such experiment, two linear synthetic peptides representing potential B-cell epitopes of HBsAg were tested for their binding affinity to pooled antisera from individuals who had recovered from hepatitis B. It was found that a synthetic peptide consisting of cyclical repeats of amino acids 139–147 had a tenfold higher affinity than cyclical repeats of amino acids 124–137. The cyclical peptide 139–147 was therefore chosen as a potential candidate for a synthetic hepatitis B vaccine.

An effective memory response for both humoral and cell-mediated immunity requires generation of a population of memory T_H cells. A successful vaccine must therefore include immunodominant T-cell epitopes. Since MHC molecules differ in their ability to present peptides to T cells, MHC polymorphism within a species influences the level of T-cell response by different individuals to different peptides. Moreover, different subpopulations of T cells probably recognize different epitopes. Experiments by E. Sercarz have identified some peptides that induce a strong helper response to an antigen and other peptides that induce immunologic suppression. These helper and suppressor peptides generally represent different, nonoverlapping amino acid sequences within an antigen. For example, immunization with the amino-terminal residues 1–17 of hen egg-white lysozyme suppressed the response to native lysozyme. By identifying suppressor peptides and eliminating them from synthetic vaccines, it might be possible to generate enhanced immunity.

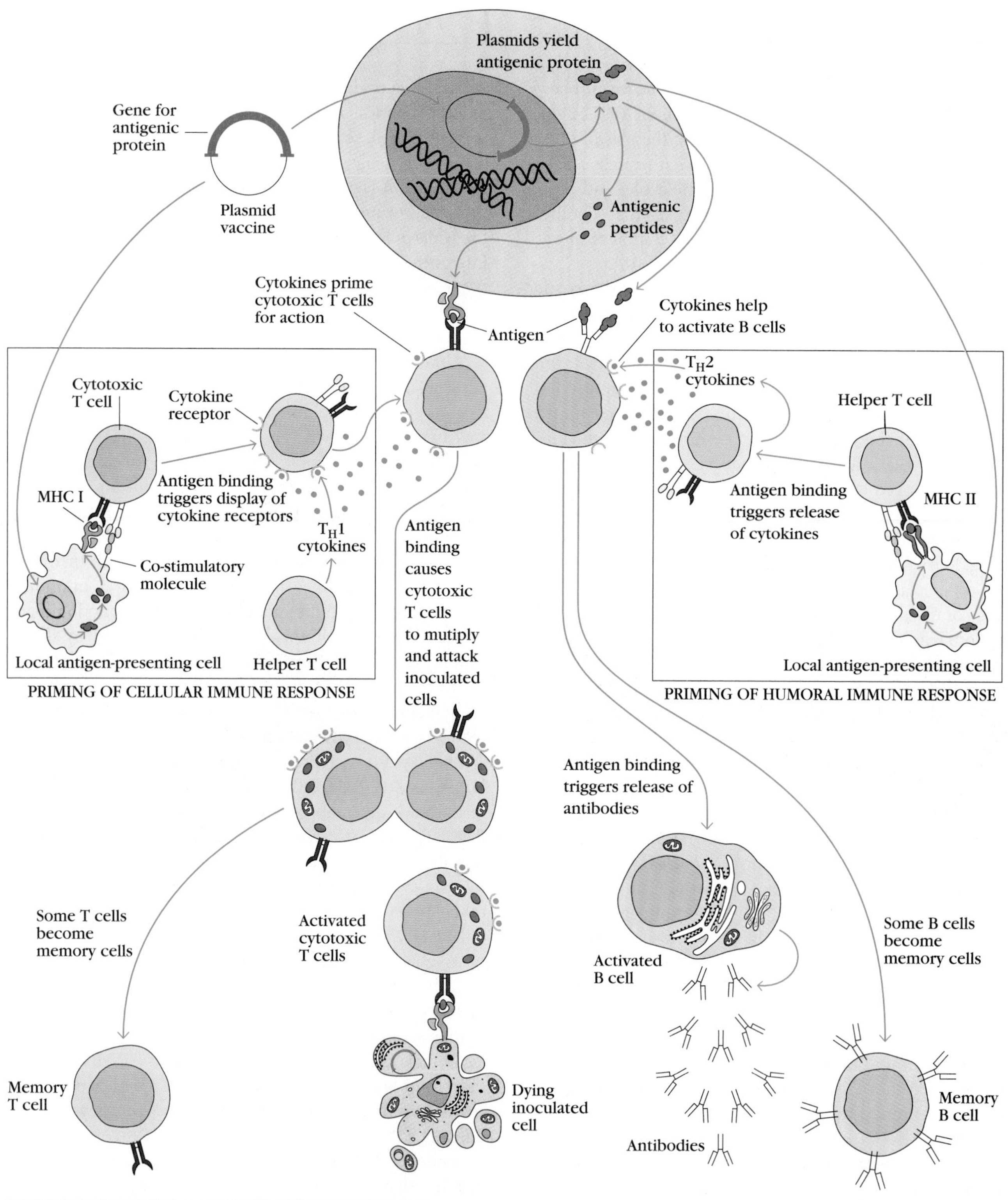

FIGURE 18-6 Use of DNA vaccines raises both humoral and cellular immunity. The injected gene is expressed in the injected muscle cell and in nearby APCs. The peptides from the protein encoded by the DNA are expressed on the surface of both cell types after processing as an endogenous antigen by the MHC class I pathway. Cells that present the antigen in the context of class I MHC molecules stimulate development of cytotoxic T cells. The protein encoded by the injected DNA is also expressed as a soluble, secreted protein, which is taken up, processed, and presented in the context of class II MHC molecules. This pathway stimulates B-cell immunity and generates antibodies and B-cell memory against the protein. [Adapted from DB Weiner and RC Kennedy, 1999, *Sci. Am.* **281:**50.]

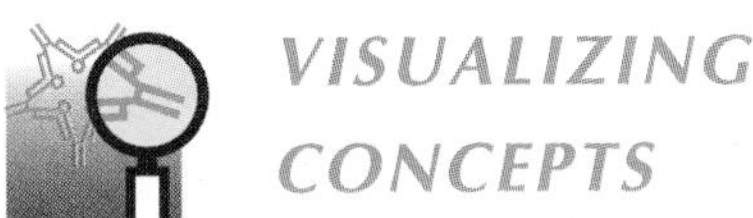

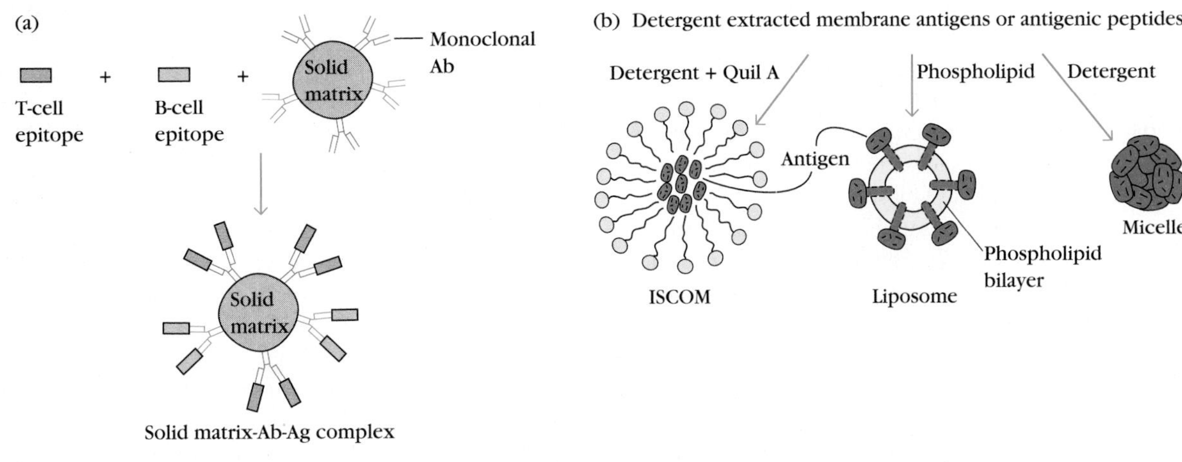

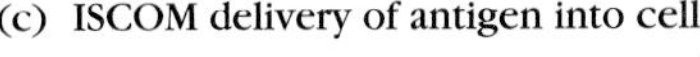

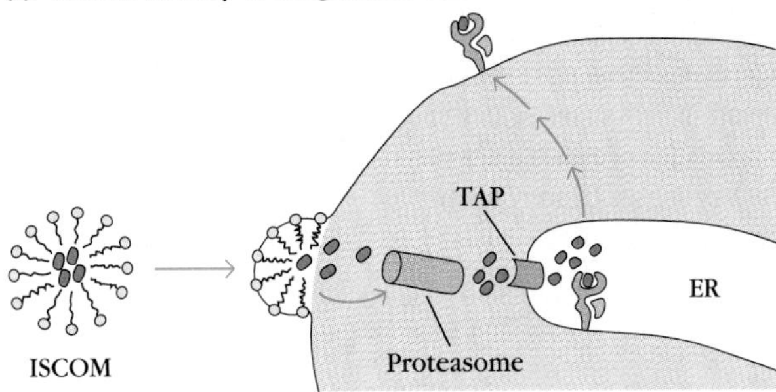

FIGURE 18-7 Multivalent subunit vaccines. (a) Solid matrix-antibody-antigen complexes can be designed to contain synthetic peptides representing both T-cell epitopes and B-cell epitopes. (b) Protein micelles, liposomes, and immunostimulating complexes (ISCOMs) can all be prepared with extracted antigens or antigenic peptides. In micelles and liposomes, the hydrophilic residues of the antigen molecules are oriented outward. In ISCOMs, the long fatty-acid tails of the external detergent layer are adjacent to the hydrophobic residues of the centrally located antigen molecules. (c) ISCOMs and liposomes can deliver antigens inside cells, so they mimic endogenous antigens. Subsequent processing by the cytosolic pathway and presentation with class I MHC molecules induces a cell-mediated response.

Multivalent Subunit Vaccines

One of the limitations of synthetic peptide vaccines and recombinant protein vaccines is that these vaccines tend to be poorly immunogenic; in addition, they tend to induce a humoral antibody response but are less likely to induce a cell-mediated response. What is needed is some method of constructing a synthetic peptide vaccine that contains both immunodominant B-cell and T-cell epitopes. Furthermore, if a CTL response is desired, the vaccine must be delivered intracellularly so that the peptides can be processed and presented together with class I MHC molecules. A number of innovative techniques are being applied to develop multivalent vaccines that can present multiple copies of a given peptide or a mixture of peptides to the immune system.

One approach is to prepare solid matrix–antibody-antigen (SMAA) complexes by attaching monoclonal antibodies to particulate solid matrices and then saturating the antibody with the desired antigen. The resulting complexes are then used as vaccines. By attaching different monoclonal antibodies to the solid matrix, it is possible to bind a mixture of peptides or proteins, composing immunodominant epitopes for both T cells and B cells, to the solid matrix (Figure 18-7a). These multivalent complexes have been shown to induce vigorous humoral and cell-mediated responses. Their particulate nature contributes to their increased immunogenicity by facilitating phagocytosis by phagocytic cells.

Another means of producing a multivalent vaccine is to use detergent to incorporate protein antigens or synthetic antigenic peptides into protein micelles, into lipid vesicles (called liposomes), or into immunostimulating complexes (Figure 18-7b). Micelles are formed by mixing proteins in detergent and then removing the detergent. The individual proteins orient themselves with their hydrophilic residues toward the aqueous environment and the hydrophobic residues at the center so as to exclude their interaction with the aqueous environment. Liposomes containing protein antigens are prepared by mixing the proteins with a suspension of phospholipids under conditions that form vesicles bounded by a bilayer. The proteins are incorporated into the bilayer with the hydrophilic residues exposed. Immunostimulating complexes (ISCOMs) are lipid carriers prepared by mixing protein or peptide antigens with detergent and a glycoside called Quil A.

Membrane proteins from various pathogens, including influenza virus, measles virus, hepatitis B virus, and HIV have been incorporated into micelles, liposomes, and ISCOMs and are currently being assessed as potential vaccines. In addition to their increased immunogenicity, liposomes and ISCOMs appear to fuse with the plasma membrane to deliver the antigen intracellularly, where it can be processed by the cytosolic pathway and thus induce a cell-mediated response (Figure 18-7c).

Summary

1. A state of immunity can be induced by passive or active immunization (see Table 18-1). Passive immunization involves transfer of preformed antibodies and provides short-term protection without the requirement for an active immune response. Active immunization is induced by natural infection or by inoculation with microbial agents or components derived from them. Active immunization induces clonal selection of lymphocytes and results in the formation of memory cells.
2. In developing a vaccine, the branch of the immune system to be activated must be considered. To induce humoral immunity, epitopes must be accessible to B-cell immunoglobulin receptors and should represent immunodominant epitopes of the infectious agent. To induce cell-mediated immunity, a vaccine capable of transient intracellular growth is desirable to extend the presentation of antigens with class I MHC molecules.
3. Three types of vaccines are currently used in humans: attenuated (avirulent) microorganisms, inactivated (killed) microorganisms, or purified macromolecules (see Table 18-4). Attenuated vaccines undergo transient growth in the recipient and therefore stimulate a more pronounced immune response and memory-cell production without the requirement for additional boosters. They do, however, pose the risk of reversion to a pathogenic state. Inactivated vaccines require repeated boosters, but pose no risk of reversion to a pathogenic state. The use of purified macromolecules, which are less complex than whole-organism vaccines, avoids certain complications due to unknown side effects. By applying recombinant DNA techniques, it is possible to produce large quantities of a defined antigen for immunization.
4. Recombinant vectors, including vaccinia virus, canarypox virus, and attenuated *S. typhimurium*, can be engineered to carry multiple genes from infectious microorganisms (see Figure 18-5). An advantage of recombinant-vector vaccines is that the engineered vector replicates in host cells, which serves to maximize cell-mediated immunity to the expressed antigens.
5. Plasmid DNA encoding a protein antigen from a pathogen has been shown to serve as an effective vaccine (see Figure 18-6). DNA vaccines induce expression of the antigen in its native state and induce both humoral and cell-mediated immunity.
6. Synthetic peptides that represent immunodominant T- or B-cell epitopes are being evaluated as vaccines for several diseases. This approach enables immunologists to produce defined vaccines that may permit selective activation of either the humoral or the cell-mediated branch of the immune system. Various types of multivalent vaccines have been devised to induce both humoral and cell-mediated immunity (see Figure 18-7).

REFERENCES

Bloom, BR. 1998. The highest attainable standard: ethical issues in AIDS vaccines. *Science* **279:**186.

Chattergoon, M, J Boyer, and DB Weiner. 1997. Genetic immunization: a new era in vaccines and immune therapeutics. *FASEB J.* **11:**754.

DiTommaso, A, et al. 1997. Acellular pertussis vaccines containing genetically detoxified pertussis toxin induce long lasting humoral and cellular responses in adults. *Vaccine* **15:**1218.

Donnelly, JJ, et al. 1995. Preclinical efficacy of a prototype DNA vaccine: enhanced protection against antigenic drift in influenza virus. *Nature Med.* **1:**583.

Dove AR, and VR Racaniello. 1997. The polio eradication effort: should vaccine eradication be next? *Science* **277:**779.

Etlinger, HM. 1992. Carrier sequence selection—one key to successful vaccines. *Immunol. Today* **13:**52.

Evans, DJ, et al. 1989. An engineered poliovirus chimera elicits broadly reactive HIV-1 neutralizing antibodies. *Nature* **339:**385.

Henderson, DA. 1976. The eradication of smallpox. *Sci. Am.* **235:**25

Kapikian, AZ, et al. 1997. Efficacy of a quadrivalent rhesus rotavirus-based human rotavirus vaccine aimed at preventing severe rotavirus diarrhea in infants and young children. *J. Inf. Dis.* **174** (Suppl 1): S65.

Milch, DR. 1989. Synthetic T and B cell recognition sites: implications for vaccine development. *Adv. Immunol.* **45:**195.

Stepanov, AV, et al. 1996. Development of novel vaccines against anthrax in man. *J. Biotechnology* **44:**155.

Steward, MW, and CR Howard. 1987. Synthetic peptides: a next generation of vaccines? *Immunol. Today* **8:**51.

Stover, CK, et al. 1991. New use of BCG for recombinant vaccines. *Nature* **351:**456.

Suhrbier, A. 1997. Multi-epitope DNA vaccines. *Immunol. and Cell Biol.* **75:**402.

Takahashi, H, et al. 1990. Induction of $CD8^+$ cytotoxic T cells by immunization with purified HIV-1 envelope protein in Iscoms. *Nature* **344:**873.

Tastemain, C. 1995. Diphtheria disaster relief. *Nature Med.* **1:**503.

Van den Dobbelsteen, GP, and EP van Rees. 1995. Mucosal immune responses to pneumococcal polysaccharides: implications for vaccination. *Trends Microbiol.* **3:**155.

Weiner, DB, and RC Kennedy. 1999. Genetic Vaccines. *Sci. Am.* **281:**50.

Weiss, R. 1992. Measles battle loses potent weapon. *Science* **258:**546.

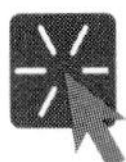

Useful Web Sites

http://www.who.int/gpv/
World Health Organization (WHO) pages on vaccines and immunization.

http://www.ecbt.org/
Every Child by Two offers information on childhood vaccination.

STUDY QUESTIONS

1. Indicate whether each of the following statements is true or false. If you think a statement is false, explain why.

a. Transplacental transfer of maternal IgG antibodies against measles confers short-term immunity on the fetus.

b. Attenuated vaccines are more likely to induce cell-mediated immunity than killed vaccines are.

c. Multivalent subunit vaccines generally induce a greater response than synthetic peptide vaccines.

d. One disadvantage of DNA vaccines is that they don't generate significant immunologic memory.

e. Macromolecules generally contain a large number of potential epitopes.

f. A DNA vaccine only induces a response to a single epitope.

2. What are the advantages and disadvantages of using attenuated organisms as vaccines?

3. A young girl who had never been immunized to tetanus stepped on a rusty nail and got a deep puncture wound. The doctor cleaned out the wound and gave the child an injection of tetanus antitoxin.

a. Why was antitoxin given instead of a booster shot of tetanus toxoid?

b. If the girl receives no further treatment and steps on a rusty nail again 3 years later, will she be immune to tetanus?

4. What are the advantages of the Sabin polio vaccine compared with the Salk vaccine?

5. In an attempt to develop a synthetic peptide vaccine, you have analyzed the amino acid sequence of a protein antigen for (a) hydrophobic peptides and (b) strongly hydrophilic peptides. How might peptides of each type be used as a vaccine to induce different immune responses?

6. Explain the phenomenon of herd immunity. How does this phenomenon relate to the appearance of certain epidemics?

7. You have identified a bacterial protein antigen that confers protective immunity to a pathogenic bacterium and have cloned the gene that encodes it. The choices are either to express the protein in yeast and use this recombinant protein as a vaccine, or to use the gene for the protein to prepare a DNA vaccine. Which approach would you take and why?

8. Explain the relationship between the incubation period of a pathogen and the approach needed to achieve effective active immunization.

9. List the three types of purified macromolecules that are currently used as vaccines.

10. The Salk polio vaccine has been recommended for use by HIV-infected children instead of the Sabin polio vaccine. Why do you think this recommendation was made?

Go to www.whfreeman.com/immunology Self-Test
Review and quiz of key terms

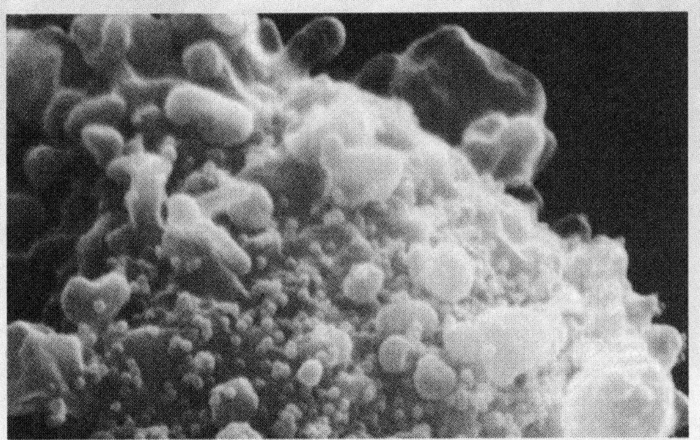

CHAPTER 19

AIDS AND OTHER IMMUNODEFICIENCIES

Primary Immunodeficiencies

AIDS and Other Acquired or Secondary Immunodeficiencies

Like any complex multi-component system, the immune system is subject to failure of some or all of its parts. This failure can have dire consequences. When the system loses its sense of self and begins to attack host cells and tissues, the result is **autoimmunity,** which is described in Chapter 20. When the system errs by failing to protect the host from disease-causing agents or from malignant cells, the result is **immunodeficiency,** which is the subject of this chapter.

A condition resulting from a genetic or developmental defect in the immune system is called a primary immunodeficiency. In such a condition, the defect is present at birth although it may not manifest itself until later in life. Secondary immunodeficiency, or acquired immunodeficiency, is the loss of immune function and results from exposure to various agents. By far the most common secondary immunodeficiency is **acquired immunodeficiency syndrome**, or **AIDS**, which results from infection with the human immunodeficiency virus 1 (HIV-1). HIV infection has reached epidemic proportions in certain populations and almost inevitably results in death. AIDS patients, like other individuals with severe immunodeficiency, are at risk of infection with so-called opportunistic agents. These are microorganisms that healthy individuals can harbor with no ill consequences but that cause disease in those with impaired immune function.

The study of immunodeficiency disorders has provided a wealth of information about the immune system by opening windows into its functional components. Recent progress in molecular immunology and in genetic analysis of immune defects has increasingly deepened our understanding of immunodeficiency and consequently of the normal workings of the immune system. The ability to dissect a given dysfunction and pinpoint its cellular and molecular origin enriches our knowledge of the immune system, and this can lead to marked improvement in the treatment of immunodeficiency and other disorders.

The first part of this chapter describes the common primary immunodeficiencies, examines progress in identifying the genetic defects that underlie these disorders, and considers approaches to their treatment, including innovative uses of gene therapy. Animal models of primary immunodeficiency are also described. The rest of this chapter describes acquired immunodeficiency, with a strong focus on HIV infection, AIDS, and the current status of therapeutic and prevention strategies for combatting this fatal acquired immunodeficiency.

Primary Immunodeficiencies

A primary immunodeficiency may affect either adaptive or innate immune functions. Deficiencies of the specific components of adaptive immunity, such as T or B cells, are thus differentiated from immunodeficiencies in which the nonspecific mediators of innate immunity, such as macrophage or complement, are impaired. Immunodeficiencies are conveniently categorized by the type or the developmental stage of the cells involved. Figure 19-1 reviews the overall cellular development in the immune system, showing the locations of defects that give rise to primary immunodeficiencies. As Chapter 2 explained, the two main cell lineages important to immune function are lymphoid and myeloid. Most defects that lead to immunodeficiencies affect either one or the other. The lymphoid cell disorders may affect T cells, B cells, or, in combined immunodeficiencies, both B and T cells. The myeloid cell disorders affect phagocytic function. Most of the primary immunodeficiencies are inherited, and the precise molecular variations and the

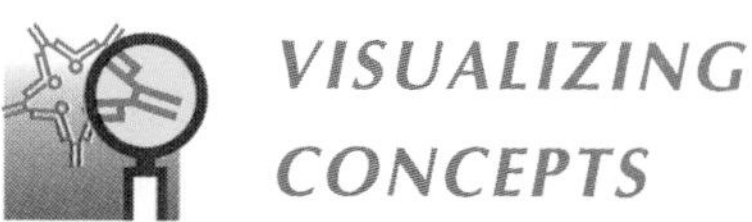

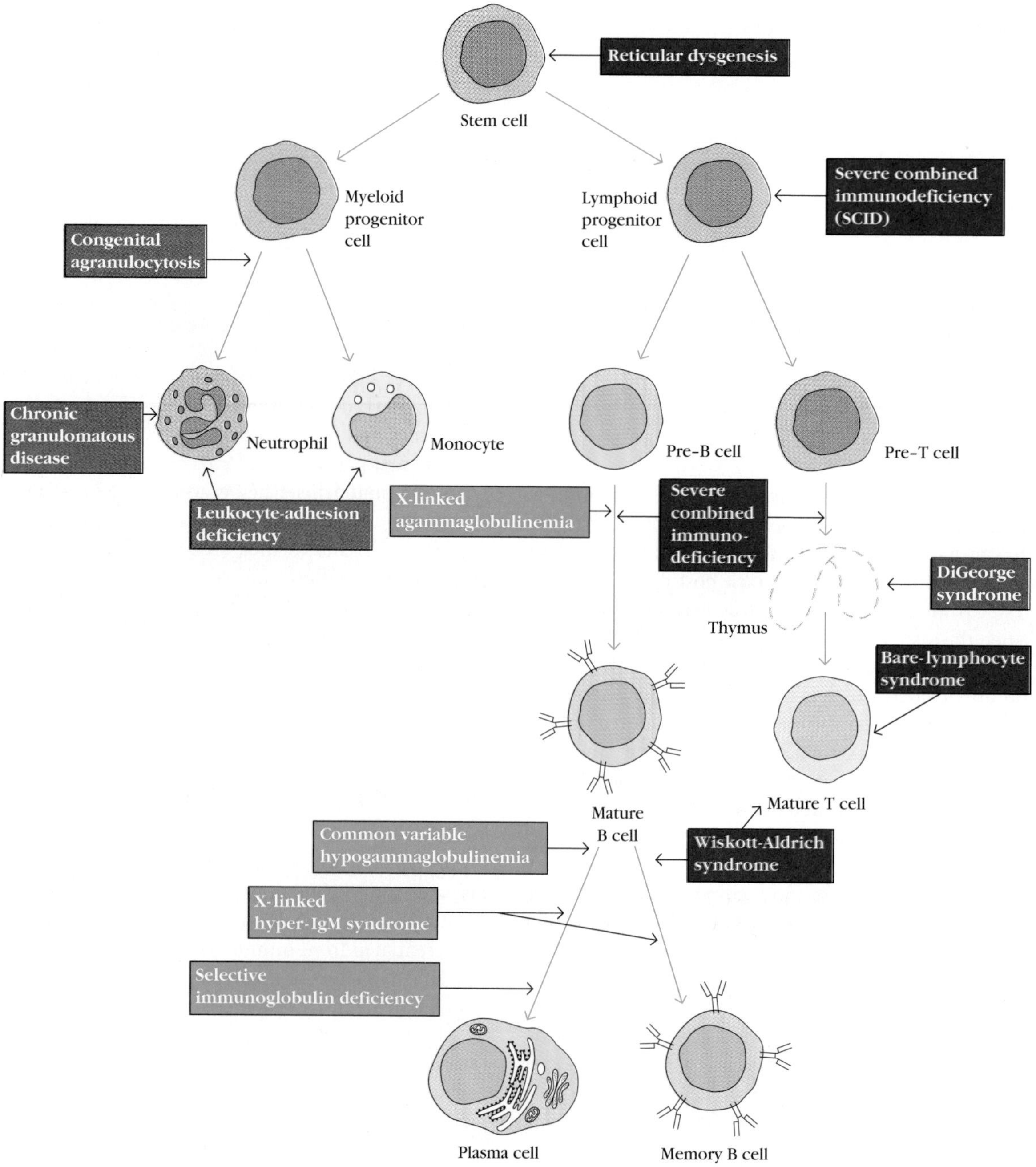

FIGURE 19-1 Congenital defects that interrupt hematopoiesis or impair functioning of immune-system cells result in various immunodeficiency diseases. (Orange boxes = phagocytic deficiencies, green = humoral deficiencies, red = cell-mediated deficiencies, and purple = combined immunodeficiencies, defects that affect more than one cell lineage.)

genetic defects that lead to many of these dysfunctions have been determined (Table 19-1 and Figure 19-2). In addition, there are immunodeficiencies that stem from developmental defects that impair proper function of an organ of the immune system.

The consequences of primary immunodeficiency depend on the number and type of immune system components involved. Defects in components early in the hematopoietic developmental scheme affect the entire immune system. In this category is reticular dysgenesis, a stem-cell defect that affects the maturation of all leukocytes; the resulting general failure of immunity leads to susceptibility to infection by a variety of microorganisms. Without aggressive treatment, the affected individual usually dies young from severe infection. In the more restricted case of defective phagocytic function, the major consequence is

TABLE 19-1 SOME PRIMARY HUMAN IMMUNODEFICIENCY DISEASES AND UNDERLYING GENETIC DEFECTS

Immunodeficiency disease	Specific defect	Impaired function	Inheritance mode*	Chromosomal defect
Severe combined immunodeficiency (SCID)	RAG-1/RAG-2 deficiency	No TCR or Ig gene rearrangement	AR	11p13
	ADA deficiency	Toxic metabolite in T and B cells	AR	20q13
	PNP deficiency		AR	14q13
	JAK-3 deficiency	Defective signals from IL-2, 4, 7, 9, 15	AR	19p13
	IL-2Rγ-deficiency		XL	Xq13
	ZAP-70 deficiency	Defective signal from TCR	AR	2q12
Bare lymphocyte syndrome	Defect in MHC class II gene promoter	No class II MHC molecules	AR	16p13
Wiskott-Aldrich syndrome (WAS)	Cytoskeletal protein (CD43)	Defective T cells and platelets	XL	Xp11
Interferon gamma receptor	IFN-γ–receptor defect	Impaired immunity to mycobacteria	AR	6q23
DiGeorge syndrome	Thymic aplasia	T- and B-cell development	AD	22q11
Ataxia telangiectasia	Defective cell-cycle kinase	Low IgA, IgE	AR	11q22
Gammaglobulinemias	X-linked agammaglobulinemia	Bruton's tyrosine kinase (Btk); no mature B cells	XL	Xq21
	X-linked hyper-IgM syndrome	Defective CD40 ligand	XL	Xq26
	Common variable immunodeficiency	Low IgG, IgA; variable IgM	Complex	
	Selective IgA deficiency	Low or no IgA	Complex	
Chronic granulomatous disease	Cyt p91^{phox}	No oxidative burst for bacterial killing	XL	Xp21
	Cyt p67^{phox}		AR	1q25
	Cyt p22^{phox}		AR	16q24
Chediak-Higashi syndrome	Defective intracellular transport protein (LYST)	Inability to lyse bacteria	AR	1q42
Leukocyte-adhesion defect	Defective integrin β2 (CD18)	Leukocyte extravasation	AR	21q22

*AR = autosomal recessive; AD = autosomal dominant; XL = X linked; "Complex" indicates conditions for which precise genetic data are not available and that may involve several interacting loci.

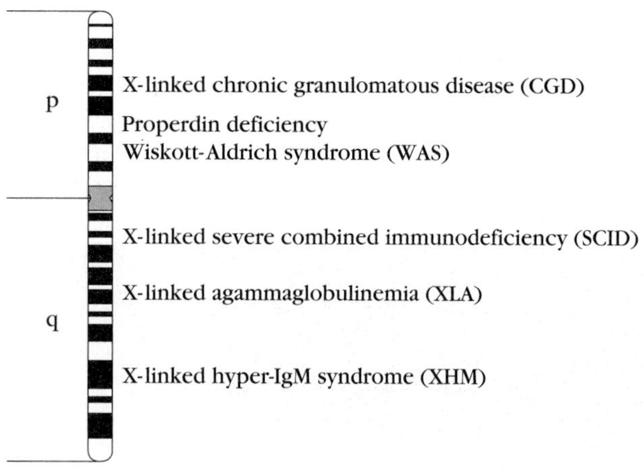

FIGURE 19-2 Several X-linked immunodeficiency diseases result from defects in loci on the X chromosome. [Based on JW Belmont, 1995, *Trends Genet.* **11**:112.]

susceptibility to bacterial infection. Defects in more highly differentiated compartments of the immune system have consequences that are more specific and usually less severe. For example, an individual with selective IgA deficiency may enjoy a normal life span, troubled only by a greater than normal susceptibility to infections of the respiratory and genitourinary tracts.

Defects in the Lymphoid Lineage

Lymphoid immunodeficiencies may involve B cells, T cells, or both of these lineages. The combined forms of lymphoid immunodeficiency, which affect both lineages, are generally lethal within the first few years of life; these arise from defects early in developmental pathways. These are less common than certain less severe conditions that result from defects in more highly differentiated cells. For example, X-linked agammaglobulinemia, which affects B cell signal transduction, occurs at a rate of 1 in 200,000 persons. Selective IgA deficiency, which affects only the synthesis of IgA, occurs at a rate of 1 in 700.

B-cell immunodeficiency disorders make up a diverse spectrum of diseases that ranges from the complete absence of mature recirculating B cells, plasma cells, and immunoglobulin to the selective absence of only certain classes of immunoglobulins. Patients with these disorders usually are subject to recurrent bacterial infections but display normal immunity to most viral and fungal infections, because the T-cell branch of the immune system is largely unaffected. Most common in patients with humoral immunodeficiencies are infections by such encapsulated bacteria as staphylococci, streptococci, and pneumococci, because antibody is critical for the opsonization and clearance of these organisms.

Because of the central role of T cells in the immune system, a T-cell deficiency can affect both the humoral and the cell-mediated responses. The impact on the cell-mediated system can be severe, with a reduction in both delayed-type hypersensitive responses and cell-mediated cytotoxicity. Whereas defects in the humoral system are associated primarily with infections by encapsulated bacteria, defects in the cell-mediated system are associated with increased susceptibility to viral, protozoan, and fungal infections. Intracellular pathogens such as *Candida albicans*, *Pneumocystis carinii*, and *Mycobacteria* are often implicated, reflecting the importance of T cells in eliminating intracellular pathogens. Infections with viruses that are rarely pathogenic for the normal individual (such as cytomegalovirus or even an attenuated measles vaccine) may be life threatening for those with impaired cell-mediated immunity. Defects that cause decreased T-cell counts generally also affect the humoral system, because of the requirement for T_H cells in B-cell activation. Generally there is some decrease in antibody levels, particularly in the production of specific antibody after immunization.

As one might expect, combined deficiencies of the humoral and cell-mediated branches are the most serious of the immunodeficiency disorders. The onset of infections begins early in infancy, and the prognosis for these infants is early death unless therapeutic intervention reconstitutes their defective immune system. As described below, there are increasing numbers of options for the treatment of immunodeficiencies.

The immunodeficiencies that affect lymphoid function have in common the inability to mount or sustain a complete immune response against specific agents. A variety of failures can lead to such immunodeficiency. Defective intercellular communication may be rooted in deleterious mutations of genes that encode cell surface receptors or signal-transduction molecules; defects in the mechanisms of gene rearrangement and other functions may prevent normal B- or T-cell responses. Figure 19-3 is an overview of the molecules involved in the more well-described interactions among T cells and B cells that give rise to specific responses, with a focus on proteins in which defects leading to immunodeficiency have been identified.

Severe Combined Immunodeficiency (SCID)

The family of disorders termed SCID stems from defects in lymphoid development that affect either T cells or both T and B cells. Several forms of human SCID arise from different genetic defects (see Table 19-1). The first described form of human SCID was an autosomal recessive disorder. That is, the gene responsible is not encoded on the X or Y chromosome and only homozygotes are affected. This was revealed from the inheritance pattern and the fact that males and females are equally affected. There is also an X-linked form (therefore occurring predominantly in males), also called primary lymphopenic immunologic deficiency, which is characterized by agammaglobulinemia (absence of immunoglobulin in the circulation). Not all forms of SCID in-

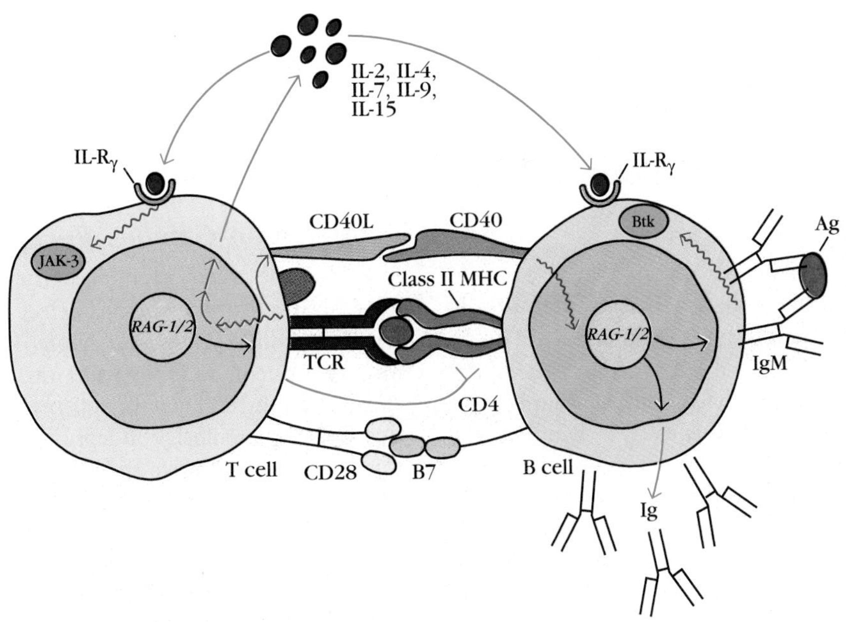

FIGURE 19-3 Defects in cell interaction and signaling can lead to severe immunodeficiency. The interaction of T cell and B cell is shown here with a number of the components important to the intra- and extracellular signaling pathways. A number of primary immunodeficiencies are rooted in defects in these interactions. SCID may result from defects in (1) the recombination-activating genes (*RAG-1* and *-2*) required for synthesis of the functional immunoglobulins and T-cell receptors that characterize mature B and T cells; (2) the γ chain of receptors for IL-2,4,7,9, and 15 (IL-Rγ); (3) JAK-3, which transduces signals from the gamma chain of the cytokine receptor; or (4) expression of the class II MHC molecule (bare lymphocyte syndrome). XLA results from defective transduction of activating signals from the cell-surface IgM by Bruton's tyrosine kinase (Btk). XHM results from defects in CD40L that preclude normal maturation of B cells. [Adapted from BA Smart and HD Ochs, 1997, *Curr. Opin. Pediatr.* **9**:570.]

clude agammaglobulinemia, but they do have common features despite differences in the underlying genetic defects. Clinically, SCID is characterized by a very low number of circulating lymphocytes (levels of other blood cells are normal). There is a failure to mount immune responses mediated by T cells. The thymus does not develop, and the few circulating T cells in the SCID patient do not respond to stimulation by mitogens, indicating that they cannot proliferate in response to antigens. Myeloid and erythroid (red-blood-cell precursors) cells appear normal in number and function, indicating that only lymphoid cells are depleted in SCID.

SCID results in severe recurrent infections and is usually fatal in the early years of life. Although both the T and B lineages may be affected, the initial manifestation of SCID in infants is almost always infection by agents, such as fungi or viruses, that are normally dealt with by T-cell immunity. The B cell defect is not evident in the first few months of life, because babies are protected by antibodies passively obtained from transplacental circulation or from mother's milk. SCID infants suffer from chronic diarrhea, pneumonia, and skin, mouth, and throat lesions as well as a host of other opportunistic infections. The immune system is so compromised that even live attenuated vaccines (such as the Sabin polio vaccine) can cause infection and disease. The life span of a SCID patient can be prolonged by avoidance of all potentially harmful microorganisms. Patients have been kept alive by confinement in a sterile atmosphere that prevents exposure to harmful microorganisms. It takes an extraordinary effort to maintain no direct contact with other persons or with unfiltered air; food or any object that comes in contact with the sequestered SCID patient must first be sterilized. Such confinement is a temporary measure, pending treatment.

The search for defects that underlie SCID has revealed several different causes for this general failure of immunity. In a survey of 108 infants with SCID carried out by Rebecca Buckley, Jennifer Puck, and their colleagues, the most prevalent defect (found in 49 of the infants) was due to mutations that impair the function of the common gamma chain of the IL-2 receptor (IL-2Rγ; see Figure 12-7). Defects in this chain impede signaling through receptors for IL-4, -7, -9, and -15 as well as the IL-2 receptor, because this chain is present in receptors for all of these cytokines. The next most common defect (16 infants) found in the survey was in the gene for the enzyme adenosine deaminase (ADA). ADA is one of the enzymes in the purine catabolic pathway, catalyzing the conversion of adenosine to inosine. Activity of ADA is especially high in lymphocytes, and its deficiency results in accumulation of metabolic byproducts that are toxic to the cells. Five of the infants had defects in the Janus kinase 3 (JAK-3), which is involved in T-cell signal transduction from the IL-2 receptor (see Figure 12-10). The remainder either were classified as autosomal recessive defects not related to known IL-2Rγ or JAK-3 mutations or were of unknown origin, with no apparent genetic defect or family history of immunodeficiency.

There are several other known defects that give rise to SCID. There is a defect that is characterized by depletion of $CD8^+$ T cells and involves the tyrosine kinase ZAP-70, an important element in T-cell signal transduction (see Figures 10-11 and 10-12). Infants with defects in ZAP-70 may have normal levels of immunoglobulin and $CD4^+$ lymphocytes; however, their $CD4^+$ T cells are nonfunctional. A deficiency in the enzyme purine nucleoside phosphorylase (PNP) causes immunodeficiency by a mechanism similar to the ADA defect, with accumulation of toxic metabolites in lymphoid cells. As described in Chapters 5 and 9, both immunoglobulin and T-cell–receptor genes undergo rearrangement to express the active forms of these molecules. A defect in the genes that encode mediators of the rearrangement processes (recombination-activating proteins RAG-1 and RAG-2) precludes development of B and T cells with functional receptors and leads to SCID.

A defect leading to general failure of immunity similar to SCID is failure to transcribe the genes that encode class II MHC molecules. Without these molecules, the patient's lymphocytes cannot participate in cellular interactions with T helper cells. This immunodeficiency is also called the "bare-lymphocyte syndrome." Molecular studies of the bare-lymphocyte syndrome revealed a defective interaction between a 5′ promoter sequence of the gene for the class II MHC molecule and a DNA-binding protein necessary for gene transcription. A defect in MHC class I gene function was identified in a patient with SCID-like symptoms. This rare variant of immunodeficiency was ascribed to mutation in the TAP genes that are vital to antigen processing by class I MHC molecules (see Chapter 8). This defect causes a deficit in CD8-mediated immunity, characterized by susceptibility to viral infection.

Wiskott-Aldrich Syndrome (WAS)

This X-linked disorder is an immunodeficiency that increases in severity with age and usually results in fatal infection or lymphoid malignancy. Initially, T and B lymphocytes are present in normal numbers, and WAS first manifests itself by defective responses to bacterial polysaccharides and by lower-than-average IgM levels. Other responses and effector mechanisms are normal in the early stages of the syndrome. As the WAS sufferer ages, there are recurrent bacterial infections and a gradual loss of humoral and cellular responses. The syndrome includes thrombocytopenia (lowered platelet count; the existing platelets are smaller than usual and have a short half-life), which may lead to fatal bleeding. Eczema (skin rashes) in varying degrees of severity may also occur, usually beginning around one year of age. The defect in WAS has been mapped to the short arm of the X chromosome (see Table 19-1) and involves a cytoskeletal glycoprotein present in lymphoid cells called sialophorin (CD43). The function of this protein is not known.

Interferon-Gamma–Receptor Defect

A recently described immunodeficiency that falls into the mixed-cell category involves a defect in the receptor for interferon gamma (IFN-γ, see Chapter 12). This deficiency was found in patients suffering from infection with atypical mycobacteria (intracellular organisms related to the bacteria that cause tuberculosis and leprosy). Most of those carrying this autosomal recessive trait are from families with a history of inbreeding. The susceptibility to infection with mycobacteria is selective in that those who survive these infections are not unusually susceptible to other agents, including other intracellular bacteria. This immunodeficiency points to a specific role for IFN-γ and its receptor in protection from infection with mycobacteria.

Whereas SCID and the related combined immunodeficiencies affect T cells or all lymphoid cells, other primary immunodeficiencies affect B-cell function and result in the reduction or absence of some or all classes of immunoglobulins. While the underlying defects have been identified for some of these, little information exists concerning the exact cause of some of the more common deficiencies, such as common variable immunodeficiency and selective IgA deficiency.

X-Linked Agammaglobulinemia

A B-cell defect called X-linked agammaglobulinemia (XLA) or Bruton's hypogammaglobulinemia is characterized by extremely low IgG levels and by the absence of other immunoglobulin classes. Individuals with XLA have no peripheral B cells and suffer from recurrent bacterial infections, beginning at about nine months of age. A palliative treatment for this condition is periodic administration of immunoglobulin, but patients seldom survive past their teens. There is a defect in B-cell signal transduction in this disorder, due to a defect in a transduction molecule called Bruton's tyrosine kinase (Btk), after the investigator who described the syndrome. B cells in the XLA patient remain in the pre-B stage with H chains rearranged but L chains in their germline configuration. (The Clinical Focus in Chapter 11 describes the discovery of this immunodeficiency and its underlying defect in detail.)

X-Linked Hyper-IgM Syndrome

A peculiar immunoglobulin deficiency first thought to result from a B-cell defect has recently been shown to result instead from a defect in a T-cell surface molecule. X-linked hyper-IgM (XHM) syndrome is characterized by a deficiency of IgG, IgA, and IgE and elevated levels of IgM, sometimes as high as 10 mg/ml (normal IgM concentration is 1.5 mg/ml). XHM syndrome is generally inherited as an X-linked recessive disorder (see Figure 19-2), but some forms appear to be acquired and affect both men and women. Affected individuals have high counts of IgM-secreting plasma cells in their peripheral blood and lymphoid tissue. In addition, XHM patients often have high levels of autoantibodies to neutrophils, platelets, and red blood cells. Children with XHM suffer recurrent infections, especially respiratory infections caused by the opportunistic pathogen *Pneumocystis carinii.* The infections observed in XHM are more severe than expected for a deficiency characterized by low levels of immunoglobulins.

Although individuals with XHM have normal numbers of B cells expressing membrane-bound IgM or IgD, they appear to lack B cells expressing membrane-bound IgG, IgA, or IgE. The defect in XHM is in the gene encoding the CD40 ligand (CD40L), which maps to the X chromosome. T_H cells from patients with XHM fail to express functional CD40L on their membrane. Since an interaction between CD40 on the B cell and CD40L on the T_H cell is required for B-cell activation, the absence of this co-stimulatory signal inhibits the B-cell response to T-dependent antigens (see Figures 19-3 and 11-10). The B-cell response to T-independent antigens, however, is unaffected by this defect, accounting for the production of IgM antibodies. As discussed in Chapter 11, class switching and formation of memory B cells both require contact with T_H cells by a CD40–CD40L interaction. The absence of this interaction in XHM results in the loss of class switching to IgG, IgA, or IgE isotypes and in a failure to produce memory B cells. In addition, XHM individuals fail to produce germinal centers during a humoral response, which highlights the role of the CD40–CD40L interaction in the generation of germinal centers.

Common Variable Immunodeficiency (CVI)

CVI is characterized by a profound decrease in numbers of antibody-producing plasma cells, low levels of most immunoglobulin isotypes (hypogammaglobulinemia), and recurrent infections. The condition is usually manifested later in life than other deficiencies and is sometimes called late onset or acquired hypogammaglobulinemia. However, CVI has a genetic component and is considered a primary immunodeficiency, although the exact pattern of inheritance is not known. Because the manifestations are very similar to those of acquired hypogammaglobulinemia, there is some confusion between the two forms (see below). Infections in CVI sufferers are most frequently bacterial and can be controlled by administration of immunoglobulin. In CVI patients, B cells fail to mature into plasma cells; however in vitro studies show that CVI B cells are capable of maturing in response to appropriate differentiation signals. The underlying defect in CVI is not known, but must involve either an in vivo blockage of the maturation of B cells to the plasma-cell stage or their inability to produce the secreted form of immunoglobulins.

Selective Deficiencies of Immunoglobulin Classes

A number of immunodeficiency states are characterized by significantly lowered amounts of specific immunoglobulin isotypes. Of these, IgA deficiency is by far the most common. There are family-association data showing that IgA deficiency prevails in the same families as CVI, suggesting a relationship between these conditions. The spectrum of clinical symptoms of IgA deficiency is broad; many of those affected are asymptomatic, while others suffer from an assortment of serious problems. Recurrent respiratory and genitourinary tract infections resulting from lack of secreted IgA on mucosal surfaces are predicted and do occur. In addition, problems such as intestinal malabsorption, allergic disease, and autoimmune disorders may also be associated with low IgA levels. The reasons for this variability in the clinical profile of IgA deficiency are not clear but may relate to the ability of some, but not all, patients to substitute IgM for IgA as a mucosal antibody. The defect in IgA deficiency is related to the inability of IgA B cells to undergo normal differentiation to the plasma-cell stage. IgG2 and IgG4 may also be deficient in IgA deficient patients. No causative defect in IgA genes has been identified, and the surface IgA molecules on these patients' B cells appear to be expressed normally. A gene outside of the immunoglobulin gene complex is suspected to be responsible for this fairly common syndrome.

A number of other immunoglobulin deficiencies have been reported but these are rarer. An IgM deficiency has been identified as an autosomal recessive trait. Victims of this condition are subject to severe infection by agents such as meningococcus, which causes fatal disease. IgM deficiency may be accompanied by various malignancies or by autoimmune disease. IgG deficiencies are also rare. These are often not noticed until adulthood and can be effectively treated by administration of immunoglobulin.

Ataxia Telangiectasia

Although not classified primarily as an immunodeficiency, ataxia telangiectasia is a disease syndrome that includes deficiency of IgA and sometimes of IgE. The syndrome is characterized by difficulty in maintaining balance (ataxia) and by the appearance of broken capillaries (telangiectasia) in the eyes. The primary defect appears to be in a kinase involved in regulation of the cell cycle. The relationship between the immune deficiency and the other defects in ataxia telangiectasia remains obscure.

Immune Disorders Involving the Thymus

Several immunodeficiency syndromes are grounded in failure of the thymus to undergo normal development. Thymic malfunction has a profound effect on T-cell function; all populations of T cells, including helper, cytolytic, and regulatory varieties, are affected. Immunity to viruses and fungi is especially compromised in those suffering from these conditions.

DiGeorge syndrome, or congenital thymic aplasia, in its most severe form is the complete absence of a thymus. This developmental defect, which is associated with the deletion in the embryo of a region on chromosome 22, causes immunodeficiency along with characteristic facial abnormalities, hypoparathyroidism, and congenital heart disease (Figure 19-4). The stage at which the causative developmental defect occurs has been determined, and the syndrome is sometimes called the *third and fourth pharyngeal pouch syndrome* to reflect its precise embryonic origin. The immune defect includes a profound depression of T-cell numbers and absence of T-cell responses. Although B cells are present in normal numbers, affected individuals do not produce antibody in response to immunization with specific antigens. Thymic transplantation is of some value for correcting the T-cell defects, but many DiGeorge patients have such severe heart disease that their chances for long-term survival are poor, even if the immune defects are corrected.

Whereas the DiGeorge syndrome results from an intrauterine or developmental anomaly, thymic hypoplasia, or the Nezelof syndrome, is an inherited disorder. The mode of inheritance for this rare disease is not known and its presentation varies, making it somewhat difficult to diagnose. As the name implies, thymic hypoplasia is a defect in which a vestigial thymus is unable to serve its function in T-cell development. In some patients, B cells are normal, whereas in others a B-cell deficiency is secondary to the T-cell defect.

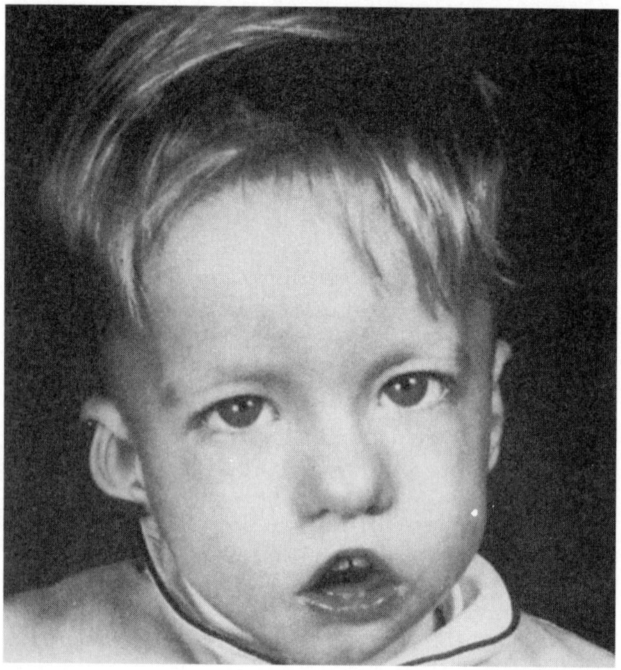

FIGURE 19-4 A child with DiGeorge syndrome showing characteristic dysplasia of ears and mouth and abnormally long distance between the eyes. [R Kretschmer et al, 1968, *New Engl. J. Med.* **279**:1295; photograph courtesy of FS Rosen.]

Affected individuals suffer from chronic diarrhea, viral and fungal infections, and a general failure to thrive.

Defects in the Myeloid Lineage

Immunodeficiencies of the lymphoid lineage affect adaptive immunity. By contrast, defects in the myeloid cell lineage affect the innate immune functions (see Figure 19-1). Most of these defects result in impaired phagocytic processes that are manifested by recurrent microbial infection of greater or lesser severity. There are several stages at which the phagocytic processes may be faulty; these include cell motility, adherence to and phagocytosis of organisms, and killing by macrophages.

Reduction in Neutrophil Count

As described in Chapter 2, neutrophils are circulating granulocytes with phagocytic function. Quantitative deficiencies in neutrophils can range from an almost complete absence of cells, called agranulocytosis, to a reduction in the concentration of peripheral blood neutrophils below 1500/mm^3, called granulocytopenia or neutropenia. These quantitative deficiencies may result from congenital defects or may be acquired through extrinsic factors. Acquired neutropenias are much more common than congenital ones.

Congenital neutropenia is often due to a genetic defect that affects the myeloid progenitor stem cell; it results in reduced production of neutrophils during hematopoiesis. In congenital agranulocytosis, myeloid stem cells are present in the bone marrow but rarely differentiate beyond the promyelocyte stage. As a result, children born with this condition show severe neutropenia with counts of less than 200 neutrophils/mm^3. These children suffer from frequent bacterial infections beginning as early as the first month of life; normal infants are protected at this age by maternal antibody as well as by innate immune mechanisms, including neutrophils. Experimental evidence suggests that this genetic defect results in decreased production of granulocyte colony-stimulating factor (G-CSF) and thus in a failure of the myeloid stem cell to differentiate along the granulocytic lineage (see Figure 2-1).

Neutrophils have a short life span, and their precursors must divide rapidly in the bone marrow to maintain levels of these cells in the circulation. For this reason, agents such as radiation and certain drugs (e.g., chemotherapeutic drugs) that specifically damage rapidly dividing cells are likely to cause neutropenia. Occasionally, neutropenia develops in such autoimmune diseases as Sjögren's syndrome or systemic lupus erythematosus; in these conditions, autoantibodies destroy the neutrophils. Transient neutropenia often develops after certain bacterial or viral infections, but neutrophil counts return to normal as the infection is cleared.

Chronic Granulomatous Disease (CGD)

CGD is a genetic disease that has at least two distinct forms: an X-linked form that occurs in about 70% of patients and an autosomal recessive form found in the rest. This disease is rooted in a defect in the oxidative pathway by which phagocytes generate hydrogen peroxide and the resulting reactive products, such as hypochlorous acid, that kill phagocytosed bacteria. CGD sufferers undergo excessive inflammatory reactions that result in gingivitis, swollen lymph nodes, and nonmalignant granulomas (lumpy subcutaneous cell masses); they are also susceptibile to bacterial and fungal infection. CGD patients are not subject to infection by those bacteria, such as pneumococcus, that generate their own hydrogen peroxide. In this case, the myeloperoxidase in the host cell can use the bacterial hydrogen peroxide to generate enough hypochlorous acid to thwart infection. Several related defects may lead to CGD; these include a missing or defective cytochrome (cyt b_{558}) that functions in an oxidative pathway and defects in proteins (phagocyte oxidases, or phox) that stabilize the cytochrome. In addition to the general defect in the killer function of phagocytes, there is also a decrease in the ability of mononuclear cells to serve as APCs. Both processing and presentation of antigen are impaired. Increased amounts of antigen are required to trigger T-cell help when mononuclear cells from CGD patients are used as APCs.

The addition of IFN-γ has been shown to restore function to CGD granulocytes and monocytes in vitro. This observation prompted clinical trials of IFN-γ for CGD patients. Encouraging increases in oxidative function and restoration of cytoplasmic cytochrome have been reported in these patients. In addition, knowledge of the precise gene defects underlying CGD makes it a candidate for gene therapy, and replacement of the defective cytochrome has had promising results (see below)

Chediak-Higashi Syndrome

This autosomal recessive disease is characterized by recurrent bacterial infections, partial oculo-cutaneous albinism (lack of skin and eye pigment), and aggressive but nonmalignant infiltration of organs by lymphoid cells. Phagocytes from patients with this immune defect contain giant granules but do not have the ability to kill bacteria. The molecular basis of the defect is a mutation in a protein (LYST) involved in the regulation of intracellular trafficking. The mutation impairs the targeting of proteins to secretory lysosomes, which makes them unable to lyse bacteria.

Leukocyte Adhesion Deficiency (LAD)

As described in Chapter 15, cell-surface molecules belonging to the integrin family of proteins function as adhesion molecules and are required to facilitate cellular interaction. Three of these, LFA-1, Mac-1 and gp150/95 (CD11a, b, and c, respectively) have a common β chain (CD18) and are variably present on different monocytic cells; CD11a is also expressed on B cells (Table 19-2). An immunodeficiency related to

TABLE 19-2 PROPERTIES OF INTEGRIN MOLECULES THAT ARE ABSENT IN LEUKOCYTE-ADHESION DEFICIENCY

	Integrin molecules*		
Property	LFA-1	CR3	CR4
CD designation	CD11a/CD18	CD11b/CD18	CD11c/CD18
Subunit composition	αLβ2	αMβ2	αXβ2
Subunit molecular mass (kDa)			
α chain	175,000	165,000	150,000
β chain	95,000	95,000	95,000
Cellular expression	Lymphocytes Monocytes Macrophages Granulocytes Natural killer cells	Monocytes Macrophages Granulocytes Natural killer cells	Monocytes Macrophages Granulocytes
Ligand	ICAM-1 ICAM-2	C3bi	C3bi
Functions inhibited with monoclonal antibody	Extravasation CTL killing T-B conjugate formation ADCC	Opsonization Granulocyte adherence, aggregation, and chemotaxis ADCC	Granulocyte adherence and aggregation

*CR3 = type 3 complement receptor, also known as Mac-1; CR4 = type 4 complement receptor, also known as gp150/90. LFA-1, CR3, and CR4 are heterodimers containing a common β chain but different α chains designated L, M, and X, respectively.

dysfunction of the adhesion molecules is rooted in a defect localized to the common β chain and affects expression of all three of the molecules that use this chain. This defect, called leukocyte adhesion deficiency (LAD), causes susceptibility to infection with both Gram-positive and Gram-negative bacteria as well as various fungi. Impairment of adhesion of leukocytes to vascular endothelium limits recruitment of cells to sites of inflammation. Viral immunity is somewhat impaired, as would be predicted from the defective T-B cell cooperation caused by the adhesion defect. LAD varies in its severity; some affected individuals die within a few years, whereas others may survive into their forties. The reason for the variable disease phenotype in this disorder is not known. LAD is the subject of a Clinical Focus in Chapter 15.

Defects in the Complement System

Immunodeficiency diseases resulting from defects in the complement system are described in Chapter 13. Many complement deficiencies are associated with increased susceptibility to bacterial infections and/or immune-complex diseases. One of these complement disorders, a deficiency in properdin, which stabilizes the C3 convertase in the alternative complement pathway, is caused by a defect in a gene located on the X chromosome (see Figure 19-2).

Treatment of Immunodeficiency

Although there are no cures for immunodeficiency disorders, there are several treatment possibilities. In addition to the drastic option of total isolation from exposure to any microbial agent, treatment options for the immunodeficiencies include:

- replacement of a missing protein
- replacement of a missing cell type or lineage
- replacement of a missing or defective gene

Administration of the missing protein immunoglobulin is the classic course of treatment for disorders that impair antibody production. Pooled human gamma globulin given either intravenously or subcutaneously protects against recurrent infection in many types of immunodeficiency. Maintenance of reasonably high levels of serum immunoglobulin (5 mg/ml serum) will prevent most common infections in the agammaglobulinemic patient. This is generally accomplished by the administration of immunoglobulin that has been selected for antibodies directed against a particular organism. Recent advances in the preparation of human monoclonal antibodies and in the ability to genetically engineer chimeric antibodies with mouse V regions and human derived C regions make it possible to prepare antibodies specific for important pathogens (see Chapter 5). Advances in molecular biology make it possible to clone the genes that encode other immunologically important proteins, such as cytokines, and to express these genes in vitro, using bacterial or eukaryotic expression systems. The availability of such proteins allows new modes of therapy in which immunologically important proteins may be replaced or their concentrations increased in the patient. For example, the administration of recombinant IFN-γ has proven effective for patients with CGD, and the use of recombinant IL-2 may help to restore immune function in AIDS patients.

Cell replacement as therapy for immunodeficiencies has been made possible by recent progress in bone-marrow transplantation (see Chapter 21). Replacement of stem cells with those from an immunocompetent donor allows development of a functional immune system (see Clinical Focus Chapter 2). High rates of success have been reported for those who are fortunate enough to have an HLA-identical donor. Careful matching of patients with donors and the ability to manipulate stem-cell populations to select $CD34^+$ precursor cells continues to minimize the risk in this procedure, even when no ideal donor exists. These procedures have been highly successful with SCID infants when haploidentical (complete match of one HLA gene set or haplotype) donor marrow is used. T cells are depleted and $CD34^+$ stem cells are enriched before introducing the donor bone marrow into the SCID infant. Because this therapy has been used only in recent years, it is not known whether transplantation cures the immunodeficiency permanently. A variation of bone-marrow transplantation is the injection of paternal $CD34^+$ cells in utero when the birth of an infant with SCID is expected. Two infants born after this procedure had normal T-cell function and did not develop the infections that characterize SCID.

If a single gene defect has been identified, as in adenosine deaminase deficiency or chronic granulomatous disease, replacement of the defective gene may be a treatment option. Clinical tests of such therapy are underway for SCID caused by ADA deficiency and for chronic granulomatous disease with defective $p67^{phox}$, with promising initial results. Disease remission for up to 18 months was seen in the SCID patients and up to 6 months in the CGD patients. A similar procedure was used in both trials. It begins with obtaining cells ($CD34^+$ stem cells are usually selected for these procedures) from the patient and transfecting them with a normal copy of the defective gene. The transfected cells are then returned to the patient. As this treatment improves, it will become applicable to a number of immunodeficiencies for which a genetic defect is well defined. As mentioned above these include defects in genes that encode the γ chain of the IL-2 receptor, JAK-3, and ZAP-70, all of which give rise to SCID.

Animal Models of Primary Immunodeficiency

Immunologists use two well-studied animal models of primary immunodeficiency for a variety of experimental purposes. One of these is the athymic, or nude, mouse; the other is the severe combined immunodeficiency, or SCID, mouse.

Nude (Athymic) Mice

A genetic trait designated *nu,* which is controlled by a recessive gene on chromosome 11, was discovered in certain mice. Mice homozygous for this trait (*nu/nu*) are hairless and, in addition, lack a thymus (Figure 19-5). Heterozygotic, *nu*/+, litter mates have hair and a normal thymus. It is not known whether the hairlessness and the absence of a thymus are caused by the same gene. It is possible that two very closely linked genes control these defects, which, although unrelated, appear together in this mutant mouse. A gene that controls development may be involved, since the pathway that leads to the differential development of the thymus is related to the one that controls the skin epithelial cells. The *nu/nu* mouse cannot easily survive; under normal conditions, the mortality is 100% within 25 weeks and 50% die within the first two weeks after birth. Therefore, when these animals are to be used for experimental purposes, they must be maintained under conditions that protect them from infection. Precautions include use of sterilized food, water, cages, and bedding. The cages are protected from dust by placing them in a laminar flow rack or by the use of air filters fitted over the individual cages.

Nude mice lack cell-mediated immune responses, and they are unable to make antibodies to most antigens. The immunodeficiency in the nude mouse can be reversed by a thymic transplant. Because they can permanently tolerate both allografts and xenografts, they have a number of practical experimental uses. For example, hybridomas or solid tumors from any origin may be grown as ascites or as implanted tumors in a nude mouse. It is known that the nude mouse does not completely lack T cells; rather, it has a limited population that increases with age. The source of these T cells is not known; an intriguing possibility is that there is an extrathymic source of mature T cells. However, this is unlikely, because nude mice do have a vestigial thymus. The majority of cells in the circulation of a nude mouse carry T-cell receptors of the $\gamma\delta$ type instead of the $\alpha\beta$ type, which prevails in the circulation of a normal mouse.

The SCID Mouse

In 1983, Melvin and Gayle Bosma and their colleagues described an autosomal recessive mutation in mice that gave rise to a severe deficiency in mature lymphocytes. They designated the trait SCID because of its similarity to human severe combined immunodeficiency. The SCID mouse was shown to have early B- and T-lineage cells, but there was a virtual absence of lymphoid cells in the thymus, spleen, lymph nodes, and gut tissue, the usual locations of functional T and B cells. The precursor T and B cells in the SCID mouse appeared to be unable to differentiate into mature functional B and T lymphocytes. Inbred mouse lines carrying the SCID defect have been derived and studied in great detail. The SCID mouse can neither make antibody nor carry out DTH or graft-rejection reactions. If the animals are not kept in an extremely clean environment, they succumb to infection early in life. Cells other than lymphocytes develop normally in the SCID mouse; red blood cells, monocytes, and granulocytes are present and functional. SCID mice may be rendered immunologically competent by transplantation of stem cells from normal mice.

The mutation in a DNA protein kinase that causes mouse SCID is a so-called "leaky" mutation, because a certain number of SCID mice do produce immunoglobulin. About half of these leaky SCID mice can also reject skin allografts. This finding suggests that the defective enzyme can function partly in T- and B-cell development, allowing normal differentiation of a small percentage of precursor cells. More recently, immunodeficient SCID-like mice have been developed by deletion of the recombination-activating enzymes (RAG-1 or RAG-2) responsible for the rearrangement of immunoglobulin or T-cell–receptor genes in both B- and T-cell precursors (RAG knockout mice). This gives rise to a defect in both B and T cells of the mouse; neither can rearrange the genes for their receptor and thus neither proceeds along a normal developmental path. Because cells with abnormal rearrangements are eliminated in vivo, both B and T cells are absent from the lymphoid organs of the RAG knockout mouse.

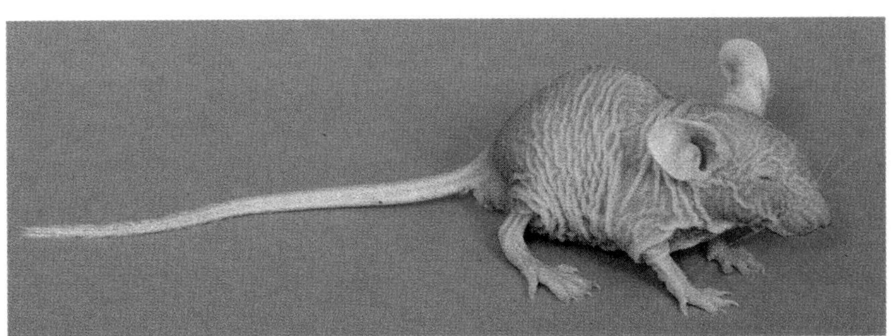

FIGURE 19-5 A nude mouse (*nu/nu*). This defect leads to absence of a thymus or a vestigial thymus and cell-mediated immunodeficiency. [Courtesy of the Jackson Laboratory, Bar Harbor Maine.]

In addition to providing a window into possible causes of combined T- and B-cell immunodeficiency, the SCID mouse has proven extremely useful in studies of cellular immunology. Because its rejection mechanisms do not operate, the SCID mouse can be used for studies on cells or organs from various origins. For example, immune precursor cells from human sources may be used to reestablish the SCID mouse's immune system. These human cells can develop in a normal fashion and, as a result, the SCID mouse circulation will contain immunoglobulin of human origin. In one important application, these SCID mice are infected with HIV-1. Although normal mice are not susceptible to HIV-1 infection, the SCID mouse reconstituted with human lymphoid tissue (SCID-Hu mouse) provides an animal model in which to test therapeutic or prophylactic strategies against HIV infection of the transplanted human lymphoid tissue.

In addition to the nude and SCID mice, gene knockout techniques now allow the creation of mouse strains deficient in other genes important to immune function. This tool allows determination of the consequences of deleting any gene that is suspected of playing a role in immunodeficiency.

AIDS and Other Acquired or Secondary Immunodeficiencies

As described above, a variety of defects in the immune system give rise to immunodeficiency. In addition to the primary immunodeficiencies, there are also acquired, or secondary, immunodeficiencies. One that has been known for some time is called acquired hypogammaglobulinemia. (As mentioned above, this condition is sometimes confused with common variable immunodeficiency, a condition that shows genetic predisposition.). The origin of acquired hypogammaglobulinemia is unknown, and its major symptom, recurrent infection, manifests itself in young adults. The patients generally have very low but detectable levels of total immunoglobulin. T-cell numbers and function may be normal, but there are some cases with T-cell defects and these may grow more severe as the disease progresses. The disease is generally treated by gammaglobulin therapy, allowing patients to survive into their seventh and eighth decades. Unlike similar deficiencies described above, there is no evidence for genetic transmission of this disease. Mothers with acquired hypogammaglobulinemia deliver normal infants. However, at birth the infants will be deficient in circulating immunoglobulin, because the deficiency in maternal circulation is reflected in the infant.

Another form of secondary immunodeficiency, known as agent-induced immunodeficiency, results from exposure to any of a number of chemical and biological agents that induce an immunodeficient state. Certain of these are drugs used to combat autoimmune diseases such as rheumatoid arthritis or lupus erythematosis. Corticosteroids, which are commonly used for autoimmune disorders, interfere with the immune response in order to relieve disease symptoms and thus induce an immunodeficient state in those treated. Similarly, a state of immunodeficiency is deliberately induced in transplantation patients who are given immunosuppressive drugs, such as cyclosporin A, in order to blunt the attack of the immune system on transplanted organs. As will be described in Chapter 21, there are recent efforts to use more specific means of inducing tolerance to allografts to circumvent the unwanted side effects of general immunosuppression. The mechanism of action of the immunosuppressive agents varies; T cells appear to be the favored target. In addition, cytotoxic drugs or radiation treatments given to treat various forms of cancer frequently damage the dividing cells in the body, including those of the immune system, and induce a state of immunodeficiency as an unwanted consequence. Patients undergoing such therapy must be monitored closely and treated with antibiotics or gammaglobulin if infection appears.

The AIDS Epidemic

In recent years, all other forms of immunodeficiency have been overshadowed by an epidemic of severe immunodeficiency caused by the infectious agent called human immunodeficiency virus 1, or HIV-1. The disease that HIV-1 causes, acquired immunodeficiency syndrome (AIDS) was first reported in the United States in 1981 in Los Angeles, New York, and San Francisco. A group of patients displayed unusual infections, including the opportunistic fungal pathogen *Pneumocystis carinii,* which causes a pneumonia called PCP (*P. carinii* pneumonia) in persons with immunodeficiency. In addition to PCP, some patients had Kaposi's sarcoma, an extremely rare skin tumor, as well as other, rarely encountered opportunistic infections. More complete evaluation of the patients showed that they had in common a marked deficiency in cellular immune responses and a significant decrease in the subpopulation of T cells that carry the CD4 marker (T helper cells.) When epidemiologists examined the background of the first patients with this new syndrome, it was found that the majority of those afflicted were homosexual males. As the number of AIDS cases increased and the disease was recognized throughout the world, persons found to be at high risk for AIDS were homosexual males, promiscuous heterosexual individuals of either sex and their partners, intravenous drug users, persons who received blood or blood products prior to 1985, and infants born to HIV-infected mothers.

Since its discovery in 1981, AIDS has increased to epidemic proportions throughout the world. As of December 1998, the cumulative total number of persons in the United States reported to have AIDS was 688,200, and of these approximately 420,000 have died. Although reporting of AIDS cases is mandatory, many states do not require cases of HIV infection that has not yet progressed to AIDS to be reported. Therefore, there is no official count of the number of HIV-infected individuals; about 1 million Americans are estimated to be infected. Although the death rate from AIDS has decreased in recent years because of improved treatments, AIDS

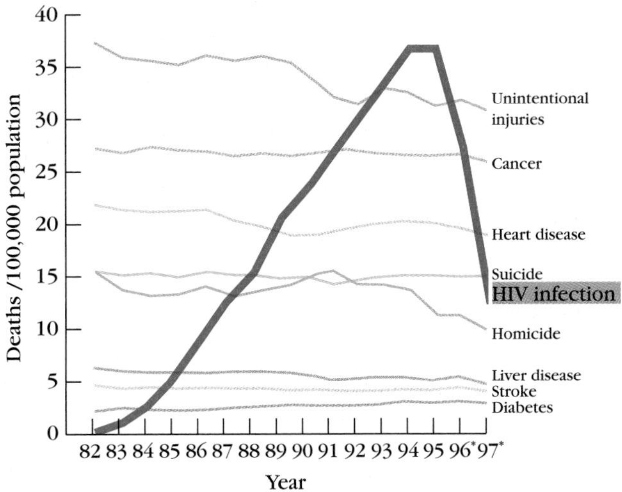

FIGURE 19-6 Death rates of the leading causes of death in persons aged 25–44 years in the United States for the years 1982–1997 (* = preliminary data). The heavy line shows that the death rate per 100,000 persons caused by AIDS surpassed any other other cause of death for those in this age range during the period 1993 to 1995. The recent decrease in AIDS deaths in the United States is attributed to improvements in anti-HIV drug therapy, which prolongs the lives of patients. [National Vital Statistics Report, 1999, vol. 47(19).]

remains among the leading killers of persons in the 25–44-year-old age range in this country (Figure 19-6). The decrease in the number of yearly AIDS deaths is encouraging, but does not indicate an end to the epidemic in this country; there were 48,269 newly reported cases of AIDS in 1998.

The magnitude of the AIDS epidemic in the United States is dwarfed by figures for other parts of the world. The global distribution of those afflicted with AIDS is shown in Figure 19-7. In sub-Saharan Africa there were an estimated 22.5 million persons with AIDS at the end of

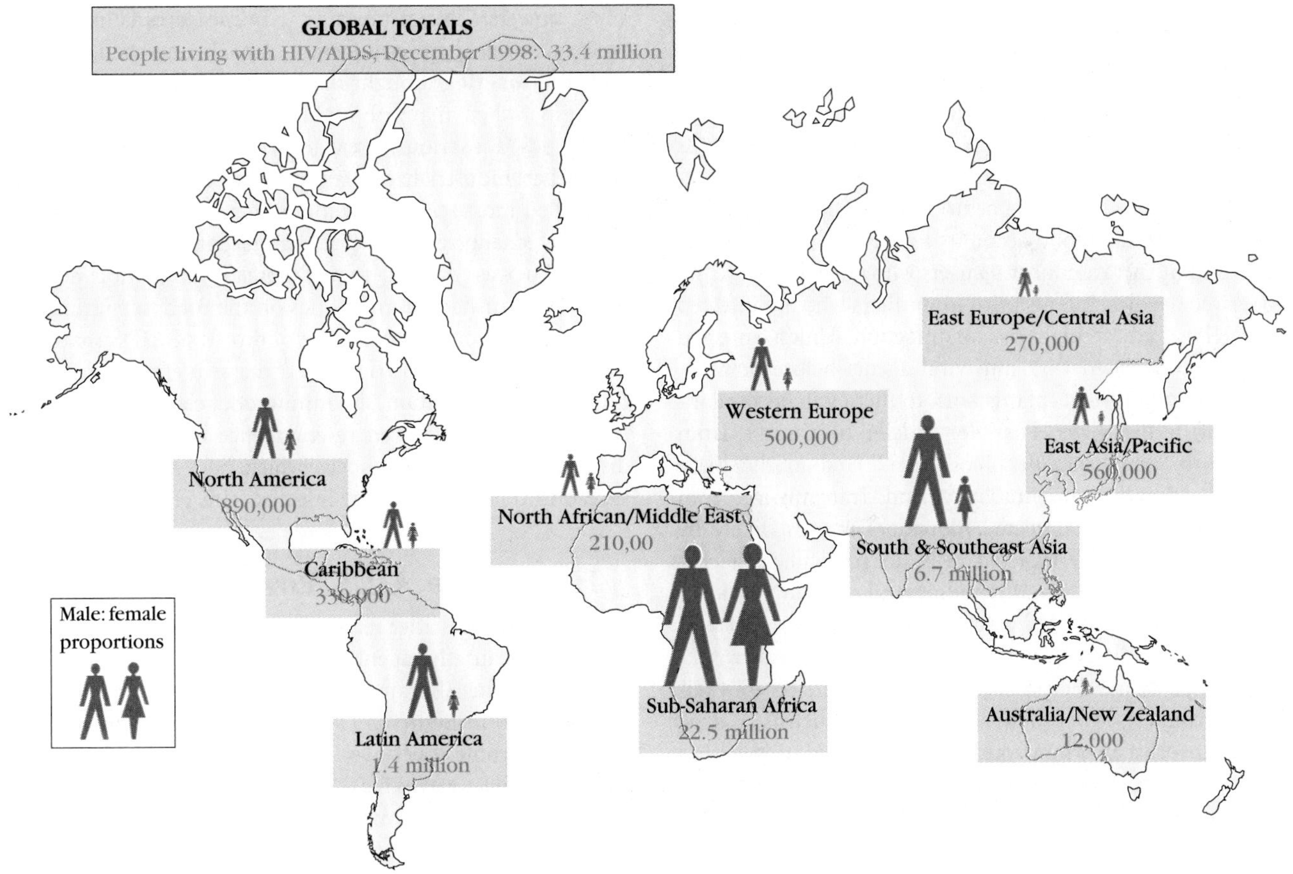

GLOBAL TOTALS
People living with HIV/AIDS, December 1998: 33.4 million

East Europe/Central Asia
270,000

Western Europe
500,000

East Asia/Pacific
560,000

North America
890,000

North African/Middle East
210,00

Caribbean
330,000

South & Southeast Asia
6.7 million

Male: female proportions

Sub-Saharan Africa
22.5 million

Australia/New Zealand
12,000

Latin America
1.4 million

FIGURE 19-7 The global AIDS epidemic. The estimated worldwide distribution of AIDS cases as of December 1998. There were approximately 33.4 million persons living with AIDS as of December 1998, most of these were in sub-Saharan Africa and Southeast Asia. In North America and Western Europe about 80% of those affected were men, whereas in Africa nearly equal numbers of women and men have AIDS. [HIV/AIDS UNAIDS: Report on the Global Epidemic, 1998.]

1998, and in South and Southeast Asia there were another 6.7 million at this time. There are an estimated 33.4 million persons worldwide with AIDS; this number includes over 5 million children. In addition, there are over 8 million children who have been orphaned by the death of their parents from AIDS. Recent estimates from the World Health Organization indicate the occurrence of 5.8 million new HIV infections in 1997, or an average of 16,000 persons infected each day during that year.

The initial group of AIDS patients in the United States and Western Europe was predominantly white and male. Although this remains the group predominantly affected, more recently the distribution in the United States has shifted to include a larger proportion of women (20% in 1996 versus 6% in 1985) and an increasing proportion of minorities (39% black and Hispanic in 1996 versus 11% in 1985). Worldwide, the number of AIDS patients distributes more equally between males and females, and in sub-Saharan Africa, which has the highest incidence of AIDS, about 50% of those afflicted are females.

Transmission of HIV-1

Although the precise mechanism by which HIV-1 infects an individual is not known, epidemiological data indicate that common means of transmission include homosexual and heterosexual intercourse, receipt of infected blood or blood products, and passage from mothers to infants. Before tests for HIV in the blood supply were routinely used, patients who received blood transfusions and hemophiliacs who received blood products were at risk for HIV-1 infection. Exposure to infected blood accounts for the high incidence of AIDS among intravenous drug users who normally share hypodermic needles. Infants born to mothers who are infected with HIV-1 are at high risk of infection. Unless infected mothers are treated with anti-viral agents before delivery, approximately 30% of infants born to them will become infected with the virus. Possible vehicles of passage from mother to infant include blood transferred in the birth process and milk in the nursing period. Transmission from an infected to an uninfected individual is most likely by transmission of HIV-infected cells, in particular, macrophages, dendritic cells, and lymphocytes.

In the worldwide epidemic, it is estimated that 75% of the cases of HIV transmission are attributable to heterosexual contact. While the probability of transmission by vaginal intercourse is lower than by other means, such as IV drug use or receptive anal intercourse, the likelihood of infection is greatly enhanced by the presence of other sexually transmitted diseases (STDs). In populations where prostitution is rampant, STDs flourish and provide a powerful cofactor for the heterosexual transmission of HIV-1. Reasons for this increased infection rate include the lesions and open sores present in many STDs, which favor the transfer of HIV-infected blood during intercourse. In addition, infection with the STD agents leads to immune stimulation, and activated lymphocytes are more readily infected by HIV-1 than are resting lymphocytes.

While the AIDS epidemic has engendered an understandable fear of infection among most informed individuals, there are also exaggerated claims of the ease with which HIV infection may be passed on. At present, there is little or no evidence that casual contact with or touching an infected person can spread HIV-1 infection. Airborne transmission has never been observed to cause infection. In virtually every well-documented case of HIV-1 infection, there is evidence for contact with blood, milk, semen, or vaginal fluid from an infected individual. Research workers and medical professionals who take reasonable precautions have a very low incidence of AIDS, despite repeated contact with infected materials. The risk of transmitting HIV infection can be minimized by simple precautionary measures, including the avoidance of any practice that could allow exposure of broken or abraded skin or any mucosal membrane to blood from a potentially infected person. The use of condoms when having sex with individuals of unknown infection status is highly recommended. One factor contributing to the spread of HIV is the long period after infection during which no clinical signs may appear but during which the infected individual may infect others. Thus, universal use of precautionary measures is important whenever and wherever infection status is uncertain.

It is a sobering thought that the epidemic of AIDS came at a time when many thought that infectious diseases no longer posed a serious threat to people in the United States and other industrialized nations. Vaccines and antibiotics controlled most serious infectious agents. The virtual eradication of smallpox in the world had recently been celebrated, and polio was yielding to widespread vaccination efforts; these were considered milestones on the road to elimination of most infectious diseases. The outbreak of AIDS shattered this complacency and triggered a massive effort to combat this disease. In addition, the immunodeficiency that characterizes AIDS has allowed re-emergence of other infectious diseases, such as tuberculosis, which have the potential to spread into populations not infected with HIV.

HIV-1: The AIDS Virus

Within a few years after recognition of AIDS as an infectious disease, the causative agent was discovered and characterized by efforts in the laboratories of Luc Montagnier in Paris and Robert Gallo in Bethesda (Figure 19-8). This immunodeficiency syndrome was novel in that it was caused by a type of virus called a **retrovirus.** Retroviruses carry their genetic information in the form of RNA. When the virus enters a cell, the RNA is reverse transcribed to DNA by a virally encoded enzyme, reverse transcriptase (RT). As the name implies, RT reverses the normal transcription process and makes a DNA copy of the viral RNA genome. This copy, which is called a **provirus,** is integrated into the cell genome

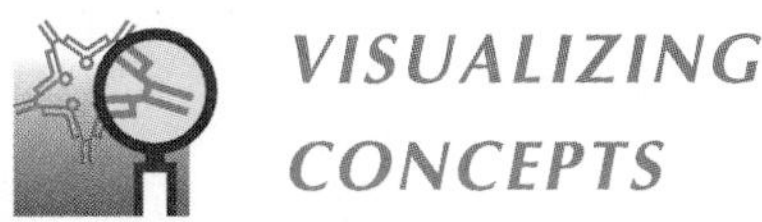

VISUALIZING CONCEPTS

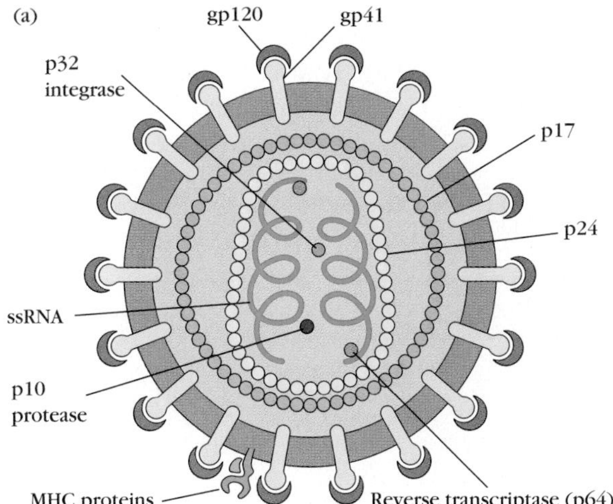

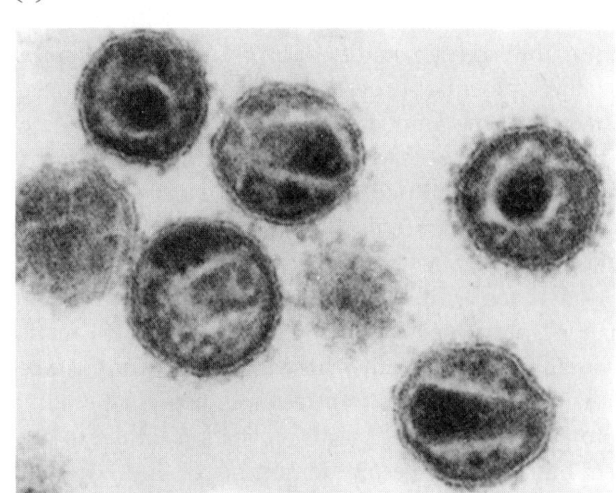

FIGURE 19-8 Structure of HIV. (a) Cross-sectional schematic diagram of HIV virion. Each virion expresses 72 glycoprotein projections composed of gp120 and gp41. The gp41 molecule is a transmembrane molecule that crosses the lipid bilayer of the viral envelope. Gp120 is associated with gp41 and serves as the viral receptor for CD4 on host cells. The viral envelope derives from the host cell and contains some host-cell membrane proteins, including class I and class II MHC molecules. Within the envelope is the viral core, or nucleocapsid, which includes a layer of a protein called p17 and an inner layer of a protein called p24. The HIV genome consists of two copies of single-stranded RNA, which are associated with two molecules of reverse transcriptase (p64) and nucleoid proteins p10, a protease, and p32, an integrase. (b) Electron micrograph of HIV virions magnified 200,000 times. The glycoprotein projections are faintly visible as "knobs" extending from the periphery of each virion. [Part (a) adapted from BM Peterlin and PA Luciw, 1988, *AIDS* **2:**S29; part (b) from a micrograph by Hans Geldenblom of the Robert Koch Institute (Berlin), in RC Gallo and L Montagnier, 1988, *Sci. Am.* **259**(6):41.]

and is replicated along with the cell DNA. When the provirus is expressed to form new virions, the cell lyses. Alternatively, the provirus may remain latent in the cell until some regulatory signal starts the expression process.

Only one other human retrovirus, human T-cell lymphotropic virus I, or HTLV-I, had been described before HIV-1. This retrovirus is endemic in the southern part of Japan and in the Caribbean. Although most individuals infected with HTLV-I display no clinical signs of disease, a small percentage develop serious illness, either adult T-cell leukemia, which is agggressive and usually fatal, or a disabling progressive neurologic disorder called HTLV-I–associated myelopathy (called tropical spastic paraparesis in early reports). Although comparisons of their genomic sequences revealed that HIV-1 is not a close relative of HTLV-I, similarities in overall characteristics led to use of the name HTLV-III for the AIDS virus in early reports. There is also a related human virus called HIV-2, which is less pathogenic in humans than HIV-1. HIV-2 is similar to viruses isolated from monkeys; it infects certain nonhuman primates that are not infected by HIV-1.

Viruses related to HIV-1 have been found in nonhuman primates. These viruses, variants of simian immunodeficiency virus, or SIV, cause immunodeficiency disease in certain infected monkeys. Normally, SIV strains cause no disease in their normal host but produce immunodeficiency similar to AIDS when injected into another species. For example, the virus from African green monkeys (SIV_{agm}) is present in a high percentage of normal healthy African green monkeys in the wild. However, when SIV_{agm} is injected into macaques, it causes a severe, often lethal immunodeficiency.

A number of other animal retroviruses more or less similar to HIV-1 have been reported. These include the feline and bovine immunodeficiency viruses and the mouse leukemia virus. Study of these animal viruses has yielded information concerning the general nature of retrovirus action, but specific information about HIV-1 cannot be gained by infecting animals because HIV-1 does not replicate in them. Only the chimpanzee supports infection with HIV-1 at a level sufficient to be useful in vaccine trials, but infected chimpanzees only rarely develop AIDS, which limits the value of this model in the study of viral pathogenesis. In addition, the number of chimpanzees available for such studies is low and both the expense and the ethical issues involved in experiments with chimpanzees preclude widespread use of this infection model. The SCID mouse (see above) reconstituted with human lymphoid tissue for infection with HIV-1 has been useful for certain studies of HIV-1 infection, especially in the development of drugs to combat viral replication.

Reasons for the limited host range of HIV-1 include not only the cell-surface receptors required for entry of the virus into the host cell but dependence of the virus on host-cell factors for early events in its replication process, such as transcription and splicing of viral messages. For example, mouse cells transfected with genes that mediate expression of the human receptors for HIV-1 will not support HIV-1 replication because they lack other host factors. By contrast, cells from hamsters or rabbits transfected to express the human receptors support levels of virus replication similar to those seen in human cells. Despite some progress in understanding the factors needed for HIV-1 infection, no clear candidate for an animal model of HIV-1 infection exists. This lack of a suitable infection model hampers efforts to develop both drugs and vaccines to combat AIDS.

In Vitro Studies of the AIDS Virus

The AIDS virus can infect human T cells in culture, replicating itself and in many cases causing the lysis of the cell host (Figure 19-9). Much has been learned about the life cycle of HIV-1 from in vitro studies. The various proteins encoded by the viral genome have been characterized and the function of many of them is known (Figure 19-10).

The first step in HIV infection is viral attachment and entry into the target cell. HIV-1 infects T cells that carry the CD4 antigen on their surface; in addition, certain HIV strains will infect monocytes and other cells that have CD4 on their surface. The preference for $CD4^+$ cells is due to a high-affinity interaction between a coat (envelope or env) protein of HIV-1 and cell-surface CD4. Although the virus binds to CD4 on the cell surface, this interaction alone is not sufficient for entry and productive infection. Expression of other cell-surface molecules, coreceptors present on T cells and monocytes, is required for HIV-1 infection. The infection of a T cell, depicted in Figure 19-11a, is assisted by the T-cell coreceptor CXCR4 (in initial reports, this molecule was called fusin). An analogous receptor called CCR5 functions for the monocyte or macrophage.

After the virus has entered the cell, the RNA genome of the virus is reverse transcribed and a cDNA copy (provirus) integrates into the host genome. The integrated provirus is transcribed and the various viral RNA messages spliced and translated into proteins, which along with a complete new copy of the RNA genome are used to form new viral particles (Figure 19-11b). The gag proteins of the virus are cleaved by the viral protease into the forms that make up the nuclear capsid (see Figure 19-10) in a mature infectious viral particle. As will be described below, different stages in this viral replication process can be targeted by anti-viral drugs.

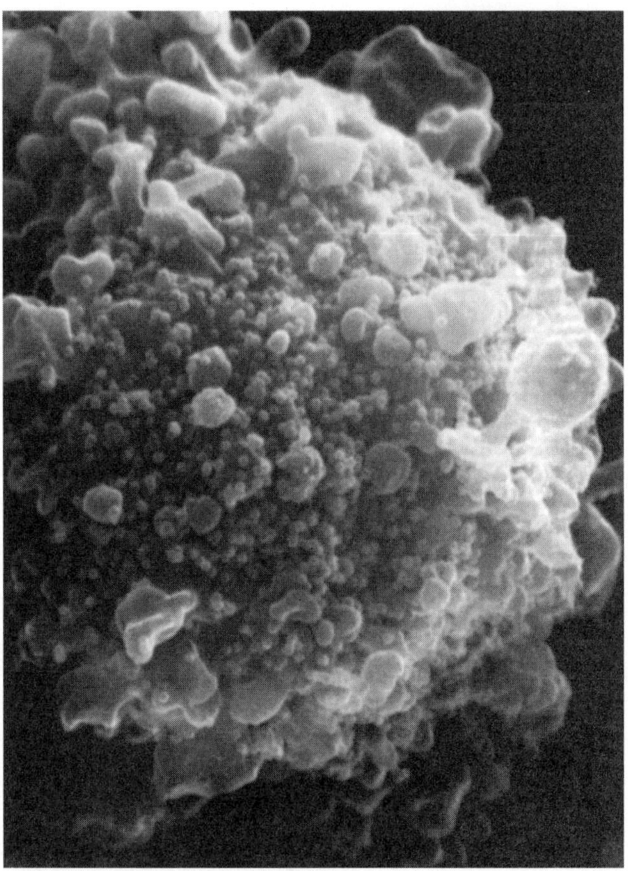

FIGURE 19-9 Once the HIV provirus has been activated, buds representing newly formed viral particles can be observed on the surface of an infected T cell. The extensive cell damage resulting from budding and release of virions leads to the death of infected cells. [Courtesy of RC Gallo, 1988, *J. Acquired Immune Deficiency Syndromes* **1**:521.]

The discovery that CXCR4 and CCR5 serve as coreceptors for HIV-1 on T cells and macrophages, respectively, explained why some strains of HIV-1 preferentially infect T cells (T-tropic strains) while others prefer macrophages (M-tropic strains). A T-tropic strain uses CXCR4, while the M-tropic strains use CCR5. This use of different coreceptors also helped to explain the different roles of cytokines and chemokines in virus replication. It was known from in vitro studies that certain chemokines had a negative effect on virus replication while certain pro-inflammatory cytokines had a positive effect. Both of the HIV coreceptors, CCR5 and CXCR4, function as receptors for chemokines (see Table 15-2). Because the receptors cannot bind simultaneously to HIV-1 and to their chemokine ligand, there is competition for the receptor between the virus and the normal ligand (Figure 19-11c), and the

Go to www.whfreeman.com/immunology Molecular Visualization
Viral Antigens *See Introduction and HIV gp120.*

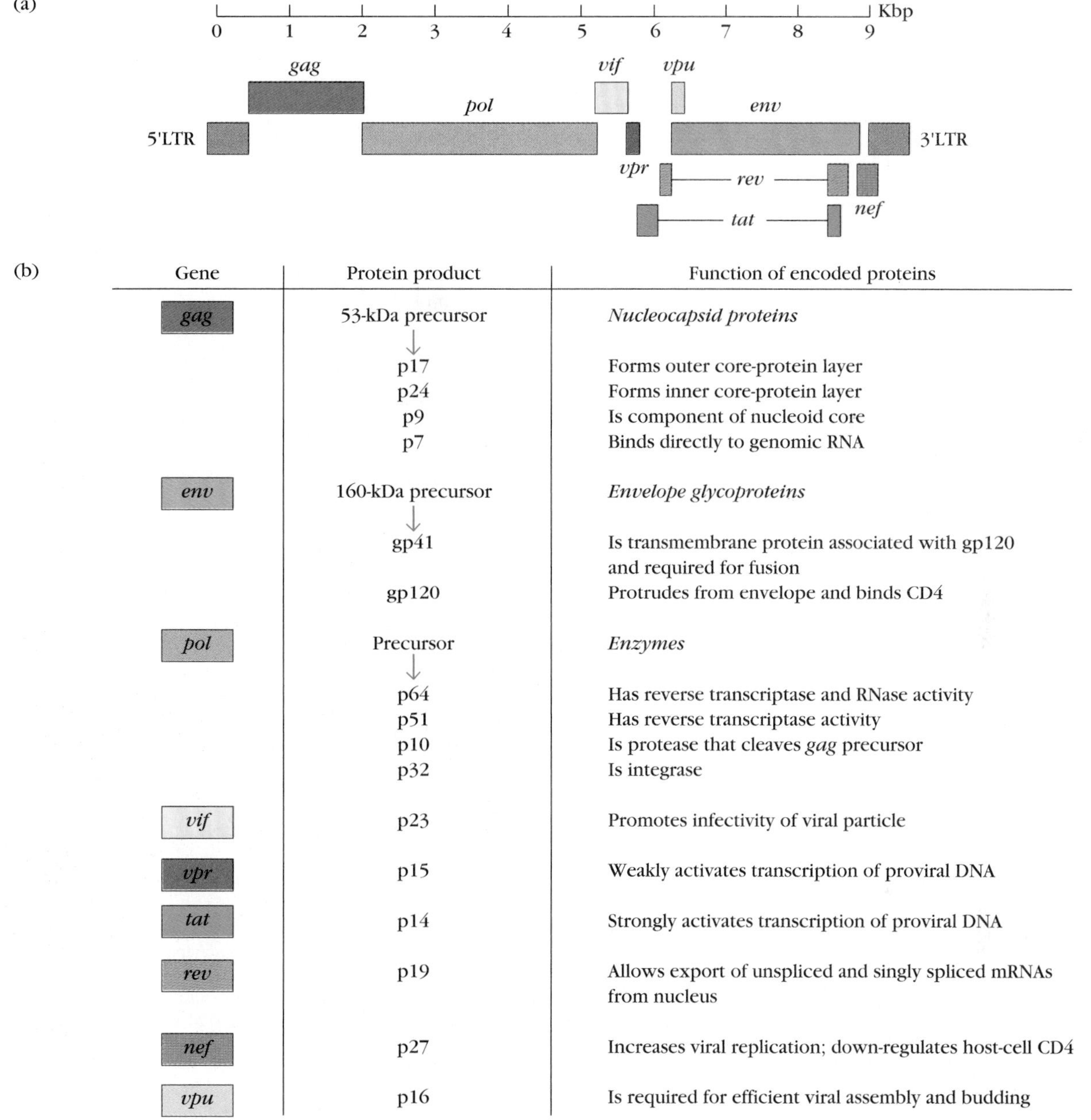

Gene	Protein product	Function of encoded proteins
gag	53-kDa precursor ↓	*Nucleocapsid proteins*
	p17	Forms outer core-protein layer
	p24	Forms inner core-protein layer
	p9	Is component of nucleoid core
	p7	Binds directly to genomic RNA
env	160-kDa precursor ↓	*Envelope glycoproteins*
	gp41	Is transmembrane protein associated with gp120 and required for fusion
	gp120	Protrudes from envelope and binds CD4
pol	Precursor ↓	*Enzymes*
	p64	Has reverse transcriptase and RNase activity
	p51	Has reverse transcriptase activity
	p10	Is protease that cleaves *gag* precursor
	p32	Is integrase
vif	p23	Promotes infectivity of viral particle
vpr	p15	Weakly activates transcription of proviral DNA
tat	p14	Strongly activates transcription of proviral DNA
rev	p19	Allows export of unspliced and singly spliced mRNAs from nucleus
nef	p27	Increases viral replication; down-regulates host-cell CD4
vpu	p16	Is required for efficient viral assembly and budding

FIGURE 19-10 Genetic organization of HIV-1 (a) and functions of encoded proteins (b). The three major genes—*gag, pol,* and *env*—encode polyprotein precursors that are cleaved to yield the nucleocapsid core proteins, enzymes required for replication, and envelope core proteins. Of the remaining six genes, three (*tat, rev,* and *nef*) encode regulatory proteins that play a major role in controlling expression; two (*vif* and *vpu*) encode proteins required for virion maturation; and one (*vpr*) encodes a weak transcriptional activator. The 5′ long terminal repeat (LTR) contains sequences to which various regulatory proteins bind. The organization of the HIV-2 and SIV genomes are very similar, except that the *vpu* gene is replaced by *vpx* in both of these.

chemokine can block viral entry into the host cell. Whereas the chemokines compete with HIV for usage of the coreceptor and thus inhibit viral entry, the pro-inflammatory cytokines induce greater expression of the chemokine receptors on the cell surface, making the cells more susceptible to viral entry.

HIV-1 infection of T cells with certain strains of virus leads to the formation of giant cells or syncytia. These are formed by the fusion of a group of cells caused by the interaction of the viral envelope protein gp120 on the surface of infected cells with CD4 and the coreceptors on the surface of other cells, infected or not. After the initial binding, the action of other cell-adhesion molecules welds the cells together in a large multinuclear mass with a characteristic fused ballooning membrane which eventually bursts. Formation of syncytia may be blocked by antibodies to some of the epitopes of the CD4 molecule, by soluble forms of the CD4 molecule

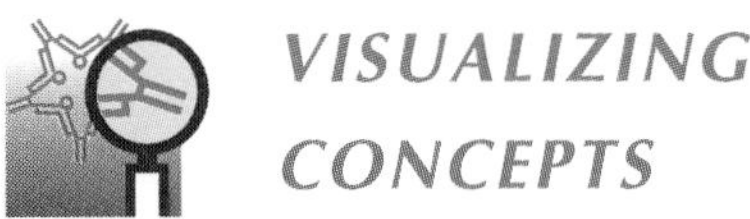

VISUALIZING CONCEPTS

(a) Infection of target cell

(b) Activation of provirus

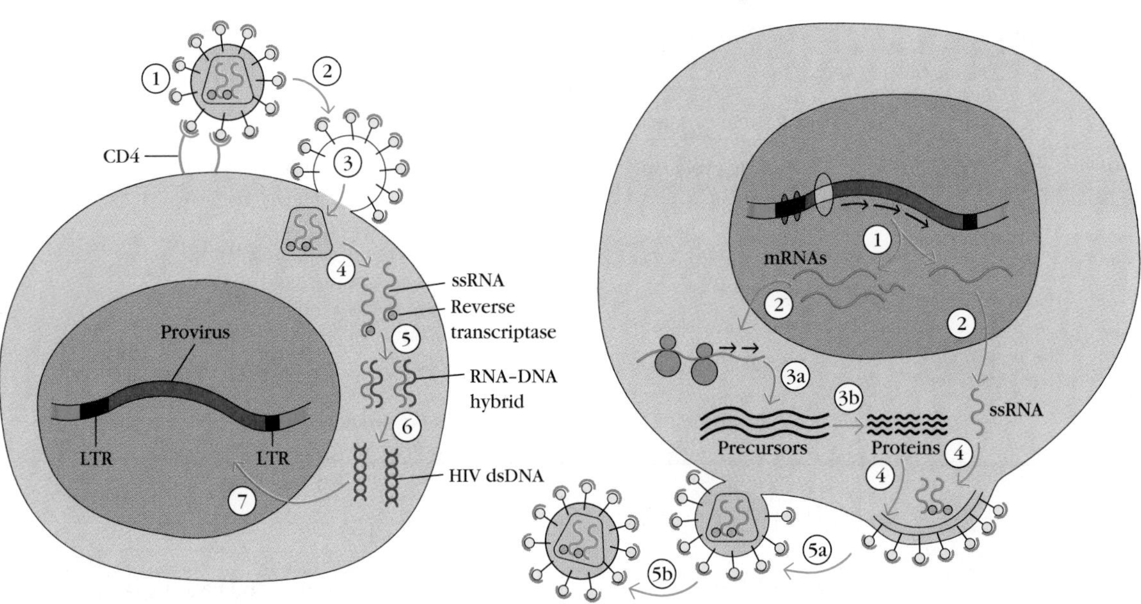

(1) HIV gp120 binds to CD4 on target cell.

(2) Fusogenic domain in gp41 and CXCR4, a G-protein-linked receptor in the target-cell membrane, mediate fusion.

(3) Nucleocapsid containing viral genome and enzymes enters cells.

(4) Viral genome and enzymes are released following removal of core proteins.

(5) Viral reverse transcriptase catalyzes reverse transcription of ssRNA, forming RNA-DNA hybrids.

(6) Original RNA template is partially degraded by ribonuclease H, followed by synthesis of second DNA strand to yield HIV dsDNA.

(7) The viral dsDNA is then translocated to the nucleus and integrated into the host chromosomal DNA by the viral integrase enzyme.

(1) Transcription factors stimulate transcription of proviral DNA into genomic ssRNA and, after processing, several mRNAs.

(2) Viral RNA is exported to cytoplasm.

(3a) Host-cell ribosomes catalyze synthesis of viral precursor proteins.

(3b) Viral protease cleaves precursors into viral proteins.

(4) HIV ssRNA and proteins assemble beneath the host-cell membrane, into which gp41 and gp120 are inserted.

(5a) The membrane buds out, forming the viral envelope.

(5b) Released viral particles complete maturation; incorporated precursor proteins are cleaved by viral protease present in viral particles.

(c)

CXCR4
SDF-1
CD4
T cell
CCR5
RANTES, MIP-1α, MIP-1β
CD4
Monocyte

FIGURE 19-11 Overview of HIV infection of target cells and activation of provirus. (a) Following entry of HIV into cells and formation of dsDNA, integration of the viral DNA into the host-cell genome creates the provirus. (b) The provirus remains latent until events in the infected cell trigger its activation, leading to formation and release of viral particles. (c) Although CD4 binds to the envelope glycoprotein of HIV-1, a second receptor is necessary for entry and infection. The T-cell–tropic strains of HIV-1 use the coreceptor CXCR4, while the macrophage-tropic strains use CCR5. Both are receptors for chemokines, and their normal ligands can block HIV infection of the cell.

Go to www.whfreeman.com/immunology Animation
Retrovirus

(prepared by in vitro expression of a CD4 gene genetically engineered to lack the transmembrane portion), and by antibodies to cell-adhesion molecules. Individual isolates of HIV-1 differ in their ability to induce syncytia formation.

Isolates of HIV-1 from different sources were formerly classified as syncytia-inducing (SI) or non–syncytium-inducing (NSI). In most cases, these differences correlated with the ability of the virus to infect T cells or macrophages: T-tropic strains were SI, whereas M-tropic strains were NSI. More recent classifications of HIV-1 are based on which coreceptor the virus uses; there is good but not absolute correlation between the use of CXCR4, which is present on T cells, and syncytia-inducing ability. The NSI strains use CCR5, which is present on monocytes. Studies of the viral envelope protein gp120 identified a region called the V3 loop, which plays a role in the choice of receptors used by the virus. A recent study by Mark Goldsmith and Bruce Chesebro and their colleagues indicates that a single amino acid difference in this region of gp120 may be sufficient to determine which receptor is used.

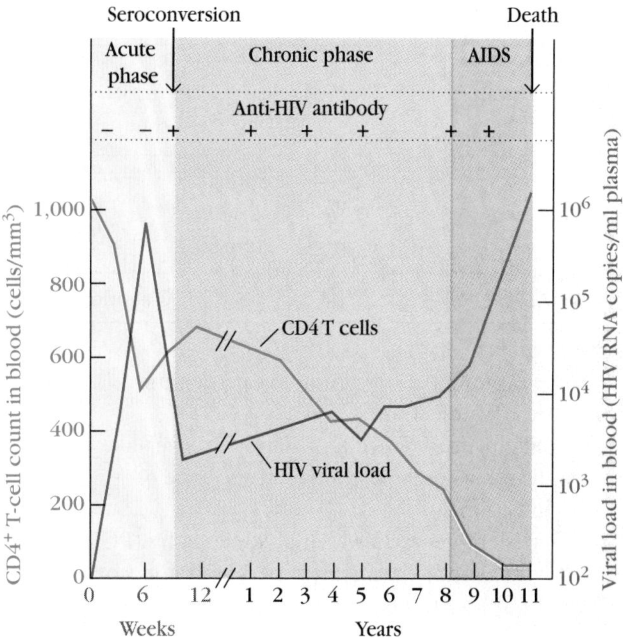

FIGURE 19-12 Serologic profile of HIV infection showing three stages in the infection process. Soon after infection, viral RNA is detectable in the serum. However, HIV infection is most commonly detected by the presence of anti-HIV antibodies after seroconversion, which normally occurs within a few months after infection. Clinical symptoms indicative of AIDS generally do not appear for at least 8 years after infection, but this interval is variable. The onset of clinical AIDS is usually signaled by a decrease in T-cell numbers and an increase in viral load. [Adapted from A Fauci et al, 1996, *Annals Int. Med.* **124**:654.]

Clinical and Immunologic Consequences of HIV-1 Infection

Isolation of HIV-1 and its growth in culture has allowed purification of viral proteins and the development of tests for infection with the virus. The most commonly used test is for the presence of antibodies directed against proteins of HIV-1. These generally appear in the serum of infected individuals by three months after the infection has occurred. When the antibodies appear, the individual is said to have seroconverted or to be seropositive for HIV-1. Although the precise course of HIV-1 infection and disease onset varies considerably in different patients, a general scheme for the progression of AIDS can be constructed (Figure 19-12). The course of HIV-1 infection begins with no detectable anti-HIV-1 antibodies or virus and progresses to the full AIDS syndrome. Diagnosis of AIDS includes evidence for infection with HIV-1 (presence of antibodies or virus in blood), greatly diminished numbers of $CD4^+$ T cells (<200 cells/mm^3), impaired or absent delayed-hypersensitivity reactions, and the occurrence of opportunistic infections (Table 19-3). Patients with AIDS generally succumb to tuberculosis, pneumonia, severe wasting diarrhea, or various malignancies. The time between acquisition of the virus and death from the immunodeficiency averages nine to twelve years. In the period between infection and severe disease, there may be few symptoms. Primary infection in a minority of patients may be symptomatic with fever, lymphadenopathy (swollen lymph nodes), and a rash, but these symptoms generally do not persist more than a few weeks. Most commonly, primary infection goes unnoticed and is followed by a long chronic phase, during which the infected individual shows little or no overt sign of HIV-1 infection.

The first overt indication of AIDS may be opportunistic infection with the fungus *Candida albicans,* which causes the appearance of sores in the mouth (thrush) or, in women, a vulvovaginal yeast infection that does not respond to treatment. A persistent hacking cough caused by *P. carinii* infection of the lungs may also be an early indicator. A rise in the level of circulating HIV-1 in the plasma and concomitant drop in the number of $CD4^+$ T cells generally previews this first appearance of symptoms. Some relation between the $CD4^+$ T-cell number and the type of infection experienced by the patient has been established (see Table 19-3). Of intense interest to immunologists are the events that take place between the initial confrontation with HIV-1 and the takeover and collapse of the host immune system. Understanding how the immune system holds HIV-1 in check during this chronic phase can lead to the design of effective therapeutic and preventive strategies.

Research into the pathogenesic process that underlies the progression of HIV infection to AIDS has revealed a dynamic interplay between the virus and the immune system. The initial infection event causes dissemination of virus to lymphoid organs and a resultant strong immune response. This response, which involves both antibody and cytotoxic $CD8^+$ T lymphocytes, keeps viral replication in check; after the initial burst of viremia (high levels of virus in the circulation), the viral level in the circulation achieves a steady state. Although

TABLE 19-3 CLINICAL DIAGNOSIS OF HIV-INFECTED INDIVIDUALS

	Clinical categories*		
$CD4^+$ T-cell count	A	B	C
≥500/µl	A1	B1	**C1**
200–499/µl	A2	B2	**C2**
<200µl	**A3**	**B3**	**C3**

Classification of AIDS indicator disease

Category A	Category C
Asymptomatic: no symptoms at the time of HIV infection	Candidiasis of bronchi, tracheae, or lungs
Acute primary infection: glandular fever-like illness lasting a few weeks at the time of infection	Candidiasis, esophageal
Persistent generalized lymphadenopathy (PGL): lymph-node enlargement persisting for 3 or more months with no evidence of infection	Cervical cancer (invasive)
	Coccidioidomycosis, disseminated or extrapulmonary
	Cryptococcosis, extrapulmonary
	Cryptosporidiosis, chronic intestinal (>1 month duration)
	Cytomegalovirus disease (other than liver, spleen, or nodes)
	Cytomegalovirus retinitis (with loss of vision)
	Encephalopathy, HIV-related
	Herpes simplex: chronic ulcer(s) (>1 month duration), bronchitis, pneumonitis, or esophagitis
Category B	Histoplasmosis, disseminated or extrapulmonary
Bacillary angiomatosis	Isosporiasis, chronic intestinal (>1 month duration)
Candidiasis, oropharyngeal (thrush)	Kaposi's sarcoma
Candidiasis, vulvovaginal: persistent, frequent, or poorly responsive to therapy	Lymphoma, Burkitt's
Cervical dysplasia (moderate or severe)/cervical carcinoma in situ	Lymphoma, immunoblastic
Constitutional symptoms such as fever (>38.5°C) or diarrhea lasting >1 month	Lymphoma, primary of brain
Hairy leukoplakia, oral	*Mycobacterium avium* complex or *M. Kansasii,* disseminated or extrapulmonary
Herpes zoster (shingles) involving at least two distinct episodes or more than one dermatome	*Mycobacterium tuberculosis,* any site
Idiopathic thrombocytopenic purpura	*Mycobacterium,* other or unidentified species, disseminated or extrapulmonary
Listeriosis	*Pneumocystis carinii* pneumonia
Pelvic inflammatory disease, particularly by tubo-ovarian abscess	Progressive multifocal leukoencephalopathy
Peripheral neuropathy	*Salmonella* septicemia (recurrent)
	Toxoplasmosis of brain
	Wasting syndrome due to HIV

*All categories shown in bold type are considered AIDS. For Category A diagnosis, no condition in categories B or C can be present; for category B, no category C condition can be present.

SOURCE: CDC guidelines for AIDS diagnosis, 1993 revision.

the infected individual normally has no clinical signs of disease at this stage, viral replication continues and virus can be detected in circulation by sensitive PCR assays for viral RNA. These PCR-based assays, which measure **viral load** (the number of copies of viral genome in the plasma), have assumed a major role in determination of the patient's status and prognosis. Even when the level of virus in the circulation is stable, large amounts of virus are produced in infected $CD4^+$ T cells; as many as 10^9 virions are released every day and continually infect and destroy additional host T cells (Figure 19-13a). Despite this high rate of replication, the virus is kept in check by the immune system throughout the chronic phase of infection, and the level of virus in circulation from about six months after infection is a good predictor of the course of disease. Low levels of virus in this period correlate with a longer time in which the infected individual remains free of opportunistic infection. But the virus inevitably breaks through host immune defenses, resulting in an increase in viral load, a decrease in $CD4^+$ T cell numbers, increased opportunistic infection, and eventual death of the patient.

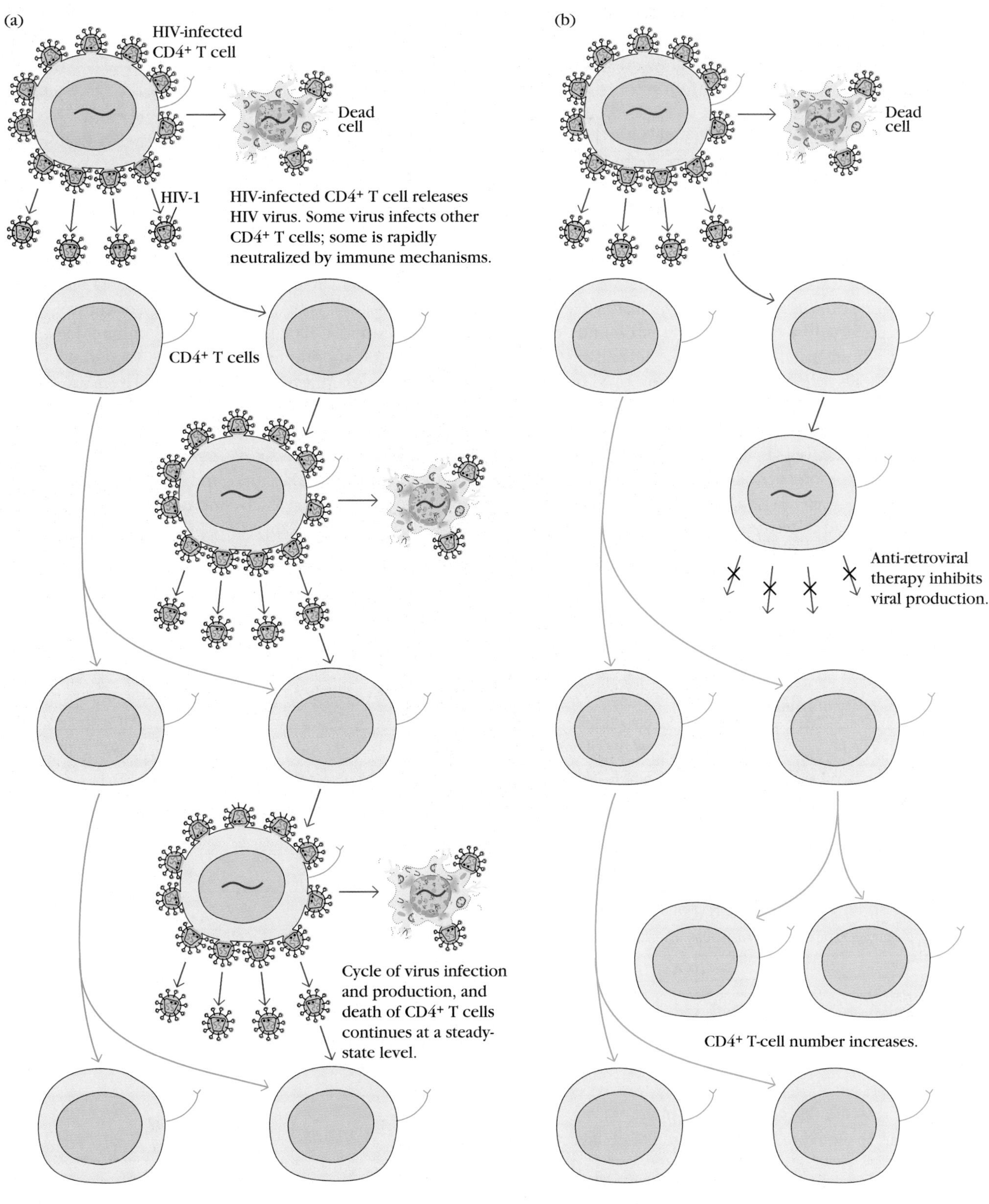

FIGURE 19-13 Production of virus by $CD4^+$ T cells and maintenance of a steady state of viral load and T-cell number. (a) A dynamic relationship exists between the number of $CD4^+$ cells and the amount of virus produced. As virus is produced, new $CD4^+$ cells are infected, and these infected cells have a half-life of 1.5 days. In progression to full AIDS, the viral load increases and the $CD4^+$ T-cell count decreases before onset of opportunistic infections. (b) If the viral load is decreased by anti-retroviral treatment, the $CD4^+$ T-cell number increases almost immediately.

While the viral load in plasma remains fairly stable throughout the period of chronic HIV infection, examination of the lymph nodes has revealed a different story. Fragments of nodes obtained by biopsy from infected subjects showed high levels of infected cells at all stages of infection; in many cases, the structure of the lymph node had been completely destroyed by virus long before plasma viral load increased above the steady-state level.

The decrease in $CD4^+$ T cells is the hallmark of AIDS. Several explanations have been advanced for the depletion of these cells in patients. In early studies, direct viral infection and destruction of $CD4^+$ T cells was discounted as the primary cause, because the large numbers of circulating HIV-infected T cells predicted by the model were not found. More recent studies indicate that the reason for the difficulty in finding the infected cells is that they are so rapidly killed by HIV; the half-life of an actively infected $CD4^+$ T cell is less than 1.5 days. There are smaller numbers of $CD4^+$ T cells that become infected but do not actively replicate virus. These latently infected cells persist for long periods, and the integrated proviral DNA replicates in cell division along with cell DNA. Studies in which viral load is decreased by anti-retroviral therapy show a concurrent increase in $CD4^+$ T cell numbers (Figure 19-13b). These data support a model of dynamic interaction between virus and T cells, with simultaneous high levels of viral production and rapid depletion of infected $CD4^+$ T cells. While other mechanisms for depletion of $CD4^+$ T cells may be envisioned, infection with HIV remains the prime suspect.

Not only depletion of $CD4^+$ T cells, but other immunologic consequences can be measured in HIV-infected individuals during the progression to AIDS. These include a decrease or absence of delayed hypersensitivity to antigens to which the individual normally reacts. Serum levels of immunoglobulins, especially IgG and IgA, show a sharp increase in the AIDS patient. This increase probably relates to the T-cell depletion, with a consequent lack of control over B-cell proliferation. Cellular parameters of immunologic response, such as the proliferative response to mitogens, to antigens, or to alloantigens, all show a marked decrease. Generally, the HIV-infected individual loses the ability to mount T-cell responses in a predictable sequence: responses to specific antigens (for example, influenza virus) are first lost, then response to alloantigens declines, and lastly, the response to mitogens such as concanavalin A or phytohemagglutinin can no longer be detected. Table 19-4 lists some immune abnormalities in AIDS.

TABLE 19-4 IMMUNOLOGIC ABNORMALITIES ASSOCIATED WITH HIV INFECTION

Stage of infection	Typical abnormalities observed
	Lymph node structure
Early	Infection and destruction of dendritic cells; some structural disruption
Late	Extensive damage and tissue necrosis; loss of folicular dendritic cells and germinal centers; inability to trap antigens or support activation of T and B cells
	T helper (T_H) cells
Early	No in vitro proliferative response to specific antigen
Late	Decrease in T_H-cell numbers and corresponding helper activities; no response to T-cell mitogens or alloantigens
	Antibody production
Early	Enhanced nonspecific IgG and IgA production but reduced IgM synthesis
Late	No proliferation of B cells specific for HIV-1: no detectable anti-HIV antibodies in some patients
	Cytokine production
Early	Increased levels of some cytokines
Late	Shift in cytokine production from T_H1 subset to T_H2 subset
	Delayed-type hypersensitivity
Early	Highly significant reduction in proliferative capacity of T_{DTH} cells and reduction in skin-test reactivity
Late	Elimination of DTH response; complete absence of skin-test reactivity
	T cytotoxic (T_C) cells
Early	Normal reactivity
Late	Reduction but not elimination of CTL activity due to impaired ability to generate CTLs from T_C cells

HIV-1 infected individuals often display dysfunction of the central and peripheral nervous systems. HIV-1 infects cells in the central nervous system (CNS). Specific viral DNA and RNA sequences have been detected by HIV-1 probes in the brains of children and adults with AIDS, suggesting that viral replication occurs there. Quantitative comparison of specimens from brain, lymph node, spleen, and lung of AIDS patients with progressive encephalopathy indicated that the brain was heavily infected. A frequent complication in later stages of HIV infection is AIDS dementia complex, a neurological syndrome characterized by abnormalities in cognition, motor performance, and behavior. Whether AIDS dementia and other clinical and histopathological effects observed in the CNS of HIV-infected individuals are a direct effect of viral antigens on the brain, a consequence of immune responses to the virus, or a result of infection by opportunistic agents remains unknown.

Therapeutic Agents to Combat AIDS

Development of a vaccine to prevent the spread of AIDS is the highest priority for immunologists, but it is also critical to develop drugs and therapies that can reverse the effects of HIV-1 in infected individuals. The number of HIV-infected persons is estimated to be close to 1 million in the United States alone; for all of these individuals to develop AIDS would be an enormous human tragedy. There are several possible strategies for development of effective anti-viral drugs. The life cycle of HIV shows several susceptible points that might be blocked by pharmaceutical agents (Figure 19-14). The key to success of such therapies is that they must be specific for HIV-1 and interfere minimally with normal cell processes. Thus far, two types of antiviral agents have found their way into common usage. The first success in treatment was with drugs that interfere with the reverse transcription of viral RNA to cDNA; several drugs in common use operate at this step. A second stage of viral replication that has proved amenable to blockade is the step at which precursor proteins are cleaved into the units needed for construction of a new mature virion. This step requires the action of a specific viral protease, which can be inhibited by chemical agents; this precludes the formation of infectious viral particles.

Several antiretroviral drugs are now in widespread use (Table 19-5) that either interfere with reverse transcription or inhibit the viral protease. The prototype of the drugs that interfere with reverse transcription is zidovudine, or AZT. The introduction of AZT, a nucleoside analog, into the growing cDNA chain of the retrovirus causes termination of the chain. AZT is effective in some but not all patients, but its efficacy is limited also because long-term use has several adverse side affects and because resistant viral mutants develop in treated patients. The administered AZT is used not only by the HIV-1 reverse transcriptase but also by human DNA polymerase. The incorporation of AZT into the DNA of host cells kills them. Precursors of red blood cells are especially sensitive to AZT, which thus causes anemia in addition to other side effects. In addition to drugs such as AZT, which interfere with reverse transcription by inserting a nucleoside analog into the growing cDNA chain, there are also drugs such as Nevirapine, which inhibit the action of the reverse transcriptase enzyme (see Table 19-5).

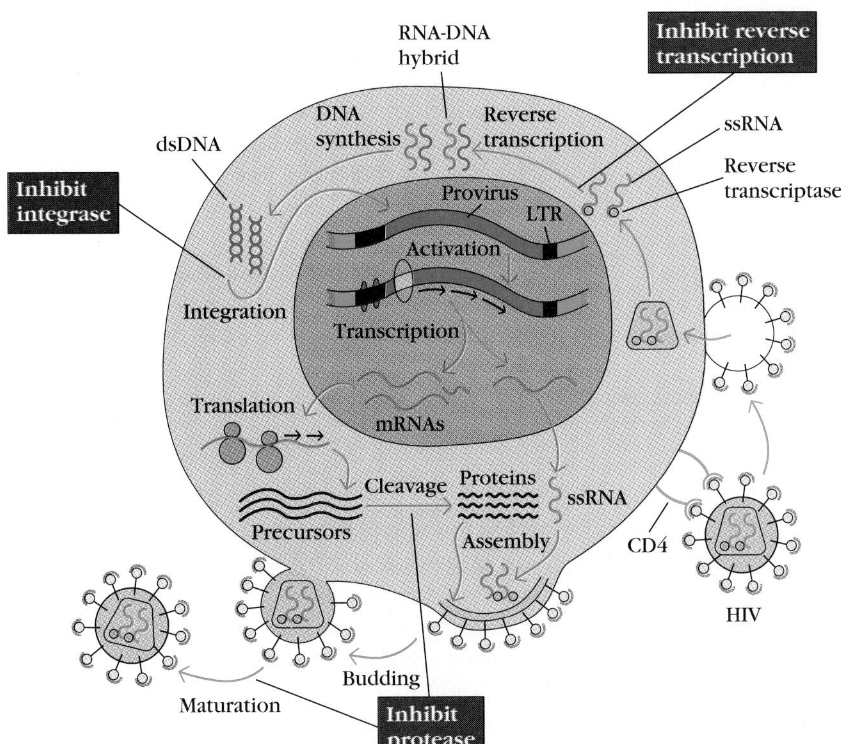

FIGURE 19-14 Stages in the viral replication cycle that provide targets for therapeutic antiretroviral drugs. At present, the licensed drugs with anti-HIV activity block the step of reverse transcription of viral RNA to cDNA or inhibit the viral protease necessary to cleave viral precursor proteins into the proteins needed to assemble a new virion and complete its maturation to infectious virus.

Go to www.whfreeman.com/immunology Molecular Visualization
HIV-1 Reverse Transcriptase

TABLE 19-5 SOME ANTI-HIV DRUGS IN CLINICAL USE

Generic name (other names)	Typical dosage	Some potential side effects
	Reverse transcriptase inhibitors: Nucleoside analog	
Didanosine (Videx, ddl)	2 pills, 2 times a day on empty stomach	Nausea, diarrhea, pancreatic inflammation, peripheral neuropathy
Lamivudine (Epivir, 3TC)	1 pill, 2 times a day	Usually none
Stavudine (Zerit, d4T)	1 pill, 2 times a day	Peripheral neuropathy
Zalcitabine (HIVID, ddC)	1 pill, 3 times a day	Peripheral neuropathy, mouth inflammation, pancreatic inflammation
Zidovudine (Retrovir, AZT)	1 pill, 2 times a day	Nausea, headache, anemia, neutropenia (reduced levels of neutrophil white blood cells), weakness, insomnia
Pill containing lamivudine and zidovudine (Combivir)	1 pill, 2 times a day	Same as for zidovudine
	Reverse transcriptase inhibitors: Nonnucleoside analogues	
Delavirdine (Rescriptor)	4 pills, 3 times a day (mixed into water); not within an hour of antacids or didanosine	Rash, headache, hepatitis
Nevirapine (Viramune)	1 pill, 2 times a day	Rash, hepatitis
	Protease inhibitors	
Indinavir (Crixivan)	2 pills, 3 times a day on empty stomach or with a low-fat snack and not within 2 hours of didanosine	Kidney stones, nausea, headache, blurred vision, dizziness, rash, metallic taste in mouth, abnormal distribution of fat, elevated triglyceride and cholesterol levels, glucose intolerance
Nelfinavir (Viracept)	3 pills, 3 times a day with some food	Diarrhea, abnormal distribution of fat, elevated triglyceride and cholesterol levels, glucose intolerance
Ritonavir (Norvir)	6 pills, 2 times a day (or 4 pills, 2 times a day if taken with saquinavir) with food and not within 2 hours of didanosine	Nausea, vomiting, diarrhea, abdominal pain, headache, prickling sensation in skin, hepatitis, weakness, abnormal distribution of fat, elevated triglyceride and cholesterol levels, glucose intolerance
Saquinavir (Invirase, a hard-gel capsule; Fortovase, a soft-gel capsule)	6 pills, 3 times a day (or 2 pills, 2 times a day if taken with ritonavir) with a large meal	Nausea, diarrhea, headache, abnormal distribution of fat, elevated triglyceride and cholesterol levels, glucose intolerance

SOURCE: JG Bartlett and RD Moore, 1998, Improving HIV therapy, *Sci. Am.* **279**(1):87.

Use of the second class of successful drugs, called protease inhibitors, in conjunction with AZT and/or other nucleoside analogs has proven effective. Current treatment for AIDS is a combination therapy, using regimens designated HAART (highly active anti-retroviral therapy). In most cases, this combines the use of two nucleoside analogs and one protease inhibitor. This strategy appears to overcome the ability of the virus to rapidly produce mutants that are drug resistant. In many cases, HAART has lowered viral load to levels that are not detectable by current methods and has improved the health of AIDS patients to the point that they can again function at a normal level. The decrease in the number of AIDS deaths in the United States in recent years (see Figure 19-6) is attributed to this advance in therapy. Despite the optimism engendered by success with HAART, present drawbacks include a strict time schedule of administration and the large number of pills to be taken every day. In addition, there may be serious side effects (see Table 19-5) that, in some patients, may be too severe to allow use of HAART.

The success of HAART in treating AIDS has opened discussion of whether it might be possible to eradicate all of the virus from an infected individual and thus actually cure AIDS. Most AIDS experts are not convinced that this is possible, mainly because of the persistence of latently infected $CD4^+$ T cells and macrophages, which can serve as a reservoir of infectious virus if the provirus should be activated. Even with a viral load beneath the level of detection by PCR assays, the immune system may not recover sufficiently to clear virus should it begin to replicate in response to some activation signal. In addition, virus may persist in sites such as the brain, not readily penetrated by the antiretroviral drugs, even though the virus in circulation is undetectable. The use of immune modulators, such as recombinant IL-2, in conjunction with HAART is being examined as a strategy to help reconstitute the immune system and restore normal immune function.

In addition to the drugs in widespread use, others are in various stages of development. One class of drugs that appears promising are those that interfere with integration of the viral DNA into the host genome (see Figure 19-14). Others being considered act at the stage of viral attachment to the host cell. It should be stressed that the development of any drug to the point at which it can be used for patients is a long and arduous procedure. The drugs that pass the rigorous tests for safety and efficacy represent a small fraction of those that receive initial consideration.

TABLE 19-6 WHY AIDS DOES NOT FIT THE PARADIGM FOR CLASSIC VACCINE DEVELOPMENT

Classic vaccines mimic natural immunity against reinfection generally seen in individuals recovered from infection; there are no recovered AIDS patients.

Most vaccines protect against disease, not against infection; HIV infection may remain latent for long periods before causing AIDS.

Most vaccines protect for years against viruses that change very little over time; HIV-1 mutates at a rapid rate and efficiently selects mutant forms that evade immunity.

Most effective vaccines are whole-killed or live-attenuated organisms; killed HIV-1 does not retain antigenicity and the use of a live retrovirus vaccine raises safety issues.

Most vaccines protect against infections that are infrequently encountered; HIV may be encountered daily by individuals at high risk.

Most vaccines protect against infections through mucosal surfaces of the respiratory or gastrointestinal tract; the great majority of HIV infection is through the genital tract.

Most vaccines are tested for safety and efficacy in an animal model before trials with human volunteers; there is no suitable animal model for HIV/AIDS at present.

SOURCE: Adapted from AS Fauci, 1996, An HIV vaccine: breaking the paradigms, *Proc. Am. Assoc. Phys.* **108:**6.

Vaccines to Prevent AIDS

The AIDS epidemic continues to rage despite the advances in therapeutic approaches outlined above. The present expense of HAART (as much as $15,000 per year), the strict regimen required, and the possibility of side effects precludes universal application. Even if eradication of the virus in individuals treated with combination therapy becomes possible, it will not greatly influence the epidemic in the developing countries, which include the majority of AIDS victims. It is likely that effective, inexpensive, and well-tolerated drugs will be developed in the future, but at present it appears that the best option to stop the spread of AIDS is a safe, effective vaccine that prevents infection and progression to disease. Why do we not have an AIDS vaccine? The best answer to this question is to examine the special conditions that must be addressed in developing a safe, effective vaccine for this disease (Table 19-6).

Most effective vaccines mimic the natural state of infection. Those recovered from most diseases are immune from subsequent attacks. The infection by HIV-1 and progression to immunodeficiency syndrome flourishes even in the presence of circulating antibodies directed against proteins of the virus. Immunity may hold the virus in check for a time, but as mentioned above, it rarely exceeds 12 years. In a rare subset of infected individuals called long-term nonprogressors, the period of infection without disease is longer and even indefinite. However, the exact state of immunity (which antibodies are present and what type of cellular immunity is active) in these individuals is not clear or consistent and therefore difficult to duplicate for vaccine development. More to the point, most long-term nonprogressors have mutations in genes encoding cell coreceptors that slow the progress of viral attack on their immune system, rather than an immune response that is holding HIV replication in check.

Most vaccines prevent disease, not infection. Polio and influenza vaccines hold the virus produced by infected cells in check so that it does not cause harm to the host, and it is then cleared. HIV-1 does not fit this model, because it integrates into the host genome and may remain latent for long periods. As described above in the context of treatment strategies, eradication of a retrovirus is not a simple matter. Clearance of a retrovirus is a difficult goal for a vaccine; every copy of the virus and every infected cell, including those latently infected, must be eradicated from the host. However even without complete eradication, an HIV vaccine may benefit the infected individual; furthermore, such a vaccine would help to control the spread of infection, because those with low viral load are less likely to be infectious.

Most vaccines prevent infection by viruses that show little variation. The instability of its genome differentiates HIV-1 from most viruses for which successful vaccines have been developed. With the exception of influenza, for which the vaccines must be changed periodically, most viruses that can be controlled by immunization show only minor variability in structure. For comparison, consider that the rhinoviruses that cause the common cold have more than 100 subtypes; therefore no effective vaccine has been developed. HIV-1 shows variation in most viral antigens; and the rate of replication may be as high as 10^9 viruses per day. This variability along with the high rate of replication allows the production of viruses with multiple mutations; some of these allow escape from immunity. The fact that significant differences in viral envelope protein sequences have been seen in viral isolates taken from the same patient at different times indicates that variation occurs and that some of the variants replicate, presumably because they have learned to evade host immune defenses. Data showing that antibody from advanced AIDS patients will not neutralize virus isolated from that patient, but will kill other strains of HIV-1, argues that HIV-1 does evade the immune system by mutation of proteins targeted by antibody.

The majority of successful vaccines are live-attenuated or heat-killed organisms. While there are exceptions to this, notably the recombinant protein used for hepatitis B vaccine and the conjugate used for *Haemophilus influenzae* B vaccine (see Chapter 18), most of the widely used vaccines are attenuated organisms. The development of a live-attenuated retrovirus vaccine from animal viruses engineered to include HIV antigens is a possible route. However, the use of live vaccines is predicated on the supposition that the immunity raised will clear the vaccine virus from the host. This is not easily done for a retrovirus, which integrates into the host genome. A massive testing effort would have to assure the safety of a live retroviral vaccine, which could cause chronic host infection.

For most viruses, the frequency of exposure to infection is rare or seasonal. In many high-risk individuals, such as commercial sex workers, monogamous sexual partners of HIV-infected subjects, and intravenous drug users, the virus is encountered frequently and, potentially, in large doses. An AIDS vaccine is thus asked to prevent infection against a constant attack by the virus and/or massive doses of virus; this is not normally the case with other viruses for which immunization has proved successful.

Most vaccines protect against respiratory or gastrointestinal infection. In addition to the frequency of exposure to HIV, which may be extraordinarily high for some high-risk individuals, there is also the question of route. The majority of successful vaccines protect against viruses that are encountered in the respiratory and gastrointestinal tracts; the most common route of HIV-1 infection is by the genital tract. It is not known whether the immunity established by conventional vaccination procedures will protect against infection by this route. Furthermore, the lack of a completely relevant animal model precludes an in-depth test of protection against challenge by the genital route.

Development of most vaccines through to clinical trials relies upon animal experiments. Testing a vaccine for safety and efficacy normally involves challenge of an animal with the virus under conditions similar to those encountered in the human. In this way, the correlates of protective immunity are established. For example, if high titers of $CD8^+$ T cells and neutralizing antibody are necessary for protection in an animal, then $CD8^+$ T-cell immunity and antibody should be measured in human trials of the vaccine. Thus far, animal studies of HIV infection and disease have not yielded consistent information about immune responses that are protective against infection or that prevent progression to disease. While there are extensive data from studies of various SIV strains in different types of monkeys, no unifying conclusion can be drawn at this point. Most results involve a specific virus in a particular host and are not easily extrapolated to universal concepts, because they depend upon host factors as well the relationships between the immunizing and challenge strains of virus.

In studies of vaccine candidates that have progressed to human trials, the results thus far are disappointing. In a group of individuals inoculated with the gp120 molecules from different HIV-1 strains or with a placebo vaccine, 18 subjects became infected over the course of the first two years of the study. Sixteen of those infected were in the group receiving the vaccine and only 2 were in the group that received a placebo. Although antibody was demonstrated, the vaccinated individuals were not protected by these viral envelope glycoproteins.

In addition to factors listed above, behavioral and social issues influence the development and testing of candidate AIDS vaccines. Counseling concerning safe sexual practice must be part of the care given to volunteers in a vaccine trial. Will this influence the results? Would a lowering of the infection rate in all groups taking part in the trial preclude seeing a meaningful difference in the infection rate between the vaccine and the placebo groups? A further consideration is the fact that anyone successfully immunized against the AIDS virus will become seropositive and will test positive in the standard screening assays for infection. What ramifications will this have? What type of tests must be carried out to ascertain whether the immunized individual is actually infected?

It is clear that development of an AIDS vaccine is not a simple exercise in classic vaccine development. More research is needed to understand how this viral attack against

TABLE 19-7 VACCINE STRATEGIES UNDER STUDY

Vaccine constituents	Status	Advantages	Disadvantages
Vaccines eliciting anti-HIV antibodies			
Viral surface proteins, such as gp120	In phase I and II trials, which examine safety	Safe and simple to prepare	Vaccine-elicited antibodies have failed to recognize HIV from patients
Whole, killed HIV	Not under study in humans	Should present HIV surface proteins in a relatively natural conformation; simple to prepare	Slight risk that preparations might include some active virus; inactivated virus might shed its proteins and become ineffective
Pseudovirions (artificial viruses containing HIV surface proteins)	Close to phase I trials	Present HIV surface proteins in a relatively natural conformation	Difficult to produce and to ensure long-term stability
Vaccines eliciting cellular responses			
Live vector viruses (non-HIV viruses engineered to carry genes encoding HIV proteins)	In phase II trials	Makers can control amount and kinds of viral proteins produced	Complicated to prepare; current vaccines elicit modest immune response
Naked DNA containing one or more HIV genes	In phase I trials	Simple and inexpensive to prepare	Some worry that integration of HIV genes into human cells could harm patients
HIV peptides (protein fragments)	In phase I trials	Simple to prepare	Do not elicit strong immune response
Vaccines eliciting antibody and cellular responses			
Combinations of elements, such as pure gp120 protein plus canarypox vector	In phase II trials	Should stimulate both arms of the immune response at once	Complicated to prepare
Live, attenuated HIV	Not under study in humans; being assessed in nonhuman primates	Most closely mimics HIV; may interfere with ability of infectious HIV to replicate	Vaccine virus could potentially cause AIDS

SOURCE: D Baltimore and C Heilman, "HIV vaccines: prospects and challenges," 1998, *Sci. Am.* **279** (1):101.

the immune system can be thwarted. While much has been written about the subject and large-scale initiatives are proposed, the path to an effective vaccine is not obvious. It is only certain that all data must be carefully analyzed and that all possible means of creating immunity must be tested. This is one of the greatest public health challenges of our time. An intense and cooperative effort must be launched to devise, test, and deliver a safe and effective vaccine for AIDS. The status of current efforts in AIDS vaccine development is summarized in Table 19-7.

Summary

1. Immunodeficiency results from the failure of one or more components of the immune system. Primary immunodeficiencies are caused by genetic or developmental defects, secondary immunodeficiencies arise from a variety of causes, including X-radiation, treatment with cytolytic and immunosuppressive drugs, and infections, notably with HIV-1.

2. Immunodeficiency may be classified by the cell types involved; it may affect either the lymphoid or the myeloid cell lineages or both (see Figure 19-1). The gene defects that underlie primary immunodeficiency are being identified, providing a more precise classification (see Figure 19-2 and Table 19-1).
3. Lymphoid immunodeficiencies may affect either T cells, B cells, or both. Many immunodeficiencies are caused by genetic defects in molecules involved in signal transduction or in cellular communication (see Figure 19-3). Failure of thymic development results in severe immunodeficiency and can hinder normal development of B cells, because of the lack of cellular cooperation.
4. Severe combined immunodeficiency or SCID is caused by a variety of defects across the lymphoid lineage and is usually fatal. Selective immunoglobulin deficiencies, which are less severe, occur as a result of defects in specific, more highly differentiated cell types.
5. Myeloid immunodeficiency causes impaired phagocytic function. Those affected suffer from increased susceptibility to bacterial infection.
6. Immunodeficiency may be treated by replacement of the defective or missing protein, cells, or gene. Administration of human immunoglobulin is the most common treatment; increasingly, bone-marrow transplantation is used and experimental gene-therapy strategies are being tested.
7. There are several animal models for immunodeficiency. The most commonly used are nude (see Figure 19-5) and SCID mice. Gene knockout mice provide a tool to study the effects of specific genes on immune function.
8. The most common secondary or acquired immunodeficiency is caused by a human retrovirus, human immunodeficiency virus 1 (HIV-1; see Figures 19-8 and 19-11). This has given rise to an epidemic of the disease called AIDS (see Figure 19-7), which is characterized by loss of $CD4^+$ T cells and profound immunodeficiency.
9. HIV-1 infection is spread mainly by sexual contact, passage of blood or blood products, and from HIV-infected mother to infant. Infection with HIV-1 leads to death from opportunistic infection (see Table 19-3), usually within 10 years of infection.
10. AIDS is treated with anti-retroviral drugs that are nucleoside analogs or inhibitors of the viral protease (see Figure 19-14 and Table 19-5). There are barriers to the development of an effective vaccine that would prevent HIV infection or forestall development of disease in infected individuals (see Table 19-6); there is an extensive research effort to find a safe effective vaccine (see Table 19-7).

REFERENCES

Ameisen, JC, et al. 1995. The relevance of apoptosis to AIDS pathogenesis. *Trends Cell Biol.* **5**:27.

Bemiller, LS, et al. 1995. Safety and effectiveness of long-term interferon gamma therapy in patients with chronic granulomatous disease. *Blood Cells, Molecules, and Diseases* **21**:239–247.

Berger, EA. 1997. HIV-1 entry and tropism: the chemokine receptor connection. *AIDS* **11**(Supp A):S3.

Blanchard, A, L Montagnier, and ML Gougeon. 1997. Influence of microbial infections on the progression of HIV disease. *Trends Microbiol.* **5**:326.

Buckley, RH, et al. 1997. Human severe combined immunodeficiency: genetic, phenotypic, and functional diversity in one hundred eight infants. *J. Pediatr.* **130**:378.

Burton, DR, and JP Moore. 1998. Why do we not have an HIV vaccine and how can we make one? *Nature Med.* (Vaccine Supplement) **4**:495.

Carmichael, C. 1997. Prevention and treatment of common HIV-associated opportunistic complications. *Primary Care; Clinics in Office Practice* **24**:561.

Coffin, JM, SH Hughe, and H Varmus, eds. 1997. *Retroviruses.* Cold Spring Harbor Laboratory Press, New York.

Cohen, OJ, A Kinter, and AS Fauci. 1997. Host factors in the pathogenesis of HIV disease. *Immunol. Rev.* **159**:31.

Cohen, OJ, et al. 1997. Studies on lymphoid tissue from HIV-infected individuals: implications for the design of therapeutic strategies. *Springer Sem. Immunopathol.* **18**:305.

Connor, RI, et al. 1998. Imunological and virological analyses of persons infected by human immunodeficiency virus type 1 while participating in trials of recombinant gp120 subunit vaccines. *J. Virology* **72**:1552.

Defeating AIDS: What Will It Take? Scientific American Special Report, July 1998, p. 81.

Doms, RW, and JP Moore. 1997. HIV-1 coreceptor use: a molecular window into viral tropism. pp. III-25–36. In BTM Korber et al, eds., *HIV Molecular Immunology Database 1997.* Theoretical Biology and Biophysics, Los Alamos National Laboratories. Los Alamos, NM.

Elder, ME. 1997. SCID due to ZAP-70 deficiency. *J. Pediatr. Hematol. Oncol.* **19**:546.

Fauci, AS. 1996. An HIV vaccine: breaking the paradigms. *Proc. Assoc. Am. Phys.* **108**:6.

Feng, Y, et al. 1996. HIV-1 entry cofactor: functional cDNA cloning of a seven-transmembrane G protein–coupled receptor. *Science* **272**:872.

Fischer, A, et al. 1997. Naturally occurring primary deficiencies of the immune system. *Annu. Rev. Immunol.* **15**:93.

Flake, AW, et al. 1996. Treatment of X-linked severe combined immunodeficiency by in utero transplantation of paternal bone marrow. *N. Eng. J. Med.* **335**:1806.

Hilleman, MR, 1996. Strategies for the achievement of prophylactic vaccination against HIV. *Antibiotics and Chemotherapy* **48**:161.

Ho, D, et al. 1995. Rapid turnover of plasma virions and CD4 lymphocytes in HIV-1 infection. *Nature* **373**:123.

Kaneshima, H. 1996. HIV-1–associated pathology in hematolymphoid organs and the experimental evaluation in the SCID-hu mouse. *Int. J. Hematol.* **63**:253.

Leonard, WJ. 1997. Genetic effects on immunity. Protein tyrosine kinases: disease loci for inherited immunodeficiencies. *Curr. Opin. Immunol.* **9**:525.

Levy, J. 1998. *HIV and the Pathogenesis of AIDS*, 2nd ed. American Society for Microbiology. Washington, DC.

Malech, HL, et al. 1997. Prolonged production of NADPH oxidase-corrected granulocytes after gene therapy of chronic granulomatous disease. *Proc. Natl. Acad. Sci. USA* **94**:12133.

Malech, HL, and WM Nauseef. 1997. Primary inherited defects in neutrophil function: etiology and treatment. *Semin. Hematol.* **34**:279.

Markert, ML, et al. 1997. Complete DiGeorge syndrome: persistence of profound immunodeficiency. *J. Pediatr.* **132**(1):15.

Onodera, M, et al. 1998. Successful peripheral T-lymphocyte–directed gene transfer for a patient with severe combined immune deficiency caused by adenosine deaminase deficiency. *Blood* **91**:30.

Puck, JM. 1997. Primary immunodeficiency diseases. *JAMA* **278**:1835.

Resta, R, and LF Thompson. 1997. SCID: the role of adenosine deaminase deficiency. *Immunol. Today* **18**:371.

Rosen, FS, MD Cooper, and RJ Wedgwood. 1995. The primary immunodeficiencies. *N. Engl. J. Med.* **333**:431.

Russell, SM, et al. 1995. Mutation of Jak3 in a patient with SCID: essential role of Jak3 in lymphoid development. *Science* **270**:797.

Smart, BA, and HD Ochs. 1997. The molecular basis and treatment of primary immunodeficiency disorders. *Curr. Opin. Pediatr.* **9**:570.

Speck, RF, et al. 1997. Selective employment of chemokine receptors as human immunodeficiency virus type 1 coreceptors determined by individual amino acids within the envelope V3 loop. *J. Virol.* **71**:7136.

Steimle, V, W Reith, and B Mach. 1996. Major histocompatibility complex class II deficiency: a disease of gene regulation. *Adv. Immunol.* **61**:327.

Stine, GT, 1998. *Acquired Immunodeficiency Syndrome: Biological, Medical, Social and Legal Issues,* 3rd ed. Prentice-Hall.

Wei, X, et al. 1995. Viral dynamics in human immunodeficiency virus type 1 infection. *Nature* **373**:117.

Weil, WM, et al. 1997. Genetic correction of p67^{phox}-deficient chronic granulomatous disease using peripheral blood progenitor cells as a target for retrovirus mediated gene transfer. *Blood* **89**:1754.

Useful Web Sites

http://www.scid.net/
The SCID home page contains links to periodicals and databases with information about SCID.

http://www.nhgri.nih.gov/DIR/LGT/SCID/
This site from the National Insitute for Human Genome Research includes a database of mutations in X-linked SCID.

http://hivinsite.ucsf.edu
Information about the global AIDS epidemic can be accessed from this site.

http://www.cdc.gov
Up-to-date information concerning AIDS epidemiology in the United States can be obtained at this site.

ftp://nlmpubs.nlm.nih.gov/aids/adatabases/drugs.txt
A listing with detailed information for several hundred drugs under development for HIV infection and opportunistic infections associated with AIDS; maintained by the National Library of Medicine.

http://www.niaid.nih.gov/daids/vaccine/abtvaccines.htm
Information about AIDS vaccines from the National Institute of Allergy and Infectious Diseases, NIH. Includes links to documents about vaccines in general.

STUDY QUESTIONS

1. Indicate whether each of the following statements is true or false. If you think a statement is false, explain why.

a. DiGeorge syndrome is a congenital birth defect resulting in absence of the thymus.

b. X-linked agammaglobulinemia (XLA) is a combined B-cell and T-cell immunodeficiency disease.

c. The hallmark of a phagocytic deficiency is increased susceptibility to viral infections.

d. In chronic granulomatous disease, the underlying defect is in a cytochrome or an associated protein.

e. Gamma-globulin injections are given to treat individuals with X-linked agammaglobulinemia.

f. Multiple defects have been identified in human SCID.

g. Mice with the SCID defect lack functional B and T lymphocytes.

h. Mice with SCID-like phenotype can be produced by knockout of RAG genes.

i. Children born with SCID often manifest increased infections by encapsulated bacteria in the first months of life.

j. Failure to express class II MHC molecules in bare-lymphocyte syndrome affects cell-mediated immunity only.

2. Granulocytes from patients with leukocyte-adhesion deficiency (LAD) express greatly reduced amounts of three integrin molecules designated CR3, CR4, and LFA-1.

a. What is the nature of the defect that results in decreased expression or in no expression of these receptors in LAD patients?

b. What is the normal function of the integrin molecule LFA-1? Give specific examples.

3. Immunologists have studied the defect in SCID mice in an effort to understand the molecular basis for severe combined immunodeficiency in humans. In both SCID mice and humans with this disorder, mature B and T cells fail to develop.

a. In what way do rearranged Ig heavy-chain genes in SCID mice differ from those in normal mice?

b. In SCID mice, rearrangement of κ light-chain DNA is not attempted. Explain why.

Go to www.whfreeman.com/immunology 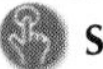 Self-Test
Review and quiz of key terms

c. If you introduced a rearranged, functional μ heavy-chain gene into progenitor B cells of SCID mice, would the κ light-chain DNA undergo a normal rearrangement? Explain your answer.

4. The accompanying figure outlines some of the steps in the development of immune-system cells. The numbered arrows indicate the cell type whose function is defective or the developmental step that does not occur in particular immunodeficiency diseases. Identify the defective cell type or developmental step associated with each of the following diseases. Use each number only once.

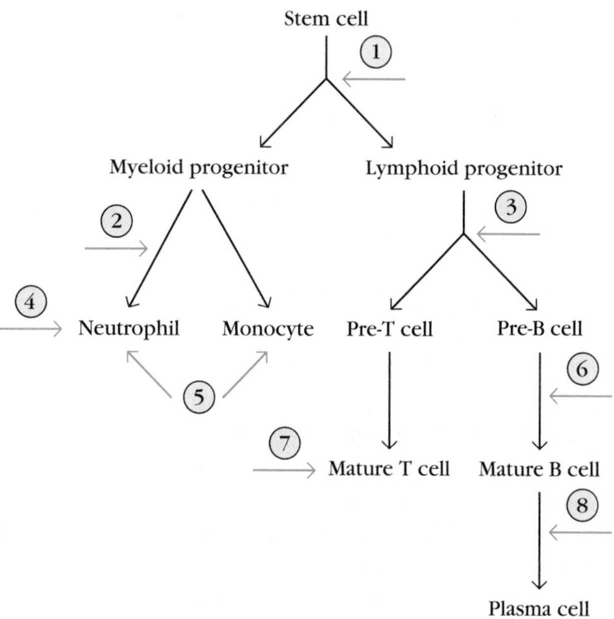

a. Chronic granulomatous disease

b. Severe combined immunodeficiency disease (SCID)

c. Congenital agranulocytosis

d. Reticular dysgenesis

e. Common variable hypogammaglobulinemia

f. X-linked agammaglobulinemia

g. Leukocyte-adhesion deficiency (LAD)

h. Bare-lymphocyte syndrome

5. Indicate whether each of the following statements is true or false. If you think a statement is false, explain why.

a. HIV-1 and HIV-2 are more closely related to each other than to SIV.

b. HIV-1 causes immune suppression in both humans and chimpanzees.

c. SIV is endemic in the African green monkey.

d. The anti-HIV drugs zidovudine and indinavir both act on the same point in the viral replication cycle.

e. T-cell activation increases transcription of the HIV proviral genome.

f. Patients with advanced stages of AIDS always have detectable antibody to HIV.

g. The polymerase chain reaction is a sensitive test used to detect antibodies to HIV.

h. If HAART is successful, viral load will decrease.

6. Various mechanisms have been proposed to account for the decrease in the numbers of $CD4^+$ T cells in HIV-infected individuals. What seems to be the most likely reason for depletion of $CD4^+$ T cells?

7. Would you expect the viral load in the blood of HIV-infected individuals in the chronic phase of HIV-1 infection to vary?

8. If viral load begins to increase in the blood of an HIV-infected individual and the level of $CD4^+$ T cells decrease, what would this indicate about the infection?

9. Why do clinicians monitor the level of skin-test reactivity in HIV-infected individuals? What change might you expect to see in skin-test reactivity with progression into AIDS?

10. Certain chemokines have been shown to suppress infection of cells by HIV, and pro-inflammatory cytokines enhance cell infection. What is the explanation for this?

11. Treatments with combinations of anti-HIV drugs (HAART) have reduced virus levels significantly in some treated patients and delayed the onset of AIDS. If an AIDS patient becomes free of opportunistic infection and has no detectable virus in in the circulation, can that person be considered cured?

12. Suppose you are a physician who has two HIV-infected patients. Patient BW has a fungal infection (candidiasis) in the mouth, and patient LS has a *Mycobacterium* infection. The $CD4^+$ T-cell counts of both patients are about 250 per mm^3. Would you diagnose either patient or both of them as having AIDS?

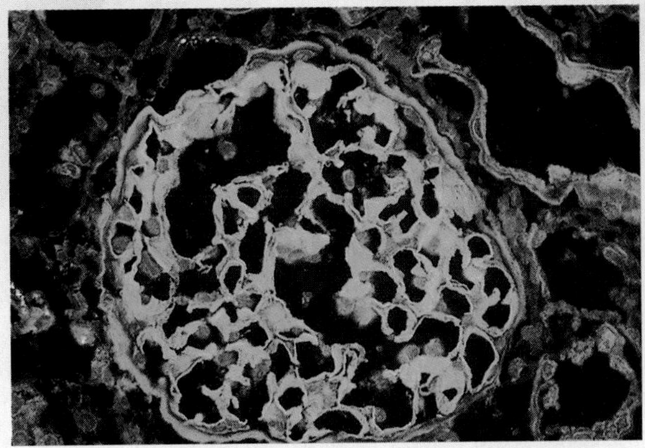

CHAPTER 20
AUTOIMMUNITY

Early in this century, Paul Ehrlich realized that the immune system could go awry and, instead of reacting against foreign antigens, could focus its attack on self-antigens. He termed this condition "horror autotoxicus." We now understand that, while mechanisms of self-tolerance normally protect an individual from potentially self-reactive lymphocytes, there are failures. They result in an inappropriate response of the immune system against self-components, and that is termed **autoimmunity**. In the 1960s, it was believed that all self-reactive lymphocytes were eliminated during their development and that a failure to eliminate these lymphocytes led to autoimmune consequences. Since the late 1970s, a broad body of experimental evidence has countered that belief, revealing that not all self-reactive lymphocytes are deleted during T-cell and B-cell maturation. Instead, normal healthy individuals have been shown to possess mature, recirculating, self-reactive lymphocytes. Since the presence of these self-reactive lymphocytes does not inevitably result in autoimmune reactions, their activity must be regulated in normal individuals through clonal anergy or clonal suppression. A breakdown in this regulation can lead to activation of self-reactive clones of T or B cells, generating humoral or cell-mediated responses against self-antigens. These reactions can cause serious damage to cells and organs, sometimes with fatal consequences.

Sometimes the damage to self-cells or organs is caused by antibodies; in other cases, T cells are the culprit. For example, a common form of autoimmunity is tissue injury by mechanisms similar to type II hypersensitivity reactions. As we saw in Chapter 16, type II hypersensitivity reactions involve antibody-mediated destruction of cells. Autoimmune hemolytic anemia is an excellent example of such an autoimmune disease. In this disease, antigens on red blood cells are recognized by auto-antibodies, which results in the destruction of the blood cells, which in turn results in anemia. Auto-antibodies also are the major offender in Hashimoto's thyroiditis, in which antibodies reactive with tissue-specific antigens such as thyroid peroxidase and thyroglobulin cause severe tissue destruction. Other autoimmune diseases that involve auto-antibodies are listed in Table 20-1.

Many autoimmune diseases are characterized by tissue destruction mediated directly by T cells. A well known example of this is rheumatoid arthritis, in which self-reactive T cells attack the tissue in joints, causing an inflammatory response that results in swelling and tissue destruction. Additionally, diseases such as insulin-dependent diabetes mellitus and multiple sclerosis are primarily due to the action of self-reactive T cells (see Table 20-1).

This chapter describes some common human autoimmune diseases. These can be divided into two broad categories: organ-specific and systemic autoimmune disease (Table 20-1). Such diseases affect 5%–7% of the human population, often causing chronic debilitating illnesses. Several experimental animal models used to study autoimmunity and various mechanisms that may contribute to induction of autoimmune reactions also are described. Finally, current and experimental therapies for treating autoimmune diseases are described.

TABLE 20-1 SOME AUTOIMMUNE DISEASES IN HUMANS

Disease	Self-antigen	Immune response
	Organ-specific autoimmune diseases	
Addison's disease	Adrenal cells	Auto-antibodies
Autoimmune hemolytic anemia	RBC membrane proteins	Auto-antibodies
Goodpasture's syndrome	Renal and lung basement membranes	Auto-antibodies
Graves' disease	Thyroid-stimulating hormone receptor	Auto-antibody (stimulating)
Hashimoto's thyroiditis	Thyroid proteins and cells	T_{DTH} cells, auto-antibodies
Idiopathic thrombocyopenia purpura	Platelet membrane proteins	Auto-antibodies
Insulin-dependent diabetes mellitus	Pancreatic beta cells	T_{DTH} cells, auto-antibodies
Myasthenia gravis	Acetylcholine receptors	Auto-antibody (blocking)
Myocardial infarction	Heart	Auto-antibodies
Pernicious anemia	Gastric parietal cells; intrinsic factor	Auto-antibody
Poststreptococcal glomerulonephritis	Kidney	Antigen-antibody complexes
Spontaneous infertility	Sperm	Auto-antibodies
	Systemic autoimmune disease	
Ankylosing spondylitis	Vertebrae	Immune complexes
Multiple sclerosis	Brain or white matter	T_{DTH} and T_C cells, auto-antibodies
Rheumatoid arthritis	Connective tissue, IgG	Auto-antibodies, immune complexes
Scleroderma	Nuclei, heart, lungs, gastrointestinal tract, kidney	Auto-antibodies
Sjogren's syndrome	Salivary gland, liver, kidney, thryoid	Auto-antibodies
Systemic lupus erythematosus (SLE)	DNA, nuclear protein, RBC and platelet membranes	Auto-antobidies, immune complexes

Organ-Specific Autoimmune Diseases

In an organ-specific autoimmune disease, the immune response is directed to a target antigen unique to a single organ or gland, so that the manifestations are largely limited to that organ. The cells of the target organs may be damaged directly by humoral or cell-mediated mechanisms. Alternatively, the antibodies may overstimulate or block the normal function of the target organ.

Diseases Mediated by Direct Cellular Damage

Autoimmune diseases involving direct cellular damage occur when lymphocytes or antibodies bind to cell-membrane antigens, causing cellular lysis and/or an inflammatory response in the affected organ. Gradually, the damaged cellular structure is replaced by connective tissue, and the function of the organ declines. This section briefly describes a few examples of this type of autoimmune disease.

Hashimoto's Thyroiditis

In Hashimoto's thyroiditis, which is most frequently seen in middle-aged women, an individual produces auto-antibodies and sensitized T_{DTH} cells specific for thyroid antigens. The DTH response is characterized by an intense infiltration of the thyroid gland by lymphocytes, macrophages, and plasma cells, which form lymphocytic follicles and germinal centers (Figure 20-1). The ensuing inflammatory response causes a goiter, or visible enlargement of the thyroid gland. Antibodies are formed to a number of thyroid proteins, including thyroglobulin and thyroid peroxidase, both of which are involved in the uptake of iodine. Binding of the auto-antibodies to these proteins interferes with iodine uptake and leads to decreased production of thyroid hormones (hypothyroidism).

Autoimmune Anemias

Autoimmune anemias include pernicious anemia, autoimmune hemolytic anemia, and drug-induced hemolytic anemia. Pernicious anemia is caused by auto-antibodies to a membrane-bound intestinal protein on gastric parietal cells, called intrinsic factor, that facilitates uptake of vitamin B_{12} from the small intestine. Binding of the auto-antibody to intrinsic factor blocks the intrinsic factor–mediated absorption of vitamin B_{12}. In the absence of sufficient vitamin B_{12}, which is necessary for proper hematopoiesis, the number of functional mature red blood cells decreases below normal. Pernicious anemia is treated with injections of vitamin B_{12}, thus circumventing the defect in its absorption.

An individual with autoimmune hemolytic anemia makes auto-antibody to RBC antigens, triggering complement-mediated lysis or antibody-mediated opsonization and phagocytosis of the red blood cells. One form of autoimmune anemia is drug-induced: when certain drugs such as penicillin or the anti-hypertensive agent methyldopa interact with red blood cells, the cells become antigenic. The immunodiagnostic test for autoimmune hemolytic anemias generally involves a Coombs test, in which the red cells are incubated with an anti–human IgG antiserum. If IgG auto-antibodies are present on the red cells, the cells are agglutinated by the antiserum.

Goodpasture's Syndrome

In **Goodpasture's syndrome**, auto-antibodies specific for certain basement-membrane antigens bind to the basement membranes of the kidney glomeruli and the alveoli of the lungs. Subsequent complement activation leads to direct cellular damage and an ensuing inflammatory response mediated by a buildup of complement split products. Damage to the glomerular and alveolar basement membranes leads to progressive kidney damage and pulmonary hemorrhage, death ensues often within several months of the onset of symptoms. Biopsies from patients with Goodpasture's syndrome stained with fluorescent-labeled anti-IgG and anti-C3b reveal linear deposits of IgG and C3b along the basement membranes (Figure 20-2).

Insulin-Dependent Diabetes Mellitus

A disease afflicting 0.2% of the population, **insulin-dependent diabetes mellitus (IDDM)** is caused by an autoimmune attack on the pancreas. The attack is directed against specialized insulin-producing cells (beta cells) that are located in spherical clusters, called the islets of Langerhans, scattered throughout the pancreas. The autoimmune attack destroys beta cells, resulting in decreased production of insulin and

(a)

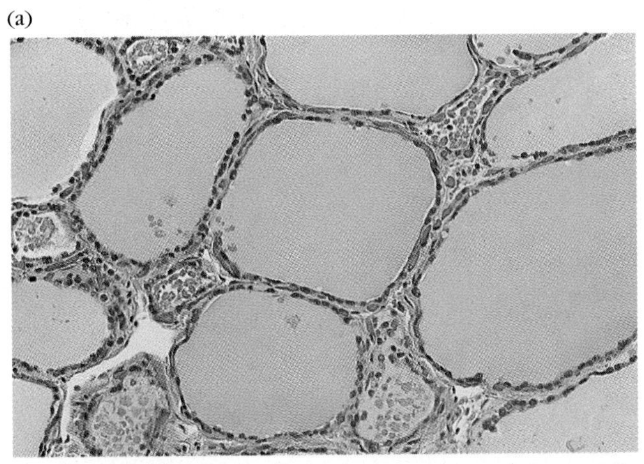

(b)

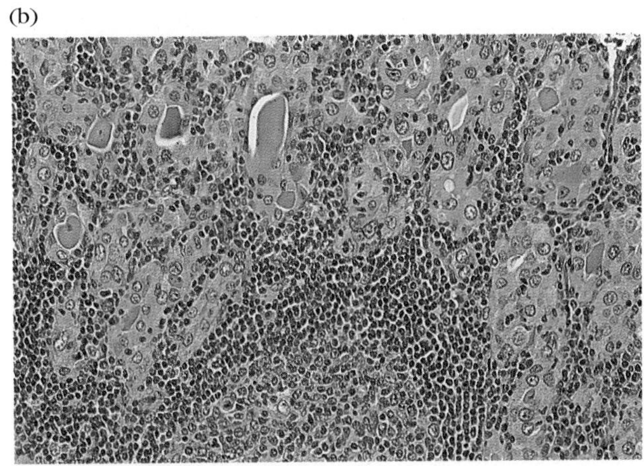

FIGURE 20-1 Photomicrographs of (a) normal thyroid gland showing a follicle lined by cuboidal follicular epithelial cells and (b) gland in Hashimoto's thyroiditis showing intense lymphocyte infiltration. [From Web Path, courtesy of EC Klatt, University of Utah.]

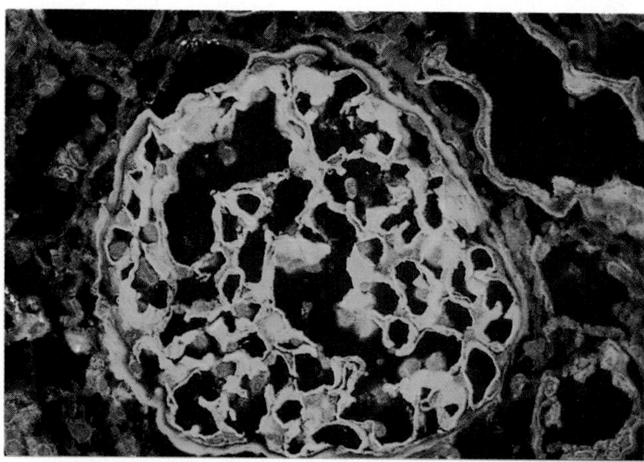

FIGURE 20-2 Fluorescent anti-IgG staining of a kidney biopsy from a patient with Goodpasture's syndrome reveals linear deposits of auto-antibody along the basement membrane. [From Web Path, courtesy of EC Klatt, University of Utah.]

consequently increased levels of blood glucose. Several factors are important in the destruction of beta cells. First, activated CTLs migrate into an islet and begin to attack the insulin producing cells. Local cytokine production released during this response include IFN-γ, TNF-α, and IL-1. Auto-antibody production also can be a contributing factor in IDDM. The first CTL infiltration and activation of macrophages, frequently referred to as insulitis (Figure 20-3), is followed by cytokine release and the presence of auto-antibodies, which leads to a cell-mediated DTH response. The subsequent beta-cell destruction is thought to be mediated by cytokines released during the DTH response and by lytic enzymes released from the activated macrophages. Auto-antibodies to beta cells may contribute to cell destruction by facilitating either antibody-plus-complement lysis or antibody-dependent cell-mediated cytotoxicity (ADCC).

The abnormalities in glucose metabolism that are caused by the destruction of islet beta cells result in serious metabolic problems that include ketoacidosis and increased urine production. The late stages of the disease are often characterized by atherosclerotic vascular lesions—which in turn cause gangrene of the extremities due to impeded vascular flow—renal failure, and blindness. Clearly, diabetes is a disease that, if not properly treated, can result in death. The most common therapy for diabetes is daily administration of insulin. This is quite helpful in managing the disease, but, because sporadic doses are not the same as metabolically regulated continuous and controlled release of the hormone, periodically injected doses of insulin do not totally alleviate the problems caused by the disease. Another complicating feature of diabetes is that people who suffer from it can go undetected for several years and thus suffer irreparable loss of pancreatic tissue.

Diseases Mediated by Stimulating or Blocking Auto-Antibodies

In some autoimmune diseases, antibodies act as agonists, binding to hormone receptors in lieu of the normal ligand and stimulating inappropriate activity. This usually leads to an overproduction of mediators or an increase in cell growth. In other autoimmune conditions, auto-antibodies bind to hormone receptors but act as antagonists, blocking receptor function. This generally causes impaired secretion of mediators and gradual atrophy of the affected organ.

Graves' Disease

The production of thyroid hormones is carefully regulated by thyroid-stimulating hormone (TSH), which is produced by the pituitary gland. Binding of TSH to a receptor on thyroid cells activates adenylate cyclase and stimulates the synthesis of two thyroid hormones, thyroxine and triiodothyronine. A patient with **Graves' disease** produces

(a)

(b)

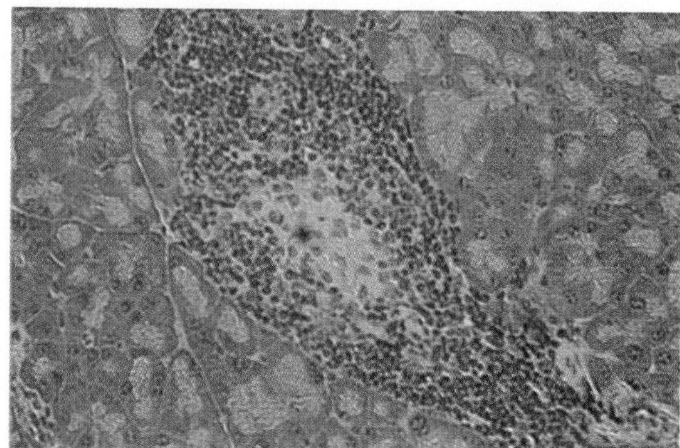

FIGURE 20-3 Photomicrographs of an islet of Langerhans (a) in pancreas from a normal mouse and (b) one in pancreas from a mouse with a disease resembling insulin-dependent diabetes mellitus. Note the lymphocyte infiltration into the islet (insulitis) in (b). [From MA Atkinson and NK Maclaren, 1990, *Sci. Am.* **263**(1):62.]

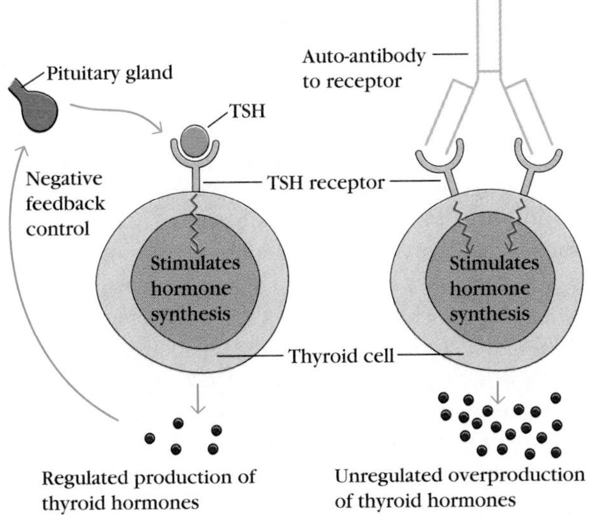

FIGURE 20-4 In Graves' disease, binding of auto-antibodies to the receptor for thyroid-stimulating hormone (TSH) induces unregulated activation of the thyroid, leading to overproduction of the thyroid hormones (purple dots).

auto-antibodies to the receptor for TSH. Binding of these auto-antibodies to the receptor mimics the normal action of TSH, activating adenylate cyclase and resulting in production of the thyroid hormones. Unlike TSH, however, the auto-antibodies are not regulated, and consequently they overstimulate the thyroid. For this reason these auto-antibodies are called long-acting thyroid-stimulating (LATS) antibodies (Figure 20-4).

Myasthenia Gravis

Myasthenia gravis is the prototype autoimmune disease mediated by blocking antibodies. A patient with this disease produces auto-antibodies to the acetylcholine receptors on the motor end-plates of muscles. Binding of these auto-antibodies to the receptors blocks the normal binding of acetylcholine and also induces complement-mediated degradation of the receptors, resulting in progressive weakening of the skeletal muscles (Figure 20-5). Ultimately, the antibodies destroy the receptors. The early signs of this disease include drooping eyelids and inability to retract the corners of the mouth, which gives the appearance of snarling.

Systemic Autoimmune Diseases

In systemic autoimmune diseases, the response is directed toward a broad range of target antigens and involves a number of organs and tissues. These diseases reflect a general defect in immune regulation that results in hyperactive T cells and B cells. Tissue damage is widespread, both from cell-mediated immune responses and from direct cellular damage caused by auto-antibodies or by accumulation of immune complexes.

Systemic Lupus Erythematosus

One of the best examples of a systemic autoimmune disease is **systemic lupus erythematosus** (SLE), which typically appears in women between 20 and 40 years of age; the ratio of female to male patients is 10:1. SLE is characterized by fever, weakness, arthritis, skin rashes, pleurisy, and kidney

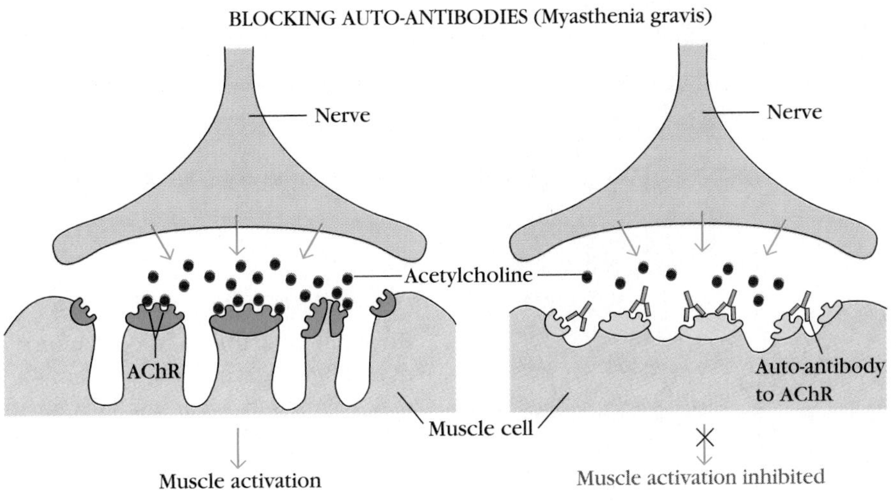

FIGURE 20-5 In myasthenia gravis, binding of auto-antibodies to the acetylcholine receptor (*right*) blocks the normal binding of acetylcholine (burgandy dots) and subsequent muscle activation (*left*). In addition, the anti-AChR auto-antibody activates complement, which damages the muscle end-plate; the number of acetylcholine receptors declines as the disease progresses. AChR = acetylcholine receptor.

dysfunction (Figure 20-6). Lupus is more frequent in African-American and Hispanic women than in Caucasians, although it is not known why this is so. Affected individuals may produce auto-antibodies to a vast array of tissue antigens, such as DNA, histones, RBCs, platelets, leukocytes, and clotting factors; interaction of these auto-antibodies with their specific antigens produces various symptoms. Auto-antibody specific for RBCs and platelets, for example, can lead to complement-mediated lysis, resulting in hemolytic anemia and thrombocytopenia, respectively. When immune complexes of auto-antibodies with various nuclear antigens are deposited along the walls of small blood vessels, a type III hypersensitive reaction develops. The complexes activate the complement system and generate membrane-attack complexes and complement split products that damage the wall of the blood vessel, resulting in vasculitis and glomerulonephritis.

Excessive complement activation in patients with severe SLE produces elevated serum levels of the complement split products C3a and C5a, which may be three to four times higher than normal. C5a induces increased expression of the type 3 complement receptor (CR3) on neutrophils, facilitating neutrophil aggregation and attachment to the vascular endothelium. As neutrophils attach to small blood vessels, the number of circulating neutrophils declines (neutropenia) and various occlusions of the small blood vessels develop (vasculitis). These occlusions can lead to widespread tissue damage.

Laboratory diagnosis of SLE focuses on the characteristic antinuclear antibodies, which are directed against double-stranded or single-stranded DNA, nucleoprotein, histones, and nucleolar RNA. Indirect immunofluorescent staining with serum from SLE patients produces various characteristic nucleus-staining patterns.

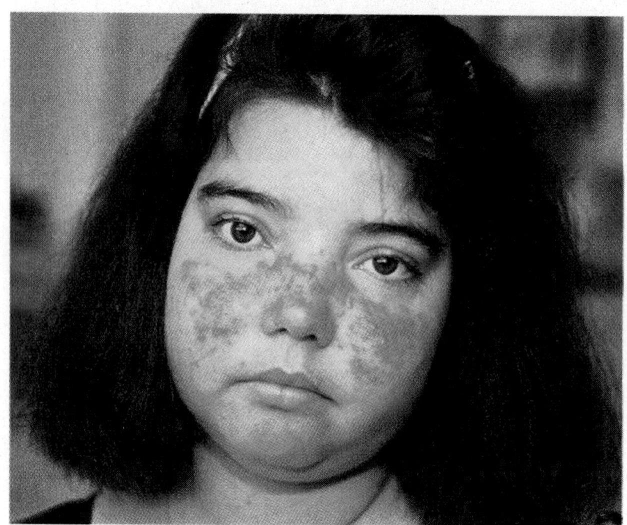

FIGURE 20-6 Characteristic "butterfly" rash over the cheeks of a young girl with systemic lupus erythematosus. [From L Steinman, 1993, *Sci. Am.* **269**(3):80.]

Multiple Sclerosis

Multiple sclerosis (MS), an autoimmune disease that affects the central nervous system, is the most common cause of neurologic disability associated with disease in Western countries. The symptoms may be mild, such as numbness in the limbs, or severe, such as paralysis or loss of vision. Most people with MS are diagnosed between the ages of 20 and 40. Individuals with this disease produce autoreactive T cells that participate in the formation of inflammatory lesions along the myelin sheath of nerve fibers. The cerebrospinal fluid of patients with active MS contains activated T lymphocytes, which infiltrate the brain tissue and cause characteristic inflammatory lesions, destroying the myelin. Since myelin functions to insulate the nerve fibers, a breakdown in the myelin sheath leads to numerous neurologic dysfunctions.

Epidemiological studies indicate that MS is more common in the Northern hemisphere and, interestingly, in the United States. Populations who live north of the 37th parallel have a prevalence of 110–140 cases per 100,000, while those who live south of the 37th parallel show a prevalence of 57–78 per 100,000. And if an individual from south of the 37th parallel moves to north of it, she assumes a new risk if the move occurs before 15 years of age. These provocative data suggest that there is an environmental component of the risk of contracting MS. This is not the entire story, however, since genetic influences also are important. While the average person in the United States has about one chance in 1,000 of developing MS, close relatives of people with MS, such as children or siblings, have a one in 100 to one in 50 chance of developing MS. The identical twin of a person with MS has a one in 3 chance of developing the disease. These data point strongly to the genetic component of the disease. And, as is described in the later Clinical Focus, MS affects women two to three times more frequently than men.

The cause of MS, like most autoimmune diseases, is not well understood. However, there are some suggestions that infection by certain viruses may predispose one to MS. Certainly some viruses can cause demyelinating diseases, and it is tempting to speculate that virus infection plays a significant role in MS, but no definitive data at present implicate a particular virus.

Rheumatoid Arthritis

Rheumatoid arthritis is a common autoimmune disorder, most often affecting women from 40 to 60 years old. The major symptom is chronic inflammation of the joints, although the hematologic, cardiovascular, and respiratory systems frequently are also affected. Many individuals with rheumatoid arthritis produce a group of auto-antibodies, called **rheumatoid factors**, that are reactive with determinants in the Fc region of IgG. The classic rheumatoid factor is an IgM antibody with that reactivity. Such auto-antibodies bind to normal circulating IgG, forming IgM-IgG complexes that are deposited in the joints. These immune complexes can activate the complement cascade, resulting in a type III hypersensitive reaction, which leads to chronic inflammation of the joints.

Scleroderma

Scleroderma is an autoimmune disease that can have local effects on the skin or more widespread systemic effects on internal organs and the vasculature. The most commonly identified symptom of scleroderma is a gradual tightening of the skin, usually in the extremities, such as hands, feet, and face. The term *scleroderma* literally means "hard skin;" it is a chronic degenerative disease that leads to the overproduction of collagen in connective tissue. The localized form of the disease results in thickening of the skin and tightness in the face and hands. Many individuals affected with the localized form develop CREST syndrome. The term *CREST* is an acronym for five symptoms that commonly occur together: *c*alcinosis, a painful calcium deposit in the skin, *R*eynaud's phenomenon, abnormal blood flow in response to cold or stress, *e*sophageal dysfunction, problems with swallowing, *s*clerodactyly, tightening of the skin; and *t*elangiectasia, the formation of red spots on the hands, palms, forearms, face, and lips. These five symptoms frequently appear after the first localized skin effects. Most patients who develop CREST do not develop the systemic form of the disease. The more severe systemic form attacks internal organs such as kidneys, lungs, heart, gastrointestinal tract, and joints, as well as the skin. This form of the disease can be quite painful and sometimes leads to premature death.

Scleroderma is a rather rare disease. In the United States there are about 150,000 individuals who have scleroderma. About 80% of these cases are women, most of whom became afflicted in the prime of life, between the ages of 35 and 54. The cause of the disease is unknown but very recent data suggest that, at least in some instances, scleroderma may not in fact be an autoimmune disease in the strictest definition of the term. In a recently published study, Nelson and others demonstrated the presence of abnormally large numbers of fetal cells in the blood of women who have scleroderma. In this study, 40 women with sons were examined, 17 of which had scleroderma. An assay for the Y chromosome in blood from these women detected 11.1 male cells/ 16 ml of blood in the scleroderma patients, but only 0.38 cells/16 ml in the others. These data suggest that scleroderma might actually be the result of the fetal cells' immune response to the mother, like what is observed in graft versus host disease, or GVHD (see Chapter 21). These results, along with earlier results that demonstrated the persistence of fetal cells in the maternal circulation for as long as 27 years, may well explain the sex linkage of the disease, but what about scleroderma in women who have not had children and in men? It turns out that, just as fetal cells can enter the maternal circulation, so maternal cells can be found in the fetus. So it is possible that, in women without children and in men, maternal cells may well be the culprit. Whether this is the cause of all cases of scleroderma remains to be determined, but it does open up a new and exciting area of exploration in this poorly understood disease.

Animal Models for Autoimmune Disease

Animal models for autoimmune diseases have contributed valuable insights into the mechanism of autoimmunity, to our understanding of autoimmunity in humans, and to potential treatments. Autoimmunity develops spontaneously in certain inbred strains of animals; autoimmunity can also be induced by certain experimental manipulations (Table 20-2).

Spontaneous Autoimmunity in Animals

A number of autoimmune diseases that develop spontaneously in animals exhibit important clinical and pathologic similarities to certain autoimmune diseases in humans. Certain inbred mouse strains have been particularly valuable models for illuminating the immunologic defects involved in the development of autoimmunity.

New Zealand Black (NZB) mice and F_1 hybrids of NZB and New Zealand White (NZW) mice spontaneously develop autoimmune diseases that closely resemble systemic lupus erythematosus. NZB mice spontaneously develop autoimmune hemolytic anemia between 2 and 4 months of age, at which time various auto-antibodies can be detected, including antibodies to erythrocytes, nuclear proteins, DNA, and T lymphocytes. F_1 hybrid animals develop glomerulonephritis from immune-complex deposits in the kidney and die prematurely by 18 months. As is true of SLE in humans, the incidence of autoimmunity in the (NZB × NZW)F_1 hybrids is greater in females.

An accelerated and severe form of systemic autoimmune disease resembling systemic lupus erythematosus develops in a mouse strain called MRL/*lpr*/*lpr*. These mice are homozygous for a gene called *lpr*, which has been identified as a defective *fas* gene. The *fas*-gene product is a cell-surface protein belonging to the TNF family of cysteine-rich membrane receptors (see Figure 12-6d). When the normal Fas protein interacts with its ligand, it transduces a signal that leads to apoptotic death of the Fas-bearing cells. This mechanism may operate in destruction of target cells by some CTLs (see Figure 14-9). Fas is known also to be essential in the death of hyperactivated peripheral $CD4^+$ cells. Normally, when mature peripheral T cells become activated, they are induced to express Fas antigen, these Fas-bearing cells are

TABLE 20-2 EXPERIMENTAL ANIMAL MODELS OF AUTOIMMUNE DISEASES

Animal model	Possible human disease counterpart	Inducing antigen	Disease transferred by T cells
Spontaneous autoimmune disease			
Nonobese diabetic (NOD) mouse	Insulin-dependent diabetes mellitus (IDDM)	Unknown	Yes
(NZB × NZW) F_1 mouse	Systemic lupus erythematosus (SLE)	Unknown	Yes
Obese-strain chicken	Hashimoto's thyroiditis	Thyroglobulin	Yes
Experimentally induced autoimmune disease*			
Experimental autoimmune myasthenia gravis (EAMG)	Myasthenia gravis	Acetylcholine receptor	Yes
Experimental autoimmune encephalomyelitis (EAE)	Multiple sclerosis (MS)	Myelin basic protein (MBP); proteolipid protein (PLP)	Yes
Autoimmune arthritis (AA)	Rheumatoid arthritis	*M. tuberculosis* (proteoglycans)	Yes
Experimental autoimmune thyroiditis (EAT)	Hashimoto's thyroiditis	Thyroglobulin	Yes

*These diseases can be induced by injecting appropriate animals with the indicated antigen in complete Freund's adjuvant. Except for autoimmune arthritis, the antigens used correspond to the self-antigens associated with the human-disease counterpart. Rheumatoid arthritis involves reaction to proteoglycans, which are self-antigens associated with connective tissue.

quite likely to come into contact with a neighboring activated cell bearing Fas ligand and be induced to die. It is also possible that Fas ligand can engage Fas from the same cell, inducing a cellular suicide. In the absence of Fas, mature peripheral T cells do not die, and these activated cells continue to proliferate and produce cytokines that result in grossly enlarged lymph nodes and spleen. Defects in *fas* expression similar to that found in the *lpr* mouse are observed in humans, and these can have severe consequences. However there is no link between *fas* expression and SLE in humans, which suggests that the *lpr* mouse may not be a true model for SLE.

Another important animal model is the nonobese diabetic (NOD) mouse, which spontaneously develops a form of diabetes that resembles human insulin-dependent diabetes mellitus (IDDM). Like the human disease, the NOD mouse disease begins with lymphocytic infiltration into the islets of the pancreas. Also, as in IDDM, there is a strong association between certain MHC alleles and the development of diabetes in these mice. Experiments with these mice have shown that T cells from diabetic mice can transfer diabetes to nondiabetic recipients. For example, when the immune system of normal mice is destroyed by lethal doses of x-rays and then is reconstituted with an injection of bone marrow cells from NOD mice, the reconstituted mice develop diabetes. Conversely, when the immune system of still healthy NOD mice is destroyed by x-irradiation and then reconstituted with normal bone marrow cells, the NOD mice do not develop diabetes. Various studies have demonstrated a pivotal role for $CD4^+$ T cells in the NOD mouse, and recent evidence implicates the T_H1 subset in disease development.

Several other spontaneous autoimmune diseases have been discovered in animals that have served as models for similar human diseases. Among these are Obese-strain chickens, which develop both humoral and cell-mediated reactivity to thyroglobulin resembling that seen in Hashimoto's thyroiditis.

Experimentally Induced Autoimmunity in Animals

Autoimmune dysfunctions similar to certain human autoimmune diseases can be induced experimentally in some animals (see Table 20-2). One of the first such animal models was discovered serendipitously in 1973 when rabbits were immunized with acetylcholine receptors purified from electric eels. The animals soon developed muscular weakness similar to that seen in myasthenia gravis. This experimental autoimmune myasthenia gravis (EAMG) was shown to result when antibodies to the acetylcholine receptor blocked muscle stimulation by acetylcholine in the synapse. Within a year, this animal model had proved its value with the discovery that auto-antibodies to the acetylcholine receptor were the cause of myasthenia gravis in humans.

Experimental autoimmune encephalomyelitis (EAE) is another animal model that has greatly improved understanding of autoimmunity. This is one of the best studied models of autoimmune disease. EAE is mediated solely by T cells and can be induced in a variety of species by immunization with myelin basic protein (MBP) or proteolipid protein (PLP) in complete Freund's adjuvant (Figure 20-7). Within 2–3 weeks the animals develop cellular infiltration of the myelin sheaths of the central nervous system, resulting in demyelination and paralysis. Most of the animals die, but others have milder symptoms, and some animals develop a chronic form of the disease that resembles chronic relapsing and remitting MS in humans. Those that recover are resistant to the development of disease from a subsequent injection of MBP and adjuvant.

The mouse EAE model provides a system for testing treatments for human MS. For example, because MBP- or PLP-specific T-cell clones are found in the periphery, it is assumed that these clones must have escaped negative selection in the thymus. Recent mouse experiments have suggested that orally administered MBP may make these antigen-specific peripheral T cell clones self-tolerant. These studies have paved the way for clinical trials in MS patients.

Experimental autoimmune thyroiditis (EAT) can be induced in a number of animals by immunizing with thyroglobulin in complete Freund's adjuvant. Both humoral antibodies and T_{DTH} cells directed against the thyroglobulin develop, resulting in thyroid inflammation. EAT appears to best mimic Hashimoto's thyroiditis. In contrast to both EAE and EAT, which are induced by immunizing with self-antigens, autoimmune arthritis (AA) is induced by immunizing rats with *Mycobacterium tuberculosis* in complete Freund's adjuvant. These animals develop an arthritis whose features are similar to those of rheumatoid arthritis in humans.

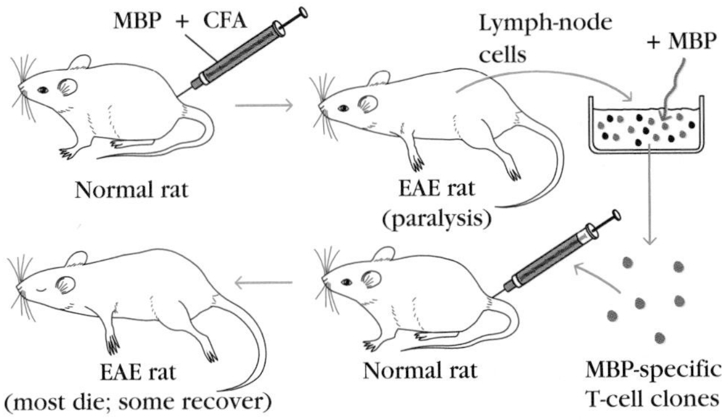

FIGURE 20-7 Experimental autoimmune encephalomyelitis (EAE) can be induced in rats by injecting them with myelin basic protein (MBP) in complete Freud's adjuvant (CFA). MBP-specific T-cell clones can be generated by culturing lymph-node cells from EAE rats with MBP. When these T cells are injected into normal animals, most develop EAE and die, although a few recover.

Evidence Implicating the CD4$^+$ T Cell, MHC, and TCR in Autoimmunity

The inappropriate response to self-antigens that characterizes all autoimmune diseases can involve either the humoral or the cell-mediated branch. Identifying the defects underlying human autoimmune diseases has been difficult, while characterizing the immune defects in the various animal models has been more successful. Each of the animal models has implicated the CD4$^+$ T cell as the primary mediator of autoimmune disease. For example, the evidence is quite strong that, in mice, EAE is caused by CD4$^+$ T_H1 cells specific for the immunizing antigen. The disease can be transferred from one animal into another by T cells from animals immunized with either MBP or PLP or by cloned T-cell lines from such animals. It also has been shown that disease can be prevented by treating animals with anti-CD4 antibodies. These data are compelling evidence for the involvement of CD4 in the establishment of EAE.

T-cell recognition of antigen, of course, involves a trimolecular complex of the T-cell receptor, an MHC molecule, and antigenic peptide (see Figure 9-16). Thus, an individual susceptible to autoimmunity must possess MHC molecules and T-cell receptors capable of binding self-antigens.

Role of CD4$^+$ T Cells and T_H1/T_H2 Balance

Autoimmune T-cell clones have been obtained from all of the animal models listed in Table 20-2 by culturing lymphocytes from the autoimmune animals in the presence of various T-cell growth factors and by inducing proliferation of specific autoimmune clones with the various autoantigens. For example, when lymph-node cells from EAE rats are cultured in vitro with myelin basic protein (MBP), clones of activated T cells emerge. When sufficient numbers of these MBP-specific T-cell clones are injected intravenously into normal syngeneic animals, the cells penetrate the blood-brain barrier and induce demyelination; EAE develops within 5 days (see Figure 20-7).

A similar experimental protocol has been used to isolate T-cell clones specific for thyroglobulin and for *M. tuberculosis* from EAT and AA animals, respectively. In each case, the T-cell clone induces the experimental autoimmune disease in normal animals. Examination of these T cells has revealed that they bear the CD4 membrane marker. In a number of animal models for autoimmune diseases it has been possible to reverse the autoimmunity by depleting the T-cell population with antibody directed against CD4. For example, weekly injections of anti-CD4 monoclonal antibody abolished the autoimmune symptoms in (NZB × NZW) F_1 mice and in mice with EAE.

Most cases of organ-specific autoimmune disease develop as a consequence of self-reactive $CD4^+$ T cells. Analysis of these $CD4^+$ T cells has revealed that the T_H1/T_H2 balance can affect whether autoimmunity develops. T_H1 cells have been implicated in the development of autoimmunity, whereas, in a number of cases, T_H2 cells not only protect against the induction of disease but also against progression of established disease. In EAE, for example, immunohistologic studies revealed the presence of T_H1 cytokines (IL-2, TNF-β, and IFN-γ) in the central nervous system tissues at the height of the disease. In addition, the MBP-specific $CD4^+$ T-cell clones generated from animals with EAE, as shown in Figure 20-7, can be separated into T_H1 and T_H2 clones. Experiments have shown that only the T_H1 clones transfer EAE to normal healthy mice, whereas the T_H2 clones not only do not transfer EAE to normal healthy mice but also protect the mice against induction of EAE by subsequent immunization with MBP plus adjuvant.

Experiments that assessed the role of various cytokines or cytokine inhibitors on the development of EAE have provided further evidence for the different roles of T_H1 and T_H2 cells in autoimmunity. When mice were injected with IL-4 at the time of immunization with MBP plus adjuvant, the development of EAE was inhibited, whereas administration of IL-12 had the opposite effect, promoting the development of EAE. As noted in Chapter 13, IL-4 promotes development of T_H2 cells and IL-12 promotes development of T_H1 cells (see Figure 12-12). Thus, the observed effects of IL-4 and IL-12 on EAE development are consistent with a role for T_H1 cells in the genesis of autoimmunity.

Association with the MHC

Several types of studies have supported an association between expression of a particular MHC allele and susceptibility to autoimmunity, and this issue is covered in detail in Chapter 7. The strongest association between an HLA allele and an autoimmune disease is seen in ankylosing spondylitis, an inflammatory disease of vertebral joints. Individuals who have *HLA-B27* have a 90 times greater likelihood of developing ankylosing spondylitis than individuals with a different *HLA-B* allele. However, the existence of such an association should not be interpreted to imply that the expression of a particular MHC allele has caused the disease, because the relationship between MHC alleles and development of autoimmune disease is complex. It is interesting to note that, unlike many other autoimmune diseases, 90% of the cases of ankylosing spondylitis are male.

Association with the T-Cell Receptor

The presence of T-cell receptors containing particular V_α and V_β domains also has been linked to a number of autoimmune diseases, including experimental EAE and its human counterpart, multiple sclerosis. In one approach, T cells specific for various encephalitogenic peptides of MBP were cloned and their T-cell receptors analyzed. For example, T-cell clones were obtained from PL/J mice by culturing their T cells with the acetylated amino-terminal nonapeptide of MBP presented in association with a class II IA^u MHC molecule. Analysis of the T-cell receptors on these clones revealed a restricted repertoire of V_α and V_β domains: 100% of the T-cell clones expressed V_α 4.3, and 80% of the T-cell clones expressed V_β 8.2. In human autoimmune diseases, evidence for restricted TCR expression has been obtained for both multiple sclerosis and myasthenia gravis. The preferential expression of TCR variable-region genes in these autoimmune T-cell clones suggests that a single epitope might induce the clonal expansion of a small number of pathogenic T cells.

Proposed Mechanisms for Induction of Autoimmunity

A variety of mechanisms have been proposed to account for the T-cell–mediated generation of autoimmune diseases (Figure 20-8). Evidence exists for each of these mechanisms, and it is likely that autoimmunity does not develop from a single event but rather from a number of different events.

In addition, susceptibility to many autoimmune diseases differs between the two sexes. As noted earlier, Hashimoto's thyroiditis, systemic lupus erythematosus, multiple sclerosis, rheumatoid arthritis, and scleroderma preferentially affect women. Factors that have been proposed to account for this preferential susceptibility, such as hormonal differences between the sexes and the potential effects of fetal cells in the maternal circulation during pregnancy, are discussed in the Clinical Focus.

Release of Sequestered Antigens

As discussed in Chapter 10, the induction of self-tolerance in T cells is thought to result from exposure of immature thymocytes to self-antigens and the subsequent clonal deletion of those that are self-reactive. Any tissue antigens that are sequestered from the circulation, and therefore are not seen by the developing T cells in the thymus, will not induce self-tolerance. Exposure of mature T cells to such normally sequestered antigens at a later time might result in their activation.

Myelin basic protein (MBP) is an example of an antigen normally sequestered from the immune system, in this case by the blood-brain barrier. In the EAE model, animals are injected directly with MBP, together with adjuvant, under conditions that maximize immune exposure. In this type of animal model, the immune system is exposed to sequestered self-antigens under nonphysiologic conditions; however, trauma to tissues following either an accident or a viral or bacterial infection might also release sequestered antigens

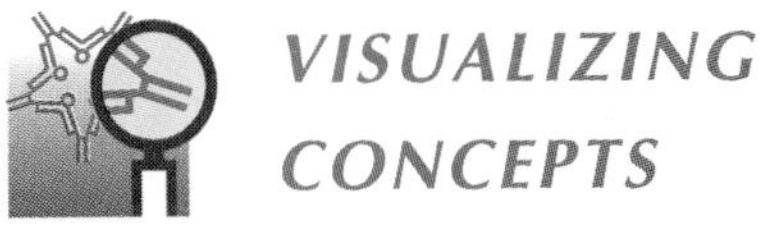

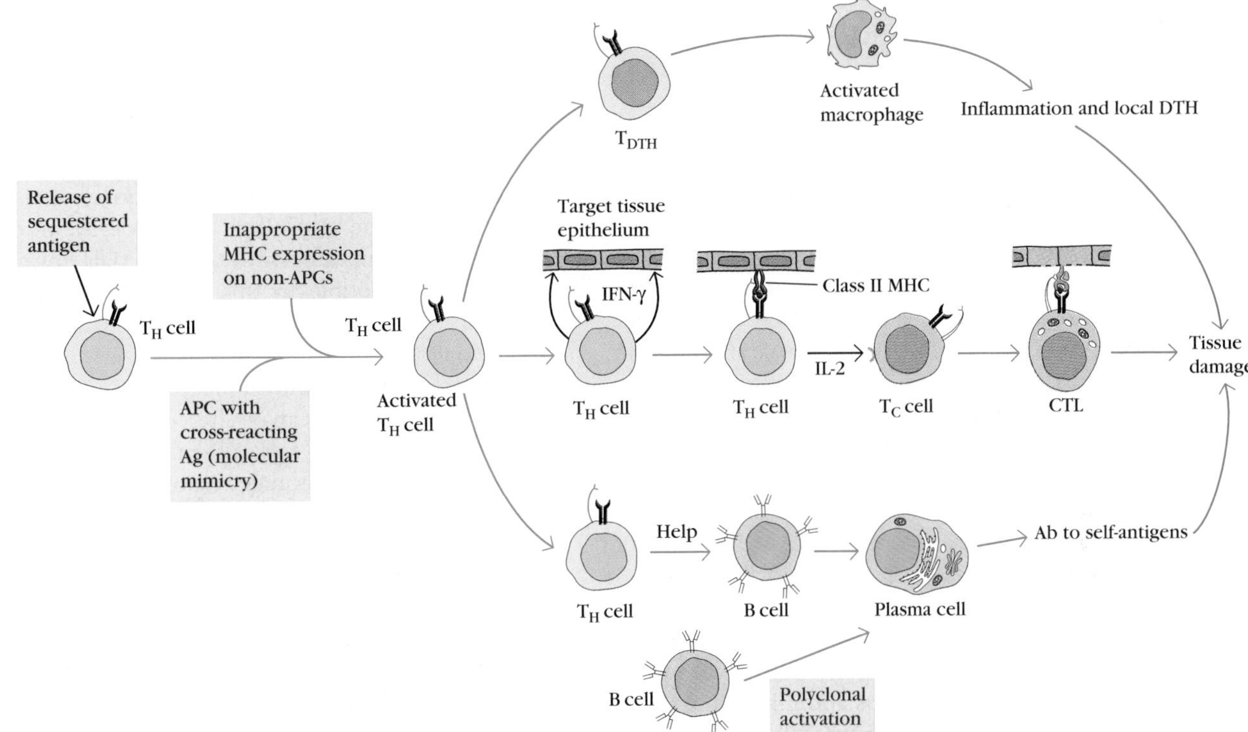

FIGURE 20-8 Proposed mechanisms for inducing autoimmune responses. Normal thymic selection appears to generate some self-reactive T_H cells; abnormalities in this process may generate even more self-reactive T_H cells. Activation of these self-reactive T cells in various ways, as well as polyclonal activation of B cells, is thought to induce an autoimmune response, in this case resulting in tissue damage. In all likelihood, several mechanisms are involved in each autoimmune disease. [Adapted from V Kumar et al, 1989, *Annu. Rev. Immunol.* **7**:657.]

into the circulation. A few tissue antigens are known to fall into this category. For example, sperm arise late in development and are sequestered from the circulation. However, after a vasectomy, some sperm antigens are released into the circulation and can induce auto-antibody formation in some men. Similarly, the release of lens protein after eye damage or of heart-muscle antigens after myocardial infarction has been shown to lead on occasion to the formation of auto-antibodies.

Data indicate that injection of normally sequestered antigens directly into the thymus can reverse the development of tissue-specific autoimmune disease in animal models. For instance, intrathymic injection of pancreatic islet beta cells prevented development of autoimmunity in NOD mice. Moreover, EAE was prevented in susceptible rats by prior injection of MBP directly into the thymus. In these experiments, exposure of immature T cells to self-antigens that normally are not present in the thymus presumably led to tolerance to these antigens.

Molecular Mimicry

For several reasons, the notion that microbial or viral agents might play a role in autoimmunity is very attractive. It is well accepted that migrant human populations acquire the diseases of the area to which they move and that the incidence of autoimmunity has increased dramatically as populations have become more mobile. This, coupled with the fact that a number of viruses and bacteria have been shown to possess antigenic determinants that are identical or similar to normal host-cell components led Michael Oldstone to propose that a pathogen may express a region of protein that

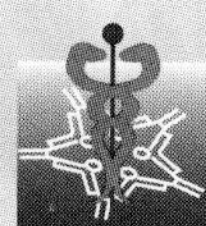

CLINICAL FOCUS

WHY ARE WOMEN MORE SUSCEPTIBLE THAN MEN TO AUTOIMMUNITY? GENDER DIFFERENCES IN AUTOIMMUNE DISEASE

Of the nearly 9 million individuals in the United States with autoimmune disease, approximately 6.7 million are women. This predisposition to autoimmunity is more apparent in some diseases than others. For example, the female:male ratio of individuals who suffer from diseases such as multiple sclerosis (MS) or rheumatoid arthritis (RA) is approximately two or three females to one male, and there are nine women for every one male afflicted with systemic lupus erythmatosus (SLE). However, these statistics do not tell the entire story, since, in some diseases, MS for example, the severity of the disease can be worse in men than in women. The fact that women are more susceptible to autoimmune disease has been recognized for several years but the reasons for this increased risk are not entirely understood. Here some of the possible explanations are considered.

Although it may seem unlikely, considerable evidence suggests there are significant gender differences in immune responses in both humans and mice. Immunization studies in both mice and humans suggest that females produce a higher titer of antibodies than males. In fact, females in general tend to mount more vigorous immune responses. In humans, this is particularly apparent in young females. Women tend to have higher levels of $CD4^+$ T cells and significantly higher levels of serum IgM.

In mice, whose gender differences are easier to study, there is a large body of literature documenting gender difference in immune responses. Female mice are much more likely than male mice to develop T_H1 responses and, in infections to which pro-inflammatory T_H1 responses are beneficial, are more likely to be resistant to the infection. An excellent example of this is infection by viruses such as vesicular stomatitis virus (VSV), herpes simplex virus (HSV), and Theiler's murine encephalomyelitis virus (TMEV). Clearance of these viruses is enhanced by T_H1 responses. In some cases, however, a pro-inflammatory response can be deleterious. For example, a T_H1 response to lymphocytic choriomeningitis virus (LCMV) correlates with more severe disease and significant pathology. Thus, female mice are more likely to succumb to infection with LCMV. The fact that gender is important in LCMV infection is underscored by experiments demonstrating that castrated male mice behave like females and are more likely to succumb to infection than their non-castrated male littermates.

Another disease in which gender plays a role is infection by coxsackie virus Type B-3 (CVB-3), an etiological agent of immune myocarditis. Male mice are much more susceptible to this disease than females. CVB-3 induces a predominant T_H1 response in males, while females, contrary to the situations described above, respond by mounting a protective T_H2 response. The response by females can be altered by injecting them with testosterone, which makes them susceptible to the disease. Additionally, the male response can be altered by injecting them with estradiol, which makes them resistant to the virus. These data in mice are consistent with the possibility that basic differences may well exist between men and women in their responses to pathogens. We must stress, however, that the particular gender differences observed in mice may not extend to human populations.

How do these gender differences arise? It appears, at least in part, that they can be traced to sex hormones. The evidence cited above that estradiol or testosterone can alter the outcome of infection by CVB-3 suggests a critical role for sex hormones. In humans it appears that estrogen on its own does not play a significant role in the etiology of either RA or MS, but there are indications that it may be important in SLE. This is suggested by data indicating that estrogen can stimulate auto-antibody production in SLE-prone mice and these effects can be modulated by an anti-estrogenic compound. Such data imply that, at least in mice, estrogen is capable of triggering SLE-like autoimmunity. Additionally, androgens such as testosterone clearly play an important role in some autoimmune diseases. Female NOD mice are much more susceptible to spontaneous diabetes and castration significantly increases the susceptibility of male NOD mice. Female SJL mice are more likely to be susceptible to EAE, a mouse MS-like disease. This indicates that testosterone may well be effective in ameliorating some autoimmune responses and so may be protective against several autoimmune diseases, including MS, diabetes, SLE, and Sjogren's syndrome.

Why do sex steroids affect immune responses? This is not well understood, but it is likely that these hormones, which circulate throughout the body, alter immune responses by altering patterns of gene expression. The sex steroids, a highly lipophilic group of compounds, function by passing through the cell membrane and binding a cytoplasmic receptor. Each hormone has a cognate receptor and binding of hormone to receptor leads to the activation and, in some instances, repression of gene expression. This is mediated by the binding of the receptor/hormone complex receptor to a specific DNA sequence and acting as a transcriptional modulator. Thus, estrogen enters a cell, binds to the estrogen receptor, and induces the binding of the estrogen receptor to a specific DNA sequence, which in turn results in the modulation of transcription. Therefore, in cells that contain hormone receptors, sex hormones can regulate gene expression. Thus it is highly likely that sex steroids play an important role in the immune system through their receptors. Whether various cells of the immune system contain hormone receptors is not well known at present; to understand how sex hormones mediate immune responses, clearly we must determine which cells express which hormone receptors.

Hormonal effects on immune responses may not be limited to steroidal sex hormones. Prolactin, a hormone that is expressed in higher levels in women than in men, is not a member of the lipophilic sex steroid family that includes estrogen, progesterone, and testosterone. But prolactin secretion (by the anterior pituitary) is stimulated by estrogen, thus explaining the higher levels of prolactin in women and the very high levels observed during pregnancy. Prolactin can have a profound influence on immune responses, as demonstrated in mice by removal of the anterior pituitary: this results in a severe immunosuppression, which can be entirely reversed by treatment with exogenous prolactin. The presence of prolactin receptors on peripheral T and B cells in humans is further evidence that this hormone may play a role in regulating immune responses. In fact, some evidence suggests that prolactin may tend to turn cells towards T_H1-dominated immune responses.

Pregnancy may give us a clue to how sex plays a role in regulating immune response. It is clear that, while women normally mount a normal response to foreign antigens, during pregnancy it is critical that the mother tolerate the fetus (which is, in fact, a foreign graft). This makes it very likely that the female immune system undergoes important modifications during pregnancy. Recall that women normally tend to mount more T_H1-like responses than T_H2 responses. During pregnancy, however, women mount more T_H2-like responses. It is thought that pregnancy-associated levels of sex steroids may promote an anti-inflammatory environment. In this regard, it is notable that diseases enhanced by T_H2-like responses, such as SLE, which has a strong antibody-mediated component, can be exacerbated during pregnancy, while diseases that involve inflammatory responses, such as RA and MS, sometimes are ameliorated in pregnant women.

Another effect of pregnancy is the presence of fetal cells in the maternal circulation (see the description of scleroderma on page 503). It is known that fetal cells can persist in the maternal circulation for decades, so these long-lived fetal cells may play a significant role in the development of autoimmune disease. Furthermore, the exchange of cells during pregnancy is bi-directional (cells of the mother may also appear in the fetal circulatory system), and this has led some to postulate that the presence of mother's cells in the male circulation could be a contributing factor in autoimmune disease.

In summary, women and men differ significantly in their ability to mount an immune response. Women mount more robust immune responses, and these responses tend to be more T_H1-like. It has been reported that estrogen is immunostimulatory; this may be due, in part, to the ability of the hormone to regulate specific gene expression through the estrogen receptor. Furthermore, the incidence of autoimmune diseases is sharply higher in women than in men. These observations have generated the compelling hypothesis that the tendency of females to mount more T_H1-like responses may, in part, explain differences in susceptibility to autoimmunity. Since this type of response is pro-inflammatory, it may enhance the development of autoimmunity. Whether the bias towards a T_H1 response is due to differences in sex steroids between males and females is less certain, but surely, in the next several years, experiments that explore this idea are likely to be pursued vigorously.

NOTE: The data discussed in this Clinical Focus were extracted from a letter to Science (CC Whitacre, SC Reingold, and PA O'Looney, 1999, Science 283:1277) from the Task Force on Gender, MS, and Autoimmunity, a group convened by the National Multiple Sclerosis Society to begin a dialog on issues of gender and autoimmune disease. Science also has established a Web site (http://www.sciencemag.org/feature/data/983519.shl) that contains more detailed data concerning autoimmunity and gender.

resembles a particular self-component in conformation or primary sequence. Such molecular mimicry appears in a wide variety of organisms (Table 20-3). In one study, 600 different monoclonal antibodies specific for 11 different viruses were tested to evaluate their reactivity with normal tissue antigens. More than 3% of the virus-specific antibodies tested also bound to normal tissue, suggesting that molecular mimicry is a fairly common phenomenon.

Molecular mimicry has been suggested as one mechanism that leads to autoimmunity. One of the best examples of this type of autoimmune reaction is post-rabies encephalitis, which used to develop in some individuals who had received the rabies vaccine. In the past, the rabies virus was grown in rabbit brain-cell cultures, and preparations of the vaccine included antigens derived from the rabbit brain cells. In a vaccinated person, these rabbit brain-cell antigens could induce formation of antibodies and activated T cells, which could cross-react with the recipient's own brain cells, leading to encephalitis. Cross-reacting antibodies are also thought to be the cause of heart damage in rheumatic fever, which can sometimes develop after a *Streptococcus* infection. In this case, the antibodies are to streptococcal antigens, but they cross-react with the heart muscle.

Mimicry Between MBP and Viral Peptides

Since the encephalitogenic MBP peptides are known, the extent to which they are mimicked by proteins from other organisms can be assessed. For example, one MBP peptide (61–69) is highly homologous with a peptide in the P3 protein of the measles virus (see Table 20-3). In one study, the sequence of another encephalitogenic MBP peptide (66–75) was compared with the known sequences of a large number of viral proteins. This computer analysis revealed sequence homologies between this MBP peptide and a number of peptides from animal viruses, including influenza, polyoma, adenovirus, Rous sarcoma, Abelson leukemia, poliomyelitis, Epstein-Barr, and hepatitis B viruses.

TABLE 20-3 MOLECULAR MIMICRY BETWEEN PROTEINS OF INFECTIOUS ORGANISMS AND HUMAN HOST PROTEINS

Protein*	Residue†	Sequence‡
Human cytomegalovirus IE2	79	P D P L G R P D E D
HLA-DR molecule	60	V T E L G R P D A E
Poliovirus VP2	70	S T T K E S R G T T
Acetylcholine receptor	176	T V I K E S R G T K
Papilloma virus E2	76	S L H L E S L K D S
Insulin receptor	66	V Y G L E S L K D L
Rabies virus glycoprotein	147	T K E S L V I I S
Insulin receptor	764	N K E S L V I S E
Klebsiella pneumoniae nitrogenase	186	S R Q T D R E D E
HLA-B27 molecule	70	K A Q T D R E D L
Adenovirus 12 E1B	384	L R R G M F R P S Q C N
α-Gliadin	206	L G Q G S F R P S Q Q N
Human immunodeficiency virus p24	160	G V E T T T P S
Human IgG constant region	466	G V E T T T P S
Measles virus P3	13	L E C I R A L K
Corticotropin	18	L E C I R A C K
Measles virus P3	31	E I S D N L G Q E
Myelin basic protein	61	E I S F K L G Q E

*In each pair, the human protein is listed second. The proteins in each pair have been shown to exhibit immunologic cross-reactivity.

†Each number indicates the position in the intact protein of the amino-terminal amino acid in the listed sequence.

‡Amino acid residues are indicated by single-letter code. Identical residues are shown in blue.

SOURCE: Adapted from MBA Oldstone, 1987, *Cell* **50**:819.

One peptide from the polymerase enzyme of the hepatitis B virus was particularly striking, exhibiting 60% homology with a sequence in the encephalitogenic MBP peptide. To test the hypothesis that molecular mimicry can generate autoimmunity, rabbits were immunized with this hepatitis B virus peptide. The peptide was shown to induce both the formation of antibody and the proliferation of T cells that cross-reacted with MBP; in addition, central nervous system tissue from the immunized rabbits showed cellular infiltration characteristic of EAE.

These findings suggest that infection with certain viruses expressing epitopes that mimic sequestered self-components, such as myelin basic protein, may induce autoimmunity to those components. Susceptibility to this type of autoimmunity may also be influenced by the MHC haplotype of the individual, since certain class I and class II MHC molecules may be more effective than others in presenting the homologous peptide for T-cell activation.

Another particularly compelling example of molecular mimicry comes from studies of herpes stromal keratinitis (HSK). In these studies, investigators showed that prior infection of mice with herpes simplex virus Type 1 leads to a disease known as herpes stromal keratinitis (HSK), an autoimmune-like disease in which T cells specific for a particular viral peptide attack corneal tissue, thus causing blindness. These data demonstrated very clearly that a particular epitope of HSV-1 is responsible for the disease and that mutant strains of HSV-1 that lack this epitope do not cause HSK. The data provide strong evidence for molecular mimicry in the development of a particular autoimmune disease.

Inappropriate Expression of Class II MHC Molecules

The pancreatic beta cells of individuals with insulin-dependent diabetes mellitus (IDDM) express high levels of both class I and class II MHC molecules, whereas healthy beta cells express lower levels of class I and do not express class II at all. Similarly, thyroid acinar cells from those with Graves' disease have been shown to express class II MHC molecules on their membranes. This inappropriate expression of class II MHC molecules, which are normally expressed only on antigen-presenting cells, may serve to sensitize T_H cells to peptides derived from the beta cells or thyroid cells, allowing activation of B cells or T_C cells or sensitization of T_{DTH} cells against self-antigens.

Other evidence suggests that certain agents can induce some cells that should not express class II MHC molecules to express them. For example, the T-cell mitogen phytohemagglutinin (PHA) has been shown to induce thyroid cells to express class II molecules. In vitro studies reveal that IFN-γ also induces increases in class II MHC molecules on a wide variety of cells, including pancreatic beta cells, intestinal epithelial cells, melanoma cells, and thyroid acinar cells. It was hypothesized that trauma or viral infection in an organ may induce a localized inflammatory response and thus increased concentrations of IFN-γ in the affected organ. If IFN-γ induces class II MHC expression on non-antigen-presenting cells, inappropriate T_H-cell activation might follow, with autoimmune consequences. It is noteworthy that SLE patients with active disease have higher serum titers of IFN-γ than patients with inactive disease. These data suggested that the increase in IFN-γ in these patients may lead to inappropriate expression of class II MHC molecules and thus to T-cell activation against a variety of autoantigens.

An interesting transgenic mouse system implicates IFN-γ and inappropriate class II MHC expression in autoimmunity. In this system, an IFN-γ transgene was genetically engineered with the insulin promoter, so that the transgenic mice secreted IFN-γ from their pancreatic beta cells (Figure 20-9a). Since IFN-γ up-regulates class II MHC expression, these transgenic mice also expressed class II MHC molecules on their pancreatic beta cells. The mice developed diabetes, which was associated with cellular infiltration of lymphocytes and inflammatory cells like the infiltration seen in autoimmune NOD mice and in patients with insulin-dependent diabetes mellitus (Figure 20-9b).

Although inappropriate class II MHC expression on pancreatic beta cells may be involved in the autoimmune reaction in these transgenic mice, other factors also may play a role. For example, IFN-γ is known to induce production of several other cytokines, including IL-1 and TNF. Therefore, the development of autoimmunity in this transgenic system may involve antigen presentation by class II MHC molecules on pancreatic beta cells together with a co-stimulatory signal, such as IL-1, that may activate self-reactive T cells. There is also some evidence to suggest that IL-1, IFN-γ, and TNF may directly impair the secretory function of human beta cells.

Polyclonal B-Cell Activation

A number of viruses and bacteria can induce nonspecific polyclonal B-cell activation. Gram-negative bacteria, cytomegalovirus, and Epstein-Barr virus (EBV) are all known to be such polyclonal activators, inducing the proliferation of numerous clones of B cells that express IgM in the absence of T_H cells. If B cells reactive to self-antigens are activated by this mechanism, auto-antibodies can appear. For instance, during infectious mononucleosis, which is caused by EBV, a variety of auto-antibodies are produced, including auto-antibodies reactive to T and B cells, rheumatoid factors, and antinuclear antibodies. Similarly, lymphocytes from patients with SLE produce large quantities of IgM in culture, suggesting that they have been polyclonally activated. Many AIDS patients also show high levels of nonspecific antibody and auto-antibodies to RBCs and platelets. These patients are often coinfected with other viruses such as EBV and cytomegalovirus, which may induce the polyclonal B-cell activation that results in auto-antibody production.

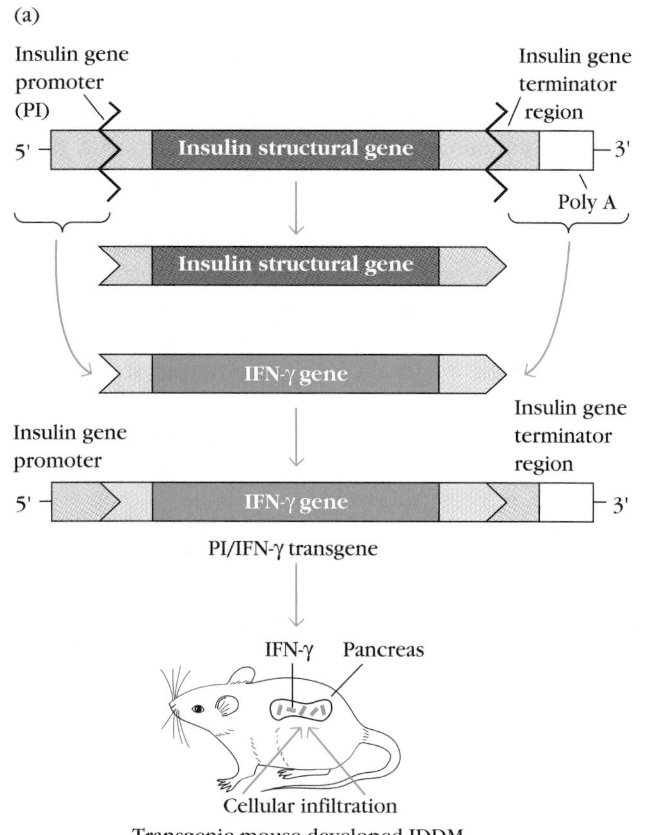

(b)

FIGURE 20-9 Insulin-dependent diabetes mellitus (IDDM) in transgenic mice. (a) Production of transgenic mice containing an IFN-γ transgene linked to the insulin promoter (PI). The transgenics, which expressed the PI/IFN-γ transgene only in the pancreas, developed symptoms characteristic of IDDM. (b) Pancreatic islets of Langerhans from a normal BALB/c mouse (*left*) and from PI/IFN-γ transgenics at 3 weeks (*right*) showing infiltration of inflammatory cells. [Part (b) from N Sarvetnick, 1988, *Cell* **52:**773.]

Treatment of Autoimmune Diseases

Ideally, treatment for autoimmune diseases should be aimed at reducing only the autoimmune response while leaving the rest of the immune system intact. To date, this ideal has not been reached.

Current Therapies

Current therapies for autoimmune diseases are not cures but merely palliatives, aimed at reducing symptoms to provide the patient with an acceptable quality of life. For the most part, these treatments provide nonspecific suppression of the immune system and thus do not distinguish between a pathologic autoimmune response and a protective immune response. Immunosuppressive drugs (e.g., corticosteroids, azathioprine, and cyclophosphamide) are often given with the intent of slowing proliferation of lymphocytes. By depressing the immune response in general, such drugs can reduce the severity of autoimmune symptoms. The general reduction in immune responsiveness, however, puts the patient at greater risk for infection or the development of cancer. A somewhat more selective approach employs **cyclosporin A** or FK506 to treat autoimmunity. Since these agents block signal transduction mediated by the T-cell receptor (see Figure 12-13), they should inhibit only antigen-activated T cells while sparing nonactivated ones.

Another therapeutic approach that has produced positive results in some cases of myasthenia gravis is removal of the thymus. Because patients with this disease often have thymic abnormalities (e.g., thymic hyperplasia or thymomas), adult thymectomy often increases the likelihood of remission of symptoms. Patients with Graves' disease, myasthenia gravis, rheumatoid arthritis, or systemic lupus erythematosus may experience short-term benefit from plasmapheresis. In this process, plasma is removed from a patient's blood by continuous-flow centrifugation. The red blood cells are then resuspended in a suitable medium and returned to the patient. Plasmapheresis has been beneficial to patients with autoimmune diseases involving antigen-antibody complexes, which are removed with the plasma. Removal of the complexes, althoughonly temporary, can result in a short-term reduction in symptoms.

Experimental Therapeutic Approaches

Studies with experimental autoimmune animal models have provided evidence that it is indeed possible to induce specific immunity to the development of autoimmunity. Several of these approaches are described in this section and outlined in Figure 20-10.

T-Cell Vaccination

T-cell vaccination has been explored as a therapy for some autoimmune diseases. The basis for this approach came from experiments with the EAE animal model. When rats were injected with low doses ($<10^4$) of cloned T cells specific for MBP, they did not develop symptoms of EAE. Instead they became resistant to the development of EAE when later challenged with a lethal dose of activated MBP-specific T cells or MBP in adjuvant. Later findings revealed that the efficacy of these autoimmune T-cell clones as a vaccine could be enhanced by crosslinking the cell-membrane components with formaldehyde or glutaraldehyde. When such crosslinked T cells were injected into animals with active EAE, permanent remission of symptoms was observed. The crosslinked T cells apparently elicit regulatory T cells specific for TCR variable-region determinants of the autoimmune clones. Presumably these regulatory T cells act to suppress the autoimmune T cells that mediate EAE.

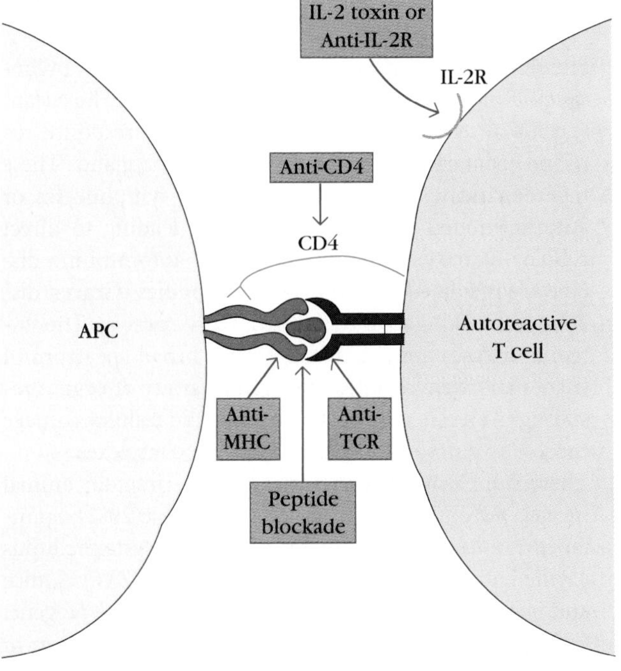

FIGURE 20-10 Some experimental agents for immunointervention in autoimmune disease.

Peptide Blockade of MHC Molecules

Identification and sequencing of various autoantigens has led to the development of new approaches to modulate autoimmune T-cell activity. In EAE, for example, the encephalitogenic peptides of MBP have been well characterized. Synthetic peptides differing by only one amino acid from their MBP counterpart have been shown to bind to the appropriate MHC molecule. Moreover, when sufficient amounts of such a peptide were administered along with the corresponding encephalitogenic MBP peptide, the clinical development of EAE was blocked. Presumably, the synthetic peptide acts as a competitor, occupying the antigen-binding cleft on MHC molecules and thus preventing binding of the MBP peptide.

In other studies, blocking peptides complexed to soluble class II MHC molecules reversed the clinical progression of EAE in mice, presumably by inducing a state of clonal anergy in the autoimmune T cells.

Monoclonal-Antibody Treatment

Monoclonal antibodies have been used successfully to treat autoimmune disease in several animal models. For example, a high percentage of (NZB × NZW) F_1 mice given weekly injections of high doses of monoclonal antibody specific for the CD4 membrane molecule recovered from their autoimmune lupus-like symptoms (Figure 20-11). Similar positive results were observed in NOD mice, in which treatment with an anti-CD4 monoclonal antibody led to disappearance of the lymphocytic infiltration and diabetic symptoms.

Because anti-CD4 monoclonal antibodies block or deplete all T_H cells, regardless of their specificity, they can threaten the overall immune responsiveness of the recipient. One remedy for this disadvantage is to try to block antigen-activated T_H cells only, since these cells are involved in the

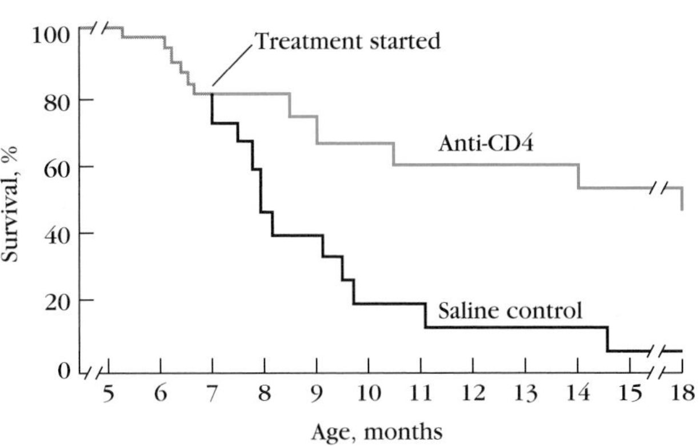

FIGURE 20-11 Weekly injections of anti-CD4 monoclonal antibody into (NZB × NZW) F_1 mice exhibiting autoimmune lupus-like symptoms significantly increased their survival rate. [Adapted from D Wofsy, 1988, *Prog. Allergy* **45:**106.]

autoimmune state. To do this, researchers have used monoclonal antibody directed against the α subunit of the high-affinity IL-2 receptor, which is expressed only by antigen-activated T_H cells. Because the IL-2R α subunit is expressed at higher levels on autoimmune T cells, monoclonal antibody to the α subunit (anti-TAC) might preferentially block autoreactive T cells. This approach was tested in adult rats injected with activated MBP-specific T cells in the presence or absence of anti-TAC. All the control rats died of EAE, whereas six of the nine treated with anti-TAC had no symptoms, and the symptoms in the other three were mild.

The association of autoimmune disease with restricted TCR expression in a number of animal models has prompted researchers to see if blockage of the preferred receptors with monoclonal antibody might be therapeutic. Injection of PL/J mice with monoclonal antibody specific for the V_β 8.2 T-cell receptor prevented induction of EAE by MBP in adjuvant. Even more promising was the finding that the anti-V_β 8.2 monoclonal antibody could also reverse the symptoms of autoimmunity in mice manifesting induced EAE (Figure 20-12) and that these mice manifested long-term remission. Clearly, the use of monoclonal antibodies as a treatment for human autoimmune diseases presents exciting possibilities.

Similarly, the association of various MHC alleles with autoimmunity (see Table 7-4), as well as the evidence for increased or inappropriate MHC expression in some autoimmune disease, offers the possibility that monoclonal antibodies against appropriate MHC molecules might retard development of autoimmunity. Moreover, since antigen-presenting cells express many different class II MHC molecules, it should theoretically be possible to selectively block an MHC molecule that is associated with autoimmunity

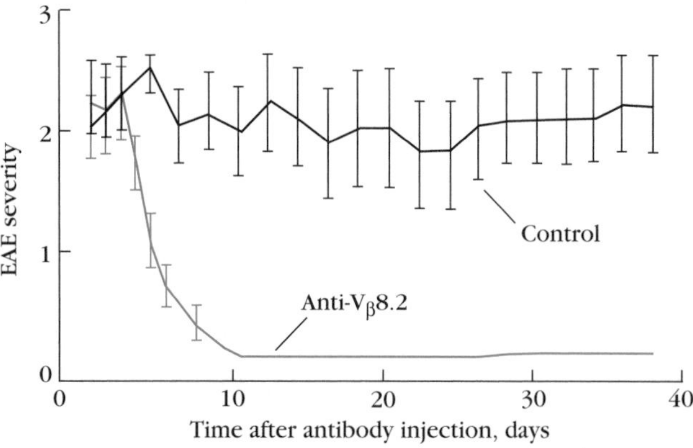

FIGURE 20-12 Injection of monoclonal antibody to the V_β 8.2 T-cell receptor into PL/J mice exhibiting EAE symptoms produced nearly complete remission of symptoms. EAE was induced by injecting mice with MBP-specific T-cell clones. EAE severity scale: 3 = total paralysis of lower limbs; 2 = partial paralysis of lower limbs; 1 = limb tail; 0 = normal (no symptoms). [Adapted from H Acha-Orbea et al, 1989, *Annu. Rev. Immunol.* **7**:371.]

while sparing the others. In one study, injecting mice with monoclonal antibodies to class II MHC molecules before injecting MBP blocked the development of EAE. If, instead, the antibody was given after the injection of MBP, development of EAE was delayed but not prevented. In nonhuman primates, monoclonal antibodies to HLA-DR and HLA-DQ have been shown to reverse EAE.

Tolerance Induction by Oral Antigens

When antigens are administered orally, they tend to induce the state of immunologic unresponsiveness called **tolerance**. For example, as mentioned earlier in this chapter, mice fed MBP do not develop EAE after subsequent injection of MBP. This finding led to a double-blind pilot trial in which 30 individuals with multiple sclerosis were fed either a placebo or 300 mg of bovine myelin every day for a year. The results of this study revealed that T cells specific for MBP were reduced in the myelin-fed group; there also was some suggestion that MS symptoms were reduced in the male recipients (although the reduction fell short of statistical significance) but not in the female recipients. While the results of oral tolerance induction in mice were promising, the data from humans do not appear to be as beneficial. However, the human clinical trials are in the early stages, and it may be that the peptides used so far were not the most effective, or perhaps the doses were not correct. Because of the promise of this approach as shown in animal studies, it is likely that more clinical trials will be conducted over the next few years.

Summary

1. Human autoimmune diseases can be divided into organ-specific and systemic diseases (see Table 20-1). The organ-specific diseases involve an autoimmune response directed primarily against a single organ or gland. These include diseases in which autoreactive lymphocytes or auto-antibodies bind to self-antigens, leading to direct cellular damage. Some organ-specific autoimmune disease are mediated by stimulating antibodies (Graves' disease) or blocking antibodies (myasthenia gravis). The systemic diseases are directed against a broad spectrum of tissues and have manifestations in a variety of organs resulting from cell-mediated responses and cellular damage caused by auto-antibodies or immune complexes.
2. There are both spontaneous and experimental animal models for autoimmune diseases (see Table 20-2). Spontaneous autoimmune diseases resembling systemic lupus erythematosus occur in NZB and (NZB × NZW) F_1 mice and in MRL/*lpr*/*lpr* mice, which have a defective *fas* gene. Other spontaneous models include a thyroiditis seen in Obese-strain chickens that parallels Hashimoto's thyroiditis and a diabetes in NOD mice that resembles human insulin-dependent diabetes mellitus. Several experimental animal models have been developed by im-

munizing animals with self-antigens in the presence of adjuvant. In experimental autoimmune myasthenia gravis (EAMG), the antigen is the acetylcholine receptor; in experimental autoimmune encephalomyelitis (EAE), the antigen is myelin basic protein; in experimental autoimmune thyroiditis (EAT), the antigen is thyroglobulin.

3. Studies with experimental autoimmune animal models have revealed a central role for $CD4^+$ T_H cells in the development of autoimmunity. In each of the experimentally induced autoimmune diseases, autoimmune T-cell clones can be isolated that induce the autoimmune disease in normal animals (see Figure 20-7). The relative number of T_H1 and T_H2 cells appears to play a pivotal role in determining whether autoimmunity develops: T_H1 cells promote the development of autoimmunity, whereas T_H2 cells appear to block development of autoimmune disease and also block the progression of the disease once it is established. The MHC haplotype of the experimental animal determines the ability to present various autoantigens to T_H cells. In addition, some autoimmune animals utilize a restricted repertoire of TCR genes, which may predispose the animal toward T-cell activity in response to a given self-antigen.
4. A variety of mechanisms have been proposed for induction of autoimmunity, including release of sequestered antigens, molecular mimicry, inappropriate class II MHC expression on cells (in some cases stimulated by IFN-γ), and polyclonal B-cell activation (see Figure 20-8). Evidence exists for each of these mechanisms, reflecting the many different pathways leading to autoimmune reactions.
5. Current therapies for autoimmune diseases include treatment with immunosuppressive drugs, thymectomy, and plasmapheresis for diseases involving immune complexes. These therapies, which are relatively nonspecific, may have significant side effects. Several more specific approaches have shown some success in various animal models for autoimmune diseases (see Figure 20-10). These include vaccination with T cells specific for a given autoantigen, administration of synthetic blocking peptides that compete with autoantigen for binding to MHC molecules, treatment with monoclonal antibodies that react with some component specifically involved in an autoimmune reaction, and induction of tolerance to autoantigens by administering them orally.

REFERENCES

Benoist, C, and D Mathis. 1998. Autoimmunity: The pathogen connection. *Nature* **394:**227.

Bianchi, DW, et al. 1996. Male fetal progenitor cells persist in maternal blood for as long as 27 years postpartum. *Proc. Natl. Acad. Sci. USA* **93:**705.

Brocke, S, et al. 1994. Infection and multiple sclerosis: a possible role for superantigens? *Trends Microbiol.* **2:**250.

Charlton, B, and KJ Lafferty. 1995. The T_H1/T_H2 balance in autoimmunity. *Curr. Opin. Immunol.* **7:**793.

Erikson, J, et al. 1998. Self-reactive B cells in nonautoimmune and autoimmune mice. *Immunol. Res.* **17:**49.

Hausmann, S, and KW Wucherpfennig. 1997. Activation of autoreactive T cells by peptides from human pathogens. *Curr. Opin. Immunol.* **9:**831.

Horwitz, MS, et al. 1998. Diabetes induced by Coxsackie virus: initiation by bystander damage and not molecular mimicry. *Nature Med.* **4:**781.

King, C, and N Sarvetnick. 1997. Organ specific autoimmunity. *Curr. Opin. Immunol.* **9:**863.

Liblau, RS, SM Singer, and HO McDevitt. 1995. T_H1 and T_H2 $CD4^+$ T cells in the pathogenesis of organ-specific autoimmune diseases. *Immunol. Today* **16:**34.

Lockshin, MD. 1998. Why women? *J. Am. Med. Womens Assoc.* **53:**4.

Nelson, JL, et al. 1998. Microchimerism and HLA-compatible relationships of pregnancy in scleroderma. *Lancet* **351:**559.

O'Garra, A, L Steinman, and K Gijbels. 1997. $CD4^+$ T-cell subsets in autoimmunity. *Curr. Opin. Immunol.* **9:**872.

Rose, NR. 1998. The role of infection in the pathogenesis of autoimmune disease. *Semin. Immunol.* **10:**5.

Silverstein, AM, and NR Rose. 1997. On the mystique of the immunological self. *Immunol. Rev.* **159:**197.

Steinman, L, JR Oskenberg, and CCA Bernard. 1992. Association of susceptibility to multiple sclerosis with TCR genes. *Immunol. Today* **13:**49.

Streilein, JW, MR Dana, and BR Ksander. 1997. Immunity causing blindness: five different paths to herpes stromal keratitis. *Immunol. Today* **18:**443.

Theofilopoulos, AN. 1995. The basis of autoimmunity. Part I: Mechanisms of aberrant self-recognition. *Immunol. Today* **16:**90.

Theofilopoulos, AN. 1995. The basis of autoimmunity. Part II: Genetic predisposition. *Immunol. Today* **16:**150.

Vyse, TJ, and BL Kotzin. 1998. Genetic susceptibility to systemic lupus erythematosus. *Annu. Rev. Immunol.* **16:**261.

Weiner, HL, et al. 1993. Double-blind pilot trial of oral tolerization with myelin antigens in multiple sclerosis. *Science* **259:**1321.

Wilder, RL. 1995. Neuroendocrine-immune system interactions and autoimmunity. *Annu. Rev. Immunol.* **13:**307.

Wucherpfennig, KW, and JL Strominger. 1995. Molecular mimicry in T-cell mediated autoimmunity: viral peptides activate human T cell clones specific for myelin basic protein. *Cell* **80:**695.

Zhao, Z-S, et al. 1998. Molecular mimicry by herpes simplex virus type-1: autoimmune disease after viral infection. *Science* **279:**1344.

Useful Web Sites

http://www.lupus.org/index.html

The site for the Lupus Foundation of America contains valuable information for patients and family members as well as current information about research in this area.

http://www.nih.gov/niams/
Home page for the National Institute for Arthritis and Musculoskeletal and Skin Diseases. This site contains links to other arthritis sites.

http://www.niddk.nih.gov/
Home page for the National Institute for Diabetes and Digestive and Kidney Diseases. This site contains an exhaustive list of links to other diabetes health-related sites.

http://www.sciencemag.org/feature/data/983519.shl
Link to a Web site that provides specific information concerning the role of gender in autoimmune disease.

STUDY QUESTIONS

1. For each of the following autoimmune diseases (a–m), select the most appropriate characteristic (1–13) listed below.

Diseases

a. ______ Experimental autoimmune encephalitis (EAE)
b. ______ Goodpasture's syndrome
c. ______ Graves' disease
d. ______ Systemic lupus erythematosus (SLE)
e. ______ Insulin-dependent diabetes mellitus (IDDM)
f. ______ Rheumatoid arthritis
g. ______ Hashimoto's thyroiditis
h. ______ Experimental autoimmune myasthenia gravis (EAMG)
i. ______ Myasthenia gravis
j. ______ Scleroderma
k. ______ Pernicious anemia
l. ______ Multiple sclerosis
m. ______ Autoimmune hemolytic anemia

Characteristics

(1) Auto-antibodies to intrinsic factor block vitamin B_{12} absorption

(2) Auto-antibodies to acetylcholine receptor

(3) T_{DTH}-cell reaction to thyroid antigens

(4) Auto-antibodies to RBC antigens

(5) T-cell response to myelin

(6) Induced by injection of myelin basic protein + complete Freund's adjuvant

(7) Auto-antibody to IgG

(8) Possible involvement of fetal cells in the initiation of disease

(9) Auto-antibodies to basement membrane

(10) Auto-antibodies to DNA and DNA-associated protein

(11) Auto-antibodies to receptor for thyroid-stimulating hormone

(12) Induced by injection of acetylcholine receptors

(13) T_{DTH}-cell response to pancreatic beta cells

2. Experimental autoimmune encephalitis (EAE) has proved to be a useful animal model of autoimmune disorders.

a. Describe how this animal model is made.

b. What is unusual about the animals that recover from EAE?

c. How has this animal model indicated a role for T cells in the development of autoimmunity?

3. Molecular mimicry is one mechanism proposed to account for the development of autoimmunity. How has induction of EAE with myelin basic protein contributed to the understanding of molecular mimicry in autoimmune disease?

4. Describe at least three different mechanisms by which a localized viral infection might contribute to the development of an organ-specific autoimmune disease.

5. Transgenic mice expressing the IFN-γ transgene linked to the insulin promoter developed diabetes.

a. Why was the insulin promoter used?

b. What is the evidence that the diabetes in these mice is due to autoimmune damage?

c. What is unusual about MHC expression in this system?

d. How might this system mimic events that might be caused by a localized viral infection in the pancreas?

6. Monoclonal antibodies have been administered for therapy in various autoimmune animal models. Which monoclonal antibodies have been used and what is the rationale for these approaches?

7. Indicate whether each of the following statements is true or false. If you think a statement is false, explain why.

a. T_H1 cells have been associated with development of autoimmunity.

b. Immunization of mice with IL-12 prevents induction of EAE by injection of myelin basic protein plus adjuvant.

c. The presence of the *HLA B27* allele is diagnostic for ankylosing spondylitis, an autoimmune disease affecting the vertebrae.

d. Individuals with pernicious anemia produce antibodies to intrinsic factor.

e. A defect in the gene encoding Fas can reduce programmed cell death by apoptosis.

8. What are some of the possible reasons why females are more susceptible to autoimmune diseases than males?

Go to www.whfreeman.com/immunology Self-Test
Review and quiz of key terms

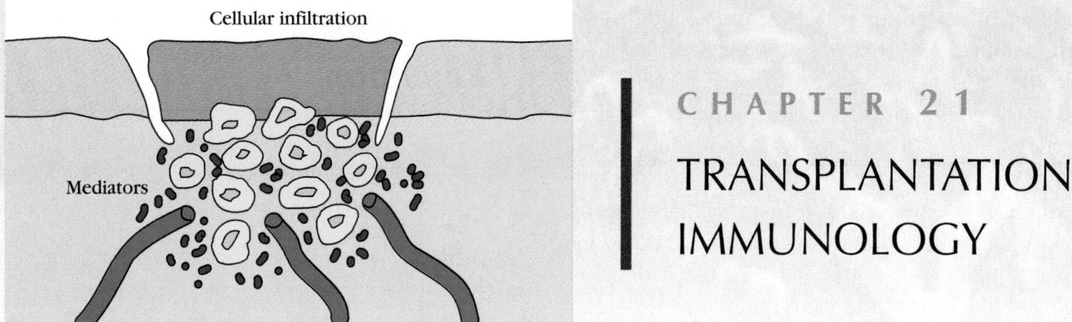

CHAPTER 21

TRANSPLANTATION IMMUNOLOGY

Immunologic Basis of Graft Rejection

Clinical Manifestations of Graft Rejection

General Immunosuppressive Therapy

Specific Immunosuppressive Therapy

Clinical Transplantation

Transplantation, as the term is used in immunology, refers to the act of transferring cells, tissues, or organs from one site to another. The desire to accomplish transplants stems from the realization that many diseases can be cured by implantation of a healthy organ, tissue, or cells (a graft) from one individual (the donor) to another in need of the transplant (the recipient or host). The development of surgical techniques that allow the facile reimplantation of organs has removed one barrier to successful transplantation, but others remain. One barrier is the lack of organs for transplantation. Although accident victims and, for some organs, living donors provide a supply of organs, there are more patients in need of transplants than there are organs available. The seriousness of the donor-organ shortage is reflected in the fact that, as of July 1999, an estimated 64,000 patients in the United States were on the waiting list for an organ transplantation. The majority of those on the list (~70%) require a kidney; at present, the waiting period for this organ averages over 800 days. While the lack of organs for transplantation is a serious issue, the most formidable barrier to making transplantation a routine medical treatment is the immune system. The immune system has evolved elaborate and effective mechanisms to protect the organism from attack by foreign agents, and these same mechanisms cause rejection of grafts from any other individual except one who is genetically identical to the recipient.

There have been several historic attempts to use organ transplantation. The first systematic study of transplantation was reported in 1908 by Alexis Carrel, who interchanged both kidneys in a series of nine cats. Some of those that received kidneys from other cats maintained urinary output for up to 25 days, but no longer, and all the cats eventually died. However, the experiment was a success in that it established the fact that a transplanted organ could carry out its normal function in the recipient. The first human kidney transplant was attempted in 1935, by a Russian surgeon. There was a mismatch of blood types between donor and recipient, which caused almost immediate rejection of the kidney, and the patient died without establishing renal function. This type of rapid immune response, which is termed hyperacute rejection, is mediated by antibodies and will be described in this chapter. The first successful human kidney transplant, which was between identical twins, was accomplished in Boston in 1954. Today, kidney, pancreas, heart, lung, liver, bone-marrow, and cornea transplantations are performed among non-identical individuals with ever-increasing frequency and success using techniques that have been developed to dampen the intensity of the immune response against the foreign organ.

The discovery of the human ABO blood groups (see Table 6-2) by Karl Landsteiner was a key event in the development of successful cell and organ transplantation. Blood transfusion, a form of transplantation, failed sporadically and sometimes disastrously until the practice of systematically matching donor and recipient for the ABO antigens was established on the basis of Landsteiner's work. The ABO system provides a simplified model of the concept that immune recognition of genetically foreign components plays a role in graft rejection (see Figure 16-13). Introduction of mismatched blood into a recipient who has antibodies (isoagglutinins) to the donor's blood-group antigen causes an immediate, often fatal response. The present practice of determining the ABO and several other blood-group antigens for all blood to be used for transfusion makes negative reactions against transfused blood rare.

In addition to its obvious importance in blood transfusion, matching of the donor and recipient ABO blood groups is also critical for survival of tissue grafts, because the vascular endothelium expresses the blood-group antigens. This means that the blood vessels of the donor organ can be attacked by blood-group antibodies that are present in unmatched recipients. Matching of blood-group antigens other than ABO (eg., Rh or Lewis) is not critical for transplantation because these antigens are expressed only on red blood cells.

Several observations by P. B. Medawar in the early 1940s provided insight into the nature of graft rejection. While working with burn patients during World War II, he noticed that grafts of skin from one site to another on the same patient were readily accepted, whereas grafts from relatives were rejected. In one patient, a skin graft from a brother had been rejected; when a second graft from the same donor was attempted, the rejection reaction occurred much faster and with much greater intensity. In subsequent animal experiments, Medawar discovered that prior sensitization with unmatched donor cells led to heightened rejection of a subsequent graft. In 1945, he published a paper suggesting that graft rejection resulted from an immunologic response to the donor organ. Medawar's suggestion proved to be correct. No matter how skilled the surgeon is, a surgically successful transplant can be thwarted by an immunologic attack. The very system that evolved to recognize and destroy altered self-cells is simply performing its function by recognizing and destroying the foreign cells of a graft. Since these early findings, the sub-discipline of transplantation immunology has developed to study the immunologic basis of graft rejection and to find techniques for reducing immune-system activation, thereby promoting graft acceptance. It is noteworthy that studies of this practical aspect of immunology have resulted in giant leaps in our understanding of basic immune processes. As detailed in Chapter 7, the discovery of the major histocompatibility complex was a direct result of studies on graft rejection in humans and tumor transplantation in animals.

An immediate goal of transplantation immunology is to prevent rejection of grafts from genetically nonidentical donors. Various immunosuppressive agents developed to diminish the immunologic attack on grafts can aid as well in the survival of the transplants, but the majority of these agents have an overall immunosuppressive effect, and their long-term use is deleterious. New methods of inducing specific tolerance to the graft without suppressing other immune responses are being developed and promise longer survival of transplants. This chapter describes the mechanisms underlying graft rejection, various procedures that are used to prolong graft survival, and the obstacles that must be overcome to realize the full potential of transplantation as a clinical tool.

Immunologic Basis of Graft Rejection

The degree of immune response to a graft varies with the type of graft. The following terms are used to denote different types of transplants:

- **Autograft** is self-tissue transferred from one body site to another in the same individual. These grafts are often performed on patients with burns by transferring healthy skin to the burned area.
- **Isograft** is tissue transferred between genetically identical individuals. In inbred strains of mice, an isograft can be performed from one mouse to another syngeneic mouse. In humans, an isograft can be performed between genetically identical (monozygotic) twins.
- **Allograft** is tissue transferred between genetically different members of the same species. In mice, an allograft is performed by transferring tissue or an organ from one inbred strain to another. In humans, unless an identical twin is available, organ grafts from one individual to another are allografts.
- **Xenograft** is tissue transferred between different species (e.g., the graft of a baboon heart into a human).

Autografts and isografts are usually accepted, owing to the genetic identity between graft and host (Figure 21-1a). Because an allograft is genetically dissimilar to the host, it is often recognized as foreign by the immune system and is rejected. Obviously, xenografts exhibit the greatest genetic disparity and therefore engender a vigorous graft rejection.

Specificity and Memory of the Rejection Response

The time sequence of allograft rejection varies according to the tissue involved. In general, skin grafts are rejected faster than other tissues such as kidney or heart. Despite these time differences, the immune response culminating in graft rejection always displays the attributes of specificity and memory. If a strain-A inbred mouse is grafted with skin from strain B, primary graft rejection, known as first-set rejection, occurs (Figure 21-1b). The skin first becomes revascularized between days 3 and 7; as the reaction develops, the vascularized transplant becomes infiltrated with lymphocytes, monocytes, neutrophils, and other inflammatory cells. There is decreased vascularization of the transplanted tissue by 7–10 days, visible necrosis by 10 days, and complete rejection by 12–14 days.

Immunologic memory is demonstrated when a second strain-B graft is transferred to a previously grafted strain-A mouse. In this case, a graft-rejection reaction develops more quickly than after the first graft, with complete rejection oc-

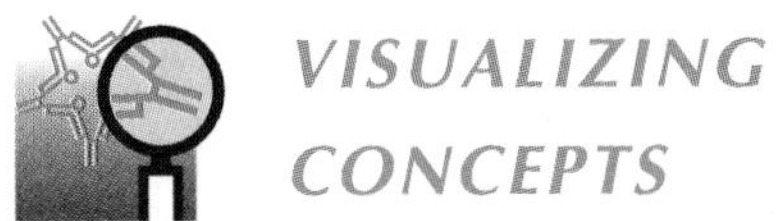
VISUALIZING
CONCEPTS
(a) Autograft acceptance
Grafted epidermis
Blood vessels
Days 3–7: Revascularization
Days 7–10: Healing
Neutrophils
Days 12–14: Resolution
(b) First-set rejection
Grafted epidermis
Days 3–7: Revascularization
Days 7–10: Cellular infiltration
Days 10–14: Thrombosis and necrosis
Necrotic tissue
Blood
clots
Damaged blood vessels
(c) Second-set rejection
Grafted epidermis
Days 3–4: Cellular infiltration
Mediators
Days 5–6: Thrombosis and necrosis
Blood clots
Necrotic tissue

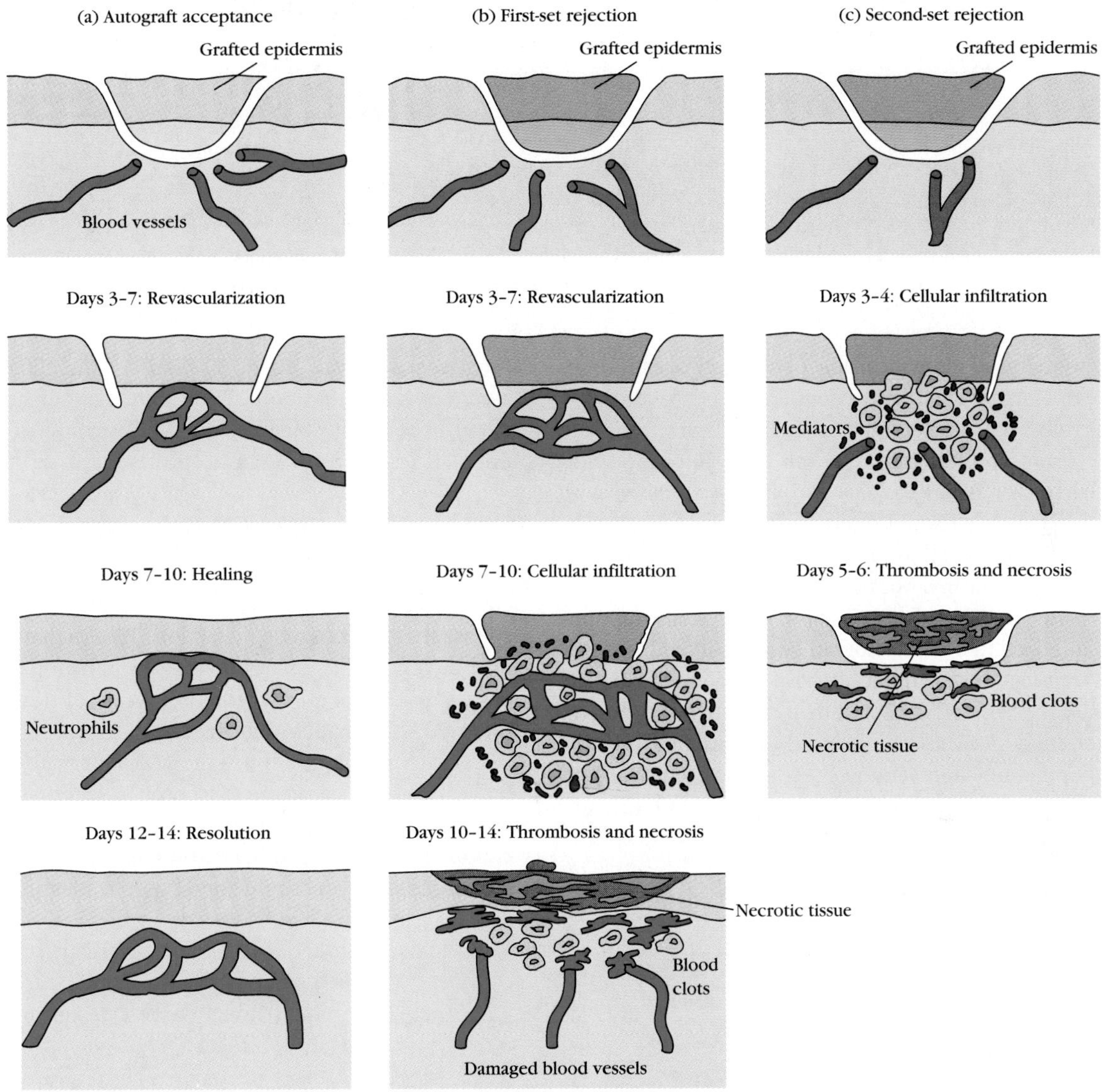

FIGURE 21-1 Schematic diagrams of the process of graft acceptance and rejection. (a) Acceptance of an autograft is completed within 12–14 days. (b) First-set rejection of an allograft begins 7–10 days after grafting, with full rejection occurring by 10–14 days. (c) Second-set rejection of an allograft begins within 3–4 days, with full rejection by 5–6 days. The cellular infiltrate that invades an allograft (b, c) contains lymphocytes, phagocytes, and other inflammatory cells.

curring within 5–6 days; this secondary response is designated second-set rejection (Figure 21-1c). The specificity of second-set rejection can be demonstrated by grafting an unrelated strain-C graft at the same time as the second strain-B graft. Rejection of the strain-C graft proceeds according to first-set rejection kinetics, whereas the strain-B graft is rejected in an accelerated second-set fashion.

Role of Cell-Mediated Responses

In the early 1950s, Avrion Mitchison showed in adoptive-transfer experiments that lymphocytes, but not serum antibody, could transfer allograft immunity. Later studies began to implicate T cells in allograft rejection. For example, nude mice, which lack a thymus and consequently lack functional

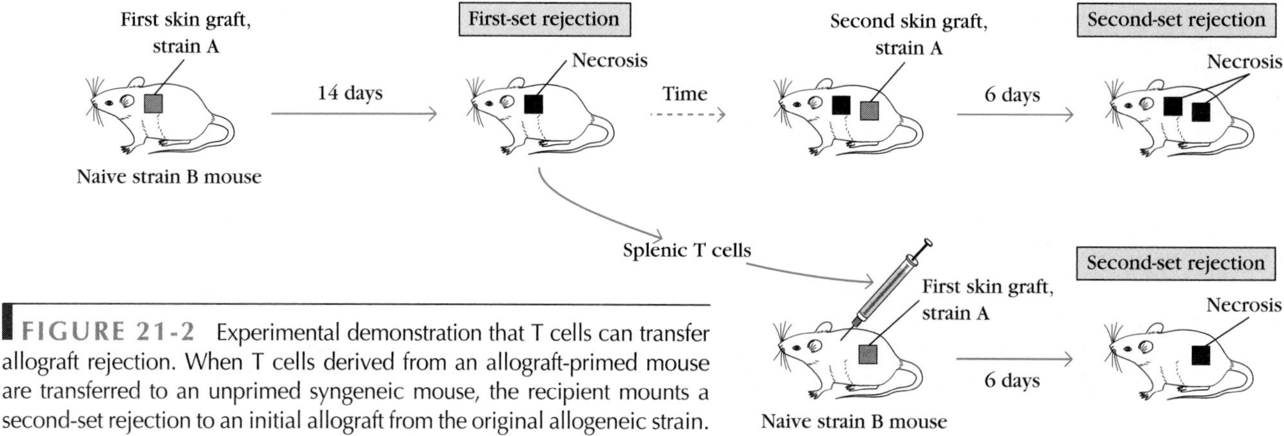

FIGURE 21-2 Experimental demonstration that T cells can transfer allograft rejection. When T cells derived from an allograft-primed mouse are transferred to an unprimed syngeneic mouse, the recipient mounts a second-set rejection to an initial allograft from the original allogeneic strain.

T cells, were found to be incapable of allograft rejection; indeed, these mice even accept xenografts. In other studies, T cells derived from an allograft-primed mouse were shown to transfer second-set allograft rejection to an unprimed syngeneic recipient, as long as that recipient was grafted with the same allogeneic tissue (Figure 21-2).

Analysis of the T-cell subpopulations involved in allograft rejection has implicated both $CD4^+$ and $CD8^+$ populations. In one study, the role of $CD4^+$ and $CD8^+$ T-cell subpopulations in rejection of skin allografts was analyzed by injecting the recipient mice with monoclonal antibodies to deplete one or both types of T cells and then measuring the rate of graft rejection. As shown in Figure 21-3, removal of the $CD8^+$ population alone had no effect on graft survival, and the graft was rejected at the same rate as in control mice (15 days). Removal of the $CD4^+$ T-cell population alone prolonged graft survival from 15 days to 30 days. However, removal of both the $CD4^+$ and the $CD8^+$ T cells resulted in

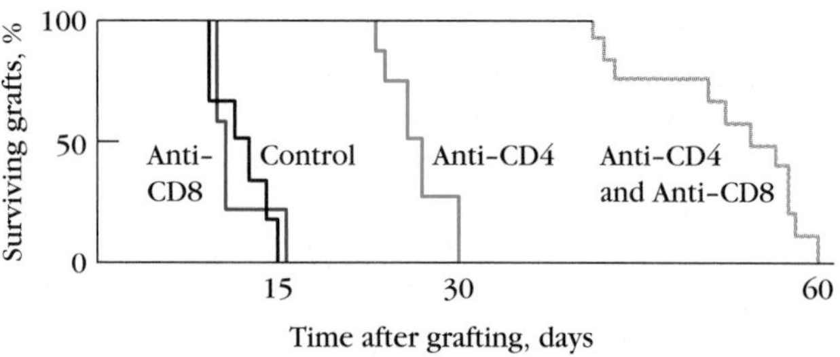

FIGURE 21-3 The role of $CD4^+$ and $CD8^+$ T cells in allograft rejection is demonstrated by the curves showing survival times of skin grafts between mice mismatched at the MHC. Animals in which the $CD8^+$ T cells were removed by treatment with an anti-CD8 monoclonal antibody (red) showed little difference from untreated control mice (black). Treatment with monoclonal anti-CD4 (blue) improved graft survival significantly, and treatment with both anti-CD4 and anti-CD8 antibody prolonged graft survival most dramatically (purple). (Adapted from SP Cobbold et al, 1986, *Nature* **323:**165.)

long-term survival (up to 60 days) of the allografts. This study indicated that both $CD4^+$ and $CD8^+$ T-cells participated in rejection and that the collaboration of both subpopulations resulted in more pronounced graft rejection.

Transplantation Antigens

Tissues that are antigenically similar are said to be **histocompatible;** such tissues do not induce an immunologic response that leads to tissue rejection. Tissues that display significant antigenic differences are histoincompatible; such tissues do induce an immune response that leads to tissue rejection. The various antigens that determine histocompatibility are encoded by more than 40 different loci, but the loci responsible for the most vigorous allograft-rejection reactions are located within the **major histocompatibility complex (MHC).** The organization of the MHC—called the H-2 complex in mice and the HLA complex in humans—was described in Chapter 7 (see Figure 7-1). Because the MHC loci are closely linked, they are usually inherited as a complete set, called a **haplotype,** from each parent.

Within an inbred strain of mice, all animals are homozygous at each MHC locus. When mice from two different inbred strains, with haplotypes *b* and *k*, for example, are mated, all the F_1 progeny inherit one haplotype from each parent (see Figure 7-2a). These F_1 offspring have the MHC type *b/k* and can accept grafts from either parent. Neither of the parental strains, however, can accept grafts from the F_1 offspring because each parent lacks one of the F_1 haplotypes. MHC inheritance in outbred populations is more complex, because the high degree of polymorphism exhibited at each MHC locus gives a high probability of heterozygosity at most loci. In matings between members of an outbred species, there is only a 25% chance that any two offspring will inherit identical MHC haplotypes (see Figure 7-2c), unless the parents share one or more haplotypes. Therefore, for purposes of organ or bone-marrow grafts, it can be assumed that there is a 25% chance of identity within the MHC between siblings. With parent-to-child grafts, the donor and recipient will always have one haplotype in common but will be mismatched for the haplotype inherited from the other parent.

Tissue Typing

Since differences in blood group and major histocompatibility antigens are responsible for the most intense graft rejection reactions, various tissue-typing procedures to identify these antigens have been developed to screen potential donor and recipient cells and assess the likelihood of tissue compatibility. Initially, donor and recipient are screened for ABO blood-group compatibility. The blood-group antigens are expressed on RBCs, epithelial cells, and endothelial cells. Antibodies produced in the recipient to any of these antigens that are present on transplanted tissue will induce antibody-mediated plus complement lysis of the incompatible donor cells.

HLA typing of potential donors and a recipient can be accomplished with a microcytotoxicity test (Figure 21-4a, b). In this test, white blood cells from the potential donors and recipient are distributed into a series of wells on a microtiter plate, and then antibodies specific for various class I and class II MHC alleles are added to different wells. After incubation, complement is added to the wells, and cytotoxicity is assessed by the uptake or exclusion of various dyes (e.g., trypan blue or eosin Y) by the cells. If the white blood cells express the MHC allele for which a particular monoclonal antibody is specific, then the cells will be lysed upon addition of complement, and these dead cells will take up a dye such as trypan blue. HLA typing based on antibody-mediated microcytotoxicity can thus indicate the presence or absence of various MHC alleles.

Even when a fully HLA-compatible donor is not available, transplantation may be successful. In this situation, a one-way mixed-lymphocyte reaction (MLR) can be used to quantify the degree of class II MHC compatibility between potential donors and a recipient (Figure 21-4c). Lymphocytes from a potential donor that have been x-irradiated or treated with mitomycin C serve as the stimulator cells, and lymphocytes from the recipient serve as responder cells. Proliferation of the recipient T cells, which indicates T cell activation, is measured by the uptake of [^{3}H]thymidine into cell DNA. The greater the class II MHC differences between the donor and recipient cells, the more [^{3}H]thymidine uptake will be observed in an MLR assay. Intense proliferation of the recipient lymphocytes indicates a poor prognosis for graft survival. The advantage of the MLR over microcytotoxicity typing is that it gives a better indication of the degree of T_H-cell activation generated in response to the class II MHC antigens of the potential graft. The disadvantage of the MLR is that it takes several days to run the assay. If the potential donor is a cadaver, for example, it is not possible to wait too long for the results of the MLR, because the organ must be used soon after removal from the cadaver. In that case, the microcytotoxicity test, which can be performed within a few hours, must be relied on.

The importance of MHC matching for acceptance of allografts is confirmed by data gathered from recipients of kidney transplants. The data in Figure 21-5 reveal that survival of kidney grafts depends primarily on donor-recipient matching of the HLA class II antigens. Matching or mismatching of the class I antigens has a lesser effect on graft survival unless there also is mismatching of the class II antigens. A two-year survival rate of 90% is seen for kidney transplants in which one or two class I HLA loci are mismatched, while transplanted kidneys with differences in the class II MHC have only a 70% chance of lasting for this period. Those with greater numbers of mismatches have a very low survival rate at one year after transplant. As described below, HLA matching is most important for kidney and bone-marrow transplants; liver and heart transplants may survive with greater mismatching.

MHC identity of donor and host is not the sole factor determining tissue acceptance. When tissue is transplanted between genetically different individuals, even if their MHC antigens are identical, the transplanted tissue can be rejected because of differences at various **minor histocompatibility loci.** As described in Chapter 10, the major histocompatibility antigens are recognized directly by T_H and T_C cells, a phenomenon termed alloreactivity. In contrast, minor histocompatibility antigens are recognized only when they are presented in the context of self-MHC molecules. The tissue rejection induced by minor histocompatibility differences is usually less vigorous than that induced by major histocompatibility differences. Still, reaction to these minor tissue differences often results in graft rejection. For this reason, successful transplantation even between HLA-identical individuals requires some degree of immune suppression.

Mechanisms Involved in Graft Rejection

Graft rejection is caused principally by a cell-mediated immune response to alloantigens (primarily, MHC molecules) expressed on cells of the graft. Both delayed-type hypersensitive and cell-mediated cytotoxicity reactions have been implicated. The process of graft rejection can be divided into two stages: (1) a sensitization phase, in which antigen-reactive lymphocytes of the recipient proliferate in response to alloantigens on the graft, and (2) an effector stage, in which immune destruction of the graft takes place.

Sensitization Stage

During the sensitization phase, $CD4^+$ and $CD8^+$ T cells recognize alloantigens expressed on cells of the foreign graft and proliferate in response. Both major and minor histocompatibility alloantigens can be recognized. In general, the response to minor histocompatibility antigens is weak, although the combined response to several minor differences

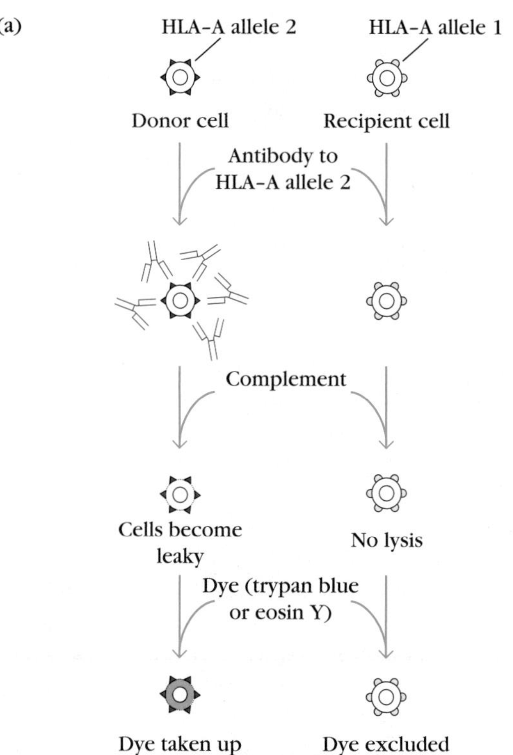

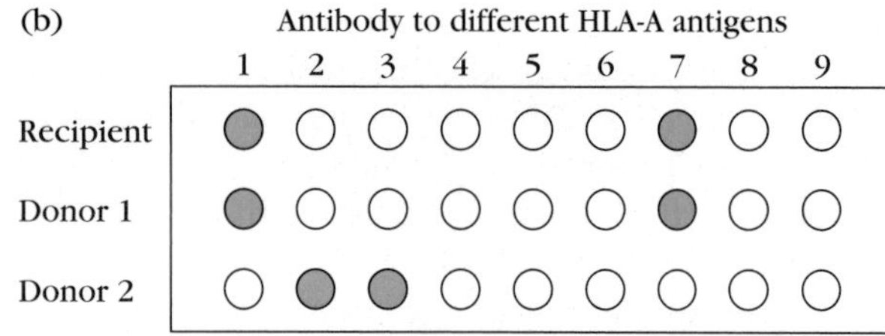

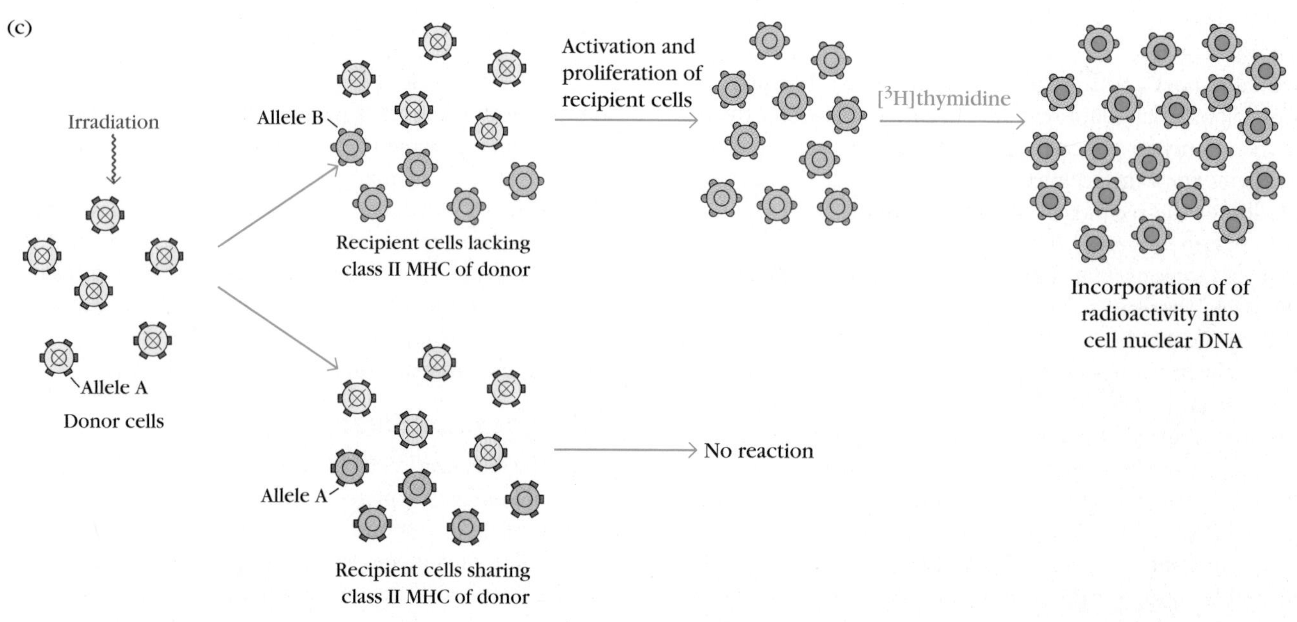

FIGURE 21-4 Typing procedures for HLA antigens. (a, b) HLA typing by microcytotoxicity. (a) White blood cells from potential donors and the recipient are added to separate wells of a microtiter plate. The example depicts the reaction of donor and recipient cells with a single antibody directed against an HLA-A antigen. The reaction sequence shows that if the antigen is present on the lymphocytes, addition of complement will cause them to become porous and unable to exclude the added dye. (b) Because cells express numerous HLA antigens, they are tested separately with a battery of antibodies specific for various HLA-A antigens. Here, donor 1 shares HLA-A antigens recognized by antisera in wells 1 and 7 with the recipient, whereas donor 2 has none of HLA-A antigens in common with the recipient. (c) Mixed lymphocyte reaction to determine identity of class II HLA antigens between a potential donor and recipient. Lymphocytes from the donor are irradiated or treated with mitomycin C to prevent cell division and then added to cells from the recipient. If the class II antigens on the two cell populations are different, the recipient cells will divide rapidly and take up large quantities of radioactive nucleotides into the newly synthesized nuclear DNA. The amount of radioactive nucleotide uptake is roughly proportionate to the MHC class II differences between the donor and recipient lymphocytes.

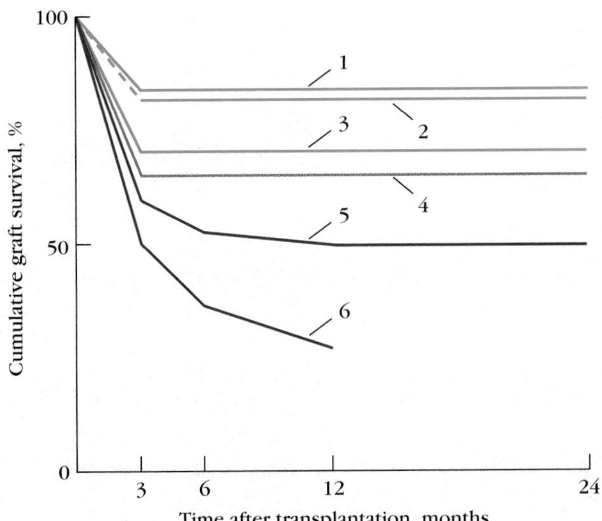

Curve no.	HLA mismatches (no.) Class I	Class II
1	0	0
2	1 or 2	0
3	3 or 4	0
4	0	1 or 2
5	1 or 2	1 or 2
6	3 or 4	1 or 2

FIGURE 21-5 The effect of HLA class I and class II antigen matching on survival of kidney grafts. Mismatching of one or two class I (HLA-A or HLA-B) antigens has little effect on graft survival. A single class II difference (line 4) has the same effect as 3 or 4 differences in class I antigens (line 3). When both class I and class II antigens are mismatched, rejection is accelerated. [Adapted from T Moen et al, 1980, *N. Engl. J. Med.* **303:**850.]

can sometimes be quite vigorous. The response to major histocompatibility antigens involves recognition of both the donor MHC molecule and an associated peptide ligand in the cleft of the MHC molecule. The peptides present in the groove of allogeneic class I MHC molecules are derived from proteins synthesized within the allogeneic cell. The peptides present in the groove of allogeneic class II MHC molecules are generally proteins taken up and processed through the endocytic pathway of the allogeneic antigen-presenting cell. In some cases, peptide fragments of allogeneic class I MHC molecules can be presented within the groove of a class II molecule.

A host T_H cell becomes activated when it interacts with an antigen-presenting cell (APC) that both expresses an appropriate antigenic ligand–MHC molecule complex and provides the requisite co-stimulatory signal. Depending upon the tissue, different populations of cells within a graft may function as APCs. Because dendritic cells are found in most tissues and because they constitutively express high levels of class II MHC molecules, dendritic cells generally serve as the major APC in grafts. APCs of host origin can also migrate into a graft and endocytose the foreign alloantigens (both major and minor histocompatibility molecules) and present them as processed peptides together with self-MHC molecules.

In some organ and tissue grafts (e.g., grafts of kidney, thymus, and pancreatic islets), a population of donor APCs called passenger leukocytes has been shown to migrate from the graft to the regional lymph nodes (Figure 21-6).

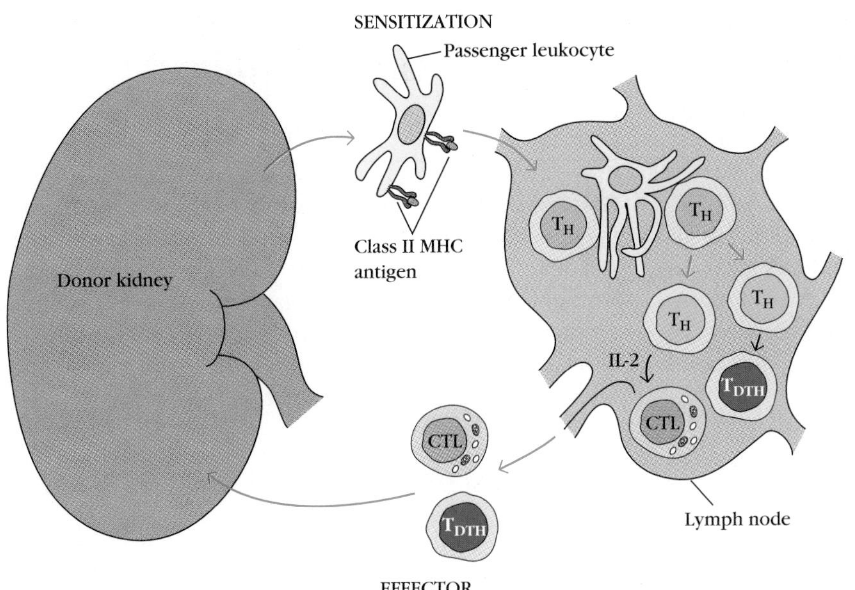

FIGURE 21-6 Migration of passenger leukocytes from a donor graft to regional lymph nodes of the recipient results in the activation of T_H cells in response to different class II MHC antigens expressed by the passenger leukocytes. These activated T_H cells then induce generation of T_{DTH} cells and/or CTLs, both of which mediate graft rejection.

These passenger leukocytes are dendritic cells, which express high levels of class II MHC molecules (together with normal levels of class I MHC molecules) and are widespread in mammalian tissues, with the chief exception of the brain. Because passenger leukocytes express the allogeneic MHC antigens of the donor graft, they are recognized as foreign and therefore stimulate immune activation of T lymphocytes in the lymph node.

Passenger leukocytes are not the only cells involved in immune stimulation. For example, they do not seem to play any role in skin grafts. Other cell types that have been implicated in alloantigen presentation to the immune system include Langerhans cells and endothelial cells lining the blood vessels. Both of these cell types express class I and class II MHC antigens.

The degree and type of immunologic response varies with the type of transplant. As will be described below, some transplants to so-called immunologically privileged sites (such as the eye and the brain) do not encounter cells of the immune system and may be tolerated despite mismatch of genetic types. This is not true for most allografts. When skin, which has no major blood vessels, is grafted, at first it does not contain functional blood vessels. As these reestablish (see Figure 21-1), host lymphocytes carried to the tissue by capillaries or lymphatics encounter the foreign antigens of the skin graft and are carried by the afferent lymphatics to regional lymph nodes. Effector lymphocytes are generated in the regional nodes and are carried by the lymphatics back to the graft to mount an immunologic attack. In kidney or heart transplants, the blood vasculature is immediately restored because it is necessary to suture the major blood vessels of the graft together with those of the host. In this case, blood-borne lymphocytes encounter the alloantigens of the graft and are carried by blood vessels to the spleen or by the lymphatics to regional lymph nodes. Here, within the spleen or lymph nodes, effector cells are generated and are then transported back to the graft by blood or lymph vessels.

Recognition of the alloantigens expressed on the cells of a graft induces vigorous T-cell proliferation in the host. This proliferation can be demonstrated in vitro in a mixed-lymphocyte reaction (see Figure 21-4c). Both dendritic cells and vascular endothelial cells from an allogeneic graft induce host T-cell proliferation. The major proliferating cell is the $CD4^+$ T cell, which recognizes class II alloantigens directly or alloantigen peptides presented by host antigen-presenting cells. This amplified population of activated T_H cells is thought to play a central role in inducing the various effector mechanisms of allograft rejection.

Effector Stage

A variety of effector mechanisms participate in allograft rejection (Figure 21-7). The most common are cell-mediated reactions involving delayed-type hypersensitivity and CTL-mediated cytotoxicity; less common mechanisms are antibody-plus-complement lysis and destruction by antibody-dependent cell-mediated cytotoxicity (ADCC). The hallmark of graft rejection involving cell-mediated reactions is an influx of T cells and macrophages into the graft. Histologically, the infiltration in many cases resembles that seen during a delayed-type hypersensitive response, in which cytokines produced by T_{DTH} cells promote macrophage infiltration (see Figure 14-15). Recognition of foreign class I alloantigens on the graft by host $CD8^+$ cells can lead to CTL-mediated killing (see Figure 14-4). In some cases, graft rejection is mediated by $CD4^+$ T cells that function as class II MHC–restricted cytotoxic cells.

In each of these effector mechanisms, cytokines secreted by T_H cells play a central role (see Figure 21-7). For example, IL-2, IFN-γ, and TNF-β have each been shown to be important mediators of graft rejection. IL-2 promotes T-cell proliferation and generally is necessary for the generation of effector CTLs (see Figure 14-1). IFN-γ is central to the development of a DTH response, promoting the influx of macrophages into the graft and their subsequent activation into more destructive cells. TNF-β has been shown to have a direct cytotoxic effect on the cells of a graft. A number of cytokines promote graft rejection by inducing expression of class I or class II MHC molecules on graft cells. The interferons (α, β, and γ), TNF-α, and TNF-β all increase class I MHC expression, and IFN-γ increases class II MHC expression as well. During a rejection episode, the levels of these cytokines increase, inducing a variety of cell types within the graft to express class I or class II MHC molecules. In rat cardiac allografts, for example, dendritic cells are initially the only cells that express class II MHC molecules. However, as an allograft reaction begins, localized production of IFN-γ in the graft induces vascular endothelial cells and myocytes to express class II MHC molecules as well, making these cells targets for CTL attack.

Clinical Manifestations of Graft Rejection

Graft rejection reactions have various time courses depending upon the type of tissue or organ grafted and the immune response involved. Hyperacute rejection reactions occur within the first 24 h after transplantation; acute rejection reactions usually begin in the first few weeks after transplantation; and chronic rejection reactions can occur from months to years after transplantation.

Hyperacute Rejection

In rare instances, a transplant is rejected so quickly that the grafted tissue never becomes vascularized. These hyperacute reactions are caused by preexisting host serum antibodies specific for antigens of the graft. The antigen-antibody com-

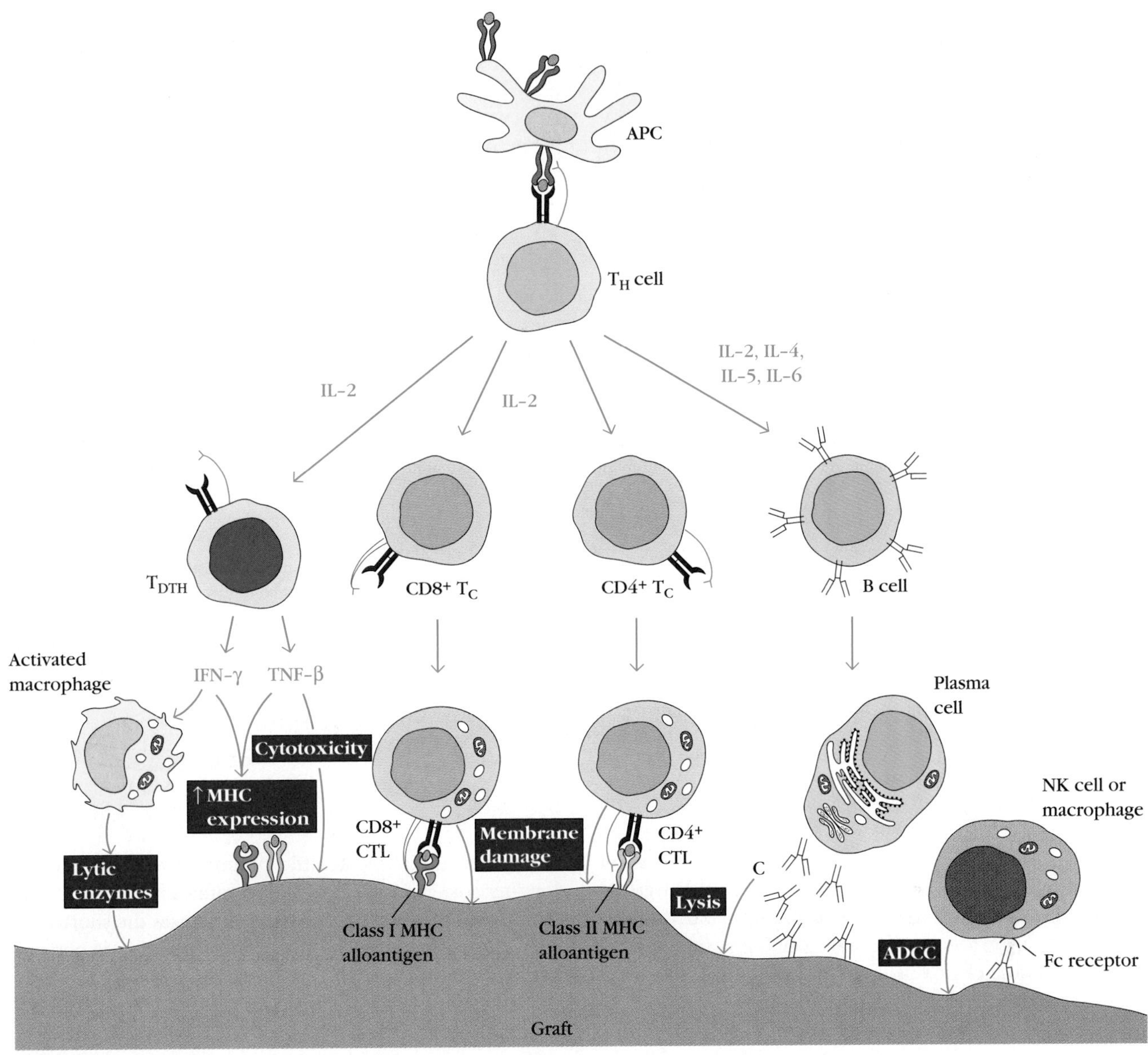

FIGURE 21-7 Effector mechanisms (purple blocks) involved in allograft rejection. The generation or activity of various effector cells depends directly or indirectly on cytokines (blue) secreted by activated T_H cells. C = complement; ADCC = antibody-dependent cell-mediated cytotoxicity.

plexes that form activate the complement system, resulting in an intense infiltration of neutrophils into the grafted tissue. The ensuing inflammatory reaction causes massive blood clots within the capillaries, preventing vascularization of the graft (Figure 21-8).

Several mechanisms can account for the presence of preexisting antibodies specific for allogeneic MHC antigens. Recipients of repeated blood transfusions sometimes develop significant levels of antibodies to MHC antigens expressed on white blood cells present in the transfused blood. If some of these MHC antigens are the same as those on a subsequent graft, then the antibodies can react with the graft, inducing a hyperacute rejection reaction. With repeated pregnancies, women are exposed to the paternal alloantigens of the fetus and may develop antibodies to these antigens. If a woman receives a graft expressing any of these same MHC antigens, it is subject to a hyperacute rejection reaction. Finally, individuals who have had a previous graft sometimes have high levels of antibodies to the allogeneic MHC antigens of that graft; these antibodies will mediate hyperacute rejection of any subsequent graft that expresses some of the same allogeneic antigens.

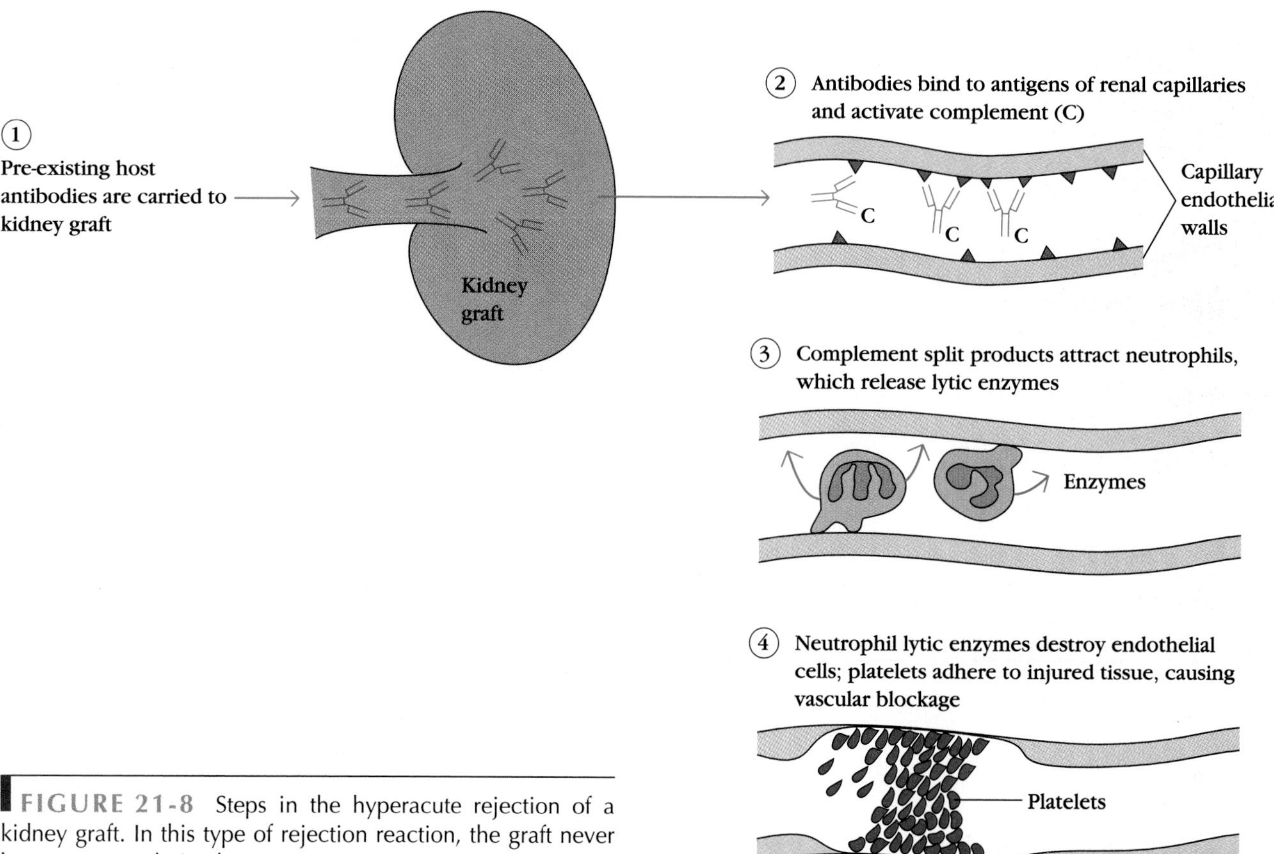

FIGURE 21-8 Steps in the hyperacute rejection of a kidney graft. In this type of rejection reaction, the graft never becomes vascularized.

In some cases, the preexisting antibodies participating in hyperacute graft rejection may be specific for blood-group antigens in the graft. If tissue typing and ABO blood-group typing are performed prior to transplantation, these preexisting antibodies can be detected and grafts that would result in hyperacute rejection can be avoided.

Acute Rejection

Cell-mediated allograft rejection manifests as an acute rejection of the graft beginning about 10 days after transplantation (see Figure 21-1b). Histopathologic examination reveals a massive infiltration of macrophages and lymphocytes at the site of tissue destruction, suggestive of T_H-cell activation and proliferation. Acute graft rejection is effected by the mechanisms described previously (see Figure 21-7).

Chronic Rejection

Chronic rejection reactions develop months or years after acute rejection reactions have subsided. The mechanisms of chronic rejection include both humoral and cell-mediated responses by the recipient. While the use of immunosuppressive drugs and the application of tissue typing methods to obtain optimum match of donor and recipient have dramatically increased survival of allografts during the first years after engraftment, little progress has been made in long-term survival. The use of immunosuppressive drugs, which are described below, greatly increases the short-term survival of the transplant, but chronic rejection is not prevented in most cases. In fact, mean survival time of a mismatched kidney after the first year has not increased significantly since the 1970s. Chronic rejection reactions are often difficult to manage with immunosuppressive drugs and may necessitate another transplantation.

General Immunosuppressive Therapy

Allogeneic transplantation requires some degree of immunosuppression if the transplant is to survive. Most of the immunosuppressive treatments that have been developed have the disadvantage of being nonspecific; that is, they result in generalized immunosuppression of responses to all antigens, not just those of the allograft, which places the recipient at increased risk of infection. In addition, many immunosuppressive measures are aimed at slowing the proliferation of activated lymphocytes. However, because any rapidly dividing nonimmune cells (e.g., epithelial cells of the gut or bone-marrow hematopoietic stem cells) are also affected, serious or even life-threatening complications can occur. Patients on long-term immunosuppressive therapy are at increased risk of cancer, hypertension, and metabolic bone disease.

Mitotic Inhibitors

Azathioprine (Imuran), a potent mitotic inhibitor, is often given just before and after transplantation to diminish T-cell proliferation in response to the alloantigens of the graft. Azathioprine acts on cells in the S phase of the cell cycle to block synthesis of inosinic acid, which is a precursor of the purines adenylic and guanylic acid. Both B-cell and T-cell proliferation is diminished in the presence of azathioprine. Functional immune assays such as the MLR, CML, and skin test show a significant decline after azathioprine treatment, indicating an overall decrease in T-cell numbers.

Two other mitotic inhibitors that are sometimes used in conjunction with other immunosuppressive agents are cyclophosphamide and methotrexate. Cyclophosphamide is an alkylating agent that inserts into the DNA helix and becomes crosslinked, leading to disruption of the DNA chain. It is especially effective against rapidly dividing cells and therefore is sometimes given at the time of grafting to block T-cell proliferation. Methotrexate acts as a folic acid antagonist to block purine biosynthesis. The fact that the mitotic inhibitors act on all rapidly dividing cells and not specifically on those involved in immune response against the allograft can lead to deleterious side reactions by thwarting division of other functional cells in the body.

Corticosteroids

As described at the end of Chapter 15, corticosteroids, such as prednisone and dexamethasone, are potent anti-inflammatory agents that exert their effects at many levels of the immune response. These drugs are often given to transplant recipients together with a mitotic inhibitor such as azathioprine to prevent acute episodes of graft rejection.

Cyclosporin A, FK506, and Rapamycin

Cyclosporin A (CsA), FK506, and rapamycin are fungal metabolites with potent immunosuppressive properties. Although chemically unrelated, CsA and FK506 have similar actions. Both drugs block activation of resting T cells by inhibiting the transcription of genes encoding IL-2 and the high-affinity IL-2 receptor (IL-2R), which are essential for activation. As shown in Figure 10–13, CsA and FK506 exert this effect by binding to cytoplasmic proteins called immunophilins, forming a complex that blocks the phosphatase activity of calcineurin. This prevents the formation and nuclear translocation of the cytoplasmic subunit NF-ATc and its subsequent assembly into NF-AT, a DNA-binding protein necessary for transcription of the genes encoding a number of molecules important to T-cell activation (see Figure 10-12). Rapamycin is structurally similar to FK506 and also binds to an immunophilin. However, the rapamycin-immunophilin complex does not inhibit calcineurin activity; instead it blocks the proliferation and differentiation of activated T_H cells in the G_1 phase of the cell cycle. All three drugs, by inhibiting T_H-cell proliferation and thus T_H-cell cytokine expression, reduce the subsequent activation of various effector populations involved in graft rejection, including T_{DTH} cells, T_C cells, NK cells, macrophages, and B cells.

The profound immunosuppressive properties of these three agents have made them a mainstay of heart, liver, kidney, and bone-marrow transplantation. Cyclosporin A has been shown to prolong graft survival in kidney, liver, heart, and heart-lung transplants. In one study of 209 kidney transplants from cadaver donors, the 1-year survival rate was 64% among recipients receiving other immunosuppressive treatments and 80% among those receiving cyclosporin A. Similar results have been obtained with liver transplants (Figure 21-9). Despite these impressive results, CsA does have some negative side effects, the most notable of which is toxicity to the kidneys. Acute nephrotoxicity is quite common, in some cases progressing to chronic nephrotoxicity and drug-induced kidney failure. FK506 and rapamycin are newer drugs, which are 10–100 times more potent as immune suppressants than CsA, and therefore can be administered at lower doses, consequently with fewer side effects than CsA.

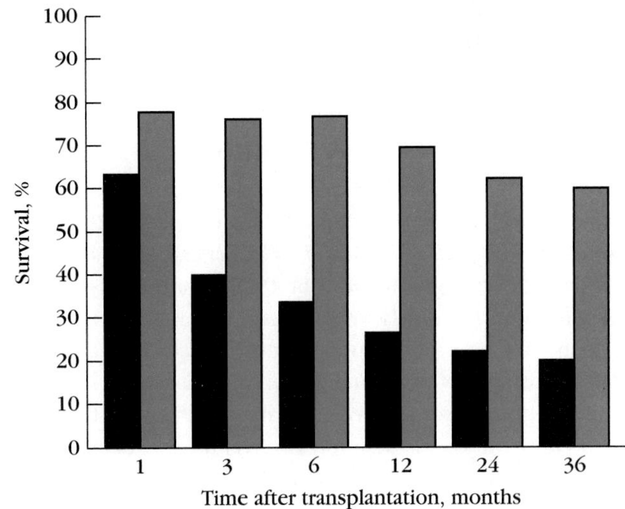

FIGURE 21-9 Comparison of the survival rate of liver transplants in 84 patients who were immunosuppressed with azathioprine and corticosteroids (black) with the survival rate in 55 patients who were immunosuppressed with cyclosporin A and corticosteroids (blue). [Adapted from SM Sabesin and JW Williams, 1987, *Hosp. Pract.* **15**(July):75.]

Total Lymphoid Irradiation

Because lymphocytes are extremely sensitive to x-rays, x-irradiation can be used to eliminate them in the transplant recipient just before grafting. In total lymphoid x-irradiation the recipient receives multiple x-ray exposures to the thymus, spleen, and lymph nodes before the transplant surgery. The typical protocol is daily x-irradiation treatments of about 200 rads per day for several weeks until a total of 3400 rads has been administered. The recipient is grafted in this immunosuppressed state. Because the bone marrow is not x-irradiated, lymphoid stem cells proliferate and renew the population of recirculating lymphocytes. These newly formed lymphocytes appear to be more tolerant to the antigens of the graft.

Specific Immunosuppressive Therapy

In addition to harmful side effects peculiar to the various immunosuppressive treatments described above, a major limitation common to all is that they lack specificity, thus producing a more-or-less generalized immunosuppression and increasing the recipient's risk for infection. What is needed ideally is an antigen-specific immunosuppressant that reduces the immune response to the alloantigens of the graft while preserving the recipient's ability to respond to other foreign antigens. Although this goal has not yet been achieved in human transplants, recent successes in animal experiments indicate that it may be possible. Specific immunosuppression to allografts has been achieved in animal experiments using antibodies or soluble ligands reactive with cell-surface molecules.

Monoclonal Antibodies to T-Cell Components or Cytokines

Monoclonal antibodies directed against various surface molecules on cells of the immune system have been used successfully to suppress T-cell activity in general or to suppress the activity of subpopulations of T cells. Results from studies with animal models suggest further that certain monoclonals may be used to suppress only T cells that are activated. Successes with animal models and planned trials with humans give reason to believe that two types of strategies involving antibodies to suppress rejection will be available eventually for clinical use. Monoclonal antibodies may be used to deplete the recipient of a certain broad or specific cell population; alternatively, they may be used to block co-stimulatory signals. In the latter case, a state of anergy is induced in those T cells that react to antigens present on the allograft.

A strategy to deplete immune cells involves use of a monoclonal antibody to the CD3 molecule of the TCR complex. Injection of such monoclonal antibodies results in a rapid depletion of mature T cells from the circulation. This depletion appears to be caused by binding of antibody-coated T cells to Fc receptors on phagocytic cells, which then phagocytose and clear the T cells from the circulation. In a further refinement of this strategy, a cytotoxic agent such as diphtheria toxin is coupled with the antibody. The cell with which the antibody reacts internalizes the toxin, causing its death. Another depletion strategy used to increase graft survival uses monoclonal antibodies specific for the high-affinity IL-2 receptor (anti-TAC). Since the high-affinity IL-2 receptor is expressed only on activated T cells, exposure to anti-TAC after the graft specifically blocks proliferation of T cells activated in response to the alloantigens of the graft.

Monoclonal antibody therapy, which was initially employed to deplete T cells in graft recipients, also has been used to treat donors' bone marrow before it is transplanted. Such treatment is designed to deplete the immunocompetent T cells in the bone-marrow transplant; these are the cells that react with the recipient tissues, causing graft-versus-host disease (described below). The efficacy of monoclonal antibodies against T cells in all strategies is maximized by selecting antibody isotypes that are good activators of the complement system.

The CD3 receptor and the high-affinity IL-2 receptor are targets present on all activated T cells; molecules present on particular T-cell subpopulations may also be targeted for immunosuppressive therapy. For example, a monoclonal antibody to CD4 has been shown to prolong graft survival. In one study, monkeys were given a single large dose of anti-CD4 just before they received a kidney transplant. Graft survival in the treated animals was markedly increased over that in untreated control animals. Interestingly, the anti-CD4 did not reduce the $CD4^+$ T-cell count, but instead appeared to induce the T cells to enter an immunosuppressed state. This is an example of a non-depleting antibody.

Other targets for monoclonal antibody therapy are the cell-surface adhesion molecules. Simultaneous treatment with monoclonal antibodies to the adhesion molecules ICAM-1 and LFA-1 for 6 days after transplantation has permitted indefinite survival of cardiac grafts between allogeneic mice. However, when either monoclonal antibody was administered alone, the cardiac transplant was rejected. The requirement that both monoclonal antibodies be given at the same time probably reflects redundancy of the adhesion molecules: LFA-1 is known to bind to ICAM-2 in addition to ICAM-1; and ICAM-1 is known to bind to Mac-1 and CD43 in addition to LFA-1. Only when all possible pairings among these adhesins are blocked at the same time is adhesion and signal transduction through this ligand pair blocked.

A potential practical difficulty with using monoclonal antibodies to prolong graft survival in humans is that they are generally of mouse origin. Many recipients develop an antibody response to the mouse monoclonal antibody, rapidly clearing it from the body. This limitation has been overcome by the construction of human monoclonal antibodies and mouse-human chimeric antibodies (see Figure 5-25 and Clinical Focus in Chapter 5).

Because cytokines appear to play an important role in allograft rejection, another strategy for prolonging graft survival is to inject animals with monoclonal antibodies specific for the implicated cytokines, particularly TNF-α, IFN-γ, and IL-2. Monoclonal antibodies to TNF-α have been shown to prolong bone-marrow transplants in mice and to reduce the incidence of graft-versus-host disease. Monoclonal antibodies to IFN-γ and to IL-2 have each been reported in some cases to prolong cardiac transplants in rats.

Agents That Block the Co-Stimulatory Signal

As described in Chapter 10, T_H-cell activation requires a co-stimulatory signal in addition to the signal mediated by the T-cell receptor. One such co-stimulatory signal is mediated by interaction of the B7 molecule on the membrane of antigen-presenting cells with the CD28 or CTLA-4 molecule on T cells (see Figure 10-14). In the absence of a co-stimulatory signal, antigen-activated T cells become anergic (see Figure 10-15). CD28 is expressed on both resting and activated T cells and binds B7 with a moderate affinity; CTLA-4 is expressed at much lower levels and only on activated T cells but binds B7 with a 20-fold higher affinity. A second pair of co-stimulatory molecules required for T-cell activation are CD40, which is present on the APC, and CD40 ligand (CD40L or CD154), which is present on the T cell.

That blocking the B7-mediated co-stimulatory signal with CTL4A after transplantation would cause the host's T cells directed against the grafted tissue to become anergic, thus enabling it to survive, was demonstrated by D. J. Lenschow, J. A. Bluestone, and colleagues. In their experiment, human pancreatic islets were transplanted into mice injected with CTLA4-Ig, a soluble fusion protein consisting of the extracellular domains of CTLA4 and the constant region of the IgG1 heavy chain. (Including the IgG1 heavy-chain constant region increases the half-life of the soluble fusion protein.) The xenogeneic graft exhibited long-term survival in treated mice but was quickly rejected in untreated controls. The fact that the soluble form of the CTLA4 receptor was able to block the rejection of the human tissue transplant in the recipient mice is evidence that blocking co-stimulatory signals in vivo is a viable strategy (Figure 21-10).

These exciting results were extended to transplantation in monkeys by Allan Kirk, David Harlan, and their colleagues. In these experiments, in which kidneys were transplanted between monkeys mismatched at both class I and class II MHC antigens, the recipients were treated for about 4 weeks after transplantation with either CTLA4-Ig or a monoclonal antibody directed against CD40L, or both in combination. Untreated control animals rejected the mismatched kidneys within 5 to 8 days; those treated with a single agent retained their grafts significantly longer, from 20 to 98 days. However, the animals given both showed no evidence of rejection at 150 days after transplantation. This suppression of allograft rejection did not lead to a state of general immunosuppression; peripheral T-cell counts remained normal and other

(a)

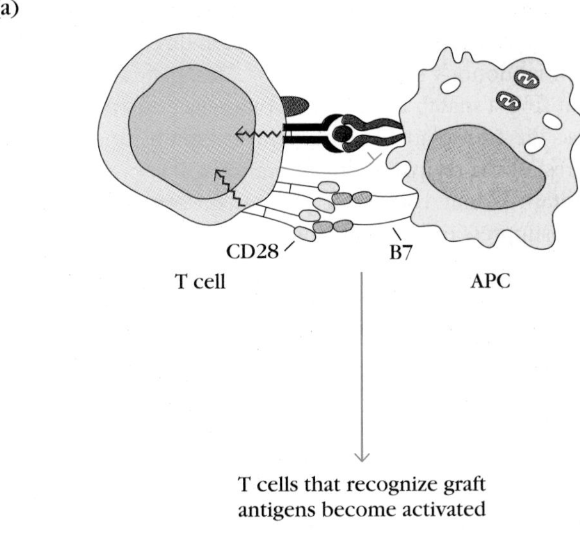

(b)

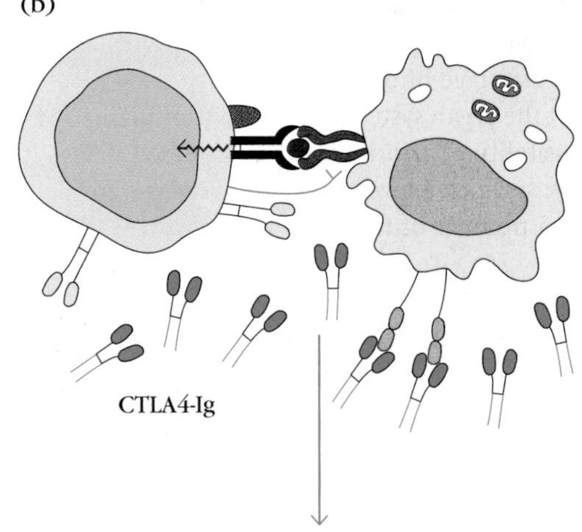

FIGURE 21-10 Blocking co-stimulatory signals at the time of transplantation can cause anergy instead of activation of the T cells reactive against the graft. T-cell activation requires both the interaction of the TCR with its ligand and the reaction of co-stimulatory receptors with their ligands (a). In (b), contact between one of the co-stimulatory receptors, CD28 on the T cell, and its ligand, B7 on the APC, is blocked by reaction of B7 with the soluble ligand CTLA4-Ig. The CTLA4 is coupled to an Ig H chain, which slows its clearance from the circulation. This process specifically suppresses graft rejection without inhibiting the immune response to other antigens.

immune functions were present, including mixed lymphocyte reactivity between donor and recipients. Human clinical trials of the procedures developed for monkeys are planned; if successful, they could revolutionize clinical transplantation procedures. The ability to block allograft rejection without general immunosuppression and without the deleterious side effects of suppressive drugs would enable recipients to lead normal lives.

Clinical Transplantation

In many cases, a transplant is the only means of therapy. Figure 21-11 summarizes the organ and cell transplants that are used routinely at the present time. In addition, certain combinations of organs, such as heart and lung or kidney and pancreas, are being transplanted simultaneously with increasing frequency. Since the first kidney transplant was performed in the 1950s, approximately 400,000 kidneys have been transplanted worldwide. The next most frequently transplanted solid organ is the liver (52,000), followed by the heart (42,000) and, more distantly, by the lung (6,000) and pancreas (2,000). Bone-marrow transplants number around 80,000. Although the clinical results of transplantation of various cells, tissues, and organs in humans have improved considerably in the past few years, major obstacles to the use of this treatment exist. As explained above, the use of immunosuppressive drugs greatly increases the short-term survival of the transplant, but medical problems arise from use of these drugs, and chronic rejection is not prevented in most cases. The need for additional transplants after rejection exacerbates the second major obstacle to the widespread use of transplantation, which is the shortage of organs.

Several of the organ systems for which transplantation offers the possibility of treatment are considered below. The frequency with which a given organ or tissue is transplanted depends on a number of factors:

- Clinical situations in which transplantation is indicated
- Availability of tissue or organs
- Difficulty in performing transplantation and in caring for post-transplantation patients
- Specific factors that aid or hinder acceptance of the particular transplant

The urgency of the transplantation may depend on the affected organ. In the case of the heart, lung, and liver, few alternative procedures can keep the patient alive when these organs cease to function. Although dialysis may be used to maintain a patient awaiting a kidney transplant, there are no comparable measures for the heart or lungs if the allograft fails. Research on artificial organs has been carried out, but no long-term successes have been reported.

Kidney Transplantation

As mentioned above, the most commonly transplanted organ is the kidney; in 1998, there were 11,990 kidney transplants performed in the United States. Major factors contributing to this number are the numerous clinical indications for kidney transplantation. Many common diseases, such as diabetes and various types of nephritis, result in kidney failure that can be alleviated by transplantation. With respect to availability, kidneys can be obtained not only from cadavers but also from living relatives or volunteers, because it is possible to donate a kidney and live a normal life with a single functioning kidney. Surgical procedures for transplantation are straightforward; technically, the kidney is simpler to reimplant than the liver or heart. Because a large number of kidney transplants have been done, patient-care procedures have been worked out in detail. Matching of blood and histocompatibility groups is advantageous in kidney transplantation because the organ is heavily vascularized, but the kidney presents no special problems that promote rejection or **graft-versus-host disease (GVHD),** as the bone marrow or liver do.

There are two major problems in serving the needs of patients waiting for a kidney. One is the short supply of available organs, and the second is the increasing number of sensitized recipients. The latter problem stems from rejection of a first transplant, which then sensitizes the individual and leads to the formation of antibodies and activation of cellular mechanisms directed against kidney antigens. Any subsequent graft containing antigens in common with the first would be quickly rejected. Therefore, detailed tissue typing procedures must be used to ascertain that the patient has no antibodies or active cellular mechanisms directed against the potential donor's kidney. In many cases, patients can never again find a match after one or two rejection episodes. Because the transplanted kidney must remain functional for the rest of the recipient's life, it is almost always necessary to maintain kidney transplant patients on some form of immunosuppression, usually for their entire lives. Unfortunately, this gives rise to complications, including risks of cancer and infection as well as other side effects such as hypertension and metabolic bone disease.

Bone-Marrow Transplants

After the kidney, bone marrow is the most frequent transplant. Since the early 1980s, bone-marrow transplantation has been increasingly adopted as a therapy for a number of malignant and nonmalignant hematologic diseases, including leukemia, lymphoma, aplastic anemia, thalassemia major, and immunodeficiency diseases, especially severe combined immunodeficiency, or SCID (see Chapter 19). The bone marrow, which is obtained from a living donor by multiple needle aspirations, consists of erythroid, myeloid,

VISUALIZING CONCEPTS

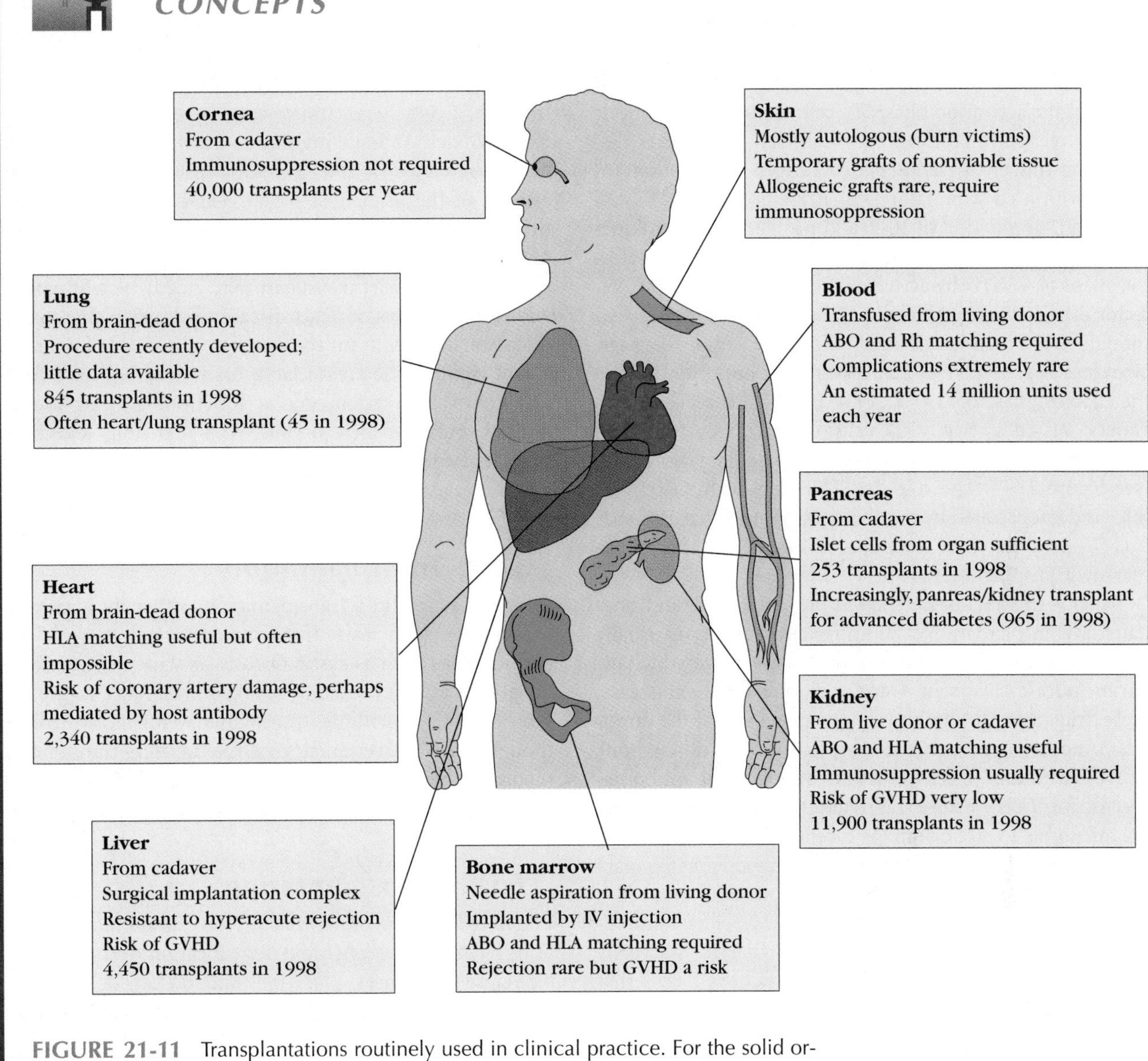

FIGURE 21-11 Transplantations routinely used in clinical practice. For the solid organs, the number of transplants performed in the United States in 1998 is indicated. Estimates are included for other transplants if available.

monocytoid, megakaryocytic, and lymphocytic lineages. The graft, usually about 10^9 cells per kilogram of host body weight, is injected intravenously into the recipient. The first successful bone marrow transplantations were performed between identical twins. However, development of the tissue-typing procedures described earlier now makes it possible to identify allogeneic donors who have HLA antigens identical or near-identical to those of the recipients. While the supply of bone marrow for transplantation is not a problem, finding a matched donor may be one.

In the usual procedure, the recipient of a bone-marrow transplant is immunologically suppressed before grafting. Leukemia patients, for example, are often treated with cyclophosphamide and total-body irradiation to kill all cancerous cells. The immune-suppressed state of the recipient makes graft rejection rare; however, because the donor bone marrow contains immunocompetent cells, the graft may reject the host, causing graft-versus-host disease. GVHD affects between 50% and 70% of bone marrow transplant patients; it develops as donor T cells recognize alloantigens on the host cells.

The activation and proliferation of these T cells and the subsequent production of cytokines generate inflammatory reactions in the skin, gastrointestinal tract, and liver. If it is severe, GVHD can result in generalized erythroderma of the skin, gastrointestinal hemorrhage, and liver failure.

GVHD has both an activation phase and an effector phase. In the activation phase, T_H cells from the donor bone marrow recognize recipient peptide-MHC complexes displayed on antigen-presenting cells. Antigen presentation, together with a co-stimulatory signal, induces donor T_H-cell activation, production of IL-2, and proliferation. Cytokines produced by the activated donor T_H cells induce the effector phase of GVHD by activating a variety of secondary effector cells, including NK cells, CTLs, and macrophages. Although CTLs can act directly to cause tissue damage, cytokines such as TNF-β may play a more important role in the effector phase of GVHD. TNF-β, which is released by a variety of cells (e.g., T_H cells, CTLs, NK cells, and macrophages), can mediate direct cytolytic damage to cells (see Figure 21-7). The role that TNF-β plays in GVHD in mice is demonstrated by the ability of monoclonal antibody to TNF-β to block the development of GVHD after bone-marrow transplantation.

Various treatments are used to prevent GVHD in bone-marrow transplantation. The transplant recipient is usually placed on a regimen of immunosuppressive drugs, which often includes cyclosporin A and methotrexate. In this case, these drugs serve to inhibit immune responses of the donor cells. Another approach has been to treat the donor bone marrow with anti-T-cell antisera or monoclonal antibodies specific for T cells before transplantation, thereby depleting the offending T cells. Complete T-cell depletion from donor bone marrow, however, increases the likelihood that the marrow will be rejected, and so the usual procedure now is a partial T-cell depletion. Apparently, a low level of donor T-cell activity, which results in a low-level GVHD, is actually beneficial because the donor cells kill any host T cells that survive the immunosuppression treatment. This prevents residual recipient cells from becoming sensitized and causing rejection of the graft. In leukemia patients, low-level GVHD also seems to result in destruction of host leukemic cells, thus making it less likely for the leukemia to recur.

Heart Transplantation

Perhaps the most dramatic form of transplantation is that of the heart, once the damaged heart has been removed, the patient must be kept alive by wholly artificial means until the transplanted heart is in place and beating. Heart-lung machines are available to circulate and aerate the patient's blood after the heart is removed. The donor's heart must be maintained in such a manner that it will begin beating when it is placed in the recipient. It has been found that a human heart can be kept viable for a limited period in ice-cold buffer solutions that effectively short circuit the electric impulses that control the rhythmic beating, which could damage the isolated organ. The surgical methods of implanting a heart have been available for a number of years. The first heart transplant was carried out in South Africa by Dr. Christian Barnard, in 1964. Since then, the one-year survival rate for transplantation of the heart has become greater than 80%. In 1998, 2,340 heart transplants were performed in the United States. An issue peculiar to heart transplantation has been a new type of atherosclerotic disease in the coronary arteries of the implanted organ. There is some possibility that host antibodies mediate injury to the vessels in the donated heart.

Although a heart transplant may greatly benefit patients with various types of heart disease or damage, there is obviously a strict limit on the number of available hearts. Accident victims who are declared brain dead but have an intact circulatory system and a functioning heart are the normal source of these organs. HLA matching is desirable but not often possible, because of the limited supply of hearts and the urgency of the procedure.

Lung Transplantation

In recent years, lung transplantation, either by itself or in conjunction with heart transplantation, has been used to treat diseases such as cystic fibrosis or acute damage to the lungs such as that caused by smoke inhalation. In 1998, 845 lung and 45 heart/lung transplants were performed. Although a 60% first-year survival rate for lung transplants is reported, there are little data concerning mechanisms and specific problems associated with them.

Liver Transplantation

The liver is a large organ that performs a number of functions related to clearance and detoxification of chemical and biological substances. Liver malfunction can be caused by damage to the organ from viral diseases such as hepatitis or by exposure to harmful chemicals as in chronic alcoholism. Damage to the liver may correct itself and the damaged tissue can regenerate after the causative injurious agent is cleared. If the liver tissue does not regenerate, damage may be fatal. The majority of liver transplants are used as a therapy for congenital abnormalities of the liver. Because the liver is large and has a complicated circulation, re-implantation of the liver initially posed a technical problem. Techniques have been developed to overcome this major surgical challenge, and successful liver transplants recently have been achieved with a one-year survival rate of approximately 65%. In 1998, 4,450 livers were transplanted in the United States. Increasingly, a liver from a single donor may be split and given to two recipients; normally, a child will receive the smaller portion and an adult the larger.

The immunology of liver transplantation is interesting because the organ appears to resist rejection by hyperacute antibody-mediated mechanisms. It has been shown that even transplantation across blood-group barriers, which would be expected to trigger hyperacute rejection, can be successful in the short term. However, leukocytes within the donor organ together with anti–blood group antibodies can mediate antibody-dependent hemolysis of recipient red blood cells if there is a mismatch of the blood groups. In addition, manifestations of GVHD have occurred in liver transplants even when donor and recipient are blood-group compatible. These reactions are obviously caused by donor lymphocytes carried by the transplanted liver.

Pancreas Transplantation

One of the more common diseases in the United States is diabetes mellitus. This disease is caused by malfunction of insulin-producing islet cells in the pancreas. Transplantation of a pancreas could provide the appropriately regulated levels of insulin necessary to make the diabetic individual normal. Recently, one-year success rates for pancreas transplantation of about 55% have been reported. Transplantation of the complete pancreas is not necessary to restore the function needed to produce insulin in a controlled fashion; transplantation of the islet cells alone could restore function. Because kidney failure is a frequent complication of advanced diabetes, there is often a need to carry out simultaneous kidney/pancreas transplants. In 1998, there were 253 pancreas transplants and 965 kidney/pancreas transplants. A group at the University of Wisconsin reports that they have overcome surgical and medical barriers to this procedure and have achieved survival rates of 87% at one year and 78% at five years for the 381 cases in their study.

Skin Grafting

Most skin transplantation in humans is done with autologous tissue. However, in cases of severe burn, grafts of foreign skin thawed from frozen deposits in tissue banks may be used. These grafts generally act as biologic dressings, because the cellular elements are no longer viable and the graft does not grow in the new host; the grafts are left in place for several days but are regularly replaced. True allogeneic skin grafting using fresh viable donor skin has been undertaken in some cases, but rejection must be prevented by the use of immunosuppressive therapy. This is not desirable because a major problem with burn victims is the high risk of infection, and immunosuppressive therapy accentuates this risk.

Xenotransplantation

While the immune system represents a formidable barrier to the use of transplantation, there has been significant progress in overcoming this obstacle. However, there has not been comparable progress in solving the complex problem of finding organs for those in need of them. The supply of available organs falls far short of the number of patients requiring transplants. As a result, a large percentage of patients will die while waiting for a transplant. The need for an alternative source of donor organs has focused attention on xenotransplantation. Nonhuman primates (chimpanzees, monkeys, and baboons) have served as the main transplant donors, and the use of the pig as a source of kidneys is under serious consideration.

The earliest transplants of chimpanzee kidney into humans date back to 1964. Since that time, sporadic attempts at kidney, heart, liver, and bone-marrow transplantation from primates into humans have been made, but none with great success. Several recent attempts have received some attention. In 1993, T. E. Starzl performed two liver transplants from baboons into patients suffering from liver failure. Both patients died, one after 26 days and the other after 70 days. In 1994, a pig liver was transplanted into a 26-year-old suffering from acute hepatic failure. The liver functioned only 30 hours before it was rejected by a hyperacute rejection reaction. In 1995, baboon bone marrow was infused into an HIV-infected man with the aim of boosting his weakened immune system with the baboon immune cells, which do not become infected with the virus. Although there were no complications from the transplant, the baboon bone marrow did not appear to establish itself in the recipient.

A major problem with xenotransplants is that immune rejection is often quite vigorous, even when recipients are treated with potent immunosuppressive drugs such as FK506 or rapamycin. The major response involves the action of humoral antibody and complement, leading to the development of a hyperacute rejection reaction. One possible approach to limiting the destruction mediated by antibody and complement is to produce transgenic donor pigs that express human decay-accelerating factor (DAF), which dissociates C3 convertase and prevents activation of C3 and C5 (see Figure 13-9d). The presence of human DAF on the cells of the implanted organ should reduce complement activity and decrease the severity of the hyperacute rejection reaction to the graft. This approach is under way, and grafts from these animals will be evaluated in human clinical trials within the next few years.

There are several reasons why pigs are under consideration as potential transplant donors. They breed rapidly, have large litters, can be housed in pathogen-free environments, and share a considerable number of anatomic and physiologic similarities with humans. Although primates are more closely related to humans than pigs are, the availability of primates as transplant donors is limited.

In addition to the problem of rejection, there is general concern that xenotransplantation has the potential of spreading pathogens from the donor to the recipient. These pathogens could potentially cause diseases, called xenozoonoses, that are fatal for humans. For example, certain viruses, including close relatives of HIV-1 found in chimpanzees and HIV-2 and herpes virus B, which occur in several primate species, cause limited pathogenesis in their primate hosts but can lead to deadly infections in humans. In addition, there is the fear that primate retroviruses (see Chapter 19) such as SIV, may recombine with human variants to produce new agents of disease. Many scientists warn of the risk of introducing new primate pathogens into the human population through xenotransplantation, and caution against moving too rapidly into this new field. The possibility of introducing new viruses into humans may be greater for transplants from closely related species, such as primates, and less in the case of more distantly related species, such as pigs, because viruses are less likely to replicate in cells from unrelated species.

Transplants to Immunologically Privileged Sites

There are certain sites in the body, called immunologically privileged sites, where an allograft can be placed without engendering a rejection reaction. These sites include the anterior chamber of the eye, the cornea, the uterus, the testes, and the brain. The cheek pouch of the Syrian hamster is also a privileged site, which has been used in experimental situations. Each of these sites is characterized by an absence of lymphatic vessels and in some cases by an absence of blood vessels as well. Consequently, the alloantigens of the graft are not able to sensitize the recipient's lymphocytes, and the graft has an increased likelihood of acceptance even when HLA antigens are not matched.

The privileged location of the cornea has allowed corneal transplants to be highly successful. The brain is an immunologically privileged site because the blood-brain barrier prevents the entry or exit of many molecules. The successful transplantation of allogeneic pancreatic islet cells into the thymus in a rat model of diabetes suggests that the thymus may also be an immunologically privileged site.

Immunologically privileged sites fail to induce an immune response because they are effectively sequestered from the cells of the immune system. This suggests the possibility of physically sequestering grafted cells. In one study, pancreatic islet cells were encapsulated in semipermeable membranes (fabricated from an acrylic copolymer) and then transplanted into diabetic mice. The islet cells survived and produced insulin. The transplanted cells were not rejected, because the recipient's immune cells could not penetrate the membrane. This novel transplant method enabled the diabetic mice to produce normal levels of insulin and is undergoing trials for treatment of human diabetics.

Summary

1. Graft rejection is an immunologic response displaying the attributes of specificity, memory, and self/nonself recognition. In hyperacute rejection, preexisting host antibodies react with graft antigens, leading to an inflammatory response that prevents vascularization of the graft and its loss within a day (see Figure 21-8). Acute graft rejection involves the cell-mediated branch of the immune system, with tissue damage mediated by T_{DTH} cells and/or CTLs (see Figure 21-7). Acute response to an allograft exhibits immunologic memory, with a more rapid second-set rejection than first-set rejection (see Figure 21-1), and this reaction can be transferred with T cells (see Figure 21-2). Chronic rejection occurs months or years after transplantation and involves both cellular and humoral immune components.
2. The immune response is generated to tissue antigens on the transplanted tissue that differ from those of the host. Although many different loci encode such antigens, antigens responsible for the most vigorous graft-rejection reactions are encoded within the major histocompatibility complex (MHC), called the HLA complex in humans. Even when a donor and a recipient have identical HLA antigens, differences in minor histocompatibility loci outside the MHC can contribute to graft rejection.
3. The degree to which a recipient and potential graft donors are matched for HLA antigens can be assessed by tissue typing. In the microcytotoxicity test, monoclonal antibodies are used to detect the presence of various class I and class II MHC antigens on donor and recipient cells (see Figure 21-4a and b). The more MHC antigens that a donor and recipient have in common, the more likely is a graft to survive (see Figure 21-5). The mixed-lymphocyte reaction (MLR) can be used to quantitatively assess the class II MHC compatibility of a recipient and potential donors (see Figure 21-4c).
4. The process of graft rejection can be divided into a sensitization stage and an effector stage (see Figure 21–6). During the sensitization stage, passenger leukocytes, derived from the donor graft, migrate from the graft to the regional lymph nodes, where they are recognized as foreign by the recipient's T_H cells, stimulating T_H-cell proliferation. After T_H-cell proliferation, a population of effector cells is generated, which migrates to the graft and mediates graft rejection.
5. In most clinical situations, graft rejection is suppressed by nonspecific immunosuppressive agents (see Figure 21-9). Nonspecific agents include mitotic inhibitors (purine analogs), corticosteroids (dexamethasone, prednisone) , fungal metabolites (cyclosporin A, FK506, rapamycin) and total lymphoid x-irradiation. However, long-term use of these agents is deleterious to the patient because of harmful side effects and the fact that the immune system is suppressed, leading to increased susceptibility to infectious diseases and cancer.
6. Experimental approaches using monoclonal antibodies offer the possibility of specific immunosuppression. These approaches include blocking proliferation of antigen-activated T cells with monoclonal antibodies to the IL-2

receptor or depletion of T-cell populations with monoclonal antibodies to CD3 or CD4. An approach that offers considerable promise is blocking the co-stimulatory signals by binding of inhibitors that interfere with the interaction of B7 and CD28 or CTLA-4 (see Figure 21-10) or those involved in the reaction CD40 with its ligand CD40L. In the absence of this co-stimulatory signal, specific antigen-activated T_H cells become anergic but other responses are not inhibited.

7. A major complication in bone-marrow transplantation is a graft-versus-host reaction mediated by the lymphocytes contained within the donor marrow. T-cell depletion from the donor marrow by antibody specific for T-cell populations reduces the risk of graft-versus-host disease. Transplantations of a variety of organs are being performed with remarkable success (see Figure 21-11). HLA typing and immunosuppressive therapy have together improved prospects for organ transplants.
8. A critical problem preventing more widespread use of transplantation is the shortage of organs available for transplantation. Although barriers remain, the possibility of using organs from non-human species (xenotransplants) is under careful consideration.
9. There are sites in the body at which tranplanted cells or organs are not rejected despite genetic mismatch between donor and recipient. These immunologically privileged sites include the cornea of the eye, brain, testes, and uterus, which have in common an absence of lymphatics.

REFERENCES

First, MR. 1998. Clinical application of immunosuppressive agents in renal transplantation. *Surg. Clin. N. Am.* **78:**61.

Goral, S, and JH Helderman. 1997. The evolution and future of immunosuppression in renal transplantation. *Sem. Nephrol.* **17:**364.

Grover, FL, et al. 1997. The past, present, and future of lung transplantation. *Am. J. Surg.* **173:**523.

Isobe, M, et al. 1992. Specific acceptance of cardiac allograft after treatment with antibodies to ICAM-1 and LFA-1. *Science* **255:**1125.

Kaufman, CL, B Gaines, and ST Ildstad. 1995. Xenotransplantation. *Annu. Rev. Immunol.* **13:**339.

Kirk, AD, et al. 1997. CTLA4-Ig and anti-CD40 ligand prevent renal allograft rejection in primates. *Proc. Natl. Scad. Sci. USA* **94:**8789.

Lacy, PE, et al. 1991. Maintenance of normoglycemia in diabetic mice by subcutaneous xenografts of encapsulated islets. *Science* **254:**1972.

Larsen, CP, and RC Pearson. 1997. The CD40 pathway in allograft rejection, acceptance, and tolerance. *Curr. Opin. Immunol.* **9:**641.

Lenschow, DJ, et al. 1992. Long-term survival of xenogeneic pancreatic islets induced by CTLA4-Ig. *Science* **257:**789.

Levy, AE, JW Alexander, and GF Babcock. 1997. A strategy for generating consistent long-term donor-specific tolerance to solid organ allografts. *Transplant Immunol.* **5:**83.

Markees, TG, et al. 1996. Tolerance to islet xenografts induced by dual manipulation of antigen presentation and co-stimulation. *Transplant. Proc.* **28:**814.

Markees, TG, et al. 1997. Prolonged survival of mouse skin allografts in recipients treated with donor splenocytes and antibody to CD40 ligand. *Transplantation* **64:**329.

Platt, JL. 1996. Xenotransplantation: recent progress and current perspectives. *Curr. Opin. Immunol.* **8:**721.

Rayhill, SC, et al. 1996. Simultaneous pancreas-kidney transplantation: recent experience at the University of Wisconsin. *Exp. Clin. Endocrinol. Diabetes* **104:**353.

Rosenberg, AS, and A Singer. 1992. Cellular basis of skin allograft rejection: an in vivo model of immune-mediated tissue destruction. *Annu. Rev. Immunol.* **10:**333.

Rowe, PM. 1996. Xenotransplantation: from animal facility to the clinic? *Mol. Med. Today* **2:**10.

Sherman, LA, and S Chattopadhyay. 1993. The molecular basis of allorecognition. *Annu. Rev. Immunol.* **11:**385.

Sigal, NH, and FJ Dumont. 1992. Cyclosporin A, FK-506, and rapamycin: pharmacologic probes of lymphocyte signal transduction. *Annu. Rev. Immunol.* **10:**519.

Steele, DJ, and H Auchincloss. 1995. Xenotransplantation. *Annu. Rev. Med.* **46:**345.

Weber, M, et al. 1998. Organ transplantation in the twenty-first century. *Urol. Clin. N. Am.* **25:**51.

Woo, S-B, SJ Lee, and MM Schubert. 1997. Graft-vs-host disease. *Crit. Rev. Oral Biol. Med.* **8:**201.

Useful Web Sites

http//www.unos.org

United Network for Organ Sharing site has information concerning all aspects of solid-organ transplantation for patients and their families, doctors, and teachers.

http://www.marrow.org

The National Marrow Donor Program Web site contains information about all aspects of bone-marrow transplantation.

STUDY QUESTIONS

1. Indicate whether each of the following statements is true or false. If you think a statement is false, explain why.

a. Acute rejection is mediated by preexisting host antibodies specific for antigens on the grafted tissue.

b. Second-set rejection is a manifestation of immunologic memory.

c. Passenger leukocytes are host dendritic cells that migrate into grafted tissue and act as antigen-presenting cells.

d. All allografts between individuals with identical HLA haplotypes will be accepted.

Go to www.whfreeman.com/immunology 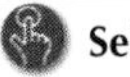 **Self-Test**
Review and quiz of key terms

e. Cytokines produced by host T_H cells activated in response to alloantigens play a major role in graft rejection.

2. You are a pediatrician treating a child who needs a kidney transplant. The child does not have an identical twin, but both parents and several siblings will donate a kidney if the MHC match with the patient is good.

a. What is the best possible MHC match that could be achieved in this situation?

b. In which relative(s) might you find it? Why?

c. What test(s) would you perform in order to find the best-matched kidney?

3. Indicate in the Response column in the table below whether a skin graft from each donor to each recipient listed would result in a rejection (R) or an acceptance (A) response. If you believe a rejection reaction would occur, then indicate in the right-hand column whether it would be a first-set rejection (FSR), occurring in 12–14 days, or a second-set rejection (SSR), occurring in 5–6 days. All the mouse strains listed in the table have different H-2 haplotypes.

4. Graft-versus-host disease(GVHD) frequently develops after certain types of transplantations.

a. Briefly outline the mechanisms involved in GVHD.

b. Under what conditions is GVHD likely to occur?

c. Some researchers have found that GVHD can be diminished by prior treatment of the graft with monoclonal antibody plus complement or with monoclonal antibody conjugated with toxins. List at least two cell-surface antigens to which monoclonal antibodies could be prepared and used for this purpose, and give the rationale for your choices.

5. A child who requires a kidney transplant has been offered a kidney from both parents and from five siblings.

a. Cells from the potential donors are screened with monoclonal antibodies to the HLA-A, -B, and -C antigens in a microcytotoxicity assay. In addition, ABO blood-group typing is performed. Based on the results in the accompanying table, a kidney graft from which donor(s) is most likely to survive?

b. Now a one-way MLR is performed using various combinations of mitomycin-treated lymphocytes. The results, expressed as counts per minute of [^{3}H]thymidine incorporated, are shown in the accompanying table; the stimulation index (ratio of the experimental value to the control in which identical leukocytes are mixed) is listed below in parentheses. Based on these data, a graft from which donor(s) is most likely to be accepted?

6. What is the biologic basis for attempting to use soluble CTL4A or anti-CD40L to block allograft rejection? Why might this be better than treating a graft recipient with CsA or FK506?

For use with Question 3:

Donor	Recipient	Response	Type of rejection
BALB/c	C3H		
BALB/c	Rat		
BALB/c	Nude mouse		
BALB/c	C3H, had previous BALB/c graft		
BALB/c	C3H, had previous C57BL/6 graft		
BALB/c	BALB/c		
BALB/c	(BALB/c × C3H)F_1		
BALB/c	(C3H × C57BL/6)F_1		
(BALB/c × C3H)F_1	BALB/c		
(BALB/c × C3H)F_1	BALB/c, had previous F_1 graft		

For use with Question 5a:

	ABO type	HLA-A type	HLA-B type	HLA-C type
Recipient	O	*A1/A2*	*B8/B12*	*Cw3*
Potential donors				
Mother	A	*A1/A2*	*B8/B12*	*Cw1/Cw3*
Father	O	*A2*	*B12/B15*	*Cw3*
Sibling A	O	*A1/A2*	*B8/B15*	*Cw3*
Sibling B	O	*A2*	*B12*	*Cw1/Cw3*
Sibling C	O	*A1/A2*	*B8/B12*	*Cw3*
Sibling D	A	*A1/A2*	*B8/B12*	*Cw3*
Sibling E	O	*A1/A2*	*B8/B15*	*Cw3*

For use with Question 5b.

	Mytomycin C–treated stimulator cells					
Responder cells	Patient	Sibling A	Sibling B	Sibling C	Sibling D	Sibling E
Patient	1,672 (1.0)	1,800 (1.1)	13,479 (8.1)	5,210 (3.1)	13,927 (8.3)	13,808 (8.3)
Sibling A	1,495 (1.6)	933 (1.0)	11,606 (12.4)	8,443 (9.1)	11,708 (12.6)	13,430 (14.4)
Sibling B	25,418 (9.9)	26,209 (10.2)	2,570 (1.0)	13,170 (5.1)	19,722 (7.7)	4,510 (1.8)
Sibling C	10,722 (6.2)	10,714 (5.9)	13,032 (7.5)	1,731 (1.0)	1,740 (1.0)	14,365 (8.3)
Sibling D	15,988 (5.1)	13,492 (4.2)	18,519 (5.9)	3,300 (1.1)	3,151 (1.0)	18,334 (5.9)
Sibling E	5,777 (6.5)	8,053 (9.1)	2,024 (2.3)	6,895 (7.8)	10,720 (12.1)	888 (1.0)

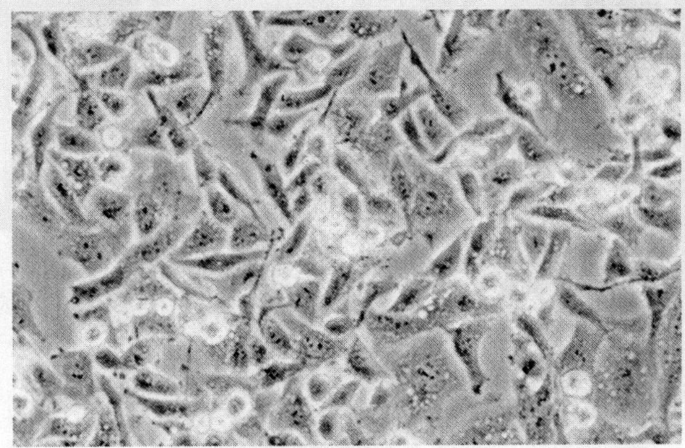

CHAPTER 22

CANCER AND THE IMMUNE SYSTEM

As the death toll from infectious disease has declined in the Western world, cancer has become the second-ranking cause of death there, led only by heart disease. Current estimates project that one person in three in the United States will develop cancer, and that one in five will die from it. From an immunologic perspective, cancer cells can be viewed as altered self-cells that have escaped normal growth-regulating mechanisms. This chapter examines the unique properties of cancer cells, paying particular attention to those properties that can be recognized by the immune system. The immune responses that develop to cancer cells, as well as the methods by which cancers manage to evade those responses, are then described. The final section describes current clinical and experimental immunotherapies for cancer.

Cancer: Origin and Terminology

In most organs and tissues of a mature animal, a balance is usually maintained between cell renewal and cell death. The various types of mature cells in the body have a given life span; as these cells die, new cells are generated by the proliferation and differentiation of various types of stem cells. Under normal circumstances, the production of new cells is so regulated that the number of any particular type of cell remains constant. Occasionally, though, cells arise that no longer responsd to normal growth-control mechanisms. These cells give rise to clones of cells that can expand to a considerable size, producing a tumor, or **neoplasm.**

A tumor that is not capable of indefinite growth and does not invade the healthy surrounding tissue extensively is **benign.** A tumor that continues to grow and becomes progressively invasive is **malignant;** the term cancer refers specifically to a malignant tumor. In addition to uncontrolled growth, malignant tumors exhibit **metastasis;** in this process, small clusters of cancerous cells dislodge from a tumor, invade the blood or lymphatic vessels, and are carried to other tissues, where they continue to proliferate. In this way a primary tumor at one site can give rise to a secondary tumor at another site (Figure 22-1).

Malignant tumors or cancers are classified according to the embryonic origin of the tissue from which the tumor is derived. Most (>80%) are **carcinomas,** tumors that arise from endodermal or ectodermal tissues such as skin or the epithelial lining of internal organs and glands. The majority of cancers of the colon, breast, prostate, and lung are carcinomas. The **leukemias** and **lymphomas** are malignant tumors of hematopoietic cells of the bone marrow and account for about 9% of cancer incidence in the United States. Leukemias proliferate as single cells, whereas lymphomas tend to grow as tumor masses. **Sarcomas,** which arise less frequently (around 1% of the incidence in the United States), are derived from mesodermal connective tissues such as bone, fat, and cartilage.

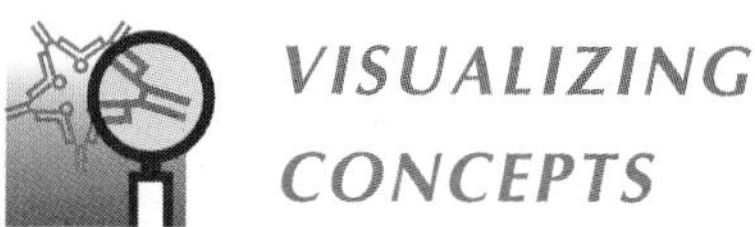

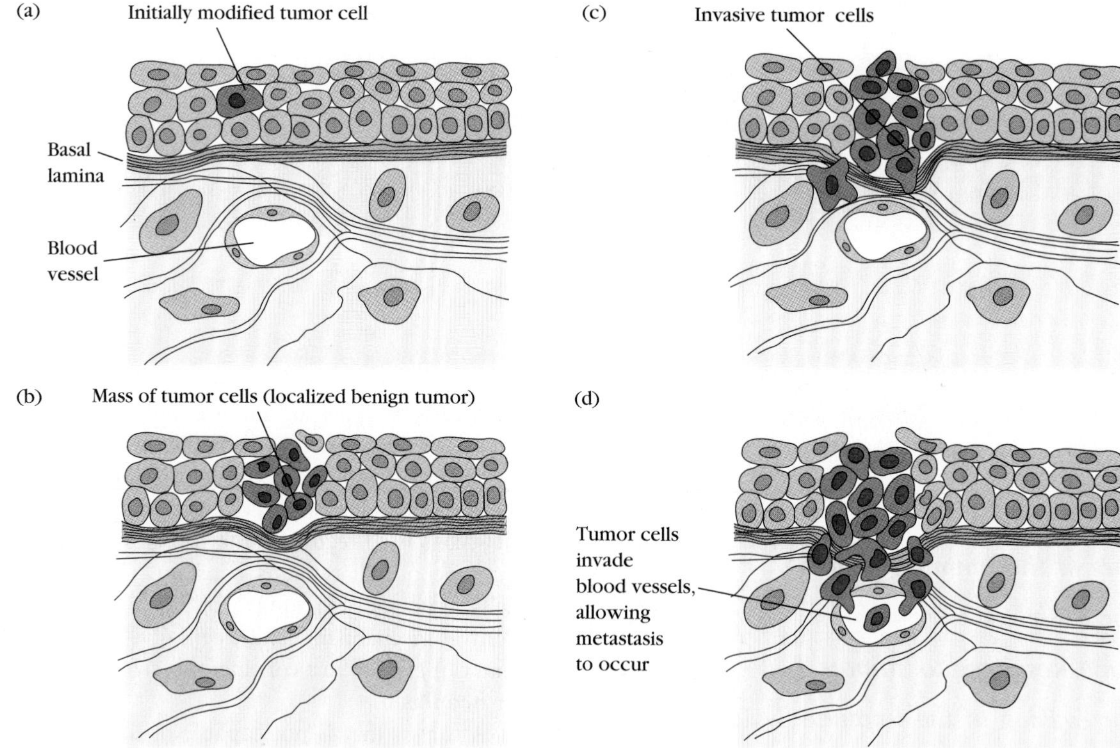

FIGURE 22-1 Tumor growth and metastasis. (a) A single cell develops altered growth properties at a tissue site. (b) The altered cell proliferates, forming a mass of localized tumor cells, or benign tumor. (c) The tumor cells become progressively more invasive, invading the underlying basal lamina. The tumor is now classified as malignant. (d) The malignant tumor metastasizes by generating small clusters of cancer cells that dislodge from the tumor and are carried by the blood or lymph to other sites in the body. [Adapted from J Darnell et al, 1990, *Molecular Cell Biology,* 2d ed., Scientific American Books.]

Malignant Transformation of Cells

Treatment of normal cultured cells with chemical carcinogens, irradiation, and certain viruses can alter their morphology and growth properties. In some cases this process, referred to as **transformation,** makes the cells able to produce tumors when they are injected into animals. Such cells are said to have undergone malignant transformation, and they often exhibit properties in vitro similar to those of cancer cells. For example, they have decreased requirements for growth factors and serum, are no longer anchorage-dependent, and grow in a density-independent fashion. Moreover, both cancer cells and transformed cells can be subcultured indefinitely; that is, for all practical purposes, they are immortal. Because of the similar properties of cancer and transformed cells, the process of malignant transformation has been studied extensively as a model of cancer induction.

Various chemical agents (e.g., DNA-alkylating reagents) and physical agents (e.g., ultraviolet light and ionizing radiation) that cause mutations have been shown to induce transformation. Induction of malignant transformation with such chemical or physical carcinogens appears to involve multiple steps and at least two distinct phases: initiation and promotion. Initiation involves changes in the genome but does not, in itself, lead to malignant transformation. After initiation, promoters stimulate cell division and lead to malignant transformation.

The importance of mutagenesis in the induction of cancer is illustrated in certain diseases, such as xeroderma pigmentosum. This rare disease is caused by a defect in the gene that encodes a DNA-repair enzyme called UV-specific endonuclease. Individuals with this disease are unable to repair UV-induced mutations and consequently develop skin cancers.

A number of DNA and RNA viruses have been shown to induce malignant transformation. Two of the best-studied DNA viruses known to cause malignant transformation are SV40 and polyoma. In both cases the viral genomes, which integrate randomly into the host chromosomal DNA, include several genes that are expressed early in the course of viral replication. SV40 encodes two early proteins called large T and little T, and polyoma encodes three early proteins called large T, middle T, and little T. Each of these proteins plays a role in the malignant transformation of virus-infected cells.

Most RNA viruses replicate in the cytoplasm and do not induce malignant transformation. The exceptions are retroviruses, which transcribe their RNA into DNA by means of a reverse transcriptase enzyme and then integrate the transcript into the host's DNA. This process is similar in the cytopathic retroviruses such as HIV-1 and HIV-2 and in the transforming retroviruses, which induce changes in the host cell that lead to malignant transformation. In some cases, retrovirus-induced transformation is related to the presence of **oncogenes,** or "cancer genes," carried by the retrovirus.

One of the best-studied transforming retroviruses is the **Rous sarcoma virus.** This virus carries an oncogene called v-*src,* which encodes a 60-kDa protein kinase (v-Src) that catalyzes the addition of phosphate to tyrosine residues on proteins. The first evidence that oncogenes alone could induce malignant transformation came from studies of the v-*src* oncogene from Rous sarcoma virus. When this oncogene was cloned and transfected into normal cells in culture, the cells underwent malignant transformation.

Oncogenes and Cancer Induction

In 1971, Howard Temin suggested that oncogenes might not be unique to transforming viruses but might also be found in normal cells; indeed, he proposed that a virus might acquire oncogenes from the genome of an infected cell. He called these cellular genes **proto-oncogenes,** or **cellular oncogenes** (c-*onc*), to distinguish them from their viral counterparts (v-*onc*). In the mid-1970s, J. M. Bishop and H. E. Varmus identified a DNA sequence in normal chicken cells that is homologous to v-*src* from Rous sarcoma virus. This cellular oncogene was designated c-*src.* Since these early discoveries, numerous cellular oncogenes have been identified.

Sequence comparisons of viral and cellular oncogenes reveal that they are highly conserved in evolution. Although most cellular oncogenes consist of a series of exons and introns, their viral counterparts consist of uninterrupted coding sequences, suggesting that the virus might have acquired the oncogene through an intermediate RNA transcript from which the intron sequences had been removed during RNA processing. The actual coding sequences of viral oncogenes and the corresponding proto-oncogenes exhibit a high degree of homology; in some cases, a single point mutation is all that distinguishes a viral oncogene from the corresponding proto-oncogene. It has now become apparent that most, if not all, oncogenes (both viral and cellular) are derived from cellular genes that encode various growth-controlling proteins. In addition, the proteins encoded by a particular oncogene and its corresponding proto-oncogene appear to have very similar functions. As described below, the conversion of a proto-oncogene into an oncogene appears in many cases to accompany a change in the level of expression of a normal growth-controlling protein.

Function of Cancer-Associated Genes

Homeostasis in normal tissue is maintained by a highly regulated process of cellular proliferation balanced by cell death. If there is an imbalance, either at the stage of cellular proliferation or at the stage of cell death, then a cancerous state will develop. Oncogenes and tumor suppressor genes have been shown to play an important role in this process, by regulating either cellular proliferation or cell death. Cancer-associated genes can be divided into three categories that reflect these different activities (Table 22-1).

Induction of Cellular Proliferation

One category of proto-oncogenes and their oncogenic counterparts encodes proteins that induce cellular proliferation. Some of these proteins function as growth factors or growth-factor receptors. Included among these are *sis,* which encodes a form of platelet-derived growth factor, and *fms, erbB,* and *neu,* which encode growth-factor receptors. In normal cells, the expression of growth factors and their receptors is carefully regulated. Usually, one population of cells secretes a growth factor that acts on another population of cells that carry the receptor for the factor, thus stimulating proliferation of the second population. Inappropriate expression of either a growth factor or its receptor can result in uncontrolled proliferation.

Other oncogenes in this category encode products that function in signal-transduction pathways or as transcription factors. The *src* and *abl* oncogenes encode tyrosine kinases, and the *ras* oncogene encodes a GTP-binding protein. The products of these genes act as signal transducers. The *myc, jun,* and *fos* oncogenes encode transcription factors. Overactivity of any of these oncogenes may result in unregulated proliferation.

Inhibition of Cellular Proliferation

A second category of cancer-associated genes—called **tumor-suppressor genes,** or anti-oncogenes—encodes proteins that

TABLE 22-1 FUNCTIONAL CLASSIFICATION OF CANCER-ASSOCIATED GENES

Type/name	Nature of gene product
Category I: Genes that induce cellular proliferation	
Growth factors	
sis	A form of platelet-derived growth factor (PDGF)
Growth-factor receptors	
fms	Receptor for colony-stimulating factor 1 (CSF-1)
erbB	Receptor for epidermal growth factor (EGF)
neu	Protein (HER2) related to EGF receptor
erbA	Receptor for thyroid hormone
Signal transducers	
src	Tyrosine kinase
abl	Tyrosine kinase
Ha-*ras*	GTP-binding protein with GTPase activity
N-*ras*	GTP-binding protein with GTPase activity
K-*ras*	GTP-binding protein with GTPase activity
Transcription factors	
jun	Component of transcription factor AP1
fos	Component of transcription factor AP1
myc	DNA-binding protein
Category II: Tumor-suppressor genes, inhibitors of cellular proliferation*	
Rb	Suppressor of retinoblastoma
p53	Nuclear phosphoprotein that inhibits formation of small-cell lung cancer and colon cancers
DCC	Suppressor of colon carcinoma
APC	Suppressor of adenomatous polyposis
NF1	Suppressor of neurofibromatosis
WT1	Suppressor of Wilm's tumor
Category III: Genes that regulate programmed cell death	
bcl-2	Suppressor of apoptosis

*The activity of the normal products of the category II genes inhibits progression of the cell cycle. Loss of a gene or its inactivation by mutation in an indicated tumor-suppressor gene is associated with development of the indicated cancers.

inhibit excessive cell proliferation. Inactivation of these results in unregulated proliferation. The prototype of this category of oncogenes is *Rb*, the retinoblastoma gene. Hereditary retinoblastoma is a rare childhood cancer, in which tumors develop from neural precursor cells in the immature retina. The affected child has inherited a mutated *Rb* allele; somatic inactivation of the remaining *Rb* allele leads to tumor growth. Probably the single most frequent genetic abnormality in human cancer is mutation in *p53*, which encodes a nuclear phosphoprotein. Over 90% of small-cell lung cancers and over 50% of breast and colon cancers have been shown to be associated with mutations in *p53*.

Regulation of Programmed Cell Death

A third category of cancer-associated genes regulates programmed cell death. These genes encode proteins that either block or induce apoptosis. Included in this category of oncogenes is *bcl-2*, an anti-apoptosis gene. This oncogene was originally discovered because of its association with B-cell follicular lymphoma. Since its discovery, *bcl-2* has been shown to play an important role in regulating cell survival during hematopoiesis and in the survival of selected B cells and T cells during maturation. Interestingly, the Epstein-Barr virus contains a gene that has sequence homology to *bcl-2* and may act in a similar manner to suppress apoptosis.

Conversion of Proto-Oncogenes to Oncogenes

In 1972, R. J. Huebner and G. J. Todaro suggested that mutations or genetic rearrangements of proto-oncogenes by carcinogens or viruses might alter the normally regulated function of these genes, converting them into potent cancer-causing oncogenes (Figure 22-2). Considerable evidence supporting this hypothesis accumulated in subsequent years. For example, some malignantly transformed cells contain multiple copies of cellular oncogenes, resulting in increased production of oncogene products. Such amplification of cellular oncogenes has been observed in cells from various types of human cancers. Several groups have identified c-*myc* oncogenes in homogeneously staining regions (HSRs) of chromosomes from cancer cells; these HSRs represent long tandem arrays of amplified genes.

In addition, some cancer cells exhibit chromosomal translocations, usually the movement of a proto-oncogene from one chromosomal site to another (Figure 22-3). In many cases of Burkitt's lymphoma, for example, c-*myc* is moved from its normal position on chromosome 8 to a position near the immunoglobulin heavy-chain enhancer on chromosome 14. As a result of this translocation, synthesis of the c-Myc protein, which functions as a transcription factor, increases.

Mutation in proto-oncogenes also has been associated with cellular transformation, and it may be a major mechanism by which chemical carcinogens or x-irradiation convert a proto-oncogene into a cancer-inducing oncogene. For instance, single-point mutations in c-*ras* have been detected in a significant fraction of several human cancers, including carcinomas of the bladder, colon, and lung. Some of these mutations appear to reduce the ability of Ras to associate with GTPase-stimulating proteins, thus prolonging its growth-activated state.

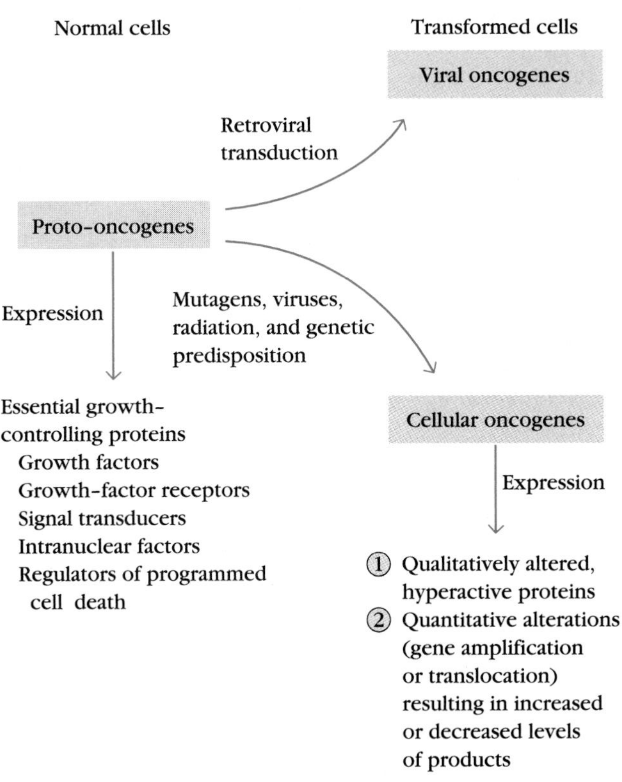

FIGURE 22-2 Conversion of proto-oncogenes into oncogenes can involve mutation, resulting in production of qualitatively different gene products, or DNA amplification or translocation, resulting in increased or decreased expression of gene products.

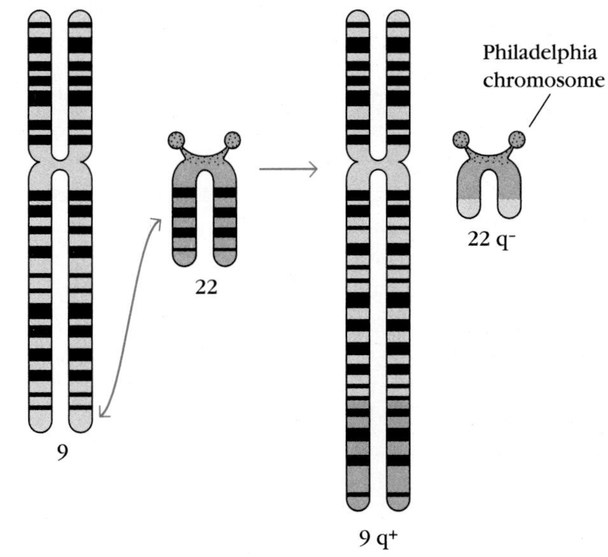

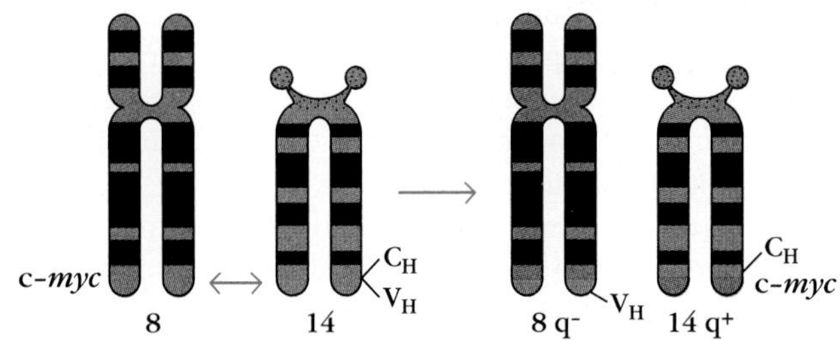

FIGURE 22-3 Chromosomal translocations in (a) chronic myelogenous leukemia (CML) and (b) Burkitt's lymphoma. Leukemic cells from all patients with CML contain the so-called Philadelphia chromosome, which results from a translocation between chromosomes 9 and 22. Cancer cells from some patients with Burkitt's lymphoma exhibit a translocation that moves part of chromosome 8 to chromosome 14. It is now known that this translocation involves c-*myc*, a cellular oncogene. Abnormalities such as these are detected by banding analysis of metaphase chromosomes. Normal chromosomes are shown on the left, and translocated chromosomes on the right.

Viral integration into the host-cell genome may in itself serve to convert a proto-oncogene into a transforming oncogene. For example, avian leukosis virus (ALV) is a retrovirus that does not carry any viral oncogenes and yet is able to transform B cells into lymphomas. This particular retrovirus has been shown to integrate within the c-*myc* proto-oncogene, which contains three exons. Exon 1 of c-*myc* has an unknown function; exons 2 and 3 encode the Myc protein. Insertion of AVL between exon 1 and exon 2 has been shown in some cases to allow the provirus promoter to increase transcription of exons 2 and 3, resulting in increased synthesis of c-Myc.

A variety of tumors have been shown to express significantly increased levels of growth factors or growth-factor receptors. Expression of the receptor for epidermal growth factor, which is encoded by c-*erbB*, has been shown to be amplified in many cancer cells. And in breast cancer, increased synthesis of the growth-factor receptor encoded by c-*neu* has been linked with a poor prognosis.

Induction of Cancer: A Multistep Process

The development from a normal cell to a cancerous cell is usually a multistep process of clonal evolution driven by a series of somatic mutations that progressively convert the cell from normal growth to a precancerous state and finally into a cancerous state.

The presence of myriad chromosomal abnormalities in precancerous and cancerous cells lends support to the role of multiple mutations in the development of cancer. This has been demonstrated in human colon cancer, which progresses in a series of well-defined morphologic stages (Figure 22-4). Colon cancer begins as small, benign tumors called adenomas in the colorectal epithelium. These precancerous tumors grow, gradually becoming increasingly disorganized in their intracellular organization until they acquire the malignant phenotype. These well-defined morphologic stages of colon cancer have been correlated with a sequence of gene changes involving inactivation or loss of three tumor-suppressor genes (*APC, DCC,* and *p53*) and activation of one cellular proliferation oncogene (K-*ras*).

Studies with transgenic mice also support the role of multiple steps in the induction of cancer. Transgenic mice expressing high levels of Bcl-2 develop a population of small resting B cells, derived from secondary lymphoid follicles, that have greatly extended life spans. Gradually these transgenic mice develop lymphomas. Analysis of lymphomas from these mice has shown that approximately half have a c-*myc* translocation to the immunoglobulin H-chain locus. The synergism of Myc and Bcl-2 is highlighted in double-transgenic mice produced by mating the *bcl-2*$^{+}$ transgenic mice with *myc*$^{+}$ transgenic mice. These mice develop leukemia very rapidly.

Tumors of the Immune System

Tumors of the immune system are classified as lymphomas or leukemias. Lymphomas proliferate as solid tumors within a lymphoid tissue such as the bone marrow, lymph nodes, or thymus; they include Hodgkin's and non-Hodgkin's lymphomas. Leukemias tend to proliferate as single cells and are detected by increased cell numbers in the blood or lymph. Leukemia can develop in lymphoid or myeloid lineages.

Historically, the leukemias were classified as acute or chronic according to the clinical progression of the disease. The acute leukemias appeared suddenly and progressed rapidly, whereas the chronic leukemias were much less aggressive and developed slowly as mild, barely symptomatic diseases. These clinical distinctions apply to untreated leukemias; with current treatments, the acute leukemias often have a good prognosis, and permanent remission can often be achieved. Now the major distinction between acute and chronic leukemias is the maturity of the cell involved. Acute leukemias tend to arise in less mature cells, whereas chronic leukemias arise in mature cells. The acute leukemias include **acute lym-**

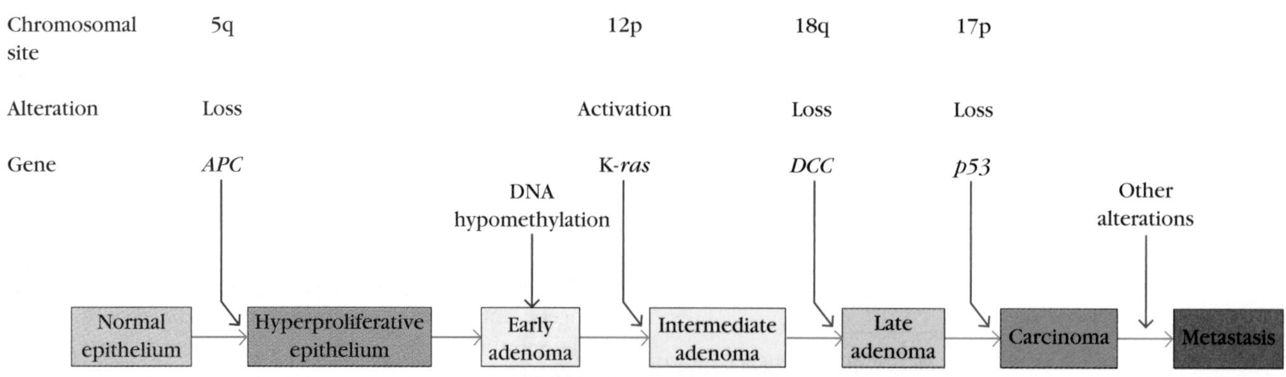

FIGURE 22-4 Model of sequential genetic alterations leading to metastatic colon cancer. Each of the stages indicated at the bottom is morphologically distinct, allowing researchers to determine the sequence of genetic alterations. [Adapted from B Vogelstein and KW Kinzler, 1993, *Trends Genet.* **9:**138.]

phocytic leukemia (ALL) and **acute myelogenous leukemia (AML);** these diseases can develop at any age and have a rapid onset. The chronic leukemias include **chronic lymphocytic leukemia** (CLL) and **chronic myelogenous leukemia (CML);** these diseases develop slowly and are seen in adults.

A number of B- and T-cell leukemias and lymphomas involve a proto-oncogene that has been translocated into the immunoglobulin genes or T-cell-receptor genes. One of the best characterized is the translocation of c-*myc* in Burkitt's lymphoma and in mouse plasmacytomas. In 75% of Burkitt's lymphoma patients, c-*myc* is translocated from chromosome 8 to the Ig heavy-chain gene cluster on chromosome 14 (see Figure 22-3b). In the remaining patients, c-*myc* remains on chromosome 8 and the κ or γ light-chain genes are translocated to a region 3′ of c-*myc*. Kappa-gene translocations from chromosome 2 to chromosome 8 occur 9% of the time, and γ-gene translocations from chromosome 22 to chromosome 8 occur 16% of the time.

Translocations of c-*myc* to the Ig heavy-chain gene cluster on chromosome 14 have been analyzed, and, in some cases, the entire c-*myc* gene is translocated head-to-head to a region near the heavy-chain enhancer. In other cases, exons 1, 2, and 3 or exons 2 and 3 of c-*myc* are translocated head-to-head to the S_μ or S_α switch site (Figure 22-5). In each case, the translocation removes the *myc* coding exons from the regulatory mechanisms operating in chromosome 8 and places them in the immunoglobulin-gene region, a very active region that is expressed constitutively in these cells. The consequences of enhancer-mediated high levels of constitutive *myc* expression in lymphoid cells have been investigated in transgenic mice. In one study, mice containing a transgene consisting of all three c-*myc* exons and the immunoglobulin heavy-chain enhancer were produced. Of 15 transgenic pups born, 13 developed lymphomas of the B-cell lineage within a few months of birth.

Tumor Antigens

The subdiscipline of tumor immunology involves the study of antigens on tumor cells and the immune response to these antigens. Two types of tumor antigens have been identified on tumor cells: **tumor-specific transplantation antigens (TSTAs)** and **tumor-associated transplantation antigens (TATAs).** Tumor-specific antigens are unique to tumor cells and do not occur on normal cells in the body. They may result from mutations in tumor cells that generate altered cellular proteins; cytosolic processing of these proteins would give rise to novel peptides that are presented with class I MHC molecules, inducing a cell-mediated response by tumor-specific CTLs (Figure 22-6). Tumor-associated antigens, which are not unique to tumor cells, may be proteins that are expressed on normal cells during fetal development when the immune system is immature and unable to respond but that normally are not expressed in the adult. Reactivation of the embryonic genes that encode these proteins in tumor cells results in their expression on the fully differentiated tumor cells. Tumor-associated antigens may also be proteins that are normally expressed at extremely low levels on normal cells but are expressed at much higher levels on tumor cells. It is now clear that the tumor antigens recognized by human T cells fall into one of four major categories:

- Antigens encoded by genes specifically expressed by tumors
- Antigens encoded by variant forms of normal genes that have been altered by mutation
- Antigens normally expressed only at certain stages of differentiation or only by certain differentiation lineages
- Antigens that are overexpressed in particular tumors

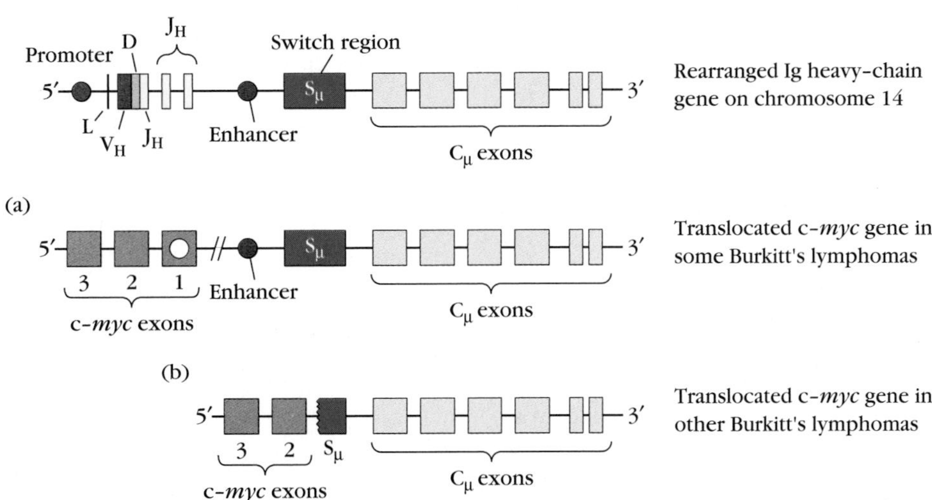

FIGURE 22-5 In many patients with Burkitt's lymphoma, the c-*myc* gene is translocated to the immunoglobulin heavy-chain gene cluster on chromosome 14. In some cases, the entire c-*myc* gene is inserted near the heavy-chain enhancer (a), but in other cases, only the coding exons (2 and 3) of c-*myc* are inserted at the S_μ switch site (b). Only exons 2 and 3 of c-*myc* are coding exons. Translocation may lead to overexpression of c-Myc.

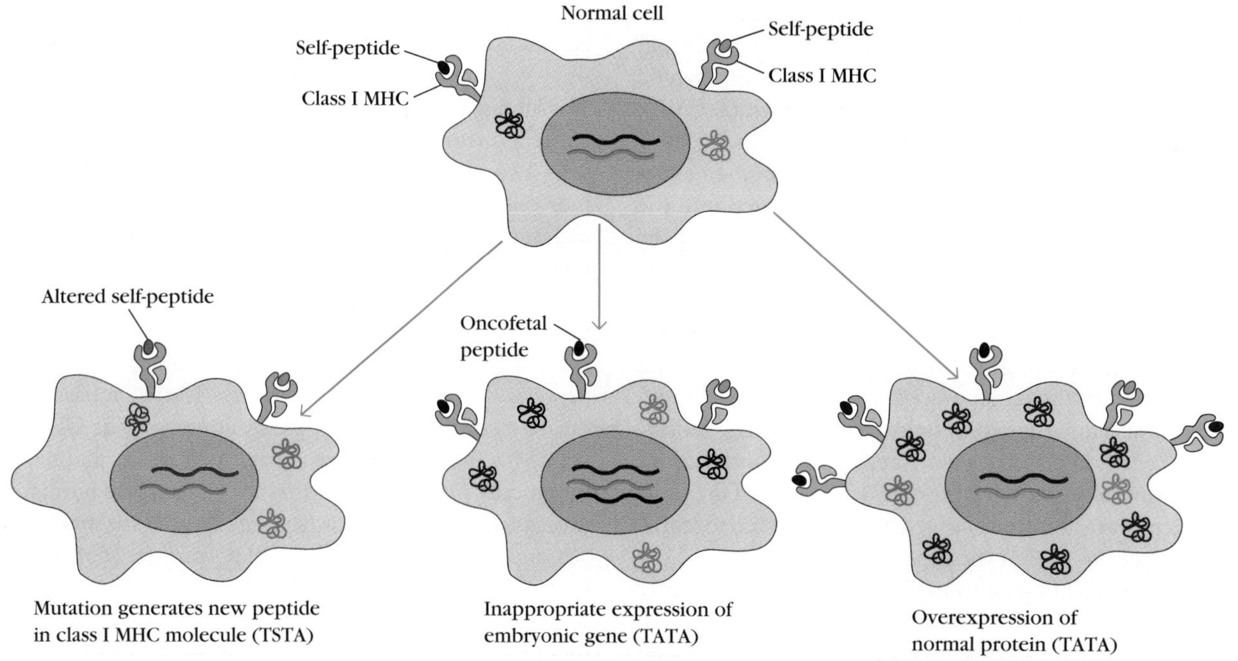

FIGURE 22-6 Different mechanisms generate tumor-specific transplantation antigens (TSTAs) and tumor-associated transplantation antigens (TATAs). The latter are more common.

Many tumor antigens are cellular proteins that give rise to peptides presented with MHC molecules; typically, these antigens have been identified by their ability to induce the proliferation of antigen-specific CTLs or helper T cells.

Tumor-Specific Antigens

Tumor-specific antigens have been identified on tumors induced with chemical or physical carcinogens and on some virally induced tumors. Demonstrating the presence of tumor-specific antigens on spontaneously occurring tumors is particularly difficult because the immune response to such tumors eliminates all of the tumor cells bearing sufficient numbers of the antigens and in this way selects for cells bearing low levels of the antigens.

Chemically or Physically Induced Tumor Antigens

Methylcholanthrene and ultraviolet light are two carcinogens that have been used extensively to generate lines of tumor cells. When syngeneic animals are injected with killed cells from a carcinogen-induced tumor-cell line, the animals develop a specific immunologic response that can protect against later challenge by live cells of the same line but not other tumor-cell lines (Table 22-2). Even when the same chemical carcinogen induces two separate tumors at differ-

TABLE 22-2 IMMUNE RESPONSE TO METHYL-CHOLANTHRENE (MCA) OR POLYOMA VIRUS (PV)*

Transplanted killed tumor cells	Live tumor cells for challenge	Tumor growth
Chemically induced		
MCA-induced sarcoma A	MCA-induced sarcoma A	–
MCA-induced sarcoma A	MCA-induced sarcoma B	+
Virally induced		
PV-induced sarcoma A	PV-induced sarcoma A	–
PV-induced sarcoma A	PV-induced sarcoma B	–
PV-induced sarcoma A	SV40-induced sarcoma C	+

*Tumors were induced either with MCA or PV, and killed cells from the induced tumors were injected into syngeneic animals, which were then challenged with live cells from the indicated tumor-cell lines. The absence of tumor growth after live challenge indicates that the immune response induced by tumor antigens on the killed cells provided protection against the live cells.

ent sites in the same animal, the tumor antigens are distinct and the immune response to one tumor does not protect against the other tumor.

The tumor-specific transplantation antigens of chemically induced tumors have been difficult to characterize because they cannot be identified by induced antibodies but only by their T-cell–mediated rejection. One experimental approach that has allowed identification of genes encoding some TSTAs is outlined in Figure 22-7. When a mouse tumorigenic cell line (tum^+), which gives rise to progressively growing tumors, is treated in vitro with a chemical mutagen, some cells are mutated so that they no longer are capable of growing into a tumor in syngeneic mice. These mutant tumor cells are designated as tum^- variants. Most tum^- variants have been shown to express TSTAs that are not expressed by the original tum^+ tumor-cell line. When tum^-

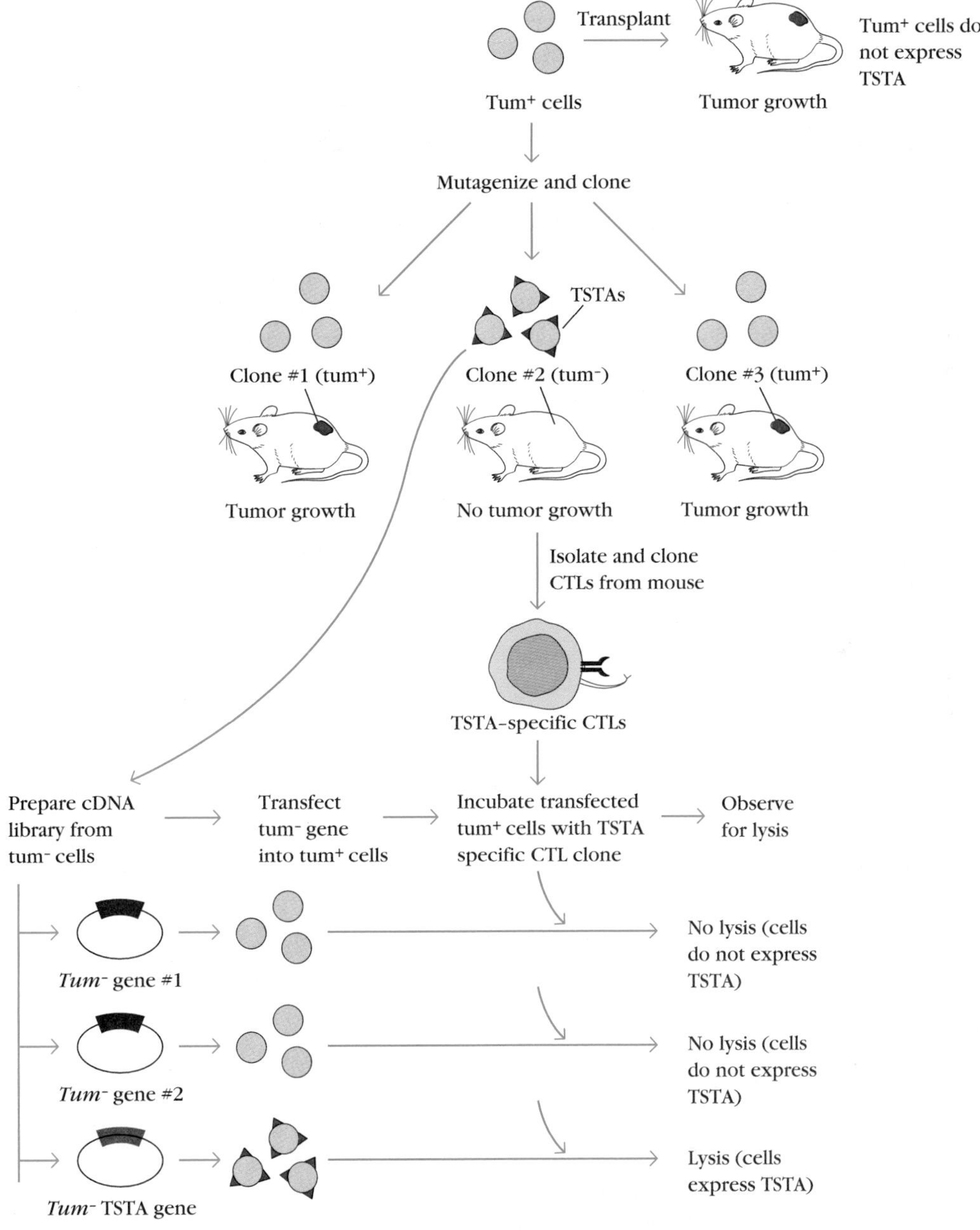

FIGURE 22-7 One procedure for identifying genes encoding tumor-specific transplantation antigens (TSTAs). Most TSTAs can be detected only by the cell-mediated rejection they elicit. In the first part of this procedure, a nontumorigenic (tum^-) cell line is generated; this cell line expresses a TSTA that is recognized by syngeneic mice, which mount a cell-mediated response against it. To isolate the gene encoding the TSTA, a cosmid gene library is prepared from the tum^- cell line, the genes are transfected into tumorigenic tum^+ cells, and the transfected cells are incubated with TSTA-specific CTLs.

cells are injected into syngeneic mice, the unique TSTAs that the tum$^-$ cells express are recognized by specific CTLs. The TSTA-specific CTLs destroy the tum$^-$ tumor cells, thus preventing tumor growth. To identify the genes encoding the TSTAs that are expressed on a tum$^-$ cell line, a cosmid DNA library is prepared from the tum$^-$ cells. Genes from the tum$^-$ cells are transfected into the original tum$^+$ cells. The transfected tum$^+$ cells are tested for the expression of the tum$^-$ TSTAs by their ability to activate cloned CTLs specific for the tum$^-$ TSTA. A number of diverse TSTAs have been identified by this method.

In the past few years, two methods have facilitated the characterization of TSTAs (Figure 22-8). In one method, peptides bound to class I MHC molecules on the membranes of the tumor cells are eluted with acid and purified by high-pressure liquid chromatography (HPLC). In some cases, sufficient peptide is eluted to allow its sequence to be deduced by Edman degradation. In a second approach, cDNA libraries are prepared from tumor cells. These cDNA libraries are transfected transiently into COS cells, which are monkey kidney cells transfected with the gene that codes for the SV40 large-T antigen. When these cells are later transfected with plasmids containing both the tumor-cell cDNA and an SV40 origin of replication, the large-T antigen stimulates plasmid replication, so that up to 10^4–10^5 plasmid copies are produced per cell. This results in high-level expression of the tumor-cell DNA.

The genes that encode some TSTAs have been shown to differ from normal cellular genes by a single-point mutation. Further characterization of TSTAs has demonstrated that many of them are not cell-membrane proteins; rather, as indicated already, they are short peptides derived from cytosolic proteins that have been processed and presented together with class I MHC molecules.

Virally Induced Tumor Antigens

In contrast to chemically induced tumors, virally induced tumors express tumor antigens shared by all tumors induced by the same virus. For example, when syngeneic mice are injected with killed cells from a particular polyoma-induced tumor, the recipients are protected against subsequent challenge with live cells from any polyoma-induced tumors (see Table 22-2). Likewise, when lymphocytes are transferred from mice with a virus-induced tumor into normal syngeneic recipients, the recipients reject subsequent transplants of all syngeneic tumors induced by the same virus. In the case of both SV40- and polyoma-induced tumors, the presence of tumor antigens is related to the neoplastic state of the cell. In humans, Burkitt's lymphoma cells have been shown to express a nuclear antigen of the Epstein-Barr virus that may indeed be a tumor-specific antigen for this type of tumor. Human papilloma virus (APV) E6 and E7 proteins are found in more than 80% of invasive cervical cancers—the clearest example of a virally encoded tumor antigen. Consequently, there is great interest in the HPVs, such as HPV-16, that are strongly linked to cervical cancer as vaccine candidates.

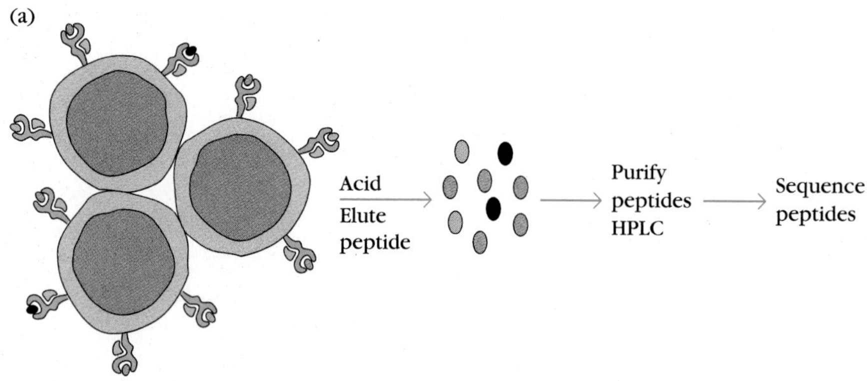

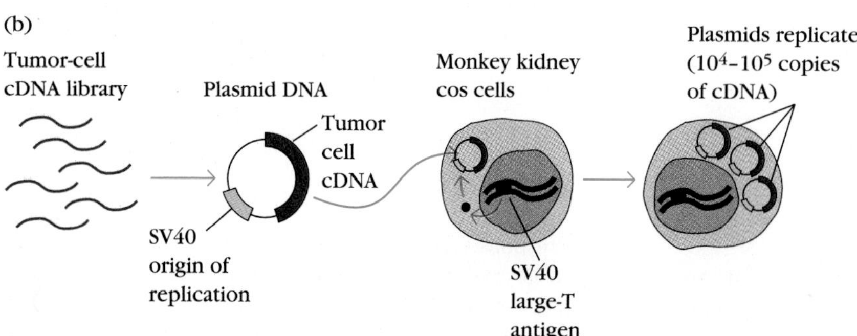

FIGURE 22-8 Two methods used to isolate tumor antigens that induce tumor-specific CTLs. See text for details.

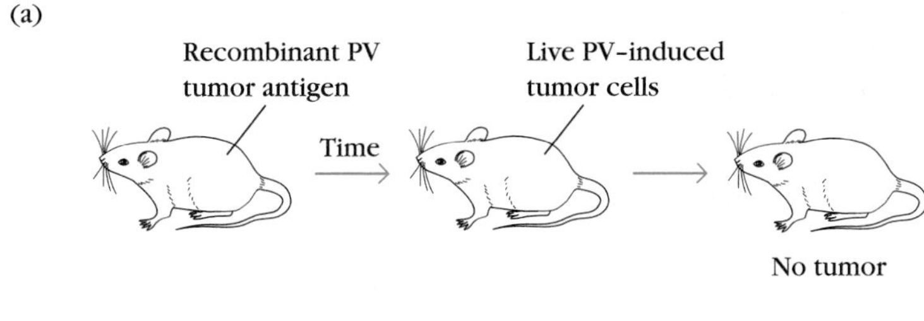

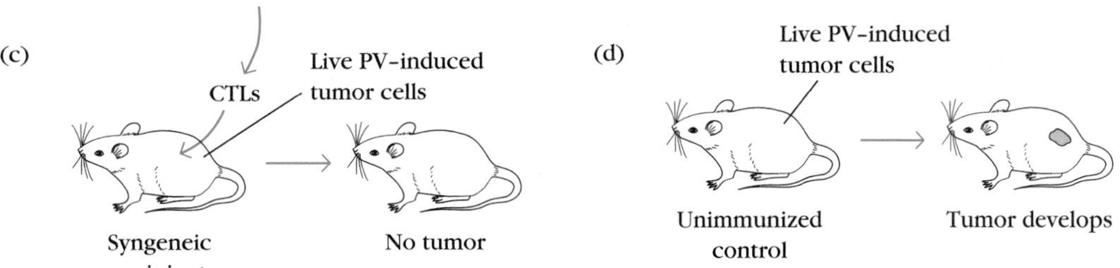

FIGURE 22-9 Experimental induction of immunity against tumor cells induced by polyoma virus (PV) has been achieved by immunizing mice with recombinant polyoma tumor antigen (a), with a vaccinia vector vaccine containing the gene encoding the PV tumor antigen (b), or with CTLs specific for the PV tumor antigen (c). Unimmunized mice (d) develop tumors when injected with live polyoma-induced tumor cells, whereas the immunized mice do not.

The potential value of these virally induced tumor antigens can be seen in animal models. In one experiment, mice immunized with a preparation of genetically engineered polyoma virus tumor antigen were shown to be immune to subsequent injections of live polyoma-induced tumor cells. In another experiment, mice were immunized with a vaccinia virus vaccine engineered with the gene encoding the polyoma tumor antigen. These mice also developed immunity, rejecting later injections of live polyoma-induced tumor cells (Figure 22-9).

Tumor-Associated Antigens

The majority of tumor antigens are not unique to tumor cells but also are present on normal cells. These tumor-associated transplantation antigens may be proteins usually expressed only on fetal cells but not on normal adult cells, or they may be proteins expressed at low levels by normal cells but at much higher levels by tumor cells. The latter category includes growth factors and growth-factor receptors, as well as oncogene-encoded proteins.

Several growth-factor receptors are expressed at significantly increased levels on tumor cells and can serve as tumor-associated antigens. For instance, a variety of tumor cells express the EGF receptor at levels 100 times greater than that in normal cells. An example of an over-expressed growth factor serving as a tumor-associated antigen is a transferrin growth factor, designated p97, which aids in the transport of iron into cells. Whereas normal cells express less than 8,000 molecules of p97 per cell, melanoma cells express 50,000–500,000 molecules of p97 per cell. The gene that encodes p97 has been cloned, and a recombinant vaccinia virus vaccine has been prepared that carries the cloned gene. When this vaccine was injected into mice, it induced both humoral and cell-mediated immune responses, which protected the mice against live melanoma cells expressing the p97 antigen. Results such as this highlight the importance of identifying tumor antigens as potential targets of tumor immunotherapy.

Oncofetal Tumor Antigens

Oncofetal tumor antigens, as the name implies, are found not only on cancerous cells but also on normal fetal cells. These antigens appear early in embryonic development, before the immune system acquires immunocompetence; if these antigens appear later on cancer cells, they are recognized as nonself and induce an immunologic response. Two well-studied oncofetal antigens are **alpha-fetoprotein (AFP)** and **carcinoembryonic antigen (CEA).**

Although the serum concentration of AFP drops from milligram levels in fetal serum to nanogram levels in normal adult serum, elevated AFP levels are found in a majority of patients with liver cancer (Table 22-3). CEA is a membrane glycoprotein found on gastrointestinal and liver cells of 2- to 6-month-old fetuses. Approximately 90% of patients with advanced colorectal cancer and 50% of patients with early colorectal cancer have increased levels of CEA in their serum; some patients with other types of cancer also exhibit increased CEA levels. However, because AFP and CEA can be found in trace amounts in some normal adults and in some noncancerous disease states, the presence of these oncofetal antigens is not diagnostic of tumors but rather serves to monitor tumor growth. If, for example, a patient has had surgery to remove a colorectal carcinoma, CEA levels are monitored after surgery. An increase in the CEA level is an indication of resumed tumor growth.

TABLE 22-3 ELEVATION OF ALPHA-FETOPROTEIN (AFP) AND CARCINOEMBRYONIC ANTIGEN (CEA) IN SERUM OF PATIENTS WITH VARIOUS DISEASES

Disease	No. of patients tested	% of patients with high AFP or CEA levels*
AFP > 400 μ/ml		
Alcoholic cirrhosis	NA	0
Hepatitis	NA	1
Hepatocellular carcinoma	NA	69
Other carcinoma	NA	0
CEA >10 ng/ml		
CEA >10 mg/ml		
Cancerous		
Breast carcinoma	125	14
Colorectal carcinoma	544	35
Gastric carcinoma	79	19
Noncarcinoma malignancy	228	2
Pancreatic carcinoma	55	35
Pulmonary carcinoma	181	26
Noncancerous		
Alcoholic cirrhosis	120	2
Cholecystitis	39	1
Nonmalignant disease	115	0
Pulmonary emphysema	49	4
Rectal polyps	90	1
Ulcerative colitis	146	5

*Although trace amounts of both AFP and CEA can be found in some healthy adults, none would have levels greater than those indicated in the table.

Oncogene Proteins as Tumor Antigens

A number of tumors have been shown to express tumor-associated antigens encoded by cellular oncogenes. These antigens are also present in normal cells encoded by the corresponding proto-oncogene. In many cases, there is no qualitative difference between the oncogene and proto-oncogene products; instead, the increased levels of the oncogene product can be recognized by the immune system. For example, as noted earlier, human breast-cancer cells exhibit elevated expression of the oncogene-encoded Neu protein, a growth-factor receptor, whereas normal adult cells express only trace amounts of Neu protein. Because of this difference in the Neu level, anti-Neu monoclonal antibodies can recognize and selectively eliminate breast-cancer cells without damaging normal cells.

TATAs on Human Melanomas

Several tumor-associated transplantation antigens have been identified on human melanomas. Five of these—MAGE-1, MAGE-3, BAGE, GAGE-1, GAGE-2—are oncofetal-type antigens. Each of these antigens is expressed on a significant proportion of human melanoma tumors, as well as on a number of other human tumors, but not on normal differentiated tissues except for the testis, where it is expressed on germ-line cells. In addition, a number of differentiation antigens expressed on normal melanocytes—including tyrosinase, gp100, Melan-A or MART-1, and gp75—are overexpressed by melanoma cells, enabling them to function as tumor-associated transplantation antigens.

Several of the human melanoma tumor antigens are shared by a number of other tumors. About 40% of human melanomas are positive for MAGE-1, and about 75% are positive for MAGE-2 or 3. In addition to melanomas, a significant percentage of glioma cell lines, breast tumors, non-small-cell lung tumors, and head or neck carcinomas express MAGE-1, 2, or 3. These shared tumor antigens could be exploited for clinical treatment. It might be possible to produce a tumor vaccine expressing the shared antigen for treatment of a number of these tumors, as described at the end of this chapter.

Immune Response to Tumors

In experimental animals, tumor antigens can be shown to induce both humoral and cell-mediated immune responses that result in the destruction of the tumor cells. In general, the cell-mediated response appears to play the major role. A number of tumors have been shown to induce tumor-specific CTLs that recognize tumor antigens presented by class I MHC on the tumor cells. However, as discussed below, expression of class I MHC molecules is decreased in a number of tumors, thereby limiting the role of specific CTLs in their destruction.

Role of NK Cells and Macrophages

The recognition of tumor cells by NK cells is not MHC restricted. Thus, the activity of these cells is not compromised by the decreased MHC expression exhibited by some tumor cells. In some cases, Fc receptors on NK cells can bind to antibody-coated tumor cells, leading to ADCC. The importance of NK cells in tumor immunity is suggested by the mutant mouse strain called beige and by **Chediak-Higashi syndrome** in humans. In each case, a genetic defect causes marked impairment of NK cells and an associated increased incidence of certain types of cancer.

Numerous observations indicate that activated macrophages also play a significant role in the immune response to tumors. For example, macrophages are often observed to cluster around tumors, and their presence is often correlated with tumor regression. Like NK cells, macrophages are not MHC restricted and express Fc receptors, enabling them to bind to antibody on tumor cells and mediate ADCC. The antitumor activity of activated macrophages is probably mediated by lytic enzymes and reactive oxygen and nitrogen intermediates. In addition, activated macrophages secrete a cytokine called tumor necrosis factor (TNF-α) that has potent antitumor activity. When TNF-α is injected into tumor-bearing animals, it has been found to induce hemorrhage and necrosis of the tumor.

Immune Surveillance Theory

The immune surveillance theory was first conceptualized in the early 1900s by Paul Ehrlich. He suggested that cancer cells frequently arise in the body but are recognized as foreign and eliminated by the immune system. Some 50 years later, Lewis Thomas suggested that the cell-mediated branch of the immune system had evolved to patrol the body and eliminate cancer cells. According to these concepts, tumors arise only if cancer cells are able to escape immune surveillance, either by reducing their expression of tumor antigens or by an impairment in the immune response to these cells.

Among the early observations that seemed to support the immune surveillance theory was the increased incidence of cancer in transplantation patients on immunosuppressive drugs. Other findings, however, were difficult to reconcile with this theory. Nude mice, for example, lack a thymus and consequently lack functional T cells. According to the immune surveillance theory, these mice should show an increase in cancer, instead, nude mice are no more susceptible to cancer than other mice. Furthermore, although individuals on immunosuppressive drugs do show an increased incidence of cancers of the immune system, other common cancers (e.g., lung, breast, and colon cancer) are not increased in these individuals, contrary to what the theory predicts. One possible explanation for the selective increase in immune-system cancers is that the immunosuppressive agents themselves may exert a direct carcinogenic effect on immune cells.

Experimental data concerning the effect of tumor-cell dosage on the ability of the immune system to respond also are incompatible with the immune surveillance theory. For example, animals injected with very low or very high doses of tumor cells develop tumors, whereas those injected with intermediate doses do not. The mechanism by which a low dose of tumor cells "sneaks through" is difficult to reconcile with the immune surveillance theory. Finally, this theory assumes that cancer cells and normal cells exhibit qualitative antigen differences. In fact, as stated earlier, many types of tumors do not express tumor-specific antigens, and any immune response that develops must be induced by quantitative differences in antigen expression by normal cells and tumor cells. However, tumors induced by viruses would be expected to express some antigens encoded by the viral genome. These antigens are qualitatively different from those expressed by normal tissues and would be expected to attract the attention of the immune system. In fact, there are many examples of specific immune responses to virally induced tumors.

Nevertheless, apart from tumors caused by viruses, the basic concept of the immune surveillance theory—that malignant tumors arise only if the immune system is somehow impaired or if the tumor cells lose their immunogenicity, enabling them to escape immune surveillance—at this time remains unproved. In spite of this, it is clear that an immune response can be generated to tumor cells, and therapeutic approaches aimed at increasing that response may serve as a defense against malignant cells.

Tumor Evasion of the Immune System

Although the immune system clearly can respond to tumor cells, the fact that so many individuals die each year from cancer suggests that the immune response to tumor cells is often ineffective. This section describes several mechanisms by which tumor cells appear to evade the immune system.

Immunologic Enhancement of Tumor Growth

Following the discovery that antibodies could be produced to tumor-specific antigens, attempts were made to protect animals against tumor growth by active immunization with tumor antigens or by passive immunization with antitumor antibodies. Much to the surprise of the researchers, these immunizations did not protect against tumor growth; in many cases, they actually enhanced growth of the tumor.

The tumor-enhancing ability of immune sera subsequently was studied in cell-mediated lympholysis (CML) reactions in vitro. Serum taken from animals with progressive tumor growth was found to block the CML reaction, whereas serum taken from animals with regressing tumors had little or no blocking activity. K. E. and I. Hellstrom extended these findings by showing that children with progressive neuroblastoma had high levels of some kind of blocking factor in their sera and that children with regressive neuroblastoma did not have such factors. Since these first reports, blocking factors have been found to be associated with a number of human tumors.

In some cases, antitumor antibody itself acts as a blocking factor. Presumably the antibody binds to tumor-specific antigens and masks the antigens from cytotoxic T cells. In many cases, the blocking factors are not antibodies alone but rather antibodies complexed with tumor antigens. Although these immune complexes have been shown to block the CTL response, the mechanism of this inhibition is not known. The complexes also may inhibit ADCC by binding to Fc receptors on NK cells or macrophages and blocking their activity.

Modulation of Tumor Antigens

Certain tumor-specific antigens have been observed to disappear from the surface of tumor cells in the presence of serum antibody and then to reappear after the antibody is no longer present. This phenomenon, called antigenic modulation, is readily observed when leukemic T cells are injected into mice previously immunized with a leukemic T-cell antigen (TL antigen). These mice develop high titers of anti-TL antibody, which binds to the TL antigen on the leukemic cells and induces capping, endocytosis, and/or shedding of the antigen-antibody complex. As long as antibody is present, these leukemic T cells fail to display the TL antigen and thus cannot be eliminated.

Reduction in Class I MHC Molecules

Since $CD8^+$ CTLs recognize only antigen associated with class I MHC molecules, any alteration in the expression of class I MHC molecules on tumor cells may exert a profound effect on the CTL-mediated immune response. Malignant transformation of cells is often associated with a reduction (or even a complete loss) of class I MHC molecules, and a number of tumors have been shown to express decreased levels of class I MHC molecules. The decrease in class I MHC expression can be accompanied by progressive tumor growth, and so the absence of MHC molecules on a tumor is generally an indication of a poor prognosis. As illustrated in Figure 22-10,

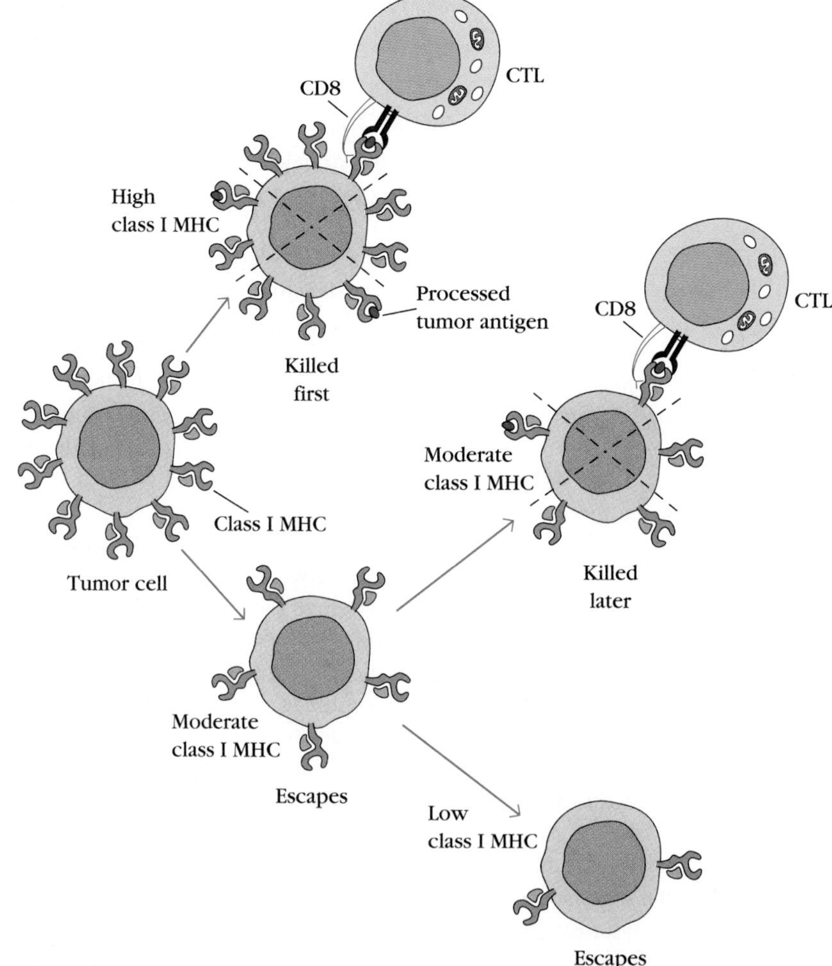

FIGURE 22-10 Down-regulation of class I MHC expression on tumor cells may allow a tumor to escape CTL-mediated recognition. The immune response may play a role in selecting for tumor cells expressing lower levels of class I MHC molecules by preferentially eliminating those cells expressing high levels of class I molecules. With time, malignant tumor cells may express progressively fewer MHC molecules and thus escape CTL-mediated destruction.

the immune response itself may play a role in selecting tumor cells with decreased class I MHC expression.

Lack of Co-Stimulatory Signal

T-cell activation requires an activating signal, triggered by recognition of a peptide–MHC molecule complex by the T-cell receptor, and a co-stimulatory signal, triggered by the interaction of B7 on antigen-presenting cells with CD28 on the T cells. Both signals are needed to induce IL-2 production and proliferation of T cells. The poor immunogenicity of many tumor cells may be due in large part to lack of the co-stimulatory molecules. Without sufficient numbers of antigen-presenting cells in the immediate vicinity of a tumor, the T cells will receive only a partial activating signal, which may lead to clonal anergy.

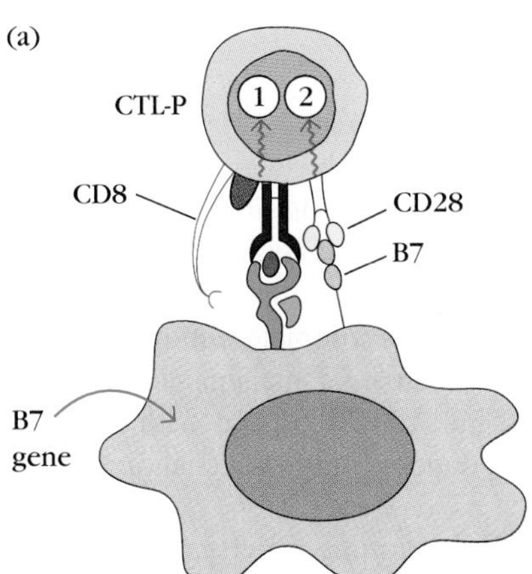

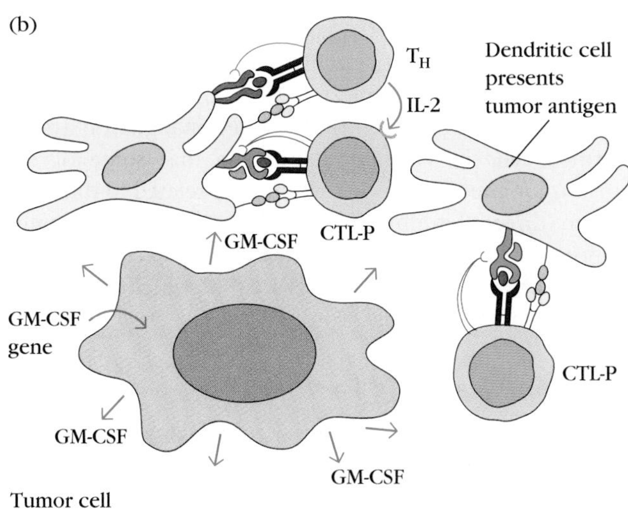

Cancer Immunotherapy

Although various immune responses can be generated to tumor cells, the response frequently is not sufficient to prevent tumor growth. One approach to cancer treatment is to augment or supplement these natural defense mechanisms. Several types of cancer immunotherapy in current use or under development are described in this concluding section.

Manipulation of Co-Stimulatory Signal

Several research groups have demonstrated that tumor immunity can be enhanced by providing the co-stimulatory signal necessary for activation of CTL precursors (CTL-Ps). When mouse CTL-Ps are incubated with melanoma cells in vitro, antigen recognition occurs, but in the absence of a co-stimulatory signal, the CTL-Ps do not proliferate and differentiate into effector CTLs. However, when the melanoma cells are transfected with the gene that encodes the B7 ligand, then the CTL-Ps differentiate into effector CTLs.

These findings offer the possibility that B7-transfected tumor cells might be used to induce a CTL response in vivo. For instance, when P. Linsley, L. Chen, and their colleagues injected melanoma-bearing mice with $B7^+$ melanoma cells, the melanomas completely regressed in more than 40% of the mice. S. Townsend and J. Allison used a similar approach to vaccinate mice against malignant melanoma. Normal mice were first immunized with irradiated, B7-transfected melanoma cells and then challenged with unaltered malignant melanoma cells. The "vaccine" was found to protect a high percentage of the mice (Figure 22-11a). It is hoped that a similar vaccine might prevent metastasis after surgical removal of a primary melanoma in human patients.

Because human melanoma antigens are shared by a number of different human tumors, it might be possible to generate a panel of B7-transfected melanoma cell lines

FIGURE 22-11 Use of transfected tumor cells for cancer immunotherapy. (a) Tumor cells transfected with the B7 gene express the co-stimulatory B7 molecule, enabling them to provide both activating signal (1) and co-stimulatory signal (2) to CTL-Ps. As a result of the combined signals, the CTL-Ps differentiate into effector CTLs, which can mediate tumor destruction. In effect, the transfected tumor cell acts as an antigen-presenting cell. (b) Transfection of tumor cells with the gene encoding GM-CSF allows the tumor cells to secrete high levels of GM-CSF. This cytokine will activate dendritic cells in the vicinity of the tumor, enabling the dendritic cells to present tumor antigens to both T_H cells and CTL-Ps.

that are typed for tumor-antigen expression and for HLA expression. In this approach, the tumor antigen(s) expressed by a patient's tumor would be determined, and then the patient would be vaccinated with an irradiated B7-transfected cell line that expresses similar tumor antigen(s).

Enhancement of APC Activity

Mouse dendritic cells cultured in GM-CSF and incubated with tumor fragments, then reinfused into the mice, have been shown to activate both $T_H$cells and CTLs specific for the tumor antigens. When the mice were subsequently challenged with live tumor cells, they displayed tumor immunity. These experiments have led to a number of approaches aimed at expanding the population of antigen-presenting cells, so that these cells can activate T_H or CTLs specific for tumor antigens.

One approach that has been tried is to transfect tumor cells with the gene encoding GM-CSF. These engineered tumor cells, when reinfused into the patient, will secrete GM-CSF, enhancing the differentiation and activation of host antigen-presenting cells, especially dendritic cells. As these dendritic cells accumulate around the tumor cells, the GM-CSF secreted by the tumor cells will enhance the presentation of tumor antigens to T_H and CTL cells by the dendritic cells (Figure 22-11b).

Another way to expand the dendritic cell population is to culture dendritic cells from peripheral-blood progenitor cells in the presence of GM-CSF, TNF-α, and IL-4. These three cytokines induce the generation of large numbers of dendritic cells. There is some hope that, if these dendritic cells are pulsed with tumor fragments and then reintroduced into the patient, they can activate $T_H$and T_C cells specific for the tumor antigens. Whether these hopes are justified will be determined by further investigation.

A number of adjuvants, including the attenuated strains of *Mycobacterium bovis* called bacillus Calmette-Guerin (BCG) and *Corynebacterium parvuum,* have been used to boost tumor immunity. These adjuvants activate macrophages, increasing their expression of various cytokines, class II MHC molecules, and the B7 co-stimulatory molecule. These activated macrophages are better activators of T_H cells, resulting in generalized increases in both humoral and cell-mediated responses. Thus far, adjuvants have shown only modest therapeutic results.

Cytokine Therapy

The isolation and cloning of the various cytokine genes has facilitated their large-scale production. A variety of experimental and clinical approaches have been developed to use recombinant cytokines, either singly or in combination, to augment the immune response against cancer. Among the cytokines that have been evaluated in cancer immunotherapy are IFN-α, β, and γ; IL-1, IL-2, IL-4, IL-5, and IL-12; GM-CSF, and TNF. Although these trials have produced occasional hopeful results, many obstacles remain to the successful use of this type of cancer immunotherapy.

The most notable obstacle is the complexity of the cytokine network itself. This complexity makes it very difficult to know precisely how intervention with a given recombinant cytokine will affect the production of other cytokines. And since some cytokines act antagonistically, it is possible that intervention with a recombinant cytokine designed to enhance a particular branch of the immune response may actually lead to suppression. In addition, cytokine immunotherapy is plagued by the difficulty of administering the cytokines locally. In some cases, systemic administration of high levels of a given cytokine has been shown to lead to serious and even life-threatening consequences. Although the results of several experimental and clinical trials of cytokine therapy for cancer are discussed here, it is important to keep in mind that this therapeutic approach is still in its infancy.

Interferons

Large quantities of purified recombinant preparations of the interferons, IFN-α, IFN-β, and IFN-γ, are now available, each of which has shown some promise in the treatment of human cancer. To date, most of the clinical trials have involved IFN-α. Daily injections of recombinant IFN-α have been shown to induce partial or complete tumor regression in some patients with hematologic malignancies such as leukemias, lymphomas, and myelomas and with solid tumors such as melanoma, Kaposi's sarcoma, renal cancer, and breast cancer.

Interferon-mediated antitumor activity may involve several mechanisms. All three types of interferon have been shown to increase class I MHC expression on tumor cells; IFN-γ has also been shown to increase class II MHC expression on macrophages. Given the evidence for decreased levels of class I MHC molecules on malignant tumors, the interferons may act by restoring MHC expression, thereby increasing CTL activity against tumors. In addition, the interferons have been shown to inhibit cell division of both normal and malignantly transformed cells in vitro. It is possible that some of the antitumor effects of the interferons are related to this ability to directly inhibit tumor-cell proliferation. Finally, IFN-γ directly or indirectly increases the activity of T_C cells, macrophages, and NK cells, all of which play a role in the immune response to tumor cells.

Tumor Necrosis Factors

In some instances, the tumor necrosis factors TNF-α and TNF-β have been shown to exhibit direct antitumor activity, killing some tumor cells and reducing the rate of proliferation of others while sparing normal cells (Figure 22-12). In the presence of TNF-α or TNF-β, a tumor un-

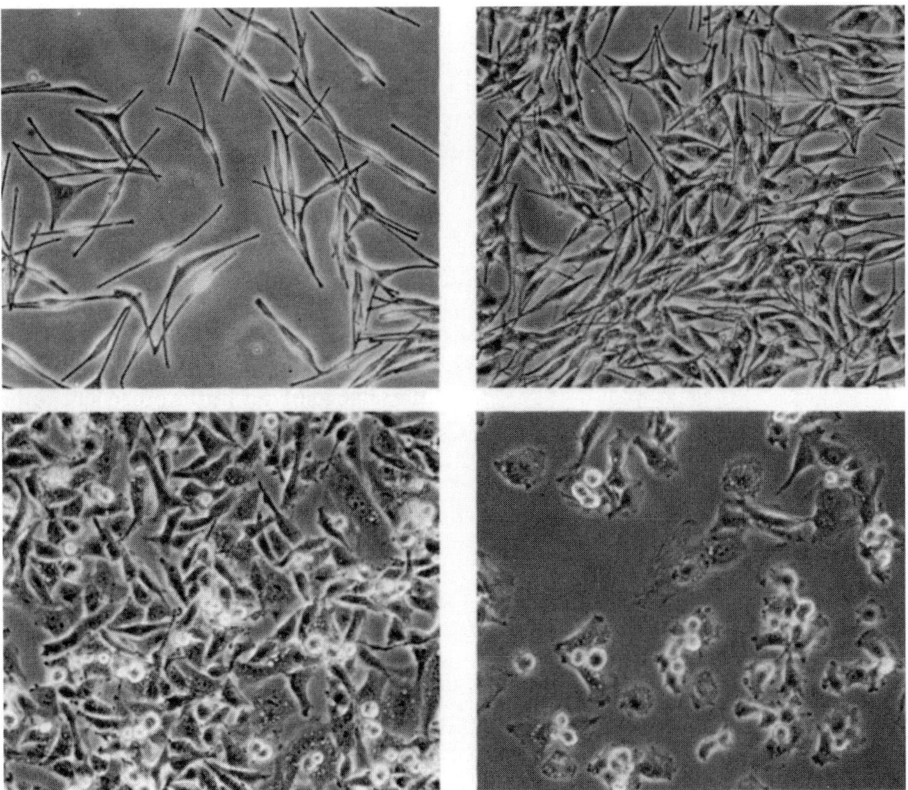

FIGURE 22-12 Photomicrographs of cultured normal melanocytes (*top*) and cultured cancerous melanoma cells (*bottom*) in the presence (*left*) and absence (*right*) of tumor necrosis factor α (TNF-α). Note that, in the presence of TNF-α, the cancer cells stop proliferating, whereas TNF-α has no inhibitory effect on proliferation of the normal cells. [From LJ Old, 1988, *Sci. Am.* **258**(5):59.]

dergoes visible hemorrhagic necrosis and regression. TNF-α has also been shown to inhibit tumor-induced vascularization (angiogenesis) by damaging the vascular endothelial cells in the vicinity of a tumor, thereby decreasing the flow of blood and oxygen that is necessary for progressive tumor growth.

In Vitro–Activated LAK and TIL Cells

Animal studies have shown that lymphocytes can be activated against tumor antigens in vitro by culturing them with x-irradiated tumor cells in the presence of IL-2 and added tumor antigens. These activated lymphocytes mediate more effective tumor destruction than untreated lymphocytes when they are reinjected into the original tumor-bearing animal. It is difficult, however, to activate in vitro enough lymphocytes with antitumor specificity to be useful in cancer therapy.

While sensitizing lymphocytes to tumor antigens by this method, S. Rosenberg discovered that, in the presence of high concentrations of cloned IL-2 but without the addition of tumor antigens, large numbers of activated lymphoid cells were generated that could kill fresh tumor cells but not normal cells. He called these cells **lymphokine-activated killer (LAK) cells.** In one study, for example, Rosenberg found that infusion of LAK cells plus recombinant IL-2 into tumor-bearing animals mediated effective tumor-cell destruction (Figure 22-13). LAK-cell populations are typically >90% activated NK cells. However, small numbers of TCR-bearing cells are present in LAK populations and it is possible that these may also contribute to their tumoricidal activity.

Because large numbers of LAK cells can be generated in vitro and because these cells are active against a wide variety of tumors, their effectiveness in human tumor immunotherapy has been evaluated in several clinical trials. In these trials, peripheral-blood lymphocytes were removed from patients with various advanced metastatic cancers and were activated in vitro to generate LAK cells. In an early study, patients were then infused with their autologous LAK cells together with IL-2. In this trial, which involved 25 patients, cancer regression was seen in some patients. Subsequently, a more extensive trial with 222 patients resulted in complete regression in 16 patients. However, a number of undesirable side effects are associated with the high levels of IL-2 required for LAK-cell activity. The most noteworthy is vascular leak syndrome, in which lymphoid cells and plasma emigrate from the peripheral blood into the tissues, leading to shock.

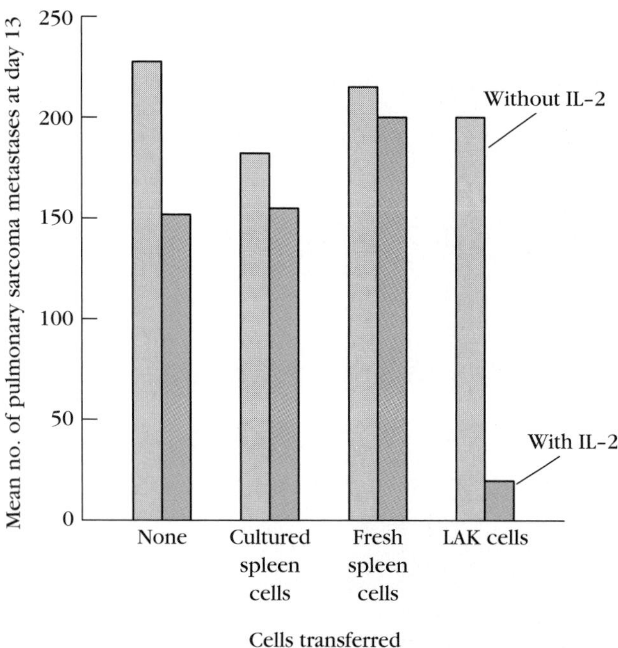

FIGURE 22-13 Experimental demonstration of tumor-destroying activity of LAK cells plus IL-2. Spleen cells or LAK cells, in the presence or absence of recombinant IL-2, were infused into mice with pulmonary sarcoma. The animals were evaluated 13 days later for the number of pulmonary sarcoma metastases. The LAK cells were prepared by isolating lymphocytes from tumor-bearing animals and incubating them in vitro with high concentrations of IL-2. Note that LAK cells caused tumor regression only when IL-2 was also infused. [Data from S Rosenberg et al, 1988, *Ann. Int. Med.*, **108:**853.]

Tumors contain lymphocytes that have infiltrated the tumor and presumably are taking part in an antitumor response. By taking small biopsy samples of tumors, one can obtain a population of these lymphocytes and expand it in vitro with IL-2. These activated **tumor-infiltrating lymphocytes** are called **TILs.** Many TILs have a wide range of antitumor activity and appear to be indistinguishable from LAK cells. However, some TILs cells have specific cytolytic activity against their autologous tumor. These tumor-specific TILs are of interest because they have increased antitumor activity and require 100-fold lower levels of IL-2 for their activity than LAK cells do. In one study, TIL populations were expanded in vitro from biopsy samples taken from patients with malignant melanoma, renal-cell carcinoma, and small-cell lung cancer. The expanded populations of TILs were reinjected into autologous patients together with continuous infusions of recombinant IL-2. Renal-cell carcinomas and malignant melanomas showed partial regression in 29% and 23% of the patients, respectively.

Monoclonal Antibodies

Monoclonal antibodies have been used in various ways as experimental immunotherapeutic agents for cancer. For example, anti-idiotype monoclonal antibodies have been used with some success in treating human B-cell lymphomas and T-cell leukemias. In one remarkable study, R. Levy and his colleagues successfully treated a 64-year-old man with terminal B-cell lymphoma. At the time of treatment, the lymphoma had metastasized to the liver, spleen, bone marrow, and peripheral blood. Because this was a B-cell cancer, the membrane-bound antibody on all the cancerous cells had the same idiotype. By the procedure outlined in Figure 22-14, these researchers produced mouse monoclonal antibody specific for the B-lymphoma idiotype. When this mouse monoclonal anti-idiotype antibody was injected into the patient, it bound specifically to the B-lymphoma cells, because these cells expressed that particular idiotype. Since B-lymphoma cells are susceptible to complement-mediated lysis, the monoclonal antibody activated the complement system and lysed the lymphoma cells without harming other cells. After four injections with this anti-idiotype monoclonal antibody, the tumors began to shrink, and this patient entered an unusually long period of complete remission.

However, this approach requires that a custom monoclonal antibody be raised for each lymphoma patient. This is prohibitively expensive and cannot be used as a general therapeutic approach for the thousands of patients diagnosed each year with B lymphoma. Recently, Levy and his colleagues have used direct immunization to recruit the immune systems of patients to an attack against their B lymphoma. In a clinical trial with 41 B-cell lymphoma patients, the genes encoding the rearranged immunoglobulin genes of the lymphomas of each patient were isolated and used to encode the synthesis of recombinant immunoglobulin that bore the idiotype typical of the patient's tumor. Each of these Igs was coupled to keyhole limpet hemocyanin (KLH), a mollusk protein that is often used as a carrier protein because of its efficient recruitment of T-cell help. The patients were immunized with their own tumor-specific antigens, the idiotypically unique immunoglobulins produced by their own lymphomas. About 50% of the patients developed anti-idiotype antibodies against their tumors. Significantly, improved clinical outcomes were seen in the 20 patients with anti-idiotype responses, but not in the others. In fact, 2 of these 20 experienced complete remission.

Despite its promise, the anti-idiotypic approach is by its very nature patient-specific. A more general monoclonal-antibody therapy for B-cell lymphoma is based on the fact that most B cells, whether normal or cancerous, bear lineage-distinctive antigens. One such determinant, CD20, has been the target of intensive efforts; a monoclonal antibody to it, raised in mice and engineered to contain mostly human sequences, has been useful in the treatment of B-cell lym-

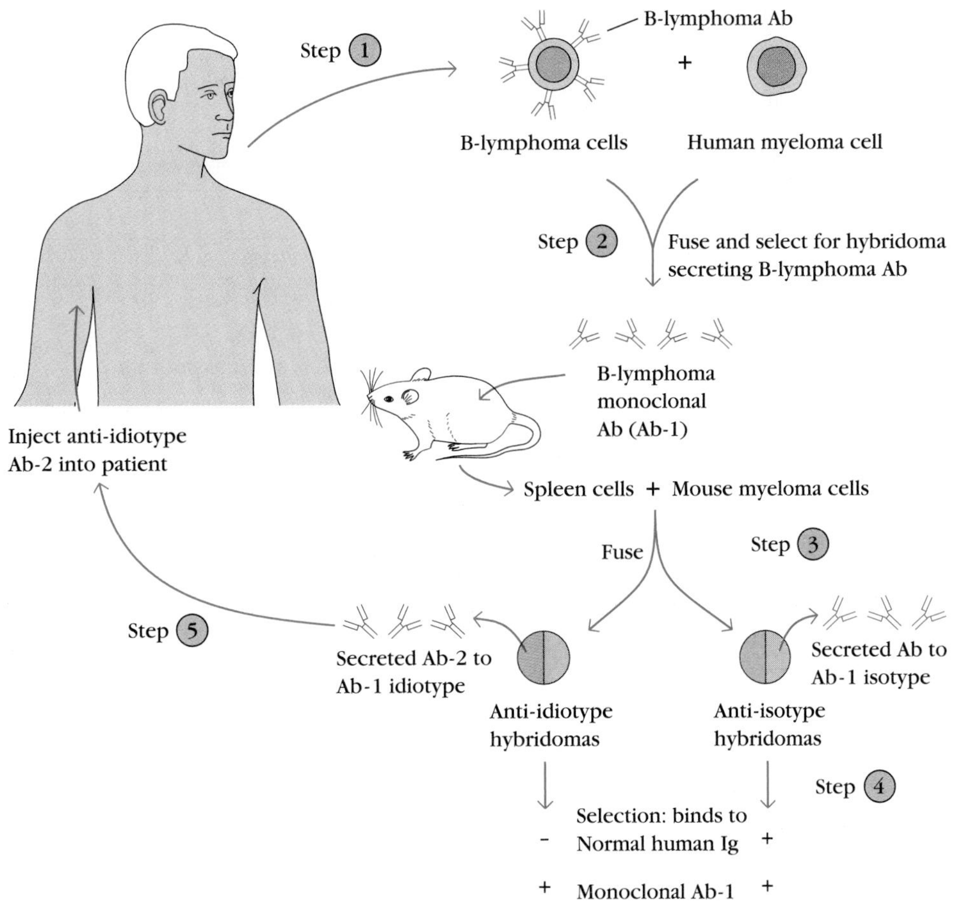

FIGURE 22-14 Treatment of B-cell lymphoma with monoclonal antibody specific for idiotypic determinants on the cancer cells. Because all the lymphoma cells are derived from a single transformed B cell, they all express membrane-bound antibody (Ab-1) with the same idiotype (i.e., the same antigenic specificity). In the procedure illustrated, monoclonal anti-idiotype antibody (Ab-2) against the B-lymphoma membrane-bound antibody was produced (steps 1–4). When this anti-idiotype antibody was injected into the patient (step 5), it bound selectively to B-lymphoma cells, which then were susceptible to complement-plus-antibody lysis.

phoma (see Clinical Focus, Chapter 5). Aside from CD20, a number of tumor-associated antigens (Table 22-4) are being tested in clinical trials for their suitability as targets for antibody-mediated anti-tumor therapy.

A variety of tumors express significantly increased levels of growth-factor receptors, which are promising targets for anti-tumor monoclonal antibodies. For example, in 25 to 30 percent of women with metastatic breast cancer, a genetic alteration of the tumor cells results in the increased expression of HER2, an epidermal-growth-factor–like receptor. An anti-HER2 monoclonal antibody was raised in mice and the genes encoding it were isolated. Except for the sequences encoding the antibody's CDRs, the mouse Ig sequences were replaced with human Ig counterparts. This prevents the generation of human anti-mouse antibodies (HAMAs) and allows the patient to receive repeated doses of the "humanized" anti-HER2 in large amounts (100 milligrams or more). Preparations of this antibody, called Herceptin, have been approved by the FDA for the treatment of HER2-receptor–bearing breast cancers (see Clinical Focus, Chapter 5). Monoclonal antibodies also have been used to prepare tumor-specific anti-tumor agents. In this approach, antibodies to tumor-specific or tumor-associated antigens are coupled with radioactive isotopes, chemotherapy drugs, or potent toxins of biological origin. In such "guided missile" therapies, the toxic agents are delivered specifically to tumor cells. This focuses the toxic effects on the tumor and spares normal tissues. Reagents known as **immunotoxins** have been constructed by coupling the inhibitor chain of a toxin (e.g., diphtheria toxin) to an antibody against a tumor-specific or tumor-associated antigen (see Figure 4-23). In vitro studies have demonstrated that these "magic bullets" can kill tumor cells without harming normal cells. Immunotoxins specific for tumor antigens in a variety of cancers (e.g., melanoma,

TABLE 22-4 SOME TUMOR ASSOCIATED-ANTIGENS UNDER EXAMINATION AS POTENTIAL TARGETS FOR MONOCLONAL ANTIBODY THERAPY

Tumor antigen	Tumor type	Target antigen
	Lymphoid cell-surface markers	
T-cell marker	T-cell leukemia/lymphoma	CD5
B-cell marker	B-cell lymphoma	CD20
Hematopoietic-cell marker	Acute myeloblastic leukemia	CD45
Anti-idiotype	B-cell lymphoma	Immunoglobulin
	Nonlymphoid tissue markers	
Cell Surface Antigens		
Carcinoembryonic antigen (CEA)	Colon cancer (some others)	Glycoprotein
MUC1	Breast cancer	Glyoprotein
Gangliosides such as GD2 and GD3	Neuroectodermal tumors	Glycolipids associated with neural tissue
Growth factor receptors		
Epidermal growth-factor receptor (EGFR)	Some lung, head, neck, and breast tumors	EGF-binding cell surface protein
HER2 (an EGF-like receptor)	Breast and ovarian tumors	Cell surface EGF-binding protein with homology to EGFR

SOURCE: Adapted from Scott and Welt, 1997, *Curr. Opin. Immunol.* **9**:717.

colorectal carcinoma, metastatic breast carcinoma, and various lymphomas and leukemias) have been evaluated in phase I or phase II clinical trials. In a number of trials, significant numbers of leukemia and lymphoma patients exhibited partial or complete remission. However in a number of cases, the clinical responses in patients with larger tumor masses were disappointing. In some of these patients, the sheer size of the tumor may render most of its cells inaccessible to the immunotoxin.

Cancer Vaccines

The generation of activated populations of T cells that recognize antigens presented by MHC molecules is a key element in the generation of anti-tumor immunity. Because of the perception that many tumor antigens might be the result of chance mutations and hence unique to a particular tumor, many early efforts to develop anticancer vaccination strategies were based on the use of the patient's own tumor cells or tumor extracts as antigens. In some clinical trials of this approach, tumor preparations derived from individual patients were mixed with bacterial adjuvants such as Bacille Calmette-Guerin (BCG) and used to immunize the patient. While there were occasional successes, these trials were plagued by inconsistent results and the usually poor ability of the vaccines to raise strong tumor-specific cytotoxic T cell responses.

Much of the recent effort in this field has been directed toward the identification of tumor antigens that are recognized by T cells. Most of the success in this effort (Table 22-5) can be credited to the application of the two approaches outlined below:

- Genetic—recombinant DNA libraries from tumors and other sources are transfected into cells expressing HLA class I molecules. The transfected cells are then tested for their ability to stimulate attack by CTLs. The transfected gene encoding the target protein antigen is identified and the antigenic peptide fragment is isolated and sequenced.
- Biochemical—MHC molecules are isolated from the cells of a particular tumor and their complex mixture of many different bound peptides are eluted and partly separated by high pressure liquid chromatography (HPLC). The many different partly purified peptide products obtained are tested individually to determine the ones that are able to sensitize human target cells for lysis by CTLs capable of reacting with the tumor. Further analysis of the peptide mixture allows the antigenic peptides to be identified and their structures determined.

A great deal of work is directed toward learning how to use these antigenic tumor peptides and other tumor anti-

TABLE 22-5 TUMOR-ASSOCIATED AND TUMOR-SPECIFIC ANTIGEN PEPTIDES RECOGNIZED BY HUMAN T CELLS

Human tumor	Protein	Peptide
Many melanomas, esophageal carcinomas, non small-cell lung carcinomas and hepatocellular carcinomas	MAGE-1	EADPTGHSY and SAYGEPRKL
Melanoma	Tyrosinase	MLLAVLYCL, YMNGTMSQV, YMDGTMSQV, and others
Colon cancer	Carcinoembryonic antigen (CEA)	YLSGANLNL
Breast and ovarian cancer	HER2/NEU	KIFGSLAFL
Head and neck squamous-cell carcinoma	Caspase 8	FPSDSWCYF
Chronic myeloid leukemia	*bcr-abl* fusion protein (product of a fusion of an Ig gene with the *abl* gene)	ATGFKQSSKALQRPVAS
Prostatic cancer	PSA	FLTPKKKLQCV and VISNDVCAQV

SOURCE: Adapted from B Van Den Eynde and P van der Bruggen, 1996, *Curr. Opin. Immunol.* **9**:684.

gens to vaccinate effectively against cancer. A major challenge is how to determine the most effective ways to present the antigens. Great hope is held for approaches that employ recombinant viral and bacterial agents to deliver genes that encode relevant tumor antigens. Infection with these vaccine vectors and the subsequent expression of the tumor antigens they bear in the appropriate cellular compartments may provide effective ways of immunogenically displaying antigenic peptides on the MHC molecules of tumor cells.

Finally, from a global perspective, viruses are a significant cause of cancer. Examples include papillomavirus-associated cervical cancer (90% of these tumors) and liver cancer induced by hepatitis virus. Cancers induced by tumor viruses are among the most promising targets for anticancer vaccines. In these tumors, virally encoded proteins act as tumor-specific antigens. In fact, as previously mentioned, two of the proteins (E6 and E7) produced by HPV, human papilloma-virus, are found in most cervical cancers. Certainly, the link between these antigens and the tumors is perhaps the closest known. Furthermore, appropriately modified forms of HPV or other viral vectors into which the E6 and E7 genes have been inserted by recombinant DNA techniques are an attractive route for the introduction and expression of genes that encode these proteins. If vaccination against cancer does prove feasible, vaccines for well-established human tumor viruses are likely to be among the first successes.

Summary

1. Tumor cells differ from normal cells in numerous ways. In particular, changes in the regulation of growth of tumor cells allow them to proliferate indefinitely, then invade the underlying tissue, and eventually metastasize to other tissues (see Figure 22-1). Normal cells can be transformed in vitro by chemical and physical carcinogens and by transforming viruses. Transformed cells exhibit altered growth properties and are sometimes capable of inducing cancer when they are injected into animals.
2. Proto-oncogenes encode proteins involved in control of normal cellular growth. The conversion of proto-oncogenes to oncogenes is one of the key steps in the induction of most human cancer. This conversion may result from mutation in an oncogene, its translocation, or its amplification (see Figure 22-2). A study of transformed cells has revealed the important role of cellular and viral oncogenes in the transformation process.
3. A number of B- and T-cell leukemias and lymphomas are associated with translocated proto-oncogenes. In its new site, the translocated gene may come under the influence of enhancers or promoters that cause its transcription at higher levels than usual (see Figure 22-5).
4. Tumor cells display tumor-specific antigens and the more common tumor-associated antigens. Among the latter are oncofetal antigens, (see Table 22-3) and increased levels

of normal oncogene products (see Figure 22-6). In contrast to tumor antigens induced by chemicals or radiation, virally encoded tumor antigens are shared by all tumors induced by the same virus.

5. The tumor antigens recognized by T cells fall into one of four major categories: antigens encoded by genes with tumor-specific expression; antigens encoded by variant forms of normal genes that have been altered by mutation; certain antigens normally expressed only at certain stages of differentiation or differentiation lineages; antigens that are overexpressed in particular tumors.
6. The use of a variety of genetic, biochemical, and immunological approaches has allowed the identification of several tumor-associated antigens (see Table 22-4). In many cases the antigen is expressed on more than one type of tumor. Common tumor antigens offer hope for the design of better therapies, detection, and monitoring, and have important implications for the possibility of anti-tumor immunization.
7. The immune response to tumors includes CTL-mediated lysis, NK-cell activity, macrophage-mediated tumor destruction, and destruction mediated by ADCC. Several cytotoxic factors, including TNF-α and TNF-β, help to mediate tumor-cell killing. Tumors may evade the immune response by modulating their tumor antigens, by reducing their expression of class I MHC molecules, and by antibody-mediated or immune complex-mediated inhibition of CTL activity.
8. Experimental cancer immunotherapy is exploring a variety of approaches. Some of these are the enhancement of the co-stimulatory signal required for T-cell activation (see Figure 22-11a), genetically engineering tumor cells to secrete cytokines that may increase the intensity of the immune response against them (see Figure 22-11b), the therapeutic use of cytokines (see Figure 22-12), and ways of increasing the activity of antigen-presenting cells.
9. A number of encouraging clinical results have been obtained with therapy using monoclonal antibodies against tumor-associated and (in a few cases) tumor-specific antigens (see Figure 22-14). Coupling of antibodies against tumor antigens with toxins, chemotherapeutic agents, or radioactive elements is being examined. The expectation is that such strategies will focus the toxic effects of these agents on the tumor and spare normal cells their deleterious effects.
10. Key elements in the design of strategies for vaccination against cancer are the identification of significant tumor antigens by genetic or biochemical approaches; the development of strategies for the effective presentation of tumor antigens; and the generation of activated populations of helper or cytotoxic T cells. In the case of the few human cancers known to be caused by clearly identified tumor viruses, vaccination against those viruses or their subunits may be effective.

REFERENCES

Aisenberg, AC. 1993. Utility of gene rearrangements in lymphoid malignancies. *Annu. Rev. Med.* **44:**75.

Allison, JP, AA Hurwitz, and DR Leach. 1995. Manipulation of costimulatory signals to enhance antitumor T-cell responses. *Curr. Opin. Immunol.* **7:**682.

Baselga J, et al. 1996. Phase II study of weekly intravenous recombinant humanized anti-p185HER2 monoclonal antibody in patients with *her2/neu*-overexpressing metastatic breast cancer. *Journal of Clinical Oncology* **14:**737.

Boon, T, et al. 1994. Tumor antigens recognized by T lymphocytes. *Annu. Rev. Immunol.* **12:**337.

Coulie, PG, et al. 1994. A new gene coding for a differentiation antigen recognized by autologous cytolytic T lymphocytes on HLA-A2 melanomas. *J. Exp. Med.* **180:**35.

Cournoyer, D, and CT Caskey. 1993. Gene therapy of the immune system. *Annu. Rev. Immunol.* **11:**297.

DeVita, VT, S Hellman, and SA Rosenberg. 1997. *Cancer Principles & Practice of Oncology,* 5th ed., Lippincott Williams & Wilkins.

Hsu, FJ, et al. 1997. Tumor-specific idiotype vaccines in the treatment of patients with B-cell lymphoma. *Blood.* **89:**3129.

Pardoll, DM. 1996. Cancer vaccines: a road map for the next decade. *Curr. Opin. Immunol.* **8:**619.

Paterson, Y, and G Ikonomidis. 1996. Recombinant *Listeria monocytogenes* cancer vaccines *Curr. Opin. Immunol.* **8:**651.

Rosenberg, SA, et al. 1994. Treatment of patients with metastatic melanoma with autologous tumor-infiltrating lymphocytes and interleukin 2. *Journal of the National Cancer Institute.* **86:**1159.

Sahin, U, O Tureci, and M Pfreundschuh. 1997. Serological identification of human tumor antigens *Curr. Opin. Immunol.* **9:**709.

Scott, AM, and S Welt. 1997. Antibody-based immunological therapies. *Curr. Opin. Immunol.* **9:**717.

Tindle, RW. 1996. Human papillomavirus vaccines for cervical cancer. *Curr. Opin. Immunol.* **8:**643.

Van Den Eynde, B, and P van der Bruggen. 1996. T cell defined tumor antigens. *Curr. Opin. Immunol.* **9:**684.

Weinberg, RA. 1996. How cancer arises. *Sci. Am.* **275**(3):62.

Useful Web Sites

http://www.oncolink.upenn.edu/
Oncolink is a site that offers comprehensive information about many types of cancer. It is a good source of information about cancer research and advances in cancer therapy. The site is regularly updated and it includes many useful links to other resources.

http://www.cancer.org/index_4up.html
This is the Web site of the American Cancer Society. It contains a great deal of information on the incidence, treatment, prevention of cancer. The site also highlights significant achievements in cancer research.

http://www.cytopathnet.org/
A good resource for information on the cytological examination of tumors and on matters related to staining patterns that are typical of the cell populations found in a number of cancers.

STUDY QUESTIONS

1. Indicate whether each of the following statements is true or false. If you think a statement is false, explain why.

a. Hereditary retinoblastoma results from overexpression of a cellular oncogene.

b. Translocation of c-*myc* gene is found in many patients with Burkitt's lymphoma.

c. Multiple copies of cellular oncogenes are sometimes observed in cancer cells.

d. Viral integration into the cellular genome may convert a proto-oncogene into a transforming oncogene.

e. All oncogenic retroviruses carry viral oncogenes.

f. The immune response against a virus-induced tumor protects against another tumor induced by the same virus.

g. LAK cells are tumor specific.

2. You are a clinical immunologist studying acute lymphoblastic leukemia (ALL). Leukemic cells from most patients with ALL have the morphology of lymphocytes but do not express cell-surface markers characteristic of mature B or T cells. You have isolated cells from ALL patients that do not express membrane Ig but do react with monoclonal antibody against a normal pre-B-cell marker (B-200). You therefore suspect that these leukemic cells are pre-B cells. How would you use genetic analysis to confirm that the leukemic cells are committed to the B-cell lineage?

3. In a recent experiment, melanoma cells were isolated from patients with early or advanced stages of malignant melanoma. At the same time, T cells specific for tetanus-toxoid antigen were isolated and cloned from each patient.

a. When early-stage melanoma cells were cultured together with tetanus-toxoid antigen and the tetanus toxoid–specific T-cell clones, the T-cell clones were observed to proliferate. This proliferation was blocked by addition of chloroquine or by addition of monoclonal antibody to HLA-DR. Proliferation was not blocked by addition of monoclonal antibody to HLA-A, -B, -DQ, or -DP. What might these findings indicate about the early-stage melanoma cells in this experimental system?

b. When the same experiment was repeated with advanced-stage melanoma cells, the tetanus-toxoid T-cell clones failed to proliferate in response to the tetanus-toxoid antigen. What might this indicate about advanced-stage melanoma cells?

c. When early and advanced malignant melanoma cells were fixed with paraformaldehyde and incubated with processed tetanus toxoid, only the early-stage melanoma cells could induce proliferation of the tetanus-toxoid-T-cell clones. What might this indicate about early-stage melanoma cells?

d. How might you confirm your hypothesis experimentally?

4. What are three likely sources of tumor antigens?

5. Various cytokines have been evaluated for use in tumor immunotherapy. Describe four mechanisms by which cytokines mediate antitumor effects and the cytokines that induce each type of effect.

6. Infusion of transfected melanoma cells into cancer patients is a promising immunotherapy.

a. Which two genes have been transfected into melanoma cells for this purpose? What is the rationale behind use of each of these genes?

b. Why might use of such transfected melanoma cells also be effective in treating other types of cancers?

Go to www.whfreeman.com/immunology Self-Test
Review and quiz of key terms

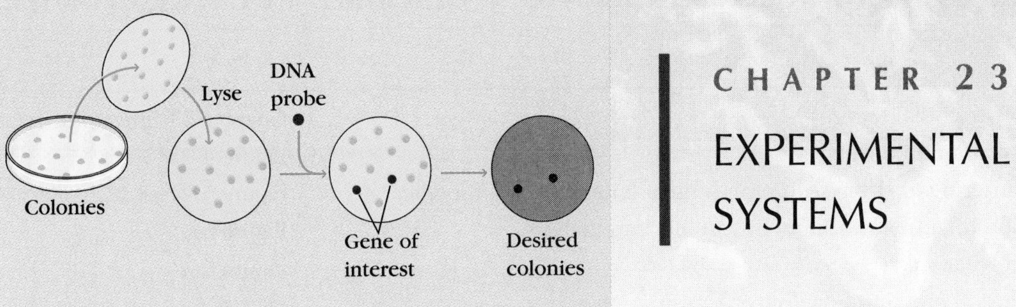

CHAPTER 23
EXPERIMENTAL SYSTEMS

Experimental Animal Models

Cell-Culture Systems

Protein Biochemistry

Recombinant DNA Technology

Analysis of DNA Regulatory Sequences

Gene Transfer into Mammalian Cells

Experimental systems of various types are used to unravel the complex cellular interactions of the immune response. The choice of experimental system influences the kinds of data that can be obtained and places certain limitations on the interpretation of those data.

In vivo systems, which involve the whole animal, provide the most natural experimental conditions. However, due to their complexity, in vivo systems have a myriad of unknown and uncontrollable cellular interactions that add ambiguity to the interpretation of data. At the other extreme are in vitro systems, in which defined populations of lymphocytes are studied under controlled and consequently repeatable conditions; in vitro systems can be simplified to the extent that individual cellular interactions can be studied effectively. Yet they have their own limitations, the most notable of which is their artificiality. For example, providing antigen to purified B cells in vitro does not stimulate maximal antibody production unless T cells are present. Therefore a study of antibody production in an artificial in vitro system that lacks T cells could lead to the incorrect conclusion that B cells do not synthesize high levels of antibodies. One must ask whether a cellular response observed in vitro reflects reality or is a product of the unique conditions of the in vitro system itself.

This chapter describes some of the experimental systems routinely used to study the immune system. It also covers some recombinant DNA techniques that have revolutionized the study of the immune system in the past decade or so. Other chapters also cover experimental systems and techniques in detail. Table 23-1 lists them and directs the reader to the appropriate location for a description.

Experimental Animal Models

The study of the immune system in vertebrates requires suitable animal models. The choice of an animal depends on its suitability for attaining a particular research goal. If large amounts of antiserum are sought, a rabbit, goat, sheep, or horse might be an appropriate experimental animal. If the goal is development of a protective vaccine, the animal chosen must be susceptible to the infectious agent so that the efficacy of the vaccine can be assessed. Mice or rabbits can be used for vaccine development if they are susceptible to the pathogen. But if growth of the infectious agent is limited to humans and primates, vaccine development may require the use of monkeys, chimpanzees, or baboons. The use of primates for research purposes must be carefully regulated to ensure that each endangered species is protected from extinction.

For most basic research in immunology, mice have been the experimental animal of choice. They are easy to handle, are genetically well characterized, and have a rapid breeding cycle. The immune system of the mouse has been characterized more extensively than that of any other species. The value of basic research in the mouse system is highlighted by the enormous impact this research has had on clinical intervention in human disease.

Inbred Strains

To control experimental variation caused by differences in the genetic backgrounds of experimental animals, immunologists

TABLE 23-1 IMMUNOLOGICAL METHODS DESCRIBED IN OTHER CHAPTERS

Method	Location
Bone-marrow transplantation	Chapter 2 Clinical Focus
Preparation of immunotoxins	Figure 4-23
Genetic engineering of chimeric mouse-human monoclonal antibodies	Figure 5-22 and Chapter 5 Clinical Focus
Determination of antibody affinity by equilibrium dialysis	Figure 6-2
Precipitation reactions	Figure 6-4
Immunodiffusion and immunoelectrophoresis	Figures 6-5, 6-6, and 6-7
Hemagglutination	Figure 6-8
Radioimmunoassay (RIA)	Figure 6-10
ELISA assays	Figure 6-11
ELISPOT assay	Figure 6-12
Western blotting	Figure 6-13
Immunoprecipitation	Figure 6-14
Immunofluorescence	Figure 6-15
Flow cytometry (FACS analysis)	Figure 6-16
Production of congenic mice	Figure 7-3
Adoptive transfer of lymphocytes to irradiated hosts	Figure 11-16
Mixed lymphocyte reaction (MLR)	Figure 14-13
Cell-mediated lympholysis (CML)	Figure 14-14
Production of vaccinia vector vaccine	Figure 18-5
Production of multivalent subunit vaccines	Figure 18-7
HLA typing	Figure 21-4

often work with inbred strains—that is, genetically identical animals produced by inbreeding. The rapid breeding cycle of mice makes them particularly well suited for the production of inbred strains, which are developed by repeated inbreeding between brother and sister littermates. In this way the heterozygosity of alleles that is normally found in randomly outbred mice is replaced by homozygosity at all loci. Repeated inbreeding for 20 generations usually yields an inbred strain whose progeny are homozygous at more than 98% of all loci. More than 150 different inbred strains of mice are available; these are designated by a series of letters and/or numbers (Table 23-2). Most of these strains are purchased by immunologists from such suppliers as Jackson Laboratory in Bar Harbor, Maine. Inbred strains have also been produced in rats, guinea pigs, hamsters, rabbits, and domestic fowl. Because inbred animals are genetically identical **(syngeneic),** their immune responses can be studied in the absence of variables introduced by individual genetic differences. Inbred strains are invaluable in the study of immunology. With inbred strains, lymphocyte subpopulations isolated from one animal can be injected into another animal of the same strain without eliciting a rejection reaction. This type of experimental system permitted immunologists to first demonstrate that lymphocytes from an antigen-primed animal could transfer immunity to an unprimed syngeneic recipient.

Adoptive-Transfer Systems

In some experiments, it is important to eliminate the immune responsiveness of the syngeneic host so that the response of only the transferred lymphocytes can be studied in isolation. This can be accomplished by a technique called **adoptive transfer:** first, exposing the syngeneic host to x-rays kills its lymphocytes; then the donor immune cells are introduced. Subjecting a mouse that will serve as host to high doses of x-rays (650–750 rads) can kill 99.99% of its lymphocytes, after which the activities of lymphocytes transplanted from the spleen of a syngeneic donor can be studied without interference from host lymphocytes. If the host's hematopoietic cells might influence an adoptive-transfer experiment, then higher x-ray levels (900–1000 rads) are used to eliminate the entire hematopoietic system. Mice irradiated with such doses will die unless reconstituted with bone marrow from a syngeneic donor.

The adoptive-transfer system has enabled immunologists to study the development of injected lymphoid stem cells in various organs of the recipient. Adoptive-transfer experiments have also facilitated the study of various populations

TABLE 23-2 SOME INBRED MOUSE STRAINS COMMONLY USED IN IMMUNOLOGY

Strain	Common substrains	Characteristics
A	A/He A/J A/WySn	High incidence of mammary tumors in some substrains
AKR	AKR/J AKR/N AKR/Cum	High incidence of leukemia *Thy 1.2* allele in AKR/Cum, and *Thy 1.1* allele in other substrains (*Thy* gene encodes a T-cell surface protein)
BALB/c	BALB/c*j* BALB/c AnN BALB/cBy	Sensitivity to radiation Used in hybridoma technology Many myeloma cell lines were generated in these mice
CBA	CBA/J CBA/H CBA/N	Gene *(rd)* causing retinal degeneration in CBA/J Gene *(xid)* causing X-linked immunodeficiency in CBA/N
C3H	C3H/He C3H/HeJ C3H/HeN	Gene *(rd)* causing retinal degeneration High incidence of mammary tumors in many substrains (these carry a mammary-tumor virus that is passed via maternal milk to offspring)
C57BL/6	C57BL/6J C57BL/6By C57BL/6N	High incidence of hepatomas after irradiation High complement activity
C57BL/10	C57BL/10J C57BL/10ScSn C57BL/10N	Very close relationship to C57BL/6 but differences in at least two loci Frequent partner in preparation of congenic mice
C57BR	C57BR/cd*j*	High frequency of pituitary and liver tumors Very resistant to x-irradiation
C57L	C57L/J C57L/N	Susceptibility to experimental autoimmune encephalomyelitis (EAE) High frequency of pituitary and reticular cell tumors
C58	C58/J C58/LwN	High incidence of leukemia
DBA/1	DBA/1J DBA/1N	High incidence of mammary tumors
DBA/2	DBA/2J DBA/2N	Low immune response to some antigens Low response to pneumococcal polysaccharide type III
HRS	HRS/J	Hairless *(hr)* gene, usually in heterozygous state
NZB	NZB/BINJ NZB/N	High incidence of autoimmune hemolytic anemia and lupus-like nephritis Autoimmune disease similar to systemic lupus erythematosus (SLE) in F_1 progeny from crosses with NZW
NZW	NZW/N	SLE-type autoimmune disease in F_1 progeny from crosses with NZB
P	P/J	High incidence of leukemia
SJL	SJL/J	High level of aggression and severe fighting to the point of death, especially in males Tendency to develop certain autoimmune diseases, most susceptible to EAE
SWR	SWR/J	Tendency to develop several autoimmune diseases, especially EAE
129	129/J 129/SvJ	High incidence of spontaneous teratocarcinoma

SOURCE: Adapted from Federation of American Societies for Experimental Biology, 1979, *Biological Handbooks,* Vol. III: Inbred and Genetically Defined Strains of Laboratory Animals.

of lymphocytes and of the cellular interactions required to generate an immune response. Such experiments, for instance, first enabled immunologists to show that a T helper cell is necessary for B-cell activation in the humoral response.

In these experiments, adoptive transfer of purified B cells or purified T cells did not produce antibody in the irradiated host. Only when both cell populations were transferred was antibody produced in response to antigen.

The Hemolytic Plaque Assay

For many years, the humoral immune response could be monitored only by quantifying antibody production by various assays based on the antigen-antibody interaction (see Chapter 6). This changed with development of the hemolytic plaque assay, counts the plasma cells in a sample. Originally developed by N. K. Jerne, A. A. Nordin, and C. Henry and later modified by other researchers, this assay has played a significant role in studies of the humoral response.

The original direct hemolytic plaque assay, which is similar in principle to a viral plaque assay, is used to measure the number of plasma cells in mice primed with sheep red blood cells (SRBCs). Spleen cells from primed mice are mixed in warm, melted agar with an excess of SRBCs (Figure 23-1a). The agar containing the cell suspension is poured into a Petri dish, whose bottom is covered with a layer of

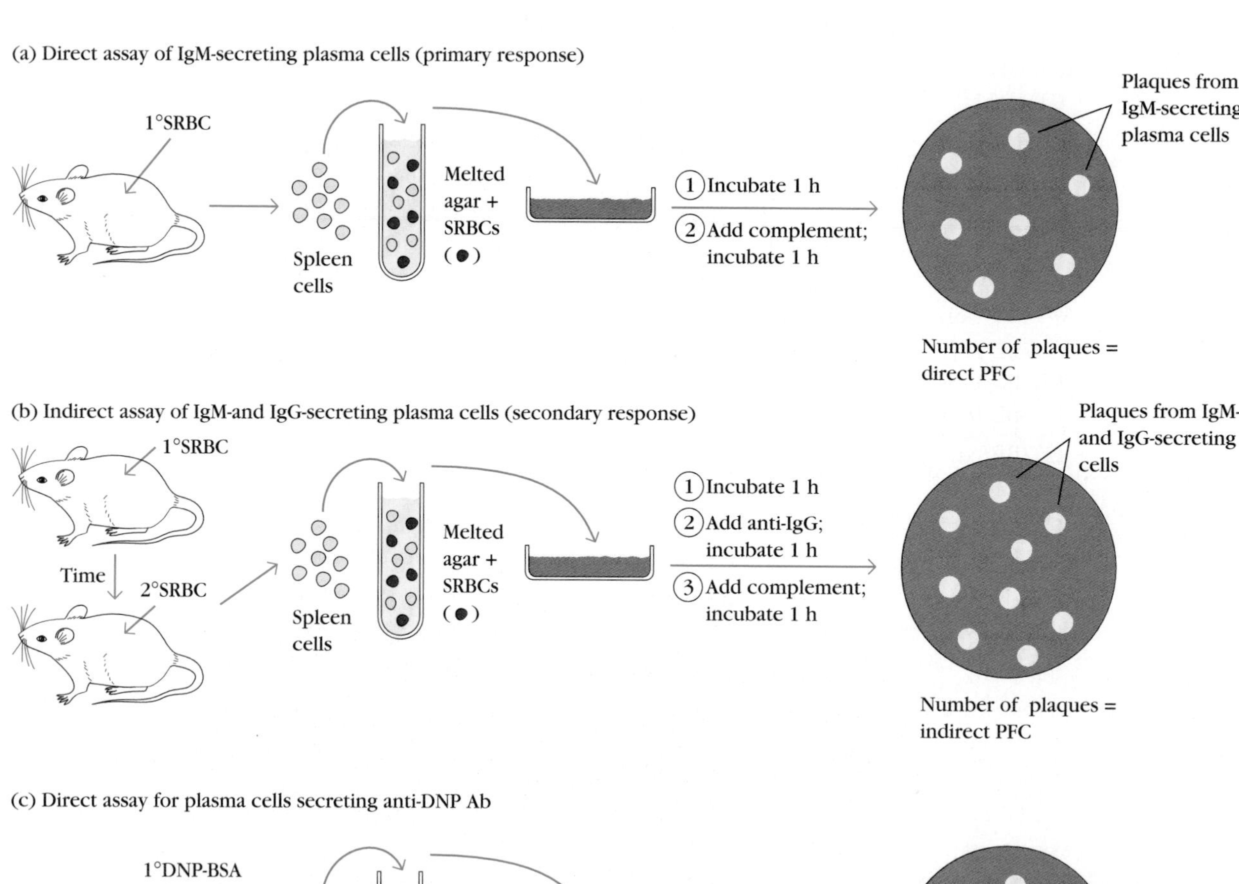

FIGURE 23-1 Hemolytic plaque assays. (a) A direct assay detects IgM-secreting plasma cells, which are predominant in a primary response. (b) In an indirect assay, which detects both IgM- and IgG-secreting plasma cells, antibodies against mouse IgG are added so that complement-mediated lysis of IgG-SRBC complexes will occur. By subtracting the direct PFC from the indirect PFC, the number of IgG-secreting plasma cells can be determined. In a secondary response, the indirect PFC is high and the direct PFC is low. (c) The response to immunization with antigens other than SRBCs can be determined with the hemolytic plaque assay if the immunizing protein or hapten is coupled to SRBCs.

hard agar, and allowed to cool and solidify. The splenic lymphocytes are thus immobilized in the agar, surrounded by a sea of SRBCs. The Petri dish is incubated for 1 h at 37°C, during which time antibody secreted by plasma cells diffuses into the agar matrix and binds to the SRBCs in the vicinity of each antibody-secreting plasma cell. Guinea-pig serum containing complement is then added. The complement reacts with the antibody bound to the SRBCs and mediates their lysis, leaving each plasma cell surrounded by a clear plaque devoid of red blood cells. The plaques are counted, and their number is the number of antibody-producing plasma cells specific for the SRBC antigen. This assay, referred to as the direct plaque-forming cells (direct PFC) assay, identifies primarily IgM-producing plasma cells.

The hemolytic plaque assay can be adapted to determine not only the number of IgM-secreting plasma cells but also the number of IgG-secreting plasma cells. In the case of IgM, complement-mediated lysis is triggered by the binding of a single pentameric IgM molecule to an SRBC. However, in the case of IgG, which exists as a monomer, complement-mediated lysis does not occur unless the Fc regions from two IgG molecules are within 30–40 nm of each other on the membrane of an SRBC. Such proximity does not normally result from the random binding of IgG secreted by a single plasma cell. Therefore, an anti-isotype antibody that reacts with the bound IgG is added to the Petri dish after the first hour of incubation. The dishes are incubated for an additional hour, at which time the complement is added, and the dishes are incubated for another hour (Figure 23-1b). This procedure, called the indirect hemolytic plaque assay (or indirect PFC), results in lysis of SRBCs to which IgM or IgG is bound. Subtraction of the number of plaques formed in the direct assay from the number formed in the indirect assay gives the number of IgG-secreting plasma cells. Since most of the antibody secreted during a primary response is IgM, the direct PFC is high and the indirect PFC is not much higher. In contrast, a secondary response leads to a low direct PFC and a much higher indirect PFC, reflecting the switch from IgM to IgG secretion.

The hemolytic plaque assay also can be modified to quantitate plasma cells that secrete antibodies directed against specific proteins, polysaccharides, or small haptens. In this case, the animal is immunized with the desired antigen, but, before the SRBCs are mixed with the isolated spleen cells, they are coated with the immunizing antigen. The induced antibody binds to these antigen-coated SRBCs, which are lysed after the complement is added (Figure 23-1c). Uncoated SRBCs can serve as a control, since they do not lyse in response to antibody secreted from the antigen-specific plasma cells.

SCID Mice and SCID-Human Mice

An autosomal recessive mutation resulting in **severe combined immunodeficiency disease (SCID)** developed spontaneously in a strain of mice called CB-17. These CB-17 SCID mice fail to develop mature T and B cells and consequently are severely compromised immunologically. This defect is due to a failure in V(D)J recombination (see Figure 5-10). SCID mice must be housed in a sterile (germ-free) environment if they are to survive, because they cannot fight off microorganisms of even low pathogenicity. The absence of functional T and B cells enables these mice to accept foreign cells and grafts from other strains of mice or even from other species.

Apart from their lack of functional T and B cells, SCID mice appear to be normal in all respects. When normal bone-marrow cells are injected into SCID mice, normal T and B cells develop, and the mice are cured of their immunodeficiency. This finding has made SCID mice a valuable model system for the study of immunodeficiency and the process of differentiation of bone-marrow stem cells into mature T or B cells.

Interest in SCID mice mushroomed when it was found that they could be used to study the human immune system. In this system, portions of human fetal liver, adult thymus, and adult lymph nodes are implanted into SCID mice (Figure 23-2). Because the mice lack mature T and B cells of their own, they do not reject the transplanted human tissue. The implanted human fetal liver contains immature lymphocytes (stem cells), which migrate to the implanted human tissues, where they mature into T and B cells, producing a **SCID-human mouse.** Because the human lymphocytes are exposed to mouse

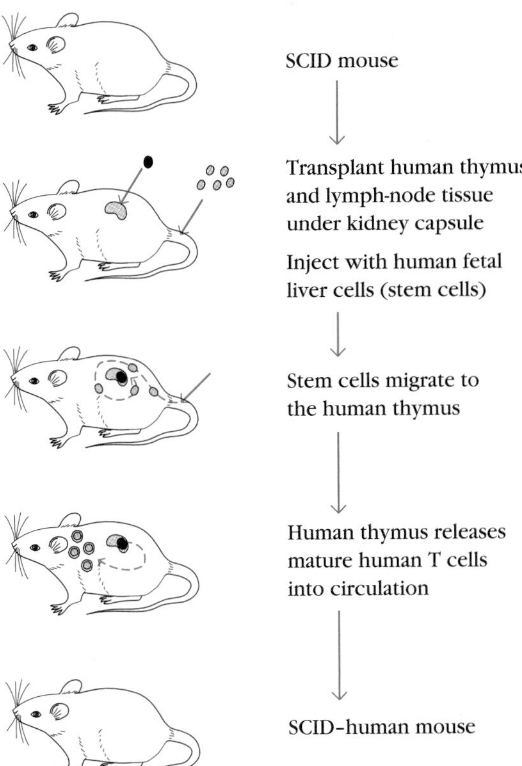

FIGURE 23-2 Production of SCID-human mouse. This system permits study of human lymphocytes within an animal model. In this example, human T-cells are transferred to SCID mouse but B-cells also can be transferred by the use of bone-marrow precursors.

antigens while they are still immature, they later recognize mouse cells as self and do not mount an immunologic response against the mouse host.

The beauty of the SCID-human mouse is that it enables one to study human lymphocytes within an animal model. This valuable system has proved useful in research on the development of various lymphoid cells and also as an important animal model in AIDS research since mouse lymphocytes cannot be infected with HIV but the lymphocytes of a SCID-human mouse are readily infected.

Cell-Culture Systems

The complexity of the cellular interactions that generate an immune response has led immunologists to rely heavily on various types of in vitro cell-culture systems. A variety of cells can be cultured, including primary lymphoid cells, cloned lymphoid cell lines, and hybrid cells.

Primary Lymphoid Cell Cultures

Primary lymphoid cell cultures can be obtained by isolating lymphocytes directly from blood or lymph or from various lymphoid organs by tissue dispersion. The lymphocytes can then be grown in a chemically defined basal medium (containing saline, sugars, amino acids, vitamins, trace elements, and other nutrients) to which various serum supplements are added. For some experiments, serum-free culture conditions are employed. Because in vitro culture techniques require from 10- to 100-fold fewer lymphocytes than do typical in vivo techniques, they have enabled immunologists to assess the functional properties of minor subpopulations of lymphocytes. It was by means of cell-culture techniques, for example, that immunologists were first able to define the functional differences between $CD4^+$ T helper cells and $CD8^+$ T cytotoxic cells.

Cell-culture techniques have also been used to identify numerous cytokines involved in the activation, growth, and differentiation of various cells involved in the immune response. Early experiments showed that media conditioned, or modified, by the growth of various lymphocytes or antigen-presenting cells would support the growth of other lymphoid cells. Conditioned media contain the secreted products from actively growing cells. Many of the individual cytokines that characterized various conditioned media have subsequently been identified and purified, and in many cases the genes that encode them have been cloned. These cytokines, which play a central role in the activation and regulation of the immune response, are described in Chapter 12 and elsewhere.

Cloned Lymphoid Cell Lines

A primary lymphoid cell culture comprises a heterogeneous group of cells that can be propagated only for a limited time. This heterogeneity can complicate the interpretation of experimental results. To avoid these problems, immunologists use cloned lymphoid cell lines and hybrid cells.

Normal mammalian cells generally have a finite life span in culture; that is, after a number of population doublings characteristic of the species and cell type, the cells stop dividing. In contrast, tumor cells or normal cells that have undergone **transformation** induced by chemical carcinogens or viruses can be propagated indefinitely in tissue culture; thus, they are said to be immortal. Such cells are referred to as **cell lines.**

The first cell line—the mouse fibroblast L cell—was derived in the 1940s from cultured mouse subcutaneous connective tissue by exposing the cultured cells to a chemical carcinogen, methylcholanthrene, over a 4-month period. In the 1950s, another important cell line, the HeLa cell, was derived by culturing human cervical cancer cells. Since these early studies, hundreds of cell lines have been established. Various techniques can be used to ensure that a cell line is derived from a single parent cell. Such a cloned cell line consists of a population of genetically identical (syngeneic) cells that can be grown indefinitely in culture.

A variety of cell lines are used in immunologic research. Table 23-3 lists some of these lines and briefly describes their properties. Some of these cell lines were derived from spontaneously occurring tumors of lymphocytes, macrophages, or other accessory cells involved in the immune response. In other cases, the cell line was induced by transformation of normal lymphoid cells with viruses such as Abelson's murine leukemia virus (A-MLV), simian virus 40 (SV40), Epstein-Barr virus (EBV), or human T-cell leukemia virus type 1(HTLV-1).

Lymphoid cell lines differ from primary lymphoid cell cultures in several important ways: They survive indefinitely in tissue culture, they show various abnormal growth properties, and they often have an abnormal number of chromosomes. Cells with more or less than the normal diploid number of chromosomes for a species are said to be aneuploid. The big advantage of cloned lymphoid cell lines is that they can be grown for extended periods in tissue culture, enabling immunologists to obtain large numbers of homogeneous cells in culture.

Until the late 1970s, immunologists did not succeed in maintaining normal T cells in tissue culture for extended periods. In 1978, a serendipitous finding led to the observation that conditioned medium containing a T-cell growth factor was required. The essential component of the conditioned medium turned out to be interleukin 2 (IL-2). By culturing normal T lymphocytes with antigen in the presence of IL-2, clones of antigen-specific T lymphocytes could be isolated. These individual clones could be propagated and studied in culture and even frozen for storage. After thawing, the clones continued to grow and express their original antigen-specific functions.

Development of cloned lymphoid cell lines has enabled immunologists to study a number of events that previously could not be examined. For example, research on the molecular events involved in activation of naive lymphocytes by antigen was hampered by the low frequency of naive B and T cells spe-

TABLE 23-3 CELL LINES COMMONLY USED IN IMMUNOLOGIC RESEARCH

Cell line	Description
L-929	Mouse fibroblast cell line; often used in DNA transfection studies and to assay tumor necrosis factor (TNF)
SP2/0	Nonsecreting mouse myeloma; often used as a fusion partner for hybridoma secretion
P3X63-Ag8.653	Nonsecreting mouse myeloma; often used as a fusion partner for hybridoma secretion
MPC 11	Mouse IgG2b-secreting myeloma
P3X63-Ag8	Mouse IgG1-secreting myeloma
MOPC 315	Mouse IgA-secreting myeloma
J558	Mouse IgA-secreting myeloma
7OZ/3	Mouse pre–B-cell lymphoma; used to study early events in B-cell differentiation
BCL 1	Mouse B-cell leukemia lymphoma that expresses membrane IgM and IgD and can be activated with mitogen to secrete IgM
CTLL-2	Mouse T-cell line whose growth is dependent on IL-2; often used to assay IL-2 production
Jurkat	Human T-cell leukemia that secretes IL-2
DO11.10	Mouse T-cell hybridoma with specificity for ovalbumin
PU 5-1.8	Mouse monocyte-macrophage line
P338 D1	Mouse monocyte-macrophage line that secretes high levels of IL-1
WEHI 265.1	Mouse monocyte line
P815	Mouse mastocytoma cells; often used as target to assess killing by cytotoxic T lymphocytes (CTLs)
YAC-1	Mouse lymphoma cells; often used as target for NK cells
HL-60	Human myeloid-leukemia cell line
COS-1	African green monkey kidney cells transformed by SV40; often used in DNA transfection studies

cific for a particular antigen; in a heterogeneous population of lymphocytes, the molecular changes occurring in one responding cell could not be detected against a background of 10^3–10^6 nonresponding cells. T- and B-cell lines with known antigenic specificity have provided immunologists with large homogeneous cell populations in which to study the membrane and intracellular events involved in antigen recognition. Similarly, the molecular-level genetic changes corresponding to different maturational stages can be studied in cell lines that appear to be "frozen" at different stages of differentiation. Cell lines have also been useful in studying the soluble factors produced by lymphoid cells. Some cell lines secrete large quantities of various cytokines; other lines express membrane receptors for particular cytokines. These cell lines have been used by immunologists to purify various cytokines and their receptors and eventually to clone their genes.

However, lymphoid cell lines have a number of limitations. Variants arise spontaneously in the course of prolonged culture, necessitating frequent subcloning to limit the cellular heterogeneity that can develop. If variants are selected in subcloning, it is possible that two subclones derived from the same parent clone may represent different subpopulations. Moreover, any cell line derived from tumor cells or transformed cells may have unknown genetic contributions characteristic of the tumor or of the transformed state; because of this possibility, researchers must be cautious when extrapolating results obtained with cell lines to the normal situation in vivo. Nevertheless, transformed cell lines have made a major contribution to the study of the immune response, and a number of molecular events discovered in experiments with transformed cell lines have later been shown to take place in normal lymphocytes.

Hybrid Lymphoid Cell Lines

In somatic-cell hybridization, immunologists fuse normal B or T lymphocytes with tumor cells, obtaining hybrid cells, or heterokaryons, containing nuclei from both parent cells. Random loss of some chromosomes and subsequent cell proliferation yield a clone of cells that contain a single nucleus with chromosomes from each of the fused cells; such a clone is called a **hybridoma.**

Historically, cell fusion was promoted with Sendai virus, but now it is generally done with polyethylene glycol. Normal antigen-primed B cells can be fused with cancerous plasma cells, called **myeloma cells** (Figure 23-3). The hybridoma

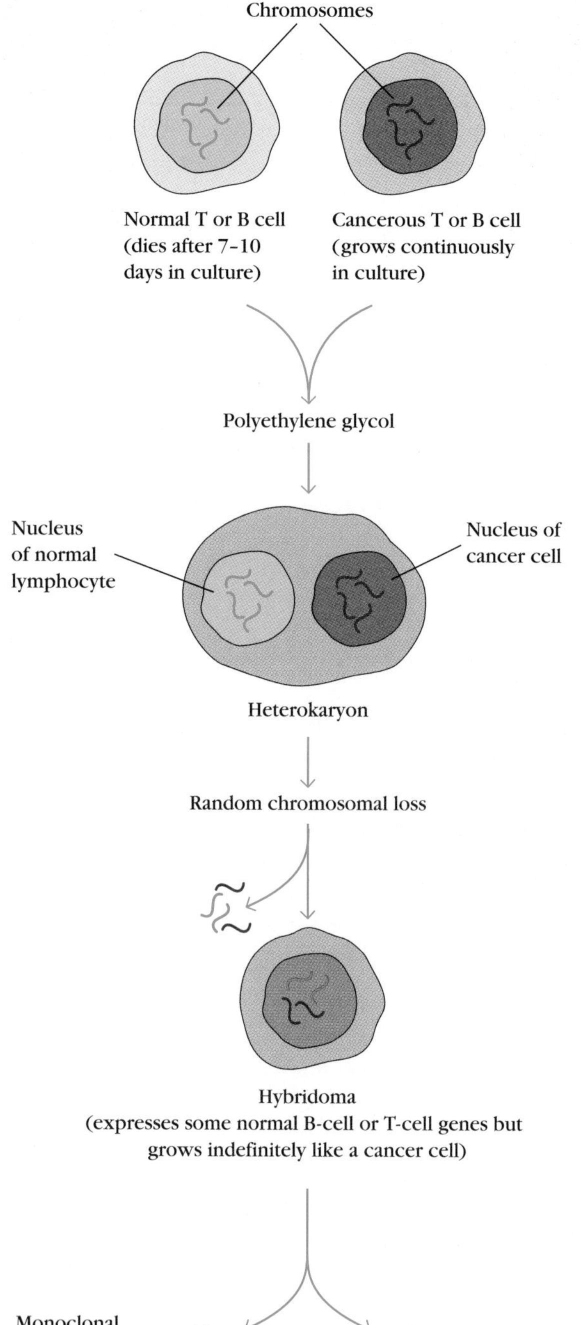

FIGURE 23-3 Production of B-cell and T-cell hybridomas by somatic-cell hybridization. The resulting hybridomas express some of the genes of the original normal B or T cell but also exhibit the immortal-growth properties of the tumor cell. This procedure is used to produce B-cell hybridomas that secrete monoclonal antibody and T-cell hybridomas that secrete various growth factors.

thus formed continues to express the antibody genes of the normal B lymphocyte but is capable of unlimited growth, a characteristic of the myeloma cell. B-cell hybridomas that secrete antibody with a single antigenic specificity, called monoclonal antibody, in reference to its derivation from a single clone, have revolutionized not only immunology but biomedical research as well as the clinical laboratory. Chapter 4 describes the production and uses of monoclonal antibodies in detail (see Figures 4-20 and 4-22).

T-cell hybridomas can also be obtained by fusing T lymphocytes with cancerous T-cell lymphomas. Again, the resulting hybridoma continues to express the genes of the normal T cell but acquires the immortal-growth properties of the cancerous T lymphoma cell. Immunologists have generated a number of stable hybridoma cell lines representing T-helper and T-cytotoxic lineages.

Protein Biochemistry

The techniques of protein biochemistry have been very important in immunology. Study of the protein biochemistry of immunoglobulins led to the determination of their structure and helped to formulate some of the early hypotheses concerning their diversification. Protein biochemistry was critical also in determining the structure of MHC molecules. Indeed, the structure of many important molecules of the immune system has been determined with the techniques of protein biochemistry. Today, some of these techniques are used in experimental immunology. For example, antibodies labeled with fluorescent or radioactive molecules allow immunologists to detect cells that bear antigens recognized by the antibody. Additionally, the ability to determine such biochemical characteristics of a protein as its size, shape, and three-dimensional structure provides essential information for understanding its function.

Radiolabeling Techniques

Radioactive labels on antigen or antibody are extremely sensitive markers for detection and quantification. There are a number of ways to introduce radioactive isotopes into proteins or peptides. Any protein or peptide that contains tyrosine residues may be labeled with radioiodine by chemical or enzymatic procedures. These reactions attach an iodine atom to the phenol ring of the tyrosine molecule. One of the enzymatic iodination techniques, which uses lactoperoxidase, can label proteins on the plasma membrane of a live cell without labeling proteins in the cytoplasm, allowing the study of cell-surface proteins without isolating them from other cell constituents.

A general radiolabeling of cell proteins may be carried out by growing the cells in a medium that contains one or more radiolabeled amino acids. The amino acids selected for this application are those most resistant to metabolic modifica-

TABLE 23-4 RADIOISOTOPES COMMONLY USED IN IMMUNOLOGY LABORATORIES

Isotope	Half-life	Radiation type*	Autoradiography†
^{125}I	60.0 da	γ	+
^{131}I	6.8 da	γ	+
^{51}Cr	27.8 da	γ	–
^{32}P	14.3 da	β	+
^{35}S	87.4 da	β	+
^{14}C	57.30 yrs	β	+
^{3}H	12.35 yrs	β	–

* γ (gamma) radiation may be detected in a solid scintillation counter. β (beta) radiation is detected in a liquid scintillation counter by its ability to convert energy to photons of light in a solution containing phosphorescent compounds.

†Radiation may also be detected by exposure to x-ray film. ^{35}S and ^{14}C must be placed in direct contact with film for detection. ^{3}H cannot be detected by normal autoradiographic techniques.

tion during cell growth so that the radioactive label will appear in the cell protein rather than in all cell constituents. Leucine marked with ^{14}C or ^{3}H, and cysteine or methionine labeled with ^{35}S, are the most commonly used amino acids for metabolic labeling of proteins. Table 23-4 lists some properties of the radioisotopes used in immunologic research.

Labeling Proteins with Biotin

In some instances direct labeling of proteins, especially with enzymes or other large molecules, as described in Chapter 6, may cause denaturation and loss of activity. A convenient labeling system has been developed which may be used in conjunction with the ELISA and ELISPOT assays described in Chapter 6. This labeling technique exploits the high affinity of the reaction between the vitamin biotin and avidin, a large molecule that may be labeled with radioactive isotopes, with fluorescent molecules, or with enzymes. Biotin is a small molecule (mol. wt. 244) that can be coupled to an antibody (or to any protein molecule) by a gentle chemical reaction that causes no loss of antibody activity. After the biotin-coupled antibody has reacted in the assay system, the labeled avidin is introduced and binding is detected according to the label on the avidin molecule (Figure 23-4). The reaction between biotin and avidin is highly specific and of such high affinity that the bond between the two molecules under most assay conditions is virtually irreversible.

Gel Electrophoresis

Separation of mixtures of biologic macromolecules according to their charge and molecular size is conveniently carried out by electrophoresis. When subjected to an electric field, a charged molecule will move toward the oppositely charged electrode. Specifically, positively charged, or cationic, molecules move toward the negative pole (cathode) and negatively charged, or anionic, molecules move in the direction of the positive pole (anode). Furthermore, when subjected to a given electrical potential, or voltage, the rate at which a charged molecule moves (its electrophoretic mobility) depends upon two factors: one is the sign and magnitude of its net electrical charge and the other is the size and shape of the molecule. All other factors being equal, if molecules are of equal size the one with higher net charge will move faster in an applied electrical field. It also follows that small molecules will move faster than large ones of the same net charge. Although there are exceptions in which the shape of a molecule may increase or decrease its frictional drag and cause atypical migration behavior, these general principles underlie all electrophoretic separations.

Because differences in size, shape, and charge are common among molecules of biological interest, electrophoresis is often the method of choice for the separation and analysis of these substances. For convenience in handling and to avoid potential distortion caused by sudden movement of the equipment or even the subtle effects of a temperature change, most electrophoretic separations are not conducted in free solution but rather in a stable supporting medium, such as a gel. A number of possible materials, such

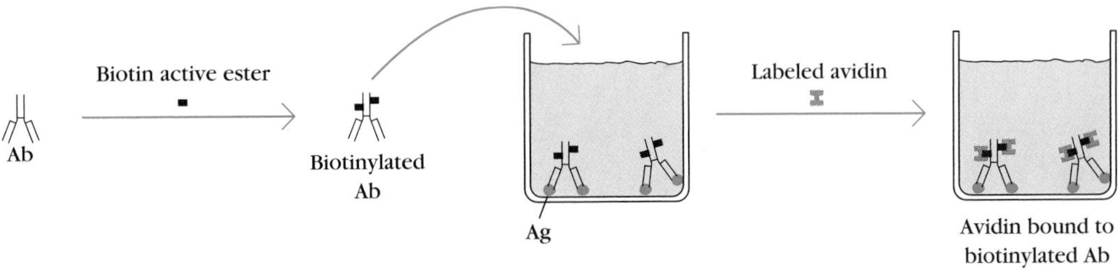

FIGURE 23-4 Labeling of antibody with biotin. An antibody preparation is mixed with a biotin ester, which reacts with the antibody. The biotin-labeled antibody can be used to detect antigens on a solid substrate such as the well of a microtiter plate. After washing away unbound antibody, the bound antibody can be detected with labeled avidin. The avidin can be radioactively labeled or linked to an enzyme that catalyzes a color reaction, as in ELISA procedures (see Figure 6-11).

as starch or agarose, are employed for the preparation of gels, but probably the most frequently used gels in the research laboratory are those prepared by the polymerization and controlled crosslinking of acrylamide to form polyacrylamide. Separation on polyacrylamide gels, commonly referred to as *p*oly*a*crylamide *g*el *e*lectrophoresis (PAGE), may be used for analysis of proteins or nucleic acids (Figure 23-5a).

In one common application, the electrophoresis of proteins through an appropriately crosslinked polyacrylamide gel is carried out in the presence of the detergent sodium dodecyl sulfate (SDS). This method, known as SDS-PAGE, provides a relatively simple and highly effective means of separating mixtures of proteins on the basis of size. The ability of SDS-PAGE to separate proteins by size, independent of their charge, is based on the fact that SDS, a negatively charged detergent, binds to protein. The amount of SDS bound is proportional to the length of the protein, and this binding destroys the characteristic tertiary and secondary structure of the protein, transforming it into a negatively charged rod. In fact, so many negatively charged SDS molecules are bound by a protein that its own intrinsic charge becomes insignificant by comparison and the net charge of any protein treated with an appropriate concentration of SDS will be negative. Therefore, treatment of a mixture of proteins with SDS transforms them into a collection of rods whose lengths and, thus, electric charges are proportional to their molecular weights. This has two extremely useful consequences. First, it is possible to separate the components of a mixture of proteins according to molecular weight. Second, because the electrophoretic mobility, or distance traveled by a species during SDS-PAGE, is inversely proportional to the logarithm of its molecular weight, that distance is a measure of its molecular weight. The gel is stained with a dye that reacts with protein to visualize the locations of the proteins. The migration distance of a protein in question is then compared with a plot of the distances migrated by a set of standard proteins (Figure 23-5b).

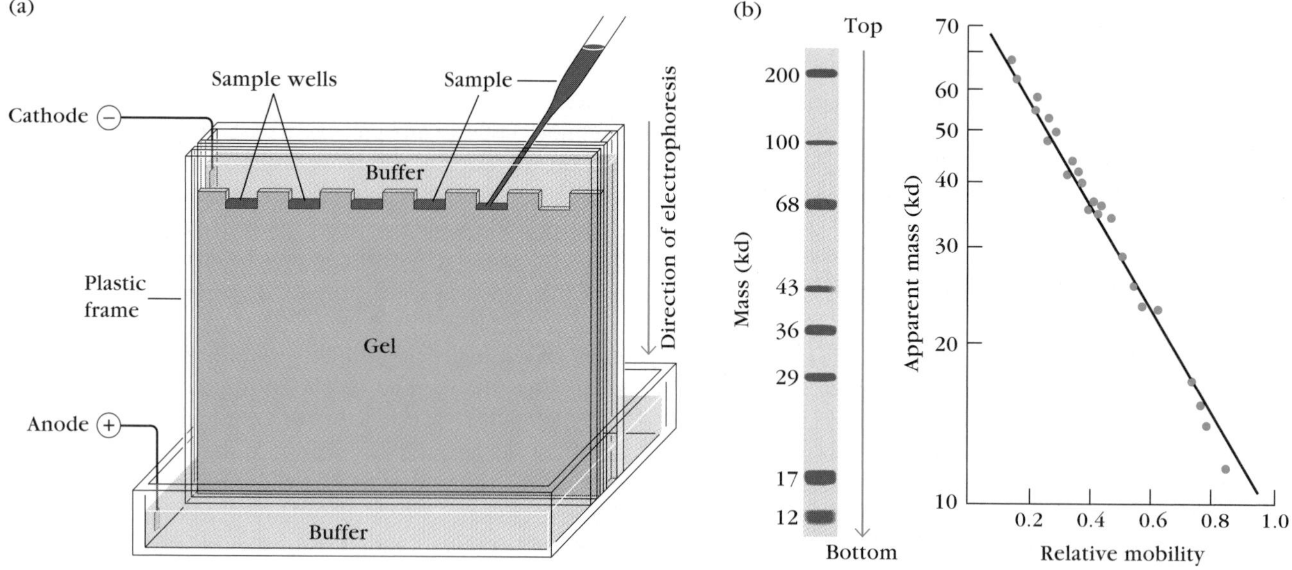

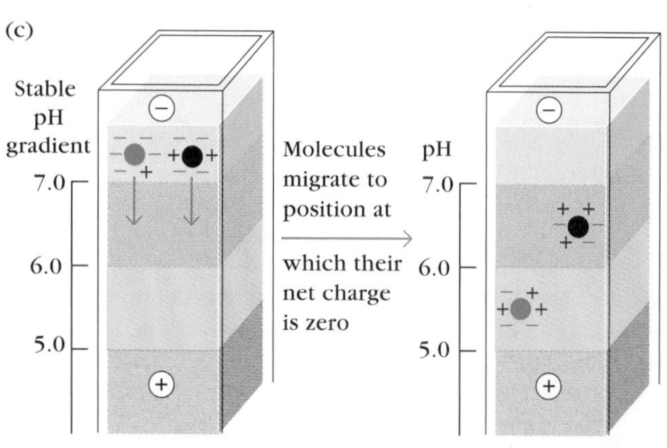

FIGURE 23-5 Gel electrophoresis. (a) A standard PAGE apparatus with cathode at the top and anode at the bottom. Samples are loaded on the top of the gel in sample wells and electrophoresis is accomplished by running a current from the cathode to the anode. (b) The electrophoretic mobility, or distance traveled by a species during SDS-PAGE, is inversely proportional to the log of its molecular weight. The molecular weight of a protein is readily determined by the log of its migration distance with a standard curve that plots the migration distances of the set of standard proteins against the logs of their molecular weights. (c) Isoelectric focusing, or IEF, separates proteins solely by charge. Proteins are placed on a stable pH gradient and subjected to electrophoresis. Each protein migrates to its isoelectric point, the point at which its net charge is zero. [Part (b) after K Weber and M Osborn, 1975, *The Proteins*, 3rd ed., vol. 1, p. 179. Academic Press.]

Another electrophoretic technique, isoelectric focusing (IEF), separates proteins solely on the basis of their charge. This method is based on the fact that a molecule will move in an electric field as long as it has a net positive or negative charge; molecules that bear equal numbers of positive and negative charges and therefore have a net charge of zero will not move. At most pH values, proteins (which characteristically bear a number of both positive and negative charges) have either a net negative or a net positive charge. However, for each protein there is a particular pH, called its isoelectric point (pI), at which that protein has equal numbers of positive and negative charges. Isoelectric focusing makes use of a gel containing substances, called carrier ampholytes, that arrange themselves into a continuous pH gradient when subjected to an electric field. When a mixture of proteins is applied to such a gel and subjected to electrophoresis, each protein moves until it reaches that point in the gradient where the pH of the gel is equal to its isoelectric point. It then stops moving because it has a net charge of zero. Isoelectric focusing is an extremely gentle and effective way of separating different proteins (Figure 23-5c).

A method known as two-dimensional gel electrophoresis (2D gel electrophoresis) combines the advantages of SDS-PAGE and isoelectric focusing in one of the most sensitive and discriminating ways of analyzing a mixture of proteins. In this method, one first subjects the mixture to isoelectric focusing on an IEF tube gel, which separates the molecules on the basis of their isoelectric points without regard to molecular weight. This is the first dimension. In the next step, one places the IEF gel lengthwise across the top of an SDS-polyacrylamide slab (that is, in place of the sample wells in Figure 23-5a) and runs SDS-PAGE. Preparatory to this step, all proteins have been reacted with SDS and therefore migrate out of the IEF gel and through the SDS-PAGE slab according to their molecular weights. This is the second dimension. The position of the proteins in the resulting 2D gel can be visualized in a number of ways. In the least sensitive the gel is stained with a protein-binding dye (such as Coomassie blue). If the proteins have been radiolabeled, the more sensitive method of autoradiography can be used. Alternatively, silver staining is a method of great sensitivity that takes advantage of the capacity of proteins to reduce silver ions to an easily visualized deposit of metallic silver. Finally, immunoblotting, the blotting of proteins onto a membrane (see Figure 6-13), can be used as a way of locating the position of specific proteins on 2D gels if an appropriate antibody is available. Figure 23-6 shows an autoradiograph of a two-dimensional gel of labeled proteins from murine thymocytes.

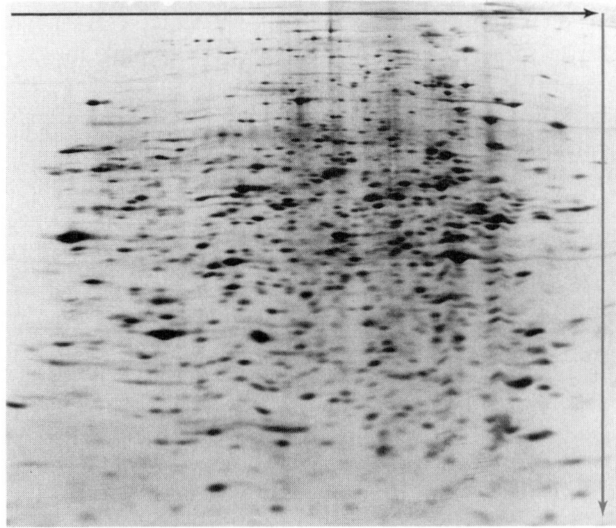

FIGURE 23-6 Two-dimensional gel electrophoresis of labeled total cell proteins from murine thymocytes. These proteins were first subjected to isoelectric focusing (direction of migration indicated by red arrow) and then the focused proteins were separated by SDS-PAGE (direction of migration indicated by blue arrow). [Courtesy of BA Osborne.]

X-Ray Crystallography

A great deal of information about the structure of cells, parts of cells, and even molecules has been obtained by light microscopy. The microscope uses a lens to focus radiation to form an image after it has passed through a specimen. However, theoretical considerations and practical limitations place constraints on the minimum dimensions that can be examined in this way. One is the limit of resolution, the smallest distance between two points at which they can still be seen as distinct. Radiation of a given wavelength cannot resolve structural features much smaller than (less than about 1/2) its wavelength. Since the shortest wavelength of visible light is around 400 nm, even the very best light microscopes have a theoretical limit of resolution of no less than 200 nm.

Because of the much shorter wavelength (0.004 nm) of the electron at the voltages normally used in the electron microscope, the theoretical limit of resolution of the electron microscope is about 0.002 nm. If it were possible to build an instrument that could actually approach this limit, the electron microscope could readily be used to determine the detailed atomic arrangement of biological molecules, since the constituent atoms are separated by distances of 0.1 nm to 0.2 nm. In practice, aberrations inherent in the operation of the magnetic lenses that are used to image the electron beam limit the resolution to about 0.1 nm (1Å). This practical limit can be reached in the examination of certain specimens, particularly metals. Other considerations, however, such as specimen preparation and contrast, limit the resolution for biological materials to about 2 nm (20 Å). To determine the arrangement of a molecule's atoms, then, we must turn to x-rays, a form of electromagnetic radiation that is readily generated in wavelengths on the order of size of interatomic distances. Even though there are no microscopes with lenses that can focus x-rays into images, x-ray crystallography can reveal molecular structure at an extraordinary level of detail.

X-ray crystallography is based on the analysis of the diffraction pattern produced when an x-ray beam passes though a crystal. When the x-rays pass through a crystal, some are scattered by the electrons in the atoms that make up the crystal. The degree to which a particular atom scatters x-rays depends upon its size. Atoms such as carbon, oxygen, or nitrogen, scatter x-rays more than do hydrogen atoms, and larger atoms, such as iron, iodide, or mercury give intense scattering. X-rays are a form of electromagnetic waves; as the scattered waves overlap, they alternately interfere with and reinforce each other. An appropriately placed detector, a sheet of x-ray film, will record a pattern of spots (the diffraction pattern) whose distribution and intensities are determined by the structure of the diffracting crystal. This relationship between crystal structure and diffraction pattern is the basis of x-ray crystallographic analysis. Here is an overview of the procedures used:

Obtain crystals of the protein of interest. To those who have not experienced the frustrations of crystallizing proteins, this may seem a trivial and incidental step of an otherwise highly sophisticated process. It is not. There is great variation from protein to protein in the conditions required to produce crystals that are of a size and geometrical formation appropriate for x-ray diffraction analysis. For example, myoglobin formed crystals over the course of several days at pH 7 in a 3 M solution of ammonium sulfate, but 1.5 M ammonium sulfate at pH 4 worked well for a human IgG1. There is no set formula that can be applied, and those who are consistently successful are persistent, determined, and, like great chefs, have a knack for making just the right "sauce." IgG2a was the first intact antibody to be crystallized; some of these crystals are shown in Figure 23-7.

Selection and mounting. Because large crystals are easier to handle and align in the x-ray beam, they are preferred. In practice, such specimens do not exceed a few millimeters in the largest dimension and are at least 0.1 mm in the smallest. Once chosen, a crystal is harvested into a capillary tube along with the solution from which the crystal was grown (the "mother liquor"). This keeps the crystal from drying and maintains its solvent content, an important consideration for maintaining the internal order of the specimen. The capillary is mounted in the diffraction apparatus and the orientation is adjusted to center the crystal in the x-ray beam.

Generating and recording a diffraction pattern. The precisely positioned crystal is then irradiated with x-rays of a known wavelength produced by accelerating electrons against the copper target of an x-ray tube. When the x-ray beam strikes the crystal, some of it goes straight through and some is scattered in directions and at intensities that reflect the detailed internal geometry of the crystal (Figure 23-8a). The diffraction of the crystal is recorded as a pattern of spots on a series of x-ray films. The positions of the spots indicate the directions of the scattered rays and the degree of blackening of the spots registers their intensity (Figure 23-8b).

Interpreting the diffraction pattern. The diffraction patterns of proteins are complex, and even a protein of modest molecular weight may yield an array of tens of thousands of spots. The core of diffraction analysis is the mathematical deduction of the detailed structure that would produce the diffraction pattern observed. One must calculate to what extent the waves scattered by each atom have combined to reinforce or cancel each other to produce the net intensity observed for each spot in the array. A difficulty arises in the interpretation of complex diffraction patterns because the waves differ with respect to phase, the timing of the period between maxima and minima. Since the pattern observed is the net result of the interaction of many waves, information about phase is critical to calculating the distribution of electron densities that is responsible. The solution of this "phase problem" always looms as a major obstacle to the derivation of a high-resolution structure of any complex molecule.

The problem is solved by derivatizing the protein modifying it by adding heavy atoms, such as mercury, and then obtaining crystals that have the same geometry as (are isomorphous with) those of the underivatized protein. The diffraction pattern of the isomorphous crystal is obtained and compared with that of the native protein. Usually, armed with a knowledge of the diffraction patterns of two or more isomorphous heavy-atom derivatives, the phases for the native protein can be calculated by reference to the characteristic diffraction patterns generated by heavy-atom land-

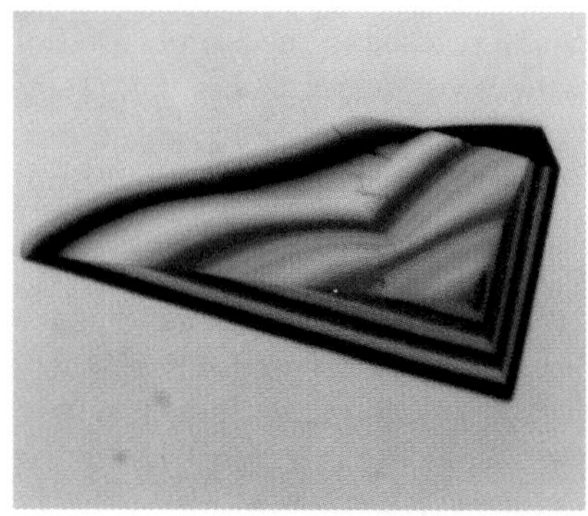

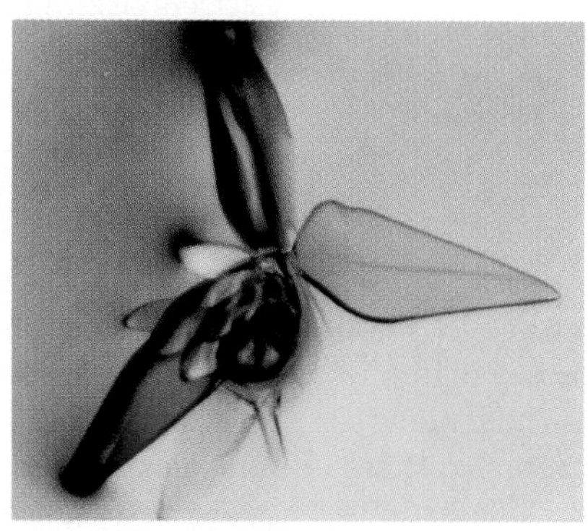

FIGURE 23-7 Crystals of murine IgG2a. [Courtesy of A McPherson.]

(a)

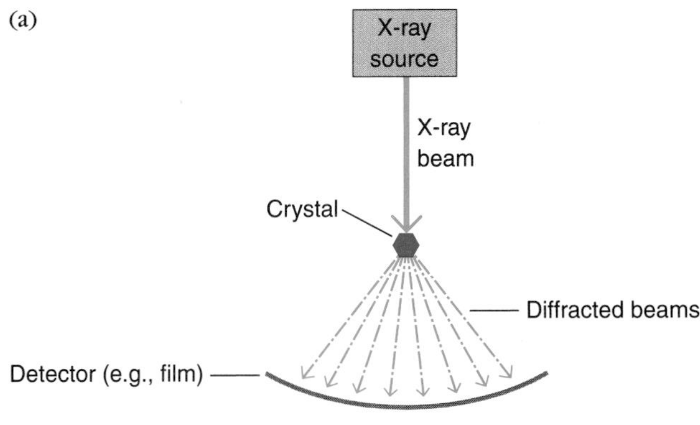

(b)

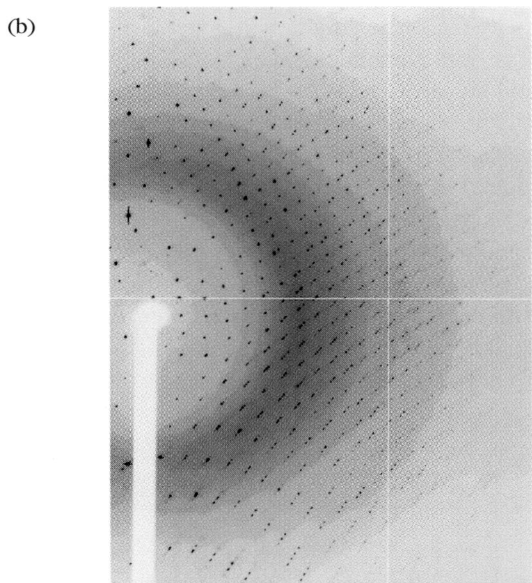

(c)

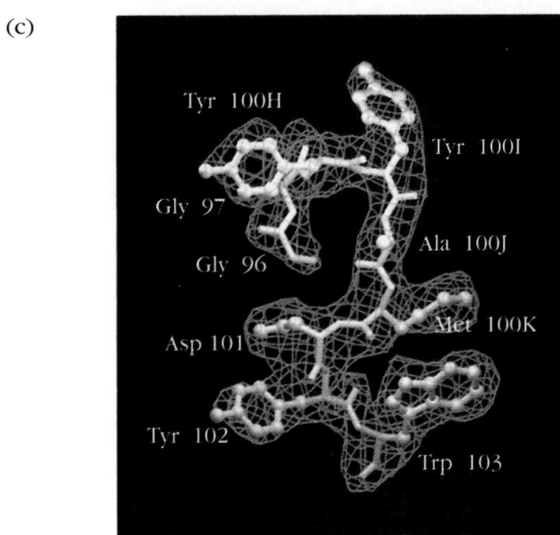

FIGURE 23-8 X-ray crystallography. (a) Schematic diagram of an x-ray crystallographic experiment in which an x-ray beam bombards the crystal and diffracted rays are detected. (b) Section of x-ray diffraction pattern of a crystal of murine IgG2a. (c) Section from the electron-density map of murine IgG2a. [Part (a) from L Stryer, 1995, *Biochemistry,* 4th ed.; parts (b) and (c) courtesy of A McPherson.]

marks. The phases established, it is possible to move on to a calculation of the distribution of electron density. This is accomplished by Fourier synthesis, a mathematical treatment particularly suited to the analysis of periodic phenomena such as those involving waves. In this case, it is used to compute the distribution of electron density along the *x, y,* and *z* axes within a unit cell of the crystal. The deduced electron density is plotted as a series of contour lines drawn in the *xy* plane on a rigid plastic transparency (or alternatively, as a layer in a computer display). A stack of such electron-density maps, each drawn for one of a number of consecutive points along the *z* axis, provides a three-dimensional representation of electronic distribution within the molecule (Figure 23-8c).

Derivation of the structure. Because the electron-density map is an indicator of the relative positions and sizes of the atoms in a molecule, it is the basis for constructing a molecular model. Traditionally, these models have been constructed manually from preformed pieces that furnish precise bond distances and angles. Increasingly, these are being replaced by sophisticated computer graphics programs. Whatever the mechanics of the process, the resolution of the model depends upon a number of factors. First of all, the ultimate resolution possible is set by the quality of the crystal and the internal order of the crystal. Even the highest-quality crystals have a degree of internal disorder that establishes a limit of resolution of about 2 Å. Second, a factor of paramount importance is the number of intensities fed into the Fourier synthesis. A relatively small number of spots may produce a low-resolution (6 Å) image that traces the course of the polypeptide chain but provides little additional structural information. On the other hand, the processing of data provided by tens of thousands of spots allows the tracing of very detailed electron-density maps. Provided one knows the amino acid sequence of the protein, such maps can guide the construction of high-resolution, three-dimensional models. Amino acid sequence data is necessary because it can be difficult, and in some cases impossible, to unambiguously distinguish among some amino acid side chains on even the most detailed electron density maps.

It should be clear that determining a structure by x-ray crystallographic analysis is not to be undertaken lightly. Aside from the artful chemistry of crystallization, a truly formidable amount of data must be collected and analyzed. As a time and labor-saving alternative to the traditionally used x-ray film plate, the field is turning to electronic detectors that determine the positions and record the intensities of the diffracted rays. The huge numbers of calculations that must be done in order to analyze the position and intensity data, as well as determine the phases, of the tens of thousands or even hundreds of thousands of reflections generated could not be undertaken without the computer. The painstaking and tedious model building and structural refinement that are necessary to realize structures of highest resolution are increasingly being written as computer-graphic algorithms. These produce tables of atomic coordinates that precisely locate each atom of the protein in three dimensions. They also allow the rapid creation and often strikingly beautiful visualization of protein structure.

Daunting as the task may be, since 1960, when the first detailed structures of proteins were deduced, the structure of several hundred proteins has been solved. These range from small and (relatively) simple proteins such as lysozyme, consisting of a single polypeptide chain, to poliovirus, an 8,500,000 dalton, stunningly complex nucleoprotein made up of RNA encased by multiple copies of four different polypeptide subunits. Of particular importance to immunologists are the large number of immunologically relevant molecules for which detailed crystal structures are now available. These include immunoglobulins, MHC proteins, and T-cell–receptor proteins.

Recombinant DNA Technology

The various techniques called recombinant DNA technology have had an impact on every area of immunologic research. Genes can be cloned, DNA can be sequenced, and recombinant proteins can be produced, supplying immunologists with defined components for study of the structure and function of the immune system at the molecular level. This section briefly describes some of the recombinant DNA techniques commonly employed in immunologic research; examples of their use have been presented throughout the book.

Restriction-Endonuclease Cleavage of DNA

A variety of bacteria produce enzymes, called restriction endonucleases, that degrade foreign DNA (e.g., bacteriophage DNA) but spare the bacterial cell DNA, which contains methylated residues. The discovery of these bacterial enzymes in the 1970s opened the way to a major technological advance in the field of molecular biology. Before the discovery of restriction endonucleases, double-stranded DNA (dsDNA) could be cut only with DNases. These enzymes do not recognize defined sites and therefore randomly cleave DNA into a variable series of small fragments, which are impossible to sort by size or sequence. In contrast, restriction endonucleases recognize and cleave DNA at specific sites, called restriction sites, which are short double-stranded segments of specific sequence containing four to eight nucleotides (Table 23-5).

A restriction endonuclease cuts both DNA strands at a specific point within its restriction site. Some enzymes, such as *Hpa*I, cut on the central axis and thus generate blunt-ended fragments. Other enzymes, such as *Eco*RI, cut the DNA at staggered points in the recognition site. In this case, the end

TABLE 23-5 SOME RESTRICTION ENZYMES AND THEIR RECOGNITION SEQUENCES

Microorganism source	Abbreviation	Sequence* 5′→3′ 3′→5′
Bacillus amyloliquefaciens H	*Bam*HI	G GATCC CCTAG G
Escherichia coli RY13	*Eco*RI	G AATTC CTTAA G
Haemophilus aegyptius	*Hae*III	GG CC CC GG
Haemophilus influenzae Rd	*Hind*III	A AGCTT TTCGA A
Haemophilus parainfluenzae	*Hpa*I	GTT AAC CAA TTG
Nocardia otitidis-caviarum	*Not*I	GC GGCCGC CGCCGG CG
Providencia stuartii 164	*Pst*I	CTGCA G G ACGTC
Staphylococcus aureus 3A	*Sau*3A	GATC CTAG

*Blue lines indicate locations of single-strand cuts within the restriction site. Enzymes that make off-center cuts produce fragments with short single-stranded extensions at their ends.

SOURCE: New England Biolabs, http://www.neb.com.

of each cleaved fragment is a short segment of single-stranded DNA, called a sticky end. When two different DNA molecules are cut with the same restriction enzyme that makes staggered cuts, the sticky ends of the fragments are complementary; under appropriate conditions, fragments from the two molecules can be joined by base pairing to generate a recombinant DNA molecule. Several hundred different restriction endonucleases have been isolated and many are available commercially, allowing researchers to purchase enzymes that cut DNA at defined restriction sites.

Cloning of DNA Sequences

The development of DNA cloning technology in the 1970s provided a means of amplifying a given DNA fragment to such an extent that unlimited amounts of identical DNA fragments (cloned DNA) could be produced.

Cloning Vectors

In DNA cloning, a given DNA fragment is inserted into an autonomously replicating DNA molecule, called a cloning vector, so that the inserted DNA is replicated with the vector. A number of different viruses have been used as vectors, including bacterial viruses, insect viruses, and mammalian retroviruses. A common bacterial virus used as a vector is bacteriophage λ. If a gene is inserted into bacteriophage λ and the resulting recombinant λ phage is used to infect *E. coli*, the inserted gene will be expressed by the bacteria.

Retroviruses, which can infect virtually any type of mammalian cell, are a common vector used to clone DNA in mammalian cells. Retroviruses are RNA viruses that contain reverse transcriptase, an enzyme that catalyzes conversion of the viral RNA genome into DNA. The viral DNA then integrates into the host chromosomal DNA, where it is retained as a provirus, replicating along with the host chromosomal DNA at each cell division. When a retrovirus is used as a vector, most of the retroviral genes are removed so that the vector cannot produce viral particles; the retroviral genes that are left include a strong promoter region, located at the 5′ end of the viral genome, in a sequence called the long terminal repeat (LTR). If a gene is inserted into such a retroviral vector and the vector is then used to infect mammalian cells, expression of the gene will be under the control of the retroviral promoter region.

Plasmids are another common type of cloning vector. A plasmid is a small, circular, extrachromosomal DNA molecule that can replicate independently in a host cell; the most common host used in DNA cloning is *E. coli*. In general, the DNA to be cloned is inserted into a plasmid that contains an antibiotic-resistance gene. After the recombinant plasmid is incubated with bacterial cells, the cells containing the recombinant plasmid can be selected by their ability to grow in the presence of the antibiotic.

Another type of vector that is often used for cloning is called a **cosmid** vector. This type of vector is a plasmid that has been genetically engineered to contain the COS sites of λ-phage DNA, a drug-resistance gene, and a replication origin. COS sites are DNA sequences that allow any DNA up to 50 kb in length to be packaged into the λ-phage head.

Cloning of cDNA and Genomic DNA

Messenger RNA (mRNA) isolated from cells can be transcribed into complementary DNA (cDNA) with the enzyme reverse transcriptase. The cDNA can be cloned by inserting it into a plasmid vector carrying a gene that confers resistance to an antibiotic, such as ampicillin. The resulting recombinant plasmid DNA is subsequently transferred into specially treated *E. coli* cells by one of several possible techniques; this transfer process is called **transfection.** If the foreign DNA is incorporated into the host cell and expressed, the cell is said to be **transformed.** When the cells are cultured on agar plates containing ampicillin, only transformed cells containing the ampicillin-resistance gene will survive and grow (Figure 23-9). A collection of DNA sequences within plasmid vectors representing all the mRNA sequences derived from a cell or tissue is called a cDNA library. A cDNA library differs from a genomic library (see below) by virtue of the fact that it contains only the sequences derived from mRNA, the sequences that represent expressed genes.

Genomic cloning, cloning of the entire genome of an animal, requires specialized vectors. *E. coli* plasmid vectors are impractical for cloning of all the genomic DNA fragments that constitute a large genome because of the low efficiency of *E. coli* transformation and the small number of transformed colonies that can be detected on a typical petri dish. Instead, cloning vectors derived from bacteriophage λ are used to clone genomic DNA fragments obtained by cleaving chromosomal DNA with restriction enzymes (Figure 23-10). Bacteriophage λ DNA is 48.5 kb long and contains a central section of about 15 kb that is not necessary for λ replication in *E. coli* and can therefore be replaced with foreign genomic DNA. As long as the recombinant DNA does not exceed the length of the original λ-phage DNA by more than 5%, it can be packaged into the λ phage head and propagated in *E. coli.* This means that somewhat more than 1.5×10^4 base pairs can be cloned in one particle of λ phage. A collection of λ clones that includes all the DNA sequences of a given species is called a genomic library. It has been calculated that about 1 million different recombinant λ-phage particles would be needed to form a genomic DNA library representing an entire mammalian genome, which contains about 3×10^9 base pairs.

Often the 20- to 25-kb stretch of DNA that can be cloned in bacteriophage λ is not long enough to include the regulatory sequences that lie outside the 5′ and 3′ ends of the direct coding sequences of a gene. As noted already, larger genomic DNA fragments—between 30 and 50 kb in length—can be cloned in a cosmid vector. A recombinant cosmid vector, although not a fully functional bacteriophage, can infect *E. coli* and replicate as a plasmid, generating a cosmid library. Recently, a larger *E. coli* virus, called bacteriophage P1 has

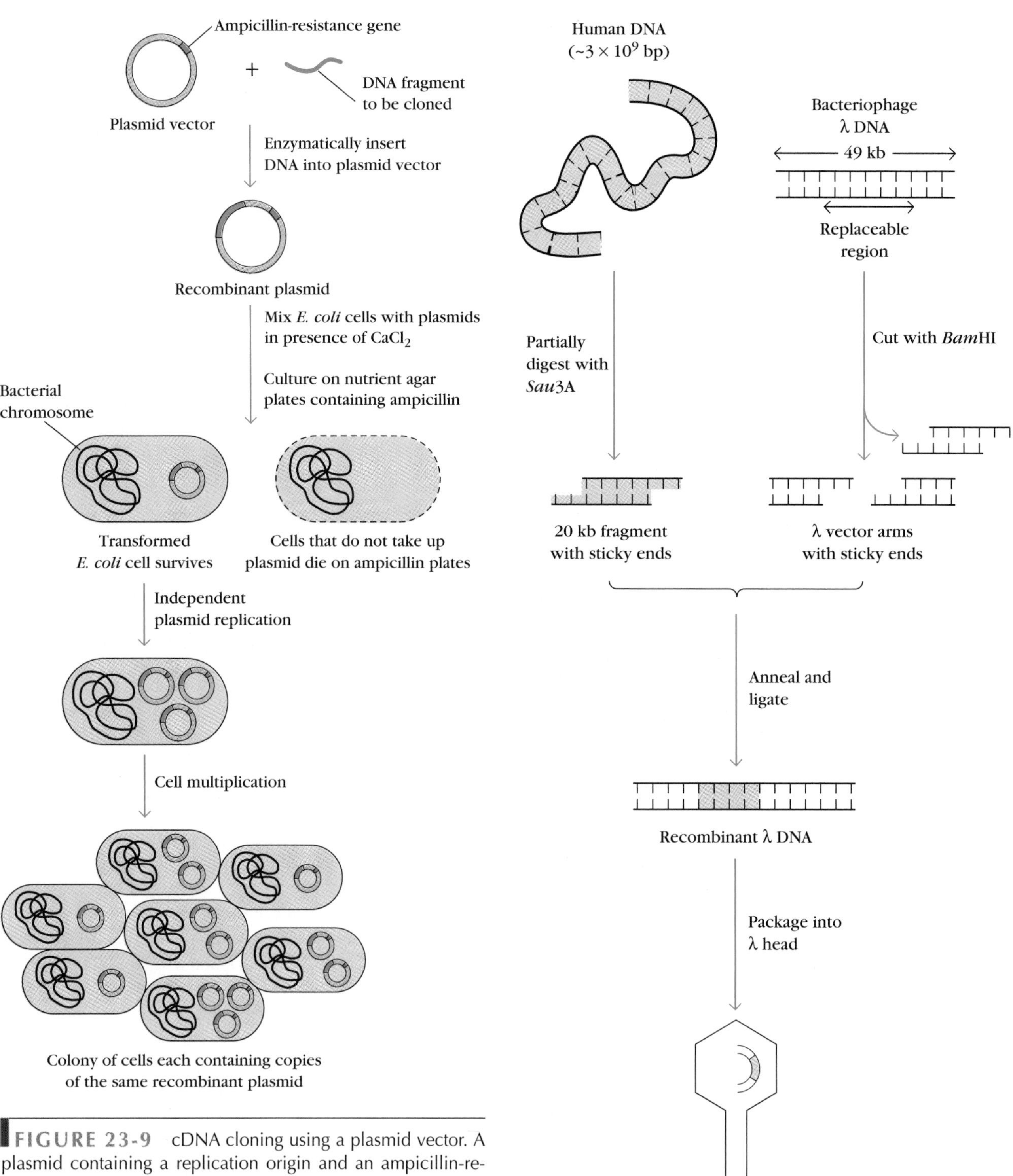

FIGURE 23-9 cDNA cloning using a plasmid vector. A plasmid containing a replication origin and an ampicillin-resistance gene is cut with a restriction endonuclease that produces blunt ends. After addition of a poly-C tail to the 3′ ends of the cDNA and of a complementary poly-G tail to the 3′ ends of the cut plasmid, the two DNAs are mixed, annealed, and joined by DNA ligase, forming the recombinant plasmid. Uptake of the recombinant plasmid into *E. coli* cells is stimulated by high concentrations of $CaCl_2$. Transformation occurs with a low frequency, but the transformed cells can be selected in the presence of ampicillin. [Adapted from H Lodish et al, 1995, *Molecular Cell Biology,* 3rd ed. Scientific American Books.]

FIGURE 23-10 Genomic DNA cloning using bacteriophage λ as the vector. Genomic DNA is partly digested with *Sau*3A, producing fragments with sticky ends. The central 15-kb region of the λ-phage DNA is cut out with *Bam*HI and discarded. These two restriction enzymes produce complementary sticky ends, so the genomic and DNA fragments can be annealed and ligated. After the resulting recombinant DNA is packaged into a λ-phage head, it can be propagated in *E. coli.*

TABLE 23-6 VECTORS AND MAXIMUM LENGTH OF DNA THAT THEY CAN CARRY

Vector type	Maximum length of cloned DNA (kb)
Plasmid	20
Bacteriophage λ	25
Cosmid	45
Bacteriophage P1	100
Yeast artificial chromosome (YAC)	>1000

been used to package DNA fragments up to 100 kb long. Even larger DNA fragments, greater than a megabase (1000 kb) in length, can be cloned in yeast artificial chromosomes, (YACs) which are linear DNA segments that can replicate in yeast cells (Table 23-6).

Selection of DNA Clones

Once a cDNA or genomic DNA library has been prepared, it can be screened to identify a particular DNA fragment by a technique called in situ hybridization. The cloned bacterial colonies, yeast colonies, or phage plaques containing the recombinant DNA are transferred onto nitrocellulose or nylon filters by replica plating (Figure 23-11). The filter is then treated with NaOH, which both lyses the bacteria and denatures the DNA, allowing single-stranded DNA (ssDNA) to bind to the filter. The filter with bound DNA then is incubated with a radioactive probe specific for the gene of interest. The probe will hybridize with DNA in the colonies or plaques on the filter that contain the sought-after gene, and they can be identified by autoradiography. The position of the positive colonies or plaques on the filter shows where the corresponding clones can be found on the original agar plate.

Various radioactive probes can be used to screen a library. In some cases, radiolabeled mRNA or cDNA serves as the probe. If the protein encoded by the gene of interest has been purified and partly sequenced, it is possible to work backward from the amino acid sequence to determine the probable nucleotide sequence of the corresponding gene. A known sequence of five or six amino acid residues is all that is needed to synthesize radiolabeled oligonucleotide probes with which to screen a cDNA or genomic library for a particular gene. To cope with the degeneracy of the genetic code, peptide segments containing amino acids encoded by a limited number of codons are usually chosen. Oligonucleotides representing all possible codons for the peptide are synthesized and used as probes to screen the DNA library.

Southern Blotting

DNA fragments generated by restriction-endonuclease cleavage can be separated on the basis of length by agarose gel electrophoresis. The shorter a fragment is, the faster it moves in the gel. An elegant technique developed by E. M. Southern can be used to identify any band containing fragments with a given gene sequence (Figure 23-12). In this technique, called **Southern blotting,** DNA is cut with restriction enzymes and the fragments are separated according to size by electrophoresis on an agarose gel. Then the gel is soaked in NaOH to denature the dsDNA, and the resulting ssDNA fragments are transferred onto a nitrocellulose or

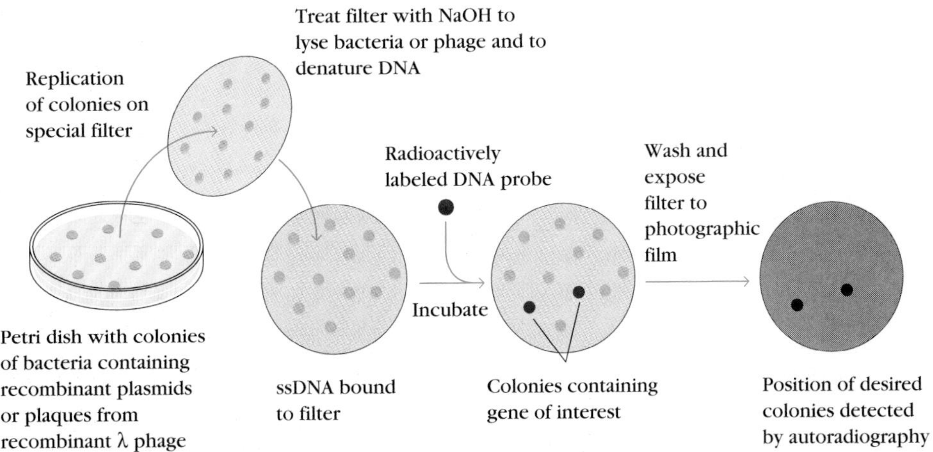

FIGURE 23-11 Selection of specific clones from a cDNA or genomic DNA library by in situ hybridization. A nitrocellulose or nylon filter is placed against the plate to pick up the bacterial colonies or phage plaques containing the cloned genes. After the filter is placed in a NaOH solution and heated, the denatured ssDNA becomes fixed to the filter. A radioactive probe specific for the gene of interest is incubated with the filter. The position of the colonies or plaques containing the desired gene is revealed by autoradiography.

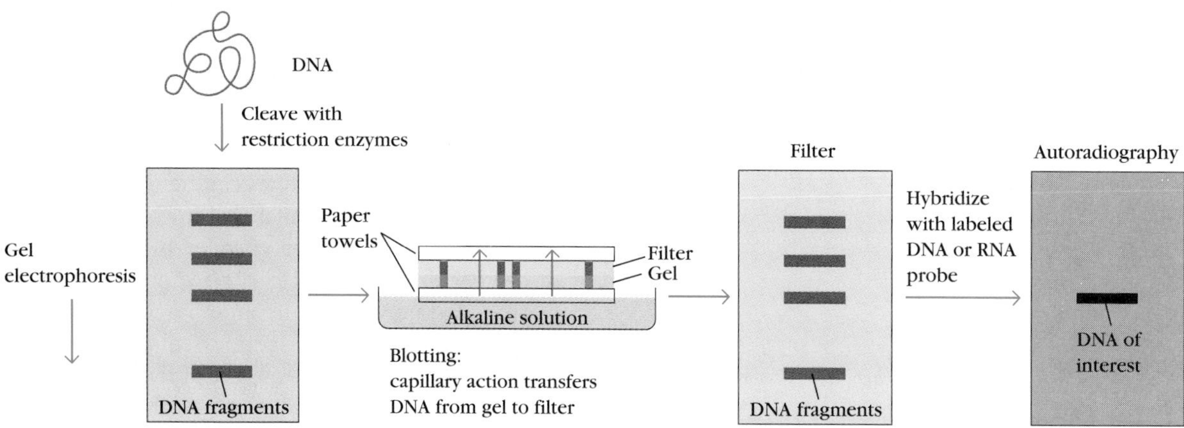

FIGURE 23-12 The Southern blot technique for detecting specific sequences in DNA fragments. The DNA fragments produced by restriction-enzyme cleavage are separated by size by agarose gel electrophoresis. The agarose gel is overlaid with a nitrocellulose or nylon filter and a thick stack of paper towels. The gel is then placed in an alkaline salt solution, which denatures the DNA. As the paper towels soak up the moisture, the solution is drawn through the gel into the filter, transferring each ssDNA band to the filter. This process is called blotting. After heating, the filter is incubated with a radiolabeled probe specific for the sequence of interest; DNA fragments that hybridize with the probe are detected by autoradiography. [Adapted from J Darnell et al, 1990, *Molecular Cell Biology,* 2nd ed., Scientific American Books.]

nylon filter by capillary action. After transfer, the filter is incubated with an appropriate radiolabeled probe specific for the gene of interest. The probe hybridizes with the ssDNA fragment containing the gene of interest, and the position of the band containing these hybridized fragments is determined by autoradiography. Southern blot analysis played a critical role in unraveling the mechanism by which diversity of antibodies and T-cell receptors is generated (see Figures 5-2 and 9-4).

Northern Blotting

Northern blotting (named for its similarity to Southern blotting) is used to detect the presence of specific mRNA molecules. In this procedure the mRNA is first denatured to ensure that it is in an unfolded, linear form. The mRNA molecules are then separated according to size by electrophoresis and transferred to a nitrocellulose filter, to which the mRNAs will adhere. The filter is then incubated with a labeled DNA probe and subjected to autoradiography. Northern blot analysis is often used to determine how much of a specific mRNA is expressed in cells under different conditions. Increased levels of mRNA will bind proportionally more of the labeled DNA probe.

Polymerase Chain Reaction

The polymerase chain reaction (PCR) is a powerful technique for amplifying specific DNA sequences even when they are present at extremely low levels in a complex mixture (Figure 23-13). The procedure requires that the DNA sequences that flank the desired DNA sequence be known, so that short oligonucleotide primers can be synthesized. The DNA mixture is denatured into single strands by a brief heat treatment. The DNA is then cooled in the presence of an excess of the oligonucleotide primers, which hybridize with the complementary ssDNA. A temperature-resistant DNA polymerase (called Taq polymerase) is then added, together with the four deoxyribonucleotide triphosphates, and each strand is copied. The newly synthesized DNA duplex is separated by heating and the cycle is repeated. In each cycle there is a doubling of the desired DNA sequence; in only 25 cycles the desired DNA sequence can be amplified about a million-fold.

The DNA amplified by the PCR can be further characterized by Southern blotting, restriction-enzyme mapping, and direct DNA sequencing. The PCR has enabled immunologists to amplify genes encoding proteins that are important in the immune response, such as MHC molecules, the T-cell receptor, and immunoglobulins.

Analysis of DNA Regulatory Sequences

The transcriptional activity of genes is regulated by promoter and enhancer sequences. These sequences are cis-acting, meaning that they regulate only genes on the same DNA molecule. The promoter sequence lies upstream from the gene it regulates and includes a TATA box, where the general transcription machinery, including RNA polymerase II, binds and begins transcription. The enhancer sequence confers a high rate of transcription on the promoter. Unlike the promoter, which always lies upstream from the gene it controls, the enhancer element can be located anywhere with respect to the gene (5′ of the promoter, 3′of the gene, or even in an intron of the gene).

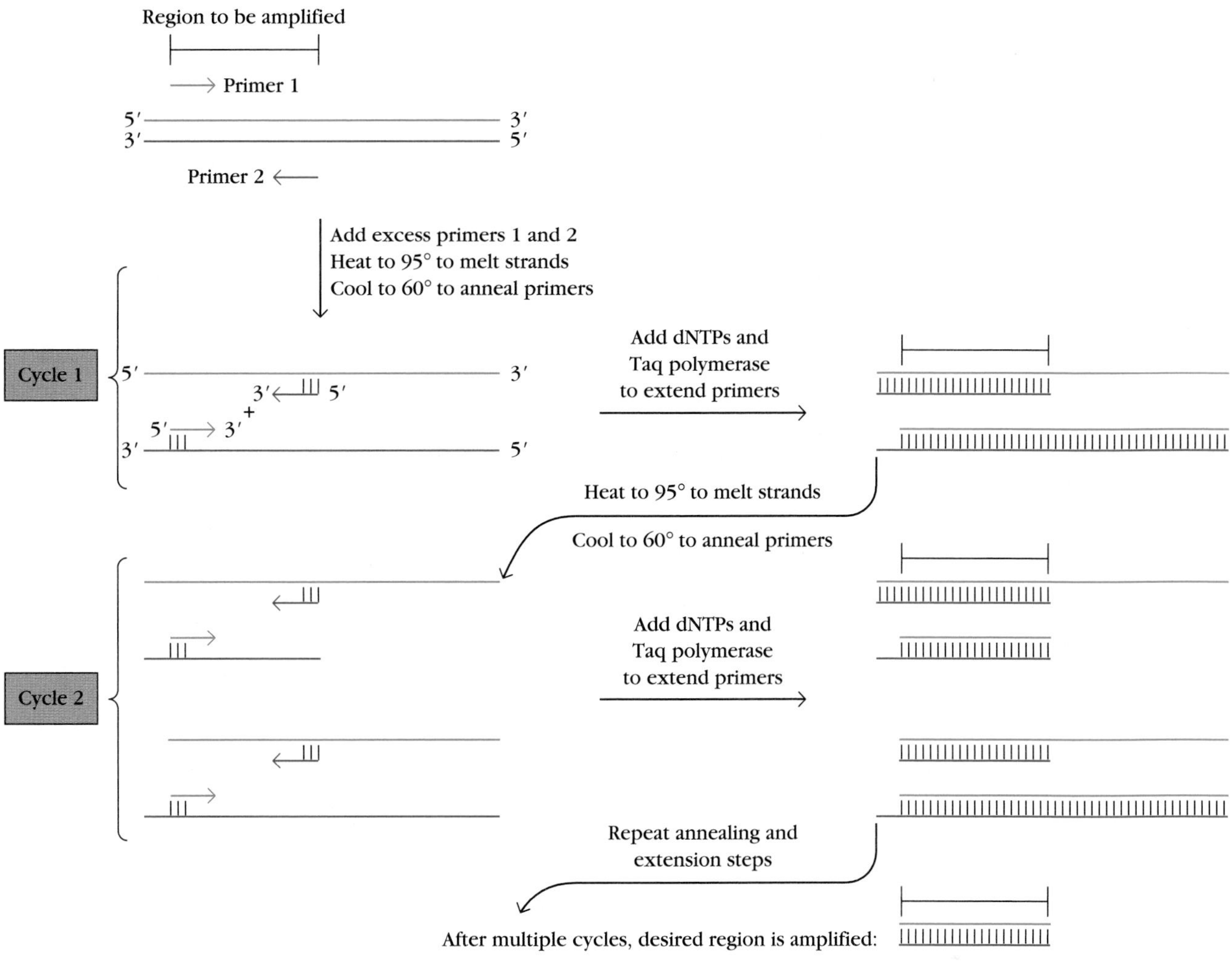

FIGURE 23-13 The polymerase chain reaction (PCR). DNA is denatured into single strands by a brief heat treatment and is then cooled in the presence of an excess of oligonucleotide primers complementary to the DNA sequences flanking the desired DNA segment. Taq polymerase, a heat-resistant DNA polymerase obtained from a thermophilic bacterium, is used to copy the DNA from the 3′ ends of the primers. Because all of the reaction components are heat stable, the heating and cooling cycle can be repeated many times, resulting in alternate DNA melting and synthesis, and rapid amplification of a given sequence. [Adapted from H Lodish et al, 1995, *Molecular Cell Biology*, 3rd ed., Scientific American Books.]

The activity of enhancer and promoter sequences is controlled by transcription factors, which are DNA-binding proteins. These proteins bind to specific nucleotide sequences within promoters and enhancers and act either to enhance or suppress their activity. Enhancer and promoter sequences and their respective DNA-binding proteins have been identified by a variety of techniques, including DNA footprinting, gel-shift analysis, and the CAT assay.

DNA Footprinting

The binding sites for DNA-binding proteins on enhancers and promoters can be identified by a technique called DNA footprinting (Figure 23-14a). In this technique, a cloned DNA fragment containing a putative enhancer or promoter sequence is first radiolabeled at the 5′ end with ^{32}P. The labeled DNA is then divided into two fractions: One fraction is incubated with a nuclear extract containing a DNA-binding protein; the other DNA fraction is not incubated with the extract. Both DNA samples are then digested with a nuclease or a chemical that makes random cuts in the phosphodiester bonds of the DNA, and the strands are separated. The resulting DNA fragments are run on a gel to separate fragments of different sizes. In the absence of DNA-binding proteins, a complete ladder of bands is obtained on the electrophoretic gel. When a protein that binds to a site on the DNA fragment is present, it covers some of the nucleotides, protecting that stretch of the DNA from digestion. The electrophoretic pattern of such protected DNA will contain blank regions (or footprints). Each footprint represents the site within an enhancer or promoter that binds a particular DNA-binding protein.

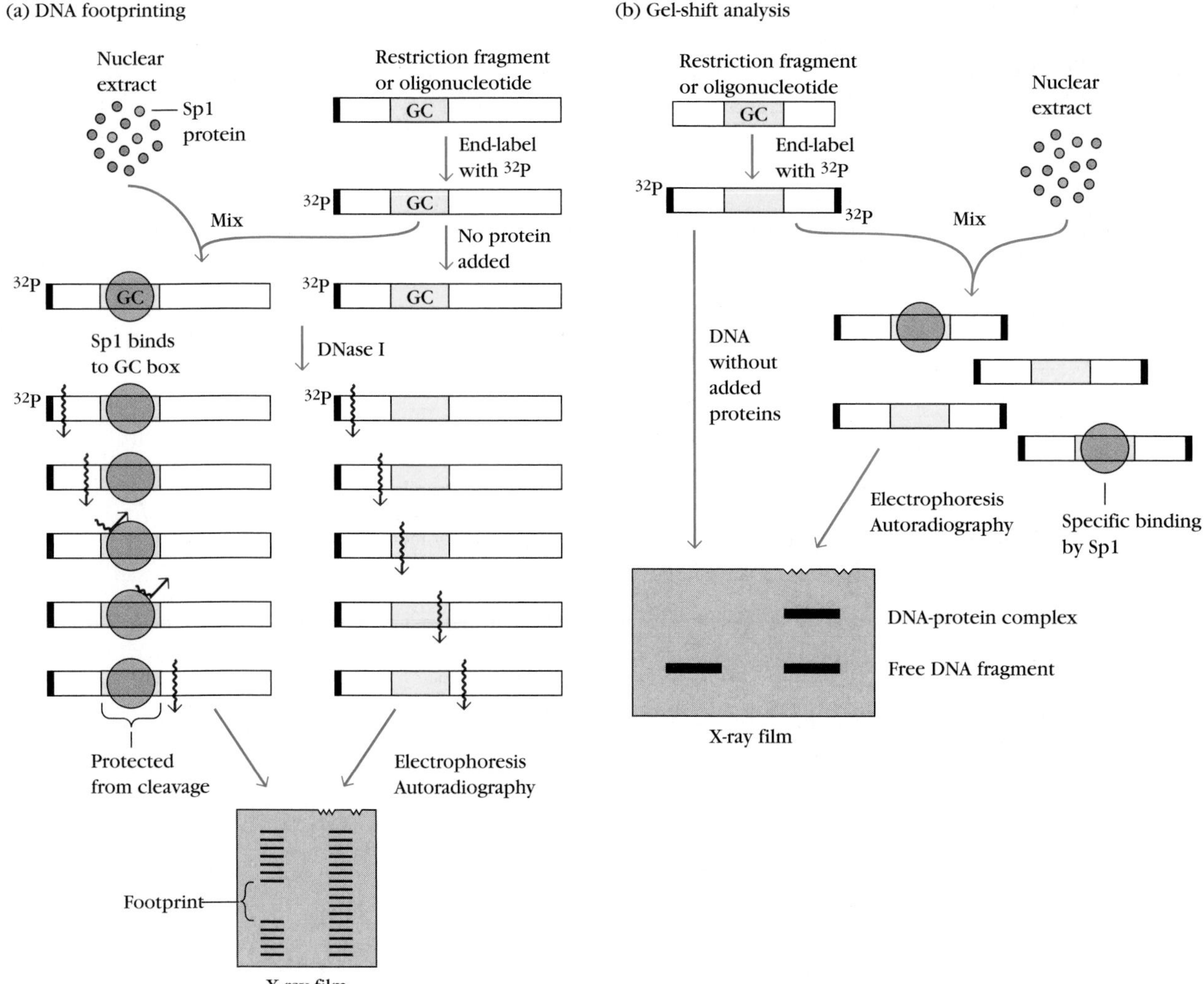

FIGURE 23-14 Identification of DNA sequences that bind protein by DNA-footprinting and gel-shift analysis. (a) In the footprinting technique, labeled DNA fragments containing a putative promoter or enhancer sequence are incubated in the presence and absence of a DNA-binding protein (e.g., Sp1 protein, which binds to a "GC box," a GC-rich region of DNA). After the samples are treated with DNase and the strands separated, the resulting fragments are electrophoresed; the gel then is subjected to autoradiography. A blank region (footprint) in the gel pattern indicates that protein has bound to the DNA. (b) In gel-shift analysis, a labeled DNA fragment is incubated with a cellular extract containing transcription factors. The electrophoretic mobility of the DNA-protein complex is slower than that of free DNA fragments. [Adapted from JD Watson et al, 1992, *Recombinant DNA,* 2nd ed., W. H. Freeman and Company.]

Gel-Shift Analysis

When a protein binds to a DNA fragment, forming a DNA-protein complex, the electrophoretic mobility of the DNA fragment in a gel is reduced, producing a shift in the position of the band containing that fragment. This phenomenon is the basis of gel-shift analysis. In this technique, radioactively labeled cloned DNA containing an enhancer or a promoter sequence is incubated with a nuclear extract containing a DNA-binding protein (Figure 23-14b). The DNA-protein complex is then electrophoresed and its electrophoretic mobility is compared with that of the cloned DNA alone. A shift in the mobility indicates that a protein is bound to the DNA, retarding its migration on the electrophoretic gel.

CAT Assay

One way to assess promoter activity is to engineer and clone a DNA sequence containing a reporter gene attached to the promoter that is being assessed. When this sequence, or construct, is introduced into eukaryotic cells, transcription will be initiated from the promoter if it is active, and the reporter gene will be transcribed and its protein product synthesized. Measuring the amount of this protein

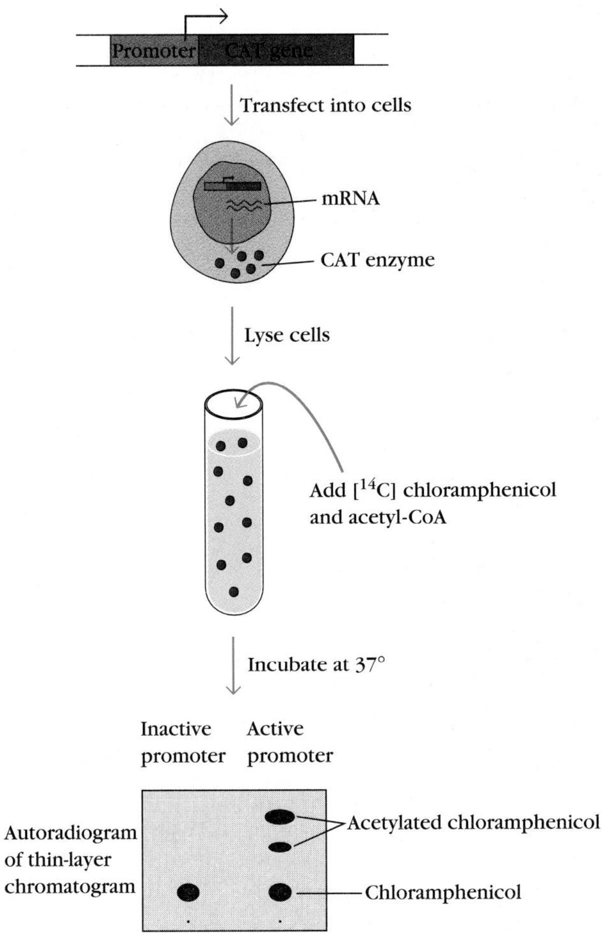

FIGURE 23-15 CAT assay for assessing functional activity of a promoter sequence. In this assay, a DNA construct consisting of the promoter of interest and the reporter gene encoding chloramphenicol acetyltransferase (CAT) is introduced (transfected) into eukaryotic cells. If the promoter is active, the CAT gene will be transcribed and the CAT enzyme will be produced within the transfected cell. The presence of the enzyme can easily be detected by lysing the cell and incubating the cell lysate with [^{14}C] chloramphenicol and acetyl-CoA. If present, the CAT enzyme will transfer the acetyl group from acetyl-CoA to the chloramphenicol, forming acetylated chloramphenicol, which can be easily detected by thin-layer chromatography. [Adapted from JD Watson et al, 1992, *Recombinant DNA,* 2nd ed., W. H. Freeman and Company.]

produced is thus a way to determine the activity of the promoter.

Most reporter genes are chosen because they encode proteins that can be easily measured, such as the enzyme chloramphenicol acetyltransferase (CAT), which transfers the acetyl group from acetyl-CoA to the antibiotic chloramphenicol (Figure 23-15). The more active the promoter is, the more CAT will be produced within the transfected cell. By introducing mutations into promoter sequences and then assaying for promoter activity with the corresponding reporter gene, conserved sequence motifs have been identified within promoters.

Gene Transfer into Mammalian Cells

A variety of genes involved in the immune response have been isolated and cloned by use of recombinant DNA techniques. The expression and regulation of these genes has been studied by introducing them into cultured mammalian cells and, more recently, into the **germ line** of animals.

Transfer of Cloned Genes into Cultured Cells

Diverse techniques have been developed for transfecting genes into cells. A common technique involves the use of a retrovirus in which a viral structural gene has been replaced with the cloned gene to be transfected. The altered retrovirus is then used as a vector for introducing the cloned gene into cultured cells. Because of the properties of retroviruses, the recombinant DNA integrates into the cellular genome with a high frequency. In an alternative method, the cloned gene of interest is complexed with calcium phosphate. The calcium phosphate–DNA complex is slowly precipitated onto the cells and the DNA is taken up by a small percentage of them. In another transfection method, called electroporation, an electric current creates pores in cell membranes through which the cloned DNA is taken up. In both of these latter methods, the transfected DNA integrates, apparently at random sites, into the DNA of a small percentage of treated cells.

Generally, the cloned DNA being transfected is engineered to contain a selectable marker gene, such as one that confers resistance to neomycin. After transfection, the cells are cultured in the presence of neomycin. Because only the transfected cells are able to grow, the small number of transfected cells in the total cell population can be identified and selected.

Transfection of cloned genes into cells has proved to be highly effective in immunologic research. By transfecting genes involved with the immune response into cells that lack those genes, the product of a specific gene can be studied apart from interacting proteins encoded by other genes. For example, transfection of MHC genes, under the control of appropriate promoters, into a mouse fibroblast cell line (L929, or simply L, cells) has enabled immunologists to study the role of MHC molecules in antigen presentation to T cells (Figure 23-16). Transfection of the gene that encodes the T-cell receptor has provided information about the antigen-MHC specificity of the T-cell receptor.

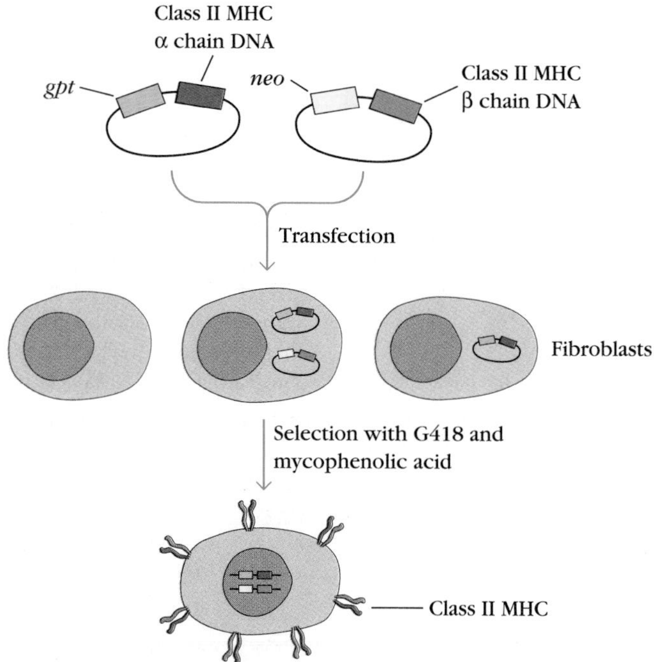

FIGURE 23-16 Transfection of the genes encoding the class II MHC α chain and β chain into mouse fibroblast L cells, which do not normally produce these proteins. Two constructs containing one of the MHC genes and a selectable gene were engineered: the α-chain gene with the guanine phosphoribosyl transferase gene (*gpt*), which confers resistance to the drug G418, and the β-chain gene with a neomycin gene (*neo*), which confers resistance to mycophenolic acid. After transfection, the cells are placed in medium containing both G418 and mycophenolic acid. Only those fibroblasts containing both the *neo* and *gpt* genes (and consequently the genes encoding the class II MHC α and β chains) will survive this selection. These fibroblasts will express both class II MHC chains on their membrane.

Transfer of Cloned Genes into Mouse Embryos

Development of techniques to introduce cloned foreign genes (called **transgenes**) into mouse embryos has permitted immunologists to study the effects of immune-system genes in vivo. If the introduced gene integrates stably into the germ-line cells, it will be transmitted to the offspring. Two techniques for producing transgenic mice are described in this section; one of these has been used to produce **knockout mice,** which cannot express a particular gene product (Table 23-7).

Transgenic Mice

The first step in producing transgenic mice is injection of foreign cloned DNA into a fertilized egg. In this technically demanding process, fertilized mouse eggs are held under suction at the end of a pipet and the transgene is microinjected into one of the pronuclei with a fine needle. The transgene integrates into the chromosomal DNA of the pronucleus and is passed on to the daughter cells of eggs that survive the process. The eggs then are implanted in the oviduct of "pseudo-pregnant" females, and transgenic pups are born after 19 or 20 days of gestation (Figure 23-17). In general the

TABLE 23-7 COMPARISON OF TRANSGENIC AND KNOCKOUT MICE

Characteristic	Transgenic mice	Knockout mice
Cells receiving DNA	Zygote	Embryonic stem (ES) cells
DNA constructs used	Natural gene or cDNA	Mutated gene
Means of delivery	Microinjection into zygote and implantation into foster mother	Transfer of ES cells to blastocyst and implantation into foster mother
Outcome	Gain of a gene	Loss of gene function

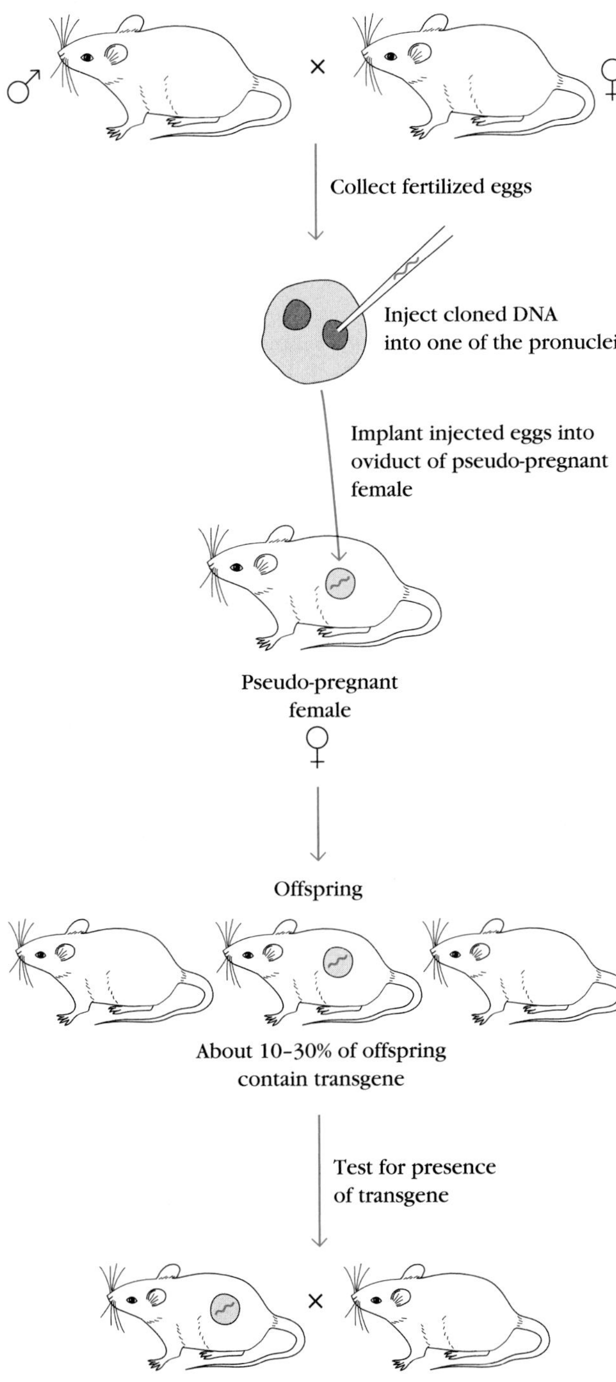

FIGURE 23-17 General procedure for producing transgenic mice. Fertilized eggs are collected from a pregnant female mouse. Cloned DNA (referred to as the transgene) is microinjected into one of the pronuclei of a fertilized egg. The eggs are then implanted into the oviduct of pseudopregnant foster mothers (obtained by mating normal females with a sterile male). The transgene will be incorporated into the chromosomal DNA of about 10%–30% of the offspring and will be expressed in all of their somatic cells. If a tissue-specific promoter is linked to a transgene, then tissue-specific expression of the transgene will result.

efficiency of this procedure is low, with only one or two transgenic mice produced for every 100 fertilized egg collected.

With transgenic mice, immunologists have been able to study the expression of a given gene in a living animal. Although all the cells in a transgenic animal contain the transgene, differences in the expression of the transgene in different tissues has shed light on mechanisms of tissue-specific gene expression. By constructing a transgene with a particular promoter, researchers can control the expression of a given transgene. For example, the metallothionein promoter is activated by zinc. Transgenic mice carrying a transgene linked to a metallothionein promoter express the transgene only if zinc is added to their water supply. Other promoters are functional only in certain tissues; the insulin promoter, for instance, promotes transcription only in pancreatic cells. Transgenic mice carrying a transgene linked to the insulin promoter, therefore, will express the transgene in the pancreas but not in other tissues.

Because a transgene is integrated into the chromosomal DNA within the one-celled mouse embryo, it will be integrated into both somatic cells and germ-line cells. The resulting transgenic mice thus can transmit the transgene to their offspring as a Mendelian trait. In this way, it has been possible to produce lines of transgenic mice in which every member of a line contains the same transgene. A variety of such transgenic lines are currently available and are widely used in immunologic research. Included among these are lines carrying transgenes that encode immunoglobulin, T-cell receptor, class I and class II MHC molecules, various foreign antigens, and a number of cytokines. Several lines carrying oncogenes as transgenes also have been produced.

Gene-Targeted Knockout Mice

One of the limitations with transgenic mice is that the transgene is integrated randomly within the genome. This means that some transgenes insert in regions of DNA that are not transcriptionally active, and hence the gene is not expressed. To circumvent this limitation, researchers have developed a technique in which a desired gene is targeted to specific sites within the germ line of a mouse. The primary use of this technique has been to replace a normal gene with a mutant allele or a disrupted form of the gene, thus knocking out the gene's function. Transgenic mice that carry such a disrupted gene, called knockout mice, have been extremely helpful to immunologists trying to understand how the removal of a particular gene product affects the immune system. A variety of knockout mice are being used in immunologic research, including mice that lack particular cytokines or MHC molecules.

Production of gene-targeted knockout mice involves the following steps:

- Isolation and culturing of embryonic stem **(ES) cells** from the inner cell mass of a mouse blastocyst
- Introduction of a mutant or disrupted gene into the

cultured ES cells and selection of homologous recombinant cells in which the gene of interest has been knocked out (i.e., replaced by a nonfunctional form of the gene)

- Injection of homologous recombinant ES cells into a recipient mouse blastocyst and surgical implantation of the blastocyst into a pseudo-pregnant mouse
- Mating of chimeric offspring heterozygous for the disrupted gene to produce homozygous knockout mice

The ES cells used in this procedure are obtained by culturing the inner cell mass of a mouse blastocyst on a feeder layer of fibroblasts or in the presence of leukemia inhibitory factor. Under these conditions, the stem cells grow but remain pluripotent and capable of later differentiating in a variety of directions, generating distinct cellular lineages (e.g., germ cells, myocardium, blood vessels, myoblasts, nerve cells). One of the advantages of ES cells is the ease with which they can be genetically manipulated. Cloned DNA containing a desired gene can be introduced into ES cells in culture by various transfection techniques. The introduced DNA will be inserted by recombination into the chromosomal DNA of a small number of ES cells.

The insertion constructs introduced into ES cells contain three genes: the target gene of interest and two selection genes, such as *neo*^{R}, which confers neomycin resistance, and the thymidine kinase gene from herpes simplex virus (*tk*^{HSV}), which confers sensitivity to gancyclovir, a cytotoxic nucleotide analog (Figure 23-18a). The construct often is engineered with the target-gene sequence disrupted by the *neo*^{R} gene and with the *tk*^{HSV} gene at one end, beyond the sequence of the target gene. Most constructs will insert at random by nonhomologous recombination rather than by gene-targeted insertion through homologous recombination. As illustrated in Figure 23-18b, a two-step selection scheme is used to obtain those ES cells that have undergone homologous recombination, whereby the disrupted gene replaces the target gene.

The ES cells obtained by this procedure are heterozygous for the knockout mutation in the target gene. These cells are

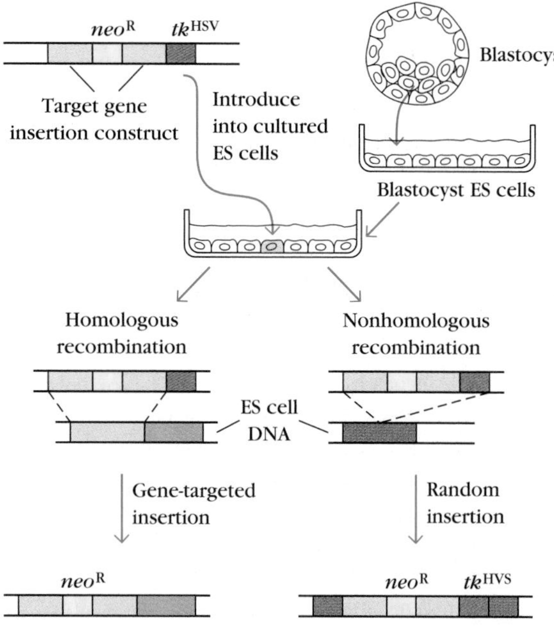

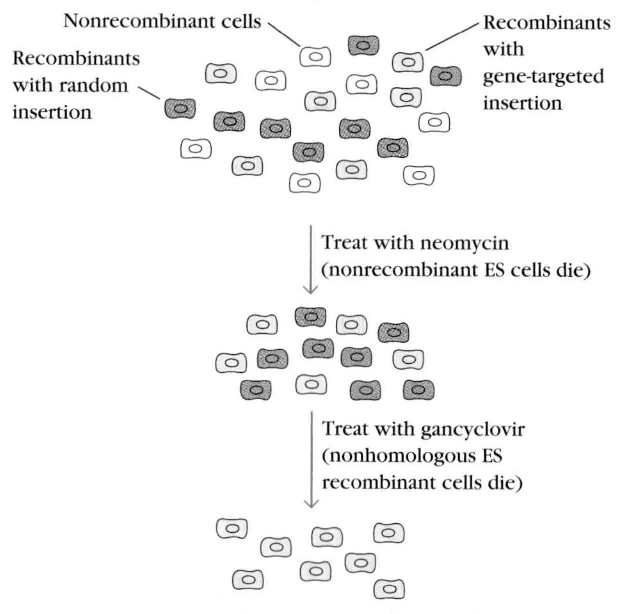

FIGURE 23-18 Formation and selection of mouse recombinant ES cells in which a particular target gene is disrupted. (a) In the engineered insertion construct, the target gene is disrupted with the *neo*^{R} gene, and the thymidine kinase *tk*^{HSV} gene is located outside the target gene. The construct is transfected into cultured ES cells. If homologous recombination occurs, only the target gene and the *neo*^{R} gene will be inserted into the chromosomal DNA of the ES cells. If nonhomologous recombination occurs, all three genes will be inserted. Recombination occurs in only about 1% of the cells, with nonhomologous recombination much more frequent than homologous recombination. (b) Selection with the neomycin-like drug G418 will kill any nonrecombinant ES cells because they lack the *neo*^{R} gene. Selection with gancyclovir will kill the nonhomologous recombinants carrying the *tk*^{HSV} gene, which confers sensitivity to gancyclovir. Only the homologous ES recombinants will survive this selection scheme. [Adapted from H Lodish et al, 1995, *Molecular Cell Biology,* 3rd ed., Scientific American Books.]

clonally expanded in cell culture and then injected into a mouse blastocyst, which subsequently is implanted into a pseudo-pregnant female. The transgenic offspring that develop are chimeric, composed of cells derived from the genetically altered ES cells and cells derived from normal cells of the host blastocyst. When the germ-line cells are derived from the genetically altered ES cells, the genetic alteration can be passed on to the offspring. If the recombinant ES cells are homozygous for black coat color (or other visible marker) and they are injected into a blastocyst homozygous for white coat color, then the chimeric progeny that carry the heterozygous knockout mutation in their germ line can be easily identified (Figure 23-19). When these are mated with each other, some of the offspring will be homozygous for the knockout mutation.

The "Knock-In" Technology

In addition to deleting a gene of choice, it also is possible to replace the endogenous gene with a mutated form of that gene. As in the strategy for knocking out a gene, DNA constructs that carry mutations in a particular gene can be exchanged for the endogenous gene. It also is possible to replace all of an endogenous gene with a DNA sequence of choice. In a recent report, for example, the CD4 gene was replaced with β-galactosidase. In these experiments, the CD4 promoter was left intact to drive the expression of β-galactosidase, which catalyzes the color change of certain reporter chemicals to blue. Using the blue color as an indicator, the experimenters could visualize cells in the developing thymus that normally transcribe CD4. Because

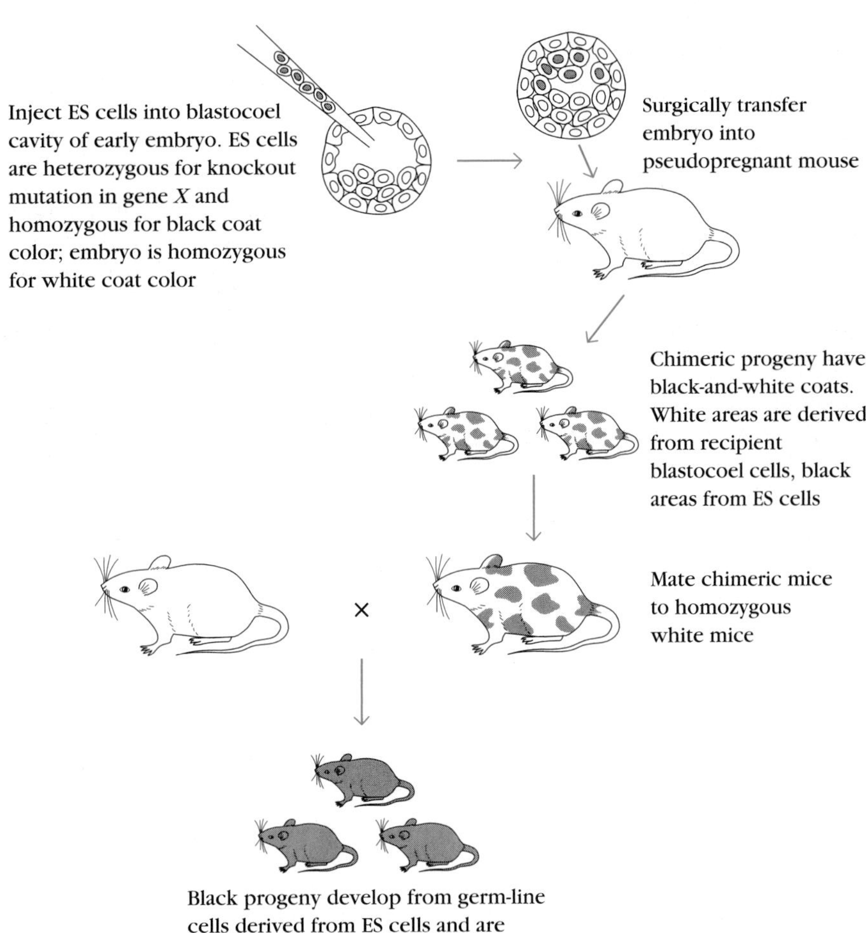

FIGURE 23-19 General procedure for producing homozygous knockout mice. ES cells homozygous for a marker gene (e.g., black coat color) and heterozygous for a disrupted target gene (see Figure 23-18) are injected into an early embryo homozygous for an alternate marker (e.g., white coat color). The chimeric transgenic offspring, which have black- and-white coats, then are mated with homozygous white mice. The all-black progeny from this mating have ES-derived cells in their germ line, which are heterozygous for the disrupted target gene. Mating of these mice with each other produces animals homozygous for the disrupted target gene, that is, knockout mice. [Adapted from MR Capecchi, 1989, *Trends Genet.* **5**:70.]

the CD4 promoter drove the expression of β-galactosidase, only those cells destined to express CD4 turned blue in the presence of the reporter chemicals. Data from these experiments were useful in tracing CD4/CD8 lineage commitment in developing T cells.

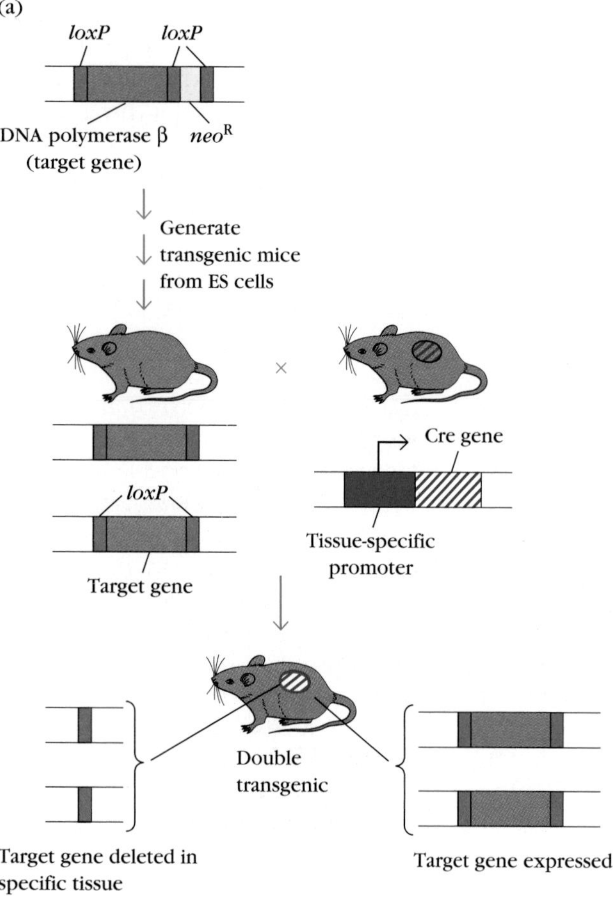

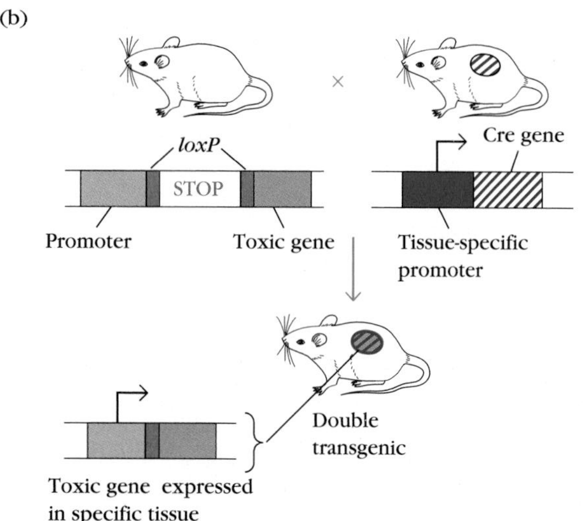

Inducible Gene Targeting—The Cre/lox System

In addition to the deletion of genes by gene targeting, recent experimental strategies have been developed that allow the specific deletion of a gene of interest in precisely the tissue of choice. These technologies rely on the use of site-specific recombinases from bacteria or yeast. The most commonly used recombinase is Cre, isolated from bacteriophage P1. Cre recognizes a specific 34-bp site in DNA known as *loxP* and, upon recognition, catalyzes a recombination. Therefore, DNA sequences that are flanked by *loxP* are recognized by Cre and the recombinational event results in the deletion of the intervening DNA sequences. In other words, animals that ubiquitously express Cre recombinase will delete all *loxP*-flanked sequences. The real innovation of this technique is that expression of the Cre recombinase gene can be controlled by the use of a tissue specific promoter. This allows tissue-specific expression of the recombinase protein and thus tissue-specific deletion of DNA flanked by *loxP*. For example, one could express Cre in B cells using the immunoglobulin promoter, and this would result in the targeted deletion of *loxP*-flanked DNA sequences only in B cells.

This technology is particularly useful when the targeted deletion of a particular gene is lethal. This is true in many circumstances. For example the DNA polymerase β gene is required for embryonic development. In experiments designed to test the Cre/*lox* system, scientists flanked the mouse DNA polymerase β gene with *loxP* and mated these

FIGURE 23-20 Gene targeting with Cre/*loxP* (a) Conditional deletion by Cre recombinase. The targeted DNA polymerase β gene is modified by flanking the gene with *loxP* sites (for simplicity, only one allele is shown). Mice are generated from ES cells by standard procedures. Mating of the *loxP*-modified-mice with a Cre transgenic will generate double transgenic mice in which the *loxP*-flanked DNA polymerase β gene will be deleted in the tissue where Cre is expressed. In this example, Cre is expressed in thymus tissue (striped) so that deletion of the *loxP*-flanked gene occurs only in the thymus (white) of the double transgenic. Other tissues and organs still express the *loxP*-flanked gene (orange). (b) Activation of gene expression using Cre/*lox*. A *loxP*-flanked translational STOP cassette is inserted between the promoter and the potentially toxic gene, and mice are generated from ES cells using standard procedures. These mice are mated to a transgenic line carrying the Cre gene driven by a tissue-specific promoter. In this example, Cre is expressed in the thymus, so that mating results in expression of the toxic gene (blue) solely in the thymus. Using this strategy, it is possible to determine the effects of expression of the potentially toxic gene in a tissue-specific fashion. [Adapted from B Sauer, 1998, *Methods* **14**:381.]

mice with mice carrying a Cre transgene under the control of a T-cell promoter (Figure 23-20a). The results of this mating are offspring that express the Cre recombinase specifically in T cells. Using such mice, the scientists were able to examine the effects of deleting the enzyme DNA polymerase β specifically in T cells. The effects of the deletion of this gene could not be examined in a conventional gene-targeting experiment, because deletion of DNA polymerase β throughout the animal would be lethal. However, with the Cre/*lox* system, it now is possible to examine the effects of the deletion of this gene in a specific tissue of the immune system.

The Cre/*lox* system also can be used to turn on gene expression in a particular tissue. Just as the lack of a particular gene may be lethal during embryonic development, the expression of a gene can be toxic. To examine tissue-specific expression of such a gene, it is possible to insert a translational stop sequence flanked by *loxP* into an intron at the beginning of the gene (Figure 23-20b). Using a tissue-specific promoter driving Cre expression, the stop sequence may be deleted in the tissue of choice and the expression of the potentially toxic gene examined in this tissue. These modifications of gene-targeting technology have been very useful in determining the effects of particular genes in cells and tissues of the immune system.

Summary

1. Inbred mouse strains allow immunologists to work routinely with syngeneic, or genetically identical, animals (see Table 23-2). With these strains, aspects of the immune response can be studied uncomplicated by unknown variables that could be introduced by genetic differences between animals.
2. In adoptive-transfer experiments, lymphocytes are transferred from one mouse to a syngeneic recipient mouse that has been exposed to a sublethal (or potentially lethal) dose of x-rays. The irradiation inactivates the immune cells of the recipient, so that one can study the response of only the transferred cells. A common technique used to determine the number of plasma cells producing antibody is the hemolytic plaque assay (see Figure 23-1). This assay can enumerate both IgM and IgG secreting plasma cells and is an excellent measure of the immune response.
3. With in vitro cell-culture systems, populations of lymphocytes can be studied under more-defined conditions than are possible with in vivo animal systems. Such systems include primary cultures of lymphoid cells, cloned lymphoid cell lines, and hybrid lymphoid cell lines (see Figure 23-3). Unlike primary cultures, cell lines are immortal and homogeneous. With cell lines, the intracellular events and cell products associated with individual subpopulations of lymphocytes can be investigated (see Table 23-3). Such studies are difficult, if not impossible, with the heterogeneous populations typical of primary cultures.
4. Biochemical techniques provide tools for labeling important proteins of the immune system. Labeling antibodies with molecules such as biotin and avidin allows accurate determination of the level of antibody response (see Figure 23-4). Gel electrophoresis is a convenient tool for determining the molecular weight of a protein (see Figures 23-5 and 23-6). Advances in protein biochemistry have led to the determination of three-dimensional structures of many immunologically important molecules such as immunoglobulins, T cell receptors, and MHC class I and class II proteins by x-ray crystallography (see Figure 23-8).
5. The ability to identify, clone, and sequence immune-system genes, using recombinant DNA techniques, has revolutionized the study of all aspects of the immune response. Both cDNA, which is prepared by transcribing mRNA with reverse transcriptase, and genomic DNA can be cloned. Generally, cDNA is cloned using a plasmid vector; the recombinant DNA containing the gene to be cloned is propagated in *E. coli* cells (see Figure 23-9). Genomic DNA can be cloned within a bacteriophage λ vector or a cosmid vector, both of which are propagated in *E. coli* (see Figure 23-10). Even larger genomic DNA fragments can be cloned within bacteriophage P1 vectors, which can replicate in *E. coli,* or yeast artificial chromosomes, which can replicate in yeast cells (see Table 23–6). Polymerase chain reaction (PCR) is a convenient tool for amplifying small quantities of DNA (see Figure 23-13).
6. Transcription of genes is regulated by promoter and enhancer sequences; the activity of these sequences is controlled by DNA-binding proteins. Footprinting and gel-shift analysis can be used to identify DNA-binding proteins and their binding sites within the promoter or enhancer sequence (see Figure 23-14). Promoter activity can be assessed by the CAT assay (see Figure 23-15).
7. Cloned genes can be transfected (transferred) into cultured cells by several methods. Commonly, immune-system genes are transfected into cells that do not normally express the gene of interest. Cloned genes also can be incorporated into the germ-line cells of mouse embryos, yielding transgenic mice, which can transmit the incorporated transgene to their offspring (see Figure 23-17). With transgenic mice, expression of a chosen gene can be studied in a living animal. Knockout mice are transgenics in which a particular target gene has been replaced by a nonfunctional form of the gene, so the gene product is not expressed (see Figure 23-18 and Table 23-7). The Cre/*lox* system provides a mechanism that allows tissue specific expression or deletion of a particular gene (see Figure 23-20).

REFERENCES

Bell, J. 1989. The polymerase chain reaction. *Immunol. Today* **10:**351.

Betz, UAK, et al. 1996 Bypass of lethality with mosaic mice generated by Cre-*loxP*-mediated recombination. *Current Biology* **6:**1307.

Camper, SA. 1987. Research applications of transgenic mice. *Biotechniques* **5:**638.

Capecchi, MR. 1989. Altering the genome by homologous recombination. *Science* **244:**1288.

Denis, KA, and ON Witte. 1989. Long-term lymphoid cultures in the study of B cell differentiation. In *Immunoglobulin Genes.* Academic Press, p. 45.

Depamphilis, ML, et al. 1988. Microinjecting DNA into mouse ova to study DNA replication and gene expression and to produce transgenic animals. *Biotechniques* **6**(7):622.

Koller, BH., and O Smithies. 1992. Altering genes in animals by gene targeting. *Annu. Rev. Immunol.* **10:**705.

McCune, JM, et al. 1988. The SCID-Hu mouse; murine model for analysis of human hematolymphoid differentiation and function. *Science* **241:**1632.

Meinl, E, et al. 1995. Immortalization of human T cells by *herpesvirus saimiri. Immunol. Today* **16:**55.

Melton, DW. 1994. Gene targeting in the mouse. *BioEssays* **16:**633.

Sauer, B. 1998. Inducible gene targeting in mice using the Cre/*lox* system. *Methods* **14:**381.

Schlessinger, D. 1990. Yeast artificial chromosomes: tools for mapping and analysis of complex genomes. *Trends Genet.* **6**(8):254.

Sharpe, AH. 1995. Analysis of lymphocyte costimulation in vivo using transgenic and knockout mice. *Curr. Opin. Immunol.* **7:**389.

Watson, J, et al. 1992. *Recombinant DNA,* 2nd ed. W. H. Freeman and Company.

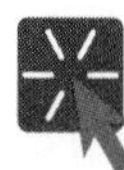

Useful Web Sites

http://www.biomednet.com/db/mkmd
Access to all known knockouts in mice, updated regularly by Current Biology. This site requires that you register, but registration is currently free.

http://www.jax.org/
Home page for The Jackson Laboratory, the major repository of inbred mice in the world.

http://www.neb.com/
Home page for New England Biolabs, a molecular biology company. Useful information concerning restriction enzymes is found at this site, under Technical Resources.

http://www.public.iastate.edu/~pedro/research_tools.html
A very useful site for molecular biology containing links to many informative sites. It is updated regularly.

Go to www.whfreeman.com/immunology **Self-Test**
Review and quiz of key terms

STUDY QUESTIONS

1. Explain why the following statements are false.

a. The amino acid sequence of a protein can be determined from the nucleotide sequence of a genomic clone encoding the protein.

b. Transgenic mice can be prepared by microinjection of DNA into a somatic-cell nucleus.

c. Primary lymphoid cultures can be propagated indefinitely and are useful in studies of specific subpopulations of lymphocytes.

2. Fill in the blanks in the following statements with the most appropriate terms:

a. In inbred mouse strains, all or nearly all genetic loci are ________________; such strains are said to be ________________.

b. SCID mice have a genetic defect that prevents development of functional ________________ and ________________ cells.

c. B-cell hybridomas are formed by fusion of ________________ with ________________. They are capable of ________________ growth and are used to produce ________________.

d. A normal lymphoid cell that undergoes ________________ can give rise to a cell line, which has an ________________ life span.

3. The gene diagrammed below contains one leader (L), three exons (E), and three introns (I). Illustrate the primary transcript, mRNA, and the protein product that could be generated from such a gene.

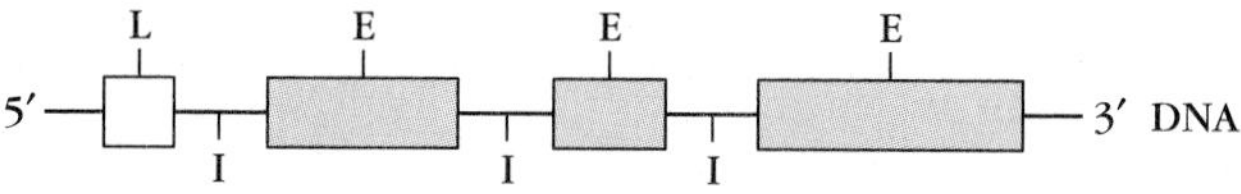

4. The term *transfection* refers to which of the following:

a. Synthesis of mRNA from a DNA template

b. Synthesis of protein based on an mRNA sequence

c. Introduction of foreign DNA into a cell

d. The process by which a normal cell becomes malignant

e. Transfer of a signal from outside a cell to inside a cell

5. Which of the following are required to carry out the PCR?

a. Short oligonucleotide primers

b. Thermostable DNA polymerase

c. Antibodies directed against the encoded protein

d. A method for heating and cooling the reaction mixture periodically

e. All of the above

6. Why is it necessary to include a selectable marker gene in transfection experiments?

7. What would be the result if a transgene were injected into one cell of a four-cell mouse zygote rather than into a fertilized mouse egg before it divides?

8. A circular plasmid was cleaved with *Eco*RI, producing a 5.4-kb band on a gel. A 5.4-kb band was also observed when the plasmid was cleaved with *Hind*III. Cleaving the plasmid with both enzymes simultaneously resulted in a single band 2.7 kb in size. Draw a diagram of this plasmid showing the relative location of its restriction sites. Explain your reasoning.

9. DNA footprinting is a suitable technique for identifying which of the following?

a. Particular mRNAs in a mixture

b. Particular tRNAs in a mixture

c. Introns within a gene

d. Protein-binding sites within DNA

e. Specific DNA sites at which restriction endonucleases cleave the nucleotide chain

10. Explain briefly how you might go about cloning a gene for interleukin 2 (IL-2). Assume that you have available a monoclonal antibody specific for IL-2.

11. You have a sample of a mouse DNA-binding protein and of the mRNA that encodes it. Assuming you have a mouse genomic library available, briefly describe how you could select a clone carrying a DNA fragment that contains the gene that encodes the binding protein.

12. What are the major differences between transgenic mice and knockout mice and in the procedures for producing them?

13. How does a knock-in mouse differ from a knockout mouse?

14. How does the Cre/*lox* technology enhance knockout and knock-in strategies?

15. For each term related to recombinant DNA technology (a–i), select the most appropriate description (1–10) listed below. Each description may be used once, more than once, or not at all.

Terms

a. ______ Yeast artificial chromosome

b. ______ Restriction endonuclease

c. ______ cDNA

d. ______ COS sites

e. ______ Retrovirus

f. ______ Plasmid

g. ______ cDNA library

h. ______ Sticky ends

i. ______ Genomic library

Descriptions

(1) Cleaves mRNA at specific sites.

(2) Cleaves double-stranded DNA at specific sites.

(3) Circular genetic element that can replicate in *E. coli* cells.

(4) Used to clone DNA in mammalian cells.

(5) Formed from action of reverse transcriptase.

(6) Collection of DNA sequences within plasmid vectors representing all of the mRNA sequences derived from a cell.

(7) Produced by action of certain DNA-cleaving enzymes.

(8) Used to clone very large DNA sequences.

(9) Used to introduce larger-than-normal DNA fragments in λ-phage vectors.

(10) Collection of λ clones that includes all the DNA sequences of a given species.

APPENDIX

CD ANTIGENS

A great deal is known about the nature, distribution, and function of CD antigens. The following table presents some essential information about each of these antigens. Because many CD antigens are known by a variety of names, synonyms are indicated in addition to the official CD designations. The molecular weight (MW) is listed for the CD antigens that are proteins but not for those that are carbohydrates or lipids. In summarizing the expression patterns for CD antigens, we have concentrated on cells of the immune system (leukocytes). However, many of these antigens are also expressed in other cell types, and we have given some examples of these as well. The description of the functions of each CD antigen also focuses on cells of the immune system, with an occasional example of functions in other cell types.

Detailed reviews of most CD antigens, which include comprehensive listings of cell expression patterns and functions of these antigens in both leukocytes and other cell types, may be found online in the CD Index at the PROW Web site (Protein Resources on the Web) of the National Library of Medicine:

http://www.ncbi.nlm.nih.gov/PROW/

These reviews are regularly updated and provide complete lists of references.

Continuing research will undoubtedly reveal new information about many of these CD antigens that will enhance and, in some cases, revise our understanding. Most immunologists believe that new ones are yet to be discovered. Therefore, for more complete information about any CD antigen or for an update on new or existing antigens, consult the PROW Web site.

An additional source of information is another Web site of the National Library of Medicine, PubMed:

http://www.ncbi.nlm.nih.gov/PubMed/medline.html

This site is an online bibliographic database that contains references, many with informative abstracts, to more than 9 million articles from a comprehensive collection of medical and biological science journals. Articles from 1966 to the present are indexed, and new references are added daily. A search engine at the Web site allows searches by key words as well as other variables, such as name of researcher or year of publication. A key-word search using the name of a particular CD antigen will provide a list of the most recent journal articles that address it. For a more comprehensive search on a particular antigen, the synonyms listed in this table can be included as alternative key words.

CD antigen	Synonyms; properties	MW in kDa	Leukocyte expression	Function
CD1a, b, c, d, e	MHC class I–like structure	43–49	Dendritic cells, B cells Langerhans cells, some thymocytes	Display of non-peptide and glycolipid antigens for T-cell responses
CD2	LFA-2, T11, E-rosette receptor; CD58-binding adhesion molecule	45–58	T cells, thymocytes, NK cells	Adhesion molecule involved in T-cell activation
CD3	T3; composed of 3 polypeptide chains: γ, δ, ϵ	γ, 25–28; δ, 20; ϵ, 20	Thymocytes, T cells, NK1-T cells	Essential role in TCR signal transduction and in cell-surface expression of the TCR
CD4	L3T4	55	MHC class II–restricted T cells, some thymocytes, monocytes/macrophages, granulocytes	Coreceptor for MHC class II–restricted T-cell activation; thymic differentiation marker for T cells; receptor for HIV

(continued)

CD antigen	Synonyms; properties	MW in kDa	Leukocyte expression	Function
CD5	Leu1, T1, Ly-1	58	Mature T cells, early thymocytes; small amounts on a subset of mature B cells (B1a B cells)	Positive or negative modulation of TCR and BCR signaling, depending on the type and developmental stage of cell displaying it
CD6	T12	105 or 130	Most peripheral T cells, thymocytes, a subset of B cells	Adhesion molecule that binds developing thymocytes to thymic epithelial cells; possible co-stimulatory molecule for mature T cells
CD7	gp40	40	Pluripotent hematopoietic cells, T cells, thymocytes	Not known
CD8	T8, Leu-2, Lty-2; a membrane-bound dimer of two chains, αβ heterodimer or αα homodimer		MHC class I–restricted T cells, some thymocytes	Coreceptor for MHC class I–restricted T cells
CD9	MRP-1, p24	24	Platelets, early B cells, activated B cells, activated T cells, eosinophils, basophils	Modulation of cell adhesion and migration; trigger of platelet activation
CD10	Common acute lymphobastic leukemia antigen (CALLA), EC 3.4.24.11 (neprilysin), enkephalinase, gp100, neutral endopeptidase (NEP), metalloendopeptidase	100	B-cell precursors, T-cell precursors, bone-marrow stromal cells	Protease
CD11a	α-L integrin chain, LFA-1 α (leukocyte function-associated molecule-1 α) chain; forms LFA-1 by association with CD18	180	Monocytes, macrophages, granulocytes, lymphocytes	Subunit of LFA-1, a membrane glycoprotein that provides cell-cell adhesion by interaction with ICAM-1 (intercellular adhesion molecule-1)
CD11b	C3biR, CR3; α chain of MAC-1 integrin; forms MAC-1 by association with CD18	165	Granulocytes, monocytes, NK cells, subset of T cells, subsets of B cells	Subunit of MAC-1, which mediates interactions of neutrophils and monocytes with stimulated endothelium, phagocytosis of particles coated with iC3b or IgG, spreading or chemotaxis of leukocytes; ligand-binding molecule that binds C3b, ICAM-1 (CD54), ICAM-2 (CD102), and fibrinogen
CD11c	α-X integrin chain, αxβ2, α chain of integrin CR4, leukocyte surface antigen, p150, 95; forms CR4 by association with CD18	145	Monocytes, macrophages, NK cells, granulocytes, subset of T cell, subset of B cells	Subunit of complex with CD18 that is similar to CD11b/CD18 complex, with which it acts cooperatively; the major form of CD11/CD18 on tissue macrophages
CD12w		90–120	Monocytes, granulocytes, platelets	Not known

CD antigen	Synonyms; properties	MW in kDa	Leukocyte expression	Function
CD13	Aminopeptidase N (APN), EC 3.4.11.2, gp 150	150	Early progenitors of granulocytes and monocytes (CFU-GM), mature granulocytes and monocytes, bone-marrow stromal cells, osteoclasts, a small number of large granular lymphocytes	Not known
CD14	LPS receptor (LPS-R)	53	Monocytes, macrophages, granulocytes (weak expression)	Receptor for endotoxin (lipopolysaccharide [LPS]), activating monocytes or neutrophils to release cytokines (TNF) and up-regulate adhesion molecules when LPS is bound
CD15	Lewis X, Lex, SSEA-1, 3-FAL, 3-FL, LNFP III, (lacto-*N*-neo-fucopentose III); poly-*N*-acetyl lactosamine carbohydrate polymer of indefinite MW	Undefined	Not known	Not known
CD15s	Sialyl Lewis X (sLex), sialylated Lewis X (SLe-x); poly-*N*-acetyl lactosamine, carbohydrate polymer of indefinite MW	Undefined	Not known	Not known
CD16	FCγRIIIA	50–80	Macrophages, NK cells, neutrophils	Subunit of low-affinity Fc receptor, involved in phagocytosis of antibody-complexed antigen and in antibody-dependent cell-mediated cytoxicity (ADCC)
CDw17	Lactosylceramide (LacCer); carbohydrate antigen		Monocytes, granulocytes, basophils, platelets, subset of peripheral B cells ($CD19^+$), tonsillar dendritic cells	Not known; ability to bind bacteria for possible role in phagocytosis
CD18	β2 integrin chain; β subunit that combines with CD11a, CD11b, or CD11c subunit to form integrins	95	All leukocytes	Adhesion and signaling in the hematopoietic system (see entries for CD11a, CD11b, and CD11c)
CD19	B4	>120	Follicular dendritic cells, B cells from earliest recognizable B-lineage cells during development to B-cell blasts but lost on maturation to plasma cells	Part of B-cell coreceptor with CD21 and CD81; a critical signal transduction molecule that regulates B-cell development, activation, and differentiation
CD20	B1, Bp35	33	B cells	Not known
CD21	C3d receptor, CR2, Epstein Barr virus receptor (EBV-R)	145 (membrane form); 130 (soluble form)	B cells, follicular dendritic cells, subset of immature thymocytes	Receptor for EBV, C3d, C3dg, and iC3b; with CD19 and CD81, part of the B-cell coreceptor, a large signal-transduction complex

(continued)

CD antigen	Synonyms; properties	MW in kDa	Leukocyte expression	Function
CD22	BL-CAM, Lyb8 in mouse	140	Surface of mature B cells, cytoplasm of late pro- and early pre-B cells	Adhesion molecule; signaling molecule
CD23	B6, BLAST-2, FcεRII, Leu-20; low-affinity IgE receptor	45	Human B cells, monocytes follicular dendritic cells	Regulation of IgE synthesis; trigger to release TNF, IL-1, IL-6, and GM-CSF from human monocytes
CD24	BA-1, heat-stable antigen (HSA) in mouse	35–45	B-cell lineage but lost at plasma-cell stage, mature granulocytes	Not known
CD25	IL-2 receptor α chain, IL-2R, Tac antigen	55	PHA-stimulated T cells; anti-IGM–stimulated B cells, LPS-stimulated monocytes/macrophages	α subunit of receptor for cytokine IL-2
CD26	EC 3.4.14.5, adenosine deaminase-binding protein (ADA-binding protein), dipeptidylpeptidase IV (DPP IV ectoenzyme)	110, 120	Mature or activated T cells, B cells, NK cells, macrophages	Co-stimulatory molecule in T-cell activation
CD27	S152, T14	55	Mature thymocytes, activated T cells and B cells, NK cells, macrophages, most peripheral T cells, memory-type B cells	Mediation of a co-stimulatory signal for T- and B-cell activation; role in murine T-cell development
CD28	T44, Tp44	≈90 (homodimeric form)	Mature $CD3^+$ thymocytes, most peripheral T cells, plasma cells	Co-stimulation of T-cell proliferation and cytokine production upon binding CD80 or CD86
CD29	β1 integrin chain, GP, platelet GPIIa, VLA-β chain	130	Leukocytes	β subunit of VLA-1 integrin
CD30	Ber-H2 antigen, Ki-1 antigen	120	Activated T cells, activated B cells, activated NK cells, monocytes	Stimulation of proliferation or induction of cell death, depending upon conditions and cell type expressing it
CD31	GPiia′, endocam, platelet endothelial cell adhesion molecule (PECAM-1)	130–140	Endothelial cells, platelets, monocytes, neutrophils, NK cells, subsets of T cells	Adhesion molecule
CD32	FCRII, FcγRII	40	B cells, granulocytes, monocytes	Receptor for Fc portion of antigen-antibody–complexed IgG molecules
CD33	gp67, p67	67	Monocytes, myeloid precursors	Sialic-acid–dependent cytoadhesion molecule, a sialoadhesin
CD34	gp105-120	40 (based on amino acid sequence)	Early lymphohematopoietic stem and progenitor cells, small-vessel endothelial cells, embryonic fibroblasts, some cells in fetal and adult nervous tissue	Cell-cell adhesion molecule

CD antigen	Synonyms; properties	MW in kDa	Leukocyte expression	Function
CD35	C3bR, C4bR, complement receptor type one (CR1), immune adherence receptor	Many forms: 160, 190, 220, 250, 165, 195, 225, 255	Erythrocytes, neutrophils, monocytes, eosinophils, B cells	Receptor for C4b/C3b-coated particles, mediating their adherence and phagocytosis; facilitator of C3b and C4b cleavage, thus limiting complement activation
CD36	GPIIIb, GPIV, OKM5-antigen, PASIV	88–113 (platelet form)	Platelets, mature monocytes/macrophages, endothelial cells	Adhesion molecule in platelet adhesion and aggregation, and in platelet-monocyte or platelet-tumor cell interaction; molecule for recognition of apoptotic neutrophils; scavenger receptor for oxidized LDL
CD37	gp52-40	40–52	B cells; low levels on T cells, neutrophils, granulocytes, and monocytes	Role in signal transduction
CD38	T10	45	Early-stage B and T cells, germinal-center B cells, plasma cells	NAD glycohydrolase
CD39	Bp50	40–52	B cells, T cells, neutrophils, granulocytes, monocytes	Role in signal transduction
CD40	Bp50	48 (monomer)	B-lineage cells (pro-B through plasma cells), macrophages, follicular dendritic cells, endothelial cells, fibroblasts, keratinocytes, $CD34^+$ hematopoietic cell progenitors	Roles in B-cell growth, differentiation, and isotype-switching; apoptosis rescue signal for germinal-center B cells; stimulation of cytokine production in macrophages and dendritic cells; up-regulation of adhesion molecules on dendritic cells
CD41	Glycoprotein IIb (GP IIb) αIIb integrin chain; forms platelet fibrinogen receptor by association with GP IIIa	αβ dimer: α, 125; β, 122	Platelets, megakaryocytes	Subunit of platelet fibrinogen receptor, which mediates platelet aggregation by acting as receptor for fibrinogen; possibly also receptor for von Willebrand factor, fibronectin, and thrombospondin
CD42a, b, c, d	a, GPIX; b, GPIb-α; c, GPIb-β; d, GPV	a, 23; b, 135, 23; c, 22; d, 85	Platelets, megakaryocytes	Adhesion of platelets to endothelium; amplification of platelet response to thrombin
CD43	gpL115, leukocyte sialoglycoprotein, leukosialin, sialophorin	95–115 in T cells; 115–135 in neutrophils	All leukocytes except most resting B cells	Possible anti-adhesive("barrier") molecule mediating repulsion between leukocytes and other cells
CD44	ECMR III, H-CAM, HUTCH-1, Hermes, Lu (In-related), Pgp-1, gp85	85	Surface of most cell types	Adhesion molecule mediating leukocyte attachment and homing to peripheral lymphoid organs and sites of inflammation
CD44R	CD44v, CD44v9; heterogeneous group of CD44 variant isoforms designated by the variant exons that they include (v2–V10 in humans)	85–250 in epithelial cells; 85–200 in lymphocytes	Epithelial cells and monocytes (constitutively), activated leukocytes	Possible role (particularly for CD44v6) in leukocyte attachment to and rolling on endothelial cells, homing to peripheral lymphoid organs and sites of inflammation

(continued)

CD antigen	Synonyms; properties	MW in kDa	Leukocyte expression	Function
CD45	Leukocyte common antigen (LCA), T200, EC 3.1.3.4.; many different isoforms with different molecular weights, eg, B220, CD45R, CD45RA, CD45RB, CD45RC, CD45RO	210, 220, 180, 200	All hematopoietic cells; different isoforms characteristic of differentiated subsets of various hematopoietic cells	Essential role in T- and B-cell antigen-receptor-mediated activation; possible role in receptor-mediated activation in other leukocytes
CD46	Membrane cofactor protein (MCP)	52–58, 35–40	Peripheral-blood lymphocytes (PBL), non-hematopoietic tissues such as salivary glands and kidney ducts	Protective barrier against inappropriate complement activation and deposition on plasma membranes
CD47	Rh-associated protein, gp42, integrin-associated protein (IAP), neurophilin, ovarian carcinoma antigen 3 (OA3)	45–60, 47–55	Most cells	Adhesion molecule; thrombospondin receptor
CD48	BCM1 in mouse, Blast-1, Hu Lym3, OX-45 in rat	45	All leukocytes except neutrophils	Adhesion molecule via its receptor, CD2
CD49a	α-1 integrin chain, very late antigen α 1 chain (VLA-1 α chain)	200	Activated T cells, monocytes, neuronal cells, smooth muscle	Integrin that associates with CD29, binds collagen, laminin-1
CD49b	α-2 integrin chain, GPIa VLA-2 α chain	160	B cells, monocytes, platelets, megakaryocytes; neuronal, epithelial, and endothelial cells; osteoclasts	Integrin that associates with CD29, binds collagen, laminin-1
CD49c	α-3 integrin chain, VLA-3 α chain	125, 30	B cells, many adherent cells	Integrin that associates with CD29, binds collagen, laminin-5, fibronectin, entactin, invasin
CD49d	α-4 integrin chain, VLA-4 α chain	145	Many cell types, including T cells, B cells, monocytes, eosinophils, basophils, mast cells, thymocytes, NK cells, dendritic cells; not on neutrophils	Cell adhesion molecule for attachment to cell surface ligands VCAM-1 ($\alpha4\beta1$ and $\alpha4\beta7$) and MAdCAM-1 ($\alpha4\beta7$), and attachment to extracellular matrix proteins fibronectin ($\alpha4\beta1$ and $\alpha4\beta7$), and thrombospondin ($\alpha4\beta1$), and for lymphocyte migration and homing; co-stimulatory molecule for T-cell activation
CD49e	α-5 integrin chain, FNR α chain, VLA-5 α chain	135	Many cell types, including memory T cells, monocytes, platelets	Integrin that associates with CD29, binds fibronoectin, invasin
CD49f	α-6 integrin chain, platelet gpI, VLA-6 α chain	125, 25	T cells, monocytes, platelets, megakaryocytes, trophoblasts	Integrin that associates with CD29, binds laminin, invasin, merosine
CD50	Intercellular molecule-3, ICAM-3	130	Leukocytes of all lineages	Co-stimulatory molecule in immune response; regulator of LFA-1/ICAM-1 and integrin-β-dependent adhesion

CD antigen	Synonyms; properties	MW in kDa	Leukocyte expression	Function
CD51	VNR-α chain, α V integrin chain, vitronectin receptor; forms α-V integrin by association with CD61	125	Platelets, megakaryocytes	Subunit of α-V integrin, which binds vitronectin, von Willebrand factor, fibronectin, thrombospondin, and probably apoptotic cells
CD52	CAMPATH-1, HE5	25–29	Thymocytes, lymphocytes, monocytes, macrophages, epithelial cells lining male reproductive tract	Not known
CD53	MRC OX44	32–42	Leukocytes	Signal transduction; crosslinking promotes activation of human B cells
CD54	Intercellular adhesion molecule-1 (ICAM-1)	90, 75–115	Activated endothelial cells, activated T cells, activated B cells, monocytes, endothelial cells	Ligand for CD11a/CD18 or CD11b/CD18; receptor for rhinoviruses and for RBCs infected with malarial parasites
CD55	Decay accelerating factor (DAF)	70, 55	Most cells	Protective barrier against inappropriate complement activation and deposition on plasma membranes
CD56	Leu-19, NKH1, neural cell adhesion molecule (NCAM)	175–220	Human NK cells, a subset of $CD4^+$ and $CD8^+$ T cells	Not known for the immune system; adhesion molecule for cells of the nervous system
CD57	HNK1, Leu-7; a carbohydrate antigen (oligosaccharide), component of many glycoproteins		NK cells; subsets of T cells, B cells, and monocytes	Not known
CD58	Lymphocyte function-associated antigen 3 (LFA-3)	55–70	Many hematopoietic and non-hematopoietic cell types	Adhesion between killer T cells and target cells, antigen-presenting cells and T cells, or thymocytes and thymic epithelial cells
CD59	IF-5Ag, H19, HRF20, MACIF, MIRL, P-18 protectin	18–25	Most hematopoietic and non-hematopoietic cell types	Inhibitor of membrane attack complex (MAC) assembly, thus protecting cells from complement mediated lysis; signaling role (as a GPI-anchored molecule) in T-cell activation; possible role in cell adhesion
CDw60	9-O-acetyl-GD3; carbohydrate modification found on some gangliosides		Subset of T cells, platelets, thymic epithelium, activated keratinocytes, synovial fibroblasts, glomeruli, smooth muscle cells, astrocytes	Possible contributor to co-stimulatory/co-mitogenic signals for T cells
CD61	CD61A, GPIIb/IIIa, β3 integrin chain	110	Platelets, megakaryocytes, macrophages	Integrin subunit, associates with CD41 (Gpllb/lla) or CD51 (vitronectin receptor)
CD62E	E-selectin, ELAM-1, LECAM-2	140	Acutely activated endothelium, chronic inflammatory lesions of skin and synovium	Adhesion molecule that mediates leukocyte rolling on activated endothelium at inflammatory sites

(continued)

CD antigen	Synonyms; properties	MW in kDa	Leukocyte expression	Function
CD62L	L-selectin, LAM-1, LECAM-1, Leu-8, MEL-14, TQ-1	65	Most peripheral-blood B cells, T cells, monocytes, granulocytes, NK cells; bone-marrow lymphocytes and myeloid cells, thymocytes	Adhesion molecule that mediates lymphocyte homing to high endothelial venules of peripheral lymphoid tissue and leukocyte rolling on activated endothelium at inflammatory sites
CD62P	P-selectin, granule membrane protein-140 (GMP-140), platelet activation–dependent granule-external membrane protein (PADGEM)	120	Endothelium, platelets, megakaryocytes	Interaction with PSGL-1 to mediate tethering and rolling of leukocytes on the surface of activated endothelial cells, the first step in leukocyte extravasation and migration toward sites of inflammation
CD63	LIMP, MLA1, PTLGP40, gp55, granulophysin lysosomal-membrane-associated glycoprotein 3 (LAMP-3), melanoma-associated antigen (ME491), neuroglandular antigen (NGA)	40–60	Platelets, endothelium, degranulated neutrophils, monocytes, macrophages endothelium	Not known
CD64	FcγRI, FCRI	72	Monocytes, macrophages, blood and germinal-center dendritic cells, PMN activated by IFN-γ or G-CSF, early myeloid-lineage cells	Phagocytosis: receptor-mediated endocytosis of IgG-antigen complexes; antigen capture for presentation to T cells; antibody-dependent cellular cytotoxicity; mediator of release by some cells of cytokines and reactive oxygen intermediates
CD65	Ceramide-dodecasaccharide, VIM-2; glycolipid		Myeloid cells	Not known
CD65s	Sialylated-CD65, VIM2; carbohydrate		Granulocytes, monocytes	Possible involvement with phagocytosis and Ca^{2+} influx
CD66a	NCA-160, biliary glycoprotein (BGP)	160–180	Granulocytes, epithelial cells	Adhesion molecule; receptor for *Neisseria gonorrheae* and *N. meningitidis;* trigger of neutrophil activation
CD66b	CD67, CGM6, NCA-95	95–100	Granulocytes	Adhesion molecule, trigger of neutrophil activation
CD66c	NCA, NCA-50/90	90	Granulocytes, epithelial cells	Adhesion molecule; trigger of neutrophil activation
CD66d	CGM1	30	Granulocytes	Unclear; receptor for *Neisseria gonorrheae* and *N. meningitidis*
CD66e	Carcinoembryonic antigen (CEA)	180–200	Epithelial cells	Unclear; possible adhesion molecule
CD66f	Pregnancy-specific b1 glycoprotein, SP-1, pregnancy-specific glycoprotein (PSG)	54–72	Fetal liver; produced in placenta and released	Unclear; possible involvement in immune regulation and protection of fetus from maternal immune system; necessary for successful pregnancy

CD antigen	Synonyms; properties	MW in kDa	Leukocyte expression	Function
CD68	gp110, macrosialin	110	Monocytes, macrophages, dendritic cells, neutrophils, basophils, mast cells, myeloid progenitor cells, subset of $CD34^+$ hematopoietic progenitor cells, activated T cells, some peripheral-blood B cells	Not known
CD69	Activation-inducer molecule (AIM), EA 1, MLR3, gp34/28, very early activation (VEA)	60	Activated leukocytes, including T cells, thymocytes, B cells, NK cells, neutrophils, eosinophils, and Langerhans cells; subset of mature thymocytes, germinal-center mantle B cells, some $CD4^+$ germinal-center T cells	Involvement in early events of lymphocyte, monocyte, and platelet activation: promotes Ca^{2+} influx, synthesis of cytokines and their receptors, induction of c-*myc* and c-*fos* proto-oncogene expression; role in promoting lysis mediated by activated NK cells
CD70	CD27-ligand, Ki-24 antigen	75, 95, 170	Activated T and B cells and macrophages	Ligand for CD27; possible role in co-stimulation of B and T cells
CD71	T9, transferrin receptor	190	All proliferating cells	Iron uptake: binds ferrotransferrin at neutral pH and internalizes complex to acidic endosomal compartment, where iron is released
CD72	Ly-19.2, Ly-32.2, Lyb-2	42	B cells (except plasma cells)	Not known
CD73	Ecto-5′-nucleotidase	69, 70, 72	Subpopulations of T and B cells, many peripheral-blood B cells, follicular dendritic cells, epithelial cells, endothelial cells	Dephosphorylation of purine and pyrimidine ribo- and deoxyribonucleoside monophosphates to their corresponding nucleosides
CD74	Class II-specific chaperone, Ii, invariant chain	33, 35, 41	B cells, activated T cells, macrophages, activated endothelial and epithelial cells	Intracellular sorting of MHC class II molecules
CDw75			B cells, subpopulation of peripheral-blood T cells, erythrocytes	Cell adhesion; ligand for CD22
CDw76	Carbohydrate antigen		B cells, subpopulation of T cells	Not known
CD77	Pk blood group antigen, Burkitt's lymphoma antigen, (BLA), ceramide trihexoside (CTH), globotriaosylceramide (Gb3); sphingolipid antigen		Germinal-center B cells	Not known
CD79a	Ig-α, MB1	40–45	B cells	Component of B-cell antigen receptor analogous to CD3, required for cell-surface expression and signal transduction

(continued)

CD antigen	Synonyms; properties	MW in kDa	Leukocyte expression	Function
CD79b	B29, Ig-β	37	B cells	Component of B-cell antigen receptor analogous to CD3, required for cell-surface expression and signal transduction
CD80	B7, B7.1, BB1	60	Activated B and T cells; macrophages	Co-stimulation of T-cell activation with CD86
CD81	Target for anti-proliferative antigen-1 (TAPA-1)	26	Broadly expressed on hematopoietic cells; expressed by endothelial and epithelial cells; absent from erythrocytes, platelets, and neutrophils	Member of CD19/CD21/Leu-13 signal-transduction complex, the B-cell coreceptor
CD82	4F9, C33, IA4, KAI1, R2	45–90	Activated/differentiated hematopoietic cells	Signal transduction: may induce T-cell spreading and pseudopod formation, modulate T-cell proliferation, and provide co-stimulatory signals for cytokine production; possible role in activation of monocytes
CD83	HB15	43	Dendritic cells, B cells, Langerhans cells	Not known
CD84	GR6	73	Monocytes, platelets, circulating B cells	Not known
CD85	GR4	110	Plasma cells, mantle-zone and germinal-center B cells, subpopulation of peripheral-blood NK cells	Possible role in T-cell activation in peripheral blood
CD86	B7.2	80	Dendritic cells, memory B cells, germinal-center B cells, monocytes	Major T cell costimulatory molecule, interacting with CD28 (stimulatory) and CTLA4 (inhibitory)
CD87	Urokinase plasminogen activator receptor (uPAR)	41–68, 35–59	T cells, NK cells, monocytes, neutrophils; non-hematopoietic cells such as vascular endothelial cells, fibroblasts, smooth muscle cells, keratinocytes, placental trophoblasts, hepatocytes	Receptor for uPA, which can convert plasminogen to plasmin; possible role in β2 integrin–dependent adherence and chemotaxis
CD88	C5a receptor, C5aR	43	Granulocytes, monocytes, dendritic cells	C5a-mediated inflammation; activation of granulocytes
CD89	Fcα-receptor R (Fcα-R), IgA Fc receptor, IgA receptor	45–70, 55–75, 70–100, 50–65	Myeloid-lineage cells from promyelocytes to neutrophils and from promonocyte to monocytes; activated eosinophils, alveolar and splenic macrophages	Induction of phagocytosis, degranulation, respiratory burst, killing of microorganisms
CD90	Thy-1	25–35	Hematopoietic stem cells, thymocytes, peripheral T cells, human lymph node HEV endothelium	Possible involvement in lymphocyte co-stimulation; possible inhibition of proliferation and differentiation of hematopoietic stem cells

CD antigen	Synonyms; properties	MW in kDa	Leukocyte expression	Function
CD91	α-2-macroglobulin receptor (ALPHA2M-R), low density lipoprotein-receptor–related protein (LRP)	515, 85	Monocytes, many non-hematopoietic cells	2-macroglobulin receptor
CDw92	GR9	70	Monocytes, granulocytes, peripheral blood lymphocytes (PBL)	Not known
CDw93	GR11	110	Monocytes, granulocytes, endothelial cells	Not known
CD94	Kp43; forms complex with NKG2-A (which contains cytoplasmic immunoreceptor tyrosine-based inhibition motifs)	70	NK cells, subsets of $CD8^+$ αβ and γδ T cells	Subunit of complex with NKG2-A that is involved in inhibition of NK cells.
CD95	APO-1, Fas antigen (Fas)	45, 90, >/200	Activated T and B cells	Mediation of apoptosis-inducing signals
CD96	T-cell activation increased late expression (TACTILE)	160	Activated T cells, NK cells	Not known
CD97	BL-KDD/F12	75–85	Activated B and T cells, monocytes, granulocytes	Binding to CD55
CD98	4F2, FRP-1, RL-388 in mouse	125	Not hematopoietic specific; activated and transformed cells; lower levels on quiescent cells	Role in regulation of cellular activation
CD99	CD99R (epitope restricted to subset of CD99 molecules), E2, *MIC2* gene product	32	Peripheral-blood lymphocytes, thymocytes	Not known
CD100		300, 120	Most hematopoietic cells except immature bone-marrow cells, RBCs, and platelets; activated T cells, germinal-center B cells	Promotion of T-cell activation and adhesion
CD101	P126, V7	240	Monocytes, granulocytes, dendritic cells, activated T cells	Possible role in T-cell activation
CD102	Intercellular adhesion molecule-2 (ICAM-2)	55–65	Vascular endothelial cells, monocytes, platelets, some populations of resting lymphocytes	Co-stimulation of immune responses; lymphocyte recirculation
CD103	HML-1, integrin αE chain	175	Intraepithelial lymphocytes (in tissues such as intestine, bronchi, inflammatory skin/breast/salivary glands), many lamina-propria T cells, some lymphocytes in peripheral blood and peripheral lymphoid organs.	Role in the tissue-specific retention of lymphocytes at basolateral surface of intestinal epithelial cells; possible accessory molecule for activation of intraepithelial lymphocytes
CD104	β4 integrin chain, tumor-specific protein 180 antigen (TSP-1180) in mouse	220	CD4 CD8 thymocytes, neuronal, epithelial, and some endothelial cells, Schwann cells, trophoblasts	Integrin that associates with CD49f, binds laminins

(continued)

CD antigen	Synonyms; properties	MW in kDa	Leukocyte expression	Function
CD105	Endoglin	180	Endothelial cells of small and large vessels, activated monocytes and tissue macrophages, stromal cells of certain tissues including bone marrow, pre-B cells in fetal marrow, erythroid precursors in fetal and adult bone marrow, syncytiotrophoblast throughout pregnancy and cytotrophoblasts transiently during first trimester	Modulator of cellular responses to TGF-β1
CD106	INCAM-110, vascular cell adhesion molecule-1 (VCAM-1)	100–110	Endothelial cells	Adhesion molecule that is ligand for VLA-4
CD107a	Lysosome-associated membrane-protein 1 (LAMP-1)	100–120	Lysosomal membrane, degranulated platelets, PHA-activated T cells, TNF-α –activated endothelium, FMLP-activated neutrophils	Not known
CD107b	Lysosome-associated membrane-protein 2 (LAMP-2)	100–120	Lysosomal membrane, degranulated platelets, TNF-α–activated endothelium, FMLP-activated neutrophils	Not known
CDw108	John-Milton-Hagen (JMH) human-blood-group antigen	76	Lymphocytes, lymphoblasts	Possible adhesion protein
CD109	8A3, E123 (7D1)	170	Activated T cells, activated platelets, vascular endothelium	Not known
CD114	CSF3R, HG-CSFR, granulocyte colony-stimulating factor receptor (G-CSFR)	150	All stages of granulocyte differentiation monocytes, mature platelets, several non-hematopoietic cell types/tissues including endothelial cells, placenta, trophoblastic cells	Specific regulator of myeloid proliferation and differentiation
CD115	C-fms, colony-stimulating factor 1R (CSF-1R), macrophage colony stimulating factor receptor (M-CSFR)	150	Monocytes, macrophages	Macrophage colony-stimulating factor (M-CSF) receptor
CD116	GM-CSF receptor α chain	80	Various myeloid cells including macrophages, neutrophils, eosinophils; dendritic cells and their precursors	Primary binding subunit of the GM-CSF receptor
CD117	C-KIT, stem cell factor receptor (SCFR)	145	Hematopoietic stem cells and progenitor cells, mast cells	Growth-factor receptor
CDw119	IFN-γR, IFN-γRa	90–100	Macrophages, monocytes, B cells, endothelium	Interferon receptor
CD120a	TNFRI, p55	50–60	Hematopoietic and non-hematopoietic cells; highest on epithelial cells	TNF receptor
CD120b	TNFRII, p75	75–85	Hematopoietic and non-hematopoietic cells	TNF receptor

CD antigen	Synonyms; properties	MW in kDa	Leukocyte expression	Function
CD121a	IL-1R, IL-1R type 1, type 1 IL-1R	80	Thymocytes, T cells	Type I interleukin-1 receptor
CDw121b	IL-1R type2, type 2 IL-1R	60–70	B cells, macrophages, monocytes	Type I interleukin-1 receptor
CD122	Interleukin-2 receptor β chain (IL-2Rβ)	70–75	T cells, B cells, NK cells, monocytes/macrophages	Critical component of IL-2– and IL-15–mediated signaling
CD123	IL-3 receptor α subunit (IL-3Rα)	70	Bone-marrow stem cells, granulocytes, monocytes, megakaryocytes	IL-3 receptor chain
CD124	IL-4R	140	Hematopoietic and non-hematopoietic cells	Receptor subunit for IL-4 and IL-13
CDw125	IL-5Rα	60	Eosinophils, activated B cells, basophils	Low-affinity receptor for IL-5; α chain of IL-5 receptor
CD126	Interleukin-6 receptor (IL-6R); associates with CD130	80	T cells, monocytes, activated B cells, hepatocytes and some other non-hematopoietic cells	Receptor for IL-6
CD127	IL-7 receptor (IL-7R), IL-7 receptor α (IL-7Rα) P90 I17 R	65–75, 90	B-cell precursors, T cells	Specific receptor for interleukin 7
CDw128a	CXCR1, interleukin-8 receptor A (IL-8RA)	58–67	Not known	Not known
CDw128b	CXCR2, interleukin-8 receptor B (IL-8RB)	58–67	Not known	Not known
CD130	gp130	~130–140	Low level on almost all cell types	Receptor subunit required for signal transduction when interleukin 6, interleukin 11, leukemia inhibitory factor, ciliary neurotrophic factor, oncostatin M, and cardiotrophin-1 bind to their receptors
CDw131	Common beta subunit	120–140 kDa	Most myeloid cells including early progenitors, early B cells	Receptor subunit required for signal transduction by IL-3, GM-CSF, and IL-5 receptors
CD132	Common cytokine receptor γ chain, common γ chain	64, 65–70	T cells, B cells, NK cells, monocytes/macrophages, neutrophils	Subunit of IL-2, IL-4, IL-7, IL-9, and IL-15 receptors
CD134	OX40	50	Activated T cells	Possible adhesion molecule co-stimulator
CD135	FMS-like tyrosine kinase 3 (flt3), Flk-2 in mice, STK-1	130	Multipotential, myelomonocytic, and primitive B-cell progenitors	Growth-factor receptor for early hematopoietic progenitors
CDw136	Macrophage-stimulating protein receptor (msp receptor), ron (p158-ron)	180	Monocytes; epithelial tissues including skin, kidney, lung, liver, intestine, and colon	Induction of migration, morphological change, and proliferation in different target cells
CDw137	4-1BB, induced by lymphocyte activation (ILA)	85	T cells, B cells, monocytes	Co-stimulator of T-cell proliferation
CD138	Heparin sulfate proteoglycan, syndecan-1	Not known	B cells	Binding to collagen type 1

(*continued*)

CD antigen	Synonyms; properties	MW in kDa	Leukocyte expression	Function
CD139		209, 228	B cells, monocytes, granulocytes, follicular dendritic cells	Not known
CD140a	PDGF receptor (PDGF-R), PDGFR, α platelet-derived growth-factor receptor (PDGFRa)	180	Some endothelial cells	Receptor for platelet-derived growth factor (PDGF)
CD140b	β platelet-derived growth factor receptor (PDGFRb)	180	Some endothelial cells	Receptor for platelet-derived growth factor (PDGF)
CD141	Fetomodulin, thrombomodulin (TM)	75	Endothelial cells, megakaryocytes, platelets, monocytes, neutrophils	Essential molecule for activation of protein C and initiation of the protein C anticoagulant pathway
CD142	Coagulation Factor III, thromboplastin, tissue factor (TF)	45–47	Inducible on monocytes and vascular endothelial cells by various inflammatory mediators	Aid in establishing environment favoring coagulation
CD143	EC 3.4.15.1, angiotensin-converting enzyme (ACE), kinase II, peptidyl dipeptidase A	170, 180, 90, 110	Endothelial cells, activated macrophages, some T cells	An enzyme, important in regulation of blood pressure, acts primarily as a peptidyl dipeptide hydrolase and is involved in the metabolism of two major vasoactive peptides, angiotensin II and bradykinin.
CD144	Cadherin-5 VE-cadherin	135	Endothelium	Control of endothelial cell-cell adhesion, permeability, and migration
CDw145		Not known	Not known	Not known
CD146	A32, MCAM, MUC18, mel-CAM, S-endo	118	Endothelium, a subpopulation of activated T cells	Potential adhesion molecule
CD147	5A11, basigin, CE9, HT7, M6, neurothelin, OX-47, extracellular-matrix metalloproteinase inducer (EMMPRIN), gp42 in mouse	50–60	All leukocytes, red blood cells, platelets, and endothelial cells	Adhesion molecule
CD148	HPTP-eta, high-cell-density–enhanced PTP 1 (DEP-1), p260	240–260, 200–250	Granulocytes, monocytes, T cells, dendritic cells, platelets	Contact inhibition of cell growth
CDw149	MEM-133	120	Peripheral-blood lymphocytes, monocytes, neutrophils, eosinophils, platelets	Not known
CDw150	IPO-3, signaling lymphocyte activation molecule (SLAM)	75–95, 70	Thymocytes, subpopulation of T cells, B cells, dendritic cells, endothelial cells	B-cell co-stimulation
CD151	PETA-3, SFA-1	32	Platelets, megakaryocytes, immature hematopoietic cells, endothelial cells	Adhesion molecule
CD152	Cytotoxic T lymphocyte–associated protein-4 (CTLA-4)	~46, ~50	Activated T cells, perhaps some activated B cells	Negative regulator of T-cell activation

CD antigen	Synonyms; properties	MW in kDa	Leukocyte expression	Function
CD153	CD30 ligand, CD30L	38–40	Activated T cells, activated macrophages, neutrophils, B cells	Ligand for CD30, may co-stimulate T cells
CD154	CD40 ligand (CD40L), T-BAM, TNF-related activation protein (TRAP), gp39	30	Activated CD4 cells	Ligand for CD40, inducer of B-cell proliferation and activation
CD155	Polio virus receptor (PVR)	80–90	Monocytes, macrophages, thymocytes, CNS neurons	Normal function unknown; receptor for poliovirus
CD156	ADAM8, MS2 human	69	Neutrophils, monocytes	Possible role in extravasation of leukocytes
CD157	BP-3/IF-7, BST-1, Mo5	42–45, 50	Granulocytes, monocytes, macrophages, some B-cell progenitors, some T-cell progenitors	Support for growth of lymphocyte progenitors
CD158a	EB6, MHC class I–specific receptors, p50.1, p58.1	58, 50	Subset of NK cells, some T cells	Regulation of NK cell–mediated cytolytic activity upon interaction with the appropriate HLA-C alleles
CD158b	GL183, MHC class I–specific receptors, p50.2, p58.2	58, 50	Subset of NK cells, some T cells	Regulation of NK cell–mediated cytolytic activity upon interaction with the appropriate HLA-C alleles
CD161	NKR-P1A	~80	Most NK cells, a subset of $CD4^+$ and $CD8^+$ T cells, thymocytes	Modulation of NK cell–mediated cytotoxicity against certain Fc-receptor–bearing targets; induction of immature thymocyte proliferation
CD162	PSGL-1	250, 160, 220	Most peripheral-blood T cells, monocytes, granulocytes, B cells	Mediation of leukocyte rolling
CD163	GHI/61, M130	130	Not known	Not known
CD164	MUC-24, multi-glycosylated core protein 24 (MGC-24v)	80	Not known	Not known
CD165	AD2, gp37	37	Peripheral lymphocytes, immature thymocytes, monocytes, most platelets, thymocytes	Adhesive interactions including adhesion between thymocytes and thymic epithelial cells
CD166	BEN, DM-GRASP, KG-CAM, neurolin, SC-1, activated-leukocyte cell-adhesion molecule (ALCAM)	100–105	Activated T cells, activated monocytes, epithelium, neurons, fibroblasts	Adhesion molecule that binds to CD6

GLOSSARY

ABO blood-group antigen Antigenic determinants of the blood-group system defined by the agglutination of red blood cells exposed to anti-A and anti-B antibodies.

Abzyme A monoclonal antibody that has catalytic activity.

Acquired immunity See **Adaptive immunity.**

Acquired immunodeficiency syndrome (AIDS) A disease caused by human immunodeficiency virus (HIV) that is marked by significant depletion of CD^4 T cells resulting in increased susceptibility to a variety of infections and cancers.

Active immunity Adaptive immunity that is induced by natural exposure to a pathogen or by **vaccination.**

Acute lymphocytic leukemia (ALL) A form of cancer in which there is uncontrolled proliferation of a cell of the lymphoid lineage. The proliferating cells usually are present in the blood.

Acute myelogenous leukemia (AML) A form of cancer in which there is uncontrolled proliferation of a cell of the myeloid lineage. The proliferating cells usually are present in the blood.

Acute-phase protein One of a group of serum proteins that increase in concentration in response to inflammation. Some **complement** components and **interferons** are acute-phase proteins.

Acute-phase response The production of certain proteins and cells that appear in the blood shortly after many infections. It is part of the host's early defense against infection and precedes the adaptive phase of the immune response (see Figure 15-11).

Adaptive immunity Host defenses that are mediated by B and T cells following exposure to antigen and that exhibit specificity, diversity, memory, and self/nonself recognition. See also **Innate immunity.**

Adjuvant A substance (e.g., Freund's adjuvant, alum, bacterial LPS) that nonspecifically enhances the immune response to an antigen (see Table 3-2).

Adoptive transfer The transfer of the ability to make or participate in an immune response by the transplantation of cells of the immune system.

Affinity The strength with which a ligand interacts with a binding site. It is represented quantitatively by the affinity constant K_a.

Affinity labeling The covalent reaction of a highly reactive analog of the antigen with the binding site of an antibody. The affinity of the binding site for the analog focuses its reactivity at the binding site.

Affinity maturation The increase in average antibody affinity for an antigen that occurs during the course of an immune response or in subsequent exposures to the antigen.

Agglutination The aggregation or clumping of particles (e.g., latex beads) or cells (e.g., red blood cells).

Agglutination inhibition The reduction of antibody-mediated clumping of particles by the addition of the soluble forms of the epitope recognized by the agglutinatin antibody.

Agglutinin A substance capable of mediating the clumping of cells or particles. In particular, a hemagglutinin causes clumping of red blood cells.

Agretope The region of a processed antigenic peptide that binds to an **MHC molecule** (see Figure 3-9).

Allele Two or more alternative forms of a gene at a particular **locus** that confer alternative characters. The presence of multiple alleles results in **polymorphism.**

Allelic exclusion A process that permits expression of only one of the allelic forms of a gene. For example, a B cell expresses only one allele for a heavy chain and one allele for a light chain (see Figure 5-13).

Allergen Noninfectious antigens that induce **hypersensitivity** reactions, most commonly IgE-mediated type I reactions.

Allergy A **hypersensitivity** reaction that can include hay fever, asthma, **serum sickness,** systemic **anaphylaxis,** or contact dermatitis.

Alloantigen Antigenic determinants present on molecules that differ among members of the same species because of genetic variation.

Allogeneic Denoting members of the same species that differ genetically.

Allograft A tissue transplant between **allogeneic** indi-viduals.

Allotype A set of **allotypic determinants** characteristic of some but not all members of a species.

Allotypic determinant An antigenic determinant that varies among members of a species. The constant regions of antibodies possess allotypic determinants (see Figure 4-17b).

Alpha-feto protein (AFP) See **Oncofetal tumor antigen.**

Altered self The idea that the binding of a nonself peptide to MHC creates a peptide-MHC structure that is different from any found in normal cells of the individual.

Alternative complement pathway Activation of **complement** that is initiated by foreign cell-surface constituents, such as microbial antigens; it is antibody independent, involves C3–C9, factors B and D, and properdin, and generates the **membrane-attack complex** (see Figure 13-2).

Alveolar macrophage A macrophage found in an aveolus of the lung.

Anaphylatoxins The **complement** split products C3a and C5a, which mediate **degranulation** of mast cells and basophils, resulting in release of mediators that induce contraction of smooth muscle and increased vascular permeability.

Anaphylaxis An immediate type I hypersensitivity reaction, which is triggered by IgE-mediated mast cell **degranulation.** Systemic anaphylaxis leads to shock and is often fatal. Localized anaphylaxis involves various types of **atopic** reactions.

Anergy A state of unresponsiveness to antigens.

Antibody A protein (immunoglobulin), consisting of two

identical heavy chains and two identical light chains, that recognizes a particular **epitope** on an antigen and facilitates clearance of that antigen (see Figure 4-2). Membrane-bound antibody is expressed by **B cells** that have not encountered antigen; secreted antibody is produced by **plasma cells.** Some antibodies are multiples of the basic four-chain structure.
Antibody-dependent cell-mediated cytotoxicity (ADCC) A cell-mediated reaction in which nonspecific cytotoxic cells that express **Fc receptors** (e.g., NK cells, neutrophils, macrophages) recognize bound antibody on a target cell and subsequently cause lysis of the target cell (see Figure 14-12).
Antigen Any substance (usually foreign) that binds specifically to an antibody or a T-cell receptor; often is used as a synonym for **immunogen.**
Antigen processing Degradation of antigens by one of two pathways yielding antigenic peptides that are displayed bound to MHC molecules on the surface of antigen-presenting cells or altered self-cells (see Figure 8-8).
Antigen-presenting cell (APC) Any cell that can process and present antigenic peptides in association with **class II MHC molecules** and deliver a **co-stimulatory signal** necessary for T-cell activation. Macrophages, dendritic cells, and B cells constitute the professional APCs (see Figure 10-18). Nonprofessional APCs, which function in antigen presentation only for short periods, include thymic epithelial cells and vascular endothelial cells.
Antigenic competition The inhibition of the immune response to one antigen by immunization with different antigen. For example, the antibody response to horse red blood cells is inhibited by prior immunization with sheep red blood cells.
Antigenic determinant The site on an antigen that is recognized and bound by a particular antibody, TCR-peptide-MHC complex, or TCR-ligand-CD1 complex; also called **epitope.**
Antigenic drift A series of spontaneous point mutations that generate minor antigenic variations in pathogens and lead to strain differences.
Antigenic peptide In general, a peptide capable of raising an immune response and in a peptide that forms a complex with MHC that can be recognized by a T-cell receptor.
Antigenic shift Sudden emergence of a new pathogen subtype possibly by genetic reassortment that has led to substantial antigenic differences.
Antigenic specificity See **Specificity, antigenic.**
Antigenicity The capacity to combine specifically with antibodies or T-cell receptor/MHC.
Anti-idiotype antibody A secondary antibody (Ab-2) that is specific for the **paratope** of a primary antibody (Ab-1) and thus mimics the **epitope** of the original antigen. It represents an internal image of the original antigen and thus might be effective as a vaccine, avoiding immunization with a pathogen.
Apoptosis Morphologic changes associated with programmed cell death, including nuclear fragmentation, blebbing, and release of apoptotic bodies, which are phagocytosed (see Figure 2-3). In contrast to **necrosis,** it does not result in damage to surrounding cells.
Appendix A well-defined pocket of organized lymphoid tissue that opens into the intestine.
Atopic Pertaining to clinical manifestations of type I (IgE-mediated) hypersensitivity, including allergic rhinitis (hay fever), eczema, asthma, and various food allergies.
Attenuate To decrease virulence of a pathogen and render it incapable of causing disease. Many vaccines are attenuated bacteria or viruses that raise protective immunity without causing harmful infection.
Autocrine A condition in which the cell acted upon by a cytokine is the source of the cytokine.
Autograft Tissue grafted from one part of the body to another in the same individual.
Autoimmunity An abnormal immune response against self-antigens.
Autologous Denoting transplanted cells, tissues, or organs derived from the same individual.
Autosomal Pertaining to all the chromosomes except the sex chromosomes.
Avidity The strength of antigen-antibody binding when multiple epitopes on an antigen interact with multiple binding sites of an antibody. See also **Affinity.**

B7-1 A 60-kDa protein, also known as CD80, that is a co-stimulatory ligand for CD28 and an inhibitory ligand when it interacts with CTLA-4.
B7-2 An 80-kDa protein, also known as CD86, that is a co-stimulatory ligand for CD28 and an inhibitory ligand when it interacts with CTLA-4.
B220 A form of CD45, a protein tyrosine phosphatase.
B cell A lymphocyte that matures in the bone marrow and expresses membrane-bound antibody. After interacting with antigen, it differentiates into antibody-secreting plasma cells and memory cells.
Bacillus Calmette-Guerin See **BCG.**
Bacteremia An infection in which viable bacteria are found in the blood.
Basophil A nonphagocytic granulocyte that expresses Fc receptors for IgE (see Figure 2-10). Antigen-mediated cross-linkage of bound IgE induces **degranulation** of basophils.
B-cell coreceptor A complex of three proteins (CR2, CD19, and TAPA-1) associated with the B-cell receptor (see Figure 11-9). It is thought to amplify the activating signal induced by crosslinkage of the receptor.
B-cell receptor (BCR) Complex comprising a membrane-bound immunoglobulin molecule and two associated signal-transducing Ig-α/Ig-β molecules (see Figure 11-7).
B-cell-specific activator protein (BSAP) A transcription factor that is encoded by gene *Pax-5,* and plays an essential role in early and later stages of B-cell development.
BCG (Bacillus Calmette-Guerin) An attenuated form of *Mycobacterium bovis* used as a specific vaccine and as an adjuvant component.
β_2-microglobulin Invariant subunit that associates with the polymorphic α chain to form **class I MHC molecules;** it is not encoded by MHC genes.
Bence-Jones protein Protein found in high concentrations in the urine of patients with multiple myeloma; usually an Ig light chain or fragment thereof.
Benign Pertaining to a nonmalignant form of a neoplasm or a mild form of an illness.
Bispecific antibody Hybrid antibody made either by chemically crosslinking two different antibodies or by fusing hybridomas that produce different monoclonal antibodies.
Bone marrow The living tissue found within the hard exterior of bone.

Booster Inoculation given to stimulate immunologic memory response.
Bradykinin An endogenously produced peptide that produces an inflammatory response.
Bursa of Fabricius A **primary lymphoid organ** in birds where B-cell maturation occurs. The bone marrow is the functional equivalent in mammals.

C (constant) gene segment The 3′ coding of a rearranged immunoglobulin or T-cell receptor gene. There are multiple C gene segments in germ-line DNA, but as a result of gene rearrangement and, in some cases, RNA processing, only one segment is expressed in a given protein.
C segment An exon that encodes a domain of the constant region of an immunoglobulin molecule.
Calcineurin A calcium/calmodulin-dependent protein phosphatase.
CAMs See **Cell-adhesion molecules.**
Carcinoembryonic antigen An oncofetal antigen (found not only on cancerous cells but also on normal cells) that can be a tumor associated antigen.
Carcinoma Tumor arising from endodermal or ectodermal tissues (e.g., skin or epithelium). Most cancers ($> 80\%$) are carcinomas.
Carrier An immunogenic molecule containing antigenic determinants recognized by T cells. Conjugation of a carrier to a nonimmunogenic **hapten** renders the hapten immunogenic.
Carrier effect A **secondary immune response** to a hapten depends on use of both the **hapten** and the **carrier** used in the initial immunization.
Caspase A family of cysteine proteases that cleave after an aspartate residue. The term caspase incorporates these elements (*c*ysteine, *asp*artate, prote*ase*), which play important roles in the chain of reactions that leads to **apoptosis.**
C-C subgroup A subgroup of chemokines in which a disulfide bond links adjacent cysteines.
CD3 A polypeptide complex containing three dimers: a $\gamma\epsilon$ heterodimer, a $\epsilon\delta$ heterodimer, and either a $\zeta\zeta$ homo-dimer or $\zeta\eta$ heterodimer (see Figure 9-9). It is associated with the T-cell receptor and functions in signal transduction.
CD4 A glycoprotein that serves as a coreceptor on MHC class II-restricted T cells. Most helper T cells are $CD4^+$.
CD8 A dimeric protein that serves as a coreceptor on MHC class I-restricted T cells. Most cytotoxic T cells are $CD8^+$.
CD28 A protein on the membrane of T cells that is the receptor for co-stimulatory ligands on antigen-presenting cells.
CD40 A molecule on the surface of B cells that is the receptor for a survival signal delivered by gp39 on the surface of helper T cells. CD40 is a member of the TNF-receptor family.
CD45 A protein tyrosine phosphatase that has several different molecular forms. It is known as the leukocyte common antigen (LCA) and is found on the surface of all leukocytes.
CD antigen Cell-membrane molecule used to differentiate human leukocyte subpopulations and identified by monoclonal antibody. All monoclonal antibodies that react with the same membrane molecule are grouped into a common cluster of differentiation, or CD (see Table 2-4).
Cell line A population of cultured tumor cells or normal cells that have been subjected to chemical or viral **transformation** (see Table 23-3). Cell lines can be propagated indefinitely in culture.
Cell-adhesion molecules (CAMs) A group of cell-surface molecules that mediate intercellular adhesion. Most belong to one of four protein families: the **integrins, selectins,** mucin-like proteins, and **immunoglobulin superfamily** (see Figure 15-2).
Cell-mediated immune response Host defenses that are mediated by antigen-specific T cells and various nonspecific cells of the immune system. It protects against intracellular bacteria, viruses, and cancer and is responsible for graft rejection. Transfer of primed T cells confers this type of immunity on the recipient. See also **Humoral immune response.**
Cell-mediated lympholysis (CML) In vitro lysis of allogeneic cells or virus-infected syngeneic cells by T cells (see Figure 14-14); can be used as an assay for CTL activity or class I MHC activity.
Centroblast A proliferating germinal center B cell found in the dark zone.
Centrocyte A nonproliferating germinal center B cell found in the light zone.
Chediak-Higashi syndrome Autosomal recessive immunodeficiency caused by defect in lysosomal granules that impairs killing by NK cells.
Chemoattractant A substance that attracts leucocytes. Some chemoattractants also cause significant changes in the physiology of cells that bear receptors for them.
Chemokine Any of several secreted low-molecular-weight polypeptides that mediate **chemotaxis** for different leukocytes and regulate the expression and/or adhesiveness of leukocyte **integrins** (see Table 15-2).
Chemotactic factor An agent that can cause leukocytes to move up its concentration gradient.
Chemotaxis Directional movement of cells up the concentration gradient of some substance.
Chimera An animal or tissue composed of elements derived from genetically distinct individuals. The **SCID-human mouse** is a chimera (see Figure 23-2). Also, an antibody that contains the amino acid sequence of one species in one region and the sequence of a different species in another (for example, an antibody with a human constant region and a mouse variable region).
Chromogenic substrate A colorless substance that is transformed into colored products by an enzymatic reaction.
Chronic lymphocytic leukemia (CLL) A type of leukemia in which cancerous lymphocytes are continually produced.
Chronic myelogenous leukemia (CML) A type of leukemia in which cells of the myeloid lineage are continually produced.
Cilia Hairlike projections on epithelial cells in the respiratory and gastrointestinal tracts; cilia function to propel microbes out of the tract.
Circulating dendritic cell Dendritic cells that have acquired antigen and are migrating to secondary lymphoid tissue such as a lymph node.
Class I MHC molecules Heterodimeric membrane proteins that consist of an α chain encoded in the **MHC** associated noncovalently with **β_2-microglobulin** (see Figure 7-5a). They are expressed by nearly all nucleated cells and function to present antigen $CD8^+$ T cells. The classical class I molecules are H-2 K, D, and L in mice and HLA-A, -B, and -C in humans.
Class II MHC molecules Heterodimeric membrane proteins that consist of a noncovalently associated α and β chain, both encoded in the **MHC** (see Figure 7-5b). They are expressed by **antigen-presenting cells** and function to present antigen to $CD4^+$ T cells. The classical class II molecules are H-2 IA and IE in mice and HLA-DP, -DQ, and -DR in humans.

Class III MHC molecules Various proteins encoded in the **MHC** but distinct from class I and class II MHC molecules. They include some complement components, two steroid 21-hydroxylases, and tumor necrosis factors α and β.
Class (isotype) switching The change in the antibody class that a B cell produces.
Classical complement pathway Activation of **complement** that is initiated by antigen-antibody complexes, involves C1–C9, and generates the **membrane-attack complex** (see Figure 13-2).
Clonal anergy A physiological state in which cells are unable to be activated by antigen.
Clonal deletion The induced death of members of a clone of lymphocytes with inappropriate receptors (those that strongly react with self during development, for example).
Clonal selection The antigen mediated activation and proliferation of members of a clone of B cells that have receptors for the antigen (or for complexes of MHC and peptides derived from the antigen, in the case of T cells).
Clone Cells arising from a single progenitor cell.
Clot Coagulated mass; usually refers to coagulated blood, in which conversion of fibrinogen in the plasma to fibrin has produced a jelly-like substance containing entrapped blood cells.
Cluster of differentiation (CD) A collection of monoclonal antibodies that all recognize an antigen found on a particular differentiated cell type or types. Each of the antigens recognized by such a collection of antibodies is called a CD marker and assigned a unique identifying number.
Coding joint The sequence at the point of union of coding sequences during V(D)J rearrangement to form rearranged antibody or T-cell receptor genes.
Codominantly expressed Pertains to allelic forms of a gene that encodes protein products that are both produced in all cells in which the gene is active.
Colony-stimulating factors Proteins that are able to induce and support the growth and development of distinct hematopoietic cell lines.
Complement A group of serum proteins that participates in an enzymatic cascade, ultimately generating the cytolytic **membrane-attack complex** (see Tables 13-1 and 13-2).
Complementarity-determining region (CDR) Portions of the variable regions of antibody molecules that protrude from the V domains and have the potential to contact antigens. The antigen-binding sites of antibody molecules are composed of the CDRs.
Conformational determinants Epitopes of a protein that are composed of amino acids that are close together in the three-dimensional structure of the protein but may not be near each other in the amino acid sequence.
Congenic Denoting individuals that differ genetically at a single genetic locus or region; also called coisogenic.
Constant (C) region The nearly invariant portion of the immunoglobulin molecule that does not contain antigen-binding domains. The sequence of amino acids in the constant region determines the isotype (α, γ, δ, ϵ and μ) of heavy chains and the type (κ and λ) of light chains.
Cortex The outer or peripheral layer of an organ.
Cosmid A genetically engineered plasmid that contains the COS sites of the λ phage. Used as a cloning vector for large pieces of foreign DNA.
Co-stimulatory signal Additional signal that is required to induce proliferation of antigen-primed T cells and is generated by interaction of CD28 on T cells with B7 on antigen-presenting cells or altered self-cells (see Figures 10-17 and 14-2). In B-cell activation, an analogous signal (competence signal 2) is provided by interaction of CD40 on B cells with CD40L on activated T_H cells (see Figure 11-10).
CR1 Complement receptor 1 or CD35, cell surface receptor present on a variety of lymphoid, myeloid, and other cell types. CR1 functions include opsonization and clearance of immune complexes.
CR2 Complement receptor 2 or CD21, a cell-surface molecule present on B cells, dendritic cells, and epithelium of cervix and nasopharynx. CR2 functions in B-cell activation and is the receptor for Epstein-Barr virus.
Cross-reactivity Ability of a particular antibody or T-cell receptor to react with two or more antigens that possess a common **epitope.**
CTL See **Cytotoxic T lymphocyte.**
C-X-C subgroup A family of chemokines that contain a disulfide bridge between cysteines separated by a different amino acid residue (X).
Cyclosporin A A fungal product used as a drug to suppress allograft rejection. The compound blocks T-cell activation by interfering with transcription factors and preventing gene activation.
Cytokine Any of numerous secreted, low-molecular-weight proteins that regulate the intensity and duration of the immune response by exerting a variety of effects on lymphocytes and other immune cells (see Table 12-1).
Cytokine-specific subunit A polypeptide chain of a multimeric cytokine receptor that is involved in a stereo-specific interaction with the target cytokine. It is responsible for the specificity of the receptor for a particular cytokine.
Cytotoxic Having the ability to kill cells.
Cytotoxic T lymphocyte (CTL) An effector T cell (usually $CD8^+$) that can mediate the lysis of target cells bearing antigenic peptides complexed with an MHC molecule (see Figure 14-4). It usually arises from an antigen-activated T_C cell (see Figure 14-1).

D (diversity) gene segment That portion of a rearranged immunoglobulin heavy-chain gene or T-cell receptor gene that is situated between the V and J gene segments and encodes part of the hypervariable region. There are multiple D gene segments in germ-line DNA, but gene rearrangement leaves only one in each functional rearranged gene.
Dark zone A portion of the germinal center that is the site of rapid cell division by forms of B cells called centroblasts.
Defensins Cysteine-rich, positively charged, antimicrobial peptides that contain 25 to 35 amino acids and are found in macrophages and neutrophils.
Degranulation Discharge of the contents of cytoplasmic granules by **basophils** and **mast cells** following crosslinkage (usually by antigen) of bound IgE (see Figure 16-6). It is characteristic of type I **hypersensitivity.**
Delayed-type hypersensitivity (DTH) A type IV hypersensitive response mediated by sensitized T_{DTH} cells, which release various **cytokines** and **chemokines** (see Figure 14-15). The response generally occurs 2–3 days after T_{DTH} cells interact with antigen. It is an important part of host defense against intracellular parasites and bacteria.
Dendritic cells Professional **antigen-presenting cells** that have long membrane extensions resembling the dendrites of

nerve cells. They are found in the lymph nodes, spleen, and thymus (follicular and interdigitating dendritic cells); skin (Langerhans cells); and other tissues (interstitial dendritic cells). Because they express class II MHC and B7 co-stimulatory molecules, dendritic cells are efficient presenters of antigen to T helper cells.
Dermis Layer of skin under the epidermis that contains blood and lymph vessels, hair follicles, nerves, and nerve endings.
Diapedesis Passage of blood cells through the intact wall of a blood vessel.
Differentiation antigen A cell-surface marker that is expressed only during a particular developmental stage or by a particular cell lineage.
DiGeorge's syndrome Congenital thymic aplasia caused by deletion of a sequence on chromosome 22 during embryonic life. Consequences include immunodeficiency, facial abnormalities, and congenital heart disease.
Direct staining A variation of fluorescent antibody staining in which the primary antibody is directly conjugated to the fluorescent label.
Domain An independently folded part of a polypeptide chain that forms a structural unit within a protein. See also **Immunoglobulin fold.**
Double immunodiffusion A type of precipitation in gel analysis in which both antigen and antibody diffuse radially from wells toward each other, thereby establishing a concentration gradient. As equivalence is reached, a visible line of precipitation, a precipitin line, forms.
Double-negative (DN) cell A stage of T-cell development at which the differentiating α/β cell does not have a T-cell receptor and does not display either the CD4 or CD8 coreceptor.
Double-positive (DP) cell A stage of T-cell development at which the differentiating α/β cell displays the pre-T-cell receptor and both the CD4 or CD8 coreceptors.

E2A A transcription factor that is required for the expression of the recombinase-activating genes (RAG) as well as the expression of the lambda 5 (λ5) component of the pre–B-cell receptor during B-cell development. It is essential for B-cell development.
Early B-cell factor (EBF) A transcription factor that is essential for early B-cell development. It is necessary for the expression of RAG.
Edema Abnormal accumulation of fluid in intercellular spaces, often resulting from a failure of the lymphatic system to drain off normal leakage from the capillaries.
Effector cell Any cell capable of mediating an immune function (e.g., activated T_H cells, CTLs, and plasma cells).
Effector response Action that occurs after recognition and binding of antigen by antibody; lysis by complement proteins is an effector function.
ELISA (enzyme-linked immunosorbent assay) An assay for quantitating either antibody or antigen by use of an enzyme-linked antibody and a substrate that forms a colored reaction product (see Figure 6-11).
Endocrine Referring to regulatory secretions such as hormones or cytokines that pass from producer cell to target cell by the blood stream.
Endocytosis Process by which cells ingest extracellular macromolecules by enclosing them in a small portion of the plasma membrane, which invaginates and is pinched off to form an intracellular vesicle containing the ingested material.
Endogenous Originating within the organism or cell.
Endotoxins Certain lipopolysaccharide (LPS) components of the cell wall of gram-negative bacteria that are responsible for many of the pathogenic effects associated with these organisms. Some function as **superantigens.**
Enhancer A regulatory DNA sequence that increases the transcription of genes located 5′ or 3′ of it. Enhancers function regardless of their orientation, so that inversion of an enhancer sequence does not prevent it from acting.
Enzyme-linked immunosorbent assay See **ELISA.**
Eosinophil Motile, somewhat phagocytic granulocytes that can migrate from blood to tissue spaces. They have large numbers of IgE receptors and are highly granular. They are thought to play a role in the defense against parasitic organisms such as roundworms. See Figure 2-10.
Epidermis The outermost layer of the skin.
Epitope The portion of an antigen that is recognized and bound by an antibody or TCR/MHC combination; also called **antigenic determinant.**
Epstein-Barr virus (EBV) The causative agent of Burkitt's **lymphoma** and infectious mononucleosis. It can transform human B cells into stable **cell lines.**
Equilibrium dialysis An experimental technique that can be used to determine the affinity of an antibody for antigen and its **valency** (see Figure 6-2).
Equivalence A measure of the proportion of antibody to antigen that yields the maximum precipitate in liquids and gels (see Figure 6-4).
Equivalence zone The point or region of a gel in which the ratio of antigen to antibody is optimal for the production of an antigen-antibody precipitate.
Erythema Redness of the skin caused by engorgement of capillaries during an **inflammatory response.**
Erythroblastosis fetalis A type II hypersensitivity reaction in which maternal antibodies against fetal **Rh antigens** cause hemolysis of the erythrocytes of a newborn (see Figure 16-14); also called hemolytic disease of the newborn.
Erythropoiesis The generation of red blood cells.
Erythropoietin (EPO) A cytokine that induces the commitment of progenitor cells to the erythroid lineage.
Exocytosis Process by which cells release molecules (e.g., cytokines, lytic enzymes, degradation products) contained within a membrane-bound vesicle by fusion of the vesicle with the plasma membrane (see Figure 2-9).
Exogenous Originating outside the organism or cell.
Exon A continuous segment of DNA that encodes part of a gene product; also called coding sequence.
Exotoxins Toxic proteins secreted by gram-positive and gram-negative bacteria; some function as **superantigens.** They cause food poisoning, toxic-shock syndrome, and other disease states. See also **Immunotoxin.**
Extravasation Movement of blood cells through an unruptured vessel wall into the surrounding tissue, particularly at sites of inflammation (see Figures 15-3 and 15-7).
Exudate Fluid with a high content of protein, salts, and cellular debris that accumulates extravascularly, usually as a result of inflammation.

Fab fragment "Fragment antigen binding." A monovalent antigen-binding fragment of an immunoglobulin molecule that consists of one light chain and part of one heavy chain, linked by an interchain disulfide bond. It is obtained by brief papain digestion (see Figure 4-3).
$F(ab')_2$ fragment Two Fab units linked by disulfide bridges between fragments of the heavy chain. They are obtained by digestion of antibody with pepsin (see Figure 4-3).
Fc fragment "Fragment crystallizable." A crystallizable, non-antigen-binding fragment of an immunoglobulin molecule that consists of the carboxyl-terminal portions of both heavy chains and possesses binding sites for Fc receptors and the C1q component of complement. It is obtained by brief papain digestion (see Figure 4-3).
Fc receptor (FcR) Cell-surface receptor specific for the Fc portion of certain classes of immunoglobulin. It is present on lymphocytes, mast cells, macrophages, and other accessory cells.
FCγRII A membrane protein also known as CD32 that acts as a receptor for the Fc region of IgG.
Fibrin A filamentous protein produced by the action of thrombin on fibrinogen; fibrin is the main element in blood clotting.
Fibrinopeptide One of two small peptides of about 20 amino acids released from fibrinogen by thrombin cleavage in the conversion to fibrin.
Fibrosis A process responsible for the development of a type of scar tissue at the site of chronic inflammation.
Fimbria A general term for any fringe-like anatomic structure. Bacterial pili are fimbriae.
First-set graft rejection Process whereby an **allograft** is rejected after the first exposure to the alloantigens of the donor. Complete rejection usually occurs within 12–14 days (see Figure 21-1b). See also **Second-set graft rejection.**
Fluorescein A dye that produces brilliant green fluorescence when excited. It is widely used as a fluorescent label in many types of **immunofluorescence** analysis.
Fluorescent antibody An antibody with a **fluorochrome** conjugated to its Fc region that is used to stain cell-surface molecules or tissues; the technique is called **immunofluorescence.**
Fluorochrome A molecule that fluoresces when excited with appropriate wavelengths of light. See **immunofluorescence.**
Follicular dendritic cell A cell with extensive dendritic extensions that is found in the follicles of lymph nodes. Although they do not express MHC class II molecules, they are richly endowed with receptors for complement and Fc receptors for antibody. They are of a lineage that is distinct from MHC class II-bearing dendritic cells.
Fragmentin Enzymes present in the granules of cytotoxic lymphocytes that induce DNA fragmentation.
Framework region A relatively conserved sequence of amino acids located on either side of the hypervariable regions in the variable domains of immunoglobulin heavy and light chains (see Figure 4-8).
Freund's complete adjuvant (CFA) A water-in-oil emulsion to which heat-killed mycobacteria have been added; antigens are administered in CFA to enhance their immunogenicity.
Freund's incomplete adjuvant Freund's adjuvant lacking heat-killed mycobacteria.
Fusin A receptor present on certain human cells, including $CD4^+$ T cells, that is linked to a G protein and thought to be required for fusion of **HIV** with target cells.

G protein Heterotrimeric proteins that are active when the guanine binding site is occupied by GTP and inactive when it holds GDP. These proteins play crucial roles in a variety of signaling pathways, including those that mediate the effects of chemokines.
Gamma globulins Group of serum proteins originally characterized by having a greater electrophoretic mobility than other fractions and later shown to contain the immunoglobulins.
γ (gamma) globulin fraction The electrophoretic fraction of serum that contains most of the immunoglobulin classes.
GATA-2 gene A gene encoding a transcription factor that is essential for the development of several hematopoietic cell lineages, including the lymphoid, erythroid and myeloid lineages.
Gene locus See **Locus.**
Genome The total genetic material contained in the haploid set of chromosomes.
Genotype The combined genetic material inherited from both parents; also, the **alleles** present at one or more specific loci.
Germ line The unmodified genetic material that is transmitted from one generation to the next through the gametes. The germ line genes of an individual are those that were present in the zygote from which it arose.
Germinal center A region within lymph nodes and the spleen where B-cell activation, proliferation, and differentiation occurs (see Figure 11-17). Germinal centers are sites of intense B cell somatic mutation and selection.
Germ-line theories Theories that explain antibody diversity by postulating that all antibodies are encoded in the host chromosomes.
Goodpasture's syndrome An autoimmune disease characterized by autoantibodies specific for certain basement-membrane antigens of the glomeruli of the kidneys and the alveoli of the lungs.
Graft-versus-host disease (GVHD) A reaction that develops when a graft contains immunocompetent T cells that recognize and attack the recipient's cells.
Granulocyte Any **leukocyte** that contains cytoplasmic granules, particularly the basophil, eosinophil, and neutrophil (see Figure 2-10).
Granulocyte CSF (G-CSF) A cytokine essential for the development of cells of the granulocytic lineage.
Granulocyte-macrophage CSF (GM-CSF) A cytokine essential for the development of cells of the granulocytic and monocytic lineages.
Granuloma A tumor-like mass or nodule that arises because of a chronic **inflammatory response** and contains many activated macrophages, epithelioid cells (modified macrophages), T_{DTH} cells, and multinucleated giant cells formed by the fusion of macrophages (see Figure 14-16).
Granzyme One of a set of enzymes found in the granules of T_C cells that can help to initiate apoptosis in target cells.
Graves' disease An autoimmune disease where the individual produces auto-antibodies to the receptor for TSH.

H-2 complex Term for the **MHC** in the mouse.
Haplotype The set of **alleles** of linked genes present on one parental chromosome; commonly used in reference to the **MHC** genes.
Hapten A low-molecular-weight molecule that can be made immunogenic by conjugation to suitable carrier (see Figure 3-12).
Hapten-carrier conjugate A covalent combination of a small molecule with a large immunogenic carrier molecule or structure.

Heat-shock protein (HSP) Family of conserved proteins that increase in concentration as a response to heat or other stress to cells. HSP function in the assembly, transport and folding of other cellular proteins.
Heavy (H) chain The larger polypeptide of an antibody molecule; it is composed of one variable domain (V_H) and three or four constant domains (C_H1, C_H2, etc.). There are five major classes of heavy chains in humans (α, γ, δ, ϵ, and μ chains), which determine the **isotype** of an antibody (see Table 4-1).
Hemagglutinin See **Agglutinin.**
Hematopoiesis The formation and differentiation of blood cells (see Figure 2-1).
Hematopoietic stem cell (HSC) The cell type from which all lineages of blood cells arise.
Hematopoietic-inducing microenvironment (HIM) An anatomical site that contains all of the cells and cellular factors required for the generation and development of blood cells.
Hematopoietins Growth factors that support the growth and development of blood cells (see Figures 12-4, 12-6).
Hemolysis Alteration or destruction of red blood cells, which liberates hemoglobin.
Hemolytic plaque assay In vitro technique for detecting **plasma cells** by their ability to lyse antigen-sensitized erythrocytes in the presence of complement, thereby forming visible plaques (see Figure 23-1).
Hereditary angioedema Autosomal dominant deficiency in the C1 complement inhibitor that leads to localized edema; the condition can be acute if it affects the respiratory tract.
Heteroconjugates Hybrids of two different antibody molecules.
Heterologous Originating from a different species; **xenogeneic.**
High-endothelial venule (HEV) An area of a capillary venule composed of specialized cells with a plump, cuboidal ("high") shape through which lymphocytes migrate to enter various lymphoid organs (see Figure 15-4).
Hinge region The segment of an immunoglobulin heavy chain between the **Fc** and **Fab** regions. It gives flexibility to the molecule and allows the two antigen-binding sites to function independently.
Histamine An amine found in mast-cell granules that dilates capillaries and stimulates muscles of the viscera.
Histiocyte An immobilized (sometimes called "tissue fixed") macrophage found in loose connective tissue.
Histocompatibility antigens Family of proteins that determine the ability of one individual to accept tissue or cell grafts from another. The major histocompatibility antigens, which are encoded by the **MHC,** function in antigen presentation.
Histocompatible Denoting individuals whose major histocompatibility are identical. Grafts between such individuals generally are accepted.
HIV (human immunodeficiency virus) A retrovirus that infects human $CD4^+$ T cells and causes **acquired immunodeficiency syndrome (AIDS).**
HLA (human leukocyte antigen) complex Term for the **MHC** in humans.
Homing The differential migration of lymphocytes or other leukocytes to particular tissues or organs.
Homing receptor A receptor that directs various populations of lymphocytes to particular lymphoid and inflammatory tissues.
Homologous Originating from the same species; also refers to similarity in the sequences of DNA or proteins.
HTLV (human T lymphotrophic virus) A **retrovirus** that infects human $CD4^+$ T cells and causes adult T-cell leukemia.
Humanized antibody An antibody that contains the antigen-binding amino acid sequences of another species within the framework of a human immunoglobulin sequence.
Humoral Pertaining to extracellular fluid, including the plasma, lymph, and tissue fluids.
Humoral immune response Host defenses that are mediated by antibody present in the plasma, lymph, and tissue fluids. It protects against extracellular bacteria and foreign macromolecules. Transfer of antibodies confers this type of immunity on the recipient. See also **Cell-mediated immune response.**
Hybridoma A **clone** of hybrid cells formed by fusion of normal lymphocytes with **myeloma** cells; it retains the properties of the normal cell to produce antibodies or T-cell receptors but exhibits the immortal growth characteristic of myeloma cells (see Figure 23-3). Hybridomas are used to produce **monoclonal antibody.**
Hypersensitivity Exaggerated immune response that causes damage to the individual. Immediate hypersensitivity (types I, II, and III) is mediated by antibody or immune complexes, and delayed-type hypersensitivity (type IV) is mediated by T_{DTH} cells (see Table 16-1).
Hypervariable region One of three regions within the variable domain of each chain in immunoglobulins and T-cell receptors that exhibits the most sequence variability and contributes the most to the antigen-binding site; also called complementary-determining region (CDR).

Iccosomes (immune-complex–coated bodies) Particles heavily coated with immune complexes that are released from the extensions of follicular dendritic cells.
Identity The result of Ouchterlony analysis when two antigens share identical epitopes; the antiserum forms a single precipitation line with each antigen, and the two lines fuse to give a single curved line.
Idiotope A single **antigenic determinant** in the variable domains of an antibody or T-cell receptor; also called idiotypic determinant. Idiotopes are generated by the unique amino acid sequence specific for each antigen (see Figure 4-17).
Idiotype The set of antigenic determinants **(idiotopes)** characterizing a unique antibody or T-cell receptor.
Ikaros A transcription factor required for the development of all lymphoid cell lineages.
Immediate hypersensitivity An exaggerated immune response mediated by antibody (type I and II) or antigen-antibody complexes (type III) that manifests within minutes to hours after exposure of a sensitized individual to antigen (see Table 16-1).
Immune complex A macromolecular complex of antibody bound to antigen, which sometimes includes **complement** components. Deposition of immune complexes in various tissues results in type III **hypersensitivity.**
Immunity State or quality of being resistant (immune), either by virtue of previous exposure **(adaptive immunity)** or as an inherent trait **(innate immunity).**
Immunization The process of producing a state of immunity in a subject. See also **Active immunity** and **Passive immunity.**
Immunoadsorption Removal of antibody or antigen from a sample by adsorption to a solid-phase system to which the complementary antigen or antibody is bound.
Immunocompetent Denoting a mature lymphocyte that is

capable of recognizing a specific antigen and mediating an immune response.

Immunodeficiency Any deficiency in the immune response. It may result from a defect in phagocytosis, the humoral response, or the cell-mediated response. Combined immunodeficiencies affect both the humoral and cell-mediated immune response (see Figure 19-1).

Immunodominant Referring to epitopes that produce a more pronounced immune response than others do under the same conditions.

Immunoelectron microscopy A technique in which antibodies used to stain a cell or tissue are labeled with an electron-dense material and visualized with an electron microscope.

Immunoelectrophoresis A technique in which an antigen mixture is first separated into its component parts by electrophoresis and then tested by **double immunodiffusion.**

Immunofluorescence Technique of staining cells or tissues with **fluorescent antibody** and visualizing them under a fluorescent microscope (see Figure 6-15).

Immunogen A substance capable of eliciting an immune response. All immunogens are **antigens,** but some antigens (e.g., haptens) are not immunogens.

Immunogenicity The capacity of a substance to induce an immune response under a given set of conditions.

Immunoglobulin An **antibody** or a heavy or light polypeptide chain that is a part of an antibody molecule.

Immunoglobulin fold Characteristic structure in immunoglobulins that consists of a **domain** of 100–110 amino acids folded into two β pleated sheets, each containing three or four antiparallel β strands, and stabilized by an intrachain disulfide bond (see Figure 4-6).

Immunoglobulin superfamily Group of proteins that contain **immunoglobulin-fold** domains, or structurally related domains; it includes immunoglobulins, T-cell receptors, MHC molecules, and numerous other membrane molecules (see Figure 4-19).

Immunoreceptor tyrosine-based activation motif (ITAM) Amino acid sequence in the intracellular portion of signal-transducing cell-surface molecules that interacts with and activates intracellular kinases after ligand binding by the surface molecule.

Immunotoxin Highly cytotoxic agents produced by conjugating an antibody with highly toxic agent, usually a protein such as ricin (see Figure 4-23).

Incomplete antibody Antibody that binds antigen but does not induce agglutination.

Indirect staining A method of immunofluorescent staining in which the primary antibody is unlabeled and is detected with an additional fluorochrome-labeled reagent.

Inductive site Small regions of a mucus membrane that lie over organized lymphoid follicles and contain **M cells.**

Inflamed Manifesting redness, pain, heat, and swelling.

Inflammatory response A localized tissue response to injury or other trauma characterized by pain, heat, redness, and swelling. The response, which includes both localized and systemic effects, consists of altered patterns of blood flow, an influx of phagocytic and other immune cells, removal of foreign antigens, and healing of the damaged tissue (see Figures 15-12 and 15-13).

Innate immunity Nonspecific host defenses that exist prior to exposure to an antigen and involve anatomic, physiologic, endocytic and phagocytic, and inflammatory mechanisms. See also **Adaptive immunity.**

Instructional model Theory that explains antibody diversity by postulating that the antigen serves as a template for the antibody, which takes on a complementary shape.

Insulin-dependent diabetes mellitus (IDDM) An autoimmune disease caused by an autoimmune attack on the pancreas directed against specialized insulin-producing cells, called the islets of Langerhans, scattered throughout the pancreas.

Integrins A group of heterodimeric cell-adhesion molecules (e.g., LFA-1, VLA-4, and Mac-1) present on various leukocytes that bind to Ig-superfamily CAMs (e.g., ICAMs, VCAM-1) on endothelium (see Figure 15-2).

Interdigitating dendritic cells Dendritic cells found in blood and in T-cell areas of secondary lymphoid tissue and the thymic medulla.

Interferons (IFNs) Several glycoprotein **cytokines** produced and secreted by certain cells that induce an antiviral state in other cells and also help to regulate the immune response (see Table 12-1).

Interleukins (ILs) A group of **cytokines** secreted by leukocytes that primarily affect the growth and differentiation of various hematopoietic and immune-system cells (see Table 12-1).

Interstitial dendritic cells The dendritic cells that populate most organs (e.g., heart, lungs, liver, kidney, and gastrointestinal tract).

Interstitial fluid Fluid found in the spaces between cells of an organ or tissue.

Intracellular pathogens Microbial agents that grow within cells (e.g., viruses and intercellular bacteria such as *Salmonella*).

Intraepidermal lymphocytes γδ T cells found in epidermal layers.

Intraepithelial lymphocytes (IELs) γδ T cells found in the epithelial layer of organs and the gastrointestinal tract.

Intron Noncoding sequence within a gene, which is transcribed into the primary transcript but is removed during processing and so is not translated into mRNA.

Invariant (Ii) chain Component of the MHC class II protein that shows no genetic polymorphism. The Ii chain stabilizes the class II molecule before it has acquired an antigenic peptide.

In vitro Referring to experiments with living cells or cellular components performed outside the intact organism.

In vivo Referring to experiments carried out in an intact, living organism.

Isograft Graft between genetically identical individuals.

Isotype An antibody class, which is determined by the constant-region sequence of the heavy chain. The five human isotypes, designated IgA, IgD, IgE, IgG, and IgM, exhibit structural and functional differences (see Table 4-2). Also refers to the set of **isotypic determinants** that is carried by all members of a species.

Isotype switching Conversion of one antibody class **(isotype)** to another resulting from the genetic rearrangement of heavy-chain constant-region genes in B cells; also called class switching.

Isotype One of the five major kinds of heavy chains in antibody molecules (α, γ, δ, ϵ and μ).

Isotypic determinant An **antigenic determinant** within the immunoglobulin constant regions that is characteristic of a species (see Figure 4-17).

J (joining) chain A polypeptide that links the heavy chains of monomeric units of polymeric IgM and di or trimeric IgA. The linkage is by disulfide bonds between the J chain and the carboxyl-terminal cysteines of IgM or IgA heavy chains (see Figure 4-13).

J (joining) gene segment The part of a rearranged immunoglobulin or T-cell receptor gene that joins the variable region to the constant region and encodes part of the **hypervariable region.** There are multiple J gene segments in germ-line DNA, but gene rearrangement leaves only one in each functional rearranged gene.

Junctional flexibility The diversity in antibody and T-cell receptor genes created by the imprecise joining of coding sequences during the assembly of the rearranged genes.

Kaposi's sarcoma A neoplastic lesion characterized by multiple bluish nodules in the skin and hemorrhages; it is common in AIDS patients.

Kappa (κ) chain One of the two types of light chains. Lambda is the other type.

Karyotype The chromosomal constitution of a given cell.

Kinins Group of peptides released during an **inflammatory response** that act as vasodilators, inducing smooth-muscle contraction and increased vascular permeability.

Knockout mouse A form of **transgenic mouse** in which a normal gene is replaced with a mutant allele or disrupted form of the gene; as a result, the animal lacks a functional gene product (see Figures 23-18 and 23-19).

Kupffer cell A type of tissue-fixed macrophage found in liver.

Lambda (λ) chain One of the two types of light chains. Kappa is the other type.

λ5 A polypeptide that associates with **Vpre-B** to form the **surrogate light chain** of the **pre-B-cell receptor.**

Langerhans cell A type of **dendritic cell** that is found in the epidermis and bears Fc receptors.

Leader (L) peptide A short hydrophobic sequence of amino acids at the N-terminus of newly synthesized immunoglobulins; it inserts into the lipid bilayer of the vesicles that transport Ig to the cell surface. The leader is removed from the ends of mature antibody molecules by proteolysis.

Lectin pathway Pathway of complement activation initiated by binding of serum protein MBL to the mannose-containing component of microbial cell walls (see Figure 13-2).

Lepromatous leprosy Hansen's disease, a chronic contagious granulomatous condition caused by *Mycobacterium leprae.* The other form of leprosy is tuberculoid, a more benign and stable form of the disease. Both forms of leprosy infect the peripheral nervous system.

Leukemia Cancer originating in any class of hematopoietic cell that tends to proliferate as single cells within the lymph or blood.

Leukocyte A white blood cell. The category includes lymphocytes, granulocytes, platelets, monocytes, and macrophages.

Leukocyte common antigen (LCA) The leukocyte common antigen is CD45, a protein tyrosine phosphatase found on all leukocytes. There are several forms of CD45.

Leukocyte-adhesion deficiency (LAD) An inherited disease in which the leukocytes are unable to undergo adhesion-dependent migration into sites of inflammation. Recurrent bacterial infections and impaired healing of wounds are characteristic of this disease.

Leukocytosis An abnormally large number of leukocytes, usually associated with acute infection. Counts greater than $10{,}000/mm^3$ may be considered leukocytosis.

Leukopenia Reduction in the number of circulating white blood cells.

Leukotrienes Several lipid mediators of inflammation and type I hypersensitivity; also called slow reactive substance of anaphylaxis (SRS-A). They are metabolic products of arachidonic acid (see Figure 15-11).

Ligand Any molecule recognized by a **receptor.**

Light (L) chains Immunoglobulin polypeptides of the lambda or kappa type that join with heavychain polypeptides to form the antibody heterodimer.

Light zone A region of the germinal center that contains numerous follicular dendritic cells.

LPS (lipopolysaccharide) An oligomer of lipid and carbohydrate that constitutes the endotoxin of gram-negative bacteria. LPS acts as a polyclonal activator of murine B cells, inducing their division and differentiation into antibody-producing plasma cells.

Locus The specific chromosomal location of a gene.

Lymph Interstitial fluid derived from blood plasma that contains a variety of small and large molecules, lymphocytes, and some other cells. It circulates through the lymphatic vessels.

Lymph node A small **secondary lymphoid organ** that contains lymphocytes, macrophages, and dendritic cells and serves as a site for filtration of foreign antigen and for activation and proliferation of lymphocytes (see Figures 2-6 and 2-18). See also **Germinal center.**

Lymphatic system A network of vessels and nodes that conveys lymph. It returns plasma-derived interstitial fluids to the blood stream and plays an important role in the integration of the immune system.

Lymphatic vessels Thinly walled vessels through which the fluid and cells of the lymphatic system moves through the lymph nodes and ultimately into the thoracic duct, where it joins the blood stream.

Lymphoblast A proliferating lymphocyte.

Lymphocyte A mononuclear leukocyte that mediates humoral or cell-mediated immunity. See also **B cell** and **T cell.**

Lymphoid progenitor cell A cell committed to the lymphoid lineage from which all lymphocytes arise.

Lymphokine A term originally applied to cytokines secreted by lymphocytes, especially by T_H cells. It has been largely superseded by the more general term *cytokine.*

Lymphokine-activated killer (LAK) cell Anti-tumor cells generated by treating peripheral blood leukocytes of tumor patients with high concentrations of IL-2. They are derived from NK cell population.

Lymphoma A cancer of lymphoid cells that tends to proliferate as a solid tumor.

Lymphopoiesis The differentiation of lymphocytes from hematopoietic stem cells.

Lysogeny State in which a viral genome (**provirus**) is associated with the host genome in such a way that the viral genes remain unexpressed.

Lysosome A small cytoplasmic vesicle found in many types of cells that contains hydrolytic enzymes, which play an important role in the degradation of material ingested by **phagocytosis** and **endocytosis.**

Lysozyme An enzyme present in tears, saliva, and mucous secretions that digests mucopeptides in bacterial cell walls and thus functions as a nonspecific antibacterial agent. It has frequently been used as a target antigen in immunological studies.

M cells Specialized cells of the intestinal mucosa and other sites, such as the urogenital tract, that deliver antigen from the apical face of the cell to lymphocytes clustered in the pocket of its basolateral face.
Macrophage Mononuclear phagocytic leukocytes that play roles in adaptive and in innate immunity. There are many types of macrophages; some are migratory whereas others are fixed in tissues.
Macrophage CSF (M-CSF) A cytokine that supports the growth and differentiation of macrophages.
Malignant Resistant to treatment or fatal; refers to uncontrollable recurring neoplasms.
MALT (mucosal-associated lymphoid tissue) Lymphoid tissue located along the mucous membranes that line the digestive, respiratory and urogenital tracts.
Marginal zone A diffuse region of the spleen, located on the periphery of the **PALS** (periartiolar lymphoid sheath) between the **red pulp** and **white pulp,** that is rich in B cells and contains lymphoid follicles, which can develop into **germinal centers** (see Figure 2-19).
Margination Accumulation of lymphocytes at the wall of blood vessels as an early result of inflammation.
Mast cell A bone-marrow-derived cell present in a variety of tissues that resembles peripheral-blood basophils, bears **Fc receptors** for IgE, and undergoes IgE-mediated **degranulation.**
Medulla The innermost or central region of an organ.
Megakaryocyte A white blood cell that produces **platelets** by cytoplasmic budding.
Membrane-attack complex (MAC) The complex of complement components C5–C9, which is formed in the terminal steps of either the classical or the alternative complement pathway and mediates cell lysis by creating a membrane pore in the target cell.
Membrane-bound immunoglobulin A form of antibody that is bound to a cell as a transmembrane protein. It acts as the antigen-specific receptor of B cells.
Memory, immunologic The attribute of the immune system mediated by **memory cells** whereby a second encounter with an antigen induces a heightened state of immune reactivity.
Memory cells Lymphocytes generated following encounters with antigen that are characteristically long lived; they are more readily stimulated than naive lymphocytes and mediate a **secondary immune response** to subsequent encounters with the antigen.
Memory response See **Memory, immunologic.**
Mesangial cell A type of macrophage found in the kidney.
Metastasis The colonization by tumor cells of sites distant from the primary site.
MHC (major histocompatibility complex) A complex of genes encoding cell-surface molecules that are required for antigen presentation to T cells and for rapid graft rejection. It is called the H-2 complex in the mouse and the HLA complex in humans.
MHC molecules Proteins encoded by the major histocompatibility complex and classified as class I, class II, and class III MHC molecules.
MHC restriction The characteristic of T cells that permits them to recognize antigen only after it is processed and the resulting antigenic peptides are displayed in association with either a **class I** or a **class II MHC molecule.**
Microglial cell A type of macrophage found in the central nervous system.
Minor histocompatibility loci Genes outside of the MHC that encode antigens contributing to graft rejection.
Minor lymphocyte stimulating (Mls) determinants Antigenic determinants encoded by endogenous retroviruses of the murine mammary tumor virus family that are displayed on the surface of certain cells.
Mitogen Any substance that nonspecifically induces DNA synthesis and cell division, especially of lymphocytes. Common mitogens are concanavalin A, phytohemagglutinin, **LPS,** pokeweed mitogen, and various **superantigens.**
Mixed-lymphocyte reaction (MLR) In vitro T-cell proliferation in response to cells expressing allogeneic MHC molecules (see Figure 14-13); can be used as an assay for class II MHC activity.
Monoclonal Derived from a single cell.
Monoclonal antibody Homogeneous preparation of antibody molecules, produced by a single clone of B lineage cells, often a hybridoma, all of which have the same antigenic specificity (see Figure 4-22).
Monocyte A mononuclear phagocytic leukocyte that circulates briefly in the bloodstream before migrating into the tissues where it becomes a **macrophage.**
Monokine A cytokine produced by macrophages. This term has been largely superseded by the term *cytokine.*
Mucin A group of serine- and threonine-rich proteins that are heavily glycosylated. They are ligands for selectins.
Multilineage CSF (M-CSF) A cytokine that supports the differentiation and growth of a number of myeloid cell lineages.
Multiple myeloma A plasma-cell cancer.
Multiple sclerosis (MS) An autoimmune disease that affects the central nervous system. In Western countries, it is the most common cause of neurologic disability caused by disease.
Myasthenia gravis An autoimmune disease mediated by antibodies that block the acetylcholine receptors on the motor end plates of muscles, resulting in progressive weakening of the skeletal muscles.
Myeloid stem cell A cell that can give rise to many types of myeloid cells.
Myeloma cell A cancerous plasma cell.
Myeloma protein A monoclonal immunoglobulin produced by a myeloma cell.

N-addition The addition of nucleotides by terminal deoxynucleotidyl transferase during the process of D-J joining or V-to-DJ joining.
Naive Denoting mature B and T cells that have not encountered antigen; synonymous with unprimed and virgin.
Natural killer (NK) cells A class of large granular cytotoxic lymphocytes that do not have T- or B-cell receptors. They are antibody-independent killers of tumor cells and also can participate in **antibody-dependent cell-mediated cytotoxicity.**
Necrosis Morphologic changes that accompany death of individual cells or groups of cells and that release large amounts of intracellular components to the environment, leading to disruption and atrophy of tissue. See also **Apoptosis.**
Negative selection The induction of death in lymphocytes bearing receptors that react too strongly with self antigens.
Neoplasm Any new and abnormal growth; a benign or malignant tumor.
Network theory The theory that the immune system is regulated by a network of idiotype and anti-idiotype reactions involving antibodies and T-cell receptors. See also **Anti-idiotype antibody.**

Neutrophil A circulating, phagocytic granulocyte involved early in the **inflammatory response** (see Figure 2-10). It expresses **Fc receptors** and can participate in **antibody-dependent cell-mediated cytotoxicity.** Neutrophils are the most numerous white blood cells in the circulation.
Nitric oxide (NO) A gas that plays important roles in intercellular signaling.
Nitric oxide synthetase An enzyme that catalyzes the transformation of L-arginine, oxygen, and NADPH to **nitric oxide (NO),** L-citrulline, and NADP.
N-nucleotides Nucleotides added by the enzyme terminal deoxynucleotidyl transferase (TdT) to the 3′ cut ends of V, D, and J coding segments during rearrangement.
NK1-T cell A lymphocyte with some of the characteristics of T cells (it has T-cell receptors) as well as those of natural killer cells.
Nonidentity The failure to form lines of **identity** during the immunoprecipitation analysis known as **Ouchterlony analysis.**
Nonproductive rearrangement Rearrangements in which gene segments are joined out of phase so that the triplet-reading frame for translation is not preserved.
Nonsequential epitopes Epitopes that are far apart in the primary sequence of the polypeptide chain but close together in the tertiary structure of the molecule.
Northern blotting Common technique for detecting specific mRNAs in which denatured mRNAs are separated electrophoretically and then transferred to a polymer sheet, which is incubated with a radiolabeled DNA probe specific for the mRNA of interest.
N-region nucleotides See **N-nucleotides.**
Nude mouse Homozygous genetic defect (*nu/nu*) carried by an inbred mouse strain that results in the absence of the thymus and consequently a marked deficiency of T cells and cell-mediated immunity. The mice are hairless (hence, the name) and can accept grafts from other species.
Null cell A small population of peripheral-blood lymphocytes that lack the membrane markers characteristic of B and T cells. **Natural killer cells** are included in this group.

Oncofetal tumor antigen An antigen that is present during fetal development but generally is not expressed in tissues except by tumor cells. Alpha-feto protein (AFP) and carcinoembryonic antigen (CEA) are two examples that have been associated with various cancers (see Table 22-3).
Oncogene A gene that encodes a protein capable of inducing cellular **transformation.** Oncogenes derived from viruses are written v-*onc;* their counterparts **(proto-oncogenes)** in normal cells are written c-*onc.*
Oncogenic Causing cancer.
One-turn recombination signal sequences Immunoglobulin gene-recombination signal sequences separated by an intervening sequence of 12 base pairs.
Opsonin A substance (e.g., an antibody or C3b) that promotes the phagocytosis of antigens by binding to them.
Opsonization Deposition of opsonins on an antigen, thereby promoting a stable adhesive contact with an appropriate phagocytic cell (see Figure 13-12).
Osteoclast A bone macrophage.
Ouchterlony analysis A double immunodiffusion technique involving the diffusion of antigen and antibody within a gel resulting in formation of a visible band of precipitate in the region of **equivalence** (see Figure 6-6).

P-addition Addition of nucleotides from cleaved hairpin loops formed by the junction of V-D or D-J gene segments during Ig or TCR gene rearrangements.
PALS (periarteriolar lymphoid sheath) See **White pulp.**
Paracortex An area of the lymph node beneath the cortex that is populated mostly by T cells and interdigitating dendritic cells.
Paracrine Regulatory secretions, such as cytokines, that arrive by diffusion from a nearby cellular source.
Paratope The site in the variable (V) domain of an antibody or T-cell receptor that binds to an epitope on an antigen.
Parenterally Introduction of materials through blood vessels or tissues rather than through the gastrointestinal tract.
Partial identity A condition encountered in **Ouchterlony analysis** that occurs when two antigens share some epitopes but one or the other has (a) unique epitope(s). The antiserum forms a line of identity with the common epitope(s) and a curved spur with the unique epitope(s).
Passive immunity Adaptive immunity conferred by the transfer of immune products, such as antibody or sensitized T cells, from an immune individual to a nonimmune one. See also **Active immunity.**
Passive immunization The acquisition of immunity by receipt of preformed antibodies rather than by active production of antibodies after exposure to antigen.
Pathogen A disease-causing organism.
Pax-5 gene This gene encodes B-cell-specific activator protein (BSAP), an essential transcription factor for B-cell development.
Perforin Cytolytic product of CTLs that, in the presence of Ca^{2+}, polymerizes to form transmembrane pores in target cells (see Figure 14-7).
Periarteriolar lymphoid sheath (PALS) See **White pulp.**
Peyer's patches Lymphoid follicles located along the wall of the small intestine that trap antigens from the gastrointestinal tract and provide sites where B and T cells can interact with antigen.
Phagocyte Cell with the capacity to internalize and degrade microbes or particulate antigens; neutrophils and monocytes are the main phagocytes.
Phagocytosis The uptake of particulate materials by cells by engulfment (see Figure 1-13).
Phagolysosome An intracellular body formed by the fusion of a phagosome with a lysosome.
Phagosome Intracellular vacuole containing ingested particulate materials; formed by the fusion of pseudopodia around a particle undergoing **phagocytosis.**
Phycoerythrin A light-gathering plant protein that is an efficient absorber of light and a brilliant emitter of red fluorescence; it is widely used as a label for immunofluorescence.
Phylogeny The evolutionary history of a species.
Pili Hairlike projections on gram-negative bacterial cells. Among functions of pili are adhesion to cells or tissues or exchange of genetic information in bacterial conjugation.
Pinocytosis A type of **endocytosis** in which a cell ingests extracellular fluid and the materials dissolved in it.
P-K reaction Prausnitz-Kustner reaction, local skin reaction to allergen by a normal subject at the site of injected IgE from an allergic individual. (No longer used because of risk of transmitting hepatitis or AIDS).

Plaque-forming count (PFC) The number of plaques formed in the in vitro **hemolytic plaque assay,** which detects antibody-forming plasma cells.

Plasma The cell-free, fluid portion of blood, which contains all the clotting factors.

Plasma cell The antibody-secreting effector cell of the B lineage.

Plasmacytoma A plasma-cell cancer.

Plasmid A small circular extrachromasomal DNA that replicates autonomously in *E. coli.* Frequently used as a cloning vector for the introduction of small pieces of foreign DNA into bacteria.

Plasmin A serine protease formed by cleavage of plasminogen. Its major function is the hydrolysis of fibrin.

Platelet A small cytoplasmic structure, derived from megakaryocytes, that contains vasoactive substances and clotting factors important in blood coagulation, inflammation, and allergic reactions; also called thrombocyte.

P-nucleotides Nucleotides added during **P-addition.**

Polyclonal Involving or arising from more than a single clone of cells.

Polyclonal antibody A mixture of antibodies produced by a variety of B-cell clones that have recognized the same antigen. Although all of the antibodies react with the immunizing antigen, they differ from each other in amino acid sequence.

Polygenic Several nonallelic genes encode the same or similar proteins. Also any trait that is due to inheritance of more than one gene.

Poly-Ig receptor A receptor for polymeric Ig molecules (IgA or IgM) that is expressed on the basolateral surface of most mucosal epithelial cells. It transports polymeric Ig across epithelia.

Polymorphism Presence of multiple **alleles** at a specific genetic locus. The major histocompatibility complex is highly polymorphic.

Positive selection A process that permits the survival of only those T cells whose T-cell receptors recognize self-MHC.

Postcapillary venules The blood vessels that contain the layer of specialized endothelial cells across which lymphocytes migrate from the blood into a lymph node.

Pre-B cell (precursor B cell) The stage of B-cell development that follows the pro-B cell stage. Pre-B cells produce cytoplasmic μ heavy chains and most display the pre–B-cell receptor.

Pre–B-cell receptor A complex of the Igα/Igβ heterodimer with membrane-bound Ig consisting of the μ heavy chain bound to the **surrogate light chain** Vpre-B/λ5.

Precipitin An antibody that aggregates a soluble antigen, forming a macromolecular complex that yields a visible precipitate.

P-region nucleotide addition See **P-addition.**

Pre–T-cell receptor (pre-TCR) A complex of the CD3 group with a structure consisting of the T-cell receptor β chain complexed with a 33 kDa glycoprotein called the pre-Tα chain.

Primary follicle A lymphoid follicle, prior to stimulation with antigen, that contains a network of follicular dendritic cells and small resting B cells.

Primary immune response The immune response that is induced by initial exposure to an antigen, which activates naive lymphocytes. It is mediated largely by IgM antibody and sensitized T cells. It develops more slowly and to a lesser extent than a **secondary immune response** (see Figure 11-15).

Primary lymphoid organs Organs in which lymphocyte precursors mature into antigenically committed, immunocompetent cells. In mammals, the bone marrow and thymus are the primary lymphoid organs in which B-cell and T-cell maturation occur, respectively.

Pro-B cell (progenitor B cell) The earliest distinct cell of the B-cell lineage.

Productive rearrangement The joining of V(D)J gene segments in phase to produce a VJ or V(D)J unit that can be translated in its entirety.

Progenitor cell A cell that has lost the capacity for self renewal and is committed to the generation of a particular cell lineage.

Programmed cell death An induced and ordered process in which the cell actively participates in bringing about its own death.

Promoter A short sequence of DNA about 200 base pairs upstream from the transcription sequence that promotes initiation of RNA transcription in a specific direction.

Prostaglandins A group of biologically active lipid derivatives of arachidonic acid (see Figure 15-11). They mediate the inflammatory response and type I hypersensitivity reaction by inhibiting platelet aggregation, increasing vascular permeability, and inducing smooth-muscle contraction.

Proteasome A large multifunctional protease complex responsible for degradation of intracellular proteins (see Figure 8-5).

Proto-oncogene A cancer-associated gene that encodes a factor that regulates cell proliferation, survival, or death; it is required for normal cell function (see Table 22-1) but, if mutated or produced in inappropriate amounts, it becomes an oncogen, which can cause transformation of the cell (see Figure 22-2).

Provirus Viral DNA that is integrated into host-cell genome in a latent state and must undergo activation before it is transcribed, leading to formation of viral particles.

Prozone effect The apparent decrease in an antigen-antibody reaction sometimes observed as the concentration of antigen or antibody is increased.

Pseudogene Nucleotide sequence that is a stable component of the genome but is incapable of being expressed. They are thought to have been derived by mutation of ancestral active genes.

Pseudopodia Membrane protrusions that extend from motile and phagocytosing cells.

Pyrogen A fever-causing substance released by activated leukocytes.

Pyrogenic Pus producing.

Radial immunodiffusion A method for determining the relative concentration of an antigen. The antigen sample is placed in a well and allowed to diffuse into agar containing a suitable dilution of an antiserum. The area of the precipitin ring that forms around the well in the region of equivalence is proportional to the concentration of antigen.

Radioimmunoassay (RIA) A highly sensitive technique for measuring antigen or antibody that involves competitive binding of radiolabeled antigen or antibody (see Figure 6-10).

RAG (recombination-activating genes) Two closely linked genes, *RAG-1* and *RAG-2,* that encode proteins essential for the rearrangement of immunoglobulin gene segments in the assembly of a functional immunoglobulin gene.

Reactive nitrogen intermediates Highly cytotoxic antimicrobial compounds formed by the combination of oxygen and nitrogen within phagocytes such as neutrophils and macrophages.

Reactive oxygen intermediates (ROIs) Highly reactive compounds such as superoxide anion (O_2^-), hydroxyl radicals ($OH^·$), and hydrogen peroxide (H_2O_2) that are formed under many conditions in cells and tissues.

Reagin IgE antibody that mediates type I immediate **hypersensitivity.**
Receptor, cell-surface Molecule present on the cell membrane that has a high affinity for a particular ligand.
Recombinant congenic Mouse strains obtained in the process of deriving a congenic strain that differ in the portion of the gene region from the donor strain present (see Figure 7-4)
Recombination-activating genes See **RAG.**
Recombination signal sequences (RSSs) Highly conserved heptamer and nonamer nucleotide sequences that serve as signals for the gene rearrangement process and flank each germline V, D, and J segment (see Figure 5-6).
Red pulp Portion of the spleen consisting of a network of sinusoids populated by macrophages and erythrocytes (see Figure 2-19). It is the site where old and defective red blood cells are destroyed.
Relative risk Probability that an individual with a given trait (usually, but not exclusively, a genetic trait) will acquire a disease compared with those in the same population group who lack that trait.
Respiratory burst A metabolic process in activated phagocytes in which the rapid uptake of oxygen is used to produce reactive oxygen intermediates that are toxic to ingested microorganisms.
Retrovirus A type of RNA virus that uses a reverse transcriptase to produce a DNA copy of its RNA genome. HIV, which causes AIDS, and HTLV, which causes adult T-cell leukemia, are both retroviruses.
Rh antigen Any of a large number of antigens present on the surface of blood cells that constitute the Rh blood group. See also **Erythroblastosis fetalis.**
Rheumatoid arthritis A common autoimmune disorder, primarily affecting women 40 to 60 years old, causing chronic inflammation of the joints.
Rheumatoid factor Autoantibody found in the serum of individuals with rheumatoid arthritis and other connective-tissue diseases.
Rhodamine An organic dye that absorbs in the yellow-green range (515 nm) and emits a deep red fluorescence (546 nm). Because it fluoresces at a different wavelength, it is often paired with **fluorescein** in two-color **immunofluorescence** assays.
Rhogam Antibody against **Rh antigen** that is used to prevent **erythroblastosis fetalis.**
RNA splicing The processing of primary RNA transcripts to remove sequences transcribed from intronic DNA and to connect sequences transcribed from exons to generate a messenger RNA.
Rocket electrophoresis The electrophoresis of a sample of negatively charged antigen in a gel that contains antibody. The precipitate formed between antigen and antibody has the shape of a rocket, whose height is proportional to the concentration of antigen in the sample.
Rous sarcoma virus (RSV) A retrovirus that induces tumors in avian species.

Sarcoma Tumor of supporting or connective tissue.
Scatchard equation The equation, $(r/c) = K_a n - K_a r$, where r = ratio of the concentration of bound ligand to total antibody concentration, c = concentration of free ligand, and n = number of binding sites per antibody molecule, allows calculation of the affinity constants of antigen with antibody.
Schistosomiasis A disease caused by the parasitic worm *Schistoma.*
SCID (severe combined immunodeficiency) A condition in which adaptive immune responses do not occur because of a lack of B and T lymphocytes.
SCID-human mouse Immunodeficient mouse into which elements of a human immune system such as bone marrow and thymic fragments have been grafted. Such mice support the differentiation of pluripotent human hematopoietic stem cells into mature immunocytes and so are valuable for studies on lymphocyte development.
SDS-polyacrylamide gel electrophoresis (SDS-PAGE) An electrophoretic method for the separation of proteins. It employs SDS to denature proteins and give them negative charges; when SDS-denatured proteins are electrophoresed through polymerized-acrylamide gels, they separate according to their molecular weights.
Sebum Acidic secretion of sebaceous glands within the dermis.
Second-set graft rejection Acute, rapid rejection of an allograft in an individual who has received a previous graft from the same donor (see Figure 21-1c). The reaction is mediated by primed T cells.
Secondary follicle A primary follicle after antigenic stimulation; it develops into a ring of concentrically packed B cells surrounding a germinal center.
Secondary immune response The immune response that is induced by a second exposure to antigen, which activates memory lymphocytes. It occurs more rapidly and is stronger than the **primary immune response** (see Figure 11-15).
Secondary lymphoid organs Organs and tissues in which mature, immunocompetent lymphocytes encounter trapped antigens and are activated into **effector cells.** In mammals, the **lymph nodes, spleen,** and mucosal-associated lymphoid tissue **(MALT)** constitute the secondary lymphoid organs.
Secreted immunoglobulin (sIg) The form of antibody that is secreted by cells of the B lineage, especially plasma cells. This form of Ig lacks a transmembrane domain.
Secretory component A fragment of the **poly-Ig receptor** that remains bound to Ig after transcytosis across an epithelium and cleavage (see Figure 4-15).
Secretory IgA J chain-linked dimers or higher polymers of IgA that have transited epithelia and retain a bound remnant of the **poly-Ig receptor** (see Figure 4-15).
Selectin One of a group of monomeric **cell-adhesion molecules** present on leukocytes (L-selectin) and endothelium (E- and P-selectin) that bind to mucin-like CAMs (e.g., GlyCam, PSGL-1) (see Figure 15-2).
Self-tolerance Unresponsiveness to self antigens.
Sequential epitopes Two or more antigenic determinants formed by a single sequence of amino acids.
Serum Fluid portion of the blood, which is free of cells and clotting factors.
Serum sickness A type III hypersensitivity reaction that develops when antigen is administered intravenously, resulting in the formation of large amounts of antigen antibody complexes and their deposition in tissues. It often develops when individuals are immunized with antiserum derived from other species.
Severe combined immunodeficiency See **(SCID).**
Signal joint In V(D)J gene rearrangement, the sequence formed by the union of recombination signal sequences.
Signal peptide A small sequence of amino acids, also called the leader sequence, that guides the heavy or light chain through the

endoplasmic reticulum and is cleaved from the nascent chains before assembly of the finished immunoglobulin molecule.
Signal-transducing subunit The chain of a multimeric cytokine receptor that, on binding of the ligand, activates the cytokine-mediated signal-transduction pathway.
Silencers Nucleotide sequences that down-regulate transcription, operating in both directions over a distance.
Single-positive CD4$^+$ Thymocytes that express a CD4 coreceptor.
Single-positive CD8$^+$ Thymocytes that express a CD8 coreceptor.
Slow-reacting substance of anaphylaxis (SRS-A) The collective term applied to leukotrienes that mediate inflammation.
Somatic hypermutation The induced increase of mutation, 10^5- to 10^6-fold over the background rate, in the regions in and around rearranged immunoglobulin genes. In animals such as humans and mice, somatic hypermutation occurs in germinal centers.
Somatic mutation A mechanism by which point mutations are introduced into rearranged immunoglobulin variable-region genes during activation and proliferation of B cells. It contributes significantly to antibody diversity.
Somatic-variation theories Theories maintaining that the genome contains a small number of immunoglobulin genes from which a large number of antibody specificities are generated in somatic cells by mutation or recombination.
Southern blotting A common technique for detecting specific DNA sequences in which restriction-enzyme fragments are separated electrophoretically, then denatured and transferred to a polymer sheet, which is incubated with a radioactive probe specific for the sequence of interest (see Figure 23-12).
Sox-4 A transcription factor that is essential for the early stages of B-cell development.
Specificity, antigenic Capacity of antibody and T-cell receptor to recognize and interact with a single, unique **antigenic determinant.**
Spleen Secondary lymphoid organ where old erythrocytes are destroyed and blood-borne antigens are trapped and presented to lymphocytes in the PALS and marginal zone (see Figure 2-19).
STAT (signal transducer and activator of transcription) A family of transcription factors that bind to the phosphorylated tyrosine residues of certain receptors at their SH_2 domains. These molecules play an essential role in the transduction of signals from a wide variety of cytokines.
Stem cell A cell from which differentiated cells derive.
Stromal cell A nonhematopoietic cell that supports the growth and differentiation of hematopoietic cells.
Superantigen Any substance that binds to the V_β domain of the T-cell receptor and residues in the α chain of class II MHC molecules (see Figure 10-16). It induces activation of all T cells that express T-cell receptors with a particular V_β domain. It functions as potent T-cell **mitogen** and may cause food poisoning and other disorders.
Surrogate light chain The polypeptides **Vpre-B** and **λ5** that associate with mu heavy chains during the pre–B-cell stage of B-cell development to form the pre–B-cell receptor.
Switch regions In class switching, DNA sequences located in the intron 5′ of each C_H segment (except C_δ).
Synergism Occurs when the combined action of two different cytokines is greater than the sum of their actions alone.
Syngeneic Denoting genetically identical individuals.
Systemic lupus erythematosus (SLE) An autoimmune disease characterized by autoantibodies to a vast array of tissue antigens such as DNA, histones, RBCs, platelets, leukocytes, and clotting factors.

T-B conjugate The antigen-specific association between an antigen-presenting B cell and a T_H cell specific for the presented antigenic peptide.
T cell A lymphocyte that matures in the thymus and expresses a T-cell receptor, CD3, and CD4 or CD8. Several distinct T-cell subpopulations are recognized.
T-cell receptor (TCR) Antigen-binding molecule expressed on the surface of T cells and associated with **CD3.** It is a heterodimer consisting of either an α and β chain or a γ and δ chain (see Figures 9-3 and 9-9).
T cytotoxic (T_C) cells T cells that kill target cells in an antigen-specific manner.
T_{DTH} cell Generally a CD4$^+$ lymphocyte derived from a T_H cell that mediates **delayed-type hypersensitivity.**
T_H1 response This response produces a cytokine profile that supports inflammation and cell mediated responses. It is antagonistic to the T_H2 response.
T_H1 subset Subset of T helper cells responsible for the T_H1 response (see Table 12-4).
T_H2 response This response produces a cytokine profile that activates mainly immune responses that depend upon antibodies. It is antagonistic to the T_H1 response.
T_H2 subset Subset of T helper cells responsible for the T_H2 response (see Table 12-4).
T helper (T_H) cells T cells that are stimulated by antigen to provide signals that promote immune responses.
T lymphocytes (T cells) Lymphocytes that mature in the thymus and have T-cell receptors.
T suppressor (T_S) cells A population of T cells postulated to be distinct from (T_H) and (T_C) cells that suppress the humoral and cell-mediated branches of the immune system in an antigen specific manner.
TAP (transporters associated with antigen processing) Heterodimeric proteins present in the membrane of the rough endoplasmic reticulum (RER) that transport peptides into the lumen of the RER where they bind to class I MHC molecules.
Tapasin Protein associated with class I MHC molecules and TAP during processing of antigen in the cytosolic pathway.
TdT (terminal deoxynucleotidyl transferase) An enzyme that adds deoxynucleotide triphosphates to the 3′ ends of DNA.
Tertiary lymphoid tissues Tissues that normally contain few lymphoid cells, lack the elaborate organization of secondary lymphoid tissue, and import lymphoid cells during an inflammatory response.
Thoracic duct The largest of the lymphatic vessels. It returns lymph to the circulation by emptying into the left subclavian vein near the heart.
Thromboxane Lipid inflammatory mediator derived from arachidonic acid (see Figure 15-11).
Thy-1 Glycoprotein that is the earliest surface marker to appear in the T-cell lineage.
Thymocyte Developing T cells present in the thymus.
Thymus A primary lymphoid organ, located in the thoracic cavity, where T-cell maturation takes place.

Thymus-dependent antigen A soluble protein that can induce antibody production only with help of T_H cells; response to such antigens involves isotype switching, affinity maturation, and memory-cell production (see Table 11-2).
Thymus-dependent area The paracortex of a lymph node.
Thymus-independent (TI) antigen B-cell responses to TI antigens do not require the help of T cells. There are two types of TI antigens: most TI-1 antigens are polyclonal B-cell activators and act without regard to the antigenic specificity of the B cell; TI-2 antigens activate B cells by extensively crosslinking the mIg receptor, and they evoke antigen-specific responses. See Table 11-2.
Thymus-independent area The cortex of a lymph node.
Tingible-body macrophage A macrophage found in germinal centers that phagocytoses dying lymphocytes.
Titer A measure of the relative strength of an antiserum. The titer is the reciprocal of the last dilution of an antiserum capable of mediating some measurable effect such as precipitation or agglutination.
Tolerance A state of immunologic unresponsiveness to particular antigens or sets of antigens. Typically, an organism is unresponsive or tolerant to self antigens.
Tonsils Nodular structures containing a meshwork of reticular cells and fibers that contain lymphocytes, macrophages, granulocytes, and mast cells. They defend the body against antigens entering through nasal and oral routes.
Toxoid A toxin that has been altered to eliminate its toxicity but that still can function as an **immunogen.**
Trafficking The differential migration of lymphoid cells to and from different tissues.
Transcytosis The movement of antibody molecules (polymeric IgA or IgM) across epithelial layers mediated by the poly-Ig receptor.
Transfection Experimental introduction of foreign DNA into cultured cells, usually followed by expression of the genes in the introduced DNA (see Figure 23-16).
Transformation Change that a normal cell undergoes as it becomes malignant; also, permanent, heritable alteration in a cell resulting from the uptake and incorporation of foreign DNA into the genome.
Transgene A cloned foreign gene present in an animal or plant.
Transgenic mouse A mouse carrying a transgene, which has been introduced and stably incorporated into germ-line cells so that it can be passed on to progeny (see Figure 23-17). See also **Knockout mouse.**
Tuberculin Crude protein fraction isolated from supernatant of *Mycobacterium tuberculosis* cultures. It can be used in a skin test for exposure to *M. tuberculosis.*
Tuberculoid leprosy Form of leprosy that is more contained and controlled than the lepromatous form. See **Lepromatous leprosy.**
Tumor antigens Cell-surface proteins present on the surface of tumor cells that can induce a cell-mediated immune response. Some are found only on tumor cells; others are also found on normal cells (see Figure 22-6).
Tumor necrosis factors (TNFs) Two related **cytokines** produced by macrophages (TNF-α) and some T cells (TNF-β). Both factors are cytotoxic to tumor cells but not to normal cells; they also play a role in inflammatory responses.
Tumor-associated transplantation antigens (TATAs) Antigens that are expressed on particular tumors or types of tumors that are not unique to tumor cells. They are generally absent from or expressed at low levels on most normal adult cells.
Tumor-infiltrating lymphocytes (TILs) Lymphocyte populations with anti-tumor activity obtained by taking small biopsy samples of tumors and expanding them in vitro with the aid of IL-2.
Tumor-specific transplantation antigens (TSTAs) Antigens that are unique to tumor cells.
Tumor-suppressor genes Genes that encode products that inhibit excessive cell proliferation.
Two-turn recombination signal sequences Immunoglobulin gene recombination signal sequences separated by an intervening sequence of 23 base pairs.

V (variable) gene segment The 5′ coding portion of rearranged immunoglobulin and T-cell receptor genes. There are multiple V gene segments in germ-line DNA, but gene rearrangement leaves only one segment in each functional gene.
V regions The amino-terminal domain of an immunoglobulin molecule; it consists of 100–110 amino acids and contains the CDRs that make up the antigen-binding site.
V(D)J recombinase The set of enzymatic activities that collectively bring about the joining of gene segments into a rearranged V(D)J unit.
Vaccination Intentional administration of a harmless or less harmful form of a pathogen to induce a specific immune response that protects the individual against later exposure to the same pathogen.
Vaccine A preparation of antigenic material used to induce immunity against pathogenic organisms.
Valence, valency Numerical measure of combining capacity, generally equal to the number of binding sites. Antibody molecules are bivalent or multivalent, whereas T-cell receptors are univalent.
Variable (V) region Amino-terminal portion of immunoglobulin and T-cell receptor chains that are highly variable and responsible for the **antigenic specificity** of these molecules.
Variolation Inoculation with smallpox; used to describe early attempts to cause immunity to smallpox by inoculation with crusts or exudates from smallpox lesions.
Vascular addressins Tissue-specific adhesion molecules that direct the extravasation of different populations of circulating lymphocytes into particular lymphoid organs.
Veiled cell A morphologic variation of Langerhans cells that are moving from sites of antigen acquisition to secondary lymphoid tissues; the dendritic extensions that these cells wrap around themselves produce a veiled appearance.
Virgin See **Naive.**
Virulence A measure of the infectious ability of a pathogen.
Vpre-B A polypeptide chain that together with **λ5** forms the **surrogate light chain** of the **pre–B-cell receptor.**

Western blotting A common technique for detecting a protein in a mixture; the proteins are separated electrophoretically and then transferred to a polymer sheet, which is flooded with radiolabeled or enzyme-conjugated antibody specific for the protein of interest (see Figure 6-13).
Wheal and flare reaction Characteristic type I hypersensitivity response that of the skin, appearing as a sharply delineated swelling of the skin (wheal) with surrounding redness (flare).
White pulp Portion of the spleen that surrounds the arteries,

forming a periarteriolar lymphoid sheath (PALS) populated mainly by T cells (see Figure 2-49).

Xenogeneic Denoting individuals of different species.
Xenograft Graft or tissue transplanted from one species to another.
X-linked hyper-IgM syndrome An immunodeficiency disorder in which T_H cells fail to express CD40L. Patients with this disorder produce IgM but not other isotypes, they do not develop germinal centers or display somatic hypermutation, and they fail to generate memory B cells.

X-linked severe combined immunodeficiency (XSCID) Immunodeficiency resulting from inherited mutations in the common γ chain of the receptor for IL-2, 4, 7, 9 and 15 that impair its ability to transmit signals from the receptor to intracellular proteins.

ZAP-70 (ξ associated protein) A 70-kDa polypeptide that becomes an active tyrosine kinase when it binds to the ITAMs of the ξ chain and undergoes phosphorylation.

ANSWERS TO STUDY QUESTIONS

Chapter 1

1. (a) CM. (b) H and CM. (c) H and CM. (d) H and CM. (e) CM. (f) CM. (g) H. (h) CM. (i) H. (j) H. (k) CM.

2. The four immunologic attributes are specificity, diversity, memory, and self/nonself recognition. Specificity refers to the ability of certain membrane-bound molecules on a mature lymphocyte to recognize only a single antigen (or small number of closely related antigens). Rearrangement of the immunoglobulin genes during lymphocyte maturation gives rise to antigenic specificity; it also generates a vast array of different specificities, or diversity, among mature lymphocytes. The ability of the immune system to respond to nonself molecules, but (generally) not to self-molecules, results from the elimination during lymphocyte maturation of immature cells that recognize self-antigens. After exposure to a particular antigen, mature lymphocytes reactive with that antigen proliferate and differentiate, generating a larger population of memory cells with the same specificity; this expanded population can respond more rapidly and intensely after a subsequent exposure to the same antigen, thus displaying immunologic memory.

3. The secondary immune response involves an amplified population of memory cells. The response is more rapid and achieves higher levels than the primary response.

4. (a) Both antibodies and T-cell receptors display fine specificity for antigen; very small modifications in an antigen can prohibit its binding to its corresponding antibody or T-cell receptor. MHC molecules do not possess such fine specificity, and a variety of unrelated peptide antigens can be bound by the same MHC molecule. (b) Antibodies are expressed only by cells of the B-cell lineage; T-cell receptors are expressed by cells of the T-cell lineage; class I MHC molecules are expressed by virtually all nucleated cells; class II MHC molecules are expressed only by specialized cells that function as antigen-presenting cells (e.g., B cells, macrophages, and dendritic cells). (c) Antibodies can bind to protein or polysaccharide antigens; T-cell receptors recognize only peptides associated with MHC molecules; MHC molecules bind only processed peptides.

5. (a) Macrophages, B cells, dendritic cells. (b) Co-stimulatory; T_H cells. (c) II; I. (d) Exogenous; endocytic processing pathway; II. (e) Endogenous; cytoplasm; I.

6. During the inflammatory response, the diameter of the capillaries in the affected region increases (vasodilation), as does their permeability, which facilitates an influx of white blood cells, particularly phagocytes.

7. They can recognize only antigen that is associated with class I MHC molecules.

8. (a) 13. (b) 19. (c) 6. (d) 12. (e) 2. (f) 18. (g) 8. (h) 15. (i) 4. (j) 14. (k) 7. (l) 9. (m) 17. (n) 5. (o) 3. (p) 10.

9. Innate and adaptive immunity cooperate to give a complete protective response against pathogens. An example is the phagocytic cell, which takes up foreign material and processes it to form peptide antigens that are presented by the phagocyte. The presented antigens stimulate T cells that either provide help to B cells for production of antibody or stimulate cytotoxic T cells to provide protection against infected or cancerous cells. In addition, the phagocytic cells take part in inflammation, producing cytokines that attract T cells and B cells to the site.

10. Invertebrate animals may protect themselves against environmental pathogens with simple forms of innate immunity. For example, the fruit fly produces peptides with antifungal activity. These small molecules protect the insect from a fungal pathogen commonly encountered in its environment. Plant immunity is similar in that plants also produce antimicrobial peptides and a host of other agents such as oxidizing radicals and enzymes that attack microbial cell walls. One of the many differences between plant and arthropod immunity is that plants lack phagocytic responses, which are present in arthropods (see Table 1-3).

11. Consequences of mild forms of immune dysfunction include sneezing, hives, and skin rashes caused by allergies. Asthma and anaphylactic reactions are more severe consequences of allergy and can result in death. Consequences of severe immune dysfunction include susceptibility to infection by a variety of microbial pathogens if the dysfunction involves immunodeficiency, or chronic debilitating diseases, such as rheumatoid arthritis, if the dysfunction involves autoimmunity. The most common cause of immunodeficiency is infection with the retrovirus HIV-1, which leads to AIDS.

Chapter 2

1. (a) In general, $CD4^+$ T cells that recognize class II MHC molecules function as T_H cells, whereas $CD8^+$ T cells that recognize class I MHC molecules function as T_C cells. However, some functional T_H cells express CD8 and are class I restricted, and some functional T_C cells express CD4 and are class II restricted. But these are exceptions to the general pattern. (b) The bone marrow contains few pluripotent stem cells, which constitute only about 0.05% of all bone-marrow cells. (c) T_H cells recognize antigen associated with class II MHC molecules. Activation of macrophages increases their expression of class II MHC molecules. (d) Organized lymphoid follicles are also present in the tonsils, Peyer's patches, and other mucosal-associated tissue. (e) In response to infection, T_H cells and macrophages are activated and secrete various

cytokines that induce increased hematopoietic activity. The induced hematopoiesis expands the population of white blood cells that can fight the infection. (f) Unlike other types of dendritic cells, follicular dendritic cells do not express class II MHC molecules and thus do not function as antigen-presenting cells for T_H-cell activation. These cells, which are present only in lymph follicles, can trap circulating antibody-antigen complexes; this ability is thought to facilitate B-cell activation and the development of memory B cells. (g) B and T lymphocytes have antigen-binding receptors, but a small population of lymphoid cells, called null cells, do not. (h) Although many animals, such as humans and mice, generate B cells in bone marrow, others, such as some ruminants, do not.

2. (a) T_H cells in paracortical areas; B cells in germinal centers within secondary follicles located in the node cortex. (b) T_H cells in paracortical areas. (c) No areas of rapid cell proliferation, since T_H cells are required for B-cell activation. (d) B cells in secondary follicles and germinal centers.

3. Monocyte progenitor cells have receptors for M-CSF; they do not secrete it. If both M-CSF and its receptor were expressed by these cells, they could stimulate their own proliferation.

4. The primary lymphoid organs are the bone marrow (bursa of Fabricius in birds) and the thymus. These organs function as sites for B-cell and T-cell maturation, respectively.

5. The secondary lymphoid organs are the spleen, lymph nodes, and mucosal-associated lymphoid tissue (MALT) in various locations. MALT includes the tonsils, Peyer's patches, and appendix, as well as loose collections of lymphoid cells associated with the mucous membranes lining the respiratory, digestive, and urogenital tracts. All these organs trap antigen and provide sites where lymphocytes can interact with antigen and subsequently undergo clonal expansion.

6. Stem cells are capable of self-renewal and can give rise to more than one cell type, whereas progenitor cells have lost the capacity for self-renewal and are committed to a single cell lineage. Commitment of progenitor cells depends on their acquisition of responsiveness to particular growth factors.

7. Nude mice and people with DiGeorge's syndrome have a congenital defect that prevents development of the thymus. Both lack circulating T cells and cannot mount cell-mediated immune responses.

8. The thymic stroma contains epithelial cells, interdigitating dendritic cells, and macrophages, which form a three-dimensional network. These cells secrete various hormonal factors that are necessary for thymocyte growth and maturation into immunocompetent T cells. Thymic stromal cells also play a role in the selection of T cells in the thymus.

9. b: The thymus of an individual reaches its maximal size during puberty. During the adult years, the thymus gradually atrophies.

10. The lethally irradiated mice serve as an assay system for pluripotent stem cells, since only mice injected with bone-marrow samples containing pluripotent stem cells will survive. As pluripotent stem cells are successively enriched in a bone-marrow sample, the total number of cells that must be injected to restore hematopoiesis decreases (see Figure 2-6).

11. In a neonatal mouse, thymectomy eliminates T-cell maturation, causing the animal to become immunodeficient and eventually to die. In an adult mouse, thymectomy does not have a profound effect because many of the recirculating T cells have a long life span and can respond to antigenic challenge by clonal selection.

12. The bursa of Fabricius in birds is the primary site where B lymphocytes develop. Bursectomy would result in a lack of circulating B cells and humoral immunity, and it would probably be fatal.

13. After phagocytosis by macrophages, most bacteria and fungi are destroyed and broken down; the resulting antigenic peptides are displayed along with class II MHC molecules on the cell surface, where they can induce T_H-cell activation and subsequent antibody (humoral) response. In contrast, intracellular bacteria and fungi have various mechanisms for surviving in macrophages after phagocytosis. These bacteria thus do not induce an antibody response.

14. (a) True. (b) False: The marginal zone is rich in B cells, and PALS is rich in T cells. (c) True. (d) True. (e) False: The spleen is not supplied with afferent lymphatics.

15. (a) 5. (b) 10. (c) 3. (d) 6. (e) 11. (f) 4. (g) 12. (h) 15. (i) 7. (j) 2. (k) 8. (l) 13. (m) 16.

Chapter 3

1. (a) True. (b) True. (c) False: A hapten cannot stimulate an immune response unless it is conjugated with a larger protein carrier. However, the hapten can combine with pre-formed antibody specific for the hapten. (d) True. (e) False: A T cell can recognize only peptides that have been processed and presented by MHC molecules. These epitopes tend to be internal peptides. (f) True. (g) True. (h) False: Each MHC molecule binds a number of different peptides. It is not yet known what features different peptides must have in common to be able to bind to the same MHC molecule. (i) False: Immunogens are capable of stimulating a specific immune response; antigens are capable of combining specifically with the antibodies or T-cell receptors induced during an immune response. Although all immunogens exhibit antigenicity, some antigens do not exhibit immunogenicity.

2. Probably not. In order to stimulate T_H-cell proliferation, the antigenic peptide must interact with class II MHC molecules expressed by the mice. Since IA^k and IA^d are encoded by allelic MHC genes and consequently exhibit allelic differences, they would most likely not bind the same hemagglutinin peptide. Thus, a peptide that is immunogenic for mice expressing IA^k probably would not be immunogenic for mice expressing IA^d.

3. (a) The UV-inactivated vaccine would be seen as an exogenous antigen. Exogenous antigens are internalized through phagocytosis or endocytosis and then are processed in the endocytic pathway. The resulting antigenic peptides are presented by class II MHC molecules on the surface of antigen-presenting cells. Since T_C cells are generally class I MHC restricted, they would not be activated by this type of vaccine, although class II MHC-restricted T_H cells might be. (b) Because the attenuated

virus replicates within host cells, it is seen as an endogenous antigen. Endogenous antigens are processed within the cytoplasm or endoplasmic reticulum and are presented by class I MHC molecules, which are present on the membrane of most nucleated cells. Therefore, the attenuated virus would be likely to activate T_C cells, which are class I MHC restricted.

4. (a) Native BSA: Heat denaturation is likely to destroy B-cell epitopes in a globular protein, although the T-cell epitopes are generally stable to heat. (b) HEL: The immunogenicity of an antigen generally is related to its foreignness to the animal exposed. However, collagen and some other proteins highly conserved throughout evolution exhibit little foreignness across diverse species and thus often are weak antigens. (c) 150,000-MW protein: Other things being equal, larger proteins are more immunogenic than smaller ones. (d) Copolymer that includes tyrosine residues: The immunogenicity of synthetic copolymers is increased by inclusion of aromatic residues.

5. b, d.

6. (a) T. (b) T. (c) B. (d) B. (e) T. (f) T. (g) BT. (h) B. (i) BT.

Chapter 4

1. (a) True. (b) False: An $HGPRT^-$ myeloma cell lacks the enzyme for utilizing hypoxanthine. (c) True. (d) False: Multiple isotypes can appear on the surface of a single B cell. A mature B cell expresses both IgM and IgD. A memory B cell can express additional isotypes, such as IgG. (e) True. (f) True. (g) True. (h) False: Secreted serum IgM is a pentamer. Because of its larger size and valency, IgM is more effective than IgG in cross-linking bacterial surface antigens, which leads to agglutination. (i) False: Hypoxanthine allows cell growth by the salvage pathway. (j) True. (k) False: Both heavy- and light-chain variable regions contain approximately 110 amino acids. (l) False: The unfused revertant would grow in HAT medium, making it impossible to select for the hybridomas.

2. (a) The molecule would have to possess the following structural features: 2 identical heavy chains and 2 identical light chains (H_2L_2); interchain disulfide bonds joining the heavy chains (H–H) and the heavy and light chains (H–L); a series of intrachain domains containing approximately 110 amino acids and stabilized by an intra-domain disulfide bridge forming a loop of about 60 amino acids; a single constant domain in the light chains and 3 or 4 constant domains in the heavy chains. The amino-terminal domain of both the heavy and the light chains should show sequence variation. (b) The antisera to both whole human IgG and human κ chain should cross-react with the new immunoglobulin class, since both of these antisera have antibodies specific for the light chain. The new isotype would be expected to contain either kappa or lambda light chains. (c) Reduce the interchain disulfide bonds of the new isotype with mercaptoethanol and alkylation. Separate the heavy and light chains. Immunize a rabbit with the heavy chain. The rabbit antisera should react with the new isotype but not with any other known isotypes.

3. IgM and IgD differ in their constant-region domains, whereas antigenic specificity is determined by the variable-region domains. Molecules of IgM and IgD that have different C domains but identical V_H and V_L domains are found on a given B cell; thus, the cell is unispecific although it bears two isotypes.

4. Advantages of IgG compared with IgM are (1) its ability to cross the placenta and protect the developing fetus; (2) its higher serum concentration, which results in IgG antibodies binding to and neutralizing more antigen molecules and being more effective in antigen clearance; (3) its smaller size, which enables IgG to diffuse more readily into intercellular fluids. The disadvantages of IgG compared with IgM are its lower capacity to (1) agglutinate antigens and (2) activate the complement system, both of which are due to the lower valency of IgG.

5. (a) See Figures 4-2 and 4-3. The number of interchain disulfide bonds joining the heavy chains varies among IgG subclasses (see Figure 4-14). (b) Draw as a dimer containing α heavy chains. Add J chain and secretory component (see Figure 4-15a). (c) Draw as a pentamer containing μ heavy chains. The μ heavy chain contains five domains and no hinge region; the extra C_H domain replaces the hinge. Add J chain. Pentameric IgM also has additional interchain disulfide bonds joining C_H domains in the subunits and the J chain to two of the subunits (see Figure 4-13e).

6.

Property	Whole IgG	H chain	L chain	Fab	F(ab')$_2$	Fc
Binds antigen	+	+/−	+/−	+	+	−
Bivalent antigen binding	+	−	−	−	+	−
Binds to Fc receptors	+	−	−	−	−	+
Fixes complement in presence of antigen	+	−	−	−	−	−
Has V domains	+	+	+	+	+	−
Has C domains	+	+	+	+	+	+

7. (a) AL. (b) ID. (c) IS. (d) AL. (e) No antibodies will be formed.

8.

	Rabbit antisera to mouse antibody component				
	γ chain	κ chain	IgG Fab fragment	IgG Fc fragment	J chain
Mouse γ chain	Yes	No	Yes	Yes	No

(continued)

	Rabbit antisera to mouse antibody component				
	γ chain	κ chain	IgG Fab fragment	IgG Fc fragment	J chain
Mouse κ chain	No	Yes	Yes	No	No
Mouse IgM whole	No	Yes	Yes	No	Yes
Mouse IgM/Fc fragment	Yes	No	No	Yes	No

9. Myeloma cells suitable for hybridoma production (1) exhibit immortal growth, enabling the hybridoma to be cultured indefinitely; (2) are Ab^-, ensuring that the hybridoma secretes only antibody characteristic of the plasma-cell fusion partner; and (3) are $HGPRT^-$, ensuring that unfused myeloma cells cannot grow in HAT-selection medium.

10. (a) Immunoglobulin-fold domains contain approximately 110 amino acid residues, which are arranged in two antiparallel β pleated sheets, each composed of multiple β strands separated by short loops of various lengths (see Figure 4-6). Each Ig-fold domain is stabilized by an intra-domain disulfide bond between two conserved cysteine residues about 60 residues apart. (b) See Figure 4-19. The Ig-fold domain structure is thought to facilitate interactions between domains; such interactions between nonhomologous domains may allow different members of the immunoglobulin superfamily to bind to each other.

11. The hypervariable regions, also called complementarity-determining regions (CDRs), are located in the loops of the immunoglobulin folds constituting the V_H and V_L domains (see Figures 4-6 and 4-8). There are three hypervariable regions in each V_H domain, and three in each V_L domain. Residues in the hypervariable regions constitute most of the amino acids involved in antigen binding.

12. In the absence of aminopterin, you could not select for the hybridoma because both the fused and unfused cells would grow using the de novo pathway.

13. (a) Some normal cells likely would be killed. Although an immunotoxin preferentially binds to tumor cells, the Fc region of the antibody component can bind to Fc receptors on various immune-system cells. If this occurs, then the toxin would be endocytosed and kill the normal cell. One way to avoid damage to normal cells is to engineer an immunotoxin in which the toxin chain replaces the Fc region of the antibody (see Figure 5-23c). (b) No. In an immunotoxin, the binding chain of the toxin, which allows it to enter cells, is replaced by a tumor-specific antibody, which targets the toxin to tumor cells (see Figure 4-23). Thus, if the antibody is degraded, the toxin will be unable to get into normal cells and kill them.

14. The antiserum would also contain antibodies to the kappa and lambda light chains, which are present in all isotypes. To prepare an IgG-specific antiserum, the investigator needs to reduce the interchain disulfide bonds in the mouse IgG with mercaptoethanol and isolate the heavy chain. Rabbits immunized with the mouse heavy chains alone will be specific for the IgG isotype.

15. (a) Four different antigen-binding sites (indicated in boldface) and 10 different antibody molecules: $\mathbf{H_sL_s}/H_sL_s$, $\mathbf{H_mL_m}/H_mL_m$, $\mathbf{H_sL_m}/H_sL_m$, $\mathbf{H_mL_s}/H_mL_s$, H_sL_s/H_mL_m, H_sL_s/H_sL_m, H_sL_s/H_mL_s, H_mL_m/H_sL_m, H_mL_m/H_mL_s, and H_sL_m/H_mL_s. (b) Two different antigen-binding sites and three different antibody molecules: $\mathbf{H_sL_s}/H_sL_s$, $\mathbf{H_mL_s}/H_mL_s$, and H_sL_s/H_mL_s. (c) One binding site and one antibody molecule: $\mathbf{H_sL_s}/H_sL_s$.

16. (a) 3, 6, 10, 11. (b) 4. (c) 2, 9, 12. (d) 5. (e) 1, 3, 4, 7, 8, 11.

Chapter 5

1. (a) False: V_κ gene segments and C_λ are located on separate chromosomes and cannot be brought together during gene rearrangement. (b) True. (c) True. (d) True. (e) True. (f) True.

2. V_H and J_H gene segments cannot join because both are flanked by recombination signal sequences (RSSs) containing a 23-bp (2-turn) spacer (see Figure 5-6b). According to the one-turn/two-turn joining rule, signal sequences having a two-turn spacer can join only with signal sequences having a one-turn (12-bp) spacer.

3. Light chains: $500\ V_L \times 4\ J_L = 2 \times 10^3$
Heavy chains: $300\ V_H \times 15\ D_H \times 4\ J_H = 1.8 \times 10^4$
Antibody molecules: $(2 \times 10^3\ \text{LCs}) \times (1.8 \times 10^4\ \text{HCs}) = 3.6 \times 10^7$

4. (a) 1, 2, 3. (b) 3. (c) 3. (d) 5. (e) 2, 3, 4. (f) 2. (g) 5.

5. Somatic mutation contributes to the variability of all three complementarity-determining regions. Additional variability is generated in the CDR3 of both heavy and light chains by junctional flexibility, which occurs during heavy-chain D-J and V-DJ rearrangements and light-chain V-J rearrangements, by P-nucleotide addition at heavy-and light-chain variable-region joints, and by N-nucleotide addition at the heavy-chain D-J and V-DJ joints. See Table 5-3.

6. (a) R: Productive rearrangement of heavy-chain allele 1 must have occurred since the cell line expresses heavy chains encoded by this allele. (b) G: Allelic exclusion forbids heavy-chain allele 2 from undergoing either productive or nonproductive rearrangement. (c) NP: The κ genes rearrange before the λ genes. Since the cell line expresses λ light chains, both κ alleles must have undergone nonproductive rearrangement, thus permitting λ-gene rearrangement to occur. (d) NP: Same reason as given in (c) above. (e) R: Productive rearrangement of λ-chain allele 1 must have occurred since the cell line expresses λ light chains encoded by this allele. (f) G: Allelic exclusion forbids λ-chain allele 2 from undergoing either productive or nonproductive rearrangement (see Figure 5-13).

7. The κ-chain DNA must have the germ-line configuration because a productive heavy-chain rearrangement must occur before the light-chain (κ) DNA can begin to rearrange.

8. (a) No. (b) Yes. (c) No. (d) No. (e) Yes.

9. Random addition of N-nucleotides at the D-J and V-DJ junctions contributes to the diversity within the CDR3 of heavy

chains, but this process can result in a nonproductive rearrangement if the triplet reading frame is not preserved.

10. The joints between variable-region gene segments (V_L-J_L and V_H-D_H-J_H) occur in CDR3. During formation of these joints, junctional flexibility, P-nucleotide addition, and N-nucleotide addition introduce diversity. Because these processes do not affect the rest of the variable region, CDR3 exhibits the greatest diversity.

11. Four chances (see Figure 5-13).

12. (a) 5. (b) 5, 6, 9. (c) 1. (d) 4. (e) 2, 8. (f) 2, 11. (g) 3, 7. (h) 3, 10.

13. (a) 5. (b) 1. (c) 6. (d) 2. (e) 3. (f) 7. (g) 4.

Chapter 6

1. (a) True. (b) True. (c) False: Papain digestion yields monovalent Fab fragments (see Figure 4-3), which cannot crosslink antigens. (d) True. (e) True. (f) True. (g) False: It is qualitative but not quantitative. (h) False: Agglutination tests are more sensitive.

2. Coat a microtiter plate with antigens from HIV. Add serum from a patient suspected of being infected with HIV. Incubate the plate, and then wash away unbound antibodies. Add a goat anti-human immunoglobulin reagent that has been conjugated with an enzyme. Incubate the plate and wash away unbound antibody. Add substrate and observe for a colored reaction.

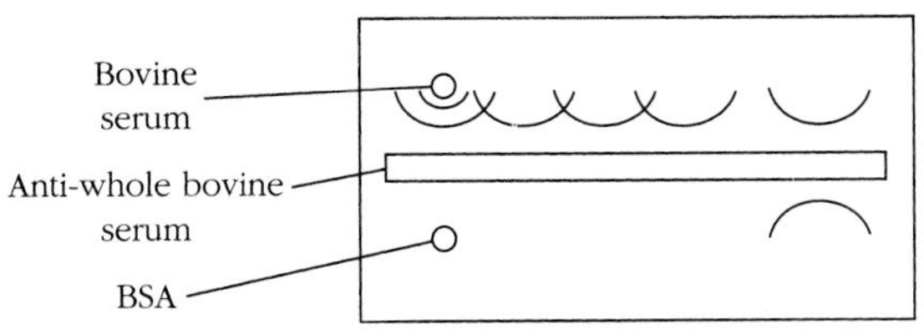

3. (a) Whole bovine serum. (b) See figure below.

4. Bottle A: H1-C1. Bottle B: H2-C2. Bottle C: H2-C1. Bottle D: H1-C2.

5. a and d: ELISA and RIA can both be used to determine the concentration of a hapten.

6. (a) A. (b) D. (c) B. (d) E. (e) F. (f) C.

7. (a) Isolate the heavy chains from the myeloma proteins of known isotype. Immunize rabbits with the isolated heavy chains to obtain antisera specific for each heavy-chain class. Then determine which of these anti-isotype antisera reacts with myeloma protein X. (b) The level of myeloma protein X could be determined by radial immunodiffusion (Mancini method) or by a more sensitive assay such as ELISA.

8. (a) Rocket electrophoresis or Mancini radial immunodiffusion with goat anti-isotype serum specific for IgG. (b) ELISA or RIA with anti-insulin antibody and radioactively labeled or enzyme-linked insulin. (c) RIA with radiolabeled IgE. (d) Immunofluorescence with fluorochrome-labeled antibody to C3. (e) Agglutination test with type-A red blood cells. (f) Ouchterlony double immunodiffusion of hamburger extract and antiserum to horsemeat. (g) Immunofluorescence with fluorochrome-labeled antibody to the syphilis spirochete.

9. b.

10. Affinity refers to the strength of the interaction between a *single* antigen-binding site in an antibody and the corresponding ligand. Avidity refers to the total effective strength of all the interactions between *multiple* antigen-binding sites in an antibody and multiple identical epitopes in a complex antigen. Because bacteria often have multiple copies of a particular epitope on their surface, the avidity of an antibody is a better measure than its affinity of its ability to combat bacteria.

11. (a) Antiserum #1 $K_0 = 1.2 \times 10^5$; antiserum #2 $K_0 = 4.5 \times 10^6$; antiserum #3 $K_0 = 4.5 \times 10^6$; (b) Each antibody has a valence of 2. (c) Antiserum #2. (d) The monoclonal antiserum #2 would be best because it recognizes a single epitope on the hormone and, therefore, would be less likely than the polyclonal antisera to cross-react with other serum proteins.

12. (a) Tube 1 contained $F(ab')_2$ fragments. Because these fragments contain two antigen-binding sites, they can crosslink and eventually agglutinate SRBCs. Activation of complement by IgG requires the presence of the Fc fragment, which is missing from $F(ab')_2$ fragments. (b) Tube 2 contained Fab fragments. Univalent Fab fragments can bind to SRBCs and inhibit subsequent agglutination by whole anti-SRBC. (c) Tube 3 contained intact antibody. (d) Tube 4 contained Fc fragments. These fragments lack antigen-binding sites and thus cannot mediate any antibody effector functions.

13. (a) In precipitation reactions, an excess of either antibody or antigen inhibits precipitate formation (see Figure 6-4b). The formation of a precipitate when equal volumes of the original undiluted solutions were mixed indicates this reaction was in the equivalence zone. The absence of precipitate with the diluted anti-X indicates that this reaction had an antigen excess. (b) In the first (undiluted) reaction, little or no protein X or anti-X would be in the supernatant. In the second (diluted) reaction, the super-natant would contain protein X, which is in excess.

Chapter 7

1. (a) True. (b) True. (c) False: Class III MHC molecules are soluble proteins that do not function in antigen presentation. They include several complement components, TNF-α, TNF-β, and two heat-shock proteins. (d) False: The offspring of heterozygous parents inherit one MHC haplotype from each parent and thus will express some molecules that differ from those of each parent; for this reason, parents and offspring are histoincompatible. In contrast, siblings have a one in four chance of being histocompatible (see Figure 7-2c). (e) True. (f) False: Most nucleated cells express class I MHC molecules, but neurons, placental cells, and sperm cells at certain stages of differentiation appear to lack class I molecules. (g) True.

2. (a) S. (b) S and C. (c) S. (d) C. (e) S and C. (f) S. (g) C.

3. (a) Strain A. (b) Strain B. (c) Strain A. (d) To introduce strain-A parental alleles at all loci except for the selected MHC.

(e) To achieve homozygosity within the MHC. (f) To identify progeny that are homozygous *b/b* within the MHC. This is achieved by selecting mice that reject grafts from strain A (see Figure 7-3).

4. (a) Liver cells: Class I K^d, K^k, D^d, D^k, L^d, and L^k.
(b) Macrophages: Class I K^d, K^k, D^d, D^k, L^d, and L^k. Class II $IA\alpha^k\beta^k$, $IA\alpha^d\beta^d$, $IA\alpha^k\beta^d$, $IA\alpha^d\beta^k$, $IE\alpha^k\beta^k$, $IE\alpha^d\beta^d$, $IE\alpha^k\beta^d$, and $IE\alpha^d\beta^k$.

5.

Transfected gene	MHC molecules expressed on the membrane of the transfected L cells					
	D^k	D^b	K^k	K^b	IA^k	IA^b
None	+	–	+	–	–	–
K^b	+	–	+	+	–	–
$IA\alpha^b$	+	–	+	–	–	–
$IA\beta^b$	+	–	+	–	–	–
$IA\alpha^b$ and $IA\beta^b$	+	–	+	–	–	+

6. (a) SLJ macrophages express the following MHC molecules: K^s, D^s, L^s, and IA^s. Because of the deletion of the *IEα* locus, IE^s is not expressed by these cells. (b) The transfected cells would express one heterologous IE molecule, $IE\alpha^k\beta^s$, and one homologous IE molecule, $IE\alpha^k\beta^k$, in addition to the molecules listed in (a).

7. See Figures 7-5, 4-2, and 4-19.

8. (a) The polymorphic residues are clustered in short stretches primarily within the membrane-distal domains of the class I and class II MHC molecules (see Figure 7-14). These regions form the peptide-binding cleft of MHC molecules. (b) MHC polymorphism is thought to arise by gene conversion of short, nearly homologous DNA sequences within unexpressed pseudogenes in the MHC to functional class I or class II genes.

9. (a) The proliferation of T_H cells and IL-2 production by them is detected in assay 1, and the killing of LCM-infected target cells by cytotoxic T lymphocytes (CTLs) is detected in assay 2. (b) Assay 1 is a functional assay for class II MHC molecules, and assay 2 is a functional assay for class I molecules. (c) Class II IA^k molecules are required in assay 1, and class I D^d molecules are required in assay 2. (d) You could transfect L cells with the IA^k gene and determine the response of the transfected cells in assay 1. Similarly, you could transfect a separate sample of L cells with the D^d gene and determine the response of the transfected cells in assay 2. In each case, a positive response would confirm the identity of the MHC molecules required for LCM-specific activity of the spleen cells. As a control in each case, L cells should be transfected with a different class I or class II MHC gene and assayed in the appropriate assay. (e) The immunized spleen cells express both IA^k and D^d molecules. Of the listed strains, only A.TL and (BALB/c × B10.A) F_1 express both of these MHC molecules, and thus these are the only strains from which the spleen cells could have been isolated.

10. It is not possible to predict. Since the peptide-binding cleft is identical, both MHC molecules should bind the same peptide. However, the amino acid differences outside the cleft might prevent recognition of the second MHC molecule by the T-cell receptor on the T_C cells.

11. Use a battery of monoclonal antibodies specific for the MHC molecules corresponding to each MHC haplotype to determine whether both strains express the same set of MHC molecules. This approach is used in tissue typing to identify potential graft donors (see Figure 21-4).

12. If RBCs expressed MHC molecules, then extensive tissue typing would be required before a blood transfusion, and only a few individuals would be acceptable donors for a given individual.

13. (a) No. Although those with the A99/B276 haplotype are at significantly increased relative risk, there is no absolute correlation between these alleles and the disease. (b) Nearly all of those with the disease will probably have the A99/B276 haplotype, but depending on the exact gene or genes responsible, this may not be a requirement for development of the disease. If the gene responsible for the disease lies between the A and B loci, then weaker associations to A99 and B276 may be observed. If the gene is located outside of the A and B regions and is linked to the haplotype only by association in a founder, then associations with other MHC genes may occur. (c) It is not possible to know how frequently the combination will occur relative to the frequency of the two individual alleles; linkage disequilibrium is difficult to predict. However, based on the data given, it may be speculated that the linkage to a disease that is fatal in individuals who have not reached reproductive years will have a negative effect on the frequency of the founder haplotype. An educated guess would be that the A99/B276 combination would be rarer than predicted on the basis of the frequency of the A99 and B276 alleles.

Chapter 8

1. By convention, antigen-presenting cells are defined as those cells that can display antigenic peptides associated with class II MHC molecules and can deliver a co-stimulatory signal to $CD4^+$ T_H cells. Target cells display peptides associated with class I MHC molecules to $CD8^+$ T_C cells.

2. (a) Self-MHC restriction is the attribute of T cells that limits their response to antigen associated with self-MHC molecules on the membrane of antigen-presenting cells or target cells. In general, $CD4^+$ T_H cells are class II MHC restricted, and $CD8^+$ T_C cells are class I MHC restricted, although a few exceptions to this pattern occur. (b) Antigen processing involves the intracellular degradation of protein antigens into peptides that associate with class I or class II MHC molecules. (c) Endogenous antigens are synthesized within altered self-cells (e.g., virus-infected cells or tumor cells), are processed in the cytosolic pathway, and are presented by class I MHC molecules to $CD8^+$ T_C cells. (d) Exogenous antigens are internalized by antigen-presenting cells, processed in the endocytic pathway, and presented by class II MHC molecules to $CD4^+$ T_H cells.

3. (a) Class I MHC molecules display only peptides derived from endogenous antigens by the cytosolic processing pathway. Since the UV-inactivated (killed) influenza virus cannot replicate in the target cells, no endogenous viral proteins are synthesized. (b) Class II MHC molecules display only peptides produced in the endocytic processing pathway, which is inhibited by chloroquine. Thus, this compound inhibits the response of class II–restricted T cells. (c) Emetine inhibits protein synthesis and thus prevents synthesis of viral proteins in target cells infected with live influenza virus. As a result, class I–restricted T cells do not respond. Since the response of class II–restricted cells does not depend on protein synthesis, their response is not inhibited by emetine.

4. (a) EN: Class I molecules associate with antigenic peptides and display them on the surface of target cells to $CD8^+$ T_C cells. (b) EX: Class II molecules associate with antigenic peptides and display them on surface of APCs to $CD4^+$ T_H cells. (c) EX: The invariant chain interacts with the peptide-binding cleft of class II MHC molecules in the rough endoplasmic reticulum, thereby preventing binding of peptides from endogenous antigens. It also assists in folding of the class II α and β chains and in movement of class II molecules from the RER to endocytic compartments. (d) EX: Lysosomal hydrolases degrade exogenous antigens into peptides; these enzymes also degrade the invariant chain associated with class II molecules, so that the peptides and MHC molecules can associate. (e) EN: TAP, a transmembrane protein located in the RER membrane, mediates transport of antigenic peptides produced in the cytosolic pathway into the RER lumen where they can associate with class I MHC molecules. (f) B: In the endogenous pathway, vesicles containing peptide–class I MHC complexes move from the RER to the Golgi complex and then on to the cell surface. In the exogenous pathway, vesicles containing the invariant chain associated with class II MHC molecules move from the RER to the Golgi and on to endocytic compartments. (g) EN: Proteasomes are large protein complexes with multiple peptidase activity that degrade intracellular proteins within the cytosol. When associated with LMP2 and LMP7, which are encoded in the MHC region, and LMP10, which is not MHC encoded, proteasomes preferentially generate peptides that associate with class I MHC molecules. (h) EX: Antigen-presenting cells internalize exogenous (external) antigens by phagocytosis or endocytosis. (i) EN: Calnexin is a protein within the RER membrane that acts as a molecular chaperone, assisting in the folding and association of newly formed class I α chains and β_2-microglobulin into heterodimers. (j) EX: After degradation of the invariant chain associated with a class II MHC molecule, a small fragment called CLIP remains bound to the peptide-binding cleft, presumably preventing premature peptide loading of the MHC molecule. Eventually, CLIP is displaced by an antigenic peptide. (k) EN: Tapasin (TAP-associated protein) brings the transporter TAP into proximity with the class I MHC molecule and allows the MHC molecule to acquire an antigenic peptide (see Figure 8-7).

5. (a) Chloroquine inhibits the endocytic processing pathway, so that the APCs cannot display peptides derived from native lysozyme. The synthetic lysozyme peptide will exchange with other peptides associated with class II molecules on the APC membrane, so that it will be displayed to the T_H cells and induce their activation. (b) Delay of chloroquine addition provides time for native lysozyme to be degraded in the endocytic pathway.

6. (a) Dendritic cells: constitutively express both class II MHC molecules and co-stimulatory signal. B cells: constitutively express class II molecules but must be activated before expressing the B7 co-stimulatory signal. Macrophages: must be activated before expressing either class II molecules or the B7 co-stimulatory signal. (b) See Table 8-1. Many nonprofessional APCs function only during sustained inflammatory responses.

7. (a) R. (b) R. (c) NR. (d) R. (e) NR. (f) R.

8. (a) Intracellular bacteria, such as members of the *Mycobacterium* family, are a major source of nonpeptide antigens; the antigens observed in combination with CD1 are lipid and glycolipid components of the bacterial cell wall. (b) Members of the CD1 family associate with β_2-micro-globulin and have structural similarity to class I MHC molecules. They are not true MHC molecules because they are not encoded within the MHC and are on a different chromosome. (c) The pathway for antigen processing taken by the CD1 molecules differs from that taken by class I MHC molecules. A major difference is that CD1 antigen processing is not inhibited in cells that are deficient in TAP, whereas class I MHC molecules cannot pre-sent antigen in TAP-deficient cells.

Chapter 9

1. (a) False: The distance between CD4 and the TCR is too great for them to coprecipitate; however, CD3 and the TCR are close enough that they will coprecipitate in response to monoclonal anti-CD3. (b) True. (c) True. (d) False: The TCR variable-region genes are located on different chromosomes from the Ig variable-region genes. (e) False: All T-cell receptors have a single binding site for peptide-MHC complexes. (f) False: Because allelic exclusion is not complete for the TCR α chain, a T cell occasionally expresses two α chains resulting from rearrangement of both α-chain alleles. (g) False: The mechanisms are very similar, but T-cell receptors do not generate diversity by somatic mutation as immunoglobulins do. (h) True.

2. Functional $\alpha\beta$ TCR genes from a T_C clone specific for one hapten on an H-2^d target cell were transfected into another T_C clone specific for a second hapten on an H-2^k target cell. Cytolysis assays revealed that the transfected T_C cells killed only target cells that presented antigen associated with the original MHC restriction element.

3. See Figure 9-3.

4. (a) CD3 is a complex of three dimers containing five different polypeptide chains. It is required for the expression of the T-cell receptor and plays a role in signal transduction across the membrane. CD3 and the T-cell receptor associate to form the TCR-CD3 membrane complex (see Figure 9-9). (b) CD4 and CD8 interact with the membrane-proximal domains of class II and class I MHC molecules, respectively, thereby increasing the avidity of the interaction between T cells and peptide-MHC complexes. CD4 and CD8 also play a role in signal transduction. (c) CD2 and other accessory molecules (LFA-1, CD28, and CD45R) bind to their ligands on antigen-presenting cells or target cells. The initial contact between a T cell and antigen-presenting cell or target cell probably is mediated by these cell-adhesion molecules.

Subsequently, the T-cell receptor interacts with peptide-MHC complexes. These molecules also may function in signal transduction.

5. (a) TCR. (b) TCR. (c) Ig. (d) TCR/Ig. (e) TCR. (f) TCR/Ig. (g) Ig.

6. (a) The three assumptions were: 1) That TCR mRNA should be associated with membrane-bound polyribosomes, like the mRNAs encoding other membrane proteins; therefore, isolation of the membrane-bound polyribosomal mRNA fraction would significantly enrich the proportion of TCR mRNA in the preparations. 2) That B cells and T cells would express many common genes, and the unique T-cell mRNAs would include those encoding the T-cell receptor; therefore, subtractive hybridization using B-cell mRNA would remove all the cDNAs common to both B and T cells, leaving the unique T-cell cDNA unhybridized. 3) That the TCR genes undergo DNA rearrangement and, therefore, can be detected by Southern blotting with cDNA probes. See Figure 9-4. (b) If they wanted to identify the IL-4 gene, they should perform subtractive hybridization using a T_H clone as an IL-4 producer and a T_C clone as a source of mRNA lacking the message for IL-4. In addition, the gene for IL-4 would not be expected to rearrange and, therefore, could not be identified by Southern-blot analysis for gene rearrangement.

7.

Gene product	cDNA source	mRNA source
IL-2	A	B
CD8	C	A or B
J chain	E	F
IL-1	D	G
CD3	A, B, or C	H

8.

Source of spleen cells from LCM-infected mice	Release of ^{51}Cr from LCM-infected target cells			
	B10.D2 (H-2^d)	B10 (H-2^b)	B10.BR (H-2^k)	(BALB/C × B10) F_1 (H-2$^{b/d}$)
B10.D2 (H-2^d)	+	–	–	+
B10 (H-2^b)	–	+	–	+
BALB/c (H-2^d)	+	–	–	+
BALB/b (H-2^b)	–	+	–	+

Chapter 10

1. (a) The immature thymocytes express both CD4 and CD8, whereas the mature CD8$^+$ thymocytes do not express CD4. To distinguish these cells, the thymocytes are double-stained with fluorochrome-labeled anti-CD4 and anti-CD8 and analyzed in a FACS. (b) See the table below.

Transgenic mouse	Immature thmocytes	Mature CD8$^+$ thymocytes
H-2^k female	+	+
H-2^k male	+	–
H-2^d female	+	–
H-2^d male	+	–

(c) Because the gene encoding the H-Y antigen is on the Y chromosome, this antigen is not present in females. Thymocytes bearing the transgenic T-cell receptor, which is H-2^k restricted, would undergo positive selection in both male and female H-2^k transgenics. However, subsequent negative selection would eliminate thymocytes bearing the transgenic receptor, which is specific for H-Y antigen, in the male H-2^k transgenics (see Figure 10-8).
(d) Because the H-2^d transgenics would not express the appropriate MHC molecules, T-cells bearing the transgenic T-cell receptor would not undergo positive selection.

2. Cyclosporin A blocks production of NF-ATc, one of the transcription factors necessary for proliferation of antigen-activated T_H cells (see Figure 10-13).

3. (a) NF-kB and NF-ATc. (b) IL-2 enhancer. See Figure 10-12.

4.

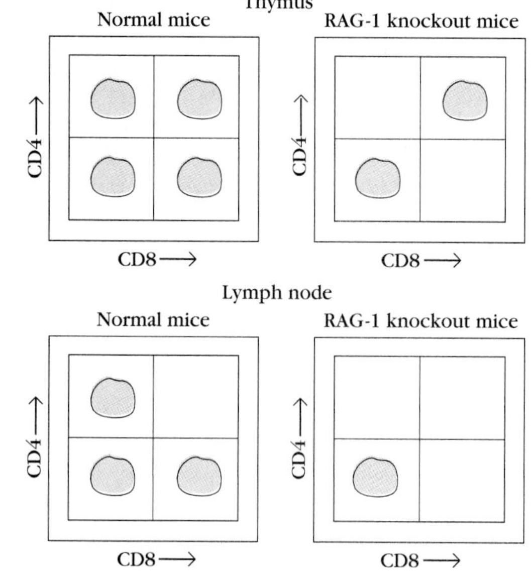

5. (a) Class I K, D, and L molecules and class II IA molecules. (b) Class I molecules only. (c) The normal H-2^b mice should have both CD4$^+$ and CD8$^+$ T cells because both class I and class II MHC molecules would be present on thymic stromal cells

during positive selection. H-2^b mice with knockout of the *IA* gene would express no class II molecules; thus, these mice would have only $CD8^+$ cells.

6. (a) Thymus donor in experiment A was H-2^d (BALB/c) and in experiment B was H-2^b (C57BL/6). (b) The haplotype of the thymus donor determines the MHC restriction of the T cells in the chimeric mice. Thus, H-2^b target cells were lysed in experiment B, in which the thymus donor was H-2^b (c) The H-2^k target cells were not lysed in either experiment because neither donor thymus expressed H-2^k MHC molecules; thus, H-2^k–reactive T cells were not positively selected in the chimeric mice.

7. (a) Protein kinases. (b) CD45. (c) B7. (d) Protein phosphatase. (e) IL-2. (f) CD28; B7. (g) CD8. (h) Class II MHC; B7. (i) CD4. (j) Phospholipase. (k) Protein kinase.

8. (a) Because the pre–T-cell receptor, which does not bind antigen, is associated with CD3, cells expressing the pre-TCR as well as the antigen-binding T-cell receptor would stain with anti-CD3. It is impossible to determine from this result how many of the CD3-staining cells are expressing complete T-cell receptors. The remaining cells are even more immature thymocytes that do not express CD3. (b) No. Because some of the CD3-staining cells express the pre-TCR or the $\gamma\delta$ TCR instead of the complete $\alpha\beta$ TCR, you cannot calculate the number of T_C cells by simple subtraction. To determine the number of T_C cells, you need fluorescent anti-CD8 antibody, which will stain only the $CD8^+$ T_C cells.

Chapter 11

1. (a) False: The V_H-D_H-J_H rearrangement occurs during the pro–B-cell stage; successful completion of heavy-chain rearrangement marks the beginning of the pre–B-cell stage, in which membrane-bound μ chains are expressed. (b) False: Immature B cells express only IgM. (c) False: TdT, which catalyzes N-nucleotide addition, is expressed only in pro-B cells. (d) True. (e) True. (f) False: Pro-B cells must interact with stromal cells to develop into pre-B cells. Progression of pre-B cells into immature B cells requires IL-7 released from stromal cells but not direct contact. (g). True. (See Figure 11-1.)

2. (a) Progenitor B cell: no cytoplasmic or membrane staining with either reagent. (b) Pre-B cell: anti-μ staining in cytoplasm and on membrane. (c) Immature B cell: anti-μ staining in cytoplasm and on membrane. (d) Mature B cell: anti-μ and anti-δ staining in cytoplasm and on membrane. (e) Plasma cell: anti-μ staining in cytoplasm; no membrane staining but pentameric IgM is secreted.

3. The B-cell coreceptor consists of three membrane proteins: TAPA-1, CR2, and CD19; the latter belongs to the Ig superfamily. The CR2 component can bind to complement-coated antigen bound to the B-cell receptor (BCR). This binding results in the phosphorylation of CD19. Src-family tyrosine kinases (Lyn and Fyn) bind to phosphorylated CD19 and can trigger signal transduction pathways that begin with phospholipase C (see Figure 11-8).

4. (a) Both single and double transgenics carried the anti-HEL transgene. Because the transgene is already rearranged, rearrangement of endogenous immunoglobulin heavy- and light-chain genes does not occur in pro-B and pre-B cells; therefore, the rearranged immunoglobulin encoded by the transgene is expressed preferentially by mature B cells. (b) Add radiolabeled HEL and use autoradiography to see whether it binds to the B-cell membrane. To determine the isotype of the membrane antibody (mIg) on these B cells, incubate the cells with fluorochrome-labeled antibodies specific for each isotype (e.g., anti-μ, anti-δ, etc.) and see which fluorescent antibodies stain the B cells. (c) So that the HEL transgene could be induced by adding Zn^{2+} to the mouse's water supply. (d) First, B cells and T cells from the double-transgenic mice and normal syngeneic mice must be separated from each other. This can be accomplished by treating a preparation of spleen cells with a fluorochrome-labeled antibody specific for CD3, which is expressed on the membrane of T cells but not B cells, and passing the treated preparation through a FACS (see Figure 6-16). This will yield a T-cell fraction and a residual fraction containing B cells and other spleen cells. After treating the residual fraction with fluorochrome-labeled anti-IgM, pass it through a FACS to obtain a B-cell fraction. Now, mix the transgenic B cells with normal syngeneic T cells (sample A), and mix the transgenic T cells with normal syngeneic B cells (sample B). Transfer each cell mixture to lethally x-irradiated, syngeneic adoptive-transfer recipients, challenge the recipients with HEL, and determine whether they produce anti-HEL serum antibodies. If the B cells are anergic, then no antibody response would occur with sample A.

5. (a) B-cell activation by soluble protein antigens requires the involvement of T_H cells. Crosslinkage of mIg on a naive B cell by thymus-dependent antigens provides competence signal 1; subsequent binding of CD40 on the B cell to CD40L on an activated T_H cell provides competence signal 2. The combined effect of these signals drives the B cell from G_0 to the G_1 stage of the cell cycle and up-regulates expression of cytokine receptors on the B cell. Binding of T_H-derived cytokines then provides a progression signal that stimulates proliferation of the activated B cells (see Figure 11-10). (b) Binding of LPS, a type 1 thymus-independent antigen, provides both competence signals 1 and 2 (see Figure 11-6). Efficient proliferation requires a cytokine-mediated progression signal.

6. (a) Light zone. (b) Paracortex. (c) Centroblasts; dark zone. (d) Centrocytes; follicular dendritic cells. (e) Light zone; T_H cells. (f) Light zone. (g) Medulla. (h) Memory B cells, plasmablasts, and plasma cells; light zone. (i) Centroblasts.

7. (a) See Table 11-2. (b) TI antigens.

8. (a) Each mIg molecule is associated with two molecules of a heterodimer called Ig-α/Ig-β forming the B-cell receptor (BCR). Both Ig-α and Ig-β have long cytoplasmic tails, which are capable of mediating signal transduction to the cell interior (see Figure 11-8). (b) B-cell activating and differentiating signals—provided by antigen binding, interaction with T_H cells, or cytokine binding—trigger intracellular signal-transduction pathways that ultimately generate active transcription factors. These then translocate to the nucleus, where they stimulate or inhibit transcription of specific genes.

9. (a) The recipient mice had a haplotype other than H-2^b. (b) The purpose of these experiments was to see the effect of a self-antigen, represented by the transgene-encoded K^b, that is expressed only in the periphery. Linking the K^b transgene to a liver-specific promoter assured that the K^b class I molecule would be

expressed in the periphery but not in the bone marrow, where immature B cells could interact with it. (c) These results suggest that exposure to self-antigens in the periphery can lead to negative selection and apoptosis (clonal deletion) in some cases (see Figure 11-14).

10. (a) True. (b) True. (c) True. (d) False: Antigenic competition will reduce the response to SRBC.

11. (a) The early stages of the response will be dominated by IgM. Although the average affinity of the antibody produced will be lower than that expected during a secondary response after challenge with the same antigen, it will be higher than that obtained during a primary response to a high dose of the antigen. (b) The antibody will tend to be largely IgG and of higher affinity than that obtained during a primary response to a low dose of the antigen. (c) The average affinity of the antibody will be of lower affinity than that obtained during the primary response to a low dose of the antigen. Most of the antibody made during the early stages of the response will be IgM. (d) The average affinity of the antibody will be higher than that of antibody made during a primary response to a high dose of the antigen, but not necessarily lower than that to of antibody made in a primary response to low doses. It will be of lower average affinity than the antibody produced during a secondary response to a low dose of the antigen. It will be mostly IgG.

12. (a) Sample B yields a single restriction fragment with each digest characteristic of unrearranged germ-line DNA. Thus, this sample is from liver cells. (b) The two fragments obtained with the *Bam*HI digest of sample C indicate that both heavy-chain alleles are rearranged, whereas no κ-chain rearrangement has occurred. Thus, this sample is from pre-B lymphoma cells. (c) The blots obtained with sample A indicate that one heavy-chain allele is rearranged and one light-chain allele is rearranged. This pattern indicates that this sample is from IgM-secreting myeloma cells.

Chapter 12

1. (a) False: The high-affinity IL-2 receptor comprises three subunits—the α, β, and γ chains—all of which are transmembrane proteins. (b) False: Anti-TAC binds to the 55-kDa α chain of the IL-2 receptor. (c) False: Although all class I and class II cytokine receptors contain two or three subunits, the receptors for IL-1, IL-8, TNF-α, TNF-β. and some other cytokines have only one chain (see Figure 12-6). (d) False: Low levels of the IL-2R β chain are expressed in resting T cells, although expression is increased greatly after activation. The α chain is expressed only by activated T cells. (e) False: The cytosolic domains of class I and class II cytokine receptors appear to be closely associated with intracellular tyrosine kinases but do not themselves possess tyrosine kinase activity. (f) True (see Figure 12-7).

2. Only antigen-activated T cells will proliferate, because they express the high-affinity IL-2 receptor, whereas resting T cells do not and therefore cannot respond to IL-2.

3. Cytokines, growth factors, and hormones are all secreted proteins that bind to receptors on target cells, eliciting various biological effects. Cytokines tend to be produced by a variety of cells, although their production is carefully regulated, and exert their effects on several cell types; most cytokines also act in an autocrine or paracrine fashion. Growth factors, unlike cytokines, are often produced constitutively. Hormones, unlike cytokines, generally act over long distances (endocrine effect) on one or a few types of target cells.

4. (a) γ chain and β chain (low level). (b) α, β, and γ chains. (c) γ chain and β chain (low level); cyclosporin A prevents the gene activation that leads to increased expression of the β and α chains. (d) γ chain and β chain (low level). (e) α, β, and γ chains. (f) β and γ chains (see Figure 12-9).

5. (a) Superantigens bind to class II MHC molecules outside of the normal peptide-binding cleft; unlike normal antigens, they are not internalized and processed by antigen-presenting cells but bind directly to class II molecules. Superantigens also bind to regions of the V_β domain of the T-cell receptor that are not involved in binding normal antigenic peptides. Superantigens exhibit specificity for one or a few V_β domains; thus, a given superantigen can activate all T cells that express the V_β domain(s) for which it is specific regardless of the antigenic specificity of the T cells. (b) A given superantigen can activate 5%–25% of T_H cells, leading to excessive production of cytokines. The high levels of cytokines are thought to cause the symptoms associated with food poisoning and toxic-shock syndrome. (c) Yes. To exert their effect, superantigens must form a ternary complex with a class II MHC molecule and T-cell receptor.

6. The receptors for IL-3, IL-5, and GM-CSF contain a common signal-transducing β chain. Cytokine binding to each of these receptors probably triggers a similar signal-transduction pathway.

7. (a) The T_H1 subset is responsible for classical cell-mediated functions (e.g., delayed-type hypersensitivity and activation of T_C cells). Viral infections and intracellular pathogens are likely to induce a T_H1 response. (b) The T_H2 subset functions primarily as a helper for B-cell activation. This subset may be best suited to respond to free-living bacteria and helminthic parasites and may mediate allergic reactions, since IL-4 and IL-5 are known to induce IgE production and eosinophil activation, respectively.

Chapter 13

1. (a) True. (b) True. (c) True. (d) True. (e) False: Enveloped viruses can be lysed by complement because their outer envelope is derived from the plasma membrane of a host cell. (f) True.

2. Serum IgM is in a planar form in which the complement-binding sites in the Fc region are not accessible. Only after binding to antigen does IgM assume a conformation in which the complement-binding sites are accessible (see Figure 13-4).

3. A C3 deficiency is more serious clinically because it impairs both the classical and alternative pathways. In contrast, with a C1 deficiency, the alternative pathway would still operate.

4. The degraded antibody would be less able to serve as an opsonin or to initiate complement activation.

5. (a) The classical pathway is initiated by immune complexes involving IgG or IgM; the alternative pathway generally is initiated by bacterial cell-wall components; and the lectin pathway is initiated by binding of mannose-binding lectin (MBL) to microbial cell-wall carbohydrates. (b) The initial reaction sequences that generate C5 convertase are the same, after the C1

step, for the classical and lectin pathways but differ between these two pathways and the alternative pathway. The terminal sequence leading from bound C5b to the MAC is the same for all three pathways. See Figure 13-2. (c) Complement activation by any of the three pathways has the *same* biological consequences because components mediating all the biological effects of complement are generated in all three.

6. (a) Innocent-bystander lysis may occur when free C5b67 binds to nearby healthy cells, including red blood cells. Binding of S protein to the free C5b67 prevents its insertion into the membrane of red blood cells and other healthy cells. In addition, red blood cells contain two membrane proteins, homologous restriction factor (HRF) and membrane inhibitor of reactive lysis (MIRL), which block the terminal sequence leading to MAC formation and thereby protect these cells from nonspecific complement-mediated lysis. (b) A defect in S protein, in the membrane-bound HRF and MIRL, or in the phospholipid membrane anchors that tether HRF and MIRL to the cell surface theoretically could lead to increased complement-mediated lysis of red blood cells. The presence of defective membrane anchors has been associated with chronic hemolytic anemia in some individuals.

7. See Table 13-6.

8. (a) 4. (b) 5. (c) 6. (d) 2. (e) 7. (f) 11. (g) 3. (h) 1. (i) 8. (j) 10. (k) 9. (l) 12.

9.

	Component knocked out						
	C1q	C4	C3	C5	C6	C9	Factor B
Complement activation							
Formation of C3 convertase in classical pathway	A	A	NE	NE	NE	NE	NE
Formation of C3 convertase in alternative pathway	NE	NE	A	NE	NE	NE	A
Formation of C5 convertase in classical pathway	A	A	A	NE	NE	NE	NE
Formation of C5 convertase in alternative pathway	NE	NE	A	NE	NE	NE	A
Effector functions							
C3b-mediated opsonization	D	D	A	NE	NE	NE	D
Neutrophil chemotaxis	D	D	D	D	D	NE	D
Cell lysis	D	D	A	A	A	A	D

Chapter 14

1. (a) True. (b) True. (c) True. (d) False: There are two pathways by which cytotoxic T cells kill target cells. One pathway is perforin dependent, and the other uses FAS ligand displayed by the CTL to induce death in FAS-expressing target cells.

2. The monoclonal antibody to LFA-1 should block formation of the CTL–target-cell conjugate. This should inhibit killing of the target cell and, therefore, should result in diminished ^{51}Cr release in the CML assay.

3.

Population 1	Population 2	Proliferation
C57BL/6 (H-2^b)	CBA (H-2^k)	1 and 2
C57BL/6 (H-2^b)	CBA (H-2^k) mitomycin C-treated	1
C57BL/6 (H-2^b)	(CBA × C57BL/6) F_1 (H-2$^{k/b}$)	1
C57BL/6 (H-2^b)	C57L (H-2^b)	Neither

4. (a) CD4$^+$ T_H cells. (b) To demonstrate the identity of the proliferating cells, you could incubate them with fluorescein-labeled anti-CD4 monoclonal antibody and rhodamine-labeled anti-CD8 monoclonal antibody. The proliferating cells will be stained only with the anti-CD4 reagent. (c) As CD4$^+$ T_H cells recognize allogeneic class II MHC molecules on the stimulator cells, they are activated and begin to secrete IL-2, which then autostimulates T_H-cell proliferation. Thus, the extent of proliferation is directly related to the level of IL-2 produced.

5. (a) Neither. (b) Both. (c) CTL. (d) CTL. (e) T_H cell. (f) CTL. (g) T_H cell. (h) CTL. (i) T_H cell. (j) T_H cell. (k) Neither. (l) Both. (m) CTL. (n) Both. (o) Both. (p) T_H cell. (q) Neither. (r) CTL. (s) T_H cell.

6.

	^{51}Cr release from LCM-infected target cells			
Source of primed spleen cells	B10.D2 (H-2^d)	B10 (H-2^b)	B10.BR (H-2^k)	(BALB/c × B10)F_1 (H-2$^{b/d}$)
B10.D2 (H-2^d)	+	–	–	+
B10 (H-2^b)	–	+	–	+
BALB/c (H-2^d)	+	–	–	+
(BALB/c × B10) (H-2$^{b/d}$)	+	+	–	+

7. To determine T_C activity specific for influenza, perform a CML reaction by incubating spleen cells from the infected mouse

with influenza-infected syngeneic target cells. To determine T_H activity, incubate the spleen cells from the infected mouse with syngeneic APCs presenting influenza peptides; measure IL-2 production.

8. NK cells mediate lysis of tumor cells and virus-infected cells by perforin-induced pore formation, as in the mechanism employed by CTLs. NK cells are able to distinguish normal cells from infected cells because normal cells express relatively high levels of class I MHC molecules, which appears to protect them from NK cells. The balance between positive signals generated by the engagement of activating receptors (NKR-P1 and others) on NK cells and negative signals induced by recognition of self MHC molecules by inhibitory receptors, such as CD94/NKG2 and the KIR family on NK cells, regulates NK-cell–mediated killing.

9. (a–e) The outcome in all cases is no lysis mediated by cytotoxic T cells. There are two pathways by which cytotoxic T cells kill target cells, one that is perforin-dependent and one that uses FasL to induce death in Fas-expressing target cells. Because both of these pathways are inoperative in the double-knockout mice, there will be no T-cell–mediated cytotoxicity.

Chapter 15

1. (a) False: Various chemokines are chemotactic for all types of leukocytes. (b) False: Integrins are expressed by various leukocytes but not by endothelial cells. (c) True. (d) True. (e) True. (f) False: Systemic effects, called the acute-phase response, are induced by cytokines generated in the localized acute inflammatory response. (g) True. (h) False: Granulomas may form in sites of chronic infection but are unlikely during an acute inflammatory response.

2. The increased expression of ICAMs on vascular endothelial cells near an inflammatory site facilitates adherence of leukocytes to the blood-vessel wall, resulting in increased migration of leukocytes into the area.

3. (a) Rolling, activation, arrest/adhesion, and transendothelial migration (see Figures 15-3a and 15-7). (b) Neutrophils generally extravasate at sites of inflammation because they bind to the cell-adhesion molecules that are induced on vascular endothelium early in the inflammatory response. (c) Different lymphocyte subsets express homing receptors that bind to tissue-specific adhesion molecules (vascular addressins) on HEVs in different lymphoid organs, on inflamed endothelium, or on venules in tertiary sites. The homing of particular lymphocytes to certain sites is facilitated by chemokines that preferentially attract different lymphocytes. Thus, differences in (1) vascular addressins, (2) homing receptors, and (3) chemokines and their receptors determine the recirculation pattern of particular lymphocyte subsets.

4. IL-1, IL-6, and TNF-α (see Table 15-3).

5. TNF-α released by activated tissue macrophages during a localized acute inflammatory response acts on vascular endothelial cells and macrophages, inducing secretion of colony-stimulating factors (CSFs), which stimulate hematopoiesis in the bone marrow. This is part of the systemic acute-phase response.

6. (a) N. (b) 1. (c) N. (d) 3. (e) N. (f) 2. (g) 3 (see Figure 15-3).

7. IFN-γ stimulates activation of macrophages, resulting in increased expression of class II MHC molecules, increased microbicidal activity, and cytokine production. The accumulation of large numbers of activated macrophages is responsible for much of the tissue damage associated with chronic inflammation. TNF-α secreted by activated macrophages also contributes to the tissue wasting common in chronic inflammation. These two cytokines act synergistically to facilitate migration of large numbers of cells to sites of chronic inflammation.

8. Binding of all these cytokines to their receptors on hepatocytes induces formation of the same transcription factor, NF-16, which stimulates transcription of acute-phase proteins.

9. (a) 7. (b) 1, 6. (c) 10, 11. (d) 2. (e) 8. (f) 4. (g) 10. (h) 9.

Chapter 16

1. (a) False: IgE is increased. (b) False: IL-4 increases IgE production. (c) True. (d) False: Antihistamines are helpful in type I hypersensitivity, which involves release of histamine by mast-cell degranulation. Because type III hypersensitivity primarily involves immune-complex deposition, antihistamines are ineffective. (e) False: Most pollen allergens contain multiple allergenic components. (f) False: Unlike IgG, IgE cannot pass through the placenta. (g) True. (h) True.

2. (a) The complete antibodies would cross-link FcεRI molecules on the membrane of mast cells and basophils, resulting in their activation and degranulation. The released mediators would induce vasodilation, smooth-muscle contraction, and a local wheal and flare reaction. Because the Fab fragment is monovalent, it cannot crosslink FcεRI molecules and thus cannot induce degranulation. However, this type of antireceptor antibody could bind to FcεRI and might thereby block binding of IgE to the receptors. (b) The response induced by complete anti-FcεRI antibodies does not depend on allergen-specific IgE and thus would be similar in allergic and nonallergic mice. Injection of Fab fragments of anti-FcεRI might prevent allergic mice from reacting to an allergen if these fragments block binding of IgE to mast cells and basophils.

3. Engineer chimeric monoclonal antibodies to snake venom that contain mouse variable regions but human heavy- and light-chain constant regions (see Figure 5-22).

4. (a) Type I hypersensitivity: localized atopic reaction that results from allergen crosslinkage of fixed IgE on skin mast cells, inducing degranulation and mediator release. (b) Type III hypersensitivity: immune complexes of antibody and insect antigens form and are deposited locally, causing an Arthus-type reaction resulting from complement activation and complement split products. (c) Type IV hypersensitivity: sensitized T_{DTH} cells release their mediators, inducing macrophage accumulation and activation. Tissue damage results from lysosomal enzymes released by the macrophages.

Immunologic event	Hypersensitivity			
	Type I	Type II	Type III	Type IV
IgE-mediated degranulation of mast cells	+			
Lysis of antibody-coated blood cells by complement		+		
Tissue destruction in response to poison oak				+
C3a- and C5a-mediated mast-cell degranulation		(some)	+	
Chemotaxis of neutrophils			+	
Chemotaxis of eosinophils	+			
Activation of macrophages by IFN-γ				+
Deposition of antigen-antibody complexes on basement membranes of capillaries			+	
Sudden death due to vascular collapse (shock) shortly after injection or ingestion of antigen	+			

5. (a) IV. (b) All four types. (c) I and III. (d) IV. (e) I. (f) II. (g) I. (h) I. (i) II. (j) II. (k) I.

6. Answer to Question 6 is shown above.

Chapter 17

1. (a) Because the infected target cells expressed H-2^k MHC molecules, but the primed T cells were H-2^b restricted. (b) Because the influenza nucleoprotein is processed by the endogenous processing pathway and the resulting peptides are presented by class I MHC molecules. (c) Probably because the transfected class I D^b molecule is only able to present peptide 365–380 and not peptide 50–63. Alternatively, peptide 50–63 may not be a T-cell epitope. (d) These results suggest that a cocktail of several immunogenic peptides would be more likely to be presented by different MHC haplotypes in humans and would provide the best vaccines for humans.

2. Nonspecific host defenses include ciliated epithelial cells, bactericidal substances in mucous secretions, complement split products activated by the alternative pathway that serve both as opsonins and as chemotactic factors, and phagocytic cells.

3. Specific host defenses include secretory IgA in the mucous secretions, IgG and IgM in the tissue fluids, the classical complement pathway, complement split products, the opsonins (IgM, IgG, and C3b), and phagocytic cells. Cytokines produced during the specific immune response, including IFN-γ, TNF, IL-1, and IL-6, contribute to the overall intensity of the inflammatory response.

4. Humoral antibody peaks within a few days of infection and binds to the influenza HA glycoprotein, blocking viral infection of host epithelial cells. Because the antibody is strain specific, its major role is in protecting against re-infection with the same strain of influenza.

5. (a) African trypanosomes are capable of antigenic shifts in the variant surface glycoprotein (VSG). The antigenic shifts are accomplished as gene segments encoding parts of the VSG are duplicated and translocated to transcriptionally active expression sites. (b) *Plasmodium* evades the immune system by continually undergoing maturational changes from sporozoite to merozoite to gametocyte, allowing the organism to continually change its surface molecules. In addition, the intracellular phases of its life cycle reduce the level of immune activation. Finally, the organism is able to slough off its circumsporozoite coat after antibody binds to it. (c) Influenza is able to evade the immune response through frequent antigenic changes in its hemagglutinin and neuraminidase glycoproteins. The antigenic changes are accomplished by the accumulation of small point mutations (antigenic drift) or through genetic reassortment of RNA between influenza virions from humans and animals (antigenic shift).

6. (a) IA^b. (b) Because antigen-specific, MHC-restricted T_H cells participate in B-cell activation.

7. (a) BCG (Bacillus Calmette-Guerin). (b) Antigenic shift; antigenic drift. (c) Gene conversion. (d) Tubercles; T_{DTH} cells; activated macrophages. (e) Toxoid. (f) Interferon α; interferon β. (g) Secretory IgA. (h) IL-12; IFN-γ.

8. One possible reason for the emergence of new pathogens is the crowding of the world's poorest populations into very small places within huge cities, because population density increases the spread of disease. Another factor is the increase in international travel. Other features of modern life that may contribute include mass distribution of food, which exposes large populations to potentially contaminated food, and unhygienic food preparation.

Chapter 18

1. (a) True. (b) True. (c) True. (d) False: Because DNA vaccines allow prolonged exposure to antigen, they are likely to generate

immunologic memory. (e) True. (f) False: A DNA vaccine contains the gene encoding an entire protein antigen, which most likely contains multiple epitopes.

2. Because attenuated organisms are capable of limited growth within host cells, they are processed by the cytosolic pathway and presented on the membrane of infected host cells together with class I MHC molecules. These vaccines, therefore, usually can induce a cell-mediated immune response. The limited growth of attenuated organisms within the host often eliminates the need for booster doses of the vaccine. Also, if the attenuated organism is able to grow along mucous membranes, then the vaccine will be able to induce the production of secretory IgA. The major disadvantage of attenuated whole-organism vaccines is that they may revert to a virulent form. They also are more unstable than other types of vaccines, requiring refrigeration to maintain their activity.

3. (a) The antitoxin was given to inactivate any toxin that might be produced if *Clostridium tetani* infected the wound. The antitoxin was necessary because the girl had not been previously immunized and, therefore, did not have circulating antibody to tetanus toxin or memory B cells specific for tetanus toxin. (b) Because of the treatment with antitoxin, the girl would not develop immunity to tetanus as a result of the first injury. Therefore, after the second injury, 3 years later, she will require another dose of antitoxin. To develop long-term immunity, she should be vaccinated with tetanus toxoid.

4. The Sabin polio vaccine is attenuated, whereas the Salk vaccine is inactivated. The Sabin vaccine thus has the usual advantages of an attenuated vaccine compared with an inactivated one (see Answer 2). Moreover, since the Sabin vaccine is capable of limited growth along the gastrointestinal tract, it induces production of secretory IgA.

5. T-cell epitopes generally are internal peptides, which commonly contain a high proportion of hydrophobic residues. In contrast, B-cell epitopes are located on an antigen's surface, where they are accessible to antibody, and contain a high proportion of hydrophilic residues. Thus, synthetic hydrophobic peptides are most likely to represent T-cell epitopes and induce cell-mediated response, whereas synthetic hydrophilic peptides are most likely to represent accessible B-cell epitopes and induce an antibody response.

6. When the majority of a population is immune to a particular pathogen—that is, there is herd immunity—then the probability of the few susceptible members of the population contacting an infected individual is very low. Thus, susceptible individuals are not likely to become infected with the pathogen. If the number of immunized individuals decreases sufficiently, most commonly because of reduction in vaccination rates, then herd immunity no longer operates to protect susceptible individuals and infection may spread rapidly in a population, leading to an epidemic.

7. In this hypothetical situation, the gene can be cloned into an expression system and the protein expressed and purified in order to test it as a recombinant protein vaccine. Alternatively, the gene can be cloned into a plasmid vector that can be injected directly and tested as a DNA vaccine. Use of the cloned gene as a DNA vaccine is more efficient, because it eliminates the steps required for preparation of the protein and its purification. However, the plasmid containing the gene for the protective antigen must be suitably purified for use in human trials. DNA vaccines have a greater ability to stimulate both the humoral and cellular arms of the immune system than protein vaccines do and thus may confer more complete immunity. The choice must also take into consideration the fact that recombinant protein vaccines are in widespread use but DNA vaccines for human use are still in early test phases.

8. Pathogens with a short incubation period (e.g., influenza virus) cause disease symptoms before a memory-cell response can be induced. Protection against such pathogens is achieved by repeated reimmunizations to maintain high levels of neutralizing antibody. For pathogens with a longer incubation period (e.g., polio virus), the memory-cell response is rapid enough to prevent development of symptoms, and high levels of neutralizing antibody at the time of infection are unnecessary.

9. Bacterial capsular polysaccharides, inactivated bacterial exotoxins (toxoids), and surface protein antigens. The latter two commonly are produced by recombinant DNA technology.

10. The attenuated Sabin vaccine can cause life-threatening infection in individuals, such as children with AIDS, whose immune systems are severely suppressed.

Chapter 19

1. (a) True. (b) False: X-linked agammaglobulinemia is characterized by a reduction in B cells and an absence of immunoglobulins. (c) False: Phagocytic defects result in recurrent bacterial and fungal infections. (d) True. (e) True. (f) True. (g) True. (h) True. (i) False: These children are usually able to eliminate common encapsulated bacteria with antibody plus complement but are susceptible to viral, protozoan, fungal, and intracellular bacterial pathogens, which are eliminated by the cell-mediated branch of the immune system. (j) False: Humoral immunity also is affected because class II-restricted T_H cells must be activated for an antibody response to occur.

2. (a) Leukocyte-adhesion deficiency results from biosynthesis of a defective β chain in LFA-1, CR3, and CR4, which all contain the same β chain. (b) LFA-1 plays a role in cell adhesion by binding to ICAM-1 expressed on various types of cells. Binding of LFA-1 to ICAM-1 is involved in the interactions between T_H cells and B cells, between CTLs and target cells, and between circulating leukocytes and vascular endothelial cells.

3. (a) The rearranged heavy-chain genes in SCID mice lack the D and/or J gene segments (see Figure 5-10). (b) According to the model of allelic exclusion discussed in Chapter 5, a productive heavy-chain gene rearrangement must occur before κ-chain genes are rearranged. Since SCID mice lack productive heavy-chain rearrangement, they do not attempt κ light-chain rearrangement. (c) Yes: The rearranged μ heavy-chain gene would be transcribed to yield a functional μ heavy chain. The presence of the μ heavy chain then would induce rearrangement of the κ-chain gene (see Figure 5-13).

4. (a) 4. (b) 3. (c) 2. (d) 1. (e) 8. (f) 6. (g) 5. (h) 7.

5. (a) False: HIV-2 and SIV are more closely related. (b) False: HIV-1 infects chimpanzees but does not cause immune suppression. (c) True. (d) False, zidovudine (AZT) acts at the level of reverse transcription of the viral genome whereas indinavir is an inhibitor of the viral protease. (e) True. (f) False: Patients with advanced AIDS sometimes have no detectable serum antibody to HIV. (g) False: The PCR detects HIV proviral DNA in latently infected cells. (h) True.

6. The most likely reason for T-cell depletion in AIDS is the cytopathic effects of HIV infection. If the amount of virus in circulation is decreased by the use of antiviral agents, the number of T cells will increase.

7. No. In the chronic phase of HIV infection, viral replication and the $CD4^+$ T cell number are in a dynamic equilibrium, and the level of virus remains relatively constant.

8. An increase in the viral load and a decrease in $CD4^+$ T-cell levels indicates that HIV infection is progressing from the chronic phase into AIDS. Often infection by an opportunistic agent occurs when the viral load increases and the $CD4^+$ T-cell level drops. The disease AIDS in an HIV-1 infected individual is defined by the presence of certain opportunistic infections or by a $CD4^+$ T-cell count of less than 200 cells/mm^3 (see Table 19-3).

9. Skin-test reactivity is monitored to indicate the functional activity of T_{DTH} cells. As AIDS progresses and $CD4^+$ T cells decline, there is a decline in skin-test reactivity to common antigens.

10. Receptors for certain chemokines, such as CXCR4 and CCR5, also function as co-receptors for HIV-1. The chemokine that is the normal ligand for the receptor competes with the virus for binding to the receptor and can thus inhibit cell infection by blocking attachment of the virus. Cytokines that activate T cells stimulate infection because they increase expression of receptors used by the virus (see Figure 19-11c).

11. No. There are latently infected cells that reside in lymph nodes or in other sites. These cells can be activated and begin producing virus, thus causing a relapse of the disease. In a true cure for AIDS, the patient must be free of all cells containing HIV DNA.

12. Patient LS fits the definition of AIDS, whereas patient BW does not. The clinical diagnosis of AIDS among HIV-infected individuals depends on both the T-cell count and the presence of various indicator diseases. See Table 19-3.

Chapter 20

1. (a) 6. (b) 9. (c) 11. (d) 10. (e) 13. (f) 7. (g) 3. (h) 12. (i) 2. (j) 8. (k) 1. (l) 5. (m) 4.

2. (a) EAE is induced by injecting mice or rats with myelin basic protein in complete Freund's adjuvant. (b) The animals that recover from EAE are now resistant to EAE. If they are given a second injection of myelin basic protein in complete Freund's adjuvant, they no longer develop EAE. (c) If T cells from mice with EAE are transferred to normal syngeneic mice, the mice will develop EAE. See Figure 20-7.

3. A number of viruses have been shown to possess proteins that share sequences with myelin basic protein (MBP). Since the encephalitogenic peptides of MBP are known, it is possible to test these peptides to see whether they bear sequence homology to known viral protein sequences. Computer analysis has revealed a number of viral peptides that bear sequence homology to encephalitogenic peptides of MBP. By immunizing rabbits with these viral sequences, it was possible to induce EAE. The studies on the encephalitogenic peptides of MBP also showed that different peptides induced EAE in different strains. Thus the MHC haplotype will determine which cross-reacting viral peptides will be presented and, therefore, will influence the development of EAE.

4. (1) A virus might express an antigenic determinant that cross-reacts with a self-component. (2) A viral infection might induce localized concentrations of IFN-γ. The IFN-γ might then induce inappropriate expression of class II MHC molecules on non-antigen-presenting cells, enabling self-peptides presented together with the class II MHC molecules on these cells to activate T_H cells. (3) A virus might damage an organ, resulting in release of antigens that are normally sequestered from the immune system.

5. (a) So that the IFN-γ transgene would be expressed only by pancreatic beta cells. (b) There was a cellular infiltration of lymphocytes and macrophages similar to that seen in insulin-dependent diabetes mellitus. (c) The IFN-γ transgene induced the pancreatic beta cells to express class II MHC molecules. (d) A localized viral infection in the pancreas might result in the localized production of IFN-γ by activated T cells. The IFN-γ might then induce the inappropriate expression of class II MHC molecules by pancreatic beta cells as well as the production of other cytokines such as IL-1 or TNF. If self-peptides are presented by the class II MHC molecules, then IL-1 might provide the necessary co-stimulatory signal to activate T cells against the self-peptides. Alternatively, the TNF might also cause localized cellular damage. See Figure 20-9.

6. Anti-CD4 monoclonal antibodies have been used to block T_H activity. Monoclonal antibodies (anti-TAC) specific for the high-affinity IL-2 receptor have been tried to block activated T_H cells. The association of some autoimmune diseases with restricted expression of the T-cell receptor has prompted researchers to use monoclonal antibody specific for T-cell receptors carrying particular V domains. Finally, antibodies against specific MHC alleles associated with increased risk for autoimmunity have been tested in EAE models.

7. (a) True. (b) False: IL-12, which promotes the development of T_H1 cells, increases the autoimmune response to MBP plus adjuvant. (c) False: The presence of HLA B27 is strongly associated with susceptibility to ankylosing spondylitis but is not the only factor required for development of the disease. (d) True. (e) True.

8. The observations that women mount more robust immune responses than men and that these responses tend to be more T_H1-like may, in part, explain gender differences in susceptibility to autoimmunity. Since the T_H1 type of response is pro-inflammatory, the development of autoimmunity may be enhanced.

Chapter 21

1. (a) False: Acute rejection is cell mediated and probably involves the first-set rejection mechanism (see Figures 21-1b and 21-7). (b) True. (c) False: Passenger leukocytes are donor dendritic cells that express class I MHC molecules and high levels of class II MHC molecules. They migrate from the grafted tissue to regional lymph nodes of the recipient, where host immune cells respond to alloantigens on them (see Figure 21-6). (d) False: A graft that is matched for the major histocompatibility antigens, encoded in the HLA, may be rejected because of differences in the minor histocompatibility antigens encoded at other loci. (e) True.

2. (a) The best possible match is identity in the MHC haplotypes of donor and recipient. (b) There is a 25% chance that siblings will share identical MHC haplotypes (see Figure 7-2c). (c) Perform HLA typing using a microcytotoxicity test with monoclonal antibody to class I and class II MHC antigens (see Figure 21-4a). In addition, a one-way MLR can be performed using donor lymphocytes treated with mitomycin C as stimulator cells and untreated recipient lymphocytes as responder cells (see Figure 21-4c).

3. Answer to Question 3 is shown below.

4. (a) Graft-versus-host disease (GVHD) develops as donor T cells recognize alloantigens on cells of an immune-suppressed host. The response develops as donor T_H cells are activated in response to recipient peptide-MHC complexes displayed on antigen-presenting cells. Cytokines elaborated by these T_H cells activate a variety of effector cells, including NK cells, CTLs, and macrophages, which damage the host tissue. In addition, cytokines such as TNF may mediate direct cytolytic damage to the host cells. (b) GVHD develops when the donated organ or tissue contains immunocompetent lymphocytes and when the host is immune suppressed. (c) The donated organ or tissue could be treated with monoclonal antibodies to CD3, CD4, or the high-affinity IL-2 receptor to deplete donor T_H cells. The rationale behind this approach is to diminish T_H-cell activation in response to the alloantigens of the host. The use of anti-CD3 will deplete all T cells; the use of anti-CD4 will deplete all T_H cells; the use of anti-IL-2R will deplete only the activated T_H cells.

5. (a) Sibling C is the best potential donor based on the match of ABO blood type and all class I MHC antigens. (b) Sibling A is the best donor as indicated by the low proliferative response in a one-way MLR with the recipient. This result indicates that class II antigens are matched with those of the recipient. By these tests, sibling A would be selected to be the donor, because the class II antigens are more important in determining potential rejection.

6. The use of soluble CTLA4 or anti-CD40 ligand to promote acceptance of allografts is based on the requirement of a T cell for a co-stimulatory signal when its receptor is bound. Even if the recipient T cell recognizes the graft as foreign, the presence of CTLA4 or anti-CD40L will prevent the T cell from becoming activated because it does not receive a second signal through the CD40 or CD28 receptor (see Figure 21-10). Instead of becoming activated, T cells stimulated in the presence of these blocking molecules become anergic. The advantage of using soluble CTLA4 or anti-CD40L is that these molecules affect only those T cells involved in the reaction against the allograft. These allograft-specific T cells will become anergic, but the general population of T cells will remain normal. More general immunosuppressive measures, such as the use of CsA or FK506, cause immunodeficiency and subsequent susceptibility to infection.

Chapter 22

1. (a) False: Hereditary retinoblastoma results from inactivation of both alleles of *Rb*, a tumor-suppressor gene. (b) True. (c) True. (d) True. (e) False: Some oncogenic retroviruses do not have viral oncogenes. (f) True. (g) False: LAK cells kill a wide variety of tumor cells and are not specific for a single type of tumor.

2. Cells of the pre–B-cell lineage have rearranged the heavy-chain genes and express the μ heavy chain in their cytoplasm (see Figure 11-3). You could perform Southern-blot analysis with a C_μ probe to see whether the heavy-chain genes have rearranged. You could also perform fluorescent staining with antibody specific for the cytoplasmic μ heavy chain.

Donor	Recipient	Response	Type of rejection
BALB/c	C3H	R	FSR
BALB/c	Rat	R	FSR
BALB/c	Nude mouse	A	
BALB/c	C3H, had previous BALB/c graft	R	SSR
BALB/c	C3H, had previous C57BL/6 graft	R	FSR
BALB/c	BALB/c	A	
BALB/c	(BALB/c × C3H) F_1	A	
BALB/c	(C3H × C57BL/6) F_1	R	FSR
(BALB/c × C3H) F_1	BALB/c	R	FSR
(BALB/c × C3H) F_1	BALB/c, had previous F_1 graft	R	SSR

3. (a) Early-stage melanoma cells appear to be functioning as antigen-presenting cells, processing the antigen by the exogenous pathway and presenting the tetanus toxoid antigen together with the class II MHC DR molecule. (b) Advanced-stage melanoma cells might have a reduction in the expression of class II MHC molecules, or they might not be able to internalize and process the antigen by the exogenous route. (c) Since the paraformaldehyde-fixed early melanoma cells could present processed tetanus toxoid, they must express class II MHC molecules on their surface. (d) Stain the early and advanced melanoma cells with fluorescent monoclonal antibody specific for class II MHC molecules.

4. See Tables 22-4 and 22-5, and Figure 22-6.

5. IFN-α, IFN-β, and IFN-γ, enhance the expression of class I MHC molecules on tumor cells, thereby increasing the CTL response to tumors. IFN-γ also increases the activity of CTLs, macrophages, and NK cells, each of which plays a role in the immune response to tumors. TNF-α and TNF-β have direct antitumor activity, inducing hemorrhagic necrosis and tumor regression. IL-2 activates LAK and TIL cells, which both have antitumor activity.

6. (a) Melanoma cells transfected with the B7 gene are able to deliver the co-stimulatory signal necessary for activation of CTL precursors to effector CTLs, which then can destroy tumor cells. Melanoma cells transfected with the GM-CSF gene secrete this cytokine, which stimulates the activation and differentiation of antigen-presenting cells, especially dendritic cells, in the vicinity. The dendritic cells then can present tumor antigens to T_H cells and CTL precursors, enhancing the generation of effector CTLs (see Figure 22-11). (b) Because some of the tumor antigens on human melanomas are expressed by other types of cancers, transfected melanoma cells might be effective against other tumors carrying identical antigens.

Chapter 23

1. (a) The genomic clone contains intervening sequences (introns) that are removed during processing of the primary transcript and therefore do not specify any amino acid residues in the protein product. (b) DNA must be microinjected into a fertilized egg so that the DNA (transgene) will be passed on to all daughter cells. (c) Primary lymphoid cultures have a finite life span and contain a heterogeneous population of cells.

2. (a) Homozygous; syngeneic. (b) B; T. (c) Normal antigen-primed B cells; cancerous plasma cells (myeloma cells); unlimited; monoclonal antibodies. (d) Transformation; indefinite.

3.

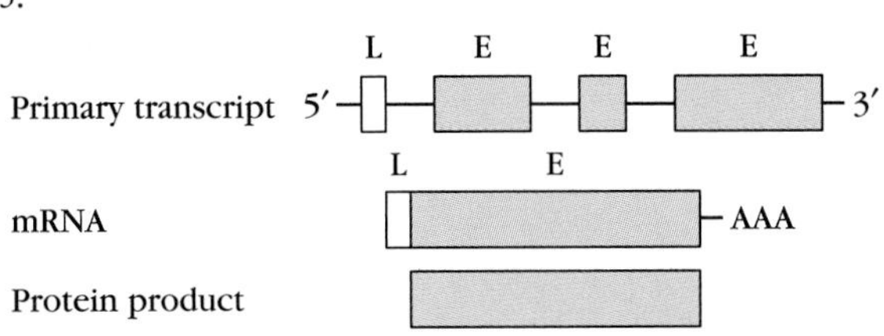

4. c.

5. a, b, d.

6. Transfected DNA integrates only into a small percentage of cells. If a selectable marker gene is also present, the small number of transfected cells will grow in the appropriate medium, whereas the much larger number of nontransfected cells will die.

7. The mouse would become a mosaic in which the transgene would have incorporated into some of the somatic cells but not all.

8. Since cleavage with each restriction enzyme alone produced a single band, the plasmid, which is circular, must contain one restriction site for each enzyme. Since simultaneous cleavage of the 5.4-kb plasmid with both enzymes yielded a single band, the fragments from each cleavage must have the same length. Thus, the restriction sites must be equidistant from each other in both directions on the plasmid, as shown in the diagram below.

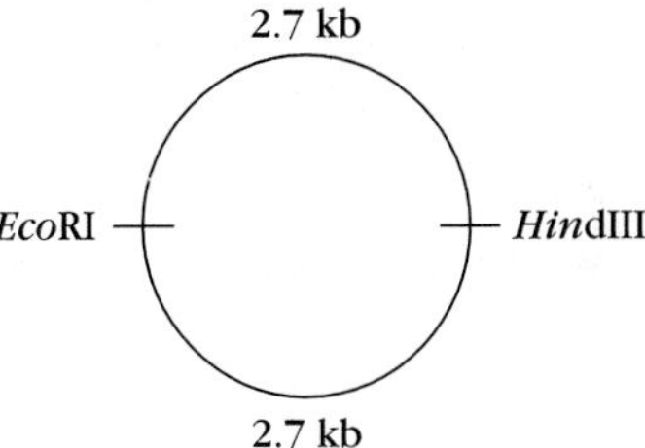

9. d.

10. Isolate mRNA from activated T cells and transcribe it into cDNA using reverse transcriptase. Insert cDNA into a suitable expression vector, such as plasmid DNA carrying an ampicillin selection gene. Transfer the recombinant plasmid DNA into *E. coli* and grow in the presence of ampicillin to select for bacteria containing the plasmid DNA. Test the bacterial culture supernatant for the presence of IL-2 by seeing whether the monoclonal antibody to IL-2 reacts with the culture supernatant. Once a bacterial culture is identified that is secreting IL-2, the cDNA can be cloned.

11. Radiolabel the mRNA and use the labeled mRNA as a probe to screen the genomic library by in situ hybridization. Re-plate and culture the selected clone, and isolate the cloned DNA from the host DNA.

12. In production of transgenic mice, a functional foreign gene is added to the genome; the process involves introducing a cloned natural gene or cDNA into a fertilized egg, which then is implanted into a pseudopregnant female. In production of knockout mice, a nonfunctional form of a mouse gene replaces the functional gene, so that the animal does not express the encoded product; the process involves selecting transfected embryonic stem (ES) cells carrying the mutated gene and injecting the ES cells into a blastocyst, which then is implanted into a pseudopregnant female.

13. Knockout mice are animals in which a particular gene or DNA sequence has been deleted, whereas knock-in mice are animals in which a piece of DNA has been exchanged for the endogenous DNA sequence.

14. The Cre/*lox* system makes it possible to specifically delete or insert a DNA sequence of choice into the tissue of choice at a particular time during development by using tissue-specific promoters to drive the change in the DNA sequence. This technology thus enhances knockout and knock-in strategies by making them more selective. Also, sometimes restricting the change in sequence to a particular tissue will allow the consequences of a particular deletion or insertion to be studied in that one tissue even though it would be lethal to the organism if present in all tissues.

15. (a) 8. (b) 2. (c) 5. (d) 9. (e) 4. (f) 3. (g) 6. (h) 7. (i) 10.

CREDITS

Line illustrations rendered by Fine Line Illustrations.

Cover Image From D. Philips, Science Source/Photo Researchers.
Preface Figure, p. xx From B. A. Osborne and S. Smith, *Journal of NIH Research,* Vol. 9, 1997, p. 35. Courtesy of Barbara Osborne, University of Massachusetts at Amherst.
Preface Figure, p. xxi, left column From J. Lescar et al., *Journal of Molecular Biology,* Vol. 267, 1997, p. 1207. Courtesy of Graham Bentley, Institute Pasteur.
Preface Figure, p. xxi, right column From D. A. Vignali and J. Strominger, *The Immunologist,* Vol. 2, 1994, p. 112.
Preface Figure, p. xxii From M. Walter et al., *Nature,* Vol. 376, 1995, p. 232. Courtesy of Mark Walter, University of Alabama.
Preface Figure, p. xxiii Adapted from A. Fauci et al., "Immunopathogenic Mechanisms of HIV Infection," *Annals of Internal Medicine,* Vol. 124, 1996, p. 654.
Part I Opener From David Scharf, Peter Arnold, Inc.
Chapter 1 Opener From N. Sharon and H. Lis, *Scientific American,* Vol. 268, January 1993, p. 85. Photograph courtesy of Kazuhiko Fujita. Micrograph by Morten H. Nielsen and Ole Werdelin.
Figure 1-1 From *Harper's Weekly,* Vol. 29, 1885, p. 836. Courtesy of the National Library of Medicine.
Figure 1-2 From N. Sharon and H. Lis, *Scientific American,* Vol. 268, January 1993, p. 85. Photograph courtesy of Kazuhiko Fujita.
Table 1-3 Data from L. Du Pasquier, "Evolution of the Immune System," in *Fundamental Immunology,* 3rd ed., W. E. Paul, ed., Raven, New York; B. Fritig, T. Heitz, and M. Legrand, "Antimicrobial Proteins in Induced Plant Defense," *Current Opinion in Immunology,* Vol. 10, 1998, p. 16; and K. Soderhall and L. Cerenius, "Role of the Prophenoloxidase-activating System in Invertebrate Immunology," *Current Opinion in Immunology,* Vol. 10, 1998, p. 23.
Figure 1-6 From A. S. Rosenthal et al., *Phagocytosis—Past and Future,* Academic Press, 1982, p. 239. Reprinted by permission.
Figure 1-12 From *Immunology: Recognition and Response,* W. E. Paul, ed., W. H. Freeman and Company, 1991, p. 49. Originally from "How T Cells See Antigen," by H. M. Grey et al., *Scientific American,* November 1989, p. 57. © 1989 by Scientific American Inc. All rights reserved. Micrograph courtesy of Morten H. Nielsen and Ole Werdelin.
Figure 1-14 From B. Lemaitre et al., *Cell,* Vol. 86, 1996, p. 973. Courtesy of Jules A. Hoffmann, University of Strasbourg.
Chapter 1 Clinical Focus Table Data from Centers for Disease Control and Prevention, National Center for Health Statistics, 1997, DHHS Publication No. (PHS)97–1790, June 1997.
Chapter 2 Opener From Lennart Nilsson, "Our Immune System: The Wars Within," *National Geographic,* June 1986, p. 718. © by Boehringer Ingelheim International. GmbH, Stockholm. Photo by Lennart Nilsson.
Figure 2-2b From M. J. Cline and D. W. Golde, "Cellular Interactions in Hematopoiesis," reprinted by permission from *Nature,* Vol. 277, 1979, p. 180. © 1979 Macmillan Magazines Ltd. Micrograph courtesy of Shirley Quan.
Figure 2-4 From B. A. Osborne and S. Smith, *Journal of NIH Research,* Vol. 9, 1997, p. 35. Courtesy of Barbara Osborne, University of Massachusetts at Amherst.
Figure 2-7b Courtesy of Dr. Joseph R. Goodman, Department of Pediatrics, University of California at San Francisco.
Figure 2-9a From Lennart Nilsson, "Our Immune System: The Wars Within," *National Geographic,* June 1986, p. 718. © by Boehringer Ingelheim International GmbH, Stockholm. Photo by Lennart Nilsson.
Figure 2-11 Reprinted from J. H. Peters et al., *Immunology Today,* Vol. 17, p. 273, © 1996, with permission of Elsevier Science.
Figure 2-12 From A. K. Szakal et al., "Isolated Follicular Dendritic Cells: Cytochemical Antigen Localization, Nomarski, SEM, and TEM Morphology," *Journal of Immunology,* Vol. 134, 1985, p. 1353. © 1985 American Association of Immunologists. Reprinted with permission.
Figure 2-13 Adapted from Lodish et al., *Molecular Cell Biology,* Third Edition, 1995, Scientific American Books.
Figure 2-14 Adapted, with permission, from W. van Ewijk, *Annual Review of Immunology,* Vol. 9, 1991, p. 591. © 1991 by Annual Reviews Inc.
Figure 2-15 From M. M. Compton and J. A. Cidlowski, *Trends in Endocrinology and Metabolism,* Vol. 3, 1992, p. 17.
Figure 2-17 From W. Bloom and D. W. Fawcett, *Textbook of Histology,* 10th Edition, 1975. © 1975, W. B. Saunders Co.
Figure 2-20b From J. Klein, *Immunology, The Science of Self-Nonself Discrimination,* p. 77. © 1982 by John Wiley Publishers. Reprinted by permission of John Wiley and Sons, Inc.
Part II Opener Reprinted with permission from K. Garcia et al., *Science,* Vol. 274, p. 209. © 1996 by the American Association for the Advancement of Science. Courtesy of K. Garcia.
Chapter 3 Opener From G. J. V. H. Nossal, *Scientific American,* Vol. 269, 1993, p. 22.
Figure 3-2 From K. C. Garcia et al., *Science,* Vol. 257, 1992, p. 502.
Figure 3-3 From A. G. Amit et al., *Science,* Vol. 233, 1986, p. 747.
Figure 3-4 From I. A. Wilson and R. L. Stanfield, *Current Opinion in Structural Biology,* Vol. 3, 1993, p. 113.
Figure 3-5 Adapted from M. Sela, "Antigenicity: Some Molecular Aspects," *Science,* Vol. 166, December 12, 1969, p. 1365. © 1969 by the American Association for the Advancement of Science.
Table 3-5 Based on K. Landsteiner, *The Specificity of Serologic Reactions,* 1962, Dover Press. Modified by J. Klein, *Immunology: The Science of Self-Nonself Discrimination,* 1982, John Wiley Publishers.

Figure 3-6 From G. J. V. H. Nossal, *Scientific American*, Vol. 269, March 1993, p. 22.
Figure 3-7a Adapted from M. Z. Atassi and A. L. Kazim, *Advanced Experimental Methods in Biology*, Vol. 98, 1978, p. 9.
Figure 3-7b Adapted from W. G. Laver et al., *Cell*, Vol. 61, 1990, p. 554.
Figure 3-8 Adapted from D. Benjamin et al., with permission from the *Annual Review of Immunology*, Vol. 2, 1984, p. 67. © 1984 by Annual Reviews Inc.
Figure 3-10 From J. Rothbard et al., *Modern Trends in Human Leukemia*, Vol. 7, 1987. Reprinted by permission of Springer-Verlag Inc.
Figure 3-11 From H. M. Grey et al., *Scientific American*, Vol. 261, May 1989, p. 59. © 1989 by Scientific American Inc. All rights reserved.
Chapter 3 Clinical Focus Figure Adapted from N. F. Adkinson, *Manual of Clinical Laboratory Immunology*, 1995, p. 85. N. Rose et al., eds., American Society of Microbiology, Washington, DC.
Figure 4-1 Adapted from A. Tiselius and E. A. Kabat, *Journal of Experimental Medicine*, Vol. 69, 1939, p. 119, with copyright permission of the Rockefeller University Press.
Table 4-3 Adapted from J. Newman, "How Breast Milk Protects Newborns", *Scientific American*, Vol. 273, June 1995, p. 76.
Figure 4-4 Adapted from H. Lodish et al., *Molecular Cell Biology*, 4th ed., 1995, p. 58. © 1995 by Scientific American Books. Reprinted by permission of W. H. Freeman and Company.
Figure 4-5 Image provided by the laboratory of Dr. Alexander McPherson. The immunoglobulin structure was determined by Harris et al., *Nature*, Vol. 360, 1992, pp. 369–372. A special thank you to the American Computing and Graphics and Visual Imaging Lab, University of California, Riverside, for help with image. The image was generated using the computer program RIBBONS. The RIBBONS reference is: M. Carson and C. E. Bugg, "An Algorithm for Ribbon Models of Proteins," *Journal of Molecular Graphics*, Vol. 4, 1986, pp. 121–122.
Figure 4–6a Adapted from M. Schiffer et al.; reprinted with permission from *Biochemistry*, Vol. 12, 1973, p. 4620. © 1973 by the American Chemical Society.
Figure 4-6b Adapted from Williams and Barclay, *Annual Review of Immunology*, Vol. 6, 1988, p. 381.
Figure 4-7a From E. W. Silverton et al., *Proceedings of the National Academy of Sciences USA*, Vol. 74, 1977, p. 5140.
Figure 4-8 Based on E. A. Kabat et al., *Sequence of Immunoglobulin Chains*, U.S. Department of Health, Education, and Welfare, 1977.
Figure 4-9a From K. C. Garcia et al., *Science*, Vol. 257, 1992, p. 502. Courtesy of Mario Amzel, Johns Hopkins University.
Figure 4-10 From J. M. Rini, W. Schulze-Gahmen, and I. A. Wilson, *Science*, Vol. 255, 1992, p. 959. Photograph courtesy of J. M. Rini, W. Schulze-Gahmen, and I. A. Wilson.
Figure 4-11 From J. Lescar et al., *Journal of Molecular Biology*, Vol. 267, 1997, p. 1207. Courtesy of Graham Bentley, Institute Pasteur.
Figure 4-12 From R. C. Valentine and N. M. Green, *Journal of Molecular Biology*, Vol. 27, 1967, p. 615. Reprinted by permission of Academic Press Inc. (London) Ltd.
Figure 4-18 Adapted from A. D. Keegan and W. E. Paul, *Immunology Today*, Vol. 13, 1992, p. 63, and M. E. Reth, *Annual Review of Immunology*, Vol. 10, 1992, p. 97.
Figure 5-2 Adapted from N. Hozumi and S. Tonegawa, *Proceedings of the National Academy of Sciences USA*, Vol. 73, 1976, p. 3628.
Figure 5-8 From K. Okazki et al., *Cell*, Vol. 49, 1987, p. 477. Reprinted by permission of Cell Press.
Figure 5-10 Adapted from F. W. Alt, *Immunology Today*, Vol. 13, 1992, p. 306. Elsevier Science Publishing Company, Inc. Reprinted by permission.
Figure 5-13 Adapted with permission from G. D. Yancopoulos and F. W. Alt, *Annual Review of Immunology*, Vol. 4, 1986, p. 339. © 1986 by Annual Reviews, Inc.
Figure 5-16 Adapted from C. Berek and C. Milstein, *Immunological Reviews*, Vol. 96, 1987, p. 23. © Munksgaard International Publishers Ltd., Copenhagen, Denmark.
Figure 5-22 Adapted from M. Verhoeyen and L. Reichmann, *BioEssays*, Vol. 8, 1988, p.74. Reprinted by permission of Cambridge University Press.
Figure 5-24 Adapted from W. D. Huse et al., *Science*, Vol. 246, 1989, p. 1275.
Table 6-1 Adapted from H. N. Eisen, *Immunology*, 3rd ed., 1990, Harper & Row Publishers.
Table 6-3 Adapted from N. R. Rose et al., eds., 1986 and 1997 editions, *Manual of Clinical Laboratory Immunology*, American Society for Microbiology, Washington, DC.
Figure 6-7b From J. S. Garvey, N. E. Cremer, and D. H. Sussdorf, *Methods in Immunology*, 3rd ed.; © 1977 by Addison-Wesley Publishing Company, Inc., Advanced Book Program. Reprinted by permission of the author.
Figure 6-8 Courtesy of Harriet C. W. Thompson, Louisiana State University Medical Center/MIP.
Figure 6-14d Courtesy of P. Groscurth, Institute of Anatomy, University of Zurich-Irchel.
Figure 6-15d From H. A. Schreuder et al., *Nature*, Vol. 386, 1997, p. 196. Courtesy of H. Schreuder, Hoechst Marion Roussel.
Figure 6-17 From A. Jenei et al., *Proceedings of the National Academy of Sciences*, Vol. 94, 1997, pp. 7269–7274. Courtesy of Attila Jenei and Sandor Damjanovich, University Medical School of Debrecen, Hungary.
Chapter 7 Opener From M. Matsumura, D. H. Fremont, P. A. Paterson, and I. A. Wilson, *Science*, Vol. 257, 1992, p. 927. Photographs courtesy of D. H. Fremont, M. Matsumura, M. Pique, and I. A. Watson.
Table 7-3 Adapted from S. Buus et al., *Science*, Vol. 235, 1987, p. 1353.
Table 7-4 Data from *SAM CD: A Comprehensive Knowledge Base of Internal Medicine,* D. C. Dale, D. D. Federman, eds., 1997, *Scientific American*, New York, NY.
Figures 7-7 and 7-8 a, b Adapted from J. H. Brown, T. S. Jerdetzky, J. C. Gorga, L. J. Stern, R. G. Urban, J. L. Strominger, and D. C. Wiley, *Nature*, Vol. 364, 1993, p. 33.
Figure 7-8c From Dessen et al., *Immunity*, Vol. 7, 1997, pp. 473–481.
Figure 7-10 a, b From D. A. Vignali and J. Strominger, *The Immunologist*, Vol. 2, 1994, p. 112.
Figure 7-11 Data from V. H. Engelhard, *Current Opinion in Immunology*, Vol. 6, 1994, p. 13.
Figure 7-12 From M. Matsumura, D. H. Fremont, P. A. Paterson, and I. A. Wilson, *Science*, Vol. 257, 1992, p. 927. Photographs courtesy of D. H. Fremont, M. Matsumura, M. Pique, and I. A. Watson.

Figure 7-13a Adapted from P. Parham; reprinted with permission from *Nature*, Vol. 360, 1992, p. 300. © 1992 Macmillan Magazines Limited.
Figure 7-13b Adapted, with permission, from M. L. Silver et al., *Nature*, Vol. 360, 1992, p. 367. © 1992 Macmillan Magazines Limited.
Figure 7-13c Adapted from D. R. Madden et al., *Cell*, Vol. 70, 1992, p. 1035. Reprinted by permission of Cell Press.
Figure 7-14a Adapted from R. Sodoyer et al., *EMBO Journal*, Vol. 3, 1984, p. 879. Published by European Molecular Biology Organization. Reprinted by permission of Oxford University Press.
Figure 7-14b Adapted, with permission, from P. Parham, *Nature*, Vol. 342, 1989, p. 617. © 1989 Macmillan Magazines Limited.
Figure 7-17 Photograph taken in the Okavango Delta, Botswana, by T. J. Kindt.
Chapter 7 Clinical Focus Figure From *SAM CD: A Comprehensive Knowledge Base of Internal Medicine*, D. C. Dale, and D. D. Federman, eds., 1997, Ch. 4:1X Figure 6b, Scientific American, New York, NY.
Figure 8-1 Adapted from A. Rosenthal and E. Shevach, *Journal of Experimental Medicine*, Vol. 138, 1974, p. 1194, by copyright permission of the Rockefeller University Press.
Figure 8-2 Adapted from P. C. Doherty and R. M. Zinkernagel, *Journal of Experimental Medicine*, Vol. 141, 1975, p. 502.
Table 8-2 Adapted from T. J. Braciale et al., *Immunological Reviews*, Vol. 98, 1987, p. 95.
Figure 8-10b From Dessen et al., *Immunity*. Vol. 7, 1997, pp. 473–481. Courtesy of Don Wiley, Harvard University.
Figure 8-11 Adapted from Melian et al., *Current Opinions in Immunology*, Vol. 8, 1996, pp. 82–88.
Chapter 9 Opener From D. N. Garboczi et al., *Nature*, Vol. 384, 1996, p. 134. Courtesy of D. N. Garboczi, NIAID, NIH.
Table 9-1 Data from P. A. H. Moss et al., *Annual Review of Immunology*, Vol. 10, 1992, p. 71.
Figure 9-2 Based on J. Kappler et al., *Journal of Experimental Medicine*, Vol. 153, 1981, p. 1198.
Figure 9-4 Based on S. Hendrick et al., *Nature*, Vol. 308, 1984, p. 149.
Figure 9-5 Adapted, with permission, from D. Raulet, *Annual Review of Immunology*, Vol. 7, 1989, p. 175; and M. Davis, *Annual Review of Biochemistry*, Vol. 59, 1990, p. 475. © 1989 and 1990, respectively, by Annual Reviews Inc.
Figure 9-11a Reprinted from S. J. Davis and P. A. van der Merve, *Immunology Today*, Vol. 17, p. 181, © 1996, permission from Elsevier Science.
Figure 9-11b From G. F. Gao et al., *Nature*, Vol. 387, 1997, pp. 630–634. Courtesy of E. Yvonne Jones, University of Oxford.
Figure 9-14a and c From D. N. Garboczi et al., *Nature*, Vol. 384, 1996, pp. 134–141. Courtesy of Don C. Wiley, Harvard University.
Figure 9-14 b and d From C. Garcia et al., *Science*, Vol. 274, 1996, p. 209. Courtesy of Chris Garcia, Scripps Research Institute.
Figure 9-15 From C. Garcia et al., *Science*, Vol. 274, 1996, p. 211. Courtesy of Chris Garcia, Scripps Research Institute.
Figure 10-1 Adapted from B. J. Fowlkes and D. M. Pardoll, *Advances in Immunology*, Vol. 44, 1989, p. 207. Reprinted by permission of Academic Press.
Table 10-3 Adapted from G. Crabtree, *Science*, Vol. 243, 1989, p. 357. © 1989 by the American Association for the Advancement of Science.
Figure 10-8 Adapted from H. Von Boehmer and P. Kisielow, *Science*, Vol. 248, 1990, p. 1370.
Figure 10-10 Adapted from A. Weiss, "T-cell Activation," in *Fundamental Immunology*, 3rd. ed., 1993, Raven, New York.
Figure 10-14 Adapted from P. S. Linsley and J. A. Ledbetter, *Annual Review of Immunology*, Vol. 11, 1993, p.191.
Chapter 10 Clinical Focus Figures First and second figures from Drappa et al., *New England Journal of Medicine*, Vol. 335, p. 1643. © 1996 by Massachusetts Medical Society. All rights reserved. Third figure adapted from G. H. Fisher et al., *Cell*, Vol. 81, 1995, p. 935.
Chapter 11 Opener From V. M. Sanders et al., "Characterization of the Physical Interaction Between Antigen-Specific B and T Cells," *Journal of Immunology*, Vol. 137, 1986, p. 2395.
Table 11-1 Adapted from D. A. Nemazee and K. Burki, *Nature*, Vol. 337, 1989, p. 562.
Table 11-3 Adapted from C. C. Goodnow, *Annual Review of Immunology*, Vol. 10, 1992, p. 489.
Figure 11-5 Adapted from D. A. Nemazee and K. Burki, reprinted from *Nature*, Vol. 337, 1989, p. 562; S. L. Tiegs et al., *Journal of Experimental Medicine*, Vol. 177, 1993, p. 1009.
Table 11-6 Adapted, with permission, from H. N. Eisen and G. W. Siskind, *Biochemistry*, Vol. 3, 1964, p. 966. © 1964 American Chemical Society.
Figure 11-8 Adapted from A. Defranco, *Fundamental Immunology*, 4th ed., p. 239, W. E. Paul, ed., Lippincott-Raven, Philadelphia and New York.
Figure 11-11 From V. M. Saunders et al., "Characterization of the Physical Interaction Between Antigen-Specific B and T cells," *Journal of Immunology*, Vol. 137, 1986, p. 2395.
Figure 11-12 From W. J. Poo et al., *Nature*, Vol. 332, 1988, p. 378. © 1988 Macmillan Magazines Ltd.
Figure 11-19 Reprinted with permission, as adapted, by C. Berek from Jacob et al., *Nature*, Vol. 354, p. 389. © 1991 Macmillan Magazines, Ltd.
Figure 11-20 Adapted from P. Gearhart in *Fundamental Immunology*, 3rd Ed., 1993, Raven, New York, p. 877.
Part III Opener From H. A. Schreuder et al., *Nature*, Vol. 386, 1997, p. 196. Courtesy of Herman Schreuder, Hoechst Marion Roussel.
Table 12-2 Adapted from E. A. Bach, M. Aguet, and R. D. Schreiber, *Annual Review of Immunology*, Vol. 15, 1997, p. 563.
Figure 12-3b Courtesy of R&D Systems.
Table 12-4 Adapted from F. Powrie and R. L. Coffman, *Immunology Today*, Vol. 14, 1993, p. 270.
Figure 12-4b From J. L. Boulay and W. E. Paul, *Current Biology*, Vol. 3, 1993, p. 573.
Figure 12-7 Adapted from K. Sugamura et al., *Annual Review of Immunology*, Vol. 14, 1996, p. 179.
Figure 12-8a Adapted from T. Kishimoto et al., *Science*, Vol. 258, 1992, p. 593. © 1992 by the American Association for the Advancement of Science.
Figure 12-10a Adapted from Bach et al., *Annual Review of Immunology*, Vol. 15, 1997, p. 563.

Figure 12-11 From M. R. Walter et al., *Nature*, Vol. 376, 1995, p. 230. Courtesy of M. Walter, University of Alabama.

Figure 12-13 From P. A. Sieling and R. L. Modlin, *Immunobiology*, Vol. 191, 1994, p. 378.

Figure 13-3a From N. C. Hughes-Jones, "The Classical Pathway," in *Immunobiology of the Complement System*, Academic Press, 1986. Originally published in H. R. Knobel et al., *European Journal of Immunology*, Vol. 5, 1975, p. 78.

Figure 13-3c From N. C. Hughes-Jones, "The Classical Pathway," in *Immunobiology of the Complement System*, Academic Press, 1986. Originally published in J. Tschopp et al., *Proceedings of the National Academy of Science USA*, Vol. 77, 1980, p. 7014.

Table 13-3 From M. K. Pangburn, "The Alternate Pathway," in *Immunobiology of the Complement System*, Academic Press, 1986.

Figure 13-4 From A. Feinstein, E. Munn, and N. Richardson, *Monographs in Allergy*, Vol. 17, 1981, p. 28, S. Karger AG, Basel; and from A. Feinstein, E. Munn, and N. Richardson, *Annals of the New York Academy of Sciences*, Vol. 190, 1981, p. 1104.

Figure 13-8a From E. R. Podack, "Assembly and Functions of the Terminal Components," *Immunobiology of the Complement System*, Academic Press, 1986.

Figure 13-8b From J. Humphrey and R. Dourmashkin, *Advances in Immunology*, Vol. 11, 1969, p. 75. Reprinted by permission of Academic Press.

Figure 13-11 From R. D. Schreiber et al., "Bacterial Activity of the Alternative Complement Pathway Generated from 11 Isolated Plasma Proteins." *Journal of Experimental Medicine*, Vol. 149, 1979, p. 870. Reproduced by copyright permission of the Rockefeller University Press.

Figure 13-12 From N. R. Cooper and G. R. Nemerow, "Complement-Dependent Mechanisms of Virus Neutralization," in *Immunobiology of the Complement System*, Academic Press, 1986, p. 155.

Figure 13-13 From N. R. Cooper and G. R. Nemerow, "Complement-Dependent Mechanisms of Virus Neutralization," in *Immunobiology of the Complement System*, Academic Press, 1986, p. 150.

Chapter 14 Opener From J. D. E. Young and Z. A. Cohn, *Scientific American*, Vol. 258, January 1988, p. 38. © 1988 by Scientific American Inc. SEM by Dr. Gilla Kaplan, The Rockefeller University.

Figure 14-3 From J. D. E. Young and Z. A. Cohn, *Scientific American*, Vol. 258, January 1988, p. 38. © 1988 by Scientific American Inc. SEM by Dr. Gilla Kaplan, The Rockefeller University.

Figure 14-4 Adapted, with permission, from P. A. Henkart, *Annual Review of Immunology*, Vol. 3, 1985, p. 31. © 1985 by Annual Reviews Inc.

Figure 14-5 Based on M. L. Dustin and T. A. Springer, *Nature*, Vol. 341, 1989, p. 619.

Figure 14-6 From J. R. Yannelli et al., "Reorientation and Fusion of Cytotoxic T Lymphocyte Granules after Interaction with Target Cells as Determined by High Resolution Cinemicrography," *The Journal of Immunology*, Vol. 136, 1986, pp. 377–382. Reprinted by permission.

Figure 14-7a From J. D. E. Young and Z. A. Cohn, *Scientific American*, Vol. 258, January 1988, p. 38. © 1988 by Scientific American Inc.

Figure 14-7b From E. R. Podack and G. Dennert, *Nature*, Vol. 301, 1983, p. 442. © 1983 Macmillan Magazines Ltd.

Figure 14-9 Adapted from Shresta et al., *Current Opinion in Immunology*, 1998, Vol. 10, p. 581.

Figure 14-17 Adapted from D. K. Dalton et al., *Science*, Vol. 259, 1993, p. 1739. © 1993 by the American Association for the Advancement of Science.

Chapter 15 Opener From S. D. Rosen and L. M. Stoolman, *Vertebrate Lectins*, 1987, Van Norstrand Reinhold.

Figure 15-1 Reprinted from A. Ager, *Trends in Cell Biology*, Vol. 4, p. 326, © 1994, with permission from Elsevier Science.

Table 15-2 Adapted from P. J. Nelson and A. M. Krensky, *Current Opinion in Immunology*, Vol. 10, 1998, p. 265, and M. Baggiolini, *Nature*, Vol. 392, 1998, p. 565.

Figure 15-4a Adapted from A. O. Anderson and N. D. Anderson, "Structure and Physiology of Lymphatic Tissues," in *Cellular Functions in Immunity and Inflammation*, J. J. Oppenheim et al., eds., Elsevier, North-Holland, 1981, p. 39. Reprinted with permission.

Figure 15-4b From S. D. Rosen and L. M. Stoolman, *Vertebrate Lectins*, 1987, Van Norstrand Reinhold.

Figure 15-4c From S. D. Rosen, *Current Opinion in Cell Biology*, Vol. 1, 1989, p. 913. Reprinted by permission of Current Science.

Table 15-4 Adapted from J. P. Girard and T. A. Springer, *Immunology Today*, Vol. 16, 1995, p. 449.

Figure 15-8 Adapted from Premack et al., *Nature Medicine*, Vol. 2, 1996, p. 1174.

Figure 15-9 Reprinted, with permission, from M. Baggiolini, *Nature*, Vol. 392, p. 565. © 1998 Macmillan Magazines Ltd.

Figure 15-15 Adapted from Research News, *Science*, Vol. 259, 1993, p. 1693.

Figure 15-16a From L. J. Old, " Tumor Necrosis Factor," *Scientific American*, Vol. 258, May 1988, p. 59.

Figure 15-16b From B. Beutler, *Hospital Practice*, April 15, 1993, p. 45.

Chapter 16 Opener From S. Burwen and B. Satir, reproduced from the *Journal of Cell Biology*, Vol. 73, 1977, p. 662, by copyright permission of the Rockefeller University Press.

Table 16-2 Based on K. Ishizaka and T. Ishizaka, *Journal of Immunology*, Vol. 99, 1967, p. 1187.

Figure 16-3 From S. Burwen and B. Satir, reproduced from the *Journal of Cell Biology*, Vol. 73, 1977, p. 662, by copyright permission of The Rockefeller University Press.

Figure 16-7 Adapted from T. Ishizaka et al., *International Archives of Allergy and Applied Immunology*, Vol. 77, 1985, p. 137. Reprinted by permission of S. Karger AG, Basel.

Figure 16-9 Adapted from G. Del Prete, *Journal of Immunology*, Vol. 140, 1988, p. 4193.

Figure 16-10 From L. M. Lichtenstein, *Scientific American*, Vol. 269, February 1993, p. 117. Used with permission.

Figure 16-12 Adapted from K. Ishizaka and T. Ishizaka in *Asthma Physiology, Immunopharmacology, and Treatment*, K. F. Austen and L. M. Lichtenstein, eds., © 1973. Academic Press.

Figure 16-16 Based on F. G. Germuth, Jr., *Journal of Experimental Medicine*, Vol. 97, 1953, p. 257.

Part IV Opener From Andrejs Liepins, Photo Researchers.

Chapter 17 Opener From M. E. Ward and P. J. Watt, *Journal of Infectious Diseases*, Vol. 126, 1972, p. 601. © 1972. Reprinted by permission of The University of Chicago Press.

Table 17-1 Data from World Health Organization, U.S. Agency for International Development, and National Institute of Allergy and Infectious Diseases.

Figure 17-2 From G. Murti, Department of Virology, St. Jude Children's Research Hospital, Memphis, TN.

Figure 17-4 Adapted from G. G. Brownlee, *Options for the Control of Influenza*, 1986, p. 47, Alan R. Liss. © 1986 by John Wiley & Sons.

Table 17-5 Adapted from M. F. Good et al., *Annual Review of Immunology*, Vol. 6, 1988, p. 633.

Figure 17-6 Adapted and reprinted, with permission, from D. C. Wiley et al., *Nature*, Vol. 289, 1981, p. 373. © 1981 Macmillan Magazines Ltd.

Figure 17-8 From M. E. Ward and P. J. Watt, *Journal of Infectious Diseases*, Vol. 126, 1972, p. 601. © 1972. Reprinted by permission of The University of Chicago Press.

Figure 17-9 Adapted from A. M. Dannenberg, *Hospital Practice*, January 15, 1993, p. 51.

Figure 17-10 Courtesy of Mark S. Klempner, New England Medical Center.

Figure 17-12a Adapted from John Donelson, *The Biology of Parasitism*, Alan R. Liss. © 1988 by John Wiley & Sons.

Figure 18-1 Data from Centers for Disease Control.

Figure 18-2 Data from Centers for Disease Control.

Figure 18-3 From M. Zanetti et al., *Immunology Today*, Vol. 8, 1987, p. 18.

Table 18-3 Adapted from the ECBT website <www.ecbt.org>; approved by the American Academy of Pediatrics.

Figure 18-4 Adapted from *Polio: The Beginning of the End*, 1997, World Health Organization, Geneva; document available from the WHO website on vaccines and vaccination <http://www.who.int/gov/>.

Figure 18-5 Adapted from B. Moss, *Immunology Today*, Vol. 6, 1985, p. 243.

Figure 18-6 Adapted from D. B. Weiner and R. C. Kennedy, *Scientific American*, Vol. 281, 1999, p. 50.

Chapter 18 Clinical Focus Figures Part (a) from A. Z. Kapikian et al., *New England Journal of Medicine*, Vol. 294, pp. 965–972. © 1976 by Massachusetts Medical Society. All rights reserved. Courtesy of Albert Z. Kapikian, NIAID, NIH. Part (b) courtesy of B. V. V. Prasad, Baylor College of Medicine.

Chapter 19 Opener From R. C. Gallo, "HIV—The Cause of AIDS," *Journal of Acquired Immune Deficiency Syndromes*, Vol. 1, 1988, p. 521. Reprinted by permission of Raven Press Ltd.

Figure 19-2 From J. W. Belmont, *Trends in Genetics*, Vol. 11, 1995, p. 112.

Figure 19-3 Adapted from B. A. Smart and H. D. Ochs, *Current Opinion in Pediatrics*, Vol. 9, 1997, p. 570.

Table 19-3 Data from CDC guidelines for AIDS diagnosis, 1993 revision.

Figure 19-4 From R. Kretschmer et al., *The New England Journal of Medicine*, Vol. 279, 1968, p. 1295. Courtesy of F. S. Rosen.

Figure 19-5 Courtesy of The Jackson Laboratory, Bar Harbor, Maine.

Table 19-5 From J. G. Bartlett and R. D. Moore, "Improving HIV therapy," *Scientific American*, Vol. 279, 1998, p. 87.

Figure 19-6 From *National Vital Statistics Report*, Vol. 47, 1999, p. 19.

Table 19-6 Adapted from A. S. Fauci, "An HIV Vaccine: Breaking the Paradigms," *Proceedings of the American Association of Physicians*, Vol. 108, 1996, p. 6.

Figure 19-7 From UNAIDS and WHO, AIDs Epidemic Update: December 1998, UNAIDS, Geneva.

Table 19-7 From D. Baltimore and C. Heilman, "HIV Vaccines: Prospects and Challenges," *Scientific American*, Vol. 279, 1998, p. 101.

Figure 19-8a Adapted from B. M. Peterlin and P. A. Luciw, *AIDS*, Vol. 2, 1988, p. S29.

Figure 19-8b From R. C. Gallo and L. Montagnier, "The AIDS Epidemic," *Scientific American*, Vol. 259, 1988, p. 41. © 1988 by Scientific American Inc. All rights reserved. Micrograph courtesy of Hans Geldenblom of the Robert Koch Institute, Berlin.

Figure 19-9 Courtesy of R. C. Gallo, *Journal of Acquired Immune Deficiency Syndromes*, Vol. 1, 1988, p. 521.

Figure 19-12 Adapted from A. Fauci et al., "Immunopathogenic Mechanisms of HIV Infection," *Annals of Internal Medicine*, Vol. 124, 1996, p. 654.

Chapter 20 Opener From J. A. Charlesworth and B. A. Pussell in *Clinical Immunology Illustrated*, J. V. Wells and D. S. Nelson, eds., Williams & Wilkins, 1986, p. 191.

Figure 20-1 From Web Path; courtesy of E. C. Klatt, M.D., University of Utah.

Figure 20-2 From Web Path; courtesy of E. C. Klatt, M.D., University of Utah.

Figure 20-3 From M. A. Atkinson and N. K. Maclaren, "What causes diabetes?" *Scientific American*, Vol. 263, January 1990, p. 62. © 1990 by Scientific American Inc. All rights reserved.

Table 20-3 Adapted from M. B. A. Oldstone, *Cell*, Vol. 50, 1987, p. 819. Reprinted by permission of Cell Press.

Figure 20-6 From L. Steinman, *Scientific American*, Vol. 269, March 1993, p. 80.

Figure 20-8 Adapted from V. Kumar et al., with permission from the *Annual Review of Immunology*, Vol. 7, 1989, p. 657. © 1989 by Annual Reviews Inc.

Figure 20-9b From N. Sarvetnick et al., *Cell*, Vol. 52, 1988, p. 773. Reprinted by permission of Cell Press.

Figure 20-11 Adapted from D. Wofsy, "Treatment of Autoimmune Diseases with Monoclonal Antibodies," *Monoclonal Antibody Therapy, Progress in Allergy*, Vol. 45, p. 106. Edited by H. Waldmann, 1988. Reprinted by permission of S. Karger AG, Basel.

Figure 20-12 Adapted, with permission, from H. Acha-Orbea, I. Steinman, and H. O. McDevitt, "T-cell Receptors in Murine Autoimmune Diseases," *Annual Review of Immunology*, Vol. 7, 1989, p. 371. © 1988 by Annual Reviews Inc. Originally published in *Cell*, Vol. 54, 1988, p. 268.

Figure 21-3 Adapted, with permission, from S. P. Cobbold, G. Martin, and H. Waldmann, *Nature*, Vol. 323, 1986, p. 165. © 1986 Macmillan Magazines Ltd.

Figure 21-5 Adapted, with permission, from T. Moen et al., *The New England Journal of Medicine*, Vol. 303, 1980, p. 850.

Figure 21-9 Adapted from S. M. Sabesin and J. W. Williams, "Current Status of Liver Transplantation," *Hospital Practice*, Vol. 15, Issue 7, 1987, p. 75. Illustration by Albert Miller. Reprinted with permission.

Chapter 22 Opener From L. J. Old, "Tumor Necrosis Factor," *Scientific American*, Vol. 258, May 1988, p. 59. © 1988 by Scientific American Inc. All rights reserved.

Figure 22-1 Adapted from J. Darnell, H. Lodish, and D. Baltimore, *Molecular Cell Biology*, 2nd ed. © 1990 by Scientific Ameri-

can Books. Reprinted by permission of W. H. Freeman and Company.
Figure 22-4 Adapted from B. Vogelstein and K. W. Kinzler, *Trends in Genetics*, Vol. 9, 1993, p. 138.
Table 22-4 Adapted from Scott and Welt, *Current Opinion in Immunology*, Vol. 9, 1997, p. 717.
Table 22-5 Adapted from B. Van Den Eynde and P. van der Bruggen, *Current Opinion in Immunology*, Vol. 9, 1996, p. 684.
Figure 22-12 From L. J. Old, "Tumor Necrosis Factor," *Scientific American*, Vol. 258, May 1988, p. 59. © 1988 by Scientific American Inc. All rights reserved.
Figure 22-13 Data from S. Rosenberg et al., *Annals of Internal Medicine*, Vol. 108, 1988, p. 853.
Table 23-2 Adapted from Federation of American Societies for Experimental Biology, *Biological Handbooks, Vol. III: Inbred and Genetically Defined Strains of Laboratory Animals*, Pergamon Press Ltd., 1979.
Table 23-5 Source: New England Biolabs, <http://www.neb.com>.
Figure 23-5b From K. Weber and M. Osborne, *The Proteins*, 3rd ed., Vol. 1, 1975, p. 179, Academic Press.
Figure 23-6 Courtesy of B. A. Osborne.
Figure 23-7 Courtesy of A. McPherson, University of California, Irvine.
Figure 23-8a From L. Stryer, *Biochemistry*, 4th ed., 1995, W. H. Freeman and Company, New York.
Figure 23-8b, c Courtesy of A. McPherson, University of California, Irvine.***Figure 23-9*** Adapted from H. Lodish et al., *Molecular Cell Biology*, 3rd ed., 1995, Scientific American Books. © 1995 by Scientific American Books.
Figure 23-12 From J. Darnell, H. Lodish, and D. Baltimore, *Molecular Cell Biology*, 2nd ed., 1990, Scientific American Books. © 1990 by Scientific American Books.
Figure 23-13 Adapted from H. Lodish et al., *Molecular Cell Biology*, 3rd ed., 1995, Scientific American Books. © 1995 by Scientific American Books.
Figure 23-14 Adapted from J. D. Watson et al., 1992, *Recombinant DNA*, 2nd ed., 1992. © 1992 by W. H. Freeman and Company.
Figure 23-15 Adapted from J. D. Watson. et al., 1992, *Recombinant DNA*, 2nd ed., 1992. © 1992 by W. H. Freeman and Company.
Figure 23-18 Adapted from H. Lodish, et al., *Molecular Cell Biology*, 3rd ed., 1995. © 1995 by Scientific American Books.
Figure 23-19 Adapted from M. R. Capecchi, *Trends in Genetics*, Vol. 5, 1989, p. 70.
Figure 23-20 Adapted from B. Sauer, *Methods*, Vol. 14, 1998, p. 381.

INDEX

Note: Page numbers in *italics* indicate illustrations; those followed by t indicate tables.